AF845955

Handbook of Practical Fine Needle Aspiration and Small Tissue Biopsies

Fan Lin • Haiyan Liu • Jun Zhang

Handbook of Practical Fine Needle Aspiration and Small Tissue Biopsies

Springer

Fan Lin
Department of Laboratory Medicine
Geisinger Health System
Danville, Pennsylvania, USA

Haiyan Liu
Department of Laboratory Medicine
Geisinger Health System
Danville, Pennsylvania, USA

Jun Zhang
Department of Laboratory Medicine
and Pathology
Mayo Clinic
Scottsdale, Arizona, USA

ISBN 978-3-319-57384-7 ISBN 978-3-319-57386-1 (eBook)
DOI 10.1007/978-3-319-57386-1

Library of Congress Control Number: 2017940478

© Springer International Publishing AG 2018
This work is subject to copyright. All rights are reserved by the Publisher, whether the whole or part of the material is concerned, specifically the rights of translation, reprinting, reuse of illustrations, recitation, broadcasting, reproduction on microfilms or in any other physical way, and transmission or information storage and retrieval, electronic adaptation, computer software, or by similar or dissimilar methodology now known or hereafter developed.
The use of general descriptive names, registered names, trademarks, service marks, etc. in this publication does not imply, even in the absence of a specific statement, that such names are exempt from the relevant protective laws and regulations and therefore free for general use.
The publisher, the authors and the editors are safe to assume that the advice and information in this book are believed to be true and accurate at the date of publication. Neither the publisher nor the authors or the editors give a warranty, express or implied, with respect to the material contained herein or for any errors or omissions that may have been made. The publisher remains neutral with regard to jurisdictional claims in published maps and institutional affiliations.

Printed on acid-free paper

This Springer imprint is published by Springer Nature
The registered company is Springer International Publishing AG
The registered company address is: Gewerbestrasse 11, 6330 Cham, Switzerland

To my loving and supportive wife Danquing,
and my sons Dustin and Benjamin

–Fan Lin

To my dear husband Shu for his support,
and my two beautiful daughters, Jenni and Vivian

–Haiyan Liu

To my wife, Peiwen for her unlimited love and support,
and my son, David for his inspiration

–Jun Zhang

Preface

Fine needle aspiration (FNA) biopsies with cellblock preparation or small tissue biopsies have become a primary modality to achieve a definitive diagnosis of a mass-like lesion of the superficial organs (such as thyroid, salivary glands, lymph nodes, breast, and soft tissue) and deep-seated organs (such as lung, pancreas, liver, kidney, adrenal, and retroperitoneum). The primary goal of this book is to address how to obtain maximal, accurate diagnostic information from the minimal available material. This book is intended to be practical, accurate, concise, and yet up-to-date and user-friendly. Some important features are summarized as follows. This book:

- Lists diagnostic pearls and pitfalls at the beginning of each chapter; these were based on the available literature and our personal practicing experience over last 20 years.
- Applies the most current WHO Classifications of Tumors for each organ.
- Delineates cytologic and histologic features with bullet points for each neoplastic and non-neoplastic lesion, including many recently introduced entities.
- Emphasizes the importance of triple tests (clinical, radiologic, and histologic/cytologic).
- Describes the utilities and pitfalls of diagnostic IHC, including over 50 IHC panels, in a tabular format and numerous recently introduced and useful diagnostic markers.
- Highlights the application of important molecular tests.
- Provides over 1400 color microphotographs.

One of the unique features of this book is the highly practical presentations of typical case scenarios seen in an anatomic pathology laboratory at the end of each chapter to re-emphasize the crucial points illustrated throughout each chapter. These are in the form of case presentations with step-by-step critical and logical analysis. Sample cases include common but challenging situations, such as evaluation of well-differentiated malignant tumors vs benign/reactive lesions, distinction of two benign entities, subclassification of a malignant tumor, identification of newly described tumor and non-tumor entities, workup of a tumor of unknown origin, and implementation of best practice in immunohistochemistry and molecular testing in a difficult case.

In short, this book will provide a unique and valuable resource in the field of cytopathology and surgical pathology, both for those currently in training and for those already in clinical practice at various skill levels. It does not seek to duplicate or completely replace other large textbooks; rather, it is a new, comprehensive yet concise and practical resource on these timely and critical topics.

Danville, PA, USA — Fan Lin, MD, PhD
Danville, PA, USA — Haiyan Liu, MD
Scottsdale, AZ, USA — Jun Zhang, MD, MS

Acknowledgments

It was a very challenging task to produce this handbook, and we wish to acknowledge the assistance and tremendous support we received. Dr. Conrad Schuerch, Chair of Geisinger Medical Laboratory, supported and encouraged this project from conception through completion. Sandy Mullay, Operations Director of Anatomic Pathology, always ensured we had the secretarial and clerical support needed throughout the project. Melissa Erb served as our project coordinator, scheduling many meetings, pulling out many interesting cases, and keeping us organized. Kathy Fenstermacher was invaluable in editing, formatting, and polishing book chapters. Without Kathy's talent and tireless effort, it would not have been possible to meet the submission deadline. Finally, we are in debt to our families and close friends for their understanding while we buried ourselves in this project for such a long period of time. We are very fortunate to have your love and incredible support.

Fan Lin, MD, PhD
Haiyan Liu, MD
Jun Zhang, MD, MS

Contents

Contributors

Fan Lin, MD, PhD Department of Laboratory Medicine, Geisinger Health System, Danville, PA, USA

Haiyan Liu, MD Department of Laboratory Medicine, Geisinger Health System, Danville, PA, USA

Jun Zhang, MD, MS Department of Laboratory Medicine and Pathology, Mayo Clinic, Scottsdale, AZ, USA

Xiaohong (Mary) Zhang, MD, PhD Department of Pathology, Geisinger Health System, Wilkes-Barre, PA, USA

1 Introduction and Application of Fine Needle Aspiration Biopsy

Fan Lin, Jun Zhang, and Haiyan Liu

Indications for Fine Needle Aspiration (FNA) Biopsy

- Mass lesion with a clinical suspicion of malignant tumor – palpable or deep-seated
- Infections – virus, fungus
- Granulomatous inflammation
- Infiltration – amyloidosis

Complications of FNA

- Pain
- Bleeding
- Faintness
- Hematoma
- Pneumothorax
- Seeding of tumor cells

Advantages of FNA

- FNA is *SAFE*.
  - *S*imple
  - *A*ccurate
  - *F*ast
  - *E*conomic

Primary Applications of FNA

- Primary diagnosis of a malignant tumor.
- Confirm a reactive/benign condition.
- Metastatic tumor of unknown primary.
- Deep-seated organ/tumor.
- Confirm a recurrent tumor.

Target Organs of FNA

Superficial Organs

- Thyroid
- Lymph node
- Salivary gland
- Soft tissue
- Breast

Deep-Seated Organs

- Liver
- Pancreas
- Lung/mediastinum
- Kidney/adrenal
- Retroperitoneum

Sensitivity and Specificity of FNA (Table 1.1)

How to Perform an FNA

Supplies

- 23- or 25-gauge, 1.0-inch or 1.5-inch needle
- Syringes – 10 mL
- Syringe holder (Fig. 1.1)

Procedure

- Stabilize the target lesion.
- Pass needle through the skin and advance into the lesion.

© Springer International Publishing AG 2018
F. Lin et al., *Handbook of Practical Fine Needle Aspiration and Small Tissue Biopsies*, DOI 10.1007/978-3-319-57386-1_1

Table 1.1 Summary of sensitivity and specificity of FNA

Organ	Sensitivity (%)	Specificity (%)
Thyroid	83	92
Breast	92.5	99.8
Salivary gland	90	95
Lymph node	90	98
Lung	89	96
Liver	85	100
Pancreas	90	100
Kidney	85	98
Adrenal gland	85	100
Soft tissue	96	96

Note: When a sample is adequate for evaluation

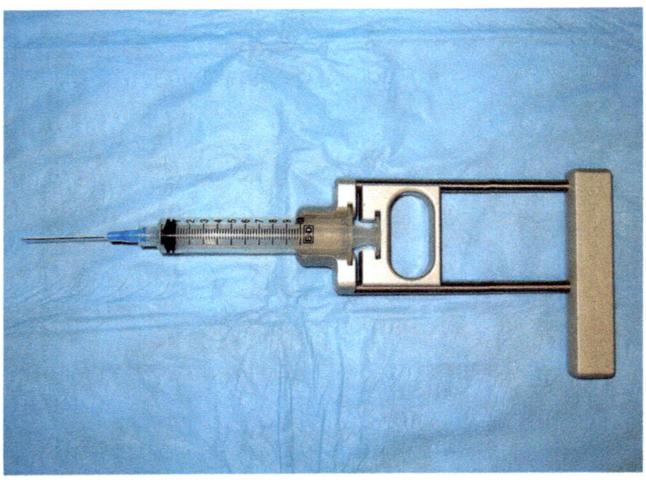

Fig. 1.1 Showing an aspiration gun (Cameco AB, Tägy, Sweden)

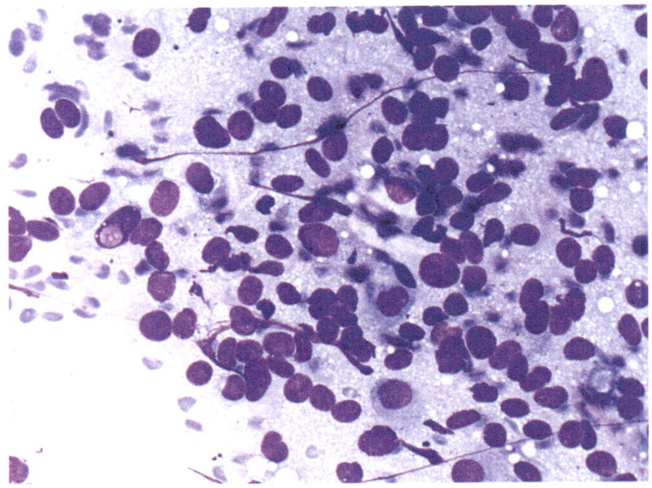

Fig. 1.2 Hypercellularity in melanoma

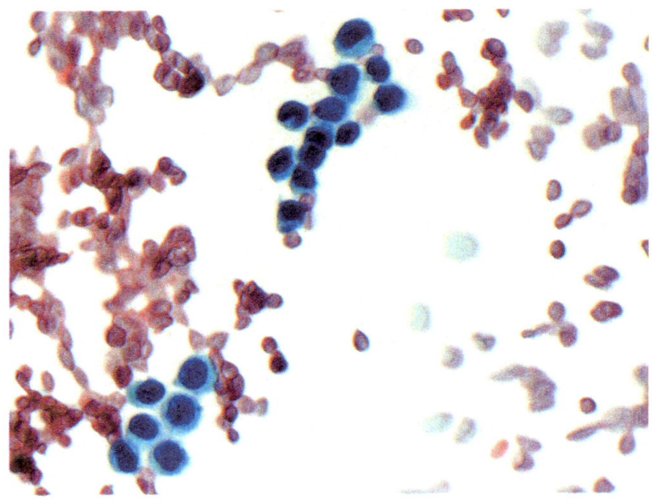

Fig. 1.3 Low cellularity in breast lobular carcinoma

- Apply suction.
- Move the needle back and forth for 10 s.
- Release suction.
- Remove the needle from patient.
- Detach the needle from the syringe.
- Fill the syringe with air and replace needle on syringe.
- Express the specimen onto microscopic slides.
- Prepare air-dried and fixed smears.

How to Interpret an FNA

Overall Cellularity

- High – lymphoma, melanoma, neuroendocrine tumor (NET) (Fig. 1.2)
- Low – lobular carcinoma, schwannoma (Fig. 1.3)

Cellular Architectures

- Papillary (Fig. 1.4)
- Tightly cohesive groups (Fig. 1.5)
- Loosely cohesive groups (Fig. 1.6)
- Acinar (Fig. 1.7)
- Glandular (Fig. 1.8)

Cell Shapes

- Epithelial (Fig. 1.9)
- Epithelioid (Fig. 1.10)
- Spindle (Fig. 1.11)
- Bizarre
- Small round cell (Fig. 1.12)
- Giant cell (Fig. 1.13)

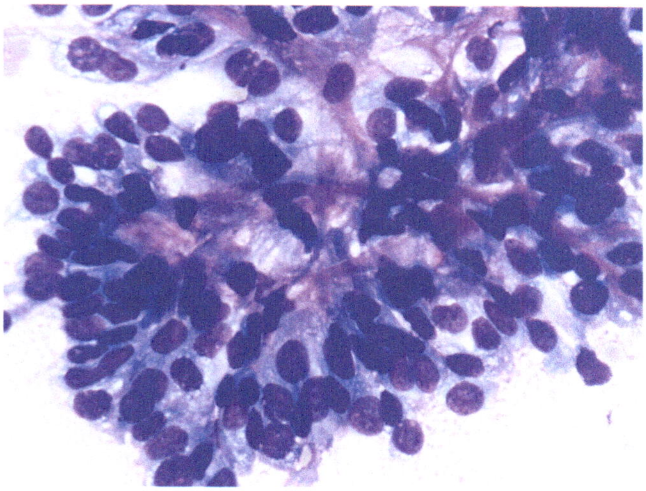

Fig. 1.4 Papillary structure in papillary RCC

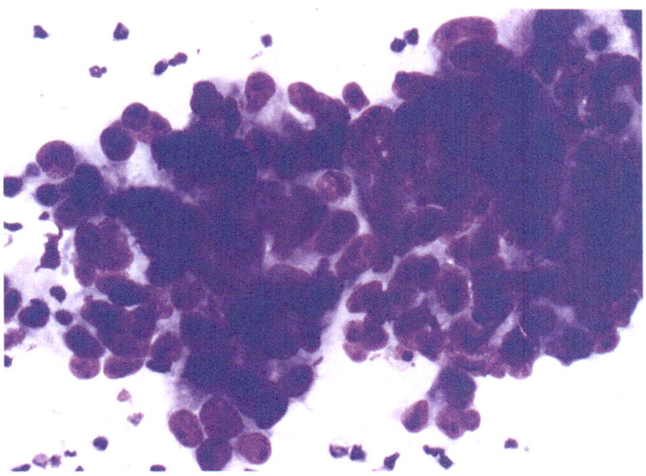

Fig. 1.5 Cohesive cellular group in medullary carcinoma of the breast

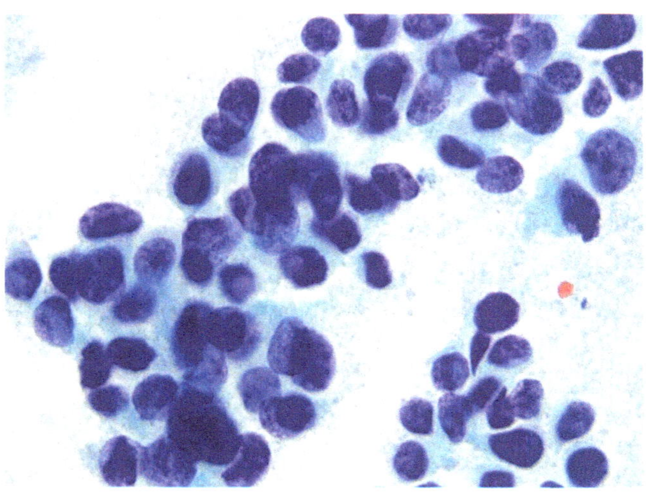

Fig. 1.6 Loosely cohesive group in breast carcinoma

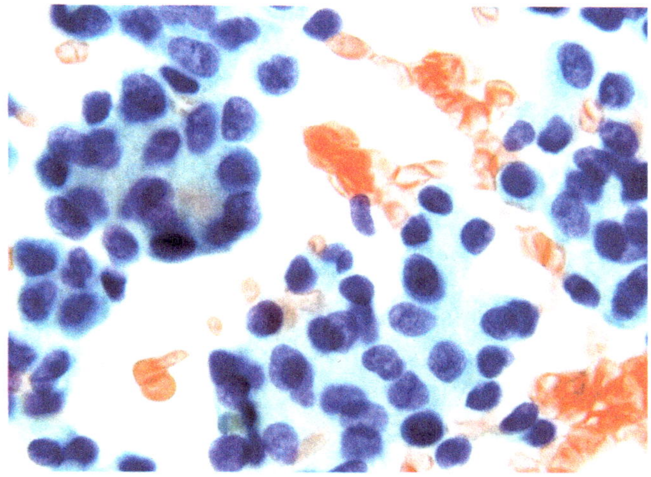

Fig. 1.7 Acinar formation in acinar cell carcinoma of the pancreas

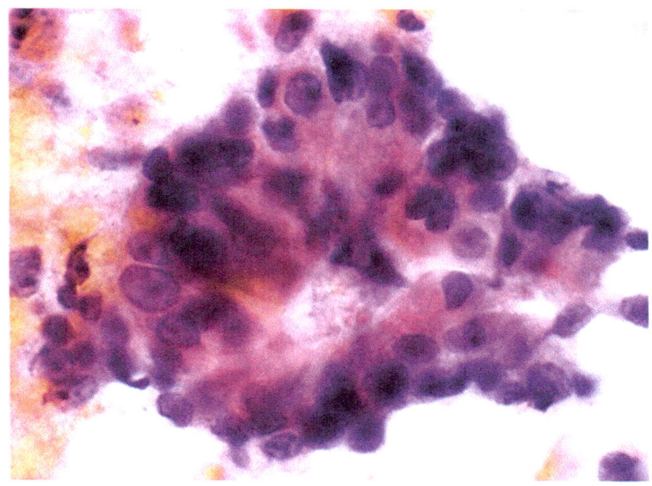

Fig. 1.8 Glandular formation in colonic ADC

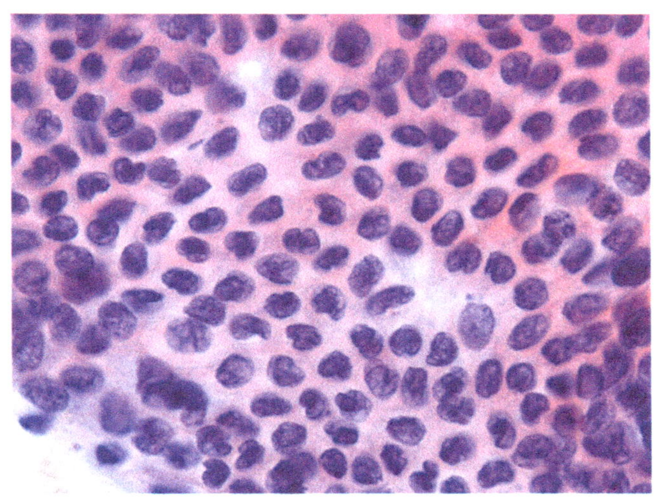

Fig. 1.9 Epithelial cells in well-differentiated ADC of the pancreas

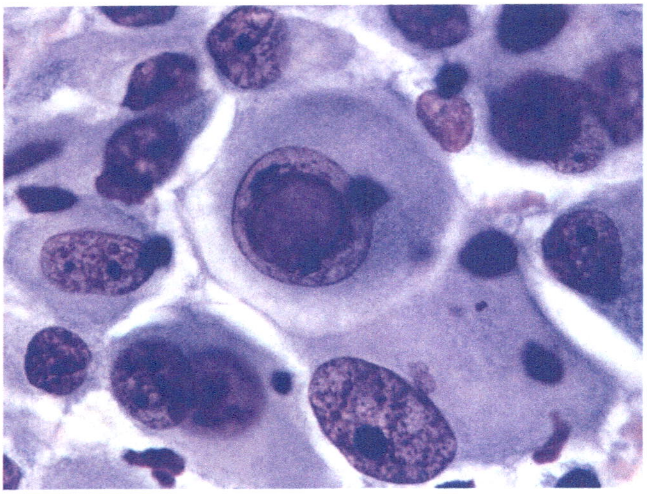

Fig. 1.10 Epithelioid cells in melanoma

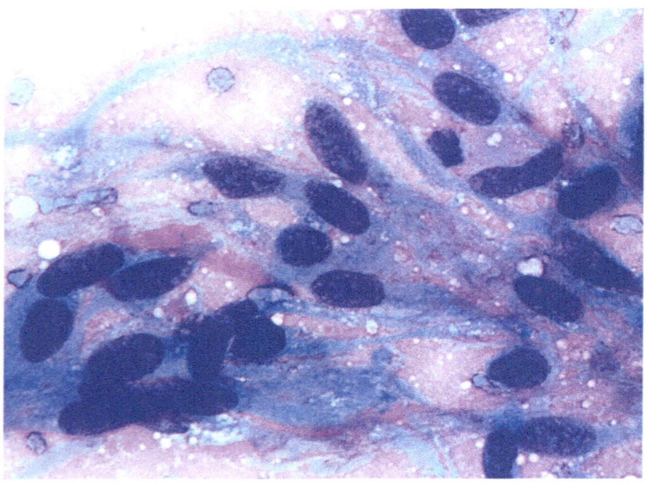

Fig. 1.11 Spindle cell in gastrointestinal stromal tumor

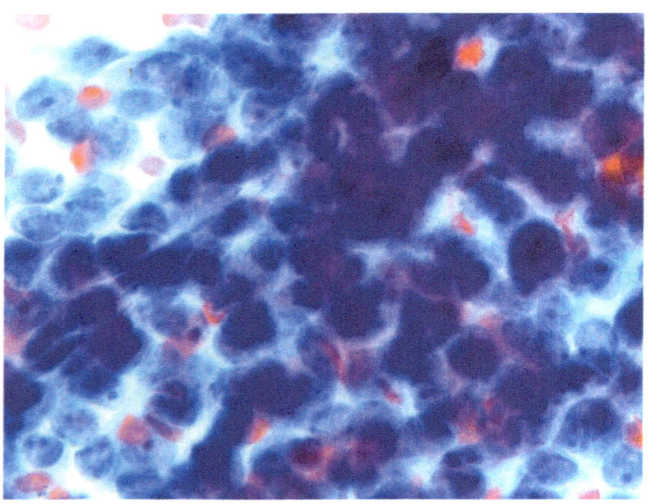

Fig. 1.12 Small blue cell in Ewing's sarcoma

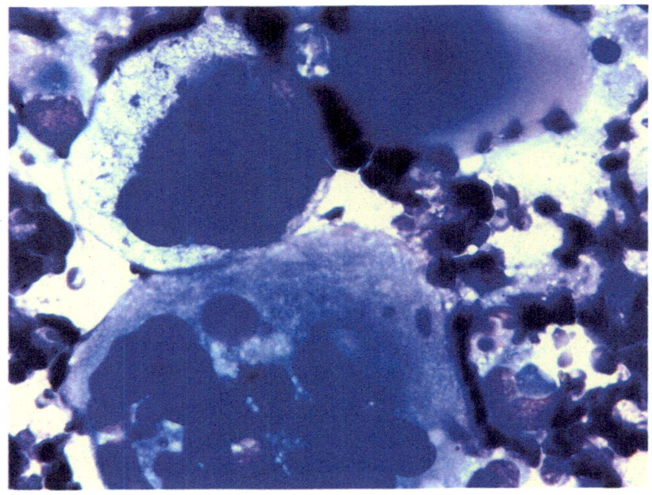

Fig. 1.13 Giant tumor cells in rhabdomyosarcoma on Diff-Quik (DQ)

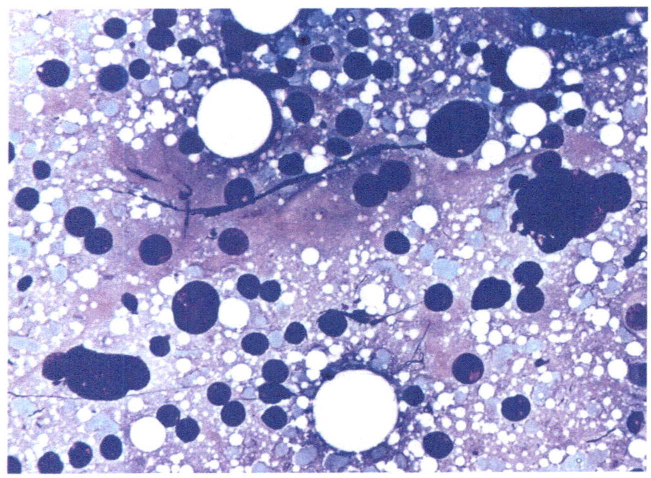

Fig. 1.14 Naked nuclei in HCC

Naked Nuclei

- Hepatocellular carcinoma (HCC) (Fig. 1.14)
- Acinar cell carcinoma
- Granular cell tumor
- Lactating adenoma
- Fibroadenoma

Nuclear Details

- Intranuclear inclusion – melanoma (Fig. 1.15), renal cell carcinoma (RCC), papillary thyroid carcinoma, HCC, and paraganglioma
- Nuclear grooves – papillary thyroid carcinoma, adult granulosa cell tumor, histiocytosis X (Fig. 1.16), solid-pseudopapillary tumor of pancreas

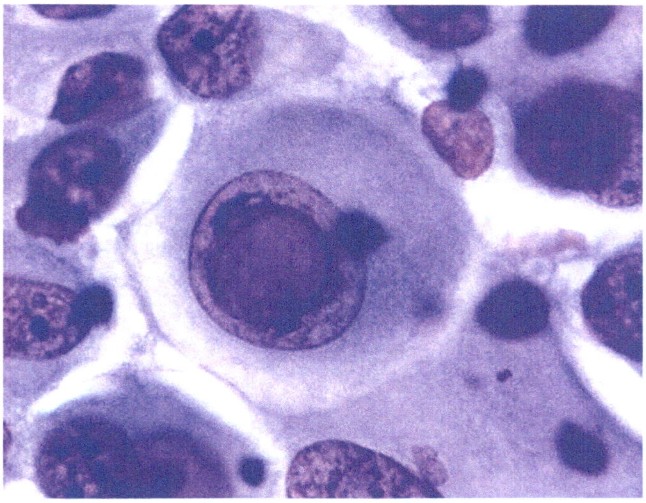

Fig. 1.15 Intranuclear inclusion in a melanoma

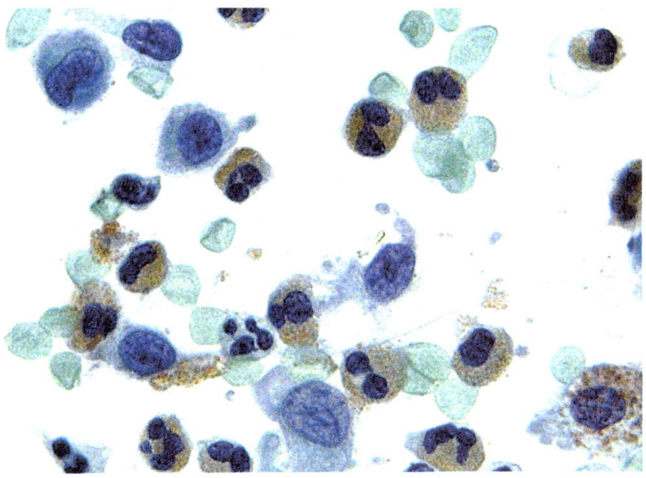

Fig. 1.16 Nuclear grooves in Langerhans cell histiocytosis

- Anisonucleosis – high-grade neoplasms (Figs. 1.17 and 1.18)
- Nuclear chromatin clearing – pancreatic carcinoma
- Prominent nucleoli – melanoma, high-grade lymphoma, HCC, high-grade RCC, adenocarcinoma (ADC), and sarcoma

Cytoplasm

- Clear – clear cell RCC (Fig. 1.19), clear cell carcinoma of the ovary and the uterus, melanoma, ADC with clear cell changes (such as pancreas), and squamous cell carcinoma (SCC) with clear cell changes
- Granular – oncocytoma (Fig. 1.20), HCC, granular cell tumor (Fig. 1.21), high-grade RCC, medullary carcinoma of the thyroid, and other NETs/carcinomas

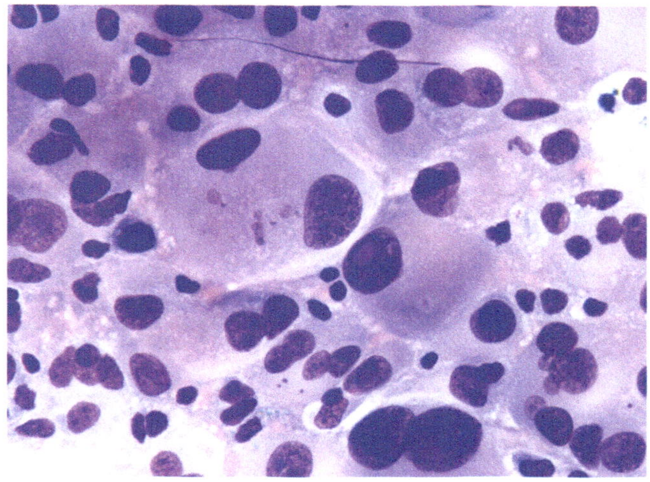

Fig. 1.17 Nuclear pleomorphism in a melanoma

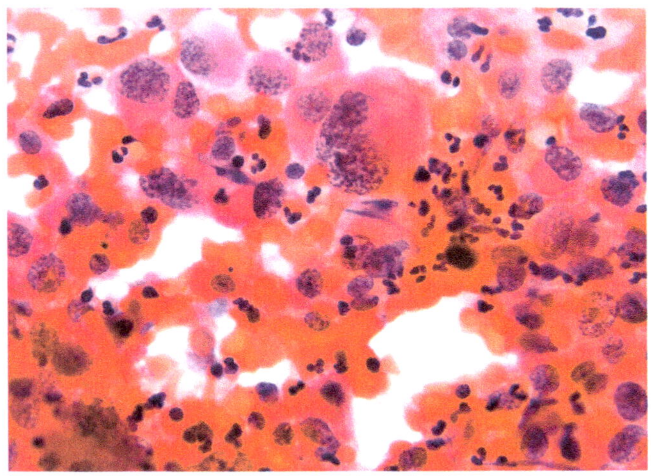

Fig. 1.18 Anaplastic carcinoma of the thyroid with marked nuclear pleomorphism

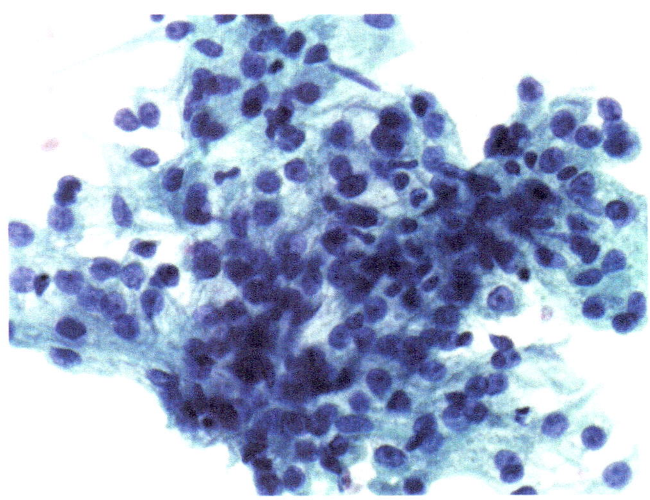

Fig. 1.19 Clear cytoplasm in a clear cell RCC

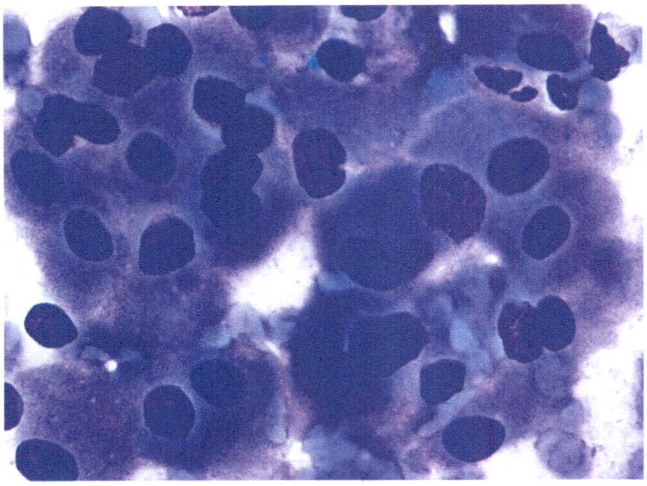

Fig. 1.20 Oncocytic cytoplasm in an oncocytoma

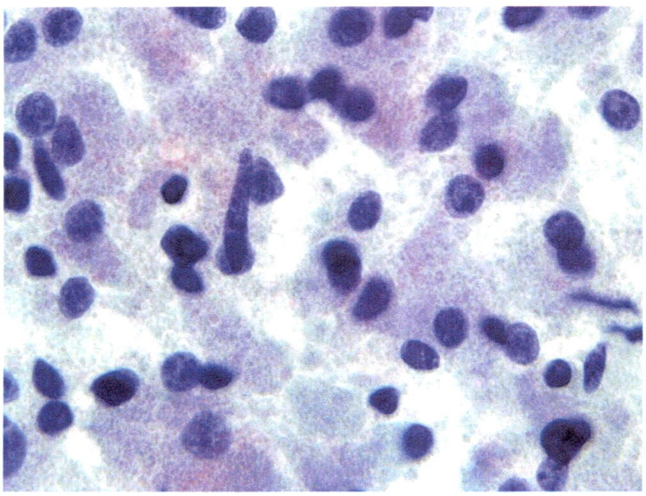

Fig. 1.21 Coarse, granular cytoplasm in a granular cell tumor

- Foamy – RCC, carcinoma of the breast, lung, and pancreas, melanoma
- Squamoid/dense – SCC (Figs. 1.22 and 1.23), papillary thyroid carcinoma, carcinoma of the lung and pancreas, and high-grade mucoepidermoid carcinoma
- Intracytoplasmic lumen – lobular carcinoma and low-grade ductal carcinoma of the breast (Fig. 1.24), signet-ring cell carcinoma, and melanoma

Background Material

- Abundant mucin – colloid carcinoma of breast and pancreas (Figs. 1.25 and 1.26) and mucoepidermoid carcinoma
- Abundant colloid – thyroid nodular goiter

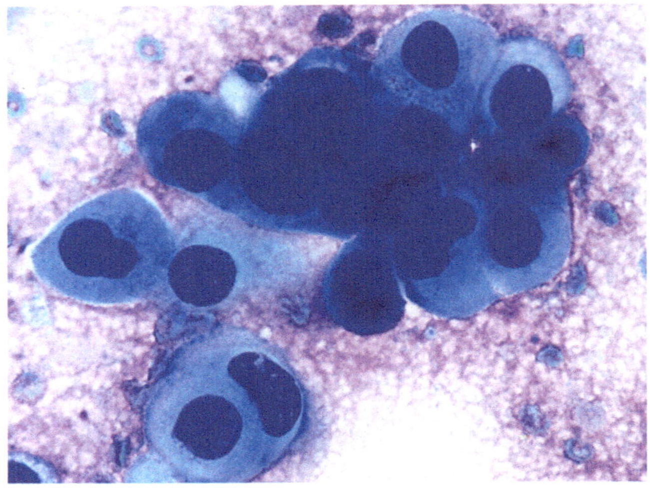

Fig. 1.22 Squamous tumor cell in a SCC on DQ

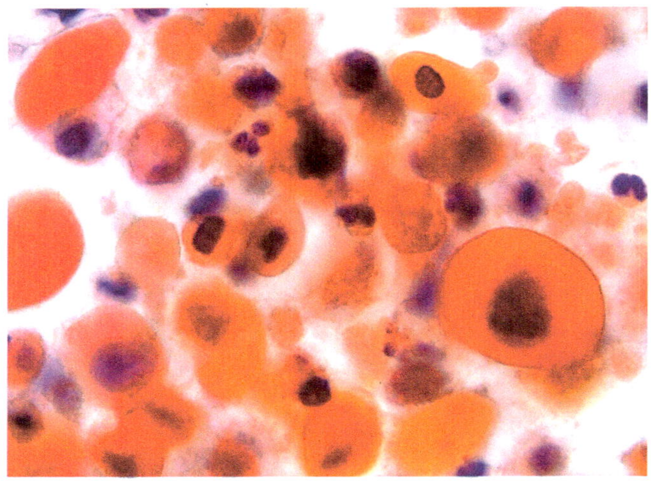

Fig. 1.23 Keratinizing squamous tumor cell in an SCC on Papanicolaou (Pap) stain

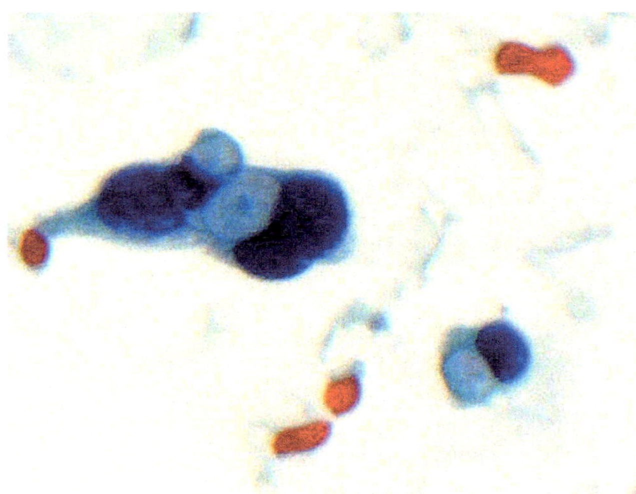

Fig. 1.24 Intracytoplasmic lumen in a breast lobular carcinoma

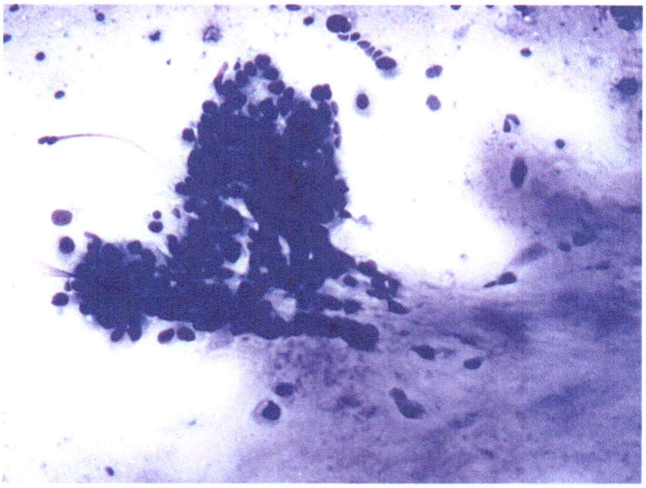

Fig. 1.25 Mucinous background in a colloid carcinoma of the breast on DQ

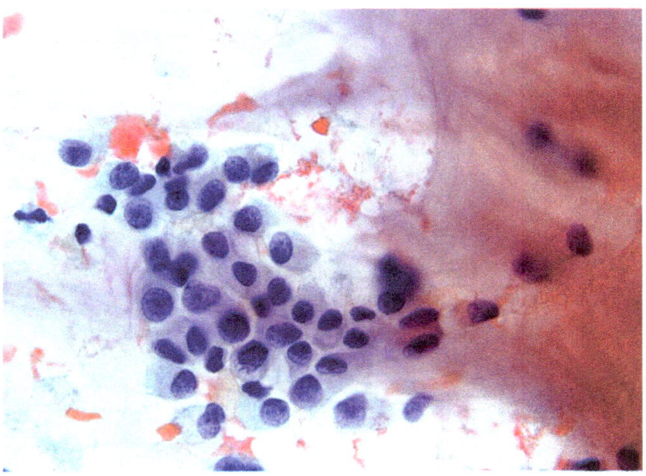

Fig. 1.26 Mucinous background in a colloid carcinoma of the breast on Pap stain

- Myxoid/chondroid – benign mixed tumor, chondrosarcoma, and myxoid and chondroid neoplasms (Figs. 1.27 and 1.28)
- Amyloid – medullary carcinoma of the thyroid, NET, and endocrine tumor of the pancreas
- Necrosis – colorectal ADC, small-cell undifferentiated carcinoma, lymphoma, and high-grade carcinoma or sarcoma
- Crushed artifact – small blue cell tumor, lymphoma, and lymphoid tissue
- Acute inflammation – infection, inflammatory process, anaplastic carcinoma of the thyroid, anaplastic large-cell lymphoma, and SCC with cystic degeneration

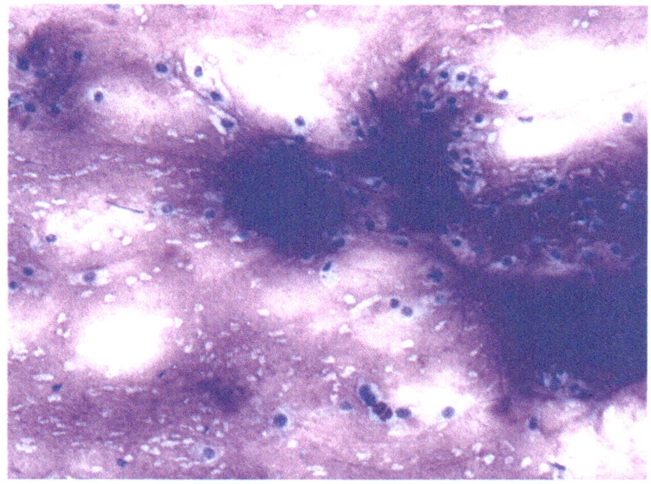

Fig. 1.27 Chondroid background in a chodorma on DQ

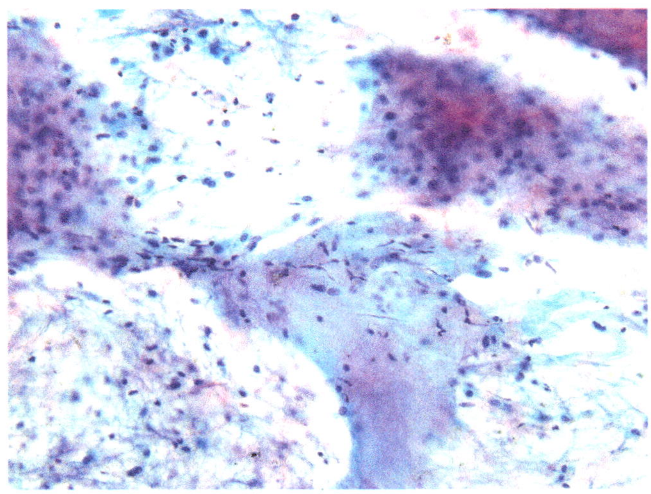

Fig. 1.28 Chondroid background in a chodorma on Pap stain

Single Cell Population

- NET (Figs. 1.29)
- Lymphoma/plasmacytoma/myeloid sarcoma (Fig. 1.30)
- Melanoma
- Sarcoma

Two Populations of Cells

- Seminoma (Figs. 1.31 and 1.32)
- Thymoma
- Hodgkin's lymphoma (Fig. 1.32)

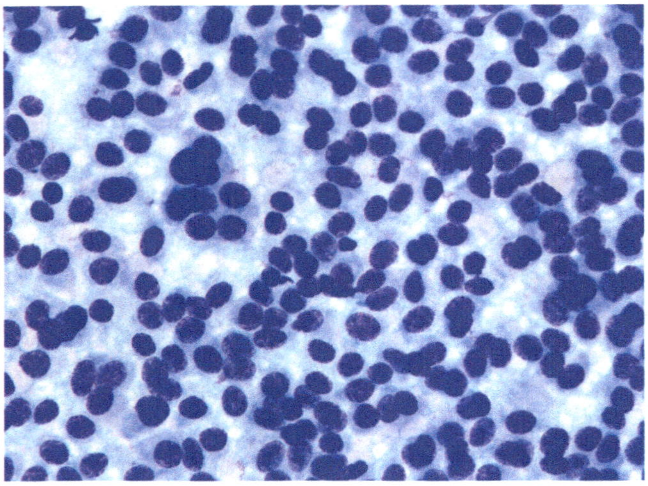

Fig. 1.29 Single cell population in a carcinoid tumor of lung on DQ

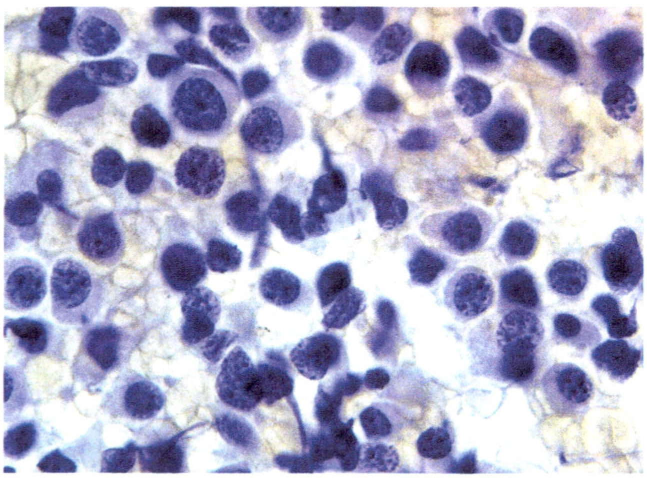

Fig. 1.30 Single cell population in a plasmacytoma on Pap stain

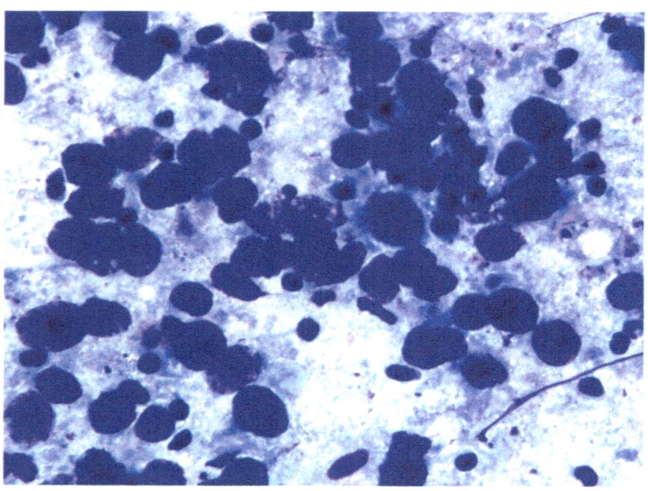

Fig. 1.31 Two populations of cells in a seminoma on DQ

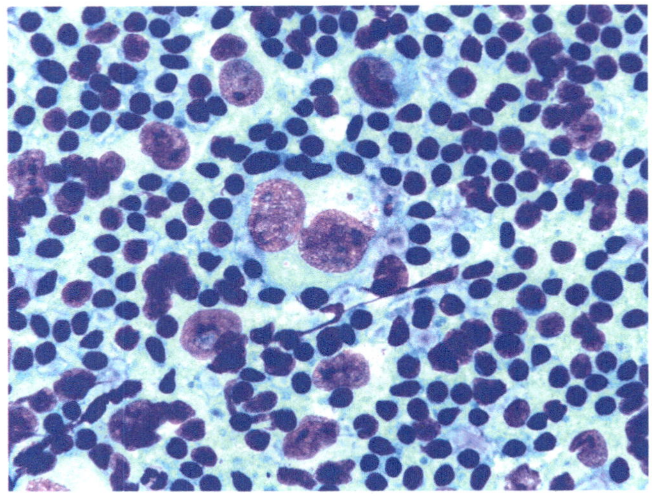

Fig. 1.32 Two populations of cells in a Hodgkin's lymphoma on DQ

- Lymphoepithelial carcinoma
- Medullary carcinoma of the colon
- Metastasis

How to Report an FNA

Category

1. Positive for malignant cells/malignant
2. Suspicious for malignant cells
3. Atypical cytology/atypical cells of undetermined significance
4. Negative for malignant cells/benign
5. Indeterminate

Specimen Adequacy

1. Adequate/satisfactory
2. Inadequate/unsatisfactory
3. Suboptimal/limited

An Example of a Formal Report of an FNA of the Thyroid

Thyroid, right, FNA
Positive for malignant cells
Papillary thyroid carcinoma
Adequately cellular specimen

Comment: Tall cell variant of papillary carcinoma of the thyroid is suspected.

Cytological Criteria of Common Neoplasms

1. *Papillary Carcinoma of Thyroid*
   Major Criteria (Fig. 1.33)
   - Nuclear enlargement
   - Nuclear overlapping
   - Nuclear clearing
   - Nuclear grooving
   - Intranuclear inclusion

   Minor Criteria
   - Squamoid cytoplasm
   - Cytoplasmic vacuoles
   - Psammoma body
   - Thick colloid
   - Multinucleated giant cells

2. *Medullary Carcinoma of the Thyroid*
   Major Criteria (Fig. 1.34)
   - Two populations of cells, epithelioid and spindle cells
   - Salt-pepper chromatin
   - Small to inconspicuous nucleoli
   - Plasmacytoid features

   Minor Criteria
   - Intranuclear inclusion
   - Granular and dense cytoplasm
   - Amyloid
   - Hyaline globules

3. *Adenoid Cystic Carcinoma of Salivary Gland*
   Major Criteria (Fig. 1.35)
   - Small uniform, basaloid cells with high nuclear-to-cytoplasmic ratio, bland nuclei, but hyperchromatic chromatin
   - Hyaline globules

   Minor Criteria
   - Usually absence of myoepithelial cells
   - Few stromal fragments
   - Exclude other entities

4. *Benign Mixed Tumor of the Salivary Gland*
   Major Criteria (Fig. 1.36)
   - Epithelial cells
   - Stromal cells
   - Metachromatic stroma
   - Spindle stromal cells
   - Plasmacytoid myoepithelial cells

   Minor Criteria
   - Epithelial cell dominant
   - Stromal cell dominant
   - Stromal acellular component dominant

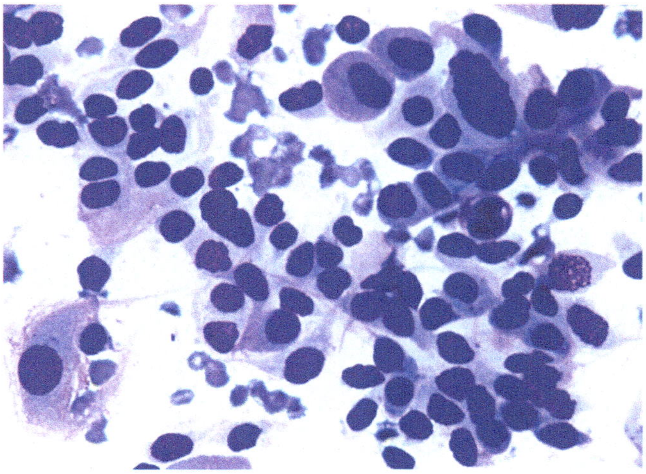

Fig. 1.34 Classic cytological features for a medullary carcinoma of the thyroid on DQ

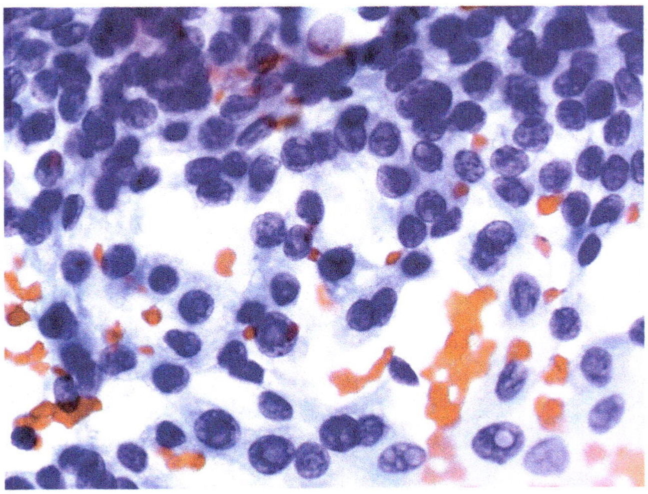

Fig. 1.33 Classic nuclear changes in a papillary carcinoma of the thyroid on Pap stain

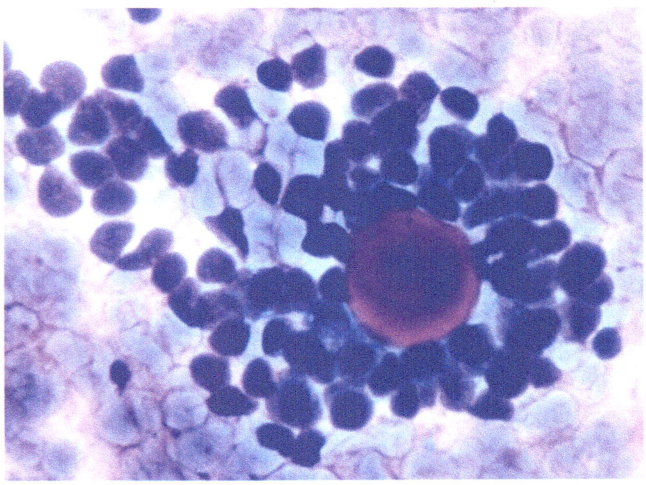

Fig. 1.35 Diagnostic hyalinizing globules in an adenoid cystic carcinoma on DQ

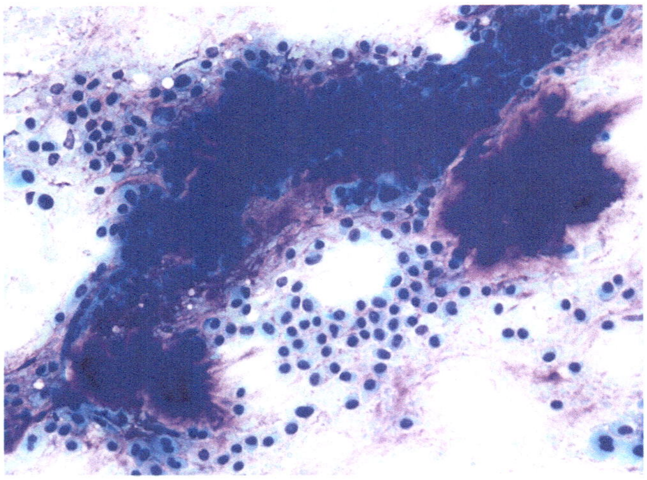

Fig. 1.36 Showing an example of benign mixed tumor on DQ

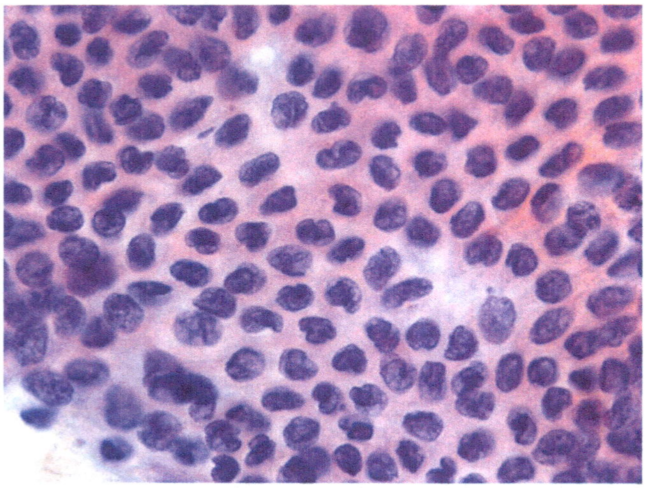

Fig. 1.37 Showing an example of well-diff ADC of the pancreas on Pap stain

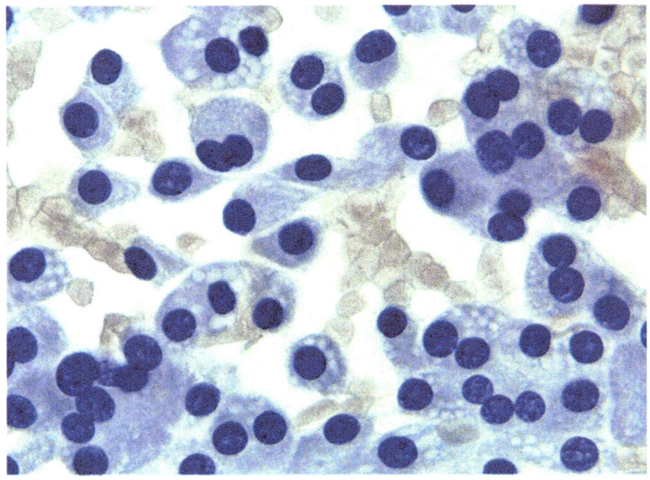

Fig. 1.38 Showing an example of pancreatic NET

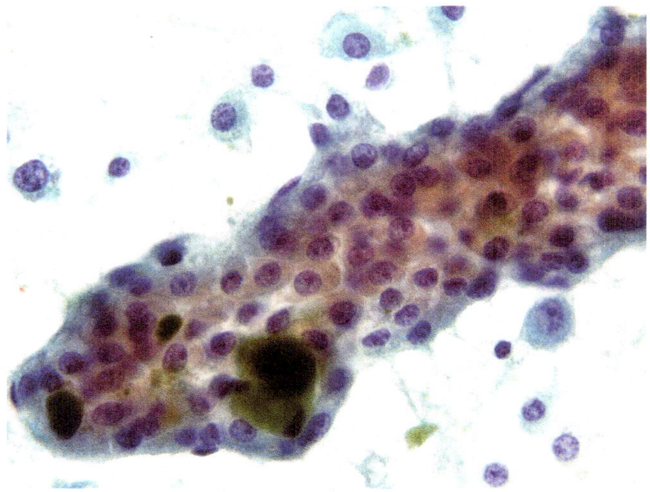

Fig. 1.39 Showing an example of HCC producing bile on Pap stain

- Myoepithelial cell dominant
- Extensive squamous metaplasia

5. *ADC of the Pancreas*

   Major Criteria (Fig. 1.37)
   - Variation in nuclear size in the same group (1:4)
   - Nuclear enlargement (>2 red blood cells [RBCs])
   - Nuclear overlapping/three dimensionality
   - Nuclear membranous irregularity

   Minor Criteria
   - Single atypical cells
   - Tumor necrosis
   - Prominent nucleoli
   - Mitosis
   - Chromatin clearing
   - Giant tumor cells
   - Hyperchromatic nuclei

6. *NET of the Pancreas*

   Major Criteria (Fig. 1.38)
   - A mixture of small cohesive groups and single cells
   - Round nuclei with salt-pepper nuclear chromatin
   - Small nucleoli
   - Plasmacytoid features
   - Binucleation

   Minor Criteria
   - Occasional large atypical cells
   - Crushed artifact
   - Focal necrosis
   - Multinucleated giant cells
   - Granular cytoplasm
   - Striped nuclei

7. *HCC*

   Major Criteria (Fig. 1.39)

- Trabecular fragment >3 cells thick and wrapped by endothelial cells or pseudoglandular formation with production of bile
- Special stain for reticulin and an immunostain for cluster of differentiation (CD)34 performed on the cell block section or core biopsy are useful

Minor Criteria

- Hypercellularity
- Many single cells
- Naked nuclei
- High nuclear-to-cytoplasmic ratio
- Few ductal cells

8. *Ductal Carcinoma of the Breast*

Major Criteria (Fig. 1.40)

- Hypercellularity
- Nuclear enlargement (>2.5 RBCs)
- Disordered, loosely cohesive epithelial group
- Single atypical cells
- Nuclear chromatin changes

Minor Criteria

- Marked nuclear atypia
- Tumor necrosis
- Mitosis
- Prominent nucleoli
- Intracytoplasmic lumens
- Foamy cytoplasm

9. *Small-Cell Carcinoma of the Lung*

Major Criteria (Figs. 1.41 and 1.42)

- Pleomorphic nuclei with salt-and-pepper nuclear chromatin
- Very high nuclear-to-cytoplasmic ratio
- Single cell necrosis and mitosis
- Inconspicuous nucleoli

Minor Criteria

- Crushed artifact
- Hypercellularity
- Many single cells
- Blue body
- Nuclear molding
- Extensive necrosis
- Marked atypical cells

10. *ADC of the Lung*

Major Criteria

- Three dimensional groups
- Glandular, tubular, acinar, or papillary formation
- Nuclear enlargement
- Chromatin clearing and clumping
- Irregular nuclear membrane
- Prominent nucleoli
- Mucinous material in the background

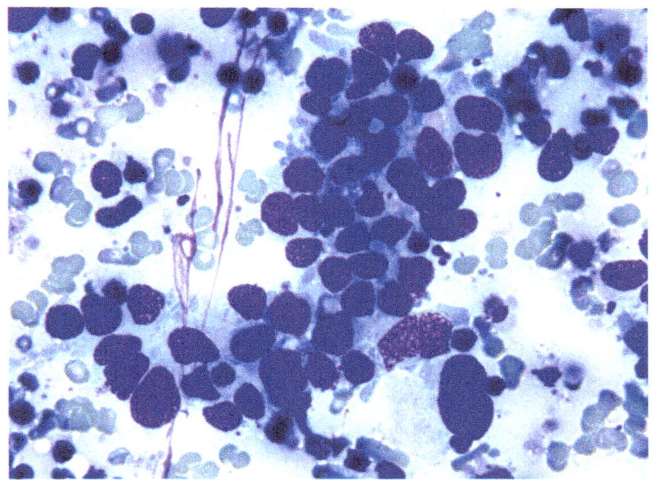

Fig. 1.41 Showing an example of small-cell carcinoma of the lung on DQ

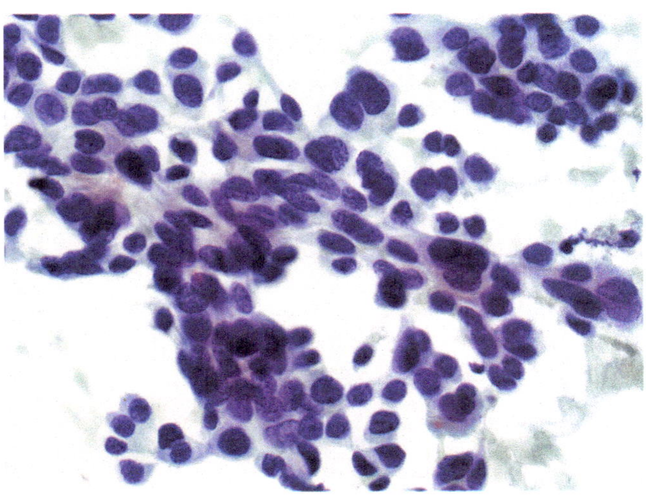

Fig. 1.40 Showing an example of breast ductal carcinoma on Pap stain

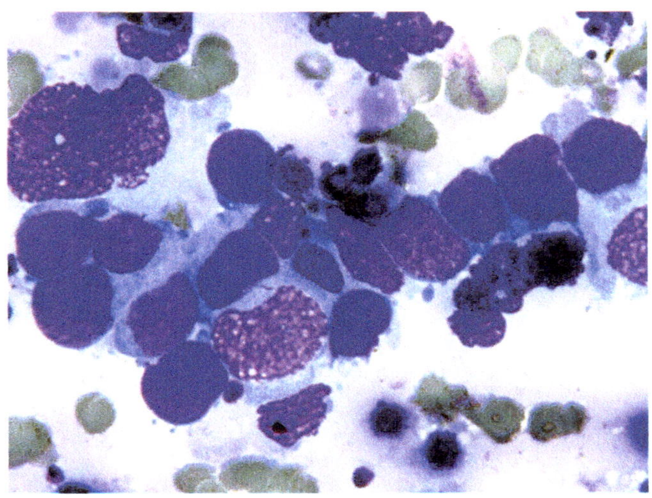

Fig. 1.42 Showing nuclear molding in a small-cell carcinoma on DQ

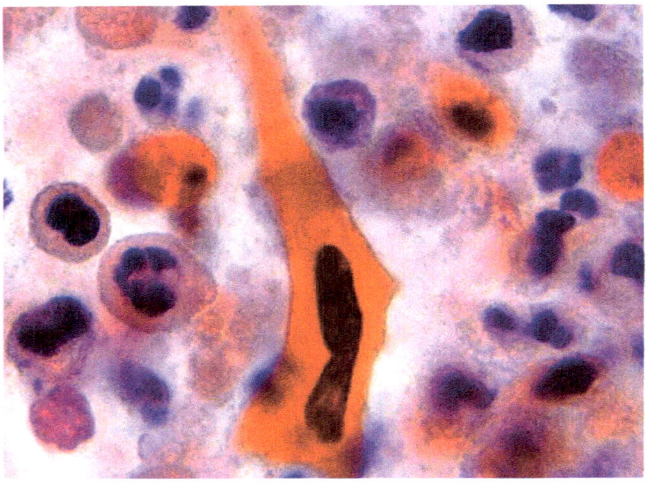

Fig. 1.43 Showing an example of well-differentiated SCC of the lung on Pap stain

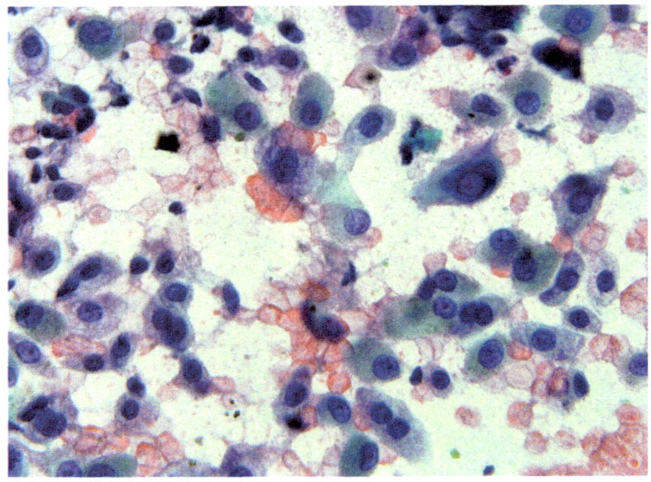

Fig. 1.44 Showing an example of melanoma with clear cytoplasm on Pap stain

Minor Criteria
- Single atypical cells with plasmacytoid features
- Mitosis
- Vacuoles in cytoplasm

11. *SCC of the Lung*

Major Criteria (Fig. 1.43)
- Two or three dimensional groups
- Keratinization
- Single atypical cells with dense cytoplasm
- Nuclear enlargement
- Small nucleoli
- Irregular nuclear membrane
- No glandular, tubular, acinar, or papillary formation
- Mucinous material in the background

Minor Criteria
- Tumor necrosis
- Mitosis
- Marked pleomorphic cells
- Bizarre cell sharps

12. *Melanoma*

Major Criteria (Fig. 1.44)
- Large epithelioid cells
- Abundant cytoplasm
- Large nuclei
- Prominent nucleoli
- Binucleation
- Intranuclear inclusion

Minor Criteria
- Two populations of cells – epithelioid and spindle
- Plasmacytoid appearance
- Marked pleomorphic cells
- Pigments

13. *Clear Cell RCC*

Major Criteria (Fig. 1.45)
- Clusters of tumor cells with vascular-rich network
- Low nuclear-to-cytoplasmic ratio

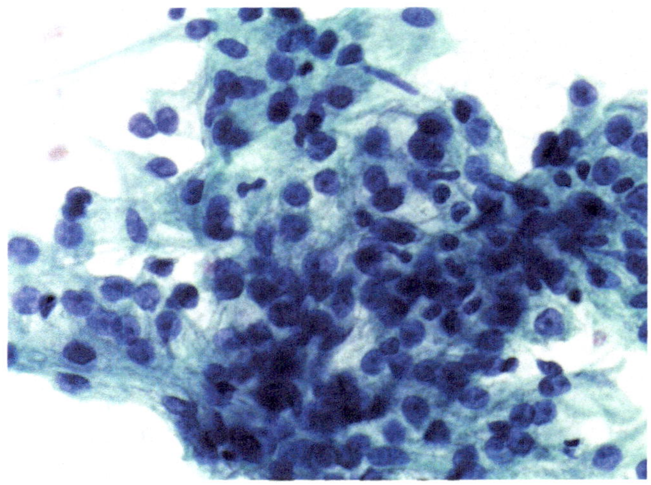

Fig. 1.45 Showing an example of clear cell RCC on Pap stain

- Clear or granular cytoplasm
- Small to prominent nucleoli
- Intranuclear inclusion

Minor Criteria
- Naked nuclei
- Mixed neutrophils, RBCs, and pigment-laden histiocytes with tumor cells

14. *Non-Hodgkin's Lymphomas*

Major Criteria (Fig. 1.46)
- Uniform population of lymphoid cells
- Classified into small, medium, and large cell size using histiocytes as a reference
- Lymphoglandular body

Minor Criteria
- Cleaved or noncleaved nuclei
- Fine granular chromatin
- Many mitoses
- Single cell or extensive necrosis

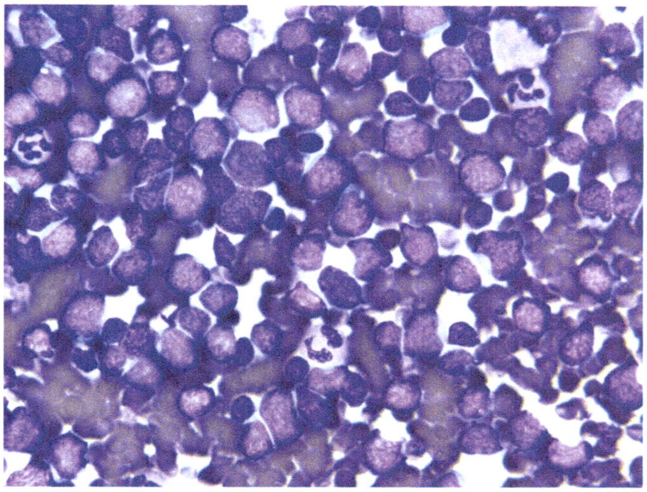

Fig. 1.46 Showing an example of lymphoblastic lymphoma on DQ

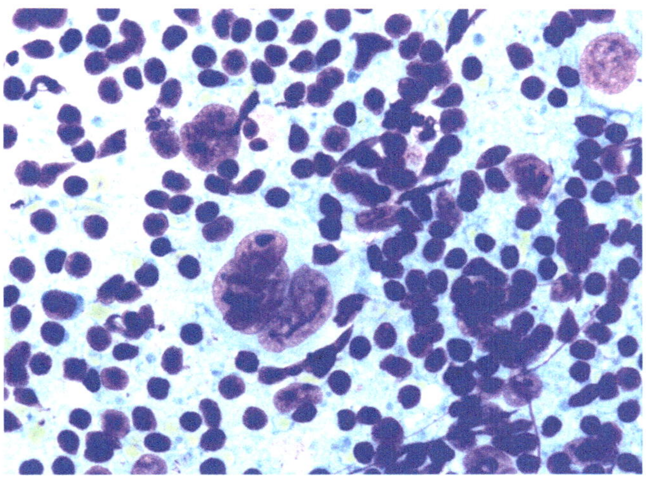

Fig. 1.47 Showing an example of Hodgkin lymphoma with Reed-Sternberg cells on DQ

- Prominent nucleoli
- Cytoplasmic vacuoles

15. *Hodgkin's Lymphoma*

    <u>*Major Criteria*</u> (Fig. 1.47)
    - Reed-Sternberg cells
    - Hodgkin's cells
    - Mixed population of small lymphoid cells, histiocytes, plasma cells, and eosinophils in the background

    <u>*Minor Criteria*</u>
    - Granulomas
    - Fibrosis
    - Necrosis

Diagnosis of lymphomas should not solely rely on cytological features; instead, it should include (1) cytomorphology, (2) immunohistochemistry (IHC), (3) flow cytometry, and (4) FISH/molecular diagnosis.

Ancillary Studies

IHC

In this section, the focus will be on the application of IHC to undifferentiated neoplasms if a cell block or a small tissue biopsy sample is available, especially carcinoma of unknown origin. The utilities of IHC on other specific entities on each organ will be delineated in each organ-based chapter.

How to Approach Undifferentiated Neoplasms/Tumors of Uncertain Origin

- *Review hematoxylin- and eosin (H&E)-stained slides.*
  Morphologic features are fundamental. The very first step is to determine if the lesion is malignant. If a benign/reactive condition is included in the differential diagnosis, caution should be taken when applying any immunostains, since IHC may or may not contribute to this process or may lead one to come to the wrong conclusion. If the lesion is malignant, it is important to review the slides and generate a broad differential diagnosis based on the morphologic features alone. One can be misled by incomplete or inaccurate clinical information.
- *Consider the basic clinical information such as age, sex, tumor location, and prior malignancy.*
  After formulating the initial differential diagnostic categories, it is time to consider the patient's age, sex, tumor location, and any prior malignancy. One should follow the statistics and focus on the common entities in that particular age group of patients and tumor location. Jumping to a conclusion of an uncommon entity in the initial diagnostic workup is not a wise choice.
- *Re-evaluate morphologic features of the tumor and predict the most likely category, such as carcinoma, melanoma, sarcoma, lymphoma, or germ cell tumor.*
  Based on the patient's age, sex, tumor location, prior malignancy, and morphologic features, one should narrow down the initial differential diagnosis to one to three options, if possible. For example: Is this a carcinoma? Is this an ADC? If it is an ADC, what is the likely primary site? Based on the tumor morphology, patient's age, and tumor location, the literature demonstrated that pathologists were able to correctly identify the tumor origin as their first choice in 50–55% of cases or as their first, second, or third choice in 67–74% of cases.

- *Determine the first diagnostic IHC panel to order.*

There are two likely scenarios. In the first, there is a clear lineage differentiation, such as an ADC/carcinoma. The next question will be: What is the likely primary site? A broad-spectrum cytokeratin cocktail (AE1/3 and CAM5.2), cytokeratin (CK)7, CK20, plus relatively organ-specific markers are recommended.

Determination of a Broad Category of Neoplasm

A cocktail of AE1/AE3 and CAM 5.2 is an effective panel of markers for identifying an epithelial lineage. AE1/AE3 by itself is insufficient to exclude an epithelial lineage. Other broad-spectrum cytokeratins containing keratin 8 and keratin 18, such as clones KL1, OSCAR, MAK6, and 5D3/LP3, are also excellent choices as a screening cytokeratin.

Leukocyte common antigen (LCA) itself is insufficient to exclude a potential diagnosis of hematopoietic neoplasm. Some diffuse large B-cell lymphomas, plasmablastic lymphomas, and anaplastic lymphomas can be negative for LCA. A combination of LCA and CD43 will cover a broad spectrum of lymphomas/myeloid sarcomas.

Vimentin is a non-specific marker; however, a vimentin-negative tumor is unlikely to be a sarcoma (with the exception of alveolar soft part sarcoma), lymphoma, or melanoma. Some carcinomas frequently co-express vimentin. A combination of S100 and sex-determining region Y-box (SOX)10 will detect nearly 100% of melanomas and greater than 80% of spindle cell/desmoplastic melanomas.

Sal-like protein 4 (SALL4) and lin-28 homolog A (LIN28) are highly sensitive and specific markers for identifying a tumor of germ cell origin. The markers for determination of a broad category of neoplasms are summarized in Table 1.2.

Tissue-Specific Markers

No single antibody is absolutely sensitive and specific for a particular tumor; however, some are especially useful when used in a small panel. Frequently used tissue-specific biomarkers are summarized in Table 1.3.

Co-expression of Cytokeratin and Vimentin

Follicular, papillary, and medullary thyroid carcinomas are nearly 100% positive for vimentin. Metaplastic breast carcinoma usually expresses both cytokeratin and vimentin in addition to high molecular weight cytokeratins and myoepithelial markers. Alveolar soft part sarcoma is a rare sarcoma which has no immunoreactivity for vimentin. Tumors that express both cytokeratin and vimentin are described in Table 1.4.

Expression of Epithelial Markers in Non-epithelial Neoplasms

Expression of cytokeratin is not restricted to epithelial neoplasms. Keratin is commonly expressed in some tumors with evidence of epithelial differentiation, such as synovial sarcomas, epithelioid sarcomas, desmoplastic small round cell tumors, chordomas, adamantinoma, and myoepithelial carcinomas. Other mesenchymal tumors can also express cytokeratin, although with a low frequency, including angiosarcomas, epithelioid hemangioendotheliomas, epithelioid leiomyosarcomas, and meningiomas. Aberrant expression of cytokeratin, which tends to be focal, has been reported in other tumors, including undifferentiated pleomorphic sarcomas, rhabdomyosarcomas, malignant rhabdoid tumors, and peripheral nerve sheath tumors, clear cell sarcomas, plasmacytomas, diffuse large B-cell lymphomas, anaplastic large-cell lymphomas, and melanomas.

Expression of Hematopoietic Markers in Non-hematopoietic Neoplasms

CD5 has been reported in thymic carcinoma, breast carcinoma, colonic ADC, pancreatic ADC, and lung ADC. CD138 is also frequently positive in SCC and can be positive in breast carcinoma, ovarian carcinoma, adrenal cortical carcinoma, and RCC.

CD56 is the most sensitive but not an entirely specific marker for neuroendocrine neoplasms, including some small-cell carcinomas which may lose expression of cytokeratins and other neuroendocrine markers but still show expression of CD56. A significant percentage of thyroid carcinomas are immunoreactive for CD56 as well, as reported in the literature. Hematopoietic markers expressed in non-hematopoietic neoplasms are listed in Table 1.5.

Table 1.2 Markers for determination of a broad category of neoplasms

Marker/Tumor	Carcinoma	Sarcoma	Melanoma	Lymphoma	GCT	Mesothelioma
CK	+	–	–	–	+/–	+
Vimentin	–/+	+	+	+	–	+/–
S100/SOX10	–/+	–	+	–	–	–
LCA/CD43	–	–	–	+	–	–
SALL4/LIN28	–	–	–	–	+	–

Note: *GCT* giant cell tumor, *CK* a broad spectrum cytokeratin, *SOX10* sex-determining region Y-box 10, *LCA* leukocyte common antigen, *CD43* cluster of differentiation 43, *SALL4* sal-like protein 4, *LIN28* lin-28 homolog A, "+" >75% of cases are positive, "–" <5% of cases are positive, "+/–" 50–75% of cases are positive, "–/+" <50% of cases are positive

Table 1.3 Useful markers for identifying tumor origin

Primary site	Markers
Lung ADC	TTF1, napsin A
Breast carcinoma	GATA3, ER, GCDFP-15, TFF1, MGB
Urothelial carcinoma	GATA3, UPII/UPIII, S100P, CK5/6, CK903, p63, CK20
Squamous cell carcinoma	p40, CK5/6, p63, SOX2, desmocollin-3
RCC, clear cell type	PAX8/PAX2, RCCma, pVHL, CD10, KIM-1
Papillary RCC	P504S, RCCma, pVHL, CD10, PAX8, KIM-1
Translocational RCC	TFE3
HCC	Arg-1, glypican-3, HepPar-1, AFP
Adrenal cortical neoplasm	Mart-1, inhibin-alpha, calretinin, SF-1
Melanoma	S100, Mart-1, HMB45, MiTF, SOX10, PNL2
Merkel cell carcinoma	CK20 (perinuclear dot staining), MCPyV
Mesothelial origin	Calretinin, WT1, D2-40, CK5/6, mesothelin
Neuroendocrine origin	Chromogranin, synaptophysin, CD56,
Upper GI tract	CDH17, CDX2, CK20
Lower GI tract	CDH17, SATB2, CDX2, CK20
Intrahepatic cholangiocarcinoma	pVHL, CAIX, albumin by RNA in situ hybridization
Pancreas, acinar cell carcinoma	Glypican-3, Bcl-10, antitrypsin
Pancreas, ductal ADC	MUC5AC, CK17, maspin, S100P, IMP3
Pancreas, NET	PR, PAX8, PDX1, islet-1
Pancreas, solid pseudopapillary tumor	Nuclear beta-catenin, loss of E-cadherin, PR, CD10, vimentin
Prostate, ADC	NKX3.1, PSA, PSAP, ERG
Ovarian serous carcinoma	PAX8, ER, WT1
Ovarian clear cell carcinoma	pVHL, HNF-1B, KIM-1, PAX8
Endometrial stromal sarcoma	CD10, ER
Endometrial ADC	PAX8/PAX2, ER, vimentin
Endocervical ADC	PAX8, p16, CEA, HPV in situ hybridization, loss of PAX2
Thyroid follicular cell origin	TTF1, PAX8, thyroglobulin
Thyroid medullary carcinoma	Calcitonin, TTF1, CEA, chromogranin
Parathyroid neoplasm	PTH, GATA3, chromogranin
Hyalinizing trabecular adenoma of the thyroid	MIB-1 (unique membranous staining pattern)
Salivary duct carcinoma	AR, GCDFP-15, HER2, GATA3
Mammary analogue secretory carcinoma of the salivary gland	S100, GATA3, MGB, GCDFP15
Thymic origin	PAX8, p63, CD5
Seminoma	SALL4, OCT4, CD117, D2-40
Yolk sac tumor	SALL4, glypican-3, AFP, GATA3
Embryonal carcinoma	SALL4, LIN28, OCT4, NANOG, CD30, SOX2
Choriocarcinoma	Beta-HCG, CD10, GATA3
Sex cord-stromal tumors	SF-1, inhibin-alpha, calretinin, FOXL2
Vascular tumor	ERG, CD31, CD34, Fli-1
Synovial sarcoma	TLE1, cytokeratin
Chordoma	Cytokeratin, S100
Desmoplastic small round cell tumor	Cytokeratin, CD99, desmin, WT1 (N-terminus)
Alveolar soft part sarcoma	TFE3
Rhabdomyosarcoma	Myogenin, desmin, MyoD1
Smooth muscle tumor	SMA, MSA, desmin, calponin
Ewing sarcoma/PNET	NKX2.2, CD99, Fli-1
Myxoid and round cell liposarcoma	NY-ESO-1
Low-grade fibromyxoid sarcoma	MUC4
Epithelioid sarcoma	CD34, loss of INI1
Atypical lipomatous tumor	MDM2 (MDM2 by FISH is a more sensitive and specific test), CDK4
Histiocytosis X	CD1a, S100
Angiomyolipoma	HMB45, SMA, PNL2
Gastrointestinal stromal tumor	CD117, DOG1
Solitary fibrous tumor	STAT6, CD34, Bcl2, CD99
Myoepithelial carcinoma	Cytokeratin and myoepithelial markers. May lose INI1
Myeloid sarcoma	CD43, CD34, MPO
Follicular dendritic cell tumor	CD21, CD35
Mast cell tumor	CD117, tryptase

Note: *ADC* adenocarcinoma, *TTF1* thyroid transcription factor 1, GATA3 GATA binding protein 3, *ER* estrogen receptor, *GCDFP-15* gross cystic disease fluid protein 15, *TFF1* trefoil factor 1, *MGB* mammaglobin, *UP* uroplakin, *S100P* placental S100, *CK* cytokeratin, *SOX* sex-determining region Y-box, *RCC* renal cell carcinoma, *PAX* paired box gene, *RCCma* renal cell carcinoma marker, *pVHL* von Hippel-Lindau tumor suppressor, *CD* cluster of differentiation, *KIM-1* kidney injury molecule 1, *P504S* alpha-methylacyl-CoA racemase, *TFE3* transcription factor E3, *HCC* hepatocellular carcinoma, *Arg-1* arginase-1, *HepPar-1* hepatocyte paraffin-1, *AFP* alpha-fetoprotein, *Mart-1* melanoma-associated antigen recognized by T cells 1, *SF-1* steroidogenic factor 1, *HMB45* human melanoma black 45, *MiTF* microphthalmia-associated transcription factor, *PNL2* melanoma-associated antigen PNL2, *MCPyV* Merkel cell polyomavirus, *WT1* Wilms' Tumor 1, *D2-40* podoplanin, *GI* gastrointestinal, *CDH17* cadherin-17, *CDX2* caudal-type homeobox 2, *SATB2* special AT-rich sequence-binding protein 2, *CAIX* carbonic anhydrase IX, *MUC* mucin, maspin mammary serine protease inhibitor, *IMP3* IMP3 insulin-like growth factor II messenger RNA-binding protein 3, *NET* neuroendocrine tumor, *PR* progesterone receptor, *PDX1* pancreatic duodenal homeobox 1, *PSA* prostate-specific antigen, *PSAP* prostate-specific acid phosphatase, *ERG* ETS-related gene, *NKX3.1* NK3 homeobox 1, *HNF-1B* hepatocyte nuclear factor 1 beta, *CEA* carcinoembryonic antigen, *HPV* human papilloma virus, *MIB-1* mindbomb homolog 1, *AR* androgen receptor, *SALL4* sal-like protein 4, *LIN28* lin-28 homolog A, *OCT4* octamer-binding transcription factor 4, *NANOG* NANOG homeobox, *Beta-HCG* Beta human chorionic gonadotropin, *FOXL2* forkhead box L2, *Fli-1* friend leukemia virus integration-1, *TLE1* transducin-like enhancer of split 1, *MyoD1* myogenic differentiation 1, *SMA* smooth muscle actin, *MSA* muscle-specific actin; *PNET* primitive neuroectodermal tumor, *NKX2.2* NK2 homeobox 2, *NY-ESO-1* cancer/testis antigen 1B; *INI1* integrase interactor 1, *MDM2* mouse double minute 2 homolog, *FISH* fluorescence in site hybridization, *CDK4* cyclin-dependent kinase 4, *DOG1* discovered on GIST-1, *Bcl2* B-cell CLL/lymphoma 2, *MPO* myeloperoxidase

Table 1.4 Tumors that frequently or rarely co-express cytokeratin and vimentin

Carcinomas that frequently express both	Mesenchymal tumors that frequently express both	Carcinomas that rarely express both
RCC	Synovial sarcoma	Breast carcinoma
Anaplastic thyroid carcinoma	DPSRCT	Ovarian carcinoma
Endometrial carcinoma	Epithelioid sarcoma	GI carcinoma
Thyroid carcinomas	Epithelioid angiosarcoma	Small-cell carcinoma
Sarcomatoid carcinoma	Malignant rhabdoid tumor	Lung non-small-cell carcinoma
Mesothelioma	Leiomyosarcoma	Prostatic carcinoma
Myoepithelial carcinoma	Chordoma	
Metaplastic breast carcinoma	Adamantinoma	

Note: *RCC* renal cell carcinoma, *DPSRCT* desmoplastic small round cell tumor, *GI* gastrointestinal

Table 1.5 Expression of hematopoietic markers in non-hematopoietic neoplasms

Marker	Diagnosis
CD5	Thymic carcinoma, cholangiocarcinoma, pancreatic carcinoma
CD30	Embryonal carcinoma
CD138	Carcinoma of lung, cholangiocarcinoma, UC
CD10	RCC, HCC, ESS, choriocarcinoma
CD15	Carcinoma of lung and other organs; renal oncocytoma
CD56	Neuroendocrine carcinomas and thyroid carcinomas

Note: *CD* cluster of differentiation, *UC* urothelial carcinoma, *RCC* renal cell carcinoma, *HCC* hepatocellular carcinoma, *ESS* endometrial stromal sarcoma

Review of Selected Antibodies

The following selected antibodies are either recently described or frequently used in identifying a tumor of uncertain origin/undifferentiated neoplasm, especially a carcinoma. As well documented, every antigen can demonstrate an aberrant expression in a certain tumor. Table 1.6 summarizes the common application of these antibodies. The antibody information for the frequently used antibodies is summarized in Table 1.7.

Recommended Diagnostic IHC Panels

As aforementioned, this section will focus on carcinomas of uncertain origin, which can be separated into four main diagnostic groups: CK7+/CK20-, CK7+/CK20+, CK7-/CK20+, and CK7-/CK20-.

Table 1.6 Summary of commonly used antibodies

Marker	Common application
TTF1	Lung ADC, 80–85% Carcinoma of thyroid (follicular, papillary, and medullary carcinomas), >90% Small-cell carcinoma of lung, >90% Small-cell carcinoma of prostate, 40% Small-cell carcinoma of bladder, 40%
Napsin A	Lung ADC, 75–80% Papillary RCC, 60% Clear cell RCC, 30% Clear cell carcinoma of the ovary, >90%
CEA	Lung ADC, >90% Colorectal ADC, >90% Gastric ADC, >90% Pancreatic ADC, >90% Breast carcinoma >50% Urothelial carcinoma, 25% Medullary carcinoma of thyroid, nearly 100% Endocervical ADC, <10%
CDX2	Colorectal ADC, >90% Small intestinal ADC, >90% Neuroendocrine neoplasm of GI tract, variable Ovarian mucinous ADC, >90% Upper GI ADC, 40–50% Pancreas/biliary ADC, 10%
SATB2	Colorectal ADC, >90% Colorectal NET >70% Upper GI, pancreas, lung ADCs, <10% Osteogenic sarcomas, >90%
GATA3	Breast carcinoma, >85% Urothelial carcinoma, >80% Salivary ductal carcinomas and mammary analogue secretory carcinomas, >90% Metastatic paraganglioma, 80% 7% of anal SCCs and 19% of uterine cervical SCCs, focally positive Parathyroid neoplasm, >90% Choriocarcinoma and yolk sac tumor, >90%
ER	Breast ductal carcinoma, >80% Breast lobular carcinoma, >95% Ovarian serous carcinomas, >90% Ovarian clear cell carcinomas, >80% Endometrial ADCs, >90%
pVHL	RCCs, >90% Intrahepatic cholangiocarcinoma, 70% Salivary oncocytoma, >90% Clear cell carcinoma of the ovary, 70% Clear cell carcinoma of the uterus, 70% Normal ducts in pancreatobiliary tract, 100%
S100	Melanoma, >90% Carcinoma/breast/renal/lung, variable Neural tumors: Neurofibroma, >90% Schwannoma, >90%, diffuse and strong MPNST, 50–60%, focal staining only Granular cell tumor, >90% Liposarcoma, >90%, weak, focal Chondrosarcoma, >90%, weak Myoepithelioma, >90%

(continued)

Table 1.6 (continued)

Marker	Common application
SOX10	Melanoma, >90% Neurogenic tumor, >90% Myoepithelial cells, >90% Some salivary gland tumors, variable
HMB45	Malignant melanoma, 80–90% Epithelioid schwannoma, >90% Clear cell sarcoma of soft part, >90% Clear cell (sugar) tumor of lung, >90% Angiomyolipoma, 80–90%, focal Lymphangioleiomyomatosis, >90% Cardiac rhabdomyoma, >90%
SALL4	Nearly all germ cell tumors, >90% Hepatoid carcinoma of GI tract, >90%
OCT4	Seminoma, >90% Embryonal carcinoma, >90% Yolk sac tumor, <5%
Arginase-1	Normal liver, 100% Benign liver lesion/tumor, 100% HCC, >85% Some hepatoid carcinomas, 60%
Glypican-3	HCC, 80% Yolk sac tumor, >80% Hepatoid carcinoma, 70% Normal liver and benign hepatocellular lesions, usually negative
PAX8	Thyroid carcinomas (follicular and papillary), >90% Renal cell carcinomas, >90% Ovarian serous carcinomas, >90% Ovarian clear cell carcinomas, >80% Endometrial ADCs, >90% Nephrogenic adenomas, >80% Thymic tumors, 70% Pancreatic NET, 50%
INI1 (loss)	Malignant rhabdoid tumors, >90% Atypical teratoid/rhabdoid tumors of CNS, 90% Medullary carcinoma of the kidney, >90% Epithelioid sarcoma, 90% Epithelioid MPNST, 50% Myoepithelial carcinoma, 30–40%

Note: *TTF1* thyroid transcription factor 1, *ADC* adenocarcinoma, *RCC* renal cell carcinoma, *CEA* carcinoembryonic antigen, *CDX2* caudal-type homeobox 2, *GI* gastrointestinal, *SATB2* special AT-rich sequence-binding protein 2, *NET* neuroendocrine tumor, *GATA3* GATA binding protein 3, *SCC* squamous cell carcinoma, *ER* estrogen receptor, *pVHL* von Hippel Lindau tumor suppressor, *RCC* renal cell carcinoma, *MPNST* malignant peripheral nerve sheath tumor, *SOX10* sex-determining region Y-box 10, *HMB45* human melanoma black 45, *SALL4* sal-like protein 4, *OCT4* octamer-binding transcription factor 4, *HCC* hepatocellular carcinoma, *PAX8* paired box gene 8, *INI1* integrase interactor 1

- *Differential diagnosis of CK7+ and CK7+/focal CK20+ carcinomas.*
  When working on a tumor of unknown primary, CK7+ or CK7+/CK20+ carcinomas are nearly always included in the diagnostic consideration. The differential diagnosis usually encompasses a broad spectrum of organs and entities, such as the breast, lung, ovary, uterus, urinary bladder, upper GI tract, pancreatobiliary tract, thyroid, kidney (papillary RCC), and mesothelioma. Table 1.8 summarizes the frequently used markers in the differential diagnosis of these common entities. A significant portion of these CK7+ carcinomas also express ER, and the major differential diagnosis of CK7+/ER+ carcinomas, including tumors from the breast and gynecologic tract, is summarized in Table 1.9.
  In real practice, each individual case will have a unique presentation; therefore, it is impractical and impossible to create a specific IHC panel for every diagnostically challenging case here. However, a few potentially useful IHC panels are recommended in Tables 1.10, 1.11, 1.12, 1.13, 1.14, and 1.15.
  Caution should be taken when using a polyclonal antibody to napsin A. A significant percentage of esophageal ADCs and some pancreatic ADCs can be positive for napsin A. Less than 10% of pancreatic ADCs may show focal positivity for GATA3.
  In addition to the entities mentioned in Tables 1.9, 1.10, 1.11, 1.12, 1.13, and 1.14, many other entities can present as CK7+ or CK7+/focally CK20+ carcinomas, including anal/rectal ADCs, ampullary ADCs, common bile duct ADCs, gallbladder ADCs, small bowel ADCs, renal collecting duct carcinomas, renal medullary carcinomas, medullary thyroid carcinomas, thymic carcinomas, salivary gland carcinomas, ovarian mucinous carcinoma, and SCCs of the uterine cervix.
- *Differential diagnosis of CK7+/ER+ carcinomas.*
  ER is one of the most critical immunomarkers when working on a tumor of uncertain origin or undifferentiated neoplasm, especially in a woman. ER is frequently positive in breast carcinomas and gynecologic primaries. Therefore, ER itself plays a limited role in differential diagnosis among these carcinomas. Table 1.9 includes the most common ER-positive carcinomas when working on a tumor of uncertain origin. GATA3 and TFF1 are two recently described sensitive markers for identifying a breast origin, which is rarely positive in other gynecologic carcinomas, including endometrial ADCs, endocervical ADCs, ovarian serous carcinomas, and clear cell carcinomas. TFF1 is expressed in 80% and 90% of breast and colorectal carcinomas, respectively, whereas other carcinomas, including those of the lung, endometrium, and ovary, are rarely positive. Vimentin is expressed in 90% of endometrial ADCs and negative in other gynecologic carcinomas, with the exception in ovarian endometrioid ADCs, which showed immunoreactivity for vimentin in over 90% of cases. p16 is a useful marker in distinguishing between endometrial ADC and endocervical ADC; it tends to be diffusely and strongly positive in endocervical ADC (nearly every tumor cell) with only patchy immunoreactivity in endometrial ADC. Human papilloma virus (HPV) in situ hybridization (ISH) demonstrated positivity in the majority of endocervical ADCs. pVHL and hepatocyte nuclear factor 1 beta

Table 1.7 Summary of antibody information

Antibody	Catalog no	Vendor	Clone	AR/Temp/Time	Dilution	pH	Loc
CAM5.2	349,205	BD Biosciences	CAM5.2	CC1/95/36	1:4	8	C
CK7	307 M-95	Cell Marque	OV-TL 12/30	CC1/95/36	1:200	8	C
CK20	790-4431	Ventana	SP33	CC1/95/64	Predilute	8	C
CK5/6	790-4554	Ventana	D5 + 16B4	CC1/95/64	Predilute	8	C
p40	PC373	Millipore	Polyclonal	CC1/95/64	1:2000	8	N
S100	790-2914	Ventana	4C4.9	CC1/95/36	Predilute	8	N + C
LCA	M0701	Dako	2B11 + PD7/26	CC1/95/36	1:80	8	C
Vimentin	790-2917	Ventana	V9	CC1/95/36	Predilute	8	C
TTF1	790-4398	Ventana	8G7G3/1	CC1/95/36	Predilute	8	N
Napsin A	AC-0191	Epitomics	EP205	CC1/95/36	1:100	8	C
ER	790-4324	Ventana	SP1	CC1/95/36	Predilute	8	N
GATA3	CM405	Biocare Medical	L50-823	CC1/95/64	1:400	8	N
TFF1	E100004-RUO	Epitomics	EPR3972	CC1/95/36	1:2000	8	C
CDX2	235R-16	Cell Marque	EPR2764Y	CC1/95/36	1:600	8	N
CDH17	AC-0095RUO	Epitomics	EP86	CC1/95/36	1:100	8	M
SATB2	SC-81376	Santa Cruz	SATBA4B10	CC1/95/64	1:20	8	N
Arg-1	5222-1	Epitomics	EPR6672(B)	CC1/95/36	1:500	8	C + N
Glypican-3	261 M-98	Cell Marque	1G12	CC1/95/36	Predilute	8	C
PAX8	CP379AK	Biocare Medical	Polyclonal	CC1/95/36	1:20	8	N
SALL4	CM384C	Biocare Medical	6E3	CC1/95/64	1:100	8	N
OCT4	309 M-18	Cell Marque	MRQ-10	CC1/95/36	Predilute	8	N
pVHL	SC5575	Santa Cruz	Polyclonal	Protease 1/37/8	1:150	8	M + C
WT1	RB-9267P	Neomarkers/ Thermo	Polyclonal	CC1/95/36	1:200	8	N

Note: *AR* antigen retrieval, *Loc* localization, *CC1* cell conditioning solution 1 (Ventana), *C* cytoplasmic, *N* nuclear, *M* membranous, *CK* cytokeratin, *LCA* leukocyte common antigen, *TTF1* thyroid transcription factor 1, *ER* estrogen receptor, *GATA3* GATA binding protein 3, *TFF1* trefoil factor 1, *CDX2* caudal-type homeobox 2, *CDH17* cadherin-17, *SATB2* special AT-rich sequence-binding protein 2; *Arg-1* arginase-1, *PAX8* paired box gene 8, *SALL4* sal-like protein 4, *OCT4* octamer-binding transcription factor 4, *pVHL* von Hippel-Lindau tumor suppressor, *WT1* Wilms' tumor 1
Vendor Information: BD Biosciences, BD Biosciences, San Jose, CA; Biocare, Biocare Medical, Inc., Concord CA; Cell Marque, Cell Marque Corporation, Rocklin CA; Dako, Dako North America, Inc., Carpinteria, CA; Epitomics, Epitomics, an Abcam Company, Burlingame, CA; Millipore, EMD Millipore, Corp., Billerica, MA; Neomarkers/Thermo, Thermo Scientific, Waltham, MA; Santa Cruz, Santa Cruz Biotechnology, Inc., Santa Cruz CA; Ventana, Ventana Medical Systems, Tucson AZ

Table 1.8 Summary of CK7+ and CK7+/CK20+ epithelial neoplasms

Marker	LADC	BADC	UGI	PADC	ICC	UC	PRCC	PTC	SADC	MS
CK7	+	+	+	+	+	+	+	+	+	+
CK20	–	–	–/+	–/+	–/+	+/–	–	–	+/–	–/+
CK5/6	–	–	–	–	–	+	–	–	–	+
p40	–	–	–	–	–	+	–	–	–	–
GATA3	–	+	–	–	–	+	–	–	–	–
ER	–	+	–	–	–	–	–	–	–	–
TTF1	+	–	–	–	–	–	–	+	–	–
Napsin A	+	–	–	–	–	–	+	–	–	–
CDH17	–	–	+/–	+/–	+/–	–	–	–	+	–
CDX2	–	–	–/+	–/+	–/+	–	–	–	+	–
PAX8	–	–	–	–	–	–	+	+	–	–
RCCma	–	–	–	–	–	–	+	–/+	–	–
pVHL	–	–	–	–	+	–	+	–	–	–
Calretinin	–	–	–	–	–	–	–	–	–	+
Vimentin	–	–	–	–	–	–	+/–	+	–	+/–

Note: *CK* cytokeratin, *LADC* lung adenocarcinoma, *BADC* breast carcinoma, *UGI* upper gastrointestinal tract, *PADC* pancreatic adenocarcinoma, *ICC* intrahepatic cholangiocarcinoma, *UC* urothelial carcinoma, *PRCC* papillary renal cell carcinoma, *PTC* papillary thyroid carcinoma, *SADC* small bowel adenocarcinoma, *MS* mesothelioma, *GATA3* GATA binding protein 3, *ER* estrogen receptor, *TTF1* thyroid transcription factor 1, *CDH17* cadherin-17, *CDX2* caudal-type homeobox 2, *PAX8* paired box gene 8, *RCCma* renal cell carcinoma marker, *pVHL* von Hippel-Lindau tumor suppressor, "+" >75% of cases are positive, "–" <5% of cases are positive, "+/–" 50–75% of cases are positive, "–/+" – <50% of cases are positive

Table 1.9 Summary of CK7+/ER+ carcinomas and useful markers

Antibody	Breast CA	EMADC	ECADC	OSCA	OCCCA
GATA3	+	–	–	–	–
TFF1	+	–	–	–	–
PAX8	–	+	+/–	+	+/–
WT1	–	–	–	+	–
Vimentin	–	+	–	–	–
p16	–	Patchy +	Diffusely +	+	+/–
HPV in situ	–	–	+/–	–	–
pVHL	–	–	–	–	+/–
HNF-1B	+/–	+/–	+/–	–	+

Note: *CK* cytokeratin, *ER* estrogen receptor, *CA* carcinoma, *EMADC* endometrial adenocarcinoma, *ECADC* endocervical ADC, *OSCA* ovarian serous carcinoma, *OCCCA* ovarian clear cell carcinoma, *GATA3* GATA binding protein 3, *TFF1* trefoil factor 1, *PAX8* paired box gene 8, *WT1* Wilms' tumor 1, *HPV* human papilloma virus, *pVHL* von Hippel-Lindau tumor suppressor, *HNF-1B* hepatocyte nuclear factor 1 beta, "+" >75% of cases are positive, "-" <5% of cases are positive, "+/–" 50-75% of cases are positive, "–/+" <50% of cases are positive

Table 1.10 Lung ADC vs. breast carcinoma

Marker/diagnosis	Lung ADC	Breast carcinoma
TTF1	+	–
Napsin A	+	–
ER	–	+
GATA3	–	+
TFF1	–	+

Note: *ADC* adenocarcinoma; *TTF1* thyroid transcription factor 1, *ER* estrogen receptor, *GATA3* GATA binding protein 3, *TFF1* trefoil factor 1, "+" >75% of cases are positive, "–" <5% of cases are positive

Table 1.11 Lung ADC vs. mesothelioma

Antibody	Lung ADC	Mesothelioma
Calretinin	–	+
WT1	–	+
CK5/6	–	+
D2-40	–	+
CEA	+	–
MOC-31	+	–
TTF1	+	–

Note: *ADC* adenocarcinoma, *WT1* Wilms' tumor 1, *CK* cytokeratin, *D2-40* podoplanin, CEA carcinoembryonic antigen, *MOC-31* epithelial-related antigen clone MOC-31, *TTF1* thyroid transcription factor 1, "+" >75% of cases are positive, "–" <5% of cases are positive. In general, to render a diagnosis of mesothelioma, the tumor should be positive for at least 2 mesothelial markers and negative for 2 carcinoma markers

(HNF-1B) are helpful markers in distinguishing ovarian serous carcinoma from ovarian clear cell carcinoma. Additionally, p53 is usually diffusely and strongly positive or completely negative in serous carcinomas and only focally and weakly positive in ovarian clear cell carcinomas. KIM-1, which is not currently commercially available, is a sensitive and relatively specific marker for ovarian and uterine clear cell carcinomas; pVHL plays a

Table 1.12 Lung vs. upper GI, pancreatobiliary primary, and urinary bladder

Markers/diagnosis	Lung ADC	Upper GI ADC	Pancreatic ADC	UC
TTF1	+	–	–	–
Napsin A	+	–/+	–	–
CDH17	–	+/–	–/+	–/+
CDX2	–	–/+	–/+	–
CK20	–	–/+	–/+	+/–
MUC5AC	–	–/+	+/–	–
p40	–	–	–	+
GATA3	–	–	–	+

Note: *GI* gastrointestinal, *ADC* ADC, *UC* urothelial carcinoma, *TTF1* thyroid transcription factor 1, *CDH17* cadherin-17, *CDX2* caudal-type homeobox 2, *CK* cytokeratin, *MUC5AC* mucin 5 AC, *GATA3* GATA binding protein 3, "+" >75% of cases are positive, "–" <5% of cases are positive, "+/–" 50–75% of cases are positive, "–/+" <50% of cases are positive

Table 1.13 Breast carcinoma vs. upper GI, pancreatobiliary primary, and urinary bladder

Markers/diagnosis	Breast CA	Upper GI ADC	Pancreatic ADC	UC
ER	+	–	–	–
GATA3	+	–	–	+
CDH17	–	+/–	+/–	–/+
MUC5AC	–	–/+	+/–	–
p40	–	–	–	+
CK20	–	–/+	–/+	+/–
p63	–	–	–	+

Note: *GI* gastrointestinal, *CA* carcinoma, *ADC* adenocarcinoma, *UC* urothelial carcinoma, *ER* estrogen receptor, *GATA3* GATA binding protein 3, *CDH17* cadherin-17, *MUC5AC* mucin 5 AC, CK20 cytokeratin 20 "+" >75% of cases are positive, "–" <5% of cases are positive, "+/–" 50–75% of cases are positive, "–/+" <50% of cases are positive

Table 1.14 Lung ADC vs. gynecologic primaries

Markers/diagnosis	Lung ADC	OSC	EMADC	ECADC	OCCC
TTF1	+	–	–	–	–
Napsin A	+	–	–	–	+
PAX8	–	+	+	+	+/–
ER	–	+	+	+/–	+/–
Vimentin	–	–	+	–	–
WT1	–	+	–	–	–
pVHL	–	–	–	–	+/–
HPV in situ	–	–	–	+	–

Note: *ADC* adenocarcinoma, *OSC* ovarian serous carcinoma, *EMADC* endometrial ADC, *ECADC* endocervical ADC, *OCCC* ovarian clear cell carcinoma, *TTF1* thyroid transcription factor 1, *PAX 8* paired box gene 8, *ER* estrogen receptor, *WT1* Wilm's tumor 1, *pVHL* von Hippel-Lindau tumor suppressor, *HPV* human papilloma virus, "+" >75% of cases are positive, "–" <5% of cases are positive, "+/–" 50–75% of cases are positive. Clear cell carcinomas of the endometrium are frequently positive for napsin A as well similar role. No reliable immunomarkers are available for differentiating a uterine serous carcinoma from an ovarian serous carcinoma.

- *Differential diagnosis of CK20+/CK7- carcinomas.*
  Predominately CK20+ carcinomas include colorectal ADC (CRADC), small intestinal ADC (SADC), bladder ADC (BADC), appendiceal ADC (APADC), Merkel cell carcinoma, and salivary gland small-cell carcinoma. Perinuclear dot-staining patterns are seen in both Merkel cell carcinoma and salivary gland small-cell carcinoma. Merkel cell polyomavirus (MCPyV) was detected in approximately 80% of Merkel cell carcinomas but not in other high-grade neuroendocrine carcinomas, including salivary gland small-cell carcinomas; therefore, MCPyV is a potentially sensitive and highly specific marker for identification of Merkel cell carcinoma of the skin. CK20+ carcinomas and useful markers are summarized in Table 1.16.
- *Differential diagnosis of CK7−/CK20- carcinomas.*
  The following neoplasms usually present as CK7−/CK20- carcinomas, and some relatively tissue-specific markers may be helpful in reaching a definitive diagnosis. These tumors include but are not limited to (1) medullary carcinomas of the colon, (2) some neuroendocrine neoplasms, (3) clear cell RCCs, (4) HCCs, (5) adrenal cortical neoplasm/carcinomas, (6) germ cell tumors, (7) prostatic ADCs, and (8) SCCs. A subset of small-cell carcinomas of the lung, gastric ADCs, esophageal ADCs, and mesotheliomas can be CK7−/CK20-.
  Medullary carcinoma of the colon frequently shows loss of microsatellite instability (MSI) markers, especially MutL homolog 1 (MLH1) and postmeiotic segregation increased 2 (PMS2), and is commonly positive for CDH17, SATB2, calretinin, trefoil factor (TFF)3, and mucin 4 (MUC4). CDX2 expression tends to be weak and focal. Focal positivity (<25% of the tumor cells stained) for neuroendocrine markers such as synaptophysin can be seen. Approximately 70% of medullary carcinomas of the large bowel can be positive for calretinin.
  Neuroendocrine neoplasms/carcinomas are positive for chromogranin, synaptophysin, and CD56. Chromogranin is expressed in well to moderately differentiated neuroendocrine neoplasms/carcinomas and tends to be only focally positive in poorly differentiated neuroendocrine carcinomas/small-cell carcinomas. CD56 is a highly sensitive marker for small-cell carcinoma; however, its expression is only seen in approximately 50% of pancreatic NETs. Additionally, CD56 can be positive in non-neuroendocrine carcinomas. More recently, preliminary studies showed that approximately 50% of pancreatic NETs showed loss of expression of anti-ATRX or anti-DAXX. The expression of ATRX/DAXX is usually present in NETs from other organs. To differentiate the tissue origin of a given neuroendocrine neoplasm/carcinoma, the following markers are useful and are summarized in Table 1.17.
  Germ cell tumors are frequently negative for CK7 and CK20. SALL4 and LIN28 are excellent screening markers for germ cell tumors, which are positive in nearly 100% of seminomas, embryonal carcinomas, and yolk sac tumors, 70% of choriocarcinomas, and 50% of teratomas. D2-40 and CD117 are specific markers for seminoma; AFP and glypican-3 are specific markers for yolk sac tumors; SOX2, NANOG, and CD30 are relatively specific markers for embryonal carcinomas, although NANOG is also positive in seminomas and SOX2 may be positive in yolk sac tumors; and CD10 and beta-human chorionic gonadotropin (B-HCG) are specific markers for choriocarcinomas. GATA3 are frequently positive in cho-

Table 1.15 PRCC vs. UC vs. CDC vs. PADC

Markers/diagnosis	PRCC	UC	CDC	PADC
PAX8	+	−	+	−
RCCma	+	−	+/−	−
GATA3	−	+	−	−
p40	−	+	−	−
S100P	−	+	−	−
P504S	+	−/+	−	+
PSA	−	−	−	+
CK7	+	+	+	−

Note: *PRCC* papillary renal cell carcinoma, *UC* urothelial carcinoma, *CDC* collecting duct carcinoma, *PADC* prostatic adenocarcinoma, *PAX 8* paired box gene 8, *RCCma* renal cell carcinoma marker, *GATA3* GATA binding protein 3, *S100P* placental S100, *P504S* alpha-methylacyl-CoA racemase, *PSA* prostate-specific antigen, *CK7* cytokeratin 7, "+" >75% of cases are positive, "−" <5% of cases are positive, "+/−" 50–75% of cases are positive, "−/+" <50% of cases are positive. Urothelial carcinoma of the renal pelvis may be focally positive for PAX8

Table 1.16 Summary of CK20+ carcinomas and useful markers

Marker/ diagnosis	CRADC	SADC	BADC	Merkel	APADC	SSCC
CK7	−	−/+	−	−	−	−
CDX2	+	+	+	−	+	−
SATB2	+	−	N/A	N/A	+	N/A
CDH17	+	+	+	−	+	−
Beta-catenin (nuclear)	+	+/−	−	−	+/−	−
Synaptophysin	−	−	−	+	−	+
GATA3	−	−	+/−	−	−	−

Note: *CRADC* colorectal adenocarcinoma, *SADC* small intestinal adenocarcinoma, *BADC* bladder adenocarcinoma, *APADC* appendiceal adenocarcinoma, *SSCC* salivary gland small-cell carcinoma, *CK* cytokeratin, *CDX2* caudal-type homeobox 2, *SATB2* special AT-rich sequence-binding protein 2, *CDH17* cadherin-17, *GATA3* GATA binding protein 3, "+" >75% of cases are positive, "−" <5% of cases are positive, "+/−" 50–75% of cases are positive, "−/+" <50% of cases are positive

Table 1.17 Markers for NETs

Markers/ diagnosis	Lung	Pan	Stoma	Duo	Ileum	Appen	LC	Rec
CK7	+	+/−	+/−	−	−	−	−	−
CK20	−	−	−	−	+	+/−	+	−/+
CDX2	−	−	−	−	+	+	+/−	+/−
SATB2	−	−	−	−	−	−/+	+	+
CDH17	−	+	+	+/−	+	+	+	+
TTF1	−/+	−	−	−	−	−	−	−
PR	−	+/−	−	−	−	−	−	−
PAX8	−	+/−	−	−	−	−	−	−/+
PDX1	−	+	−	+	−	−	−	−

Note: *Pan* pancreas, *Stoma* stomach, *Duo* duodenum, *Appen* appendix, *LC* left colon, *Rec* rectum, *CK* cytokeratin, *CDX2* caudal-type homeobox 2, *SATB2* special AT-rich sequence-binding protein 2, CDH17 cadherin-17, *TTF1* thyroid transcription factor 1, *PR* progesterone receptor; *PAX8* paired box gene 8, *PDX1* pancreatic duodenal homeobox 1,"+" >75% of cases are positive, "−" <5% of cases are positive, "+/−" 50–75% of cases are positive, "−/+" <50% of cases are positive

Table 1.18 Markers for germ cell tumors

Marker	Seminoma	Embryonal CA	Yolk sac tumor	ChorioCA
SALL4	+	+	+	+/−
LIN28	+	+	+	+/−
OCT4	+	+	−	+/−
SOX2	−	+	−/+	−
NANOG	+	+	−	−
CD30	−	+	−	−
CD117	+	−	−	−
D2-40	+	−	−	−
Glypican-3	−	−	+	−
AFP	−	−	+	−
Beta-HCG	−	−	−	+
CD10	−	−	−	+

Note: *CA* carcinoma, *chorioCA* choriocarcinoma, *SALL4* sal-like protein 4, *LIN28* lin-28 homolog, *OCT4* octamer-binding transcription factor 4, *SOX2* sex-determining region Y-box 2, *NANOG* NANOG homeobox, *CD* cluster of differentiation, *D2-40* podoplanin, *AFP* alpha-fetoprotein, *beta-HCG* beta-human chorionic gonadotropin, "+" >75% of cases are positive,"−" <5% of cases are positive, "+/−" 50–75% of cases are positive, "−/+" <50% of cases are positive

riocarcinomas and yolk sac tumors. The useful markers are summarized in Table 1.18.

Over 90% of clear cell RCCs are negative for both CK7 and CK20. Co-expression of cytokeratin/vimentin is one of the important features for clear cell RCC. Five markers (PAX8, pVHL, RCCma, CD10, and KIM-1) are helpful in confirming the diagnosis of clear cell RCC. PAX8 is likely the most sensitive marker among these five markers; however, it also expresses in tumors from the thyroid, gynecologic tract, thymus, and others. RCCma has a low sensitivity of approximately 50% in detecting a high-grade clear cell RCC. Both pVHL and KIM-1 are also expressed in clear cell carcinomas of the uterus and ovary; however, KIM-1 is not commercially available yet. CD10 is a highly sensitive but not very specific marker for clear cell RCC. In general, a small panel of antibodies consisting of CAM5.2, vimentin, PAX8, pVHL, and RCCma can serve as an initial panel to confirm a metastatic clear cell RCC. When it comes to a sarcomatoid RCC, an extended panel of antibodies including cytokeratins, vimentin, PAX8, pVHL, RCCma, CD10, KIM-1, and alpha-methyl-acyl-CoA racemase (P504S) is recommended to increase the diagnostic sensitivity.

A majority of HCCs are negative for CK7 and CK20, with the exception of fibrolamellar HCC, which is usually CK7+/CK20-. Approximately 10% of HCCs may show positive staining for both CK7 and CK20. AE1/AE3 is only positive in approximately 30% of HCCs, whereas over 90% of HCCs are positive for CAM5.2 which contains keratin 8. Other cytokeratins such as 5D3, 5D3/LP34, and KL1 (containing both keratins 8 and 18) are good screening markers for HCC. Many markers are useful for identifying HCC, including arginase-1, glypican-3, HepPar-1, CD10, and polyclonal carcinoembryonic antigen (CEA). Arginase-1 is the most sensitive and specific marker for HCC, including poorly differentiated HCC, whereas HepPar-1 is a sensitive but not very specific marker for HCC since its immunoreactivity has been reported in many other carcinomas. The diagnostic sensitivity of both arginase-1 and HepPar-1 for identifying liver cell origin is over 90%. Glypican-3 is a good marker for both well-differentiated and poorly differentiated HCC, with a diagnostic sensitivity of approximately 85%. In addition, glypican-3 is not expressed in benign or reactive hepatocytes; in contrast, both arginase-1 and HepPar-1 are expressed in both benign and neoplastic hepatocytes. Both CD10 and polyclonal CEA demonstrate a canalicular staining pattern in HCC and benign liver. AFP has limited utility due to its low sensitivity of approximately 25%, but AFP is a highly sensitive marker for hepatoblastoma. Nearly all HCCs are negative for MOC-31.

Adrenal cortical neoplasm/carcinoma is another group of epithelial tumors which is usually negative for both CK7 and CK20. Mart-1, calretinin, SF-1, and inhibin-alpha are a group of sensitive and relatively specific markers for identifying adrenal cortical neoplasm/carcinomas. They are usually negative for hepatocellular markers (arginase-1, HepPar-1, and glypican-3) and RCC markers (PAX8, RCCma, CD10, CAIX, and pVHL) .

Over 90% of prostatic acinar ADCs are negative for CK7 and CK20, with the exception of prostatic ductal ADC, which is usually positive for CK7. Prostate-specific antigen (PSA) and prostate-specific acid phosphatase (PSAP) are highly sensitive and specific markers for identifying over 90% of metastatic prostatic ADCs. NK3 homeobox 1 (NKX3.1) is a highly sensitive and specific nuclear staining marker for both primary and metastatic prostatic ADCs and has been reported in virtually 100% of prostatic ADCs. NKX3.1 is a marker of choice for a metastatic prostatic ADC in a decalcified specimen. P504S is another very sensitive but not totally specific marker for prostatic ADC. ERG is a recently described specific but not very sensitive marker for prostatic ADC, with a diagnostic sensitivity of approximately 40–50%. ERG is the most sensitive marker for benign and malignant vascular tumors. SCCs frequently showed no immunoreactivity for CK7 or CK20. Many markers such as p40, CK5/6, p63, CK903, and SOX2 are indicative of squamous differentiation. CK5/6 and p40 are the most reliable markers to confirm squamous cell differentiation; however, a majority of urothelial carcinomas is also positive for both p40 and CK5/6.

Diagnostic IHC Panels Based on Histomorphology

If based on the histomorphology alone, four major morphologic types of neoplasms are usually encountered, including epithelioid cells (Table 1.19), small round cells (Table 1.20), spindle cells (Table 1.21), and pleomorphic cells (Table 1.22). Each morphologic category encompasses a wide differential diagnosis. Tables 1.19, 1.20, and 1.21 summarize the useful markers in the differential diagnosis of each category of tumor.

Alveolar soft part sarcoma may be positive for transcription factor E3 (TFE3) but negative for vimentin. Epithelioid sarcoma frequently shows loss of INI1 expression. PEComas can be patchy positive for S100 and usually positive for HMB45 and Mart-1 as well.

Application of Molecular Techniques on FNA Specimens

As our understanding of the molecular genetics of tumors is growing, the application of molecular tests on FNA specimens is accelerating. Most molecular techniques include:

- In-situ hybridization (ISH)
- Polymerase chain reaction (PCR)
- Reverse transcription-polymerase chain reaction (RT-PCR)
- Southern blotting
- Gene microarrays
- Transcriptional profiling

These techniques can be performed with FNAB specimens including direct smears, Thin Prep, or Surepath and have been used with different organ systems and different objectives to:

- Detect cancer cells.
- Render a specific diagnosis.
- Distinct benign from malignant disease.

Table 1.20 Markers for small round cell tumors

Marker/diagnosis	NB	ES/PNET	RHMS	LYM	DPSRCT	SmCC	PC
Desmin	−	−	+	−	+	−	−
Myogenin	−	−	+	−	−	−	−
CD99	−	+	−/+	+/−	+/−	−	−
NSE	+	+	−	−	−/+	+/−	−
LCA	−	−	−	+	−	−	−
S100	−	−	−	−	−	−	−
Vimentin	+	+	+	+	+	−	+
CK	−	−	−	−	+	+	−
WT1	−	−	−	−	+/−	−	−
Fli-1	−	+	−	+	−	−	−

Note: *NB* neuroblastoma, *ES/PNET* Ewing sarcoma/primitive neuroectodermal tumor, *RHMS* rhabdomyosarcoma, *LYM* lymphoblastic lymphoma, *DPSRCT* desmoplastic small round cell tumor, *SmCC* small-cell carcinoma, *PC* plasmacytoma, *CD* cluster of differentiation, *NSE* neuron-specific enolase, *LCA* leukocyte common antigen, *CK* cytokeratin, *WT1* Wilms' tumor 1; *Fli-1* friend leukemia virus integration 1, "+" >75% of cases are positive, "−" <5% of cases are positive, "+/−" 50–75% of cases are positive; "−/+" <50% of cases are positive

Table 1.19 Markers for epithelioid tumors

Diagnosis/markers	CK	S100	Myo	CD117	SMA	CD34	ERG	Mart-1
Carcinoma	+	−	−	−	−	−	−	−
Melanoma	−	+	−	−/+	−	−	−	+
Mesothelioma	+	−	−	−	−	−	−	−
Epithelioid sarcoma	+	−	−	−	−	+/−	−	−
Epithelioid angiosarcoma	− or focally +	−	−	−	−	+	+	−
Clear cell sarcoma	−	+	−	−	−	−	−	+
Epithelioid GIST	−	−	−	+	−/+	+/−	−	−
Epithelioid MPNST	− or focally +	focally +	−	−	−	−	−	−
Alveolar soft part sarcoma	−	−	−	−	−	−	−	−
PEComas	−	−	−	−	+	−	−	+/−
Chordoma	+	+	−	−	−	−	−	−

Note: *CK* cytokeratin (AE1/3+ CAM5.2), *Myo* myogenin, *CD* cluster of differentiation, *SMA* smooth muscle actin, *ERG* ETS-related gene, *Mart-1* melanoma-associated antigen recognized by T cells 1, *GIST* gastrointestinal stromal tumor, *MPNST* malignant peripheral nerve sheath tumor, *PEComas* perivascular epithelioid cell tumors, "+" >75% of cases are positive, "−" <5% of cases are positive, "+/−" 50–75% of cases are positive, "−/+" <50% of cases are positive

Table 1.21 Markers for spindle cell tumors

Diagnosis/markers	CK	S100	Vimentin	SMA	Desmin	CD34	CD117
Spindle cell carcinoma	+	–	+/–	–	–	–	–
Spindle cell melanoma	–	+	+	–	–	–	–
Neurogenic tumor	–	+	+	–	–	–	–
GIST	–	–	+	–/+	–	+/–	+
Smooth muscle tumor	–	–	+	+	+	–	–
Fibrosarcoma	–	–	+	–	–	–	–
DFSP	–	–	+	–	–	+	–
SFT	–	–	+	–	–	+	–
Synovial sarcoma	+	–	+	–	–	–	–
Kaposi sarcoma	–	–	+	–	–	+/–	–

Note: *CK* cytokeratin, *SMA* smooth muscle actin, *CD* cluster of differentiation, *GIST* gastrointestinal stromal tumor, *DFSP* dermatofibrosarcoma protuberans, *SFT* solitary fibrous tumor, "+" >75% of cases are positive, "–" <5% of cases are positive, "+/–" 50–75% of cases are positive, "–/+" <50% of cases are positive

Table 1.22 Markers for pleomorphic tumors

Diagnosis/markers	CK	Vimentin	S100	Desmin	Myogenin	SMA
Carcinoma	+	–/+	–	–	–	–
Pleomorphic sarcoma	–	+	–	–	–	–
Liposarcoma	–	+	Focally +	–	–	–
Rhabdomyosarcoma	–	+	–	+/–	+/–	+/–
Leiomyosarcoma	–	+	–	Focally +	–	+
Melanoma	–	+	+	–	–	–

Note: *CK* cytokeratin, *SMA* smooth muscle actin, "+" >75% of cases are positive, "–" <5% of cases are positive, "+/–" 50–75% of cases are positive, "–/+" <50% of cases are positive

- Determine the genetic abnormalities and genetic makeup of tumors.
- Predict response to chemotherapy.
- Perform risk assessment.
- Select patients for targeted therapy.

Interphase cytogenetic studies by ISH techniques, unlike metaphase karyotyping, allow analysis of cytogenetic alterations of individual cells independent of their ability to proliferate. ISH with chromogenic or fluorescent signals has distinct advantages over other molecular techniques because it allows comparison of cellular morphology with chromosomal alterations in cells. FNA specimens, unlike cell block sections or tissue sections, are particularly suitable for ISH. The availability of intact cells makes it possible to count hybridized signals in the nuclei without nuclear transection and the associated inaccuracy in signal counting that can occur with cell block or tissue sections. With the availability of the commercial DNA probes, fluorescence in-situ hybridization (FISH) has several clinical applications for FNA specimens.

PCR can be performed using aspirated material collected solely for molecular analysis, from cells scraped from cellular smears, or from 10-micron tissue sections of cell blocks prepared from FNAB samples. The success of the test depends on the amount of viable material available for analysis:

- PCR amplification, which allows automated enzymatic in-vitro synthesis of a target DNA sequence in millions of copies for subsequent sequence analysis, is one of the most commonly used molecular technique to demonstrate molecular alterations in FNA specimens.
- RT-PCR analysis allows for amplification of very limited quantities of transcripts. This technique is suitable for molecular analysis of limited amounts of material, such as that procured by FNA.
- Multiplex PCR allows for amplification of several target sequences simultaneously and is increasingly used for molecular analysis.

Microarray analysis has been used on FNA specimens. DNA chip or microarray technology relies on the accurate binding or hybridization of strands of DNA with their precise complementary copies where the known sequences are bound onto a solid-state substrate. These are hybridized with probes of fluorescent cDNAs or genomic sequences from test material. By analyzing the intensity of fluorescence on the chip, the expression of several thousands of genes can be determined simultaneously. The bioinformatics statistical programs were used to analyze the data generated in microarray experiments. And transcriptional profiling of using the currently available gene chips has been reported on FNA specimens from sites such as breast, lymph node, and lung.

Although some molecular tests are used for patient care, such as assessment of human epidermal growth factor receptor 2 (HER2/neu) for gene amplification in breast cancer, detection of clonality in hematopoietic neoplasms, and specific chromosomal translocations in the diagnosis of soft tissue sarcoma and hematopoietic neoplasms, most are currently investigational only.

Breast Cancer

- The FISH assay for HER2/neu gene amplification can be performed on FNAB air-dried cytology smears or cell block sections of metastatic tumors because the HER2/neu status is usually concordant among primary tumor, locoregional, and distant metastasis.
- Two kits approved by the US Food and Drug Administration (FDA) are either using an HER2/neu probe alone (Oncor, Gaithersburg, MD) or using an HER2/neu probe and a centromere 17 probe (Path Vysion, Vysis, Downers Grove, IL) .

Soft Tissue Tumors

- The specific cytogenetic alterations can be detected using karyotypic analysis, PCR, or ISH. Touch preparations of core needle biopsy and cytospin or monolayer preparations of FNA specimens of primary or recurrent sarcomas are excellent specimens for FISH testing because of the availability of single cells for analysis.
- Common and specific translocations can lead to recombination of coding sequences of different genes and result in the formation of pathologic fusion genes and expression of pathologic gene fusion products, which is valuable for making accurate diagnosis of soft tissue tumors.
- The chromosomal translocation (11;22) (q24;q12) is specific for Ewing sarcoma, peripheral neuroepithelioma, and Askin's tumor. When EWS gene is fused with the ATF-1 gene resulting from t(12;22)(q13;q12), it is specific for clear cell sarcoma; when it is fused with the WT-1 gene in t(11;22)(p13;q12), it is specific for desmoplastic small round cell tumor; when it is fused with the CHN gene in t(9;22)(q22;q12), it is specific for myxoid chondrosarcoma.
- Alveolar rhabdomyosarcoma is characterized by two tumor-specific chromosomal translocations, t(2;13)(q35;q14) and t(1;13)(p36;q14), resulting in fusions of the PAX3 and PAX7 genes, which are members of the PAX transcription factor gene family mapped to 2q35 and 1p36 with the FKRH gene mapped to 13q14.
- Synovial sarcoma is characterized by specific t(X;18)(p11;q11) translocation involving the SYT gene on chromosome 18 and 1 of the SSX genes on chromosome X, leading to functional fusion (SYT-SSX). These translocations are specific for synovial sarcoma and are particularly valuable for diagnosis of the small-cell and monophasic variants of synovial sarcoma.
- Molecular analysis of c-kit mutations can be successfully performed using FNA samples for making a diagnosis of primary and recurrent gastrointestinal stromal tumors (GIST) .

Hematopoietic Neoplasms

- In many cases cytomorphologic features in conjunction with immunophenotyping of aspirated material using flow cytometry and/or immunocytochemistry (ICC) alone may be sufficient for making a specific diagnosis.
- In selected cases of malignant lymphoma where immunophenotyping using flow cytometry and/or ICC produces confusing results, molecular tests such as Southern blotting, PCR, and FISH can be used with FNA to demonstrate the clonality.
- PCR is the most widely used for detection of immunoglobulin (Ig) heavy-chain and T-cell receptor gene rearrangements.
- FISH and PCR can be used to detect bcl-1 and bcl-2 gene rearrangements in aspirates.
- FISH performed on FNA smears using cyclin D1 and immunoglobulin heavy chain probes to demonstrate t(11;14)(q13;q32) chromosomal translocation in mantle cell lymphoma.
- FISH performed on FNA smears using bcl-2 and immunoglobulin heavy chain probes indicating t(14;18)9q32;q21) chromosomal translocation.

Thyroid Neoplasms

- FNA is routinely used to guide management of patients in the preoperative evaluation of thyroid nodules.
- In 5–10% of cases, the results are inadequate; and in 20% of cases, the findings could be indeterminate for malignancy would require thyroidectomy.
- Telomerase, RET/PTC rearrangements, and BRAF mutation have been studied with FNA of the thyroid.
- More than half of all papillary thyroid carcinomas (PTC) harbor at least one of several chimeric oncogenes, called RET/PTC, which results from gene rearrangements involving the ret. proto-oncogene on chromosome 10 resulting in the generation of novel fusion transcripts.
- Study supports the usefulness of RET/PTC RT-PCR and Southern hybridization as an ancillary test to cytology in selected cases for a definitive diagnosis of PTC.
- BRAF mutations by RT-PCR are found in 70–72% of PTC cases and highly specific; they have not been noted in benign nodules or in other thyroid malignancies and has been investigated as an adjunct to cytology for making a definitive diagnosis of PTC. BRAF mutations also established the presence of malignancy in 16% of carcinomas that could not be diagnosed conclusively by FNA alone. The use of FNA sample in evaluating RET/PTC and BRAF mutations for making a diagnosis of PTC in

indeterminate and suspicious cases of thyroid malignancies will require validation in future studies.

- The telomerase activity has been investigated in thyroid FNA samples and archival Diff-Quik stained smears to distinguish malignant from benign lesions. Telomeres are highly conserved hexameric nucleotide repeats at the ends of chromosomes. Telomerase activity and hTERT gene expression by RT-PCR are noted in malignancy and in lymphocytic thyroiditis and 40% of follicular adenomas. The occurrence of telomerase activity in benign tumors decreases the specificity of the test in the preoperative diagnosis of thyroid nodules on FNA specimens.
- Gene expression profiling by extracellular matrix and adhesion molecule cDNA arrays and real-time quantitative RT-PCR for FNA samples has been studied for the preoperative distinction of benign and malignant thyroid nodules from FNA samples and is promising and still needed to be validated in prospective trials.

Pulmonary Neoplasms

- The sensitivity of lung FNA in the diagnosis of bronchogenic carcinoma is around 80%. The need for ancillary molecular testing with lung FNA samples arises in some cases with indeterminate or suspicious cytology findings where corresponding core needle biopsy (CNB) are unavailable or when CNB could not be performed either because of technical reasons or because of the development of pneumothorax. In de-stained Papanicolaou (Pap)-stained smears (the exfoliative and transbronchial FNA cases), the multitarget FISH assay (La Vysion, Vysis), which includes probes for chromosome 6p11-q11, 7p12 (EGFR), 8q24 (myc), and 5p15.2-chromosomal loci commonly affected in non-small-cell lung carcinoma (NSCLC), has been investigated to distinguish benign from malignant lesions. The test has been reported with an overall sensitivity and specificity of 79% and 100% and has potential in clinical practice for making a definite diagnosis in selected cases of lung FNA cases.
- The c-myc E2F-1/p21 WAF1/Cip1 interactive gene expression index has been used for standardized RT-PCR testing of lung FNA with a sensitivity of 100% and specificity of 94%. The contribution of these molecular tests as an adjunct to cytology needs further validation.
- The echinoderm microtubule-associated protein-like 4-anaplastic lymphoma kinase (ALK) re-arrangements and epidermal growth factor receptor (EGFR) mutations have emerged as a leading target for the treatment of patients with NSCLC, which are commonly mutually exclusive. If there is an EGFR mutation, the presence of KRAS mutation needs to be evaluated since its presence will negate the effect of EGFR inhibitors downstream and render the treatment ineffective. RT-PCR-based assays that target specific mutations in the EGFR gene have been reported to predict good response to tyrosine kinase (TK) inhibitors and can be easily performed on FNA material to aid in the selection of patients with advanced NSCLC for therapy with EGFR inhibitors. There are reports indicating the utility of assessing EGFR gene amplification for selecting patients for EGFR inhibitor therapy; and the gene amplification tests can be performed on FNAB samples.
- The gene expression profiling of advanced NSCLC using RNA from lung FNA samples was performed and showed that transcriptional profiles were comparable with that from surgically excised tissue.

Metastatic Tumor in Lymph Node

- The ancillary molecular tests can be used to detect small metastases and is considered currently investigational.
- PCR for selected markers has been used to detect hypermethylation of CpG islands in promoter regions of MGMT, p16, and p14 as markers for micrometastases in EUS-guided lymph node FNA samples from patients with gastrointestinal and lung cancer.
- RT-PCR has also been reported to detect levels of human telomerase reverse transcriptase mRNA to identify metastasis in the lymph nodes in patients with NSCLC.
- Numerical aberrations in cyclin D1 gene copy numbers by FISH on FNA have been done in patients with previously untreated stage I and II oral squamous cell carcinoma who had not undergone radical neck dissection and showed independently predicted late cervical lymph node metastasis and that the results of such an analysis could be a valuable marker for poor prognosis, tumor aggressiveness, recurrence, and for selecting patients for elective cervical lymph node dissection.
- RT-PCR for tyrosinase, a tissue-specific enzyme that regulates melanin biosynthesis, has been done in lymph node FNAB samples to detect metastasis of melanoma.

Pancreatic Neoplasms

- K-ras oncogene mutations by mutant-enriched PCR have been investigated using FNA samples as a possible adjunct to conventional cytology for making a definite diagnosis of pancreatic adenocarcinoma. The K-ras oncogene is activated by point mutations in 75–90% of pancreatic adenocarcinoma with typical localization in codon 12. And K-ras mutations have been described in few proven cases of chronic pancreatitis.
- Semiquantitative PCR for assessment of telomerase activity as a possible ancillary test to increase the sensitivity of pancreatic FNA in patients with pancreatic adenocarcinomas.
- Comparative genomic hybridization (CGH) enables the study of global chromosomal aberrations in patient tissues without the need to culture the constituent cells. Target mutant DNA and normal DNA are tagged with different

fluorescent signals and are mixed and applied to the normal metaphase chromosome preparations. The normal and mutant DNAs compete to hybridize with their complementary chromosomal loci. Digital image scanning is then used to quantify and compare the relative amounts of differentially colored signals indicating loss or gain of DNA in a given chromosomal locus.

- The differentially expressed genes, lipocalin 2 (LCN2) and PLAT (tissue-type plasminogen activator or tPA), have been validated by RT-PCR in FNA samples and reported to be significantly increased in all pancreatic adenocarcinoma. Lipocalins are small extracellular proteins with an important role in cell proliferation and differentiation. PLAT is important in tumor angiogenesis and in the development of exocrine pancreatic cancer, contributing to the invasive phenotype. The utility of evaluating markers, such as lipocalin 2 and PLAT by RT-PCR using FNA of the pancreas for the diagnosis of pancreatic adenocarcinoma, needs further validation in future studies.

Renal Neoplasms

- MN/CA9, carbonic anhydrase family member, is upregulated by hypoxia-inducible factor 1 alpha in many cancers in response to hypoxic conditions. Its gene expression by RT-PCR in kidney FNA samples have been investigated as potential ancillary aids for making a definite diagnosis of malignancy on renal FNA. It has been established as a reliable biomarker for RCC and is present in almost all clear RCCs and in about 56% of papillary RCCs but is absent from chromophobe RCCs, oncocytomas, and normal tissue. The overall sensitivity and specificity were 68% and 100%, respectively. MN/CA9 protein expression can also be demonstrated by ICC.
- FISH was performed on kidney tumors using centromere-specific probes for chromosome Y, 7, 17, 16, 12, 8, and 3 to study chromosomal alterations in FNA and effusions of primary and metastatic renal cell carcinoma and found numerical aberrations of chromosome 3 to be most frequent in RCC.

Infectious Disease

- There are few reports discussing PCR on FNA samples from lymph nodes as an adjunct to conventional methods for the diagnosis of tuberculous lymphadenitis. An RT-PCR assay was developed to diagnose and identify the causative agent of suspected mycobacterial lymphadenitis using primers to detect *M. avium* and *M. tuberculosis*. This assay detected mycobacterial infections in 71.6% of patients; auramine staining and culture were positive in 46.3% and 41.2% of patients, respectively.
- A PCR method for the amplification of *Bartonella henselae* DNA was developed, and showed that the results of this test can be useful for making an accurate diagnosis of cat-scratch disease in FNA specimens of the lymph nodes and primary lesion in comparison to Warthin-Starry silver impregnation stains and culture and can obviate the need for excisional biopsy.
- The detection of HPV DNA in metastatic squamous cell carcinoma by PCR or in-situ hybridization can be used in selected cases to support a possible anogenital origin of the tumor, if the differential diagnosis includes tumors reported to have a low prevalence of HPV DNA such as from lung, esophagus, and skin in non-immunocompromised patients. The presence of high-risk HPV type in that case would suggest either an anogenital or a head-and-neck origin of the carcinoma.

The literature reports the excellent potential of material procured from FNA for applications in almost any type of molecular analysis, but few of the tests alone are used for patient care. However, some of these tests have the potential for clinical use in the coming years. The possible integration of molecular tests with current practice for the distinction of benign from malignant lesions in selected cases, determining the genetic makeup of tumors, and identifying specific molecular targets for typing, diagnosis, determining prognosis, and response to therapy are some of the anticipated uses of molecular tests as applied to FNA in the near future. Combining the stringent cytological criteria with ancillary molecular testing is expected to yield more discrete and diagnostic categories for research and reporting.

Abbreviations List

Abbreviation	Full Text
ADC	Adenocarcinoma
AFP	Alpha-fetoprotein
APADC	Appendiceal adenocarcinoma
Appen	Appendix
AR	Androgen receptor
AR	Antigen retrieval
Arg-1	Arginase-1
ATRX	Anti-transcriptional regulator
BADC	Breast carcinoma
BADC	Bladder adenocarcinoma
Bcl2	B-cell CLL/lymphoma 2
Beta-HCG	Beta human chorionic gonadotropin
C	Cytoplasmic
CA	Carcinoma
CAIX	Carbonic anhydrase IX
CC1	Cell conditioning solution 1 (Ventana)
CD	Cluster of differentiation
CDC	Collecting duct carcinoma
CDH17	Cadherin-17
CDK4	Cyclin-dependent kinase 4

Abbreviation	Full Text
CDX2	Caudal-type homeobox 2
CEA	Carcinoembryonic antigen
ChorioCA	Choriocarcinoma
CK	Cytokeratin
CNS	Central nervous system
CRADC	Colorectal adenocarcinoma
D2-40	Podoplanin
DAXX	Anti-death domain-associated protein 6
DFSP	Dermatofibrosarcoma protuberans
DOG1	Discovered on GIST-1
DPSRCT	Desmoplastic small round cell tumor
Duo	Duodenum
ECADC	Endocervical adenocarcinoma
EMADC	Endometrial adenocarcinoma
ER	Estrogen receptor
ERG	ETS-related gene
ESS	Endometrial stromal sarcoma
FISH	Fluorescence in site hybridization
Fli-1	Friend leukemia virus integration 1
FNA	Fine needle aspiration
FOXL2	Forkhead box L2
GATA3	GATA binding protein 3
GCDFP-15	Gross cystic disease fluid protein 15
GI	Gastrointestinal
GIST	Gastrointestinal stroma tumor
H&E	Hematoxylin and eosin
HCC	Hepatocellular carcinoma
HepPar-1	Hepatocyte paraffin-1
HMB45	Human melanoma black 45
HNF-1B	Hepatocyte nuclear factor 1 beta
HPV	Human papilloma virus
ICC	Intrahepatic cholangiocarcinoma
IHC	Immunohistochemistry
IMP3	Insulin-like growth factor II messenger RNA-binding protein-3
INI1	Integrase interactor 1
ISH	In situ hybridization
KIM-1	Kidney injury molecule 1
LADC	Lung adenocarcinoma
LC	Left colon
LCA	Leukocyte common antigen
LIN28	Lin-28 homolog A
Loc	Localization
LYM	Lymphoblastic lymphoma
M	Membranous
Mart-1	Melanoma-associated antigen recognized by T cells
Maspin	Mammary serine protease inhibitor
MCPyV	Merkel cell polyomavirus
MDM2	Mouse double minute 2 homolog
MGB	Mammaglobin
MIB-1	Mindbomb homolog 1
MiTF	Microphthalmia-associated transcription factor

Abbreviation	Full Text
MLH1	MutL homolog 1
MOC-31	Epithelial-related antigen clone MOC-31
MPNST	Malignant peripheral nerve sheath tumor
MPO	Myeloperoxidase
MS	Mesothelioma
MSA	Muscle-specific actin
MSI	Microsatellite instability
MUC	Mucin
MUC4	Mucin 4
MUC5AC	Mucin 5 AC
Myo	Myogenin
MyoD1	Myogenic differentiation 1
N	Nuclear
NANOG	NANOG homeobox
NB	Neuroblastoma
NET	Neuroendocrine tumor
NKX2.2	NK2 homeobox 2
NKX3.1	NK3 homeobox 1
NSE	Neuron-specific enolase
NY-ESO-1	Cancer/testis antigen 1B
OCCCA	Ovarian clear cell carcinoma
OCT4	Octamer-binding transcription factor 4
OSCA	Ovarian serous carcinoma
P504S	Alpha-methylacyl-CoA racemase
PADC	Pancreatic adenocarcinoma
PADC	Prostatic adenocarcinoma
Pan	Pancreas
PAX	Paired box gene
PC	Plasmacytoma
PDX1	Pancreatic duodenal homeobox 1
PECOMa	Perivascular epithelioid cell tumor
PMS2	Postmeiotic segregation increased 2
PNET	Primitive neuroectodermal tumor
PNL2	Melanoma-associated antigen PNL2
PR	Progesterone receptor
PRCC	Papillary renal cell carcinoma
PSA	Prostate-specific antigen
PSAP	Prostate-specific acid phosphatase
PTC	Papillary thyroid carcinoma
pVHL	Von Hippel-Lindau tumor suppressor
RBC	Red blood cell
RCC	Renal cell carcinoma
RCCma	Renal cell carcinoma marker
Rec	Rectum
RHMS	Rhabdomyosarcoma
S100P	Placental S00
SADC	Small bowel adenocarcinoma
SADC	Small intestinal adenocarcinoma
SALL4	Sal-like protein 4
SATB2	Special AT-rich sequence-binding protein 2
SCC	Squamous cell carcinoma
SF-1	Steroidogenic factor 1
SFT	Solitary fibrous tumor

Abbreviation	Full Text
SMA	Smooth muscle actin
SmCC	Small-cell carcinoma
SOX	Sex-determining region Y-box
SSCC	Salivary gland small-cell carcinoma
Stoma	Stomach
TFE3	Transcription factor E3
TFF1	Trefoil factor 1
TLE1	Transducin-like enhancer of split 1
TTF1	Thyroid transcription factor 1
UC	Urothelial carcinoma
UGI	Upper gastrointestinal tract
UP	Uroplakin
WT1	Wilms' tumor 1

Suggested Reading

Cytology/FNA

DeMay RM. Chapter 8. Building blocks of cytodiagnosis. In:The art and science of cytopathology, vol. 2. 2nd ed. Chicago: ASCP Press; 2010a. p. 562–619.

DeMay RM. Chapter 7. Introduction to FNA biopsy. In:The art and science of cytopathology, vol. 2. 2nd ed. Chicago: ASCP Press; 2010b. p. 536–61.

Ancillary Study: IHC

Bahrami A, Truong LD, Ro JY. Undifferentiated tumor: true identity by immunohistochemistry. Arch Pathol Lab Med. 2008;132(3):326–48.

Barbareschi M, Murer B, Colby TV, Chilosi M, Macri E, Loda M, et al. CDX-2 homeobox gene expression is a reliable marker of colorectal adenocarcinoma metastases to the lungs. Am J Surg Pathol. 2003;27(2):141–9.

Baumhoer D, Tornillo L, Stadlmann S, Roncalli M, Diamantis EK, Terracciano LM. Glypican 3 expression in human nonneoplastic, preneoplastic, and neoplastic tissues: a tissue microarray analysis of 4,387 tissue samples. Am J Clin Pathol. 2008;129(6):899–906.

Bishop JA, Sharma R, Illei PB. Napsin a and thyroid transcription factor-1 expression in carcinomas of the lung, breast, pancreas, colon, kidney, thyroid, and malignant mesothelioma. Hum Pathol. 2010;41(1):20–5.

Cao D, Guo S, Allan RW, Molberg KH, Peng Y. SALL4 is a novel sensitive and specific marker of ovarian primitive germ cell tumors and is particularly useful in distinguishing yolk sac tumor from clear cell carcinoma. Am J Surg Pathol. 2009a;33(6):894–904.

Cao D, Humphrey PA, Allan RW. SALL4 is a novel sensitive and specific marker for metastatic germ cell tumors, with particular utility in detection of metastatic yolk sac tumors. Cancer. 2009b;115(12):2640–51.

Chang A, Brimo F, Montgomery EA, Epstein JI. Use of PAX8 and GATA3 in diagnosing sarcomatoid renal cell carcinoma and sarcomatoid urothelial carcinoma. Hum Pathol. 2013;44(8):1563–8.

Chu PG, Weiss LM. Modern immunohistochemistry. New York: Cambridge University Press; 2009.

Dabbs DJ. Diagnostic immunohistochemistry. 3rd ed. Philadelphia: Churchill Livingstone Elsevier; 2010.

Dejmek A, Naucler P, Smedjeback A, Kato H, Maeda M, Yashima K, et al. Napsin a (TA02) is a useful alternative to thyroid transcription factor-1 (TTF-1) for the identification of pulmonary adenocarcinoma cells in pleural effusions. Diagn Cytopathol. 2007;35(8):493–7.

Dennis JL, Hvidsten TR, Wit EC, Komorowski J, Bell AK, Downie I, et al. Markers of adenocarcinoma characteristic of the site of origin: development of a diagnostic algorithm. Clin Cancer Res. 2005;11(10):3766–72.

DeYoung BR, Wick MR. Immunohistologic evaluation of metastatic carcinomas of unknown origin: an algorithmic approach. Semin Diagn Pathol. 2000;17(3):184–93.

Erickson LA, Papouchado B, Dimashkieh H, Zhang S, Nakamura N, Lloyd RV. Cdx2 as a marker for neuroendocrine tumors of unknown primary sites. Endocr Pathol. 2004;15(3):247–52.

Higgins JP, Kaygusuz G, Wang L, Montgomery K, Mason V, Zhu SX, et al. Placental S100 (S100P) and GATA3: markers for transitional epithelium and urothelial carcinoma discovered by complementary DNA microarray. Am J Surg Pathol. 2007;31(5):673–80.

Hornick JL, Dal Cin P, Fletcher CD. Loss of INI1 expression is characteristic of both conventional and proximal-type epithelioid sarcoma. Am J Surg Pathol. 2009;33(4):542–50.

Jones TD, Ulbright TM, Eble JN, Baldridge LA, Cheng L. OCT4 staining in testicular tumors: a sensitive and specific marker for seminoma and embryonal carcinoma. Am J Surg Pathol. 2004;28(7):935–40.

Krishna M. Diagnosis of metastatic neoplasms: an immunohistochemical approach. Arch Pathol Lab Med. 2010;134(2):207–15.

Liu A, Cheng L, Du J, Peng Y, Allan RW, Wei L, et al. Diagnostic utility of novel stem cell markers SALL4, OCT4, NANOG, SOX2, UTF1, and TCL1 in primary mediastinal germ cell tumors. Am J Surg Pathol. 2010;34(5):697–706.

Lin F, Liu H. Immunohistochemistry in undifferentiated neoplasm/tumor of uncertain origin. Arch Pathol Lab Med. 2014;138(12):1583–610.

Lin F, Liu H. Unknown primary/undifferentiated neoplasm. In: Lin F, Prichard JW, Liu H, Wilkerson M, Chen ZM, editors. Handbook of practical immunohistochemistry – frequently asked questions. 2nd ed. New York: Springer Science+Business Media; 2015. p. 119–64.

Lin F, Shi J, Liu H, Zhang J, Zhang PL, Wang HL, et al. Immunohistochemical detection of the von Hippel-Lindau gene product (pVHL) in human tissues and tumors: a diagnostic marker for metastatic renal cell carcinoma and clear cell carcinoma of the ovary and uterus. Am J Clin Pathol. 2008;129(4):592–605.

Liu H, Shi J, Wilkerson ML, Lin F. Immunohistochemical evaluation of GATA3 expression in tumors and normal tissues: a useful immunomarker for breast and urothelial carcinomas. Am J Clin Pathol. 2012;138(1):57–64.

Liu H, Shi J, Wilkerson M, Yang XJ, Lin F. Immunohistochemical evaluation of ERG expression in various benign and malignant tissues. Ann Clin Lab Sci. 2013;43(1):3–9.

Long KB, Srivastava A, Hirsch MS, Hornick JL. PAX8 expression in well-differentiated pancreatic endocrine tumors: correlation with clinicopathologic features and comparison with gastrointestinal and pulmonary carcinoid tumors. Am J Surg Pathol. 2010;34(5):723–9.

Magnusson K, de Wit M, Brennan DJ, Johnson LB, McGee SF, Lundberg E, et al. SATB2 in combination with cytokeratin 20 identifies over 95% of all colorectal carcinomas. Am J Surg Pathol. 2011;35(7):937–48.

Miettinen M, Wang ZF, Paetau A, Tan SH, Dobi A, Srivastava S, et al. ERG transcription factor as an immunohistochemical marker for vascular endothelial tumors and prostatic carcinoma. Am J Surg Pathol. 2011;35(3):432–41.

Ordóñez NG. Napsin a expression in lung and kidney neoplasia: a review and update. Adv Anat Pathol. 2012a;19(1):66–73.

Ordóñez NG. Thyroid transcription factor-1 is not expressed in squamous cell carcinomas of the lung: an immunohistochemical study with review of the literature. Appl Immunohistochem Mol Morphol. 2012b;20(6):525–30.

Ordóñez NG. Value of PAX 8 immunostaining in tumor diagnosis: a review and update. Adv Anat Pathol. 2012c;19(3):140–51.

Ordóñez NG. Value of PAX8, PAX2, napsin a, carbonic anhydrase IX, and claudin-4 immunostaining in distinguishing pleural epithelioid mesothelioma from metastatic renal cell carcinoma. Mod Pathol. 2013;26(8):1132–43.

Ordóñez NG. Value of thyroid transcription factor-1 immunostaining in tumor diagnosis: a review and update. Appl Immunohistochem Mol Morphol. 2012d;20(5):429–44.

Panarelli NC, Yantiss RK, Yeh MM, Liu Y, Chen YT. Tissue-specific cadherin CDH17 is a useful marker of gastrointestinal adenocarcinomas with higher sensitivity than CDX2. Am J Clin Pathol. 2012;138(2):211–22.

Park SY, Kim BH, Kim JH, Lee S, Kang GH. Panels of immunohistochemical markers help determine primary sites of metastatic adenocarcinoma. Arch Pathol Lab Med. 2007;131(10):1561–7.

Timek DT, Shi J, Liu H, Lin F. Arginase-1, HepPar-1, and Glypican-3 are the most effective panel of markers in distinguishing hepatocellular carcinoma from metastatic tumor on fine-needle aspiration specimens. Am J Clin Pathol. 2012;138(2):203–10.

Varadhachary GR, Abbruzzese JL, Lenzi R. Diagnostic strategies for unknown primary cancer. Cancer. 2004;100(9):1776–85.

Wang HL, Anatelli F, Zhai QJ, Adley B, Chuang ST, Yang XJ. Glypican-3 as a useful diagnostic marker that distinguishes hepatocellular carcinoma from benign hepatocellular mass lesions. Arch Pathol Lab Med. 2008;132(11):1723–8.

Wennerberg AE, Nalesnik MA, Coleman WB. Hepatocyte paraffin 1: a monoclonal antibody that reacts with hepatocytes and can be used for differential diagnosis of hepatic tumors. Am J Pathol. 1993;143(4):1050–4.

Yan BC, Gong C, Song J, Krausz T, Tretiakova M, Hyjek E, et al. Arginase-1: a new immunohistochemical marker of hepatocytes and hepatocellular neoplasms. Am J Surg Pathol. 2010;34(8):1147–54.

Ancillary Study: Molecular Analysis

Betz BL, Dixon CA, Weigelin HC, Knoepp SM, Roh MH. The use of stained cytologic direct smears for ALK gene rearrangement analysis of lung adenocarcinoma. Cancer Cytopathol. 2013;121:489–99.

Bofin AM, Ytterhus B, Martin C, O'Leary JJ, Hagmar BM. Detection and quantitation of HER-2 gene amplification and protein expression in breast carcinoma. Am J Clin Pathol. 2004;122:110–9.

Cheng L, Zhang S, Alexander R, Yao Y, MacLennan GT, Pan CX, et al. The landscape of EGFR pathways and personalized management of non-small-cell lung cancer. Future Oncol. 2011;7:519–41.

Cheung CC, Carydis B, Ezzat S, Bedard YC, Asa SL. Analysis of ret/PTC gene rearrangements refines the fine needle aspiration diagnosis of thyroid cancer. J Clin Endocrinol Metab. 2006;86:2187–90.

Cibas E, Ducatman B. Thyroid. In:Text cytology diagnostic principles and clinical correlates. 3rd ed. Philadelphia: Saunders Elsevier; 2009. p. 255.

Cohen Y, Rosenbaum E, Clark DP, et al. Mutational analysis of BRAF in fine needle aspiration biopsies of the thyroid: a potential application for the preoperative assessment of thyroid nodules. Clin Cancer Res. 2004;10:2761–5.

Dimashkieh H, Wolff DJ, Smith TM, Houser PM, Nietert PJ, Yang J. Evaluation of UroVysion and cytology for bladder cancer detection: a study of 1835 paired urine samples with clinical and histologic correlation. Cancer Cytopathol. 2013;121:591–7.

Frostad B, Martinsson T, Tani E, et al. The use of fine-needle aspiration cytology in the molecular characterization of neuroblastoma in children. Cancer (Cancer Cytopathol). 1999;87:60–8.

Kebebew E, Peng M, Reiff E, Targ O, Clark OH, McMillan A. ECM1 and TMPRSS4 are diagnostic markers of malignant thyroid neoplasms and improve the accuracy of fine needle aspiration biopsy. Ann Surg. 2005;242:353–61.

Kipp BR, Fritcher EG, del Rosario KM, Stevens CL, Sebo TJ, Halling KC. A systematic approach to identifying urothelial cells likely to be polysomic by fluorescence *in situ* hybridization. Anal Quant Cytol Histol. 2005;27:317–22.

Krishnamurthy S. Applications of molecular techniques to fine-needle aspiration. Biopsy Cancer (Cancer Cytopathol). 2007;111:106–22.

Mezzelani A, Alasio L, Bartoli C, et al. C-erbB2/neu gene and chromosome 17 analysis in breast cancer by FISH on archival cytological fine-needle aspirates. Br J Cancer. 1999;80:519–25.

Nikiforov YE. Molecular diagnostics of thyroid tumors. Arch Pathol Lab Med. 2011;135:569–77.

Nikiforova MN, Khalid A, Fasanella KE, McGrath KM, Brand RE, Chennat JS, et al. Integration of KRAS testing in the diagnosis of pancreatic cystic lesions: a clinical experience of 618 pancreatic cysts. Mod Pathol. 2013;26:1478–87.

Nizzoli R, Bozzetti C, Crafa P, et al. Immunocytochemical evaluation of HER-2/neu on fine-needle aspirates from primary breast carcinomas. Diagn Cytopathol. 2003;28:142–6.

Rhyu MS. Telomeres, telomerase and immortality. J Natl Cancer Inst. 1995;87:884–94.

Rosell R, Moran T, Queralt C, Porta R, Cardenal F, Camps C, et al. Screening for epidermal growth factor receptor mutations in lung cancer. N Engl J Med. 2009;361:958–67.

Santoro M, Carlomagno F, Hay ID, et al. Ret oncogene activation in human thyroid neoplasms is restricted to the papillary cancer subtype. J Clin Invest. 1992;89:1517–22.

Siddiqui MT, Greene KL, Clark DP, et al. Human telomerase reverse transcriptase expression in diff-Quik stained FNA samples from thyroid nodules. Diagn Mol Pathol. 2001;10:123–9.

Willmore-Payne C, Layfield LJ, Holden JA. C-KIT mutation analysis for diagnosis of gastrointestinal stromal tumors in fine needle aspiration specimens. Cancer (Cancer Cytopathol). 2005;105:165–70.

Yoder BJ, Skacel M, Hedgepeth R, Babineau D, Ulchaker JC, Liou LS, et al. Reflex UroVysion testing of bladder cancer surveillance patients with equivocal or negative urine cytology: a prospective study with focus on the natural history of anticipatory positive findings. Am J Clin Pathol. 2007;127:295–301.

Salivary Glands and Other Head and Neck Structures

2

Haiyan Liu, Jun Zhang, and Fan Lin

Summary of Pearls and Pitfalls

- The techniques and applications of biopsy of needle puncture with aspiration were first described in the1930s by Drs. Ellis and Martin at the Memorial Sloan Kettering Cancer Center. However, the widespread application of fine needle aspiration (FNA) in salivary gland and head and neck lesions has only occurred in the past 4+ decades.
- The advantages of FNA are its virtually risk-free, convenient, and yet providing sufficient information to triage patients into different treatment groups, such as surgical therapy, medical management, or follow-up without intervention.
- The limitations and pitfalls are mainly due to the considerable overlapping cyto- and histomorphology among various tumors of the salivary glands and the heterogeneity within individual tumor entities.
- Both false-positive and false-negative rates were reported in the ranges of 1–14%.
- Inadequate sampling was the most common cause of false-negative diagnosis.
- The sensitivity and specificity for rendering a benign or malignant diagnosis is high, in the range of 81–98%. However, a specific diagnosis may be challenging if not feasible at times.
- The objectives of FNA of salivary gland lesions are the following: (a) to distinguish neoplastic from nonneoplastic lesions, (b) to differentiate benign from malignant neoplasms, (c) to identify the lineage of a neoplasm, (d) to separate low-grade from high-grade malignant neoplasms, and (e) to distinguish primary vs metastatic neoplasms.
- The indications for FNA include any palpable lesions of the salivary gland or head and neck structures.
- The contraindications are few, including bleeding disorder and acute sialadenitis; the latter is due to associated significant pain.
- Complications are rare.
- Ancillary studies, especially immunohistochemistry (IHC), play a significant role in the confirmation of cell linage, especially in cytology and small biopsy specimens. With the addition of a new generation of biomarkers and molecular genetic discoveries, the diagnostic accuracy of FNA and small biopsy specimens improved significantly.
- For other head and neck structures, a specific diagnosis was usually achieved with the aid of ancillary studies, including IHC and flow cytometry studies in particular.

Normal Tissues

- Normal salivary gland tissues may be sampled, including normal acinic cells, ductal cells, and occasionally adipocytes.
- There are usually scattered clusters of acinic cells forming acini, admixed with benign ductal cells and occasional adipocytes, as illustrated in Fig. 2.1a–c.

Nonneoplastic Salivary Gland Disorders

Acute and Chronic Sialadenitis

Key Clinical Features

- Painful
- Acute: Often in the parotid gland

© Springer International Publishing AG 2018

F. Lin et al., *Handbook of Practical Fine Needle Aspiration and Small Tissue Biopsies*, DOI 10.1007/978-3-319-57386-1_2

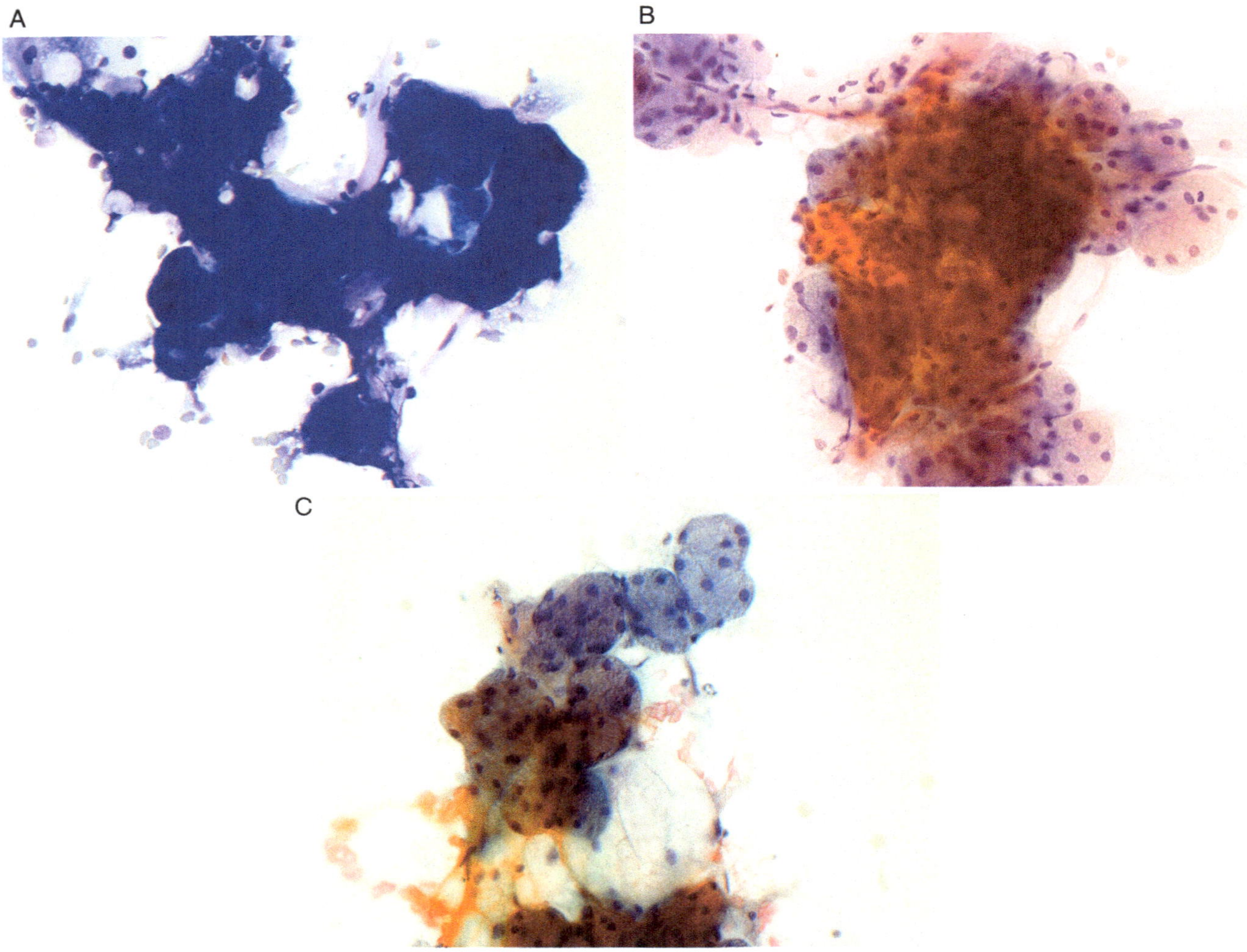

Fig. 2.1 (**a–c**) Normal salivary gland tissues. (**a**) Normal acinar and ductal unit, Diff-Quik. (**b**) Normal ductal and acinar unit, Pap stain. (**c**) Normal acinar cells and adipocytes, Pap stain

Tenderness associated with diffuse or localized swelling, may be fluctuant; usually no discrete mass

Etiology: Postoperative complication, viral or fungal infection, and bacterial infection due to obstruction (such as sialolithiasis)

- Chronic: Often in the submandibular gland

  Discrete mass

  Etiology: sialolithiasis and radiation therapy for head and neck cancer

Cytological Features

- Acute:
  1. Scant ductal elements in a background of neutrophils and necrotic debris
  2. Stone fragments if sialolithiasis is present
- Chronic:
  1. Hypocellular specimen
  2. Sparse to absent acinar cells
  3. Small sheets and tubules of ductal epithelial cells with sharp borders in a background of blood, proteinaceous debris, mature lymphocytes, and fragments of fibrous tissue (Fig. 2.2a, b)

Differential Diagnosis

- Acute: Rarely aspirated, usually a clinical diagnosis; microbiologic workup should be ordered. If a neoplastic process is suspected clinically, a repeat aspiration is warranted after the resolution of acute inflammation.
- Chronic:
  1. Lymphoepithelial sialadenitis (LESA): the presence of lymphoepithelial lesions and germinal center fragments.

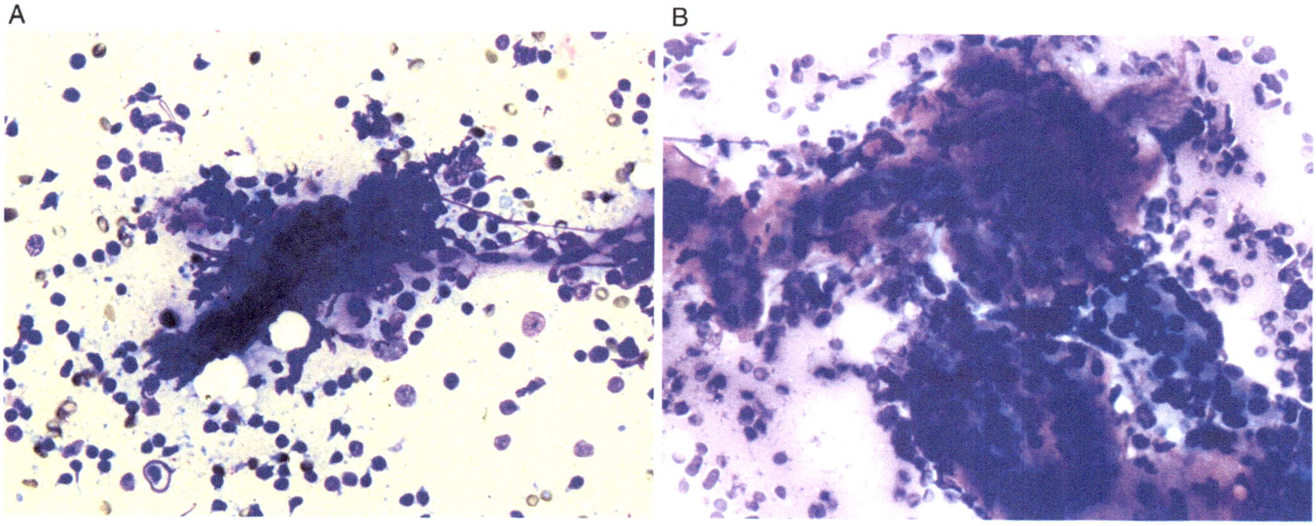

Fig. 2.2 Chronic sialadenitis. (**a**) Sparsely cellular specimen showing few reactive ductal cells, fibrous, vascular tissue, and inflammatory cells, mainly lymphocytes, Diff-Quik. (**b**) Fibrovascular stromal fragment, few benign ductal cells, inflammatory cells, and debris, Diff-Quik

2. Warthin's tumor: the presence of cohesive groups of oncocytes with lymphocytes and a cystic background.
3. Carcinoma: chronic sialadenitis is separated from carcinoma by its scant cellularity; small, angulated, tightly cohesive clusters of ductal cells; lack of marked atypia; and rare single epithelial cells in the background.

Histology

- Acute: Acute inflammation accompanied by edema and hyperemia. Peri- and intraductal collections of neutrophils are evident, with associated destruction of ductal epithelium and loss of acini. There may be microabscesses.
- Chronic: Depending on the etiologies, there are histomorphologic variations. However, the basic histology is chronic inflammatory cell infiltration, including lymphocytes, histiocytes, and plasma cells, with occasional neutrophils; stromal fibrosis; acinar atrophy of various degrees; and ductal dilatation with squamous, mucous, and oncocytic metaplasia. A granulomatous inflammatory response may be seen, with extravasation of saliva secondary to duct rupture.

Immunohistochemistry:

Rarely utilized in this setting; however, if an exuberant lymphoid population is present, flow cytometry study may be performed.

Granulomatous Sialadenitis

Key Clinical Features

- A form of chronic sialadenitis
- Caused by infection (fungi, mycobacteria, the agent of cat-scratch disease), cyst rupture, sarcoidosis or Wegener's involving the parotid gland, or rarely neoplasia (Hodgkin lymphoma, T-cell lymphoma, or metastatic carcinoma)

Cytological Features

- Aggregates of epithelioid histiocytes and multinucleated forms in a variable background of granular, necrotic cell debris and inflammation (Fig. 2.3a, b).
- In sarcoidosis: asteroid bodies, Schaumann bodies, and calcium oxalate crystals may be present.

Differential Diagnosis

The findings are not specific; an infectious etiology must be excluded by special stains and/or microbiologic cultures.

Histology

- Noncaseating granulomas are often seen in cases of sarcoidosis; in contrast, necrotizing granulomas are usually identified in cases with mycobacterial or fungal infection.
- Special stains for fungus (Grocott's methenamine silver [GMS]) and acid-fast bacilli (AFB) should be performed in cases of necrotizing granulomas.

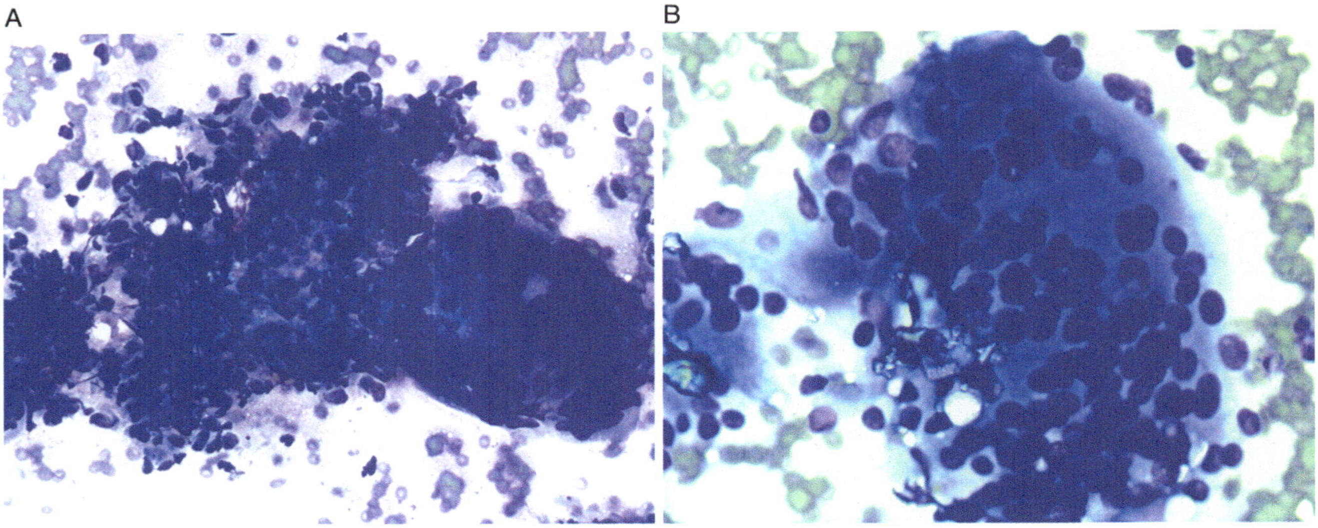

Fig. 2.3 Granulomatous sialadenitis. (**a**) Aggregate of epithelioid histiocytes and multinucleated form in a background of inflammatory cells and debris, Diff-Quik. (**b**) Multinucleated giant cell and crystal debris, Diff-Quik

- Additionally, Wegener's granulomatosis, in which necrotizing arteritis is the fundamental feature, must also be considered.
- Elastic stain may aid in identifying remnants of vessels in tissue damaged by inflammation and necrosis.

Immunohistochemistry:

Usually not applied

Lymphoepithelial Sialadenitis (Mikulicz Disease, Benign Lymphoepithelial Lesion, Myoepithelial Sialadenitis)

Clinical Features

- Women, 90%; average age at diagnosis of 50.
- Often bilateral parotid gland enlargement, painless; a minority of cases involve the submandibular gland.
- Autoimmune disorder, seen in patients with Sjogren's syndrome, or other connective tissue disorder.

Sialographic Features

- Punctate cavitary defects filled with radiopaque contrast medium, described as a "fruit-laden, branchless tree"

Cytological Features

- Cellular specimen.
- Lymphoepithelial islands and germinal center fragments in a background of a mixed population of lymphocytes, plasma cells, and tangible-body macrophages.
- Acinar cells are rarely present.

Differential Diagnosis

- Chronic sialadenitis: sparsely cellular specimen with fewer lymphocytes and germinal center fragments; no characteristic lymphoepithelial islands.
- Lymphoepithelial cyst.
- Human immunodeficiency virus (HIV)-associated cystic lymphoepithelial lesions.
- Warthin's tumor: the presence of oncocytic epithelium.
- Extranodal marginal zone B-cell lymphoma (EMZBCL) of mucosa-associated lymphoid tissue (MALT): large numbers of monocytoid B-cells present. Flow cytometry and immunocytochemistry studies should be performed.

Nonneoplastic Cysts

Squamous Epithelial-Lined Cyst

Key Clinical Features

Including congenital cysts (dermoid cyst and branchial cleft cyst) and sporadic lymphoepithelial cyst:

- Lymphoepithelial cyst: common in the parotid gland; unilateral and solitary, occasionally bilateral (HIV-associated); usually painless swelling; common in middle-aged men (no association with HIV or Sjogren's

syndrome) or children (HIV-associated is the most common presentation); facial nerve dysfunction may occur when the parotid gland is involved.
- Dermoid cyst: usually in the oral, orbital, and nasal area, occasionally in the neck; usually paramidline, can be lateral, in submandibular triangle; benign squamous epithelial cells, keratin debris, and sebaceous glands.
- Branchial cleft cyst: painless nodule located along the anterior border of the sternocleidomastoid muscle from the hyoid bone to the suprasternal notch; tender mass with secondary infection; equal male-to-female ratio, 20–40 years old.

Cytological Features

- Cellular specimen.
- Small clusters of squamous (and/or columnar) cyst lining cells in a background of keratin debris/anucleate squames, histiocytes, and mixed population of lymphocytes (Fig. 2.4a, b).
- Germinal center fragments with tangible-body macrophages may be present.
- No lymphoepithelial lesions, except in HIV-associated cases and cystic LESA. Figure 2.5a, b show a lymphoepithelial cyst in an HIV patient.

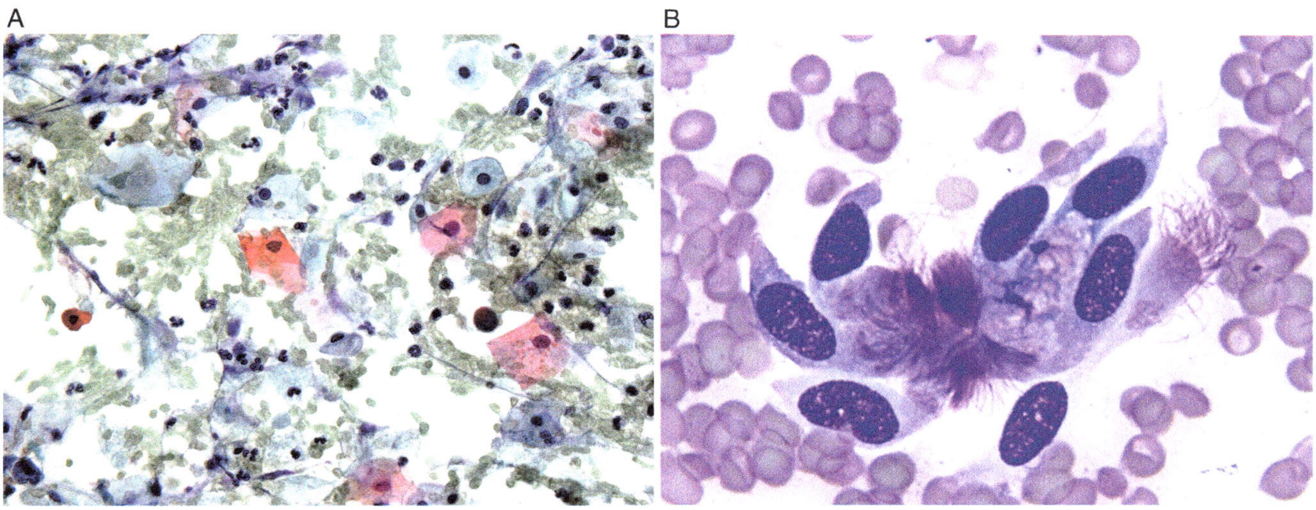

Fig. 2.4 Branchial cleft cyst. (**a**) Squamous cells, histiocytes, inflammatory cells, and debris, Pap stain. (**b**) Ciliated columnar cells, Diff-Quik

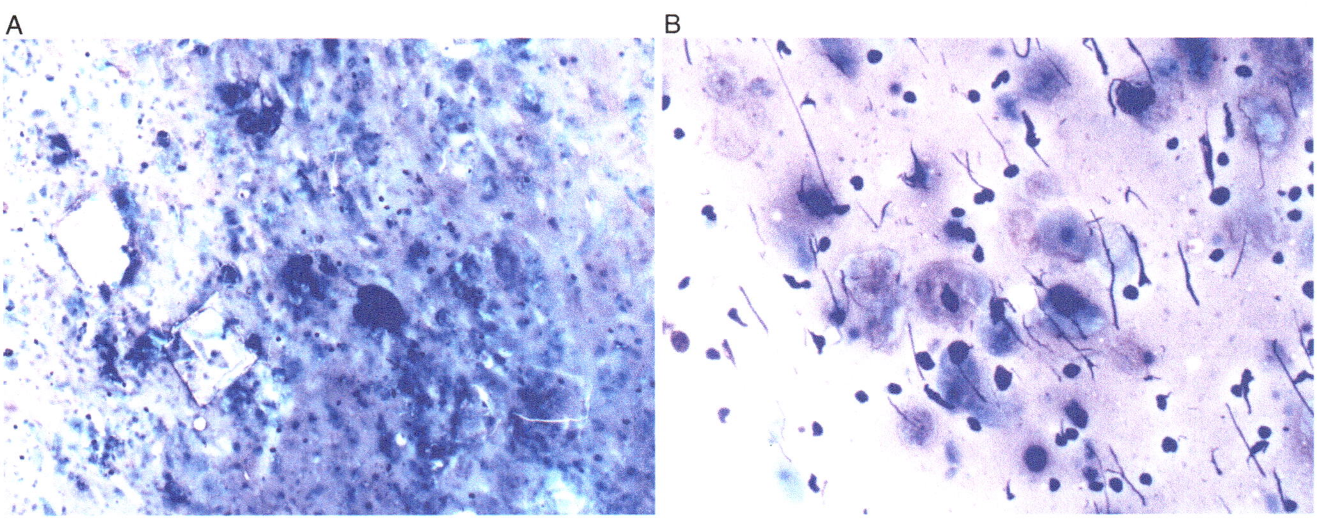

Fig. 2.5 A lymphoepithelial cyst in a patient with HIV infection. (**a**) Cyst contents with degenerated foam histiocytes, lymphocytes, squamous epithelial cells (many anucleated), rare columnar-shaped ductal epithelial cells, crystals, and mucinous debris, Diff-Quik; (**b**) cyst contents with squamous cells, lymphocytes, histiocytes, and debris, Diff-Quik

Differential Diagnosis

Cystic metastatic squamous cell carcinoma:

- Chronic sialadenitis
- Pure lymphoid lesions (intraparotid lymph node, lymphoma)
- Cystic salivary gland neoplasms (Warthin's tumor, acinic cell carcinoma [AciCC], MEC)

Histology

Lymphoepithelial Cyst:

- Usually an encapsulated, unilocular cyst with a stratified squamous epithelial lining.
- Cuboidal, columnar, mucous, and sebaceous cells may be present.
- The cyst contents can be fluid to mucoid to caseous.
- There are dense lymphoid infiltrates in the cyst wall.

Bronchial Cleft Cyst:

- Usually in the lateral neck, with histological features similar to benign lymphoepithelial cyst

Dermoid Cyst:

- Generally is midline in the floor of the mouth.
- A squamous epithelial-lined cyst with skin adnexa.

Immunohistochemistry:

Usually not applied

Mucus-Containing Cysts

Acquired cysts, including mucoceles and retention cysts, are often the result of ductal obstruction (such as a stone) or ductal disruption due to trauma.

Key Clinical Features

- Often in minor salivary glands: the submandibular and sublingual glands
- Mucocele: pseudocysts, no epithelial lining
- Mucus retention cysts: lined by squamous, columnar, or oncocytic epithelium

Cytological Features

- Histiocytes and some inflammatory cells in a background of thick mucus.
- Rare metaplastic epithelium and normal salivary gland cells may be seen.
- Calcifications and dirty debris.
- Figure 2.6a–d.

Differential Diagnosis

- Low-grade MEC
- Chronic sialadenitis with mucinous metaplasia of ducts

Histology

Mucocele:

- A pseudocyst resulting from the rupture of minor salivary gland ducts to cause mucus extravasation.
- A pool of mucin containing inflammatory cells and mucin-laden macrophages surrounded by granulation tissue without lining cells.
- The background salivary gland tissue often exhibits chronic inflammation.

Mucus Retention Cyst:

- Usually unicystic but can be a multicystic lesion with lining epithelium, including cuboidal to columnar cells, mucous cells, squamous cells, and rarely oncocytoid cells.
- The cyst contents are comprised of inspissated mucinous secretions containing scant inflammatory cells, ductal epithelial cells with or without metaplastic changes, or microliths.
- The background salivary gland tissue often exhibits chronic inflammation and possibly ectasia of adjacent ducts (in cases of multicystic lesions).
- Representative images are illustrated in Fig. 2.7a, b.

Immunohistochemistry:

Usually plays no role in this setting.

Neoplasms of the Salivary Gland

Salivary gland tumors are uncommon, with an annual incidence worldwide of 0.4–13.5/per 100,000 population, representing approximately 3% of head and neck neoplasms. The following are general features of salivary gland neoplasms:

1. Female-predominant except Warthin's tumor and high-grade carcinomas
2. Benign in a majority, the most common being pleomorphic adenoma (PA)

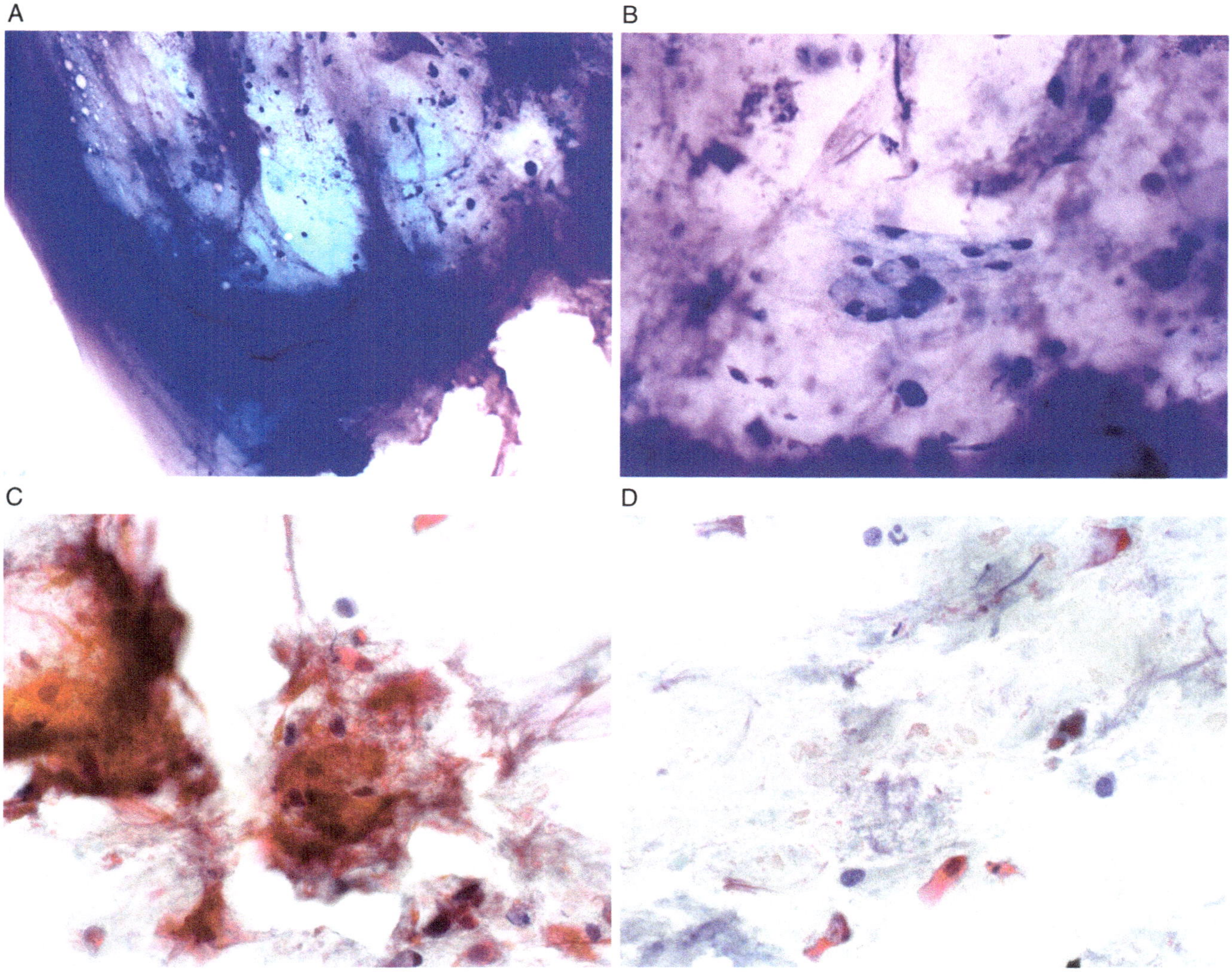

Fig. 2.6 Mucus retention cyst of the submandibular gland in setting of chronic sialadenitis, cytology. (**a**, **b**) Thick, inspissated mucinous secretion containing scant macrophages, inflammatory cells, ductal epithelial cells, and rare mucous cells, Diff-Quik. (**c**, **d**) Pap stain

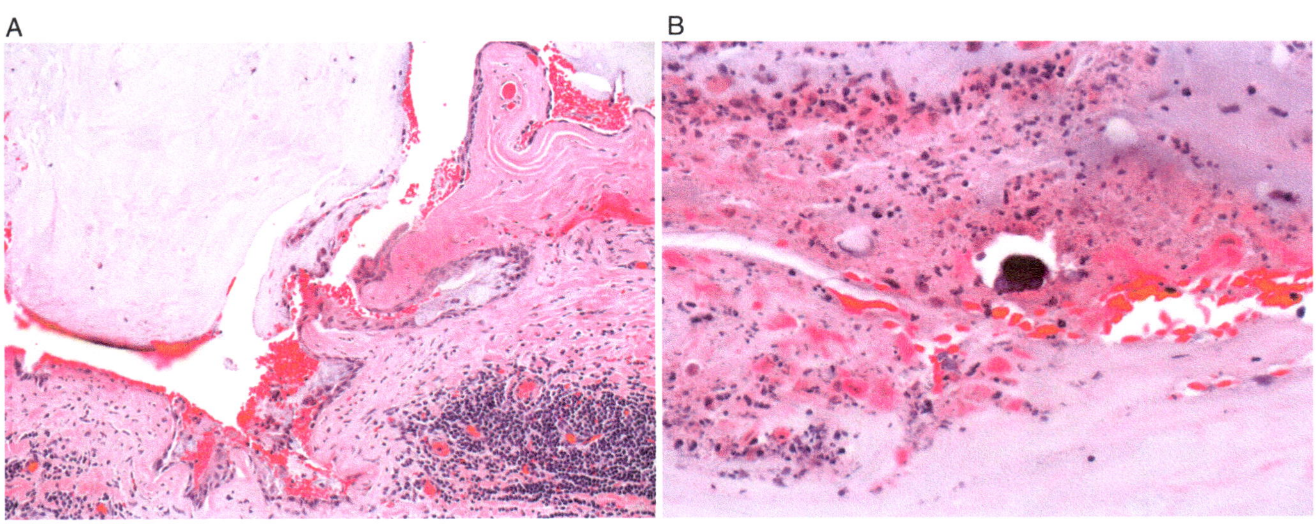

Fig. 2.7 Mucus retention cyst of the submandibular gland in setting of chronic sialadenitis, surgical resection. (**a**) True cystic space lined by ductal epithelium, showing mucous cells and focal squamoid changes, with adjacent tissue showing chronic inflammation, H&E; (**b**) the inspissated mucinous secretion containing scant macrophages, inflammatory cells, ductal epithelial cells with squamous metaplastic changes, and microlith with debris, H&E

3. Parotid gland being the most common site of tumor origin, 80% benign
4. Less commonly arising from an intraoral location; however, with the highest chance of being malignant (86–90%)
5. Rare in children; however, approaching 50% malignant in patients younger than 18
6. Bilaterality in 12% of tumors, commonly seen in AciCCs, Warthin's tumors, and oncocytomas.

Salivary gland tumors show a predilection for major or minor glands, as summarized in Table 2.1.

Salivary glands exhibit a two-tiered organization comprising luminal cells (acinar and ductal cells) and abluminal cells (myoepithelial cells and basal cells). The secretory acini and intercalated ducts are wrapped by myoepithelial cells, while the striated ducts and subsequent conducting ducts are supported by basal cells. Tumors of the salivary glands exhibit extraordinary diversity and heterogeneity in cyto- and histomorphology as well as tumor composition. For practical purposes, the common tumors of salivary glands can be categorized into four major groups:

1. Tumors with mixed luminal and myoepithelial cell differentiation, as well as abundant mesenchymal metaplasia, characterized by chondromyxoid matrix material.
2. Tumors with biphasic cell populations (luminal and abluminal cells without significant matrix material.
3. Tumors with myoepithelial/basal cell proliferation.
4. Tumors lacking myoepithelial cell differentiation.
5. See summary in Table 2.2.

The diagnostic approach for tumors of the salivary gland in cytology and small biopsy specimens aims to define the cell population of the tumor, that is, to demonstrate the presence or absence of myoepithelial cells or luminal cells and to apply newly discovered tumor-specific biomarkers or molecular cytogenetic assays to render as specific a diagnosis as possible. IHC plays a significant role in this regard, especially in cytology and small biopsy specimens. The commonly used immunomarkers for luminal or abluminal cell differentiation are summarized in Table 2.3.

Table 2.1 Summary of tumors with predilection for major or minor salivary glands (SG)

Exclusive in major SGs	Exclusive in minor SGs
Warthin's tumor	*Lip, buccal mucosa*:
AciCC	Canalicular adenoma
MASC	Cystadenoma/cystadenocarcinoma
Basal cell adenoma/ADC	Inverted papilloma
Oncocytoma/oncocytic CA	Intraductal papilloma
Epithelial-myoepithelial CA	*Palate*:
Salivary duct CA	PLGA
Lymphoepithelial	Sialadenoma papilliform
	Oral mucosa:
	Cribriform ADC of minor SGs (also tongue)
	Signet ring cell ADC

SG salivary gland, *AciCC* acinic cell carcinoma, *MASC* mammary analogue secretory carcinoma, *ADC* adenocarcinoma, *CA* carcinoma, *PLGA* polymorphous low-grade adenocarcinoma

Table 2.2 Summary of salivary gland tumors based on cell lineage or tumor composition

	Benign	Malignant
Mixed luminal and myoepithelial cells as well as abundant mesenchymal metaplasia	PA	CA ex pleomorphic adenoma
Biphasic cell populations without significant matrix material	Basal cell adenoma	Basal cell ADC Epithelial-myoepithelial CA AdCC Sialoblastoma
Myoepithelial cell differentiation only	Myoepithelioma	Myoepithelial CA
Tumors lacking myoepithelial cell differentiation	Warthin's tumor Oncocytoma Sebaceous adenoma Lymphadenoma Cystadenoma	PLGA Acinic cell CA Mucoepithelial CA MASC Salivary ductal CA Oncocytic CA Malignant sebaceous CA ADC, NOS

PA pleomorphic adenoma, *CA* carcinoma; *ADC* adenocarcinoma, *AdCC* adenoid cystic carcinoma, *PLGA* polymorphous low-grade adenocarcinoma, *MASC* mammary analogue secretory carcinoma, *NO* not otherwise specified

Table 2.3 Commonly used biomarkers for the identification of cell differentiation in salivary gland neoplasms

Markers of luminal cells	Markers of myoepithelial or basal cells
Acinar and ductal cells	*Myoepithelial and basal cells*
LMWCK, pan-cytokeratin (AE1/AE3)	HMWCK (including CK14)
	Pan-cytokeratin (AE1/AE3)
CEA	Vimentin
EMA	P63
CD117[a]	*Myoepithelial cells*
DOG1[b]	SMA
SOX10[b]	Calponin
Acinar cells	MSA
Amylase	GFAP (variable)
PAS-D	S100 protein (variable)
Ductal cells	Maspin (variable)
CK7	CD10 (variable)
GCDFP-15	SOX10 (myoepithelial cells of intercalated ducts)
pVHL	

LMWCK low molecular weight cytokeratin, *CEA* carcinoembryonic antigen, *EMA* epithelial membrane antigen, *HMWC* high molecular weight cytokeratin, *CD* cluster of differentiation, *DOG1* discovered on GIST1, *SOX* sex determining region Y box, *PAS-D* periodic acid-Schiff with diastase, *CK* cytokeratin, *GCDFP-15* gross cystic disease fluid protein-15, *pVHL* von Hippel von tumor suppressor, *SMA* α-smooth muscle actin, *MSA* muscle specific actin, *GFAP* glial fibrillary acidic protein

[a]CD117 is negative in normal salivary gland luminal cells, but positive in luminal cells of various tumors

[b]Acinar cells and intercalated ductal cells

Table 2.4 WHO histological classification of tumors of the salivary glands, 2017

Malignant tumors	Myoepithelioma
Mucoepidermoid carcinoma	Basal cell adenoma
Adenoid cystic carcinoma	Warthin's tumor
Acinic cell carcinoma	Oncocytoma
Polymorphous adenocarcinoma	Lymphadenoma
Clear cell carcinoma	Cystadenoma
Basal cell adenocarcinoma	Sialadenoma papilliferum
Intraductal carcinoma	Ductal papillomas
Adenocarcinoma, NOS	Sebaceous adenomas
Salivary duct carcinoma	Canalicular adenoma and other ductal adenomas
Myoepithelial carcinoma	*Nonneoplastic epithelial lesions*
Epithelial-myoepithelial carcinoma	Sclerosing polycystic adenosis
Carcinoma ex pleomorphic adenoma	Nodular oncocytic hyperplasia
Secretory carcinoma	Lymphoepithelial sialadenitis
Sebaceous adenocarcinoma	Intercalated duct hyperplasia
Carcinosarcoma	*Benign soft tissue lesions*
Poorly differentiated carcinoma	Hemangioma
Undifferentiated carcinoma	Lipoma/sialolipoma
Large cell neuroendocrine carcinoma	Nodular fasciitis
Small cell neuroendocrine carcinoma	*Hematolymphoid tumors*
Lymphoepithelial carcinoma	Extranodal marginal zone B-cell lymphoma of mucosa-associated lymphoid tissue (MALT Lymphoma)
Squamous cell carcinoma	
Oncocytic carcinoma	
Uncertain malignant potential	
Sialoblastoma	
Benign tumors	
Pleomorphic adenoma	

Used with permission from El-Naggar AK, Chan JKC, Grandis JR, Takata T, Slootweg PJ, eds. WHO Classification of Head and Neck Tumours. Lyon, France: IARC; 2017

The relatively tumor-specific biomarkers and the new discovery of molecular genetic abnormalities of individual tumors will be discussed under each entity.

The World Health Organization (WHO) classification of tumors of salivary glands is summarized in Table 2.4.

Benign Epithelial Tumors

Pleomorphic Adenoma (Benign Mixed Tumor)

Key Clinical Features

- The most common neoplasm of the salivary glands
- Parotid gland (the vast majority) > the minor salivary glands (especially the palate) > the submandibular gland
- In adults, 3rd to 6th decades of life, female predominant; in children and adolescents, peak at age 5–15 years, more frequent in males
- Presents as a solitary, slow-growing, well-circumscribed, painless firm mass

Key Radiological Features

- Ultrasound: typically a hypoechoic, homogenous, well-circumscribed mass with posterior acoustic enhancement.
- Magnetic resonance imaging (MRI): intermediate or low T1 signal; variable T2-weighted signal, high in cellular areas to very high in myxoid areas.
- Computed tomography (CT): typically a well-circumscribed mass of soft tissue density, either heterogeneous or homogeneous contrast enhancement.
- Radiologic findings are not specific, unable to distinguish PA from other benign tumors, such as myoepithelioma and basal cell adenoma.

Cytological Features

Three components in varying proportions:

- Ductal cells: small, cuboidal, bland nuclei may show moderate atypia.
- Myoepithelial cells: spindled or plasmacytoid, entrapped in the matrix.
- Chondromyxoid matrix: magenta on Diff-Quik and pale and gray to cyanophilic on Papanicolaou (Pap) stain.
- Occasionally, radiating, cauliflower-shaped tyrosine-rich crystals are present.
- Examples are shown in Fig. 2.8a–i.

Differential Diagnosis

- Low-grade MEC
- Adenoid cystic carcinoma (AdCC)
- Polymorphous low-grade adenocarcinoma (PLGA)
- Plasmacytoma or plasmacytoid malignant lymphoma
- Myoepithelioma

Histology

- Usually an encapsulated tumor that may be multinodular with satellite nodule.
- PA is comprised of three basic cellular components, including luminal cells, abluminal cells (myoepithelial cells), and stroma, often arranged in various proportions to produce a variety of growth patterns, such as tubular structures of luminal cells with enveloped myoepithelial

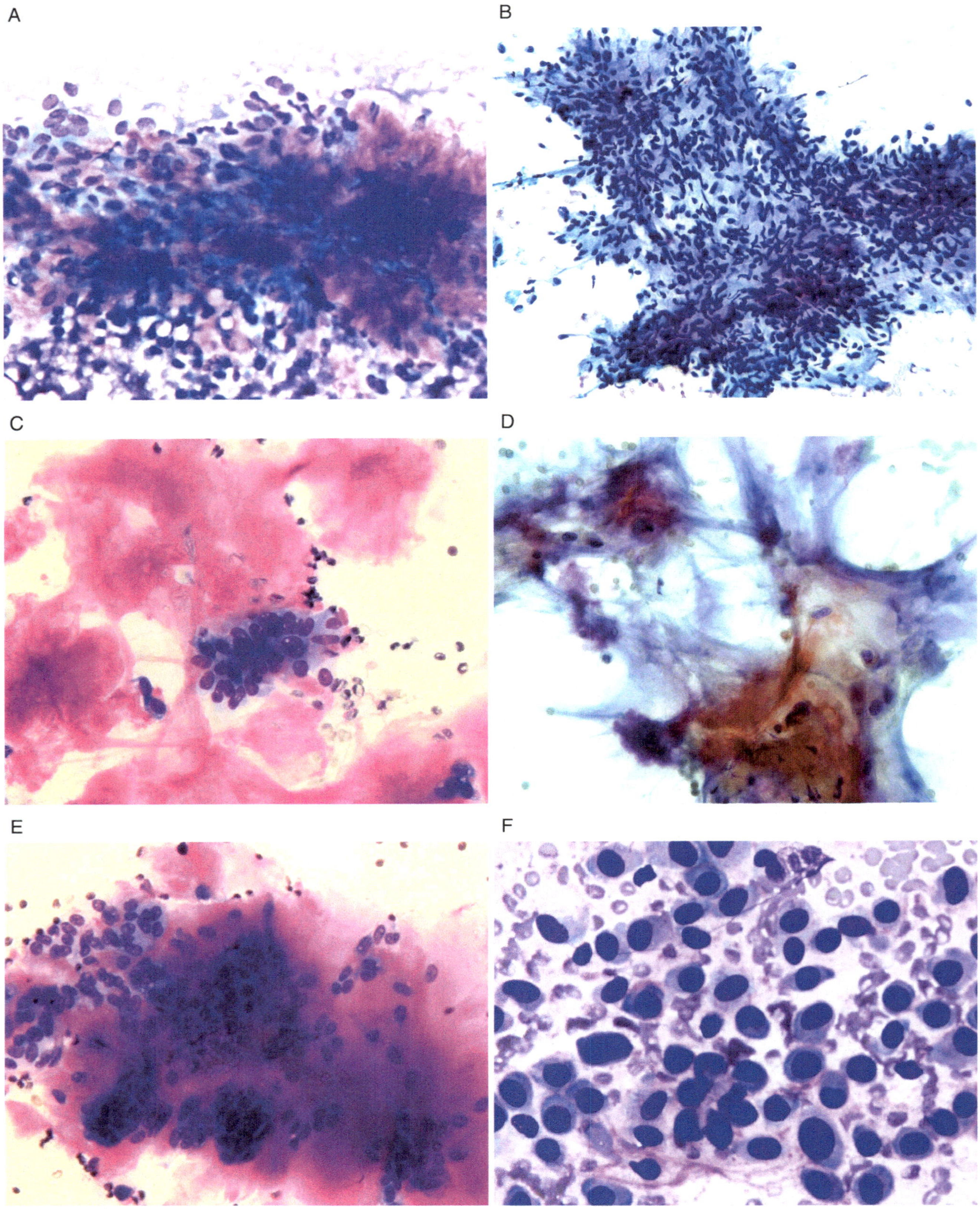

Fig. 2.8 Pleomorphic adenoma of the parotid gland, cytology. (**a**) Magenta chondromyxoid matrix with embedded and background myoepithelial cells and few ductal epithelial cells, Diff-Quik. (**b**) Pale and gray to cyanophilic chondromyxoid matrix and myoepithelial cells, Pap stain. (**c**, **d**) Abundant chondromyxoid matrix with few myoepithelial cells and ductal epithelial cells, Diff-Qiuk and Pap stain. (**e**) Magenta chondromyxoid matrix with embedded and background myoepithelial cells and few ductal epithelial cells, Diff-Qiuk. (**f**) Background myoepithelial cells, Diff-Quik. (**g**) Ductal epithelial cells, myoepithelial cells, and pale to gray matrix, Pap stain. (**h**) Tyrosine-rich crystals, Pap stain. (**i**) Cell block, H&E

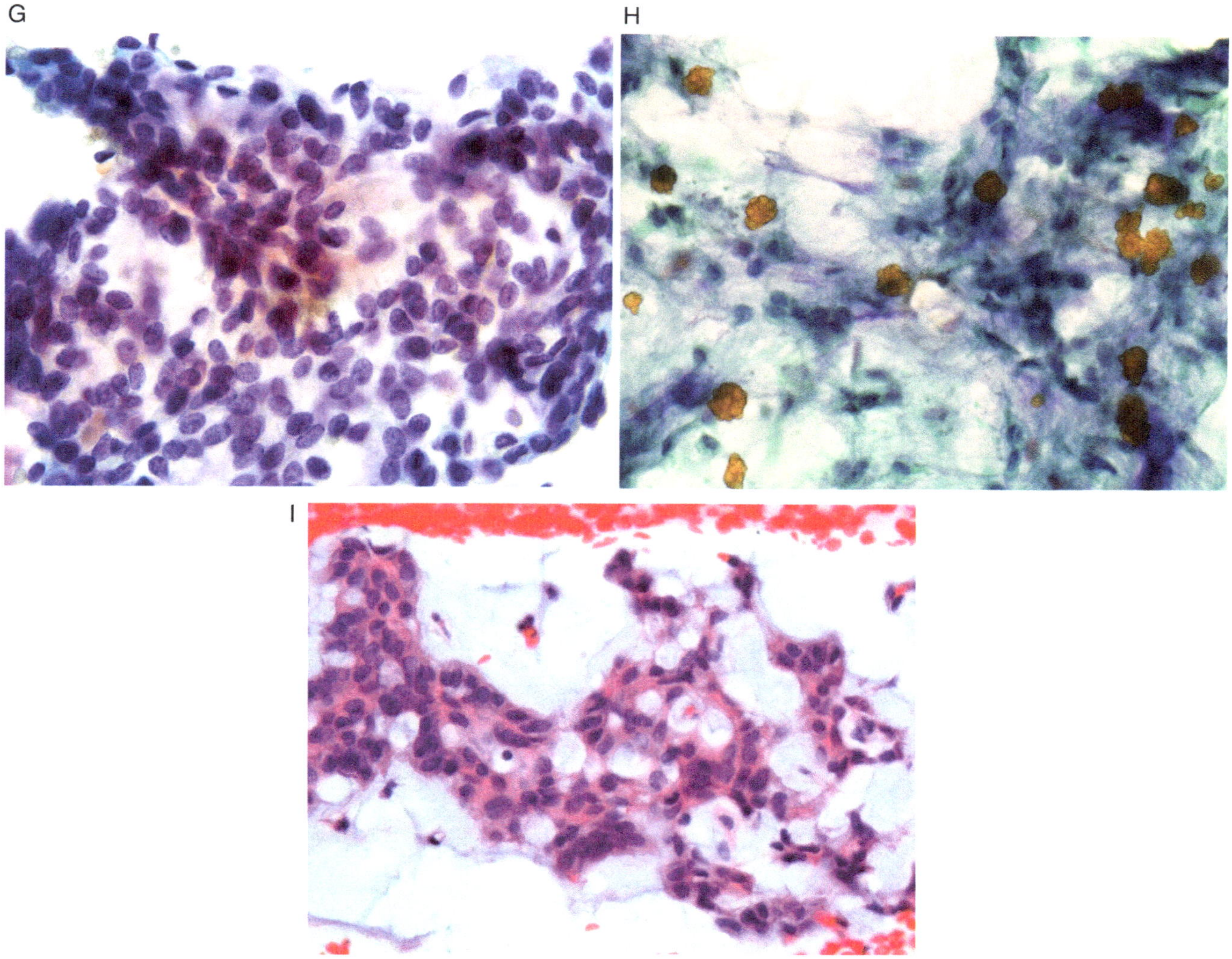

Fig. 2.8 (continued)

cells embedded in a chondromyxoid stroma or sheets, islands, and single myoepithelial cells melting into a myxoid matrix stroma. A focal pattern resembling AdCC may be seen.

- The luminal cells may undergo metaplastic changes to squamous, sebaceous, oncocytic, or clear cells or rarely to goblet or mucous cells. The latter, in association with squamous epithelium, can lead to an erroneous interpretation of MEC.
- Myoepithelial cells can be cuboidal, spindled, stellate, plasmacytoid hyaline, or hydropic clear cells and often form sheets, trabeculae, or cribriform structures.
- The identification of plasmacytoid hyaline cells is diagnostic for PA and myoepithelioma.
- Rarely skeletal muscle differentiation can be identified.
- The extracellular stroma is often a mixture of chondroid, myxoid, chondromyxoid, and hyaline matrix, rarely osseous and adipose tissues. The chondromyxoid stroma is a characteristic for PA.
- Occasional tumors may have very scant or no extracellular stroma. Those tumors can be designated as "cellular PAs."
- Elastic fibers are present in variable amounts in most PAs and especially abundant in long-standing lesions. These thick elastic fibers are diagnostically helpful because they are rare in other salivary gland tumors.
- Various histologic patterns of PAs are illustrated in Fig. 2.9a–h.

Immunohistochemistry:

- In cytology or small biopsy specimens, IHC may be applied to demonstrate the coexistence of luminal and abluminal (myoepithelial) cells.

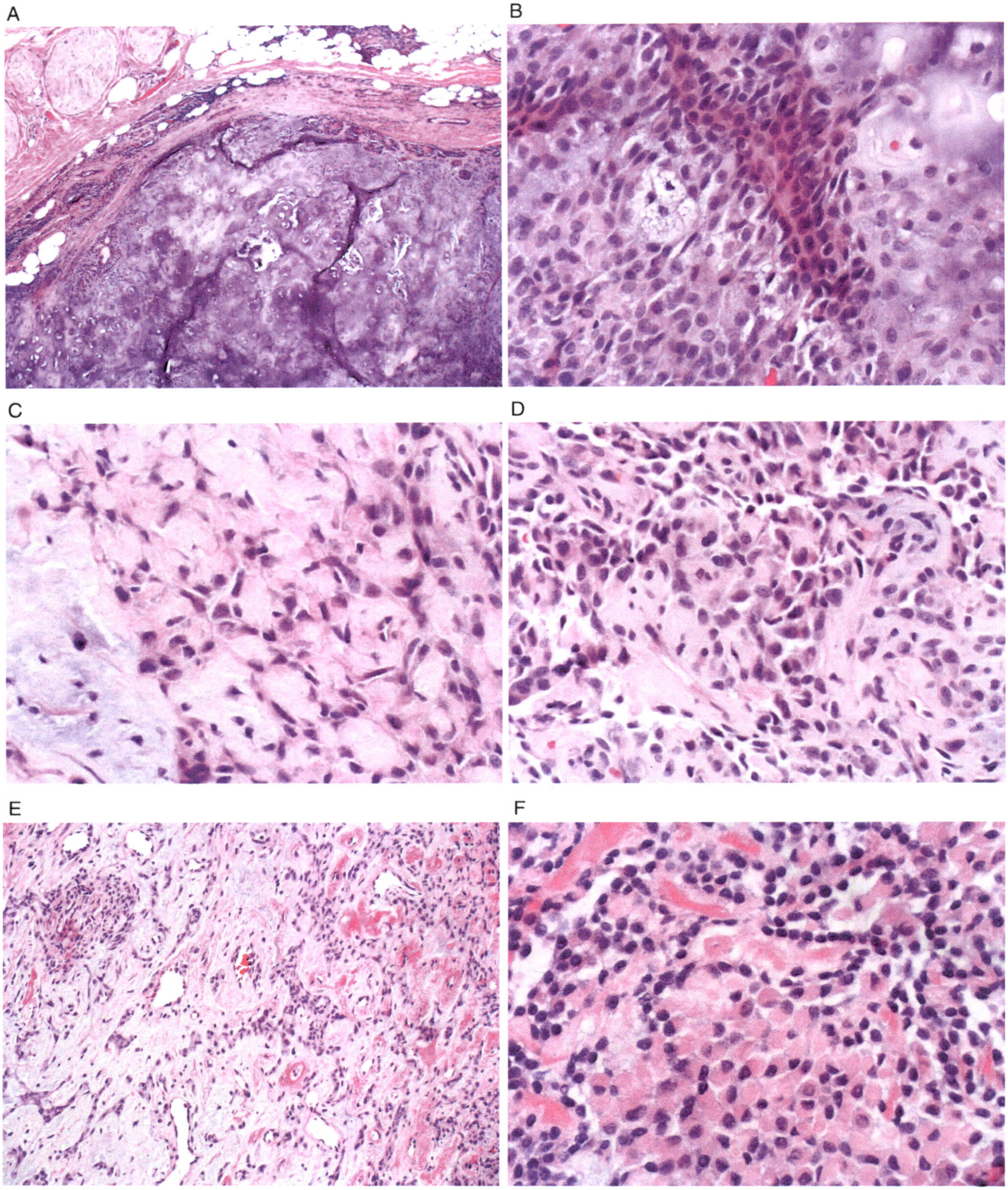

Fig. 2.9 Pleomorphic adenoma of parotid gland, histology. (**a**) Well-circumscribed, thinly encapsulated, lobulated growth pattern, H&E. (**b**) Tubular structure enveloped by myoepithelial cells, focal chondromyxoid stroma, and a few sebaceous cells seen, H&E. (**c**, **d**) Myoepithelial cells merging into chondromyxoid stroma, H&E. (**e**) Tubules and cords of cells merging into chondromyxoid stroma; focal thick elastic fibers are seen, H&E. (**f**) Plasmacytoid hyaline cells, H&E. (**g**) CD117 decorates luminal cells; (**h**) p63 highlights abluminal myoepithelial cells

G H

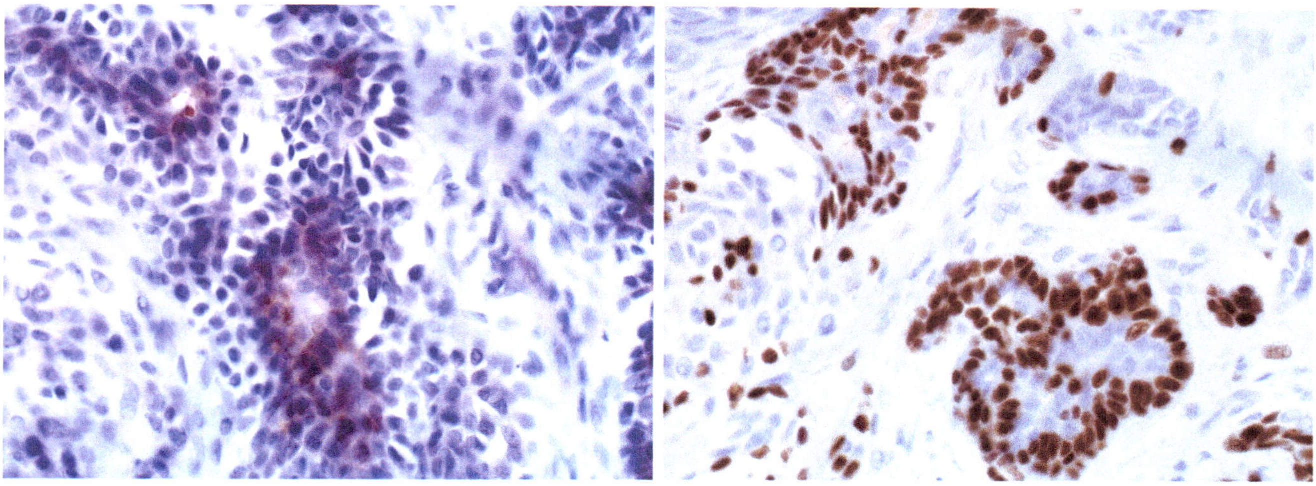

Fig. 2.9 (continued)

- The luminal cells are decorated by epithelial membrane antigen (EMA), carcinoembryonic antigen (CEA), and CD117.
- The abluminal cells are positive for p63, calponin, S100, and sex determining region Y box (SOX)10.
- Pleomorphic adenoma gene 1 (PLAG1) was reported in 94.4% of PAs, all myoepitheliomas (low intensity), 25% (2/8) of PLGAs, and one salivary ductal carcinoma ex pleomorphic adenoma, but was negative in other common salivary gland tumors including AdCC, MEC, and AciCC.
- In addition, Ki67, p53, and Bcl2 may help in the differential diagnosis of PA from AdCC. PA shows a low proliferative index (1.6%), rare p53 reactivity (1.2%), and weak Bcl2 staining; while AdCC has been reported to have a mean proliferative index of 20.5–54% depending on tumor grades, p53 of 4.3–24%, and strong diffuse staining for Bcl2.
- Discovered on GIST-1 (DOG1) was reported mostly negative in PAs.
- Representative images are shown in Fig. 2.9g, h.

The majority of PAs exhibit a translocation t(3;8)(p21;q12) involving *PLAG1* and one of several other fusion partners, commonly catenin (cadherin-associated protein), β1 (*CTNNB1*), which is the gene coding for β-catenin. This gene rearrangement is specific for PAs and its malignant counterpart, the carcinoma ex pleomorphic adenoma, leading to overexpression of PLAG1 by immunoassay. Approximately 10% of PAs show rearrangement at 12q13–15 involving high-mobility group AT hook 2 (*HMGA2*). The characteristic translocations involving *PLAG1* or *HMGA2* with associated immunoexpression of PLAG1 in PAs have also been observed in myoepitheliomas but not in basal cell adenomas.

Monomorphic Adenoma/Basal Cell Adenoma

Key Clinical Features

- Less than 5% of all salivary gland tumors, 75% in the parotid gland.
- Slightly more common in females than in males.
- Presents as an asymptomatic, solitary, slow-growing mass.
- The membranous pattern of basal cell adenoma often affects males.

Key Radiological Features

Similar to PA (benign mixed tumor)

Cytological Features

- Numerous small blue cells associated with variable amounts of collagenous stroma (Fig. 2.10a–c).
- Naked nuclei and single cells may be numerous.
- Arborizing stroma contains fibroblast-like spindle cells and capillaries.

Differential Diagnosis

- AdCC, solid variant
- Basal cell carcinoma

Histology

- Comprised of two cell types, the basaloid cells (basal cells or myoepithelial cells) and luminal cells, sharply delineated from the stroma by basement membrane-like

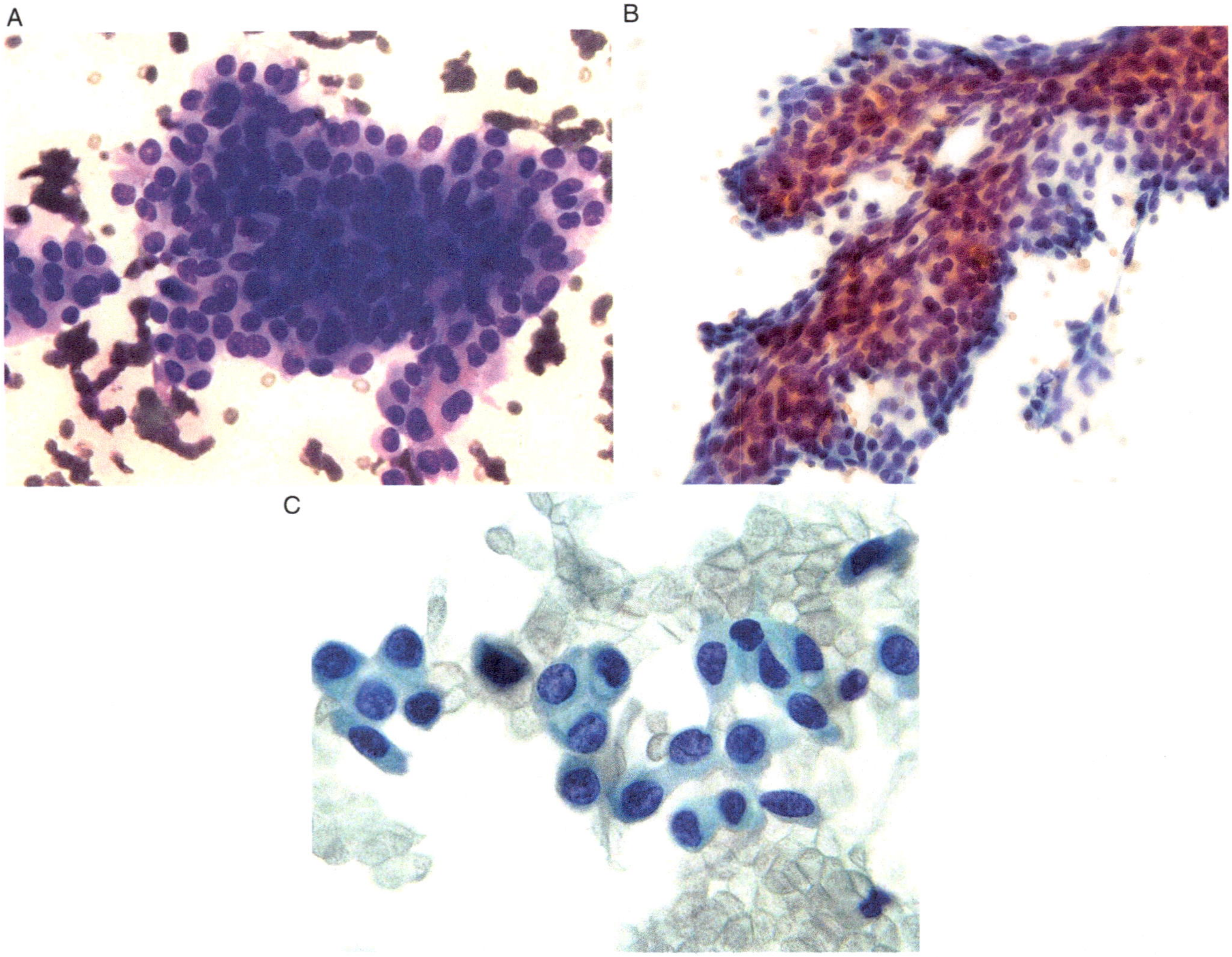

Fig. 2.10 Monomorphic adenoma (basal cell adenoma), cytology. (**a, b**) Angulated, usually sharp bordered groups of cytologically bland basaloid ductal epithelial cells with appreciable peripheral palisading and clinging of collagenous stroma, (**a**) Diff-Quik. (**b**) Pap stain. (**c**) Scattered plasmacytoid myoepithelial cells entrapped in matrix, Pap stain

material, differing greatly from the centrifugal or "melting" growth of PA.

- Chondromyxoid stroma is absent.
- The tumor cells are often predominated by basaloid cells, typically arranged in anastomosing jigsaw puzzle-like islands and trabeculae with peripheral palisading.
- Small ductal structures with luminal cell lining may be appreciated.
- Cribriform pattern is rarely present; however, the spaces lack luminal cells.
- For tumors with myoepithelial-derived stroma, there are plump spindle cells in the stroma.
- For the membranous variant of basal cell adenoma, the smooth-contoured basaloid tumor islands are surrounded by thick, eosinophilic, periodic acid-Schiff (PAS)-positive hyaline basal lamina material. This variant often grows in a multinodular fashion with entrapped normal salivary gland tissue to mimic tumor invasion.
- Representative images are illustrated in Fig. 2.11a, b.

Immunohistochemistry:

- The luminal cells are positive for CD117, CK AE1/AE3, CEA, and EMA.
- The basaloid cells are reactive to p63, calponin, glial fibrillary acidic protein (GFAP), and S100.
- For the tumors with myoepithelial-derived stroma, the plump spindle cells in the stroma are decorated by S100, not p63.
- Studies also reported nuclear expression of β-catenin in about 50% of cases, corresponding to mutations in CTNNB1 (β-catenin) in basal cell adenomas/adenocarcinomas (ADCs).
- Representative images are shown in Fig. 2.11c, d.

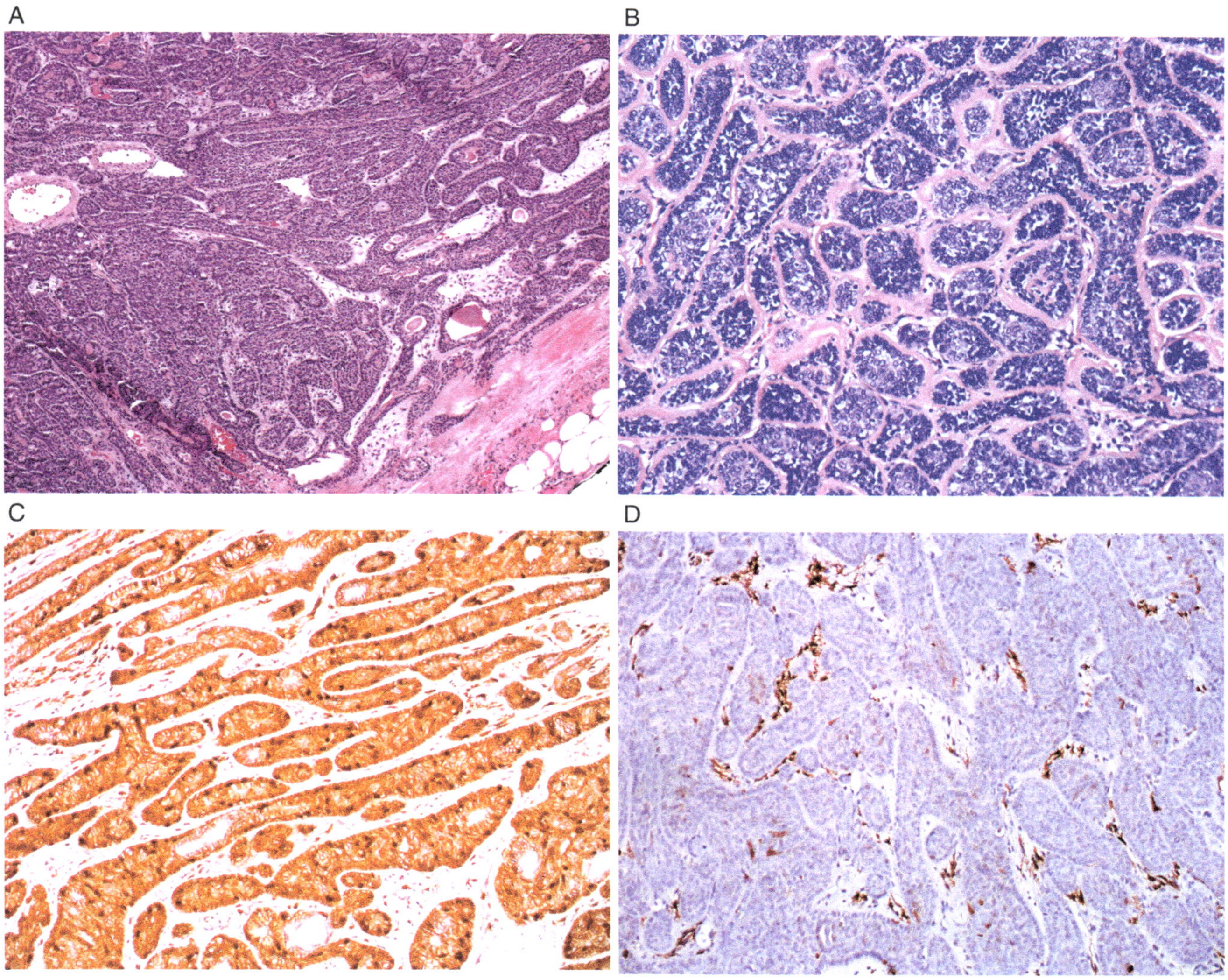

Fig. 2.11 Monomorphic adenoma (basal cell adenoma), histology. (**a**) Well-circumscribed, encapsulated border, H&E. (**b**) Jigsaw puzzle-like islands and trabecular of basaloid cells with peripheral palisading and thick basement membrane material surrounding, H&E. (**c**) Aberrant nuclear expression for β-catenin was reported in about 50% of cases. The current case shows patchy nuclear staining for β-catenin. (**d**) S100 decorates the plump spindle cells in the stroma; tumor cells are negative

Warthin's Tumor (Papillary Cystadenoma Lymphomatosum)

Key Clinical Features

- The second most common benign salivary gland tumor, exclusively in the parotid gland, occasionally in periparotid lymph nodes.
- Smokers, commonly found in males in the 6th to 7th decades of life; found in whites and Asians more frequently than in Hispanic and African Americans.
- Presents as a painless, slow-growing, fluctuant cystic mass over the angle of the mandible.
- Bilaterality (5–14%) and multifocality (12–20%) occur more frequently than others.

Key Radiological Features

- CT scanning may demonstrate a well-defined mass in the posterior inferior segment of the superficial lobe of the parotid.
- Radiosialography shows increased activity due to high mitochondrial contents in oncocytes.

Cytological Features

Three components in varying proportions:

- Oncocytic epithelium: usually in flat sheets, with abundant granular cytoplasm and may have prominent nucleoli; also seen in papillary structures

- Lymphocytes: a mixed population of lymphoid cells and germinal center fragments
- Cyst fluid: foam macrophages and debris, giving a "dirty" background
- Figure 2.12a–f

Differential Diagnosis

- Cystic salivary gland lesions: when only non-specific cyst fluid present, a repeat aspiration may be useful.
- Oncocytic neoplasms usually do not have a cystic background and have very limited lymphoid cells.
- Low-grade MEC.
- Low-grade malignant lymphoma: when lymphocytes are the most prominent elements, cell marker studies should be performed.
- Squamous cell carcinoma: squamous metaplasia with marked individual keratosis and degenerative atypia often present in Warthin's tumor and may mimic squamous cell carcinoma. In questionable cases, a repeat aspiration or concentrating any recovered fluid to search for oncocytes should be considered.
- AciCC, oncocytic variant.

Histology

- Irregular cystic structures lined by double-layer oncocytic epithelium, often with a papillary proliferation, occasionally metaplasia to squamous or mucous or ciliated cells in a lymphoid stroma.
- Germinal centers and rare granulomatous reactions may be seen.
- Representative images are shown in Fig. 2.13a–c.

Immunohistochemistry:

- The oncocytes show luminal ductal cell differentiation and are therefore positive for low molecular weight cytokeratin (LMWCK), pan-cytokeratin, EMA, and CEA.
- No myoepithelial cell differentiation is identified, leading to negative staining for p63 and calponin.
- DOG1 and SOX10 expressions are often lacking.
- S100 and mammaglobin are nonreactive.
- GATA-binding protein 3 (GATA3) is positive in 100% of cases, with weak to moderate intensity.

Oncocytoma

Key Clinical Features

- Less than 1% of all salivary gland tumors, 80–90% in the parotid
- No gender predilection, older adults, peak in the 7th–9th decades, common in Caucasians
- Multifocal and bilateral in 70% of cases
- Presents as a soft, well-circumscribed, slow-growing painless mass

Key Radiological Features

- Radiosialography: high uptake of technetium-99 m due to high mitochondrial content of oncocytes
- Ultrasound: non-specific, a hypoechoic mass with well-defined margins
- CT: a well-defined mass showing homogeneous enhancement
- MRI: T1 and T2 hypointensities with homogeneous contrast enhancement

Cytological Features

- Monotonous population of large cells with abundant densely granular cytoplasm, discernible cell borders, and occasional nucleoli (Fig. 2.14a, b.)
- Clean background without lymphocytes.
- Most are benign regardless of pleomorphism.

Differential Diagnosis

- Warthin's tumor: cohesive groups of oncocytic epithelium, lymphocytes, and a cystic background.
- AciCC: loosely cohesive groups and single cells; the tumor cells usually have round nuclei with a smooth nuclear membrane and prominent nucleoli; the cytoplasm is coarsely granular, with indistinct cell border; many naked nuclei with the same nuclear features; granular debris in the background; delicate vasculatures; may contain abundant lymphocytes.
- Malignant oncocytoma: significant cytologic atypia, mitotic activity, and necrosis.

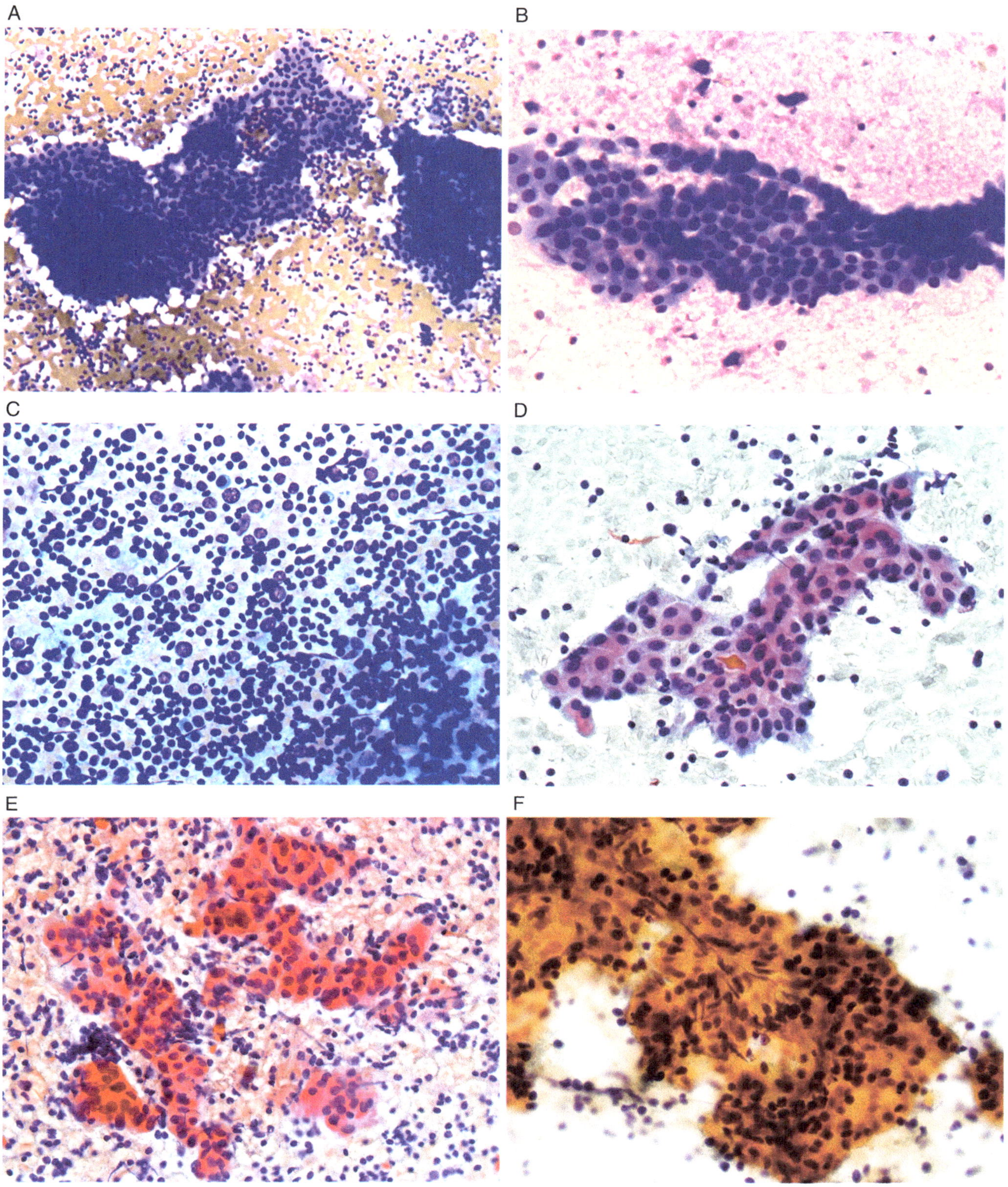

Fig. 2.12 Warthin's tumor of the parotid gland, cytology. (**a**) Sheet of oncocytic epithelium with abundant eosinophilic, granular cytoplasm and intraepithelial lymphocytes in a background of cyst debris and lymphocytes, Diff-Quik. (**b**) The oncocytes are cytologically bland in a dirty background, Diff-Quik. (**c**) A Mixed population of lymphocytes with germinal center sampling, Diff-Quik. (**d, e**) Oncocytes with an appreciable double layer in a background of lymphocytes and cystic debris, Pap stain. (**f**) Oncocytes with papillary architecture, intraepithelial and background lymphocytes, Pap stain

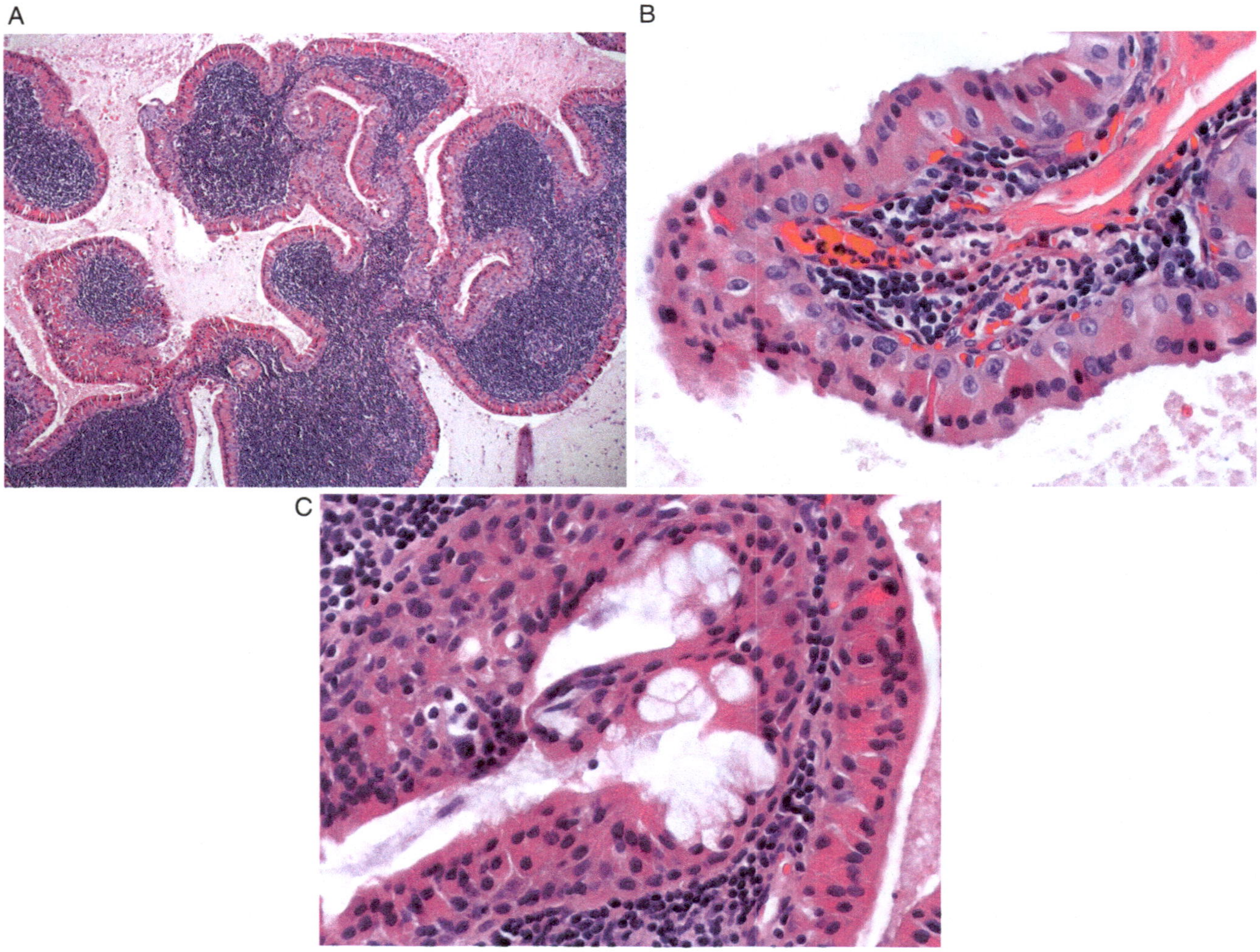

Fig. 2.13 Warthin's tumor of the parotid gland, surgical resection. (**a**) Irregular cystic structures with papillary folds of double-layered oncocytic epithelium and underlying dense lymphoid stroma, H&E. (**b**) High power showing oncocytic columnar cells with brightly eosinophilic granular cytoplasm, H&E. (**c**) Focal mucous cell metaplasia, H&E

- Metastatic renal cell carcinoma: more cytologic atypia; IHC aids differential diagnosis.
- MEC.

Histology

- Usually solid but may have a cystic component.
- The tumor cells are uniform, polygonal or cuboidal, and contain a centrally placed round nucleus with nucleoli and abundant eosinophilic granular or clear cytoplasm arranged in trabeculae, packets, sheets, or rarely glands, separated by scanty loose vascular stroma.
- Focal sebaceous, goblet cell, or squamous differentiation may be present.
- For tumors with predominant clear cells, the designation of clear cell oncocytoma is applied. Those tumors carry a higher frequency for bilaterality and recurrence.
- Oncocytoma is prone to infarction, either spontaneously or after FNA.
- Representative images are illustrated in Fig. 2.14c, d.

Immunohistochemistry:

- The diagnosis of oncocytoma is straightforward in the majority of cases; Immunohistochemical assay is not necessary.
- In cases of small biopsy or FNA cellblock material, immunohistochemical assay may be applied to confirm cell lineage.

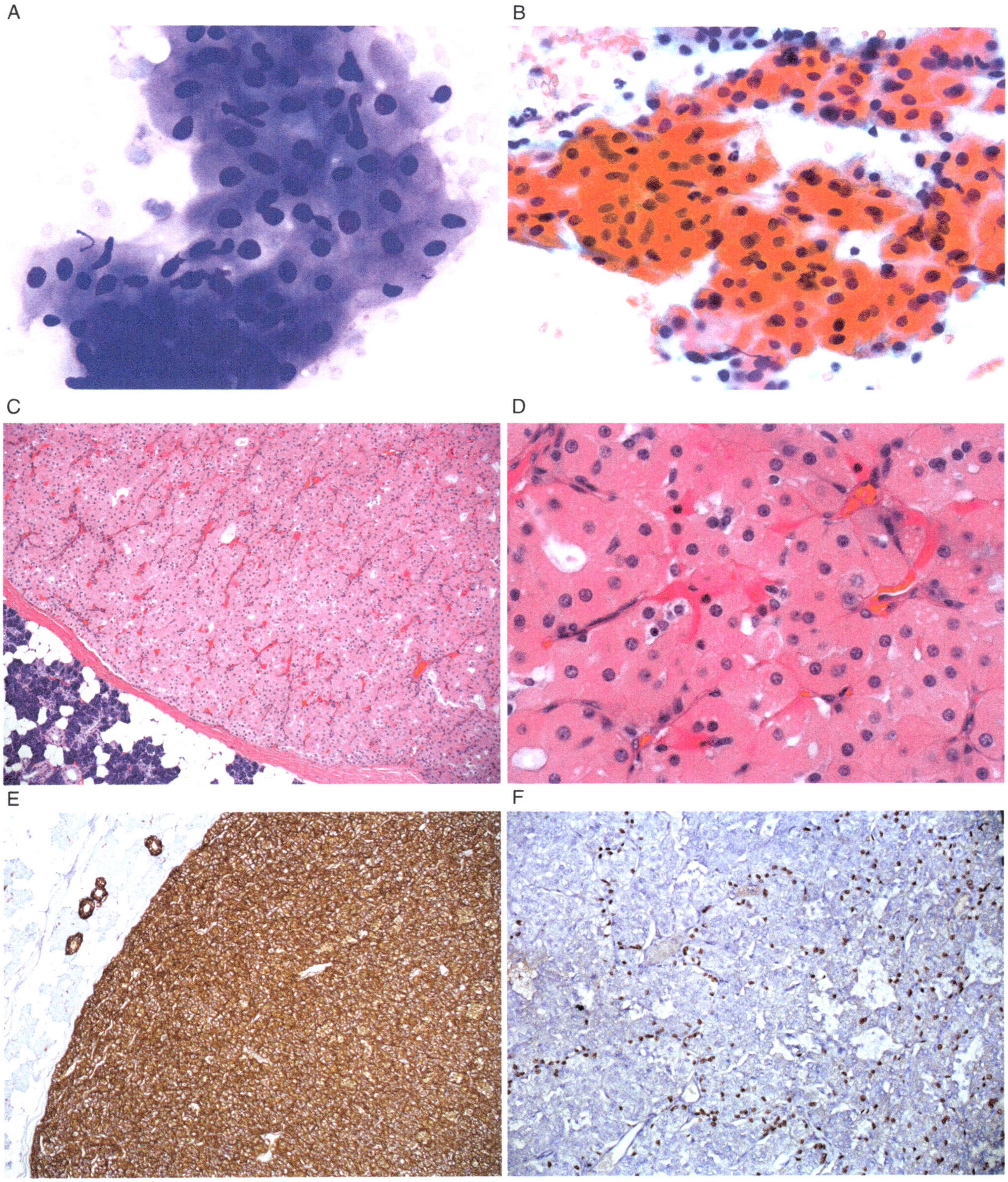

Fig. 2.14 Oncocytoma. (**a**) Population of oncocytes with abundant densely granular cytoplasm, relatively defined cell borders, and focally discernible nucleoli in a clean background without lymphocytes, Diff-Quik. (**b**) The same, Pap stain. (**c**) Well-circumscribed, thinly encapsulated border, H&E. (**d**) Polygonal oncocytes with abundant eosinophilic granular cytoplasm and central round nuclei containing distinct nucleoli, H&E. (**e**) Positive for pVHL stain, also note the normal duct in adjacent is positive for pVHL, but not the acinar cells. (**f**) Tumor cells are negative for p63, and only residual myoepithelial cells are positive

- The neoplastic oncocytes are usually positive for cytokeratin, von Hippel von tumor suppressor (pVHL), CD117, and CK20 and negative for myoepithelial markers (including p63, calponin, S100), SOX10, and DOG1.
- GATA3 is positive in 100% of cases with variable intensity.
- Representative images are illustrated in Fig. 2.14e, f.

Myoepithelioma

Key Clinical Features

- An unusual salivary gland tumor (<1% of all tumors), considered a monomorphic variant of PA.
- 50% occur in the parotid, followed by minor salivary glands (especially the palate).
- No gender predilection, mean age in early to mid-40s.
- Presents as slowly enlarging, painless masses, usually 1–5 cm in diameter.

Key Radiological Features

- Similar to PA (benign mixed tumor)

Cytological Features

- Loosely cohesive and single cells with spindled, clear cell, epithelioid, and/or plasmacytoid appearance (Fig. 2.15a)
- No matrix material or honeycombed epithelial sheets

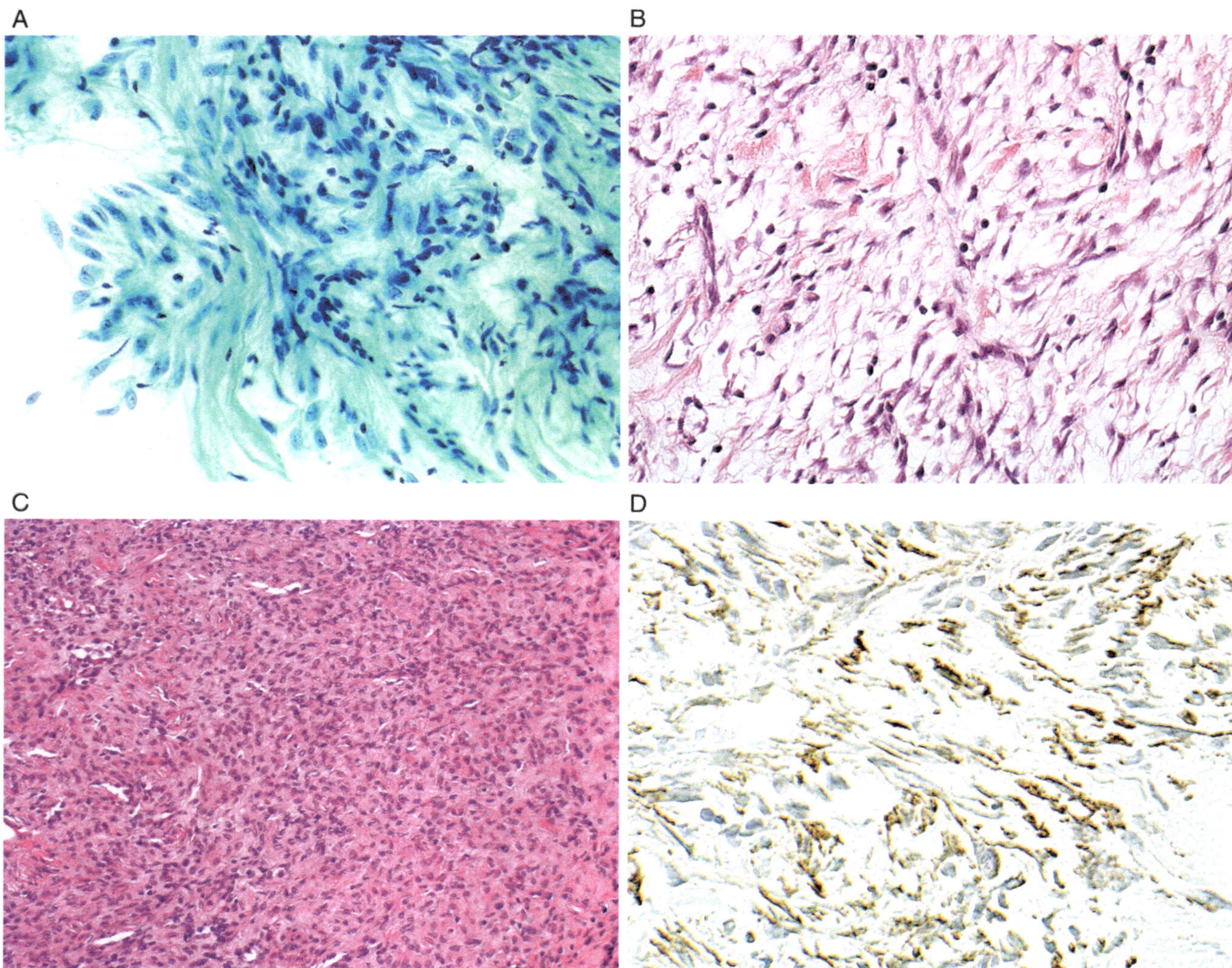

Fig. 2.15 Myoepithelioma. (**a**) Loosely cohesive clusters of fusiform, spindly to focally plump myoepithelial cells in a clean background, devoid of stroma, Pap stain. (**b**) Spindled cells in a myxoid background, H&E. (**c**) Spindled myoepithelial cells in a solid sheet, H&E. (**d**) Desmin positive, IHC

Differential Diagnosis

- Myoepithelial-rich PA: the discrimination between myoepithelial-cell-rich PA and myoepithelioma is of little biological consequence.
- Schwannoma: difficult to distinguish from spindle cell myoepithelioma morphologically; IHC has great value; positive for cytokeratin, smooth muscle actin (SMA), and calponin in myoepithelioma; S100 and SOX10 are positive in both.
- Plasmacytoma: to distinguish from plasmacytoid variant of myoepithelioma; CD38, CD138 positive; in situ hybridization for cytoplasmic immunoglobulin light chain showing restriction; negative for myoepithelial cell markers.
- Epithelial-myoepithelial carcinoma: contains epithelial component.
- Metastatic renal cell carcinoma: to distinguish from clear cell variant of myoepithelioma; paired box gene (PAX)8, carbonic anhydrase IX (CAIX), and renal cell carcinoma marker (RCCma)-positive; negative for myoepithelial cell markers.

Histology

- Usually a thinly encapsulated tumor comprising trabeculae and sheets of spindled, plasmacytoid hyaline, clear, oncocytic, or polygonal to cuboidal cells with abundant eosinophilic granular cytoplasm with delicate vasculature in the background.
- The stroma ranges from scant to myxoid, hyaline, or sclerotic.
- Radially arranged collagenous fibers and tyrosine crystals can be present, but cartilaginous matrix, characteristic of PA by definition, is not present.
- Representative images are illustrated in Fig. 2.15b, c.

Immunohistochemistry:

- The tumor cells express pan-cytokeratin (such as AE1/AE3, MNF116) and myoepithelial markers (such as calponin, actin, p63, SOX10, S100, GFAP, and CK14). However, expression of individual markers in a given tumor is highly variable.
- Expression of S100 has been reported most sensitive in almost every tumor but lacks specificity.
- Pan-cytokeratin and CK14 are expressed in nearly all tumors.
- EMA is positive in a majority of tumors.
- CEA and DOG1 are negative.
- Myoepithelioma of the soft tissues commonly exhibits Ewing sarcoma region 1-octamer-binding transcription factor 4 (*OCT4)(EWSR1-POU5F1*) or Ewing sarcoma region 1-pre-B-cell leukemia homeobox 1 (*EWSR1-PBX1*) gene fusion, but salivary gland myoepithelioma has not been well studied.
- Representative images are illustrated in Fig. 2.15d.

Sebaceous Lymphadenoma

Key Clinical Features

- A rare benign tumor of the salivary glands, commonly in parotid gland or periparotid lymph nodes
- No gender predilection, common in 6th to 8th decades
- Presents as a painless slow-growing mass or incidental finding

Key Radiologic Features

- Thin-section CT image: well-defined, inhomogeneous, low-density mass with scattered fat density areas
- Dynamic MRI: a mass lesion with areas of fat density, early enhanced and delayed washout pattern, as well as an enhanced capsule

Differential Diagnosis

- Warthin's tumor
- AciCC
- Mucoepidermoid carcinoma (MEC)
- Mammary analogue secretory carcinoma (MASC)

Cytological Features

- Sebaceous epithelial cells and lymphoid cells
- Sebaceous epithelial cells with various degrees of cytological atypia and containing cytoplasmic fine vacuoles
- Fig. 2.16a

Histology

- The microscopic appearance at low power view is similar to Warthin's tumor.
- Usually well-circumscribed or encapsulated, comprised of islands, trabeculae, duct-like structures of sebaceous glands admixed with a dense lymphoid stroma, often with lymphoid follicles
- The cells at the periphery of the cell nests and tubuloglandular structures have a basaloid appearance.
- Foci of squamous differentiation with keratinization can be seen.

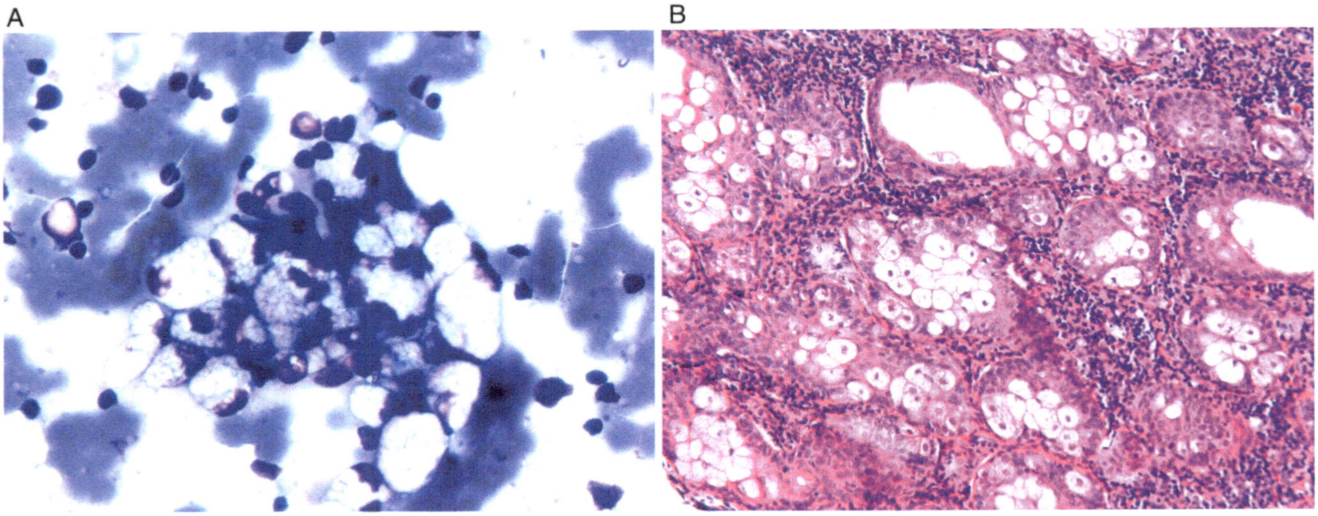

Fig. 2.16 Sebaceous lymphadenoma. (**a**) Sebaceous epithelial cells showing abundant cytoplasmic fine vacuoles and small nuclei; in addition, there are lymphocytes in background, Diff-Quik. (**b**) The tumor islands are comprised of central sebaceous cells with peripheral basaloid cells in a lymphoid background, H&E

- The lymphoid stroma often contains many reactive lymphoid follicles.
- Histiocytes and foreign-body giant cell inflammatory reactions are commonly observed, which is a feature that can be used to differentiate it from MEC.
- Rarely, the epithelial component can undergo a malignant transformation to carcinoma, such as sebaceous carcinoma or basal cell ADC.
- A representative image is shown in Fig. 2.16b.

Immunohistochemistry:

- When a MEC is in the differential, a mucincarmine stain reveals no intra- or extracellular mucin.
- The tumor shows a biphasic cell population. The luminal cells express luminal cell markers, such as pan-cytokeratin, EMA, CEA, and CK7; the peripheral cells exhibit basal cell phenotype, positive for p63 and high molecular weight cytokeratin (HMWCK), such as CK903 and CK5/CK6.
- Myoepithelial cell markers (SMA, calponin, S100) are usually negative.

Malignant Epithelial Tumors

Mucoepidermoid Carcinoma

Key Clinical Features

- Mucoepidermoid carcinoma (MEC) is the most common malignant salivary gland tumor and the most common salivary gland malignancy in children and adolescents <20 years of age.
- Female-to-male ratio 3:2, mean age in the 5th decade.
- Approximately 50% major salivary gland predominant, especially the parotid gland; also in minor salivary glands, especially the palate, mouth; and upper and lower respiratory tracts, rarely intra-bony tumors in the mandible or maxilla.
- Presents as a painless, slow-growing, firm mass of widely varying duration; pain is associated with high-grade tumors.

Key Radiological Features

- Well-visualized lower-intensity mass on T1-weighted MRI; low to intermediate signal intensity on T2-weighted MRI; however, low-grade MEC may exhibit elevated signal intensity.
- Evidence of invasion, excellent on T1-weighted images.

Cytological Features

Low-Grade MEC:

- Sparse cellular sample with a small volume of mucoid fluid.
- Foam cells and epithelial cells, may be squamous, mucinous, or intermediate, present in a background of abundant extracellular mucin.
- Chronic inflammation often presents.

High-Grade MEC:

- Cellular specimen with cytologic malignant cells with squamous features.
- Mucin-producing cells and histiocytes may be present.
- Cystic background may or may not be present.

Representative images are illustrated in Fig. 2.17a–f.

Differential Diagnosis
Low-Grade MEC:

- Warthin's tumor
- Lymphoepithelial cyst
- Chronic sialadenitis
- Sialolithiasis

High-Grade MEC:

- Salivary duct carcinoma
- Malignant mixed tumor
- Primary and metastatic squamous cell carcinomas
- Other high-grade carcinomas

Histology
MECs are composed of haphazardly arranged cystic structures or nests of epidermoid cells, mucus-secreting cells, and intermediate cells in a sclerotic and dense lymphoid stroma. The proportion of each cell type and the morphology and arrangement of the cells vary among and between tumor grades.

Low-Grade MEC:

- Usually well-circumscribed, mucin-containing cystic structures predominate.
- The lining cells are rich in bland-looking mucous cells and intermediate cells, with occasional epidermoid cells, which are often inconspicuous for intercellular bridges.
- Keratinization or keratin pearls are never seen.
- Representative images are shown in Fig. 2.18a, b.

Intermediate-Grade MEC:

- Histological features are between low-grade and high-grade MECs.
- Cystic structures are less prominent.
- Epidermoid cells are more obvious compared to low-grade tumors. The cells show more atypia.
- Representative images are shown in Fig. 2.18c, d.

High-Grade MEC:

- Usually infiltrative, solid growth pattern predominant, with only sparse mucous cells.
- The epidermoid cells show more developed squamous cell features, such as intercellular bridges and even individual cell keratinization; however, keratin pearls are rare.
- There are significant cytological atypia, mitosis, and necrosis.
- Perineural and angiolymphatic invasions are frequently seen.
- Representative images are shown in Fig. 2.18e, f.

There is no universally accepted grading system; however, WHO 2005 provided a grading system based on histologic features to classify low-, intermediate-, and high-grade tumors, as summarized in Table 2.5.

Immunohistochemistry

- The tumor cells of MEC are reactive to cytokeratin (including CK7), variably to EMA and CEA.
- S100 expression may be seen but is usually lacking.
- The intermediate, epidermoid, and clear cells are positive for p63, but negative for calponin and SMA.
- DOG1 and SOX10 are predominantly negative but reported positive in a small proportion of cases, usually focal reactivity.
- MEC shows high expression of membrane-bound mucins (MUC1, MUC4, and MUC5AC); MUC1 is often associated with high-grade MECs, while MUC4 expression is related to low-grade MECs. MUC5AC is helpful in distinguishing high-grade MEC from squamous cell carcinoma.
- GATA3 expression was reported in 41% of cases with variable staining patterns.

The specific translocation t(11;19)(q14–21;p12–13) involving *MEC translocated-1* (*MECT1*) or *CREB-regulated transcription coactivator 1* (*CRTC1*) gene at 19q13 and the mastermind-like 2 (*MAML2*) gene at 11q21 was reported in 60–70% of MECs, especially in low-grade MEC (74% of patients), associated with a favorable prognosis.

Acinic Cell Carcinoma

Key Clinical Features

- Over 80% in the parotid gland; less in minor salivary glands, especially the upper lip/vestibule, buccal mucosa and palate; uncommon in submandibular and sublingual gland
- Female-to-male ratio 3:2
- 3rd–7th decades, average age 38–46 years
- The second most common malignant salivary gland tumor in children

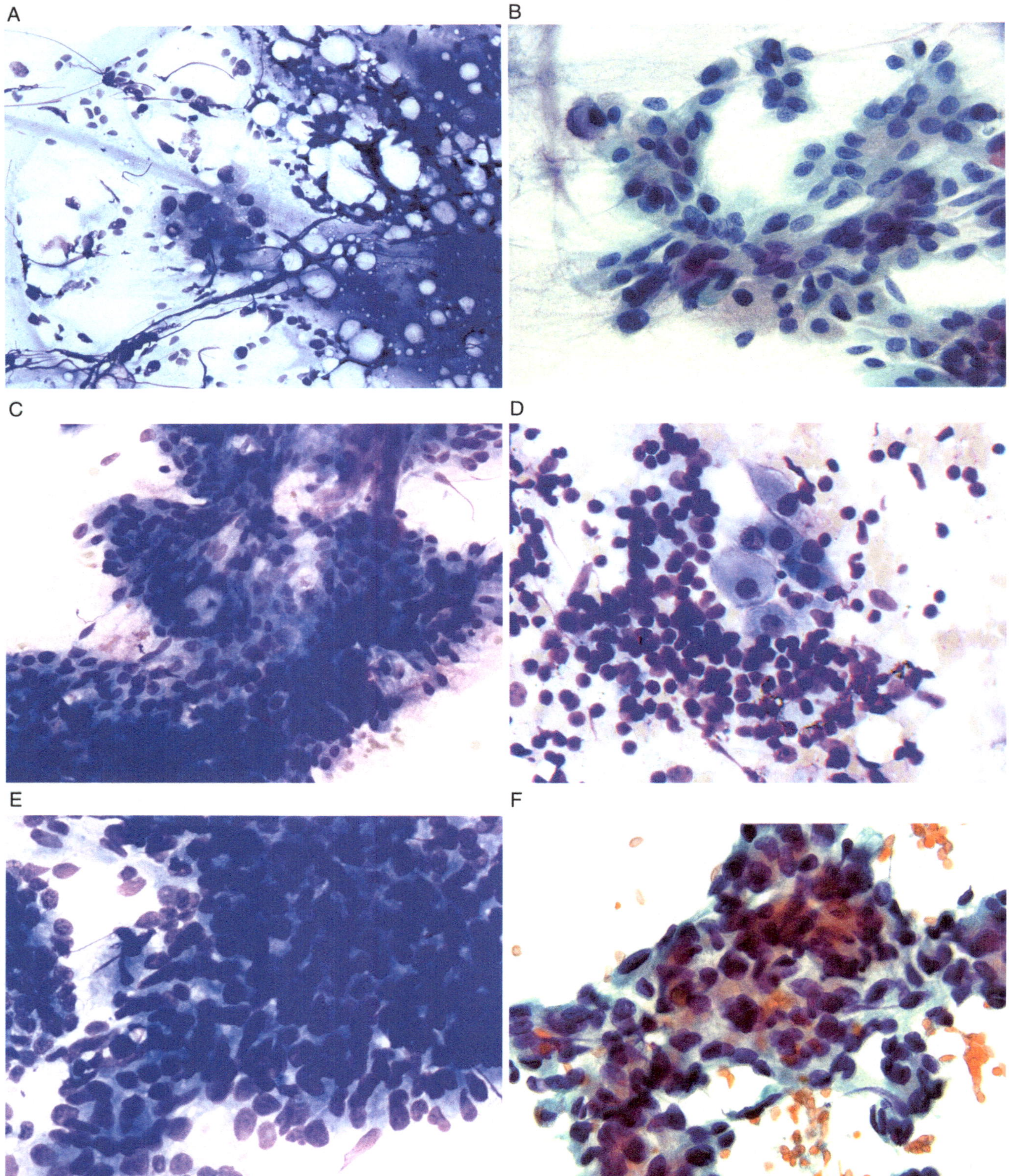

Fig. 2.17 Mucoepidermoid carcinoma, cytology. (**a**) A low-grade tumor showing cytologically bland intermediate ductal epithelial cells and mucinous cells with delicate vasculature in a background of abundant mucinous debris and few lymphocytes, Diff-Quik. (**b**) Intermediate, mucinous, and rare squamous cells with mild nuclear atypia in a background of abundant mucinous debris and few lymphocytes, Pap stain. (**c**) Cluster of intermediate cells, mucinous cells with delicate vasculature, Diff-Quik. (**d**) A few mucus cells with prominent nucleoli and intermediate cells in a background of scant mucin and lymphocytes, Diff-Quik. (**e**) Cluster of atypical intermediate and mucinous cells, Diff Quik. (**f**) A high-grade tumor showing highly atypical ductal and mucinous cells, Pap stain

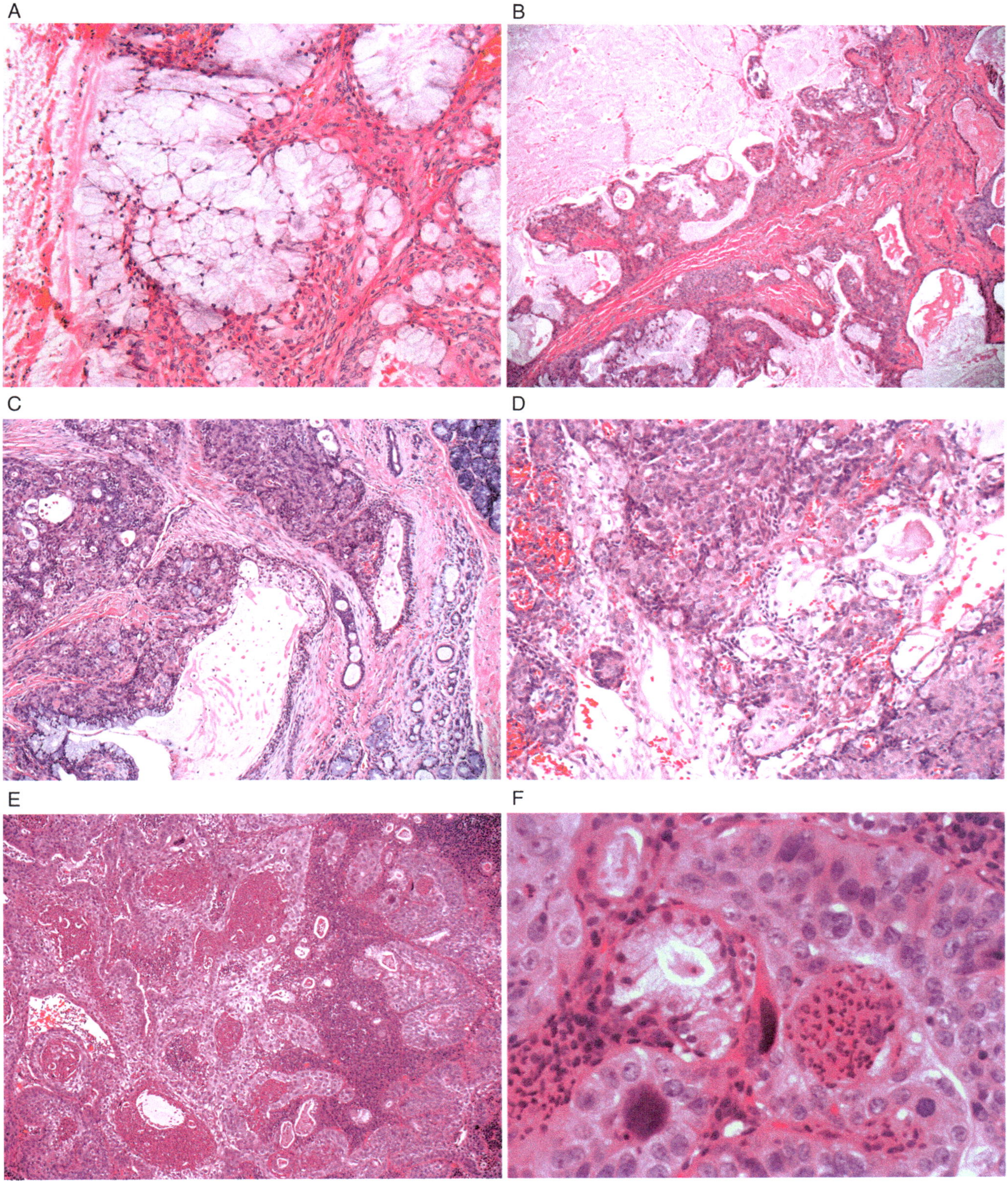

Fig. 2.18 Mucoepidermoid carcinoma, histology. (**a**, **b**) The tumor is composed mainly cystic spaces with mucus cell lining, low grade; the bland mucus cells and multiple cystic spaces containing mucinous debris are shown, H&E. (**c**, **d**) The tumor shows less mucinous cystic spaces with more solid areas and epidermoid cells, intermediate grade, H&E. (**e**, **f**) Mainly solid, squamoid, and mucinous cell proliferation with significant cytologic atypia, mucinous cystic component is minimal, high grade, H&E

Table 2.5 WHO histopathologic features, point values, and point scores used in grading mucoepidermoid carcinoma

Histopathologic features	Point values
Cystic component <20%	2
Neural invasion	2
Necrosis	3
4 or more mitoses/10 HPF	3
Anaplasia	4
Tumor grade	*Point scores*
Low	0–4
Intermediate	5–6
High	7 or more

Used with permission from Harnes L, Eveson JW, Reichart P, et al. WHO Classification of Tumours: Pathology and Genetics, Head and Neck Tumours. Lyon, France: IARC; 2005
HPF high-power field

- The 3rd most common bilateral salivary gland tumor; but the most frequent bilateral malignant salivary gland tumor
- Presents as a slow-growing mass, often painful and tender, with varying durations

Key Radiological Features

- Similar to MEC

Cytological Features

- Cellular aspirates, showing numerous large cells with abundant finely granular cytoplasm (if intact) with variably prominent nucleoli, singly or in groups; the cells are often damaged in the smearing process to yield many large naked nuclei with fine granules in background; otherwise, the background is relatively clean.
- Absence of duct cells and adipocytes (contamination from surrounding normal parenchyma may occur).
- Large tissue particles contain intact cells and transverse vessels.
- May have oncocytic or clear cell changes.
- Many histological variants; in a diagnostically difficult case, acinic cell carcinoma (AciCC) should be included.
- Figure 2.19a–d.

Differential Diagnosis

- Normal acinar tissue
- Warthin's tumor
- MEC
- Oncocytic neoplasm

Histology

- Usually circumscribed, lobulated solitary nodule, some with ill-defined, infiltrative borders with multinodular patterns.
- The tumors exhibit several cell types with a variety of growth patterns, including acinar, intercalated ductal, vacuolated, clear, and non-specific glandular cells arranged in solid/lobular, microcystic, papillary-cystic, and follicular growth patterns.
- The cytoplasmic zymogen-like granules in acinar cells are PAS-positive and diastase resistant.
- Although a single cell type or growth pattern often dominates any given tumor, a mixture of cell types and growth patterns is seen in many tumors.
- Acinic cells and intercalated duct-like cells are the most common cell types.
- Prominent lymphoid infiltrates are observed in many tumors.
- Representative images are illustrated in Fig. 2.20a, b.

Immunohistochemistry:

- AciCC shows serous acinar and intercalated duct differentiation and expresses cytokeratin (especially LMWCK), CEA, DOG1, SOX10, and characteristic cytoplasmic periodic acid-Schiff diastase (PAS-D)-positive zymogen granules.
- The majority is negative for S100; however, S100 was reported positive in 10% of cases.
- Tumor cells are negative for myoepithelial cell markers, including p63.
- In addition, pVHL expression is lacking. GATA3 expression is mostly negative.
- Representative immunostains are illustrated in Fig. 2.20c, d.
- There is no specific molecular alteration identified currently.

Adenoid Cystic Carcinoma

Key Clinical Features

- 75% of minor salivary gland tumors, especially in the palate; 25% of major salivary gland tumors, especially the submandibular gland.
- Peak in 4th–7th decades; female-to-male ratio of 3:2.
- Presents as a slow-growing mass of long duration; may be tender or painful, with facial nerve palsy.
- Mucosal ulceration is often present in minor salivary gland tumors.

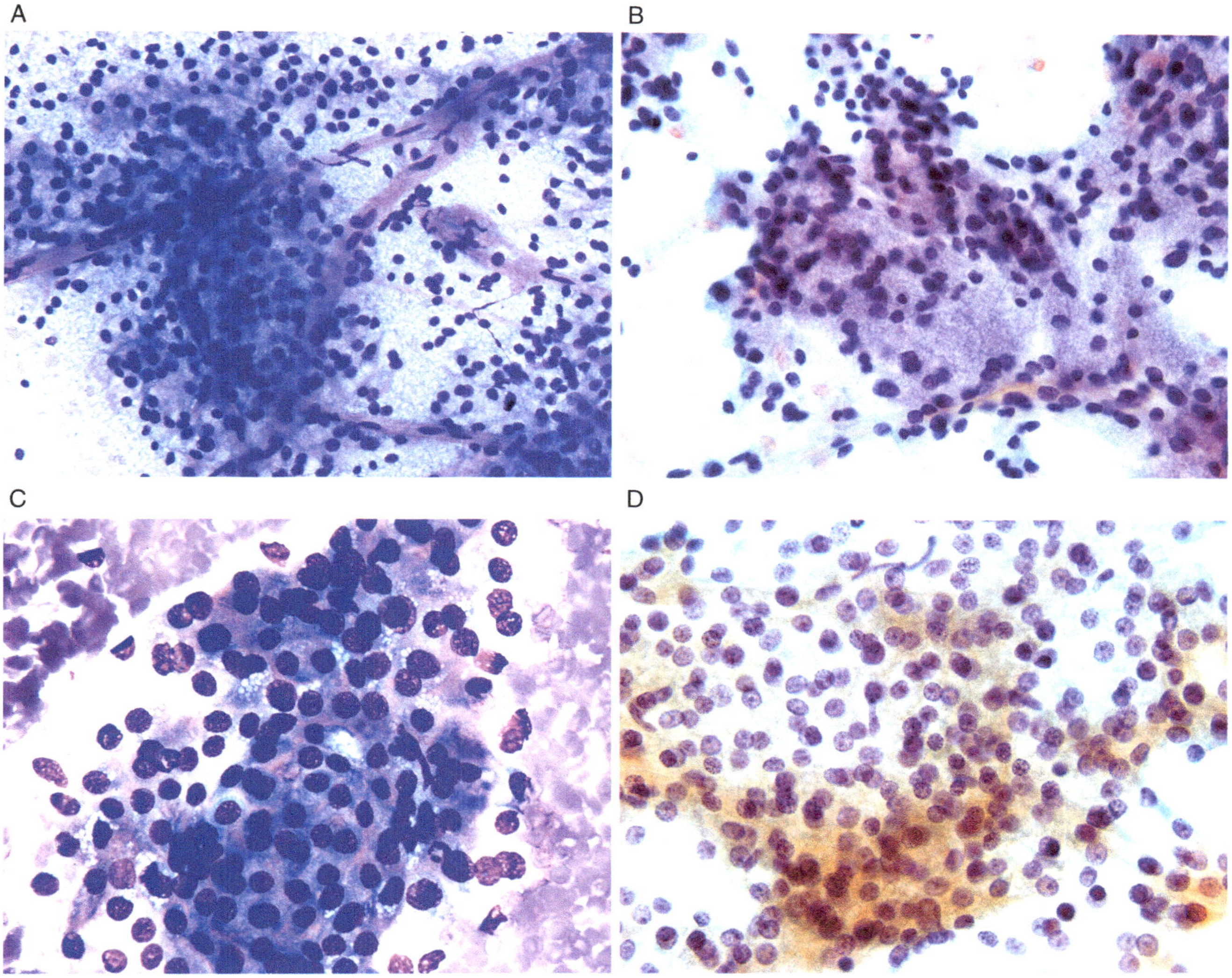

Fig. 2.19 Acinic cell carcinoma, cytology. (**a, b**) Cellular aspirate contains abundant epithelial cells with round nuclei, prominent nucleoli, and ample granular cytoplasm in background of granular debris, as well as delicate vasculature. Many naked nuclei showing similar morphology are seen. (**a**) Diff-Quik. (**b**) Pap stain. (**c, d**) Prominent nucleoli are well demonstrated; some cells show cytoplasmic vacuoles. (**c**) Diff-Quik. (**d**) Pap stain

Key Radiological Features

- Similar to MEC

Cytological Features

- Small uniform cells (usually angulated nuclei) with relatively hyperchromatic nuclear chromatin, scant cytoplasm, and inconspicuous nucleoli.
- Naked nuclei may be numerous.
- Stromal spheres or cylinders are translucent or pale on Pap-stained slide, have a sharp interface with tumor cells, and appear magenta on Diff-Quik stain.
- Lack of myoepithelial cells, spindle cells, or vessels.
- Desmoplastic stroma may contain spindle cells or vessels and mimic basal cell adenoma or PA.
- Fig. 2.21a–f.

Differential Diagnosis

- Basal cell adenoma
- PA
- Basal cell adenocarcinoma
- PLGA

Histology

- Adenoid cystic carcinomas (AdCCs) are solid, well-circumscribed tumors with invasion into adjacent salivary gland parenchyma.
- The tumor is comprised of two cell types, the inner luminal (ductal) cells and the peripheral modified myoepithelial cells. The latter is characterized by hyperchromatic, angulated nuclei often with clear cytoplasm.

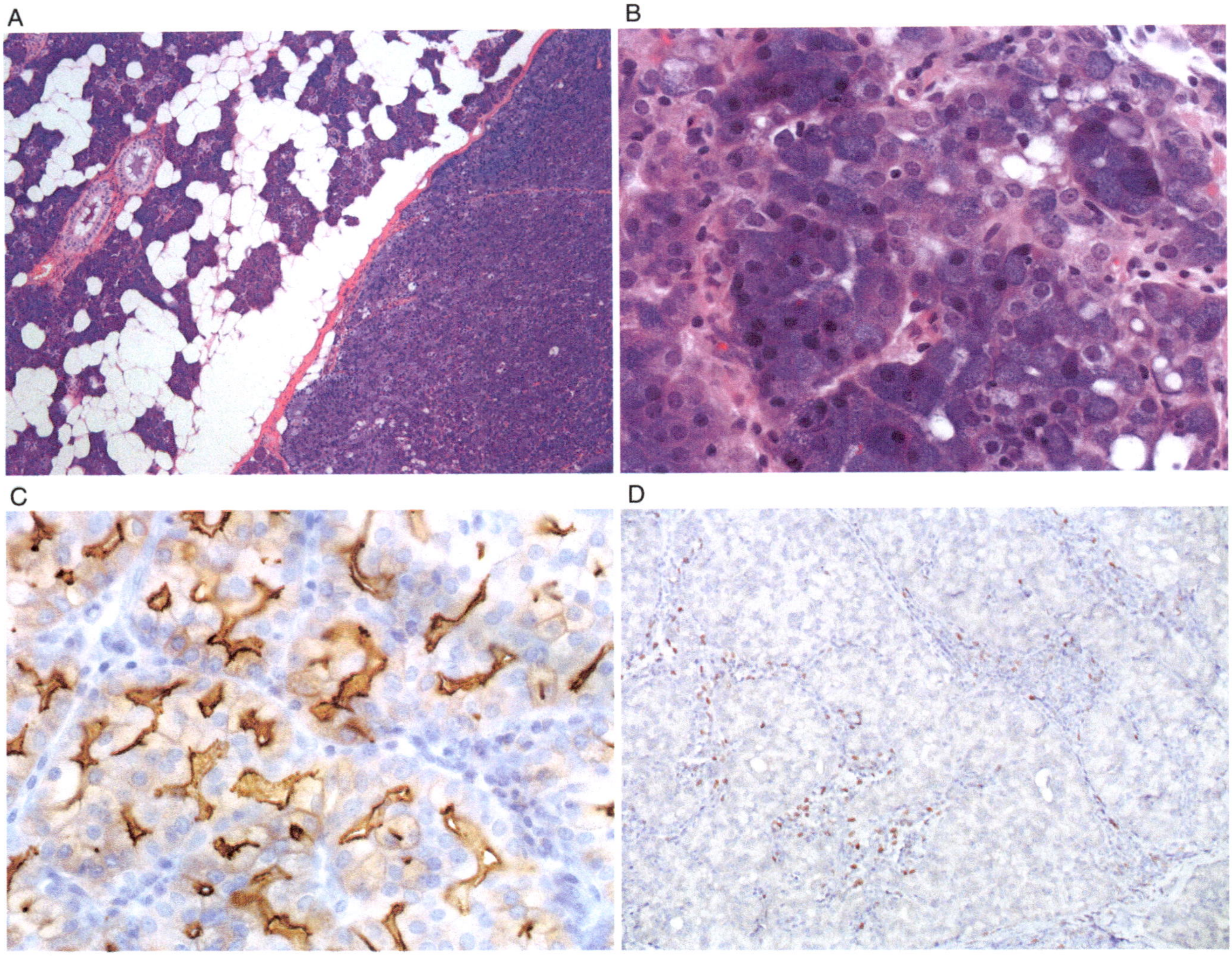

Fig. 2.20 Acinic cell carcinoma, histology, and immunophenotype. (**a**) The tumor shows well-circumscribed border, H&E. (**b**) Sheet of polygonal tumor cells containing round nuclei with prominent nucleoli and abundant cytoplasm with basophilic granules, H&E. (**c**) Positive for DOG1, showing an apical luminal membranous staining pattern; focal complete membranous staining also noted, not shown, IHC. (**d**) Negative for p63, IHC

- The tumor exhibits tubular, cribriform, and solid patterns, with the cribriform pattern being the most common.
- The hyaline or basophilic mucoid material in the cribriform pattern is characteristic.
- The stroma of the tumor is generally hyalinized.
- Perineural invasions are frequent.
- Representative images are illustrated in Fig. 2.22a–d.

Immunohistochemistry:

- The luminal cells express cytokeratins (LMWCK and pan-cytokeratin, including CK7, usually strong), CEA, EMA, and CD117; myoepithelial markers decorate the peripheral basal cells and the cells in solid areas.
- GFAP is negative.
- Estrogen receptor (ER) and progesterone receptor (PR) have been reported positive.
- DOG1 is positive in all cases, decorating both luminal and myoepithelial components.
- SOX10 expression was reported in 96% of cases.
- CD43 was reported to be preferentially expressed in AdCCs compared to PLGAs and monomorphic adenomas.
- Strong v-myb avian myeloblastosis viral oncogene homolog (MYB) immunoreactivity was reported in the majority of AdCCs.
- GATA3 expression was reported in 22% of cases with variable staining pattern.
- Representative images are illustrated in Fig. 2.22e, f.

AdCCs are characterized by the specific translocation t(6;9) *MYB* and nuclear factor 1 B-type (*NFIB*) in a majority

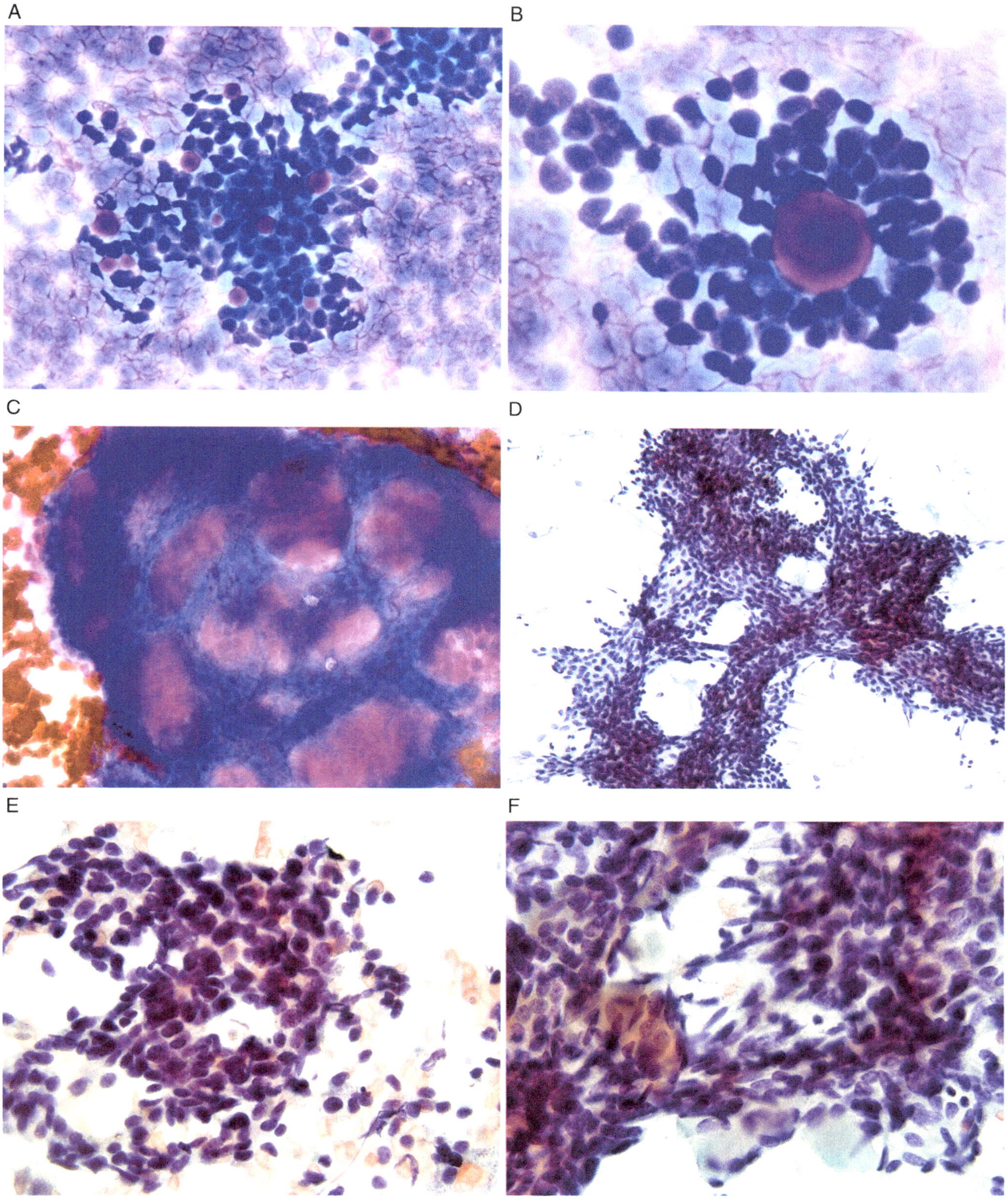

Fig. 2.21 Adenoid cystic carcinoma, cytology. (**a**) Hyperchromatic, angulated basaloid cells with hyaline globules, Diff-Quik. (**b**) High-power view of the basaloid cells and magenta hyaline globule, Diff Quik. (**c**) Three-dimensional fragment, Diff-Quik. (**d–f**) Tumor cells appear small, basaloid; the hyaline globules are translucent, presenting as empty spaces on Pap stain

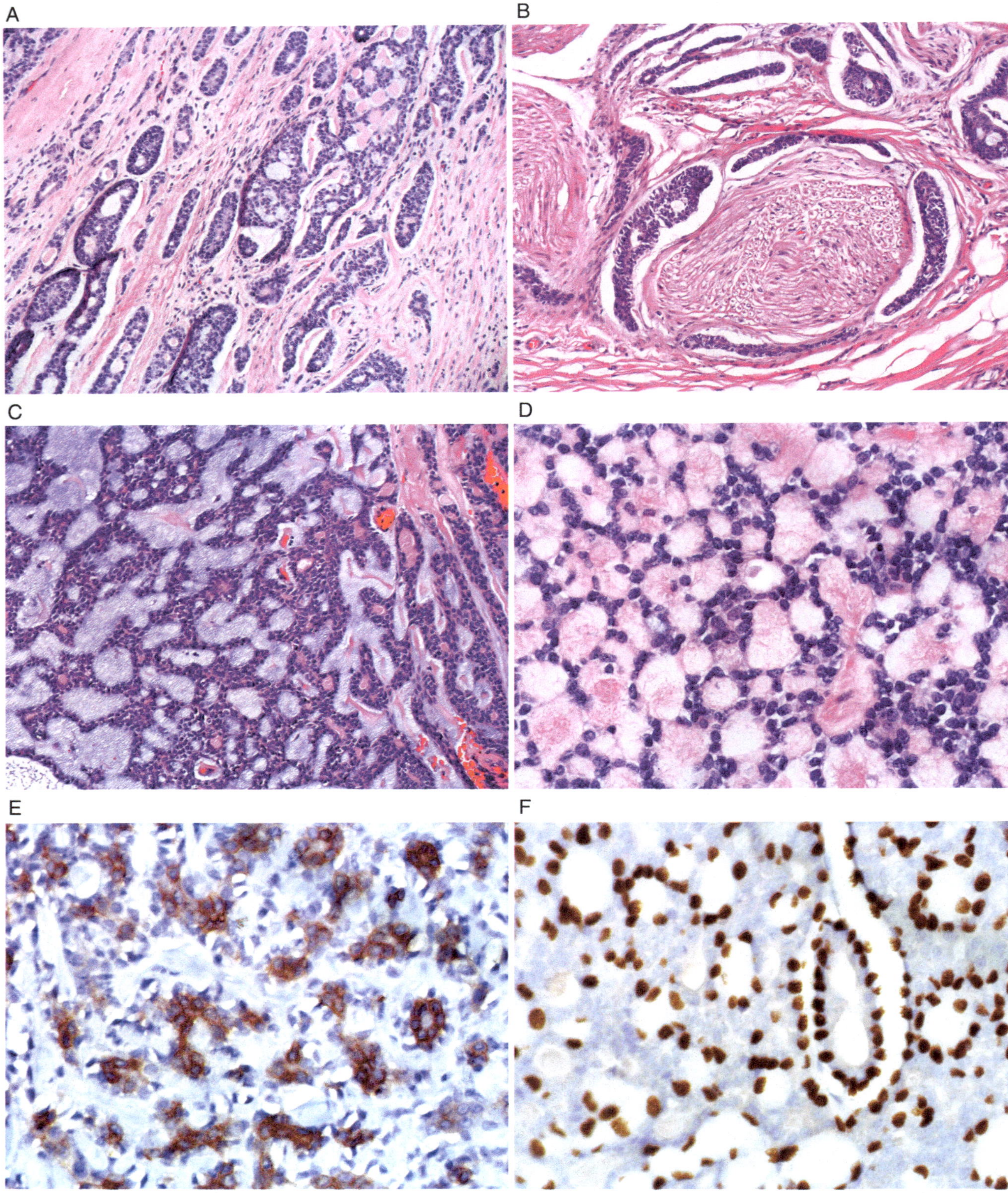

Fig. 2.22 Adenoid cystic carcinoma, histology, and immunophenotype. (**a**) The tumor shows an infiltrative border, comprised of nests, cords, and cribriform-patterned tumor cells, H&E. (**b**) Perineural invasion, H&E. (**c**) Cribriform pattern with prominent myxoid changes, H&E. (**d**) Cribriform pattern with abundant hyaline stromal globules, H&E. (**e**) CD117 decorates luminal cells, IHC. (**f**) p63 positive in the basal cells, IHC

of tumors, reported in approximately 64% of patients. The translocation t(6;9)(*MYB-NFIB*) was not observed in other salivary gland tumors, except rare PLGAs. The detection of t(6;9)(*MYB-NFIB*) by fluorescence in situ hybridization (FISH) or next-generation sequencing (NGS) can be used as a diagnostic marker for AdCCs. Immunohistochemical overexpression of MYB was observed in vast majority of AdCCs, reported in 82–85%, while all tested PAs were negative. In addition, a majority of AdCCs exhibit strong and diffuse expression for CD117 without c-kit gene mutation, therefore showing no beneficial effects for therapy with a specific tyrosine kinase receptor inhibitor (imatinib) in clinical trials.

Malignant Mixed Tumor

There are three types: metastasizing mixed tumor, carcinosarcoma, and carcinoma ex pleomorphic adenoma.

Key Clinical Features

- Carcinoma ex pleomorphic adenoma: the most common form (>95%), 6.2% of all mixed tumor; presents as a long-standing painless mass with rapid enlargement and pain or with multiple recurrences; incidence increases with the duration of tumor, 1.6% for tumors of <5 years, 9.5% for >15 years; mean age at presentation is 61 years.
- Metastasizing mixed tumor: a cytologically benign mixed tumor in a distant site; the majority of patients have a history of incomplete surgery and locoregional recurrences of benign mixed tumor; often fatal.
- Carcinosarcoma: very rare, a true malignant mixed tumor, mostly in major salivary glands, with a mean age of 58–62 years, no sex predilection.

Key Radiological Features

- Similar to MEC

Cytological Features

- Carcinoma ex pleomorphic adenoma: cellular smears, nuclear features of high-grade carcinoma, usually ductal subtype (Fig. 2.23a); elements of benign mixed tumor present.
- Metastasizing mixed tumor: typical morphology of benign mixed tumor.
- Carcinosarcoma: malignant epithelial and mesenchymal elements; the most common differentiated mesenchymal elements are chondrosarcoma and osteosarcoma.

Differential Diagnosis

Difficult to distinguish from other high-grade carcinomas, such as:

- High-grade MEC.
- Salivary duct carcinoma.
- Metastatic carcinoma.
- Primary soft tissue sarcoma: the identification of epithelial component (such as cytokeratin positive) within chondromyxoid stroma or contractile smooth muscle elements

A B

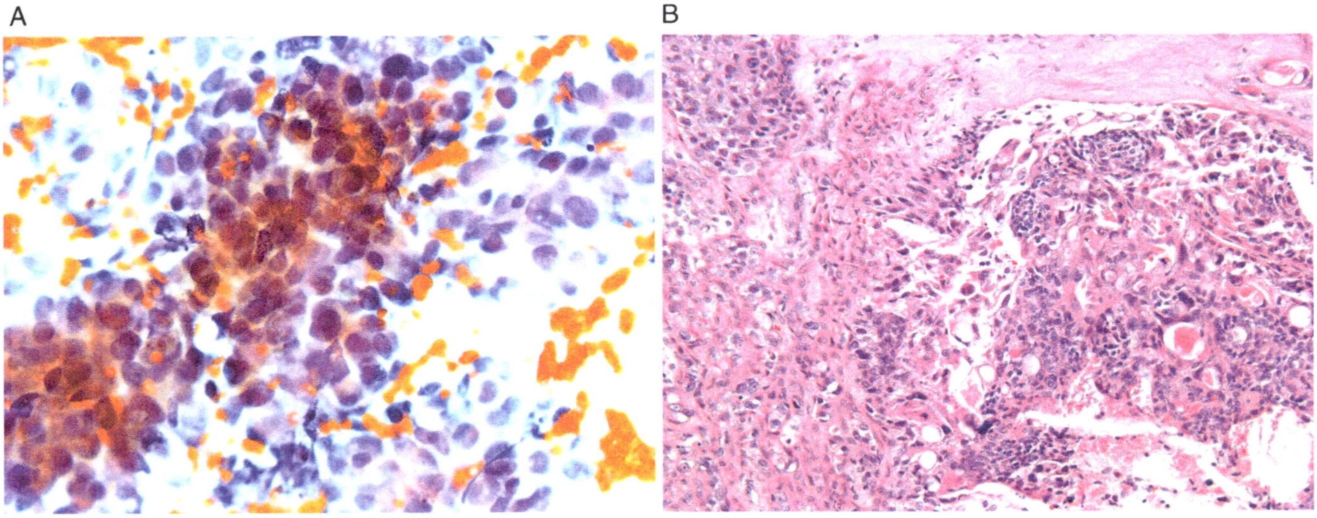

Fig. 2.23 Malignant mixed tumor. (**a**) High-grade carcinoma, ductal type, showing a cluster of highly atypical ductal cells with several mitoses, Pap stain. (**b**) Histology, high-grade carcinoma with adjacent benign mixed tumor, H&E

(positive for HHF-35, SMA, calponin) and GFAP within myoepithelial cells are features unique to salivary gland neoplasm, therefore, favoring a metastasizing PA or carcinosarcoma.

Histology

- Carcinoma ex pleomorphic adenomas are typically larger, poorly circumscribed with infiltrative borders.
- However, well-circumscribed, scar-like, or encapsulated tumors may occasionally be seen.
- Benign component (PA) may or may not be identified.
- The malignant component is usually a poorly differentiated adenocarcinoma of the ductal or NOS type or an undifferentiated carcinoma.
- Frequent mitoses and necrosis are often present.
- Carcinoma ex pleomorphic adenomas should be subclassified into noninvasive (carcinoma in situ), minimally invasive (≤1.5 mm penetration into extracapsular tissue), and invasive (>1.5 mm invasion into extracapsular tissue).
- Representative images are illustrated in Fig. 2.23b.

Immunohistochemistry:

- Carcinoma ex pleomorphic adenoma shows a similar immunophenotype to PA.
- Both luminal cell and myoepithelial cell markers are positive.
- SOX10 expression is identified in 100% of cases.
- The demonstration of overexpression for human epidermal growth factor receptor 2 (HER2) and placental S100 (S100P) may aid in the distinguishing carcinoma ex pleomorphic adenoma from atypical PA.
- Carcinoma ex pleomorphic adenoma also shows overexpression of p53 and high proliferative index (MIB-1), with a mean of 35%.
- Similar to PAs, rearrangements of chromosome 8q21 and 12q13–15 are frequent in carcinoma ex pleomorphic adenoma.

Salivary Duct Carcinoma

Key Clinical Features

- Uncommon, most frequently in the elderly, 6th–7th decades, male predominant
- Over 80% in the parotid gland
- Presents as a rapidly enlarging parotid mass associated with facial nerve palsy, pain, and cervical lymphadenopathy

Key Radiological Features

- Similar to high-grade MEC

Cytological Features

- Cytologic malignant cells with large nuclei, prominent nucleoli, and a moderate amount of cytoplasm.
- Necrotic debris in the background,
- 90% of tumors are positive for androgen receptor (AR) by IHC.
- Figure 2.24a–d.

Differential Diagnosis

- MEC
- Other high-grade carcinomas

Histology

- The salivary duct carcinomas are solid, infiltrative, with a cystic component.
- The tumor cells are pleomorphic, usually in a cribriform growth pattern with "Roman bridge" formation and comedonecrosis.
- Solid and papillary growth patterns may be seen.
- Rare micropapillary components have been reported.
- Psammoma bodies and squamous differentiation are also evident.
- Mitoses are abundant.
- A sarcomatoid growth pattern is occasionally present.
- Representative images are illustrated in Fig. 2.24e, f.

Immunohistochemistry:

- Salivary duct carcinomas are positive for AR, gross cystic disease protein-15 (GCDFP-15), GATA3, low- and high-molecular weight cytokeratin, CEA, and EMA.
- Negative for S100, ER, PR, DOG1, SOX10, and myoepithelial markers.
- Variable expression of prostatic markers (prostate-specific antigen [PSA], prostatic acid phosphatase [PAP]) has been reported.
- Representative images are illustrated in Fig. 2.24g, h.

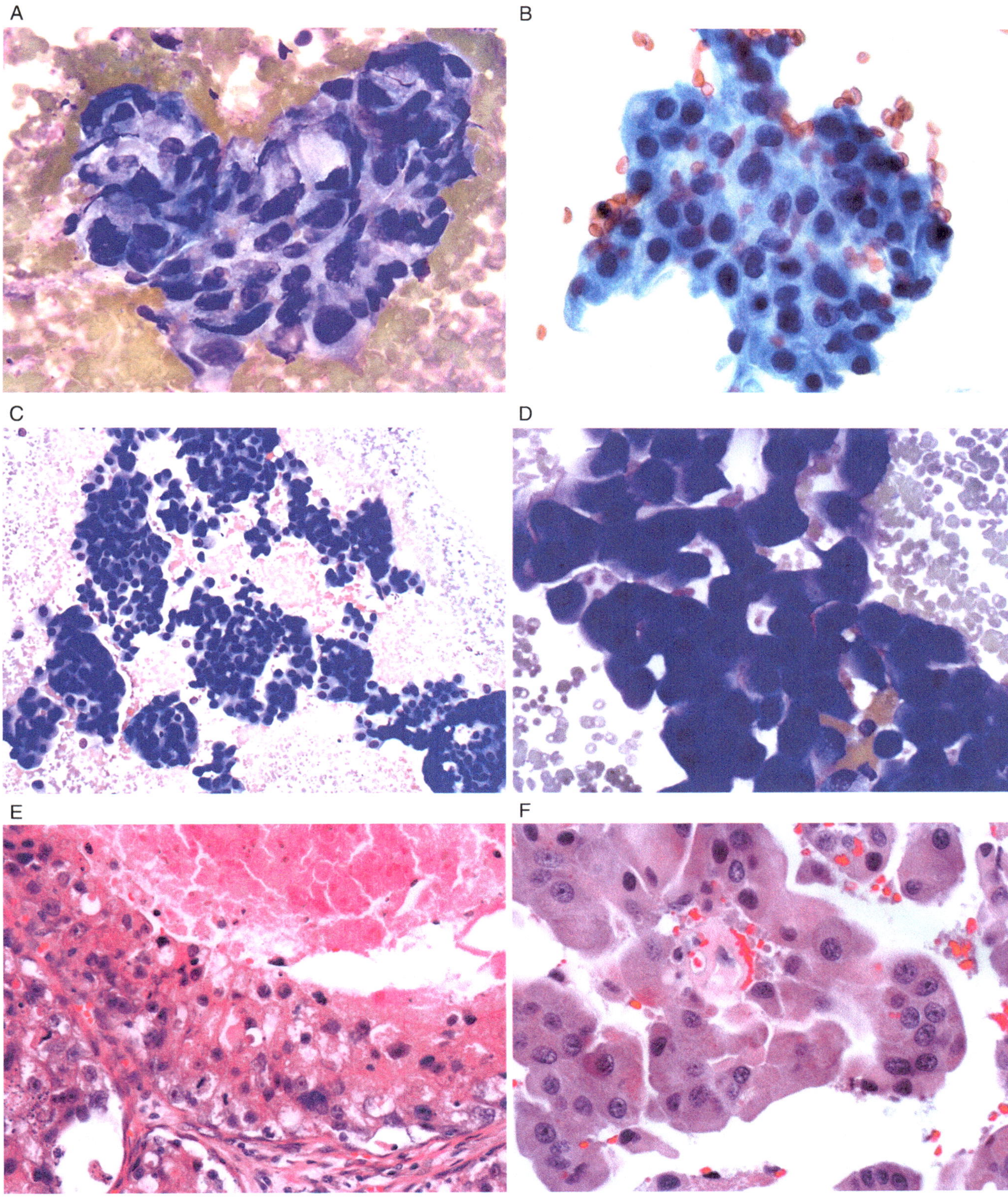

Fig. 2.24 Salivary duct carcinoma. (**a**) High-grade ductal carcinoma cells with scant necrosis in the background, Diff-Quik. (**b**) Same as A (Pap stain). (**c**, **d**) Highly atypical ductal epithelial cells, Diff-Quik. (**e**) Ductal carcinoma with comedonecrosis, H&E. (**f**) Ductal carcinoma with oncocytic features, H&E. (**g**) Nuclear staining for AR, IHC. (**h**) Positive for GCDFP-15, IHC

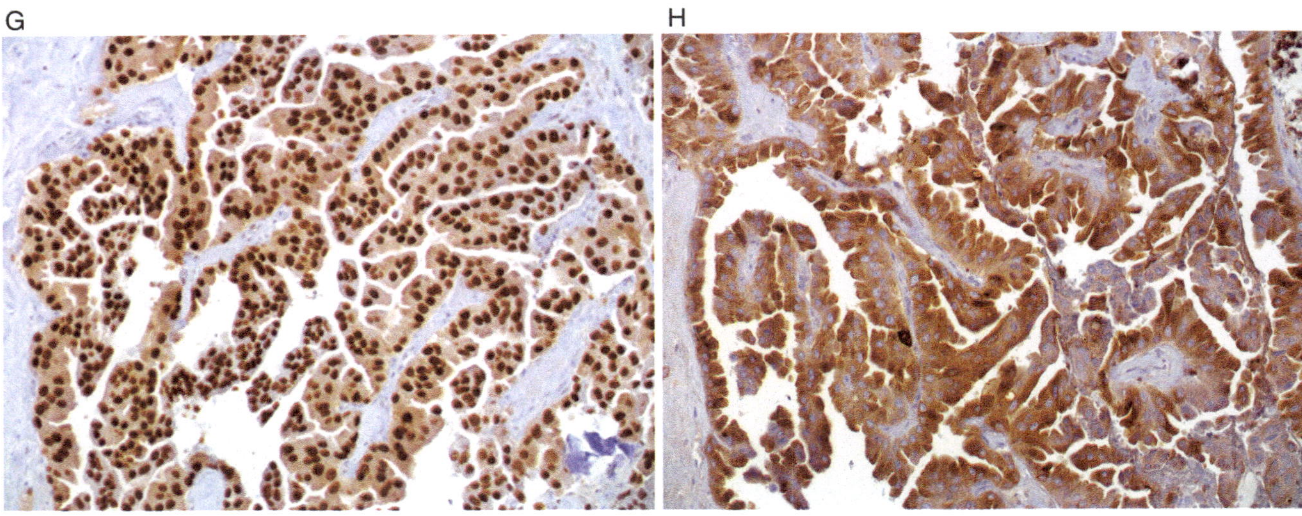

Fig. 2.24 (continued)

PLGA (Terminal Duct Carcinoma or Lobular Carcinoma)

Key Clinical Features

- The second most common intraoral malignant salivary gland tumor, accounting for 26% of all carcinomas.
- Exclusively in minor salivary glands, especially the palate (60–70%), buccal mucosa at the junction of the hard and soft palates, and upper lip.
- Peak in 5th–6th decades, but children can be affected; female predominance.
- Presents as a slow-growing, painless mass for years, with or without ulceration.

Key Radiological Features

- Similar to MEC

Cytological Features

- Uniform, small- to medium-sized cells with fine chromatin, tiny nucleoli, and moderate amounts of cytoplasm, arranged in branching papillary clusters, sheets, glands, or solid rounded groups.
- Hyaline globules are often present.
- Tyrosine crystals and a myxohyaline matrix may be present.

Differential Diagnosis

- AdCC
- PA

Histology

- Polymorphous low-grade adenocarcinoma (PLGA) is comprised of uniform, bland-looking tumor cells arranged in a variety of growth patterns, including lobular, papillary or papillary-cystic, cribriform, trabecular, and small duct-like patterns.
- Mitosis or necrosis is not typical.
- Neurotropism is common.
- Occasional foci of oncocytic, squamous, or mucous cells may be seen.
- The tumor stroma may show areas of mucinosis or hyalinization.

Immunohistochemistry:

- The tumor cells of PLGA are positive for cytokeratin, vimentin, and S100; frequently positive for CEA; occasionally positive for smooth muscle actin (SMA) and EMA.
- Negative or rarely positive for GFAP.
- Occasional cases with focal DOG1 reactivity were reported.
- Overexpression of Bcl2 is seen in the majority of cases.

- Myoepithelial markers are usually negative. GATA3 expression is not identified.

Serine/threonine-protein kinase D1 (*PRKD1*) mutations have been reported in 72.9% of PLGAs but no other salivary gland tumors, leading to overexpression of PRKD1 in PLGAs by immunoassays.

Basal Cell Adenocarcinoma

Key Clinical Features

- Rare, 2.9% of malignant salivary gland neoplasms
- 90% involve the parotid gland
- Mean age of 60 years, no sex predilection, presents as a painless swelling
- Low-grade malignancy with local destruction and a tendency for local recurrence

Key Radiological Features

- Similar to MEC

Cytological Features

The majority of cases are cytologically identical to basal cell adenoma and can only be distinguished by a histologically infiltrative growth pattern.

- A minority of cases show nuclear atypia, mitotic activity, and/or necrosis.
- Figure 2.25a, b.

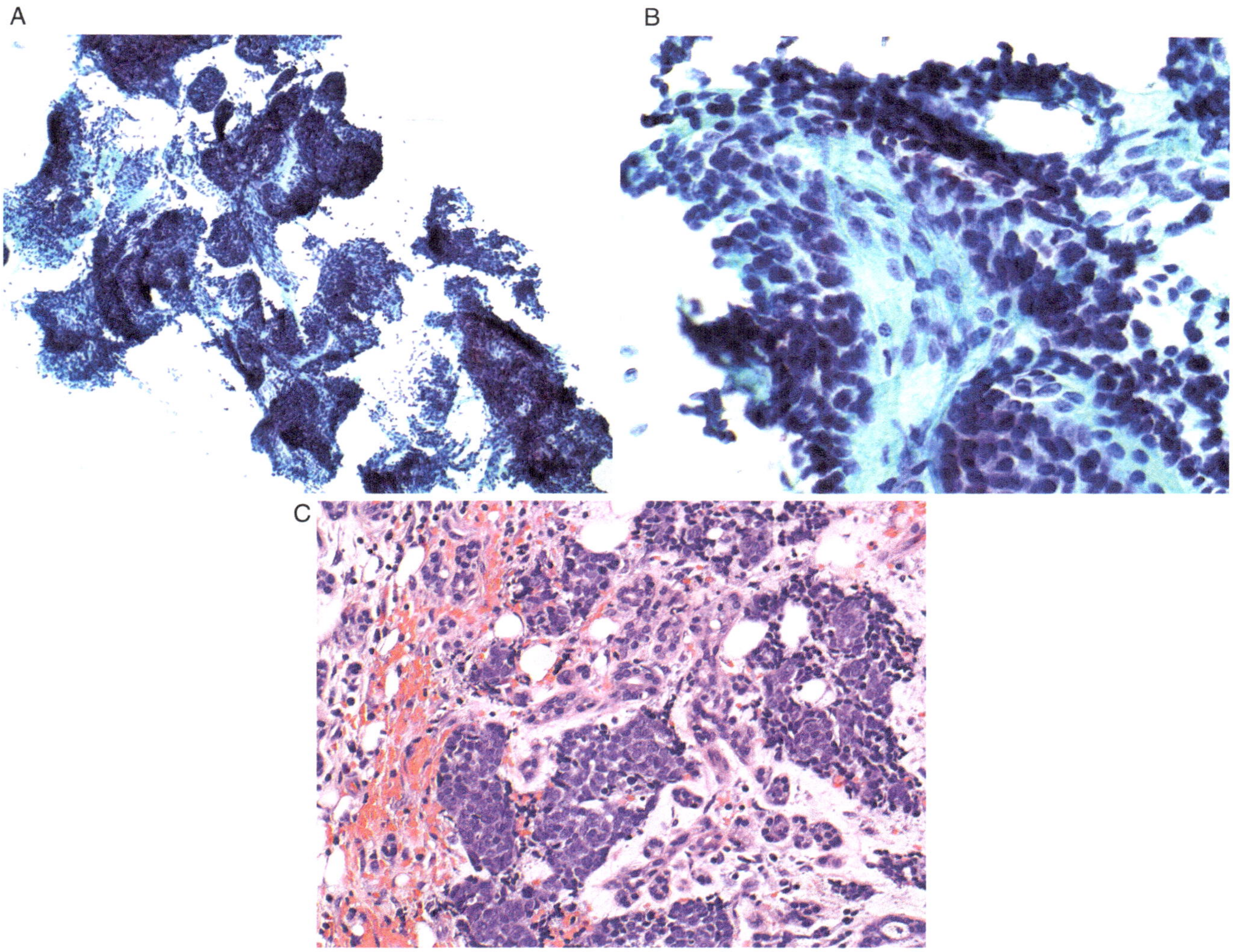

Fig. 2.25 Basal cell adenocarcinoma. (**a**, **b**) Cellular smear contains multilayered clusters, sheets, and tubular structures of small basaloid cells accompanied by arborizing stroma containing fibroblast-like spindle cells and capillaries, Pap stain. (**c**) Histology reveals atypical basaloid cells with an infiltrative growth pattern, H&E

Differential Diagnosis

- Basal cell adenoma: identical cytology
- Basaloid neoplasms (AdCC, basaloid squamous carcinoma, sebaceous carcinoma, Merkel cell carcinoma, small cell undifferentiated carcinoma)

Histology

- Basaloid epithelial cells arranged in solid, membranous, trabecular, and tubular patterns.
- The solid growth pattern is most common, featuring nests of variable-sized and variable-shaped tumor cells separated by septa or bands of collagenous stroma.
- Abundant eosinophilic, hyalinized basal lamina material forming intracellular droplets and membranes around tumor cells characterizes the membranous type.
- Peripheral tumor cell palisading is often seen.
- Rare foci of squamous differentiation may be appreciated.
- Cytological atypia and mitosis are often minimal.
- Vascular invasion and perineural invasion are evident in a quarter of cases.
- A representative image is shown in Fig. 2.25c.

Immunohistochemistry:

- Tumor cells are positive for cytokeratin and focally to S100 protein, EMA, and CEA.

Epithelial-Myoepithelial Carcinoma

Key Clinical Features

- Rare, 1% of all salivary gland neoplasms, 75% in parotid gland
- 60% in women; peak in 6th–7th decades, occasionally in children
- Presents as a painless, slow-growing mass, occasionally with pain and facial weakness
- Low-grade malignancy, with recurrence in 30–40%, as late as 28 years after initial surgery

Key Radiological Features

- Similar to MEC

Cytological Features

- Cellular specimen
- Irregular cohesive clusters of biphasic cells, including small, dark ductal cells and large clear myoepithelial cells (Fig. 2.26a, b)
- Naked nuclei and acellular hyalinized stromal material in the background

Differential Diagnosis

- AdCC
- Basal cell tumors
- Myoepithelial carcinoma
- PA
- PLGA
- Metastatic renal cell carcinoma
- Other clear cell neoplasms

Histology

- Epithelial-myoepithelial carcinomas usually exhibit a lobulated, multinodular mass with a well-circumscribed border but poorly circumscribed in minor salivary glands.
- The tumor shows a mixed tubular and solid growth pattern, with occasional papillary and cystic components.
- The presence of the bilayered duct-like structures, formed by an inner layer of eosinophilic cuboidal cells and an outer layer of myoepithelial cells with clear cytoplasm, is characteristic of this tumor.
- Rarely, the inner layer of cells may appear squamoid, spindled, or oncocytic.
- Mitoses are few; necrosis is uncommon.
- Perineural and vascular invasions are frequent.
- Representative images are illustrated in Fig. 2.26c, d.

Immunohistochemistry:

- The luminal epithelial cells are positive for cytokeratin (including CK7) EMA, and DOG1, variably for S100, and negative for myoepithelial cell markers.
- The myoepithelial cells are positive for pan-cytokeratin (often weak) and myoepithelial markers, such as p63, S100, SMA, and calponin.
- GFAP is negative.
- SOX10 expression is identified in 100% of cases, decorating both epithelial and myoepithelial tumor cells.

Primary Small Cell Carcinoma

Key Clinical Features

- Rare, 1–2% of all major and minor salivary gland malignancies, >80% of major gland cases involving the parotid gland

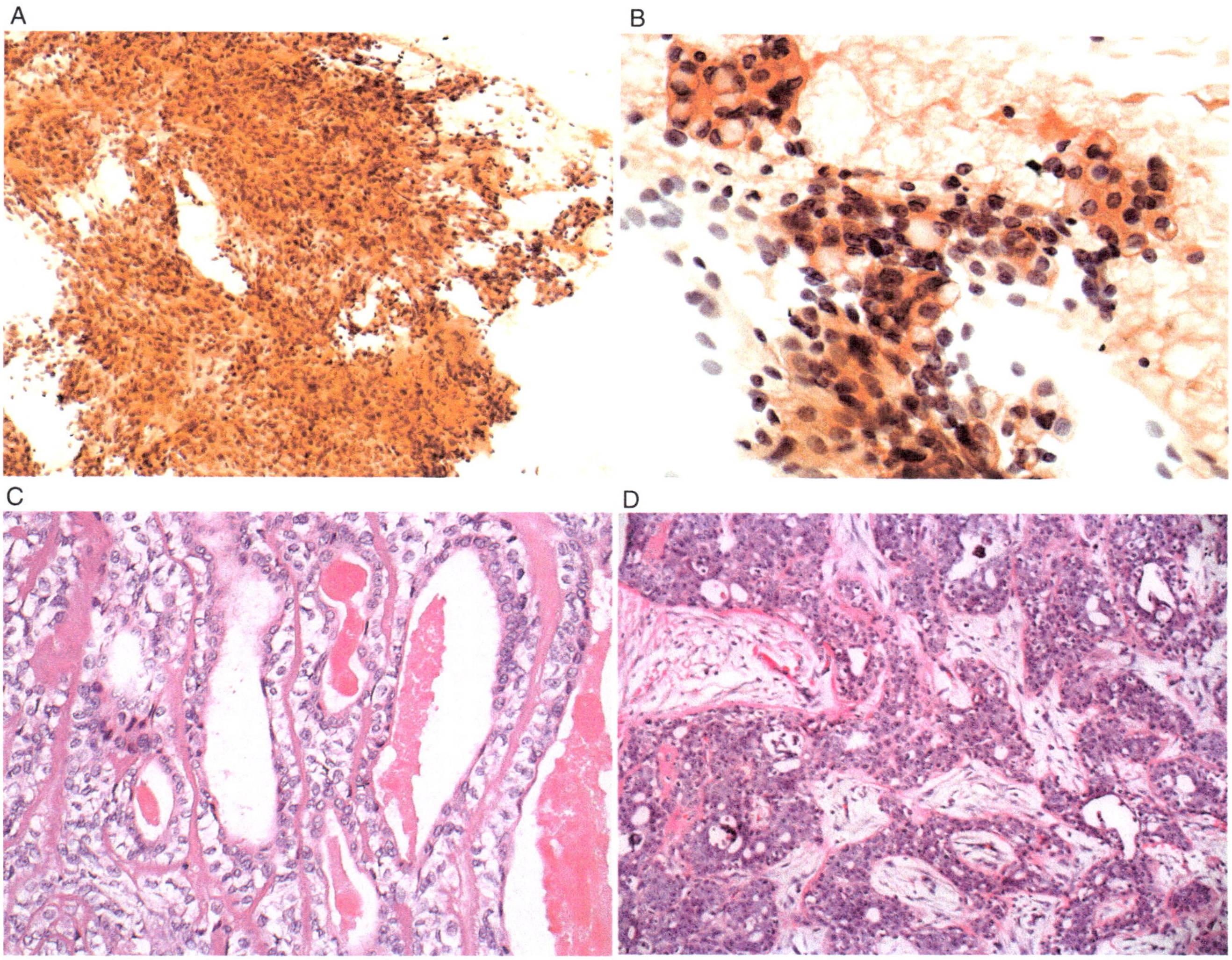

Fig. 2.26 Epithelial-myoepithelial carcinoma. (**a**) Cluster of cytologically bland myoepithelial cells and focal cuboidal ductal cells with hyalinized stromal material, Pap stain. (**b**) Mixed ductal cells, myoepithelial cells, and stromal cells, Pap stain. (**c**, **d**) Bilayered ductal structures with inner cuboidal ductal cells and peripheral myoepithelial cells are demonstrated, H&E

- Male predominant, in 5th–7th decades
- Presents as a rapidly growing, painless mass with <3 months' duration
- High-grade tumor with poor prognosis

Key Radiological Features

- Similar to high-grade MEC

Cytological Features

- Cellular specimen.
- Discohesive small cells with round-to-oval, hyperchromatic nuclei, indistinct nucleoli, high nuclear-to-cytoplasmic ratio, and nuclear molding.
- Frequent mitosis and background necrosis present.

Differential Diagnosis

- Lymphoma
- AdCC, solid variant
- Basaloid squamous cell carcinoma
- Metastatic small cell carcinoma of lung
- Merkel cell carcinoma: CK20 positive (as are primary small cell carcinomas of the salivary gland)

Histology

- Small cell carcinoma of the salivary gland is usually a poorly circumscribed tumor with an infiltrative border.

- The tumor is comprised of sheets, cords, and irregular nests of undifferentiated tumor cells with extensive necrosis, numerous mitoses, and frequent vascular as well as perineural invasions.
- The tumor cells exhibit hyperchromatic nuclei with a finely granular chromatin pattern, inconspicuous nucleoli, and scant cytoplasm with an ill-defined cell border. Nuclear molding is often seen.

Immunohistochemistry

- The tumor cells express at least one neuroendocrine marker (chromogranin A, synaptophysin, or CD56).
- Cytokeratins (including CK20) are often expressed in the majority of tumors, with a perinuclear dotlike staining pattern.
- EMA is positive in the majority.
- S100 and human melanoma black 45 (HMB45) are nonreactive.

Lymphoepithelial Carcinoma (Malignant Lymphoepithelial Lesion)

Key Clinical Features

- Rare tumor in the USA, <0.5% of all salivary gland neoplasms, 70–94% in the parotid gland
- Most common among Greenlanders, North American Inuit, and Southern Chinese
- Usually adults, with a median age of 44.5 years
- Presents as an indurated mass with or without pain; regional lymph node metastasis in 40% of patients at presentation
- Strong association with Epstein-Barr virus (EBV)

Key Radiological Features

- Similar to MEC

Cytological Features

- Syncytial sheets of large- to spindle-shaped cells with pleomorphic vesicular nuclei, large nucleoli, and frequent mitosis.
- Lymphocytes and plasma cells present in the background.

Differential Diagnosis

- Other undifferentiated carcinomas, especially metastatic nasopharyngeal carcinoma

Histology

- Lymphoepithelial carcinomas are characterized by irregular sheets, cords, or nests of epithelial tumor cells with vesicular nuclei, prominent nucleoli, and lightly eosinophilic cytoplasm without defined cell borders in a background of heavy lymphoplasmacytic infiltration, often accompanied by reactive lymphoid follicles.
- Occasional cystic formation, noncaseating granulomas, and amyloid deposits may be seen.

Immunohistochemistry

- The tumor cells are positive for pan-cytokeratin and EMA.
- The lymphocytes are reactive in nature, with a mixture of T- and B-cell labeling.
- EBV-encoded RNA (EBER) by FISH can be detected in tumor cells in endemic cases; immunostain for EBV latent membrane protein 1 (EBV LMP1) is variable.

Other Malignancies

Squamous Cell Carcinoma

Key Clinical Features

- Primary salivary gland squamous cell carcinoma is very rare; metastases are far more common than primary.
- Mainly in elderly men, with a mean age of 64 years, 2/3 in the parotid, the rest in submandibular gland.
- Often present as a cystic mass, usually with regional lymphadenopathy.

Key Radiological Features

- Similar to high-grade MEC

Cytological Features

- Highly atypical squamous epithelial cells with nuclear enlargement, nuclear membrane irregularity, prominent nucleoli, and pleomorphism
- Atypical keratinizing cells in background of necrosis and keratin debris
- Figure 2.27a–f

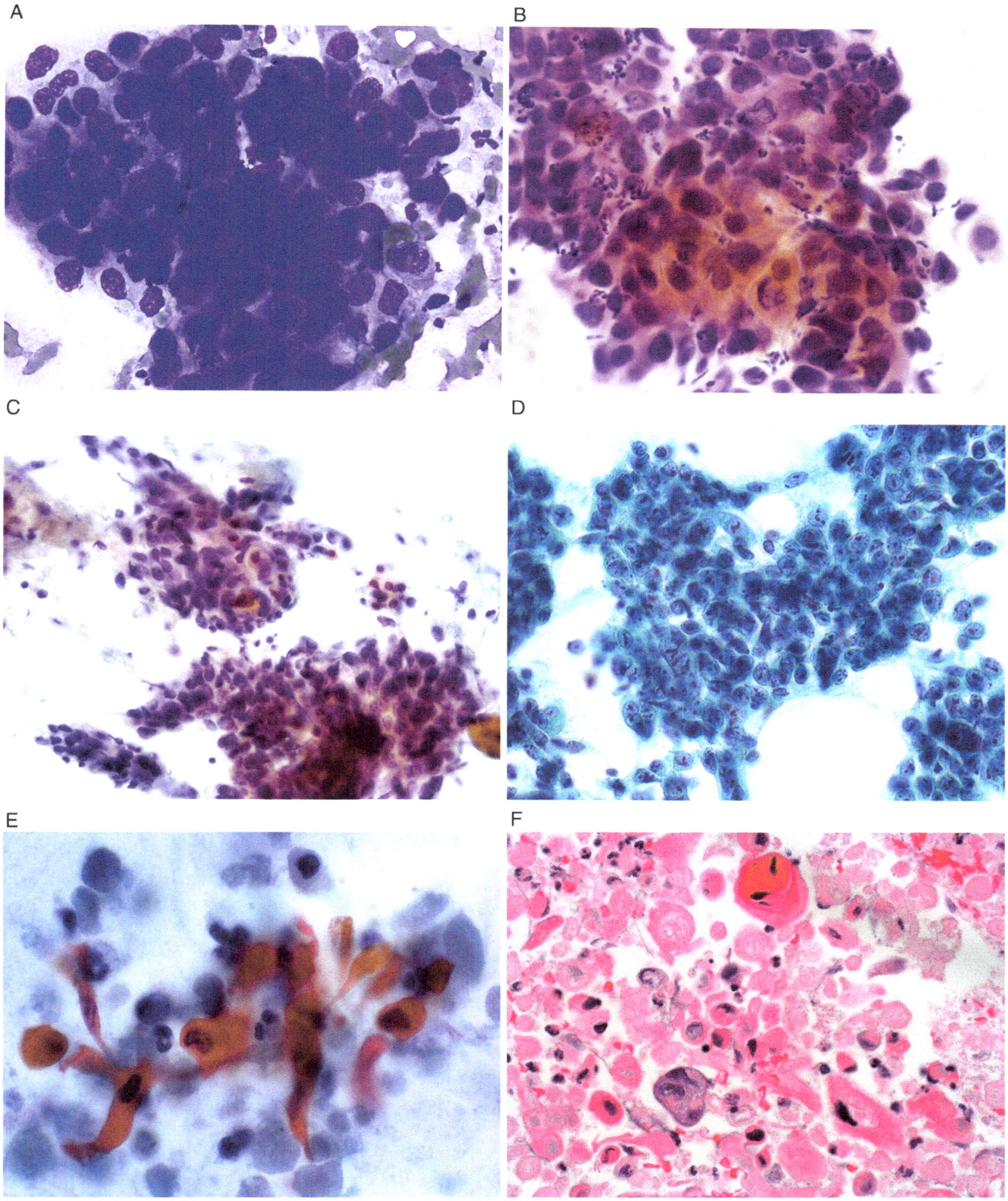

Fig. 2.27 Squamous cell carcinoma, cystic variant, of submandibular gland. (**a**) Atypical squamous epithelial cells in cluster with scant keratin debris and few neutrophils, Diff-Quik. (**b–d**) Highly atypical keratinized squamous cells, neutrophils, and necrotic debris, Pap stain. (**e**) Highly atypical keratinized squamous cells in cystic necrotic background, Pap stain. (**f**) Cell block preparation shows scattered atypical squamous cells, keratin pearls, and debris, H&E

Differential Diagnosis

- High-grade salivary gland carcinomas, such as high-grade MEC and salivary duct carcinoma

Histology

- Squamous cell carcinomas of salivary gland origin are histologically similar to those of tumors arising from elsewhere.
- The tumor is usually infiltrative in the form of irregular nests or trabeculae of tumor cells into the salivary gland parenchyma in a desmoplastic, fibrous stroma.
- Perineural invasion is often seen.

Immunohistochemistry:

- Squamous cell carcinomas of salivary gland origin show the same immunophenotype as tumors arising from anywhere else, such as positivity for HMWCK, p63, p40, and pan-cytokeratin.
- No intracytoplasmic mucin can be identified by special stain.
- SOX10 is nonreactive in poorly differentiated squamous cell carcinomas, which may aid in the differential diagnosis in the setting of a basaloid tumor of the salivary gland.

Lymphoma Involving Salivary Gland

Key Clinical Features

- 2–5% of salivary gland neoplasms, often in the parotid (50–93%) and submandibular glands.
- Primary or secondary; however, difficult to make a distinction between the two.
- MALT lymphoma (extranodal marginal zone lymphoma of mucosa-associated lymphoid tissue type) is the most common primary salivary gland lymphoma, followed by diffuse large B-cell lymphoma and follicular lymphoma; rarely, Hodgkin lymphoma.
- MALT lymphoma: female predominant (female-to-male ratio 9:1), in the 55–65-year age range; typically develop in a background of LESA or Sjogren's syndrome.

Key Radiological Features

- Similar to high-grade MEC

Cytological Features

- EMZBCL of the MALT type:
  - Small- to intermediate-size lymphocytes
  - Round to slightly irregular nuclei
  - Occasional immunoblasts
  - CD45 +, CD20 +, CD5 -, CD10 -, CD23 -, cyclin D1 -
  - Figure 2.28a, b
- Follicular lymphoma:
  - Mixed population of small, large cleaved, and large non-cleaved cells
  - CD45 +, CD20 +, CD10 +, CD5 -
- Diffuse large B-cell lymphoma:
  - Large markedly atypical lymphocytes
  - CD45 +, CD20 +, keratin -, S100 -

Differential Diagnosis

- IHC and flow cytometry studies are necessary.

Histology

- EMZBCL of the MALT type of the parotid gland is vaguely nodular, comprised of an infiltrative, heterogeneous population of atypical small lymphocytes, centrocyte-like (cleaved) lymphocytes, monocytoid B-cells, immunoblasts, lymphoplasmacytic cells, and plasma cells in a background of LESA.
- The normal salivary gland structures are often effaced with neoplastic B-cells infiltrating the glandular epithelium.
- Intranuclear inclusions (Dutcher bodies) may be seen.
- The formation of "halos," epimyoepithelial islands surrounded by monocytoid and centrocyte-like B-cells, is an early change of EMZBCL in the setting of LESA.
- Large cell transformation may be seen.

Immunohistochemistry:

- EMZBCLs are decorated by B-cell markers (CD20, PAX5, CD79a) and marginal zone cell-associated antigens (CD21, CD35).
- May be +/– for CD43 and CD11c (weak).
- The tumor cells are negative for CD5, CD10, and CD23.
- Typically, the tumor cells express immunoglobulin M (IgM), showing light chain restriction.
- Representative images are shown in Fig. 2.28c, d.

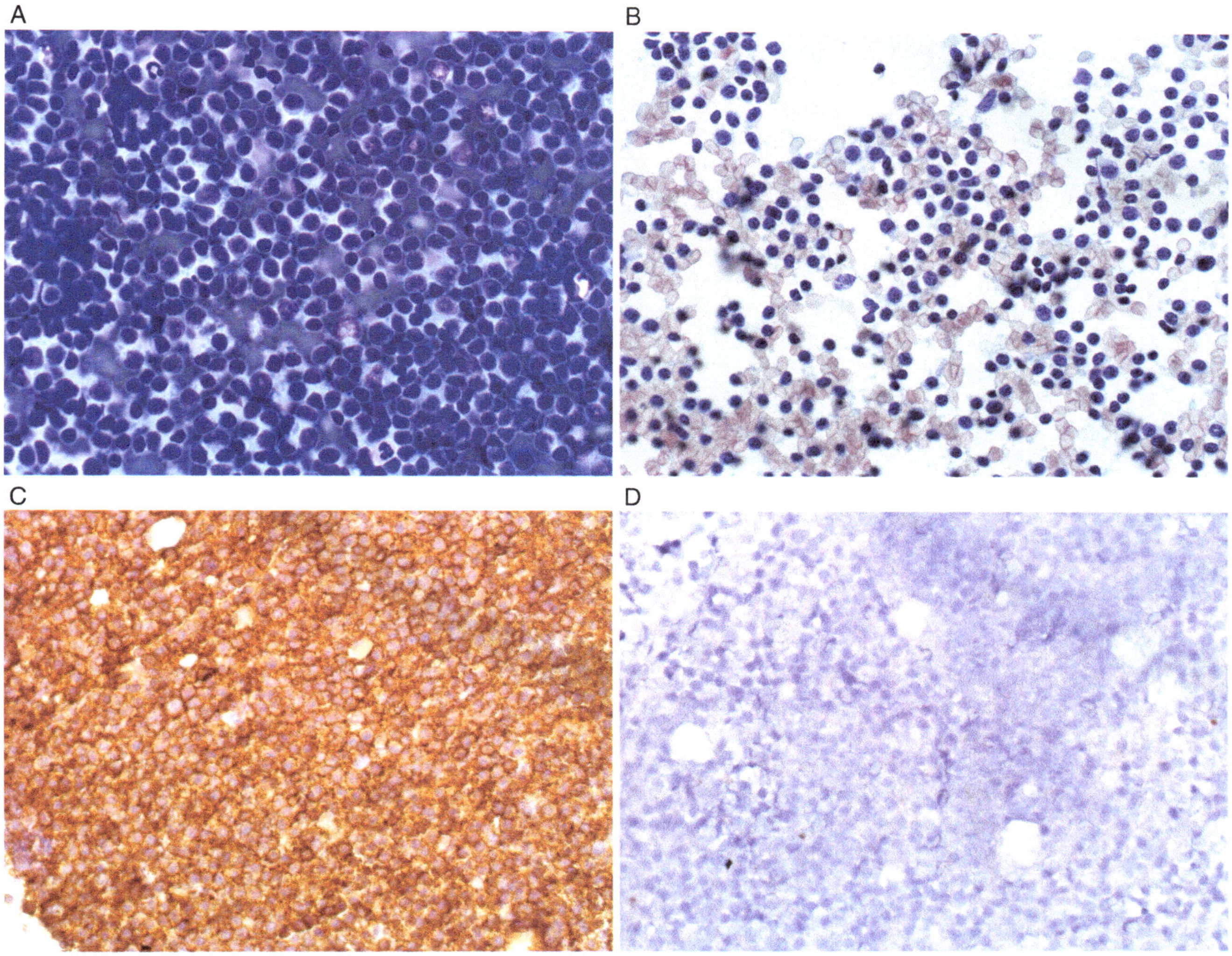

Fig. 2.28 Extranodal marginal zone B-cell lymphoma. (**a**, **b**) Monotonous population of small- to intermediate-sized atypical lymphocytes with round to slightly irregular nuclei and discernible to prominent nucleolus, Diff-Quik and Pap stain. (**c**) Positive CD20 stain, IHC. (**d**) Negative CD10, IHC

Case Presentations

Salivary gland mass-like lesions are the subjects of extremely diverse and heterogenic conditions. The histomorphology of salivary gland neoplasms is complex and overlapping. FNA of salivary gland masses/tumors represents one of the most challenging areas of cytopathology. Nevertheless, salivary gland FNA is a common practice and plays an important role in the preoperative planning of patient's management. Therefore, an algorithmic or systemic approach for the interpretation of salivary gland FNA is deemed necessary. In addition, ancillary studies, such as IHC and molecular profiling, especially with the addition of recently discovered novel biomarkers, have increased the diagnostic accuracy significantly for several specific tumor entities.

The following are goals that one should try to achieve when working on salivary gland FNAs: (1) to identify benign nonneoplastic processes, (2) to differentiate benign from malignant neoplasms, (3) to differentiate low-grade from high-grade neoplasms, (4) to differentiate primary from metastatic tumors, (5) to identify non-epithelial neoplasms, such as lymphoid disorders, spindle cell neoplasms, or melanoma.

Besides benign mixed tumors, the following working categories are proposed based on cytomorphology: (1) tumors with basaloid morphology, (2) oncocytic lesions, (3) neoplasms with a cystic background with

(continued)

or without lymphocytes, (4) high-grade carcinomas, (5) neoplasms with clear cell morphology, and (6) spindle cell lesions.

The following case scenarios are intended to illustrate the categorized approach for cytology FNA diagnosis of both common and newly described salivary gland tumors.

Case Scenario 1: Basaloid Neoplasm

Learning Objectives

1. To describe the differential cytological features of each entity of basaloid neoplasms
2. To be aware of the solid variant of AdCC
3. To be familiar with the potential utility of immunohistochemical markers in the differential diagnosis of basaloid neoplasms

Case

A 75-year-old woman presented with an enlarging right parotid mass for 3 months and pain in the recent month. Physical examination revealed a tender 3 cm mass in the right angle of jaw. FNA was performed. The smears were cellular, composed of single and clusters of small basaloid epithelial cells with hyperchromatic and angulated nuclei without discernible nucleolus in a clean background without significant matrix material, as illustrated in Fig. 2.29a, b. No peripheral palisading was appreciated in any of the clusters. Rare clusters of tumor cells showed a cribriform or tubular patterns with eosinophilic globules, as shown in Fig. 2.29c, d.

The cytological features suggest a neoplasm with basaloid morphology. The major differential considerations include a basal cell adenoma/ADC, an AdCC with significant solid pattern, and basaloid squamous cell carcinoma. Immunoassays were performed, revealing the tumor cells to be positive for p63, SOX10, and CD117 and some cells to be positive for CK7 and EMA. The solid areas showed diffuse, cytoplasmic, and membranous reactivity to CD117, while only luminal cells in cribriform or tubular components were decorated by CD117. The proliferative index (MIB-1) was estimated at 15%. Representative images are shown in Fig. 2.29e–h.

The immunoprofile suggests the biphasic differentiation of this tumor, including luminal and abluminal differentiations. Basaloid squamous cell carcinomas are tumors with one population of cell differentiation—that is, the basaloid squamous cell lineage—expressing HMWCK, p63, and p40. Histologically, basaloid squamous cell carcinomas are usually high-grade tumors comprised of larger, hyperchromatic nuclei with a coarse chromatin pattern and high rate of mitosis or apoptosis. The findings of uniform, small, angulated basaloid cells, diffuse CK7 and SOX10 positivity, relatively lower proliferative index, and parotid gland location of this tumor make a basaloid squamous cell carcinoma less likely. Basal cell adenomas or ADCs are tumors with biphasic differentiation, showing similar morphology. Distinguishing between the two is challenging at times. Invasion (local, perineural, or angiolymphatic) is the most commonly used criterion; however, this is impractical in cytology or small biopsy specimens. Biomarkers such as Ki-67, p53, and Bcl2 may play a role in this setting. In general, adenomas show a lower proliferative index than ADCs, usually <2–5%. The cyto- and histomorphological features of nested tumor cells with peripheral palisading and central cells with a larger vesicular chromatin pattern and paler cytoplasm in basal cell adenomas/ADCs, and hyperchromatic, uniform small, angulated tumor nuclei in AdCCs can be helpful in the differential diagnosis of those tumors. The AdCCs show a higher proliferative index than basal cell adenomas. Studies reported that a proliferative index (MIB-1) of 10% could be used to separate benign basal cell adenomas from malignant tumors, such as AdCCs. For the current case, a 15% mitotic index is in favor of a low-grade malignant tumor, such as an AdCC or basal cell ADC.

Overall, the findings in this case are those of a salivary gland neoplasm with basaloid morphology, in favor of an AdCC with predominant solid growth pattern or a basal cell ADC, although the former is favored due to the presence of a focal cribriform pattern with some basement membrane globules, hyperchromatic, angulated tumor nuclei, and the absence of peripheral palisading.

The differential diagnostic features of basaloid tumors of salivary gland are summarized in Table 2.6.

AdCCs are a group of tumors composed of both luminal and myoepithelial cells. The expression of c-kit, a transmembrane receptor tyrosine kinase, was reported in several normal cell types (mast cells, interstitial cells of Cajal, melanocytes, and epithelial cells of the breast); alteration in c-kit expression was seen in tumors such as mastocytosis, gastrointestinal stromal

(continued)

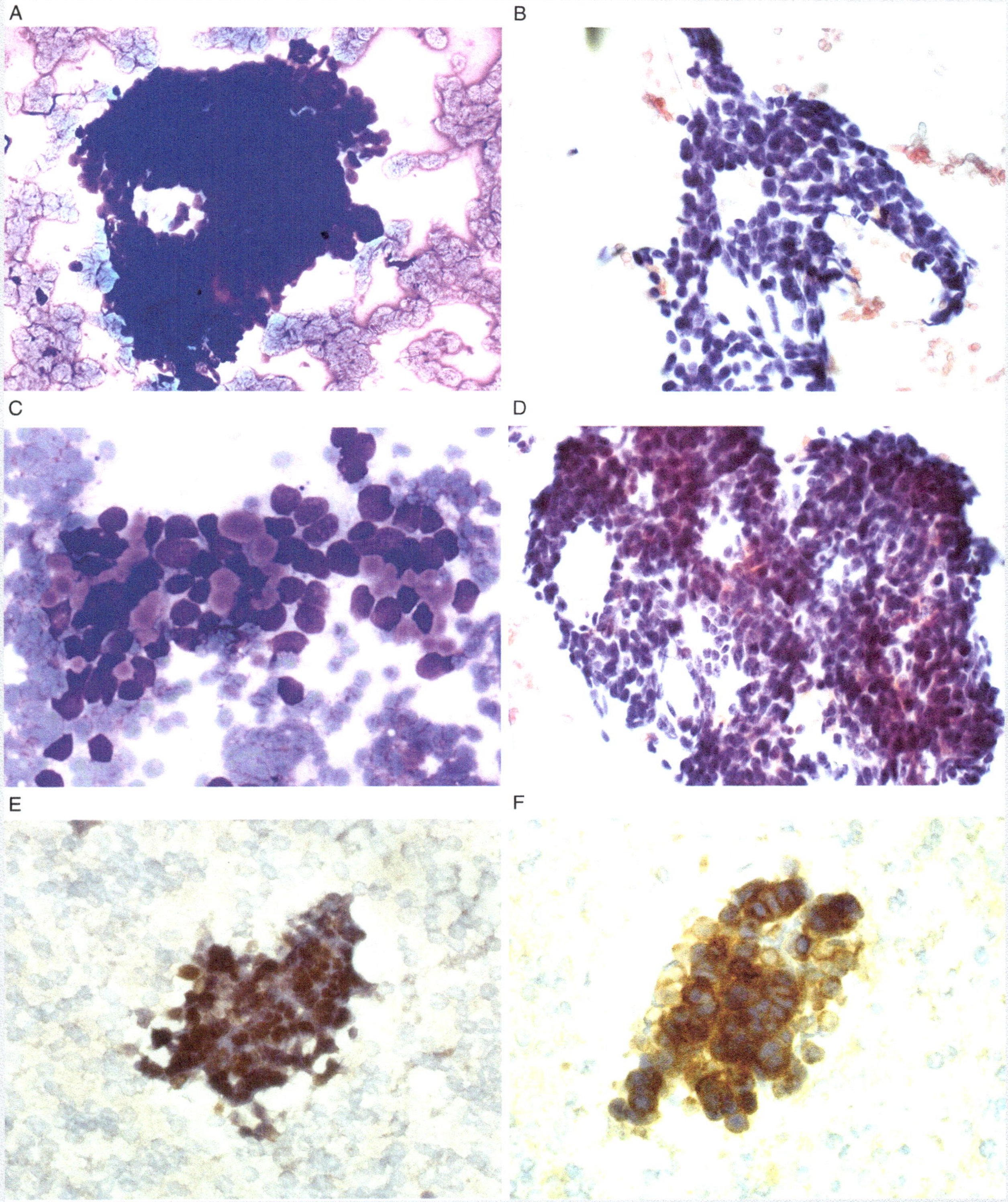

Fig. 2.29 Basaloid neoplasm, case scenario 1. (**a**) Cluster of small basaloid cells with hyperchromatic nuclei, some angulated, focal eosinophilic globule noted, Diff-Quik. (**b**) Same as A, basaloid cells with focal empty spaces, Pap stain. (**c**) Cribriform pattern with eosinophilic globules, Diff-Quik. (**d**) Same as C (Pap stain). (**e**) Positive SOX10 in some cells, IHC. (**f**) Positive for CD117, IHC. (**g**) Positive for CK7, IHC. (**h**) Focally positive for CK5/CK6, IHC

(continued)

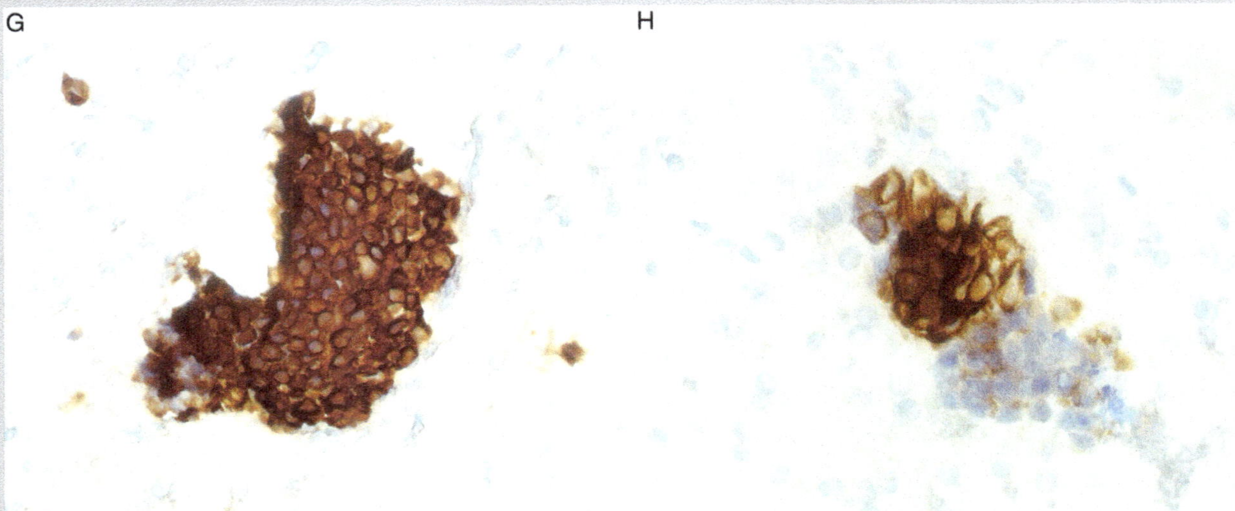

Fig. 2.29 (continued)

Table 2.6 Differential diagnosis of Basaloid tumors of salivary gland

	AdCC	BCA/BCAC	BSqCC
Cell population	Luminal and abluminal cells	Luminal and abluminal cells	Basaloid squamous cells only
Cyto-, histomorphology	Cribriform pattern with basement membrane globules; small uniform, hyperchromatic, angulated tumor nuclei	Nested tumor cells with peripheral palisading; the nuclei are oval or round with vesicular chromatin pattern and paler cytoplasm in the center of tumor nests	Nests of basaloid cells containing larger, hyperchromatic nuclei with coarse chromatin pattern and high rate of mitoses or apoptosis
CK AE1/AE3	+	+	+
Luminal cell markers (EMA, CEA, CK7, CD117, pVHL)	+	+	EMA+, CEA+; CK7−, CD117−, pVHL−
Abluminal cell Markers and others	SMA+, p63+, calponin+, SOX10+, CK14+	SMA+, p63+, calponin+, SOX10+, CK14+	HMWCK+, p63+, p40+, SOX10−
Proliferative index (MIB-1)	>10%	<3–5%/>10%	High-grade, >>10%
β-catenin	−	+ (nuclear stain)	N/A
S100P	+	−	−

AdCC adenoid cystic carcinoma, *BCA/BCAC* basal cell adenoma/basal cell ADC, *BSqCC* basaloid squamous cell carcinoma, *CK* cytokeratin, *EMA* epithelial membrane antigen, *CEA* carcinoembryonic antigen, *CD117* cluster of differentiation 117, *pVHL* von Hippel-Lindau tumor suppressor, *S100P* placental S100, *SMA* smooth muscle actin, *SOX10* sex determining region Y box 10, *HMWCK* high molecular weight cytokeratin, *N/A* not available

cell tumors, and germ cell tumors; in addition, salivary gland AdCCs were reported to express c-kit; however, the claimed diagnostic value of positive c-kit in AdCC of the salivary gland has not been substantiated. c-kit expression has been reported in salivary gland tumors with luminal cell differentiation, including basal cell adenomas/ADCs and PLGAs.

Case Scenario 2: Oncocytic Lesions

Learning Objectives

1. To describe the differential cytological features of each entity of oncocytic lesions
2. To be aware of the lymphocyte-rich variant of AciCC

(continued)

3. To be familiar with the potential utility of immunohistochemical markers in the differential diagnosis of oncocytic lesions

Case

A 67-year-old woman presented with an enlarging, painless angle of jaw mass for a couple of years. Physical examination revealed a non-tender 2.5 cm mass in the right parotid gland region. FNA was performed. The smears were highly cellular, composed of single and clusters of oncocytic cells with abundant vasculature in a background of rich lymphocytes, illustrated in Fig. 2.30a, b. The oncocytic cells were relatively uniform in appearance, with round nuclei, prominent nucleoli, and abundant eosinophilic, slightly granular cytoplasm without defined cell borders. The background was overall clean, with granular debris focally in the cellular areas. Naked nuclei with similar cytomorphology were noted, as shown in Fig. 2.30c, d.

The cytological features suggest an oncocytic lesion with abundant lymphocytes. The major differential diagnoses include an acinic carcinoma of the lymphocyte-rich variant and a Warthin's tumor. A limited panel of immunoassays and special stains were performed, as illustrated in Fig. 2.30e–h.

The tumor cells were positive for CAM5.2, DOG1, and SOX10 while negative for pVHL, CK7, and myoepithelial or basal cell markers; special stain for periodic acid-Schiff with diastase (PAS-D) revealed coarse eosinophilic cytoplasmic zymogen granules. The findings are consistent with an AciCC. The follow-up surgical resection confirmed the diagnosis, as illustrated in Fig. 2.30i.

The cytomorphology of AciCC and Warthin's tumor belongs to the group of oncocytic lesions. Both tumors may present with abundant lymphocytes. The tumor cells are oncocytic in appearance, that is, polygonal cells with slightly eccentrically located nuclei, prominent nucleoli, and abundant eosinophilic cytoplasm. However, the tumor cells of AciCCs show round nuclei with more prominent nucleoli and coarsely granular cytoplasm without defined cell borders. There are usually naked nuclei with identical features in a clean or focally granular background. On the other hand, the tumor cells of Warthin's tumors show slightly dense, eosinophilic cytoplasm with defined cell borders. No naked nuclei are seen. The background is usually dirty, with macrophages, scattered metaplastic squamous cells, and granular cystic debris. The differential immunophenotypes are summarized in Table 2.7.

The gene *anoctamin-1 (ANO-1),* also known as *discovered on GIST-1 or DOG1*, is a calcium-activated chloride channel that was initially noted by gene expression profiling specifically expressed in gastrointestinal stromal tumors (GISTs). Immunohistochemical expression of DOG1 was validated in GISTs and in squamous cell carcinomas of esophagus and head/neck. In normal salivary gland tissue, DOG1 is a marker for acinar cells and intercalated ductal luminal cells. The expression of DOG1 in salivary gland neoplasms was reported in 100% of AciCCs, 75% of AdCCs, and 47% of epithelial-myoepithelial carcinomas, with focal to very focal expression in 37% of MECs, 33% of MASCs, and 31% of PLGA, while negative in Warthin's tumor, oncocytomas, oncocytic carcinomas, and salivary ductal carcinomas. Although DOG1 expression is not specific for AciCC, its diffuse and intense staining pattern for DOG1 in conjunction with cyto-, histomorphology, as well as PAS-D-positive zymogen granules is a helpful feature to distinguish AciCC from its mimics.

Case Scenario 3: Neoplasm with Ample Eosinophilic Vacuolated Cytoplasm

Learning Objectives

1. To describe the cytological features of this entity
2. To be aware of the common differential diagnosis of this tumor
3. To be familiar with the potential utility of immunohistochemical markers in the diagnosis of this tumor

Case

A 45-year-old woman presented with a slow-growing, painless angle of jaw nodule for a couple of years. Physical examination revealed a non-tender 2.5 cm mass in the right parotid gland region. FNA was performed. The smears were highly cellular, composed of loosely cohesive clusters, "papillary" fragments, and single monotonous epithelioid cells with centrally to slightly eccentrically located, round-to-oval vesicular nuclei, discernible to prominent nucleoli, and abundant eosinophilic, vacuolated, or bubbly cytoplasm. Many tumor cells were large, round to polygonal, with well-defined cell borders; large naked nuclei with macronucleoli are not appreciated. Abundant delicate vasculatures and fine granular or cystic debris are noted in the background. No lymphocytes, mucinous material, or stromal fragments were seen. Representative images are illustrated in Fig. 2.31a–d.

(continued)

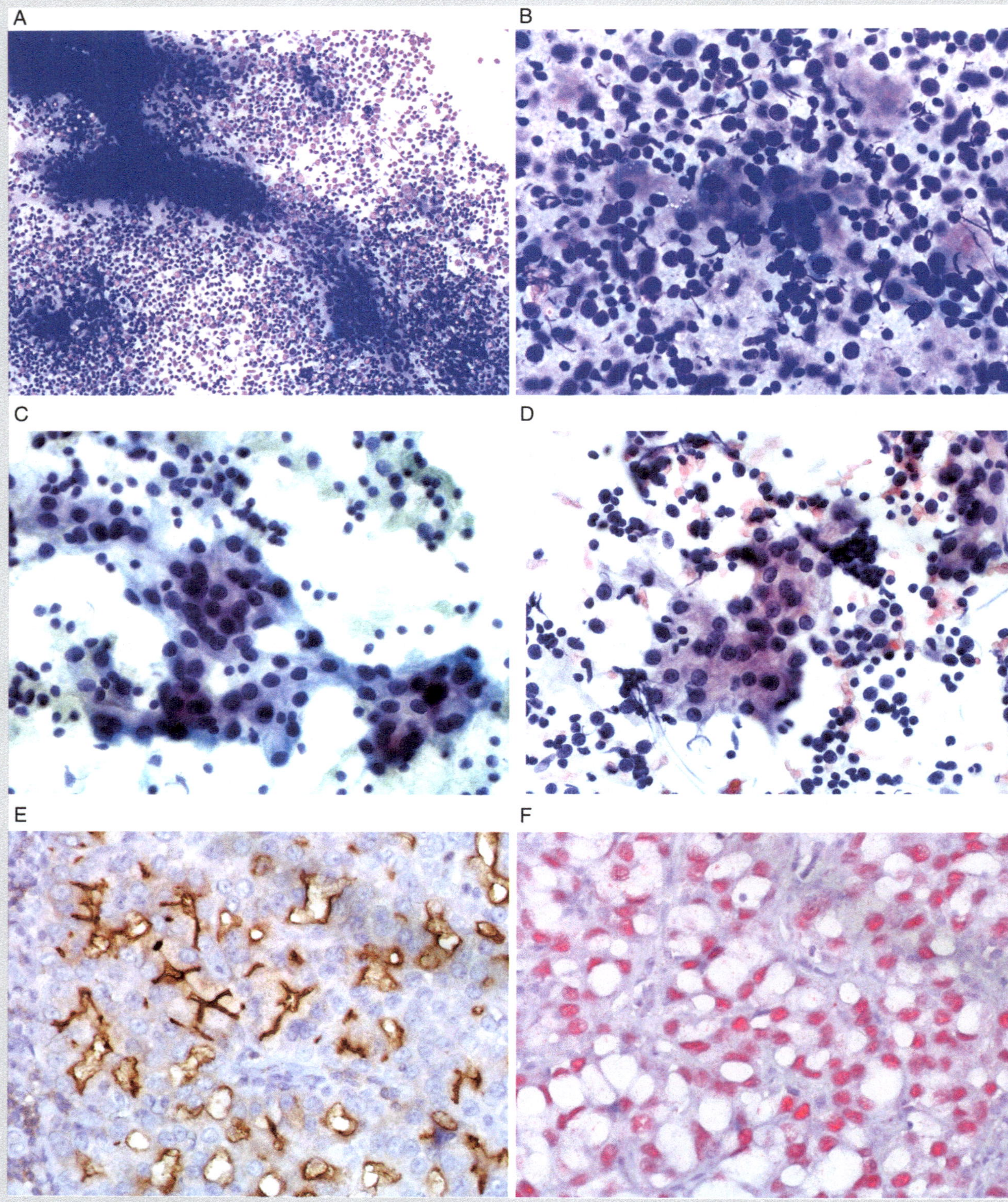

Fig. 2.30 Acinic cell carcinoma, case scenario 2. (**a**) Highly cellular smear composed of abundant lymphoid cells and clusters of oncocytic epithelial cells, Diff-Quik. (**b, c, d**) High-power view showing tumor cells with round nuclei, prominent nucleoli, and abundant granular cytoplasm; in addition, noted many naked nuclei with same cytological features, granular debris, and lymphocytes in background, (**b**) Diff-Quik. (**c, d**) Pap stain. (**e**) Positive for DOG1, showing an apical luminal membranous staining pattern, IHC. (**f**) Nuclear decoration by SOX10, IHC. (**g**) Negative pVHL, IHC. (**h**) PAS-D reveals cytoplasmic granules. (**i**) Follow-up surgical resection, H&E

(continued)

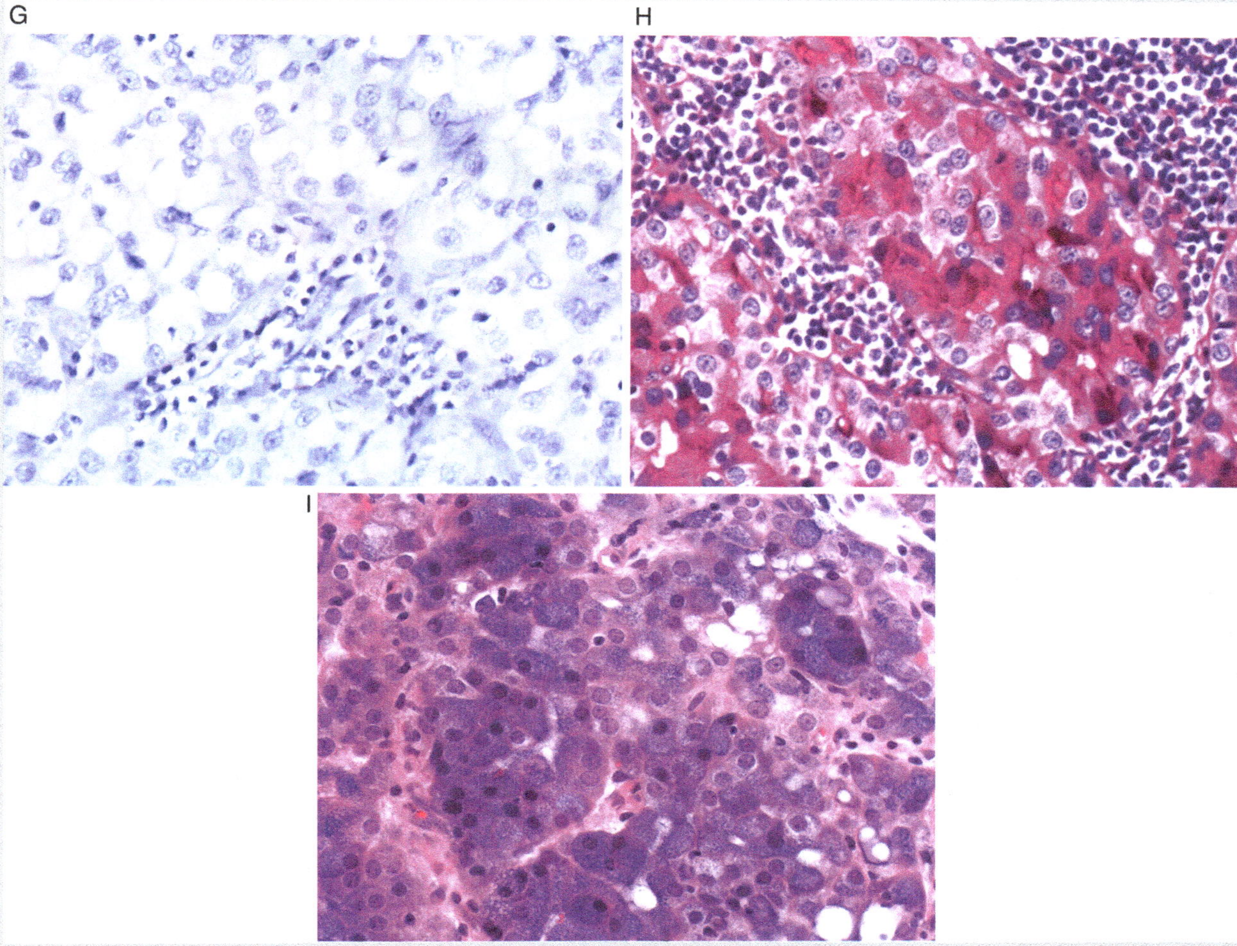

Fig. 2.30 (continued)

Table 2.7 Immunophenotype of AciCC and Warthin's tumor

Biomarkers	AciCC	Warthin's tumor
DOG1	+	−
SOX10	+	−
CEA, EMA	−	+
CK7, pVHL	−	+
PAS-D[a]	+	−
GATA3	−	+

AciCC acinic cell carcinoma, *DOG1* SOX10: pVHL: *DOG1* discovered on GIST 1, *CEA* carcinoembryonic antigen, *EMA* epithelial membrane antigen, *Ck7* cytokeratin 7, *pVHL* von Hippel-Lindau tumor suppressor, *PAS-D* periodic acid-Schiff diastase, *GATA3* GATA-binding protein 3

[a]PAS-D highlights the densely eosinophilic zymogen granules in the cytoplasm of acinic cells

The cytological features raise the differential diagnosis of MASC, AciCC, or MEC. A limited panel of immunoassays and special stains was performed, as illustrated in Fig. 2.31e–h.

The tumor cells showed strong positivity to S100 protein, vimentin, and CK AE1/AE3 and focal weak positivity to GATA3, mammaglobin, and GCDFP-15 and were negative for p63, CD68, ER, pVHL, and CK7. Special stain for PAS-D revealed no coarse eosinophilic cytoplasmic granules. The overall findings suggested a MASC. The follow-up surgical resection confirmed the diagnosis, as illustrated in Fig. 2.31i–l. FISH using LSI ETV6 (TEL) break apart rearrangement probe demonstrated split signals, indicating break of *ETV6* gene.

(continued)

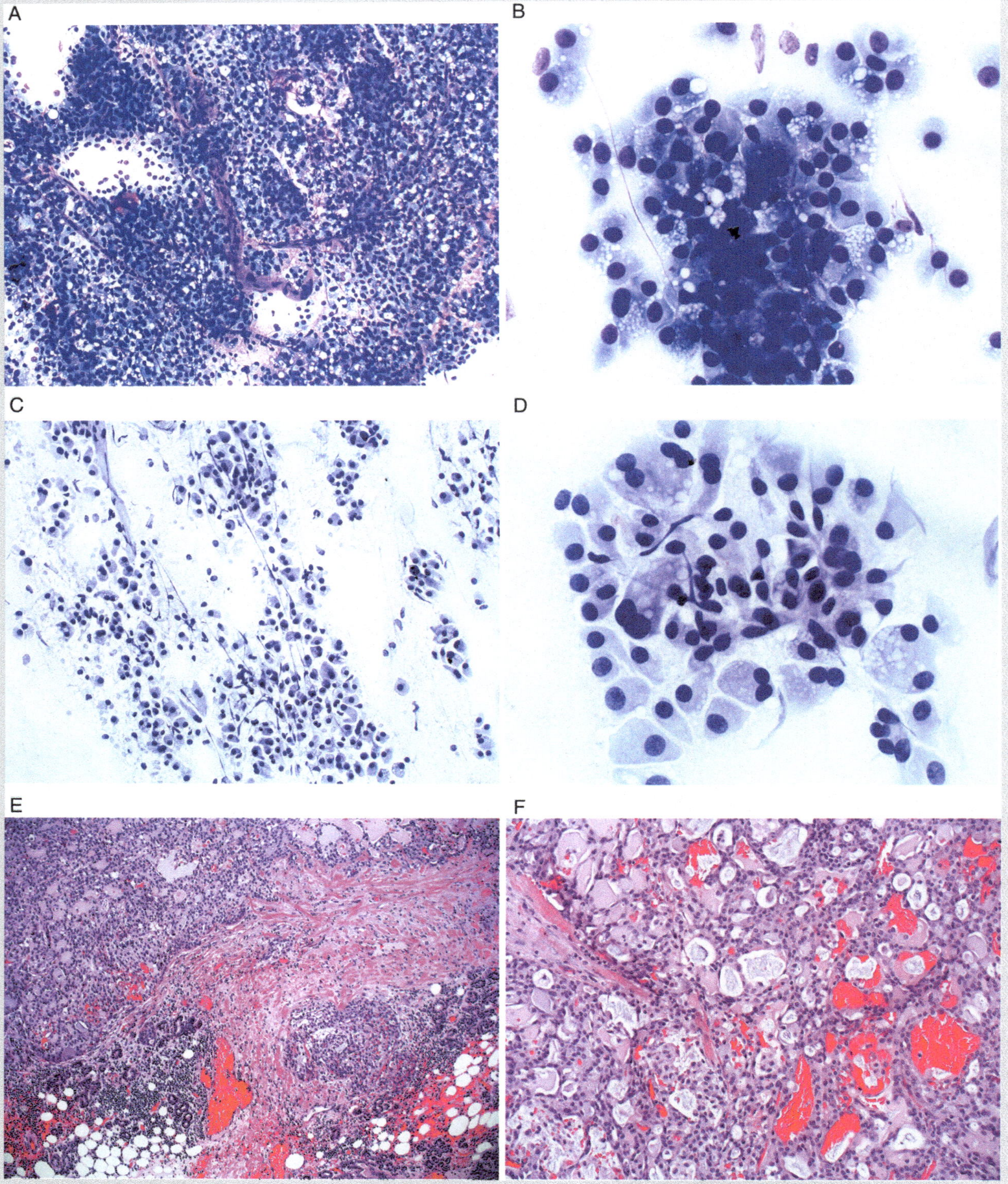

Fig. 2.31 Mammary analogue secretory carcinoma, case scenario 3. (**a**) Highly cellular smears contain loosely cohesive epithelioid cells with abundant basophilic, vacuolated cytoplasm in a background of abundant vasculature, Diff-Quik. (**b**) High magnification showing polygonal cells with round nuclei, prominent nucleoli, and abundant vacuolated, bubbly cytoplasm, Diff-Quik. (**c**, **d**) The same, in addition, granular background is noted, Pap stain. (**e**) The tumor is usually well demarcated, but has an infiltrative border, H&E. (**f**) Microcystic pattern, containing colloid-like secretions, giving an appearance of thyroid follicles, H&E. (**g**) Tumor cells contain round nuclei with prominent nucleoli and bubbly cytoplasm, H&E. (**h**) Area of solid growth, H&E. (**i**) Diffuse and strong positivity for S100, IHC. (**j**) Diffuse strong positivity for mammaglobin, IHC. (**k**) Weak to moderate positive for GATA3, IHC. (**l**) p63 is nonreactive, IHC

(continued)

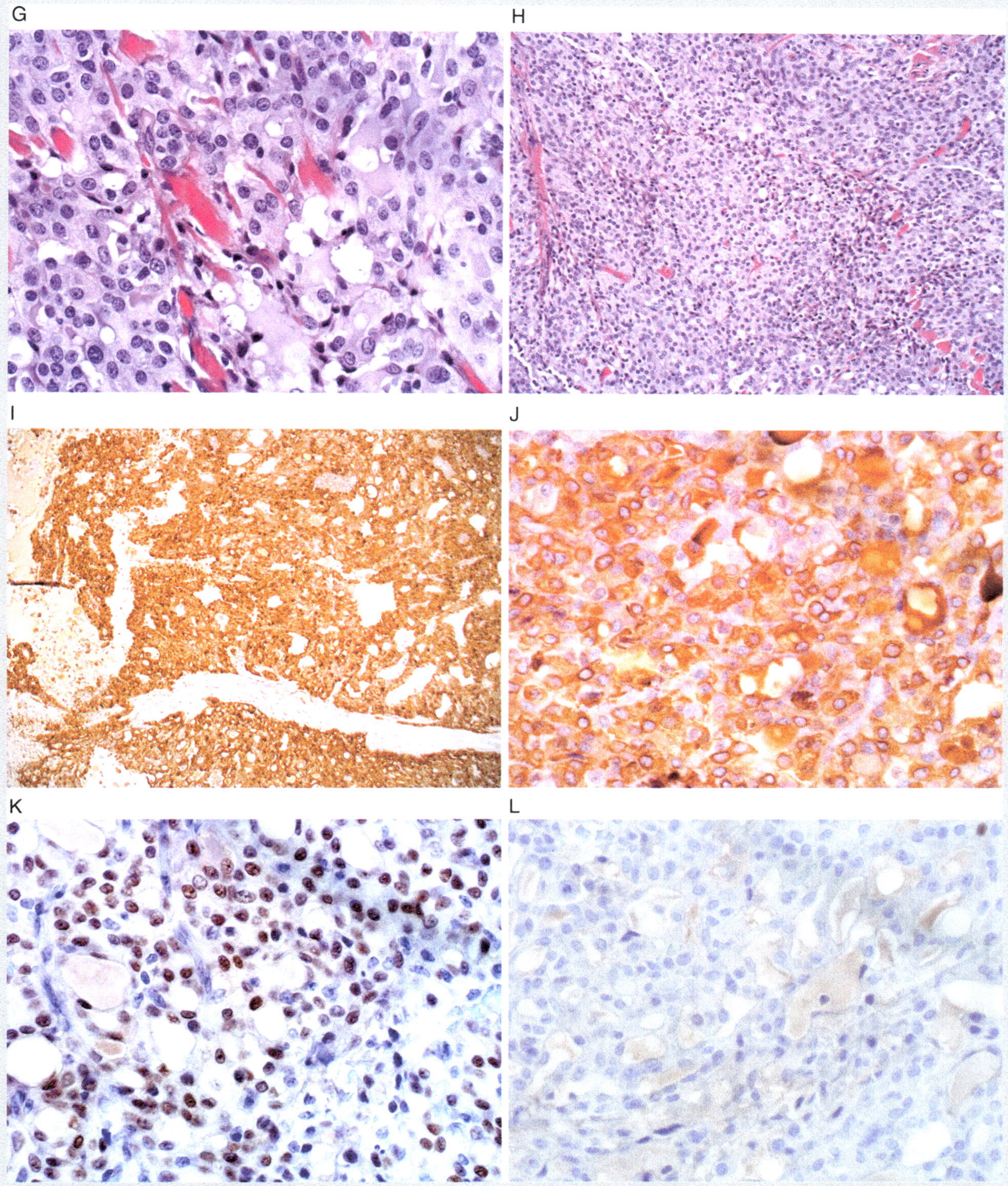

Fig. 2.31 (continued)

The *ETV6-NTRK3* fusion transcript was detected by reverse transcriptase polymerase chain reaction (RT-PCR).

MASC is a recently described salivary gland tumor harboring a recurrent balanced chromosomal translocation t(12;15)(p13;q25) leading a fusion gene between the *ETV6* gene on chromosome 12 and the *NTRK3* gene on chromosome 15. Histologically, the tumor is lobulated, usually exhibiting a well-circumscribed border without capsule, often with invasion into adjacent salivary gland tissue, and occasional extension into extraglandular tissue. The tumor cells are large, polygonal, with a centrally or slightly eccentrically located, round-to-oval vesicular nucleus, distinct single nucleolus, and ample pale to eosinophilic vacuolated or bubbly cytoplasm. Microcystic, solid, and tubular patterns have dominated the majority of cases; in addition, papillary, macrocystic, and follicular patterns are often seen. The cystic spaces or lumens of the ductal structures often contain eosinophilic or pale basophilic homogeneous colloid-like or bubbly secretions. Perineural invasion may be present; however, angiolymphatic invasion or tumor necrosis is not typically seen. Cytological features of this tumor have not been well described.

From the few published studies and our own experiences of this tumor, the FNA specimens of this tumor are usually highly cellular, composed of loosely cohesive clusters, "papillary" fragment, and single monotonous epithelioid cells with centrally to slightly eccentrically located, round-to-oval vesicular nuclei, discernible to prominent nucleoli, and abundant eosinophilic, vacuolated, or bubbly cytoplasm. Many tumor cells are large, round to polygonal, with well-defined cell borders; large naked nuclei with macronucleoli are not appreciated. Abundant delicate vasculatures and fine granular or cystic debris are noted in background; however, coarse blue-purple zymogen granules are not appreciated. No lymphocytes, mucinous material, or stromal fragments are seen. Significant nuclear hyperchromasia, nuclear pleomorphism, tumor necrosis, or mitoses are usually absent, except in cases with high-grade transformation. No lymphocytes, mucinous material, or stromal fragments are present.

Studies reported that the tumor cells express pancytokeratin, CK7, CK19, EMA, S100 protein, and vimentin, usually diffuse and strong, and also mammaglobin, STAT5a, GATA3, and GCDFP-15. The myoepithelial markers (p63, calponin, CK14, CK5/CK6, and SMA) are nonreactive. DOG1 expression is lacking, different from AciCC.

Among the common salivary gland tumors, the greatest mimic of MASC is AciCC, especially the zymogen granule-poor type. The monotonous cell population, the distinct cell borders, and the lack of PAS-D-positive, blue-purple zymogen-like cytoplasmic granules in MASC are features differentiating it from AciCC. Immunohistochemically, MASC is positive for S100, mammaglobin, CK7, vimentin, GCDFP-15 and GATA3, and negative for DOG1, ER, and PR; while AciCC is reactive to DOG1 and SOX10, and negative for CK7, S100, and mammaglobin. The differential phenotypes are summarized in Table 2.8. S100, mammaglobin, and DOG1 can serve as a screen panel before further confirmatory cytogenetic study to demonstrate the *ETV6-NTRK3* translocation in equivocal cases.

Low-grade MEC is included in the differential as well. The presences of true squamoid cells or basaloid intermediate cells and abundant intra- or extracellular mucin in low-grade MEC are helpful features. Immunohistochemically, lack of p63 expression with diffuse S100 positivity in MASC is unusual for low-grade MEC. Cytogenetic t(11;19) translocation coding for a *CRTC1-MAML2* fusion protein is identified in 50% of MECs, while no *ETV6-NTRK3* translocation identified.

Cystadenocarcinoma/ADC, NOS, is a malignant salivary gland tumor with ductal differentiation but lacking features of any specific types. It is a diagnosis of exclusion. ADC, NOS, is another differential consideration; however, the demonstration of *ETV6-NTRK3* translocation designates a tumor as MASC.

Table 2.8 Immunohistochemical phenotype of MASC and AciCC

	S100	MGB	DOG1	CK7	Vimentin	GATA3	STAT5a
AciCC	–	–	+	–	–	–	–
MASC	+	+	–/+	+	+	+	+

MASC mammary analogue secretary carcinoma, *AciCC* acinic cell carcinoma, *MGB* mammaglobin, *DOG1* discovered on GIST1, *CK7* cytokeratin 7, *GATA3* GATA-binding protein 3, *STAT5a* signal transducer and activator of transcription 5A

Abbreviations List

Abbreviation	Full text
AciCC	Acinic cell carcinoma
ADC	Adenocarcinoma
AdCC	Adenoid cystic carcinoma
AFB	Acid-fast bacilli
ANO-1	Anoctomin-1
AR	Androgen receptor
BCA	Basal cell adenoma (only in table)
BCAC	Basal cell adenocarcinoma (only in table)
BCL	B-cell CLL lymphoma
BSqCC	Basaloid squamous cell carcinoma (only in table)
CA	Carcinoma
CAIX	Carbonic anhydrase IX
CD	Cluster of differentiation
CEA	Carcinoembryonic antigen
CK	Cytokeratin
CRTC1	CREB-regulated transcription coactivator 1
CT	Computed tomography
CTNNB1	Catenin (cadherin-associated protein), beta 1
DOG1	Discovered on *GIST*-1
EBER	EBV-encoded RNA
EBV	Epstein-Barr virus
EBV LMP1	EBV latent membrane protein 1
EMA	Epithelial membrane antigen
EMBZBCL	Extranodal marginal zone B-cell lymphoma of the MALT type
ER	Estrogen receptor
EWSR1	Ewing sarcoma region 1
FISH	Fluorescence in situ hybridization
FNA	Fine needle aspiration
GATA3	GATA-binding protein 3
GCDFP-15	Gross cystic disease fluid protein-15
GFAP	Glial fibrillary acidic protein
GIST	Gastrointestinal stromal tumor
GMS	Grocott's methenamine silver
HER2	Human epidermal growth factor receptor 2
HIV	Human immunodeficiency virus
HMB45	Human melanoma black 45
HMGA2	High-mobility group AT hook 2
HMWCK	High molecular weight cytokeratin
HPF	High-power field
IgM	Immunoglobulin M
IHC	Immunohistochemistry
KIT C-kit	Same as CD117
LESA	Lymphoepithelial sialadenitis
LMWCK	Low molecular weight cytokeratin
MALT	Mucosa-associated lymphoid tissue
MAML2	Mastermind-like2 gene
MASC	Mammary analogue secretory carcinoma
MEC	Mucoepidermoid carcinoma
MECT1	Mucoepidermoid carcinoma translocated-1
MGB	Mammaglobin
MRI	Magnetic resonance imaging
MSA	Muscle specific actin
MUC	Mucin
MYB	v-myb avian myeloblastosis viral oncogene homolog
NFIB	Nuclear factor 1 B-type
NGS	Next-generation sequencing
NOS	Not otherwise specified
PA	Pleomorphic adenoma
Pap	Papanicolaou stain
PAP	Prostatic acid phosphatase
PAS	Periodic acid-Schiff
PAS-D	Periodic acid-Schiff with diastase
PAX	Paired box gene (PAX5, PAX8)
PBX1	Pre-B-cell leukemia homeobox 1
PLAG1	Pleomorphic adenoma gene 1
PLGA	Polymorphous low-grade adenocarcinoma
PLGA	Polymorphous low-grade adenocarcinoma
POUF5F1	Octamer-binding transcription factor 4 (OCT4)
PR	Progesterone receptor
PRKD1	Serine/threonine-protein kinase D1
PSA	Prostate-specific antigen
pVHL	von Hippel von tumor suppressor
RCCma	Renal cell carcinoma marker
RT-PCR	Reverse transcriptase polymerase chain reaction
S100P	Placental S100P
SG	Salivary gland (table abbr only)
SMA	Smooth muscle actin
SOX	Sex determining region Y box
STAT5a	Signal transducer and activator of transcription 5A
WHO	WorldHealth Organization

Suggested Reading

Cytology

Bibbo M, Wilbur DC. Comprehensive cytopathology. 4th ed. Philadelphia: Elsevier, Saunders; 2015.

Cibas ES, Ducatman BS. Cytology: diagnostic principles and clinical correlates. 2nd ed. Philadelphia: Saunders; 2003.

Colella G, Cannavale R, Flamminio F, Foschini MP. Fine-needle aspiration cytology of salivary gland lesions: a systematic review. J Oral Maxillofac Surg. 2010;68(9):2146–53.

DeMay RM. The art and science of cytopathology. 2nd ed. Chicago: American Society for Clinical Pathology (ASCP) Press; 2012.

Hughes JH, Volk EE, Wilbur DC, Cytopathology Resource Committee, College of American Pathologists. Pitfalls in salivary gland fine-needle aspiration cytology: lessons from the College of American Pathologists Interlaboratory Comparison

Program in Nongynecologic cytology. Arch Pathol Lab Med. 2005;129(1):26–31.
Martin HE, Ellis EB. Biopsy by needle puncture and aspiration. Ann Surg. 1930;92(2):169–81.
Schmidt RL, Hunt JP, Hall BJ, Wilson AR, Layfield LJ. A systematic review and meta-analysis of the diagnostic accuracy of frozen section for parotid gland lesions. Am J Clin Pathol. 2011;136(5):729–38.
Stewart FW. The diagnosis of tumors by aspiration. Am J Pathol. 1933;9(Suppl):801–812.3.
Yousem DM, Kraut MA, Chalian AA. Major salivary gland imaging. Radiology. 2000;216(1):19–29.

Histology

Chan JKC, Cheuk W. Tumors of the salivary glands. In: Fletcher CDM, editor. Diagnostic histopathology of tumors. 4th ed. Philadelphia: Saunders; 2013. p. 270–377.
El-Naggar AK, JKC C, Grandis JR, Takata T, Slootweg PJ. WHO classification of head and neck tumours. Lyon: IARC; 2017.
Gnepp DR. Diagnostic surgical pathology of the head and neck. 2nd ed. Philadelphia: Saunders; 2009.
Harnes L, Eveson JW, Reichart P, et al. WHO classification of tumours: pathology and genetics, head and neck tumours. Lyon: IARC; 2005.

Ancillary Studies

Abd Raboh NM, Hakim SA. Diagnostic role of DOG1 and p63 immunohistochemistry in salivary gland carcinomas. Int J Clin Exp Pathol. 2015;8(8):9214–22.
Angiero F, Sozzi D, Seramondi R, Valente MG. Epithelial-myoepithelial carcinoma of the minor salivary glands: immunohistochemical and morphological features. Anticancer Res. 2009;29(11):4703–9.
Behboudi A, Enlund F, Winnes M, Andrén Y, Nordkvist A, Leivo I, et al. Molecular classification of mucoepidermoid carcinomas-prognostic significance of the MECT1-MAML2 fusion oncogene. Genes Chromosomes Cancer. 2006;45(5):470–81.
Bishop JA. Unmasking MASC: bringing to light the unique morphologic, immunohistochemical and genetic features of the newly recognized mammary analogue secretory carcinoma of salivary glands. Head Neck Pathol. 2013;7(1):35–9.
Bishop JA, Yonescu R, Batista DA, Westra WH, Ali SZ. Cytopathologic features of mammary analogue secretory carcinoma. Cancer Cytopathol. 2013;121(5):228–33.
Brill LB 2nd, Kanner WA, Fehr A, Andrén Y, Moskaluk CA, Löning T, et al. Analysis of MYB expression and MYB-NFIB gene fusions in adenoid cystic carcinoma and other salivary neoplasms. Mod Pathol. 2011;24(9):1169–76.
Chan JK, Suster S, Wenig BM, Tsang WY, Chan JB, Lau AL. Cytokeratin 20 immunoreactivity distinguishes Merkel cell (primary cutaneous neuroendocrine) carcinomas and salivary gland small cell carcinomas from small cell carcinomas of various sites. Am J Surg Pathol. 1997;21(2):226–34.
Chandan VS, Wilbur D, Faquin WC, Khurana KK. Is c-kit (CD117) immunolocalization in cell block preparations useful in the differentiation of adenoid cystic carcinoma from pleomorphic adenoma? Cancer. 2004;102(4):207–9.
Chênevert J, Duvvuri U, Chiosea S, Dacic S, Cieply K, Kim J, et al. DOG1: a novel marker of salivary acinar and intercalated duct differentiation. Mod Pathol. 2012;25(7):919–29.
Connor A, Perez-Ordoñez B, Shago M, Skálová A, Weinreb I. Mammary analog secretory carcinoma of salivary gland origin with the ETV6 gene rearrangement by FISH: expanded morphologic and immunohistochemical spectrum of a recently described entity. Am J Surg Pathol. 2012;36(1):27–34.
Debiec-Rychter M, Van Valckenborgh I, Van den Broeck C, Hagemeijer A, Van de Ven WJ, Kas K, et al. Histologic localization of PLAG1 (pleomorphic adenoma gene 1) in pleomorphic adenoma of the salivary gland: cytogenetic evidence of common origin of phenotypically diverse cells. Lab Investig. 2001;81(9):1289–97.
do Prado RF, Consolaro A, Taveira LA. Expression of beta catenin in carcinoma in pleomorphic adenoma, pleomorphic adenoma and normal salivary gland: an immunohistochemical study. Med Oral Pathol Oral Cir Bucal. 2006;11(3):E247–51.
Edwards PC, Bhuiya T, Kelsch RD. C-kit expression in the salivary gland neoplasms adenoid cystic carcinoma, polymorphous low-grade adenocarcinoma, and monomorphic adenoma. Oral Surg Oral Med Oral Pathol Oral Radiol Endod. 2003;95(5):586–93.
Foo WC, Jo V, Krane JF. Utility of Myb, CD117 and PLAG1 Immunocytochemistry in fine needle aspiration diagnosis of salivary gland neoplasms. J Am Soc Cytopathol. 2013;2(suppl):S51–2.
Genelhu MC, Gobbi H, Arantes DC, Cardoso SV, Cassali GD. Immunolocalization of beta-catenin in pleomorphic adenomas and carcinomas ex-pleomorphic adenomas of salivary glands. Appl Immunohistochem Mol Morphol. 2007;15(3):273–8.
Griffith CC, Stelow EB, Saqi A, Khalbuss WE, Schneider F, Chiosea SI, et al. The cytological features of mammary analogue secretory carcinoma: a series of 6 molecularly confirmed cases. Cancer Cytopathol. 2013;121(5):234–41.
Jazaerly T, Bandyopadhyay S, Almardini N, Husain M. Diagnosis of sebaceous lymphadenoma by fine needle aspiration in a patient with Cowden syndrome: case report and review of the literature. Cytojournal. 2014;11:25.
Jung MJ, Kim SY, Nam SY, Roh JL, Choi SH, Lee JH, et al. Aspiration cytology of mammary analogue secretory carcinoma of the salivary gland. Diagn Cytopathol. 2015;43(4):287–93.
Jung MJ, Roh JL, Choi SH, Nam SY, Kim SY, Lee SW, et al. Basal cell adenocarcinoma of the salivary gland: a morphological and immunohistochemical comparison with basal cell adenoma with and without capsular invasion. Diagn Pathol. 2013;8:171.
Kas K, Voz ML, Roijer E, Aström AK, Meyen E, Stenman G, et al. Promoter swapping between the genes for a novel zinc finger protein and beta-catenin in pleiomorphic adenomas with t(3;8)(p21;q12) translocations. Nat Genet. 1997;15:170–4.
Kawahara A, Harada H, Abe H, Yamaguchi T, Taira T, Nakashima K, et al. Nuclear β-catenin expression in basal cell adenomas of salivary gland. J Oral Pathol Med. 2011;40(6):460–6.
Kawahara A, Taira T, Abe H, Takase Y, Kurita T, Sadashima E, et al. Diagnostic utility of phosphorylated signal transducer and activator of transcription 5 immunostaining in the diagnosis of mammary analogue secretory carcinoma of the salivary gland: a comparative study of salivary gland cancers. Cancer Cytopathol. 2015;123(10):603–11.
Levine P, Fried K, Krevitt LD, Wang B, Wenig BM. Aspiration biopsy of mammary analogue secretory carcinoma of accessory parotid gland: another diagnostic dilemma in matrix-containing tumors of the salivary glands. Diagn Cytopathol. 2014;42(1):49–53.
Lin F, Liu H. Immunohistochemistry in undifferentiated neoplasm/tumor of uncertain origin. Arch Pathol Lab Med. 2014;138(12):1583–610.
Mariano FV, dos Santos HT, Azañero WD, da Cunha IW, Coutinho-Camilo CM, de Almeida OP, et al. Mammary analogue secretory carcinoma of salivary glands is a lipid-rich tumour, and adipophilin can be valuable in its identification. Histopathology. 2013;63(4):558–67.
Matsuyama A, Hisaoka M, Nagao Y, Hashimoto H. Aberrant PLAG1 expression in pleomorphic adenomas of the salivary gland: a molecular genetic and immunohistochemical study. Virchows Arch. 2011;458(5):583–92.

Mino M, Pilch BZ, Faquin WC. Expression of KIT (CD117) in neoplasms of the head and neck: an ancillary marker for adenoid cystic carcinoma. Mod Pathol. 2003;16(12):1224–31.

Mitani Y, Li J, Rao PH, Zhao YJ, Bell D, Lippman SM, et al. Comprehensive analysis of the MYB-NFIB gene fusion in salivary adenoid cystic carcinoma: incidence, variability, and clinicopathologic significance. Clin Cancer Res. 2010;16(19):4722–31.

Mitani Y, Rao PH, Futreal PA, Roberts DB, Stephens PJ, Zhao YJ, et al. Novel chromosomal rearrangements and break points at the t(6;9) in salivary adenoid cystic carcinoma: association with MYB-NFIB chimeric fusion, MYB expression, and clinical outcome. Clin Cancer Res. 2011;17(22):7003–14.

Nagao T, Sugano I, Ishida Y, Hasegawa M, Matsuzaki O, Konno A, et al. Basal cell adenocarcinoma of the salivary glands: comparison with basal cell adenoma through assessment of cell proliferation, apoptosis, and expression of p53 and bcl-2. Cancer. 1998;82(3):439–47.

Nikitakis NG, Tosios KI, Papanikolaou VS, Rivera H, Papanicolaou SI, Ioffe OB. Immunohistochemical expression of cytokeratins 7 and 20 in malignant salivary gland tumors. Mod Pathol. 2004;17(4):407–15.

Ohtomo R, Mori T, Shibata S, Tsuta K, Maeshima AM, Akazawa C, et al. SOX10 is a novel marker of acinus and intercalated duct differentiation in salivary gland tumors: a clue to the histogenesis for tumor diagnosis. Mod Pathol. 2013;26(8):1041–50.

Ozolek JA, Bastacky SI, Myers EN, Hunt JL. Immunophenotypic comparison of salivary gland oncocytoma and metastatic renal cell carcinoma. Laryngoscope. 2005;115(6):1097–100.

Patel KR, Solomon IH, El-Mofty SK, Lewis JS Jr, Chernock RD. Mammaglobin and S-100 immunoreactivity in salivary gland carcinomas other than mammary analogue secretory carcinoma. Hum Pathol. 2013;44(11):2501–8.

Penner CR, Folpe AL, Budnick SD. C-kit expression distinguishes salivary gland adenoid cystic carcinoma from polymorphous low-grade adenocarcinoma. Mod Pathol. 2002;15(7):687–91.

Persson M, Andren Y, Mark J, Horlings HM, Persson F, Stenman G. Recurrent fusion of MYB and NFIB transcription factor genes in carcinomas of the breast and head and neck. Proc Natl Acad Sci U S A. 2009a;106:18740–4.

Persson F, Andren Y, Winnes M, Wedell B, Nordkvist A, Gudnadottir G, et al. High-resolution genomic profiling of adenomas and carcinomas of the salivary glands reveals amplification, rearrangement, and fusion of HMGA2. Genes Chromosomes Cancer. 2009b;48(1):69–82.

Pinto A, Nosé V, Rojas C, Fan YS, Gomez-Fernandez C. Searching for mammary analogue [corrected] secretory carcinoma of salivary gland among its mimics. Mod Pathol. 2014;27(1):30–7.

Pusztaszeri MP, García JJ, Faquin WC. Salivary gland FNA: new markers and new opportunities for improved diagnosis. Cancer Cytopathol. 2016;124(5):307–16.

Rotellini M, Palomba A, Baroni G, Franchi A. Diagnostic utility of PLAG1 immunohistochemical determination in salivary gland tumors. Appl Immunohistochem Mol Morphol. 2014;22(5):390–4.

Schmitt AC, Cohen C, Siddiqui MT. Expression of SOX10 in salivary gland oncocytic neoplasms: a review and a comparative analysis with other immunohistochemical markers. Acta Cytol. 2015;59(5):384–90.

Schmitt AC, McCormick R, Cohen C, Siddiqui MT. DOG1, p63, and S100 protein: a novel immunohistochemical panel in the differential diagnosis of oncocytic salivary gland neoplasms in fine- needle aspiration cell blocks. J Am Soc Cytopathol. 2014;3(6):303–8.

Schuerch C, Zhu S. Salivary glands and head and neck. In: Lin F, Prichard JW, Liu H, Wilkerson M, Chen ZE, editors. Handbook of practical immunohistochemistry: frequent asked questions. 2nd ed. New York: Springer Science+Business Media; 2015. p. 287–311.

Schwartz LE, Begum S, Westra WH, Bishop JA. GATA3 immunohistochemical expression in salivary gland neoplasms. Head Neck Pathol. 2013;7(4):311–5.

Sedassari BT, Dos Santos HT, Mariano FV, da Silva Lascane NA, Altemani A, Sousa S. Carcinoma ex pleomorphic adenoma of minor salivary glands with major epithelial-myoepithelial component: clinicopathologic and immunohistochemical study of 3 cases. Ann Diagn Pathol. 2015;19(3):164–8.

Seethala RR, Thompson LD, Gnepp DR, Barnes EL, Skalova A, Montone K, et al. Lymphadenoma of the salivary gland: clinicopathological and immunohistochemical analysis of 33 tumors. Mod Pathol. 2012;25(1):26–35.

Shah AA, Wenig BM, LeGallo RD, Mills SE, Stelow EB. Morphology in conjunction with immunohistochemistry is sufficient for the diagnosis of mammary analogue secretory carcinoma. Head Neck Pathol. 2015;9(1):85–95.

Skalova A. Mammary analogue secretory carcinoma of salivary gland origin: an update and expanded morphologic and immunohistochemical spectrum of recently described entity. Head Neck Pathol. 2013;7(Suppl 1):S30–6.

Skálová A, Simpson RH, Lehtonen H, Leivo I. Assessment of proliferative activity using the MIB1 antibody help to distinguish polymorphous low grade adenocarcinoma from adenoid cystic carcinoma of salivary glands. Pathol Res Pract. 1997;193(10):695–703.

Skálová A, Vanecek T, Sima R, Laco J, Weinreb I, Perez-Ordonez B, et al. Mammary analogue secretory carcinoma of salivary glands, containing the ETV6-NTRK3 fusion gene: a hitherto undescribed salivary gland tumor entity. Am J Surg Pathol. 2010;34(5):599–608.

Tognon C, Knezevich SR, Huntsman D, Roskelley CD, Melnyk N, Mathers JA, et al. Expression of the ETV6-NTRK3 gene fusion as a primary event in human secretory breast carcinoma. Cancer Cell. 2002;2(5):367–76.

Tonon G, Modi S, Wu L, Kubo A, Coxon AB, Komiya, et al. t(11;19)(q21;p13) translocation in mucoepidermoid carcinoma creates a novel fusion product that disrupts a notch signaling pathway. Nat Genet. 2003;33(2):208–13.

Urano M, Nagao T, Miyabe S, Ishibashi K, Higuchi K, Kuroda M. Characterization of mammary analogue secretory carcinoma of the salivary gland: discrimination from its mimics by the presence of the ETV6-NTRK3 translocation and novel surrogate markers. Hum Pathol. 2015;46(1):94–103.

Voz ML, Astrom AK, Kas K, Mark J, Stenman G, Van de Ven WJ. The recurrent translocation t(5;8)(p13;q12) in pleomorphic adenomas results in upregulation of PLAG1 gene expression under control of the LIFR promoter. Oncogene. 1998;16(11):1409–16.

Woo VL, Bhuiya T, Kelsch R. Assessment of CD43 expression in adenoid cystic carcinomas, polymorphous low-grade adenocarcinomas, and monomorphic adenomas. Oral Surg Oral Med Oral Pathol Oral Radiol Endod. 2006;102(4):495–500.

Thyroid and Parathyroid Glands

3

Fan Lin, Haiyan Liu, and Jun Zhang

Summary of Pearls and Pitfalls

- Based on the *Bethesda System for Reporting Thyroid Cytopathology*, the terminology "follicular lesion" is no longer recommended in routine practice. Instead, a distinct subcategory of "Atypia of Undetermined Significance/Follicular Lesion of Undetermined Significance" (AUS/FLUS) was recommended.
- Focal nuclear pleomorphism of the follicular cells is frequently seen in a lymphocytic/Hashimoto's thyroiditis; one should avoid overdiagnosing this change as "Atypia of Undetermined Significance."
- When a fine-needle aspiration (FNA) smear is composed of a mixture of epithelioid and spindle cells singly and in loosely cohesive groups, and absence of colloid, regardless of the cellularity, a medullary carcinoma should be included in the diagnostic consideration.
- Hyalinizing trabecular neoplasm is an uncommon lesion and shares many important cytological features with papillary carcinoma of the thyroid, including nuclear grooves and intranuclear pseudoinclusions. When the follicular cells appear to be elongated and a hyaline matrix-like material between cellular components is present, it is necessary to exclude a hyalinizing trabecular neoplasm before a definitive diagnosis of papillary carcinoma is rendered. An immunostain for mindbomb E3 ubiquitin protein ligase 1 (MIB-1 clone[Ki-67]) with distinctive membranous staining pattern is useful in confirming the diagnosis.
- If abundant acute inflammation is present, in addition to an acute inflammatory process, undifferentiated (anaplastic) carcinoma of the thyroid should be included in the diagnostic consideration. Paired box gene 8 (PAX8) is positive in 50% of the tumors; in contrast, both thyroid transcription factor 1 (TTF1) and thyroglobulin are usually negative.
- The vast majority of cystic lesions of the thyroid are benign; however, cystic papillary carcinoma of the thyroid or metastatic squamous cell carcinoma with cystic degeneration may mimic a benign cystic lesion.
- Parathyroid adenoma/neoplasm should be excluded if colloid is absent and numerous small naked nuclei and vascular-rich stroma are seen. Clear cell or oncocytic changes are common.
- If the neoplastic cells are morphologically unlike follicular cells and colloid is absent in the background, a rare primary tumor or a metastasis should be considered. The most common metastases in the thyroid are renal cell (clear cell) carcinoma, melanoma, and adenocarcinoma of the lung, breast, and stomach.
- If a mixture of histiocyte-like cells and lymphoid cells is present, Langerhans cell histiocytosis, follicular dendritic cell tumors, and other rare histiocytic lesions should be considered.

Modified from the 2004 World Health Organization (WHO) Classification of Thyroid and Parathyroid Tumors[1]

Thyroid

Benign Nonneoplastic Lesions

- Acute thyroiditis
- Granulomatous thyroiditis/subacute thyroiditis

[1]Modified with permission from DeLellis RA, Williams ED. Tumors of the thyroid and parathyroid. In: DeLellis RA, Lloyd RV, Heitz PU, Eng C, editors. WHO classification of tumours. Pathology and genetics tumours of endocrine organs. Lyon, France: IARC Press; 2004:49–136.

© Springer International Publishing AG 2018
F. Lin et al., *Handbook of Practical Fine Needle Aspiration and Small Tissue Biopsies*, DOI 10.1007/978-3-319-57386-1_3

- Hashimoto's thyroiditis/lymphocytic thyroiditis
- Nodular goiter
- Graves' disease

Neoplasms

Follicular Neoplasms

- Follicular adenoma
- Follicular carcinoma

Hurthle Cell Neoplasms

- Hurthle cell adenoma
- Hurthle cell carcinoma

Other Neoplasms

- Papillary carcinoma
- Medullary carcinoma
- Poorly (insular) differentiated carcinoma
- Undifferentiated (anaplastic) carcinoma
- Hyalinizing trabecular neoplasm

Uncommon and Rare Lesions

Squamous cell carcinoma
Mucoepidermoid carcinoma
Sclerosing mucoepidermoid carcinoma with eosinophilia
Mucinous carcinoma
Spindle cell tumor with thymus-like differentiation
Carcinoma showing thymus-like differentiation
Lymphoma and plasmacytoma
Angiosarcoma
Smooth muscle tumor
Peripheral nerve sheath tumor
Solitary fibrous tumor
Follicular dendritic cell tumor
Langerhans cell histiocytosis
Teratoma
Ectopic thymoma
Second tumors

- Kidney
- Skin (melanoma)
- Lung adenocarcinoma
- Breast carcinoma
- Gastric adenocarcinoma
- Squamous cell carcinoma of the head and neck

Parathyroid

Parathyroid adenoma
Parathyroid carcinoma

The Bethesda System for Reporting Thyroid Cytopathology

FNA biopsy plays a crucial role in the assessment and triage of a thyroid nodule, and it has resulted in a significant reduction in unnecessary surgeries for patients with a benign lesion. However, some of the diagnostic categories and terminologies are inconsistent from one laboratory to another, which has created ambiguity and confusion among pathologists and clinicians. To clarify the potential misunderstanding and improve clarity of communication, the *Bethesda System for Reporting Thyroid Cytopathology* was introduced and published as an atlas in 2010. Six diagnostic categories and the associated risk of malignancy and recommended clinical management for each category were recommended as summarized in Table 3.1 below.

Perhaps the most important change was to introduce a distinct subcategory of "Atypia of Undetermined Significance/Follicular Lesion of Undetermined Significance." This subcategory of lesions was defined as cellular components (follicular cells, lymphoid cells, and others) with architectural and/or nuclear atypia that is not sufficient to be classified as suspicious for a follicular neoplasm/Hurthle cell neoplasm, suspicious for malignancy, or malignancy. Also, the atypia cannot be confidently classified as benign change. The risk of malignancy in this category is about 5–15%, and a repeat FNA in a reasonable interval was suggested.

Normal Thyroid

Colloid

Colloid is the key diagnostic component for thyroid disease. Colloid appears to be light blue or blue-purple on a Diff-Quik (DQ)-stained slide (Fig. 3.1) and light purple to pink on Papanicolaou (Pap) stain (Fig. 3.2). Comparing the two staining methods, colloid is easier to observe on DQ stain. In the presence of blood and the absence of follicular cells, thin colloid can be difficult to differentiate from serum. The finding of even few follicular cells is an important clue to confirm the presence of thin or watery colloid. In general, two types of colloid are seen: one is thin or watery colloid (Fig. 3.3) and the other is thick or inspissated colloid (Fig. 3.4). When watery colloid falls off the slide, it resembles a spider web (Fig. 3.5).

Table 3.1 Summary of the Bethesda System for Reporting Thyroid Cytopathology

Diagnostic category	Diagnosis	Risk of malignancy (%)	Recommended management
Non-diagnostic or unsatisfactory	Cyst fluid only [a]Virtually acellular specimen	–	Repeat FNA with ultrasound guidance
Benign	Benign follicular nodule Lymphocytic (Hashimoto's) thyroiditis Granulomatous thyroiditis	0–3	Clinical follow-up
Atypia of Undetermined Significance/ Follicular Lesion of Undetermined Significance	Atypical follicular cells	5–15	Repeat FNA
Follicular neoplasm or suspicious for follicular neoplasm	Follicular neoplasm Hurthle cell neoplasm	15–30	Lobectomy
Suspicious for malignancy	Suspicious for papillary carcinoma, medullary carcinoma, metastatic carcinoma, lymphoma, and others	60–75	Lobectomy or near-total thyroidectomy
Malignant	Papillary thyroid carcinoma (PTC) Medullary thyroid carcinoma Poorly differentiated thyroid carcinoma Anaplastic thyroid carcinoma Squamous cell carcinoma Non-Hodgkin's lymphoma Metastatic carcinoma Others	97–99	Near-total thyroidectomy

Used with permission from Ali SZ and Cibas ES, editors. The Bethesda System for Reporting Thyroid Cytopathology. New York: Springer Science+Business Media; 2010

[a]In general, an adequate specimen should contain a minimum of six groups of well-visualized follicular cells with at least ten cells per group, preferably on a single slide, with the exception of these special circumstances: (1) colloid nodule, (2) solid nodules with cytologic atypia, and (3) solid nodules with inflammation such as lymphocytic thyroiditis or abscess

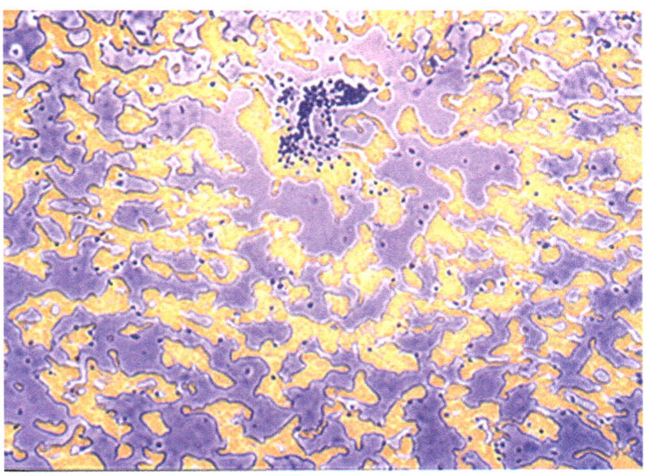

Fig. 3.1 Watery colloid on DQ stain

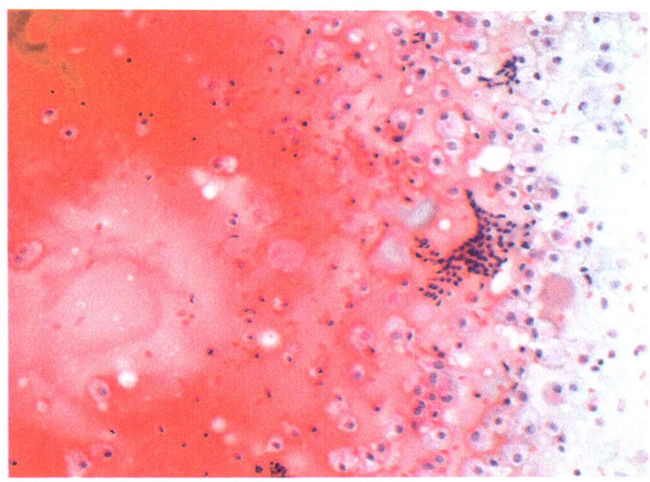

Fig. 3.2 Watery colloid on Pap stain

Follicular Cells

Follicular cells are cuboids and uniform in size, with a honeycomb arrangement. Nuclei are round, 6–9 um, with small to inconspicuous nucleoli, fine nuclear chromatin with even distribution, and a smooth nuclear contour (Fig. 3.6).

In general, an adequate specimen should contain a minimum of six groups of well-visualized follicular cells with at least ten cells per group, preferably on a single slide, with the exception of these special circumstances: (1) colloid nodule, (2) solid nodules with cytologic atypia, and (3) solid nodules with inflammation such as lymphocytic thyroiditis or abscess.

Hurthle Cells

A subtype of follicular cells, slightly larger than normal follicular cells, with abundant granular cytoplasm, small to conspicuous nucleoli, and binucleation; they appear light purple on DQ stain and orange to pink on Pap stain (Fig. 3.7).

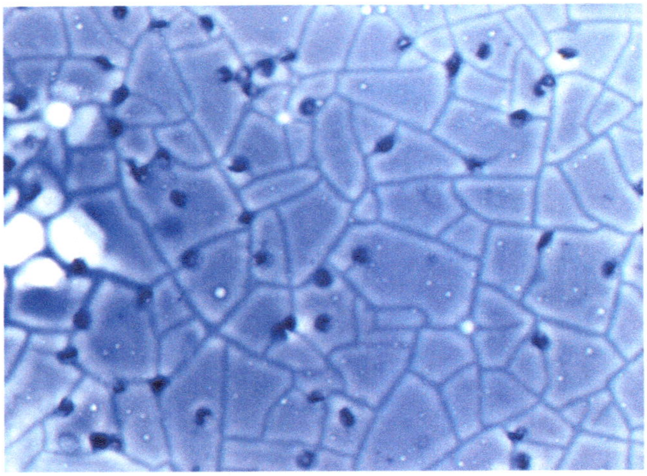

Fig. 3.3 Colloid on DQ stain with cracked glass window appearance

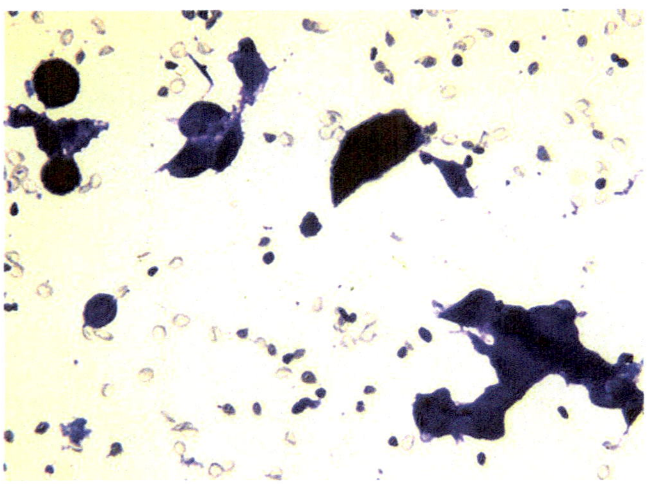

Fig. 3.4 Thick colloid with *dark blue* staining on DQ stain

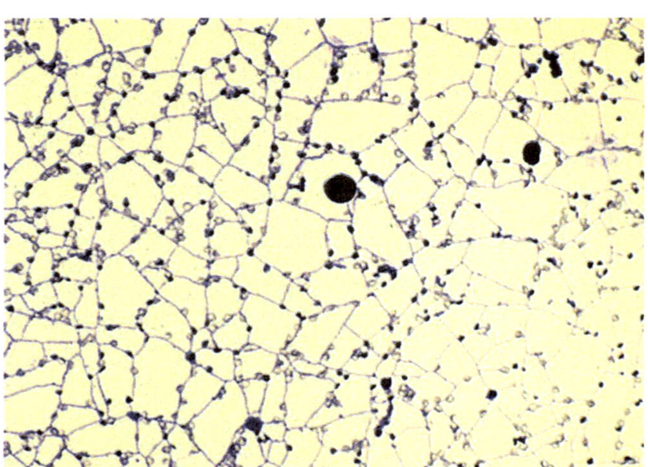

Fig. 3.5 Colloid fell off the slide, with spiderweb appearance on DQ stain

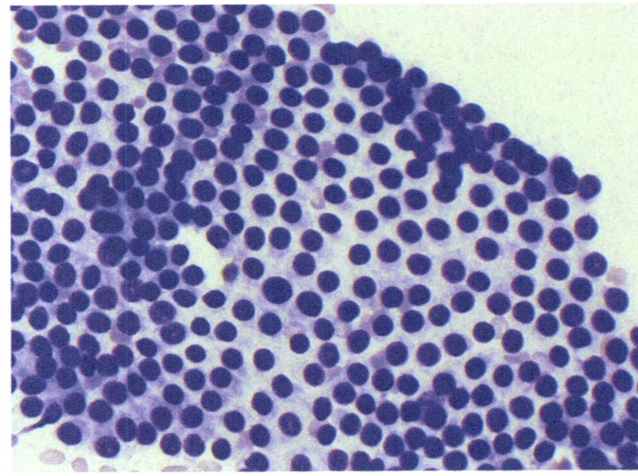

Fig. 3.6 Benign follicular cells with uniform size and orderly arrangement on DQ stain

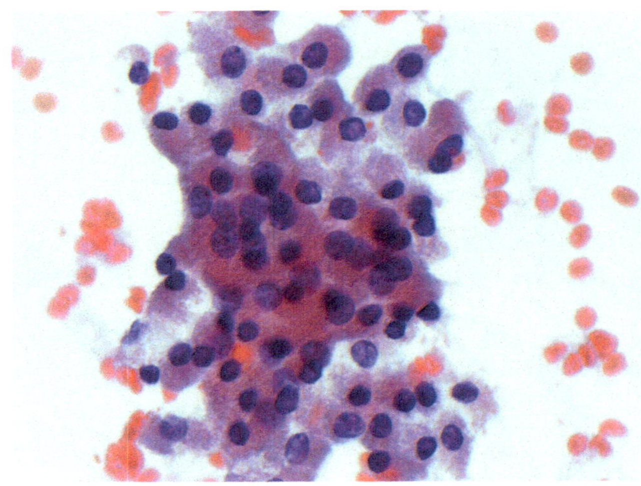

Fig. 3.7 Hurthle cells with large nuclei and abundant eosinophilic granular cytoplasm

Flame Cells

A subtype of follicular cells, with abundant cytoplasm with cytoplasmic fine vacuoles; they appear purple-pink on DQ stain (Fig. 3.8). They reflect the hyperfunctional status of the thyroid, such as in Graves' disease. They can be seen in nodular goiter and subacute thyroiditis as well.

Respiratory Epithelial Cells

During the aspiration procedure, the needle may accidentally enter the trachea, and the aspirate may contain respiratory epithelial cells (Fig. 3.9).

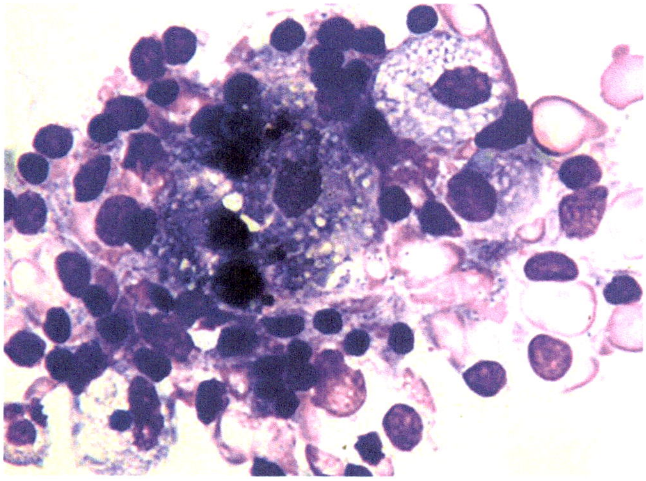

Fig. 3.8 Flame cells frequently seen in nodular goiter with hyperthyroid function

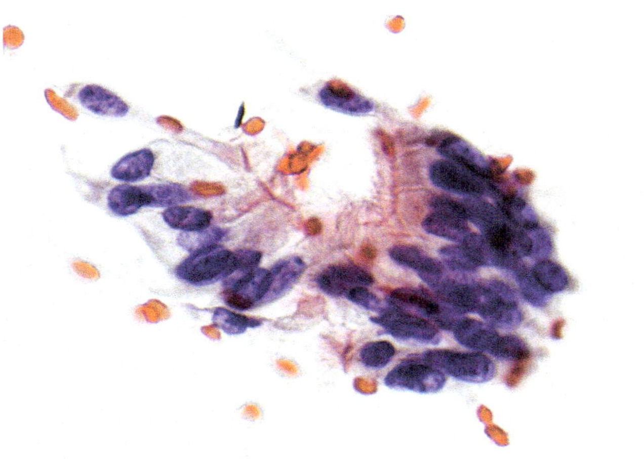

Fig. 3.9 Ciliated columnar respiratory epithelial cells when a needle accidentally enters the trachea

Benign Thyroid Lesions

Acute Thyroiditis

Clinical Features

- Rare, caused by bacteria and fungus.
- Fever and neck pain.
- Biopsy is generally unnecessary because of the obvious clinical presentation. If a nodular lesion is formed, then a neoplastic lesion, especially an anaplastic carcinoma, should be included in the diagnostic consideration.

Cytological Features

- Numerous acute inflammatory and histiocytes (Fig. 3.10a, b)
- Only few follicular cells
- Necrotic debris or granulomatous inflammation
- Fungus or bacteria can be seen on a special stain (Fig. 3.11)

Histologic Features

- Acute inflammation with abscess formation and tissue necrosis

Differential Diagnosis

- Anaplastic carcinoma

Granulomatous (de Quervain) Thyroiditis/ Subacute Thyroiditis

Clinical Features

- Caused by viral infection and a self-limiting process
- More common in young female
- Painful or painless diffuse thyroid enlargement

Cytological Features

- Granulomatous inflammation with multinucleated giant cells; some giant cells may engulf colloid.
- Many giant cells may contain many nuclei (many more nuclei than multinucleated giant cells seen in PTC).
- Acute and chronic inflammatory cells.
- Few follicular cells.

Histologic Features

- Usually multiple non-caseating granulomas associated with marked inflammation
- Granulomas containing foreign-body giant cells, which may engulf colloid (Figs. 3.12 and 3.13)
- Thyroid follicles surrounded by granulomas and inflammation
- Patchy fibrosis

Differential Diagnosis

- Tuberculosis
- Sarcoidosis
- Mycoses

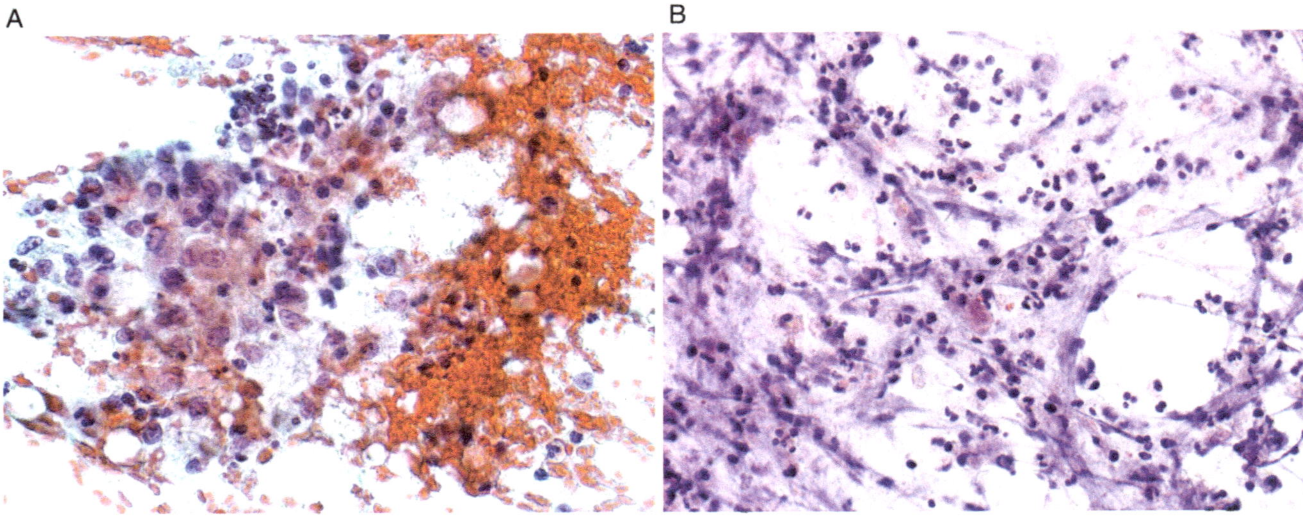

Fig. 3.10 Acute inflammatory cells, histiocytes, and necrotic debris in acute thyroiditis (Pap stain)

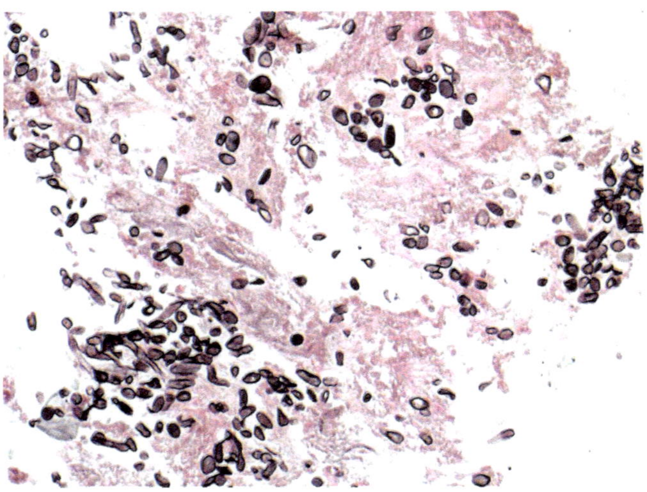

Fig. 3.11 Fungal elements in acute thyroiditis (Grocott's methenamine silver [GMS] stain)

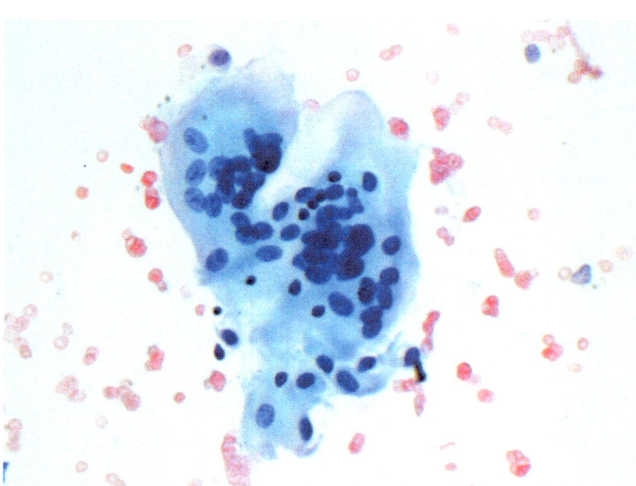

Fig. 3.12 A large multinucleated giant cell in subacute thyroiditis

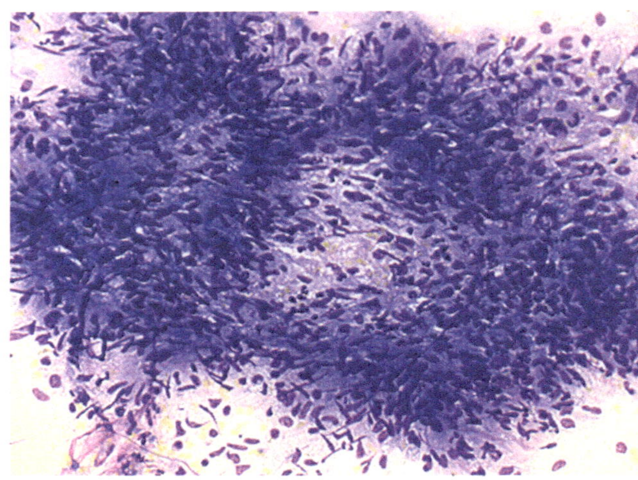

Fig. 3.13 Epithelioid histiocytes in chronic granulomatous inflammation (DQ stain)

Hashimoto's Thyroiditis/Lymphocytic Thyroiditis

Clinical Features

- An autoimmune-related disease.
- More common in middle-aged women.
- Present with firm and diffuse enlargement of the thyroid.
- Normal thyroid function in early stage and hypothyroidism in late stage.
- Serological tests are positive for anti-thyroglobulin, anti-mitochondrial antibody, and anti-oxidase antibody.

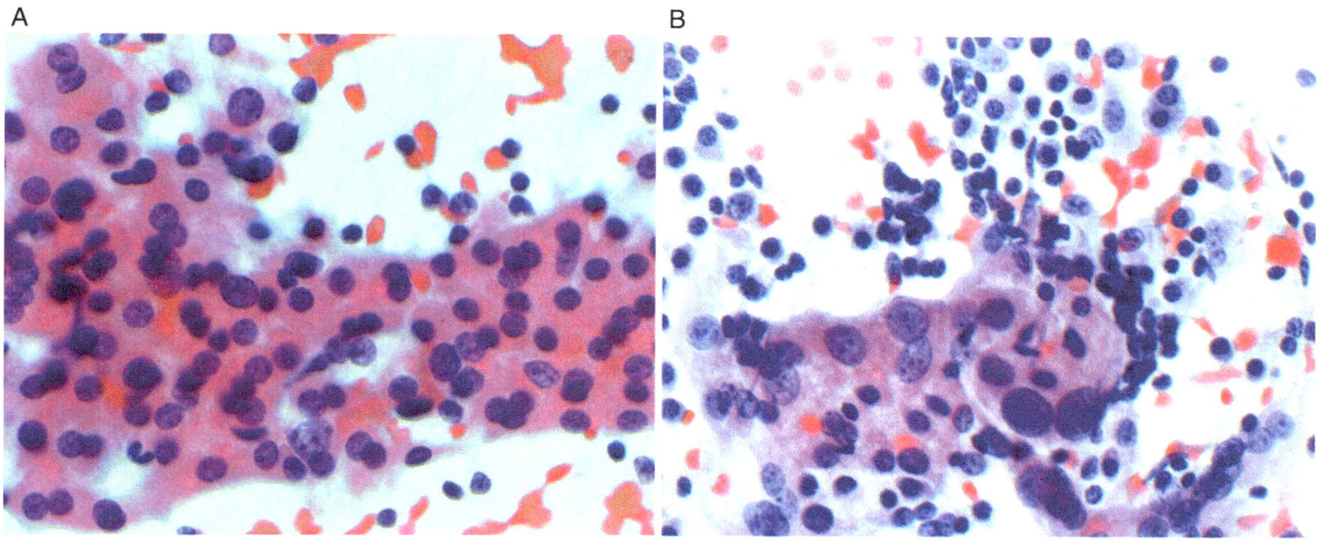

Fig. 3.14 Infiltration of lymphoid cells within Hurthle cells in Hashimoto's thyroiditis (Pap stain and DQ stain)

Cytological Features

- Infiltration of lymphocytes in Hurthle cells (Fig. 3.14a, b).
- Acute and chronic inflammatory cells with plasma cells.
- Multinucleated giant cells.
- Granulomatous inflammation.
- Reduced numbers of follicular cells dependent upon of the stage of the disease. It can be divided into three phases: (1) florid lymphoid phase, predominately a mixed population of lymphoid cells with sparse Hurthle cells and follicular cells; (2) cellular phase, proliferation of Hurthle cells; and (3) fibrotic phase, fibrotic tissue, scant Hurthle cells and lymphoid cells, and squamous cells (squamous metaplasia).
- Reactive atypical follicular cells/Hurthle cells; may mimic papillary carcinoma.
- May coexist with papillary carcinoma, especially papillary microcarcinoma.

Histologic Features

- Typically diffuse involvement of the thyroid both grossly and microscopically but can be a localized process with a distinct nodular involvement.
- Thyroid follicles with oncocytic changes and epithelial atrophy.
- Lymphoplasmacytic infiltration of the stroma with many large lymphoid follicles, which contain prominent germinal centers (Fig. 3.15a–c).
- Lymphoplasmacytic cells infiltrating oncocytic follicular cells.
- Lymphoid cells, plasma cells, histiocytes, and scattered granulomas.
- Patchy fibrosis or extensive fibrosis with dense hyaline-type collagens.
- Squamous metaplasia is common.
- Cystic formation may be present.
- Reactive atypical follicles, which may mimic PTC (Fig. 3.15d).

Immunohistochemistry

- Reactive oncocytic follicular cells may be positive for galectin-3 and Hector Battifora mesothelial epitope-1 (HBME-1) but usually negative for cytokeratin (CK) 19 and tumor-associated calcium signal transducer 2 (TROP2).

Differential Diagnosis

- Papillary carcinoma
- Hurthle cell neoplasm
- Lymphoma
- Riedel's thyroiditis

Nodular Goiter

Clinical Features

- The most common benign lesion
- More common in middle-aged women

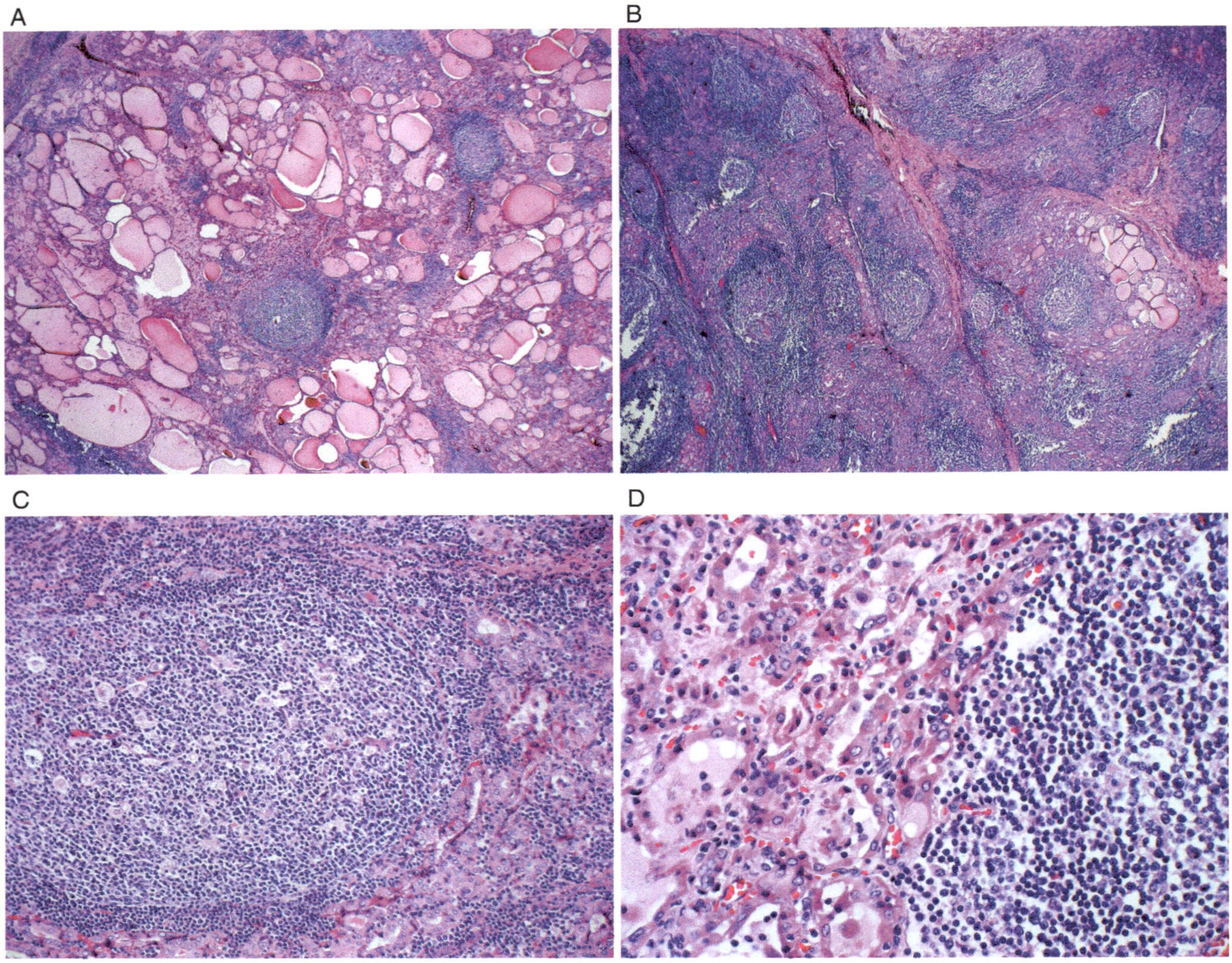

Fig. 3.15 Histologic sections of Hashimoto's thyroiditis with oncocytic follicular cells with lymphoid cell infiltration (**a**, **b**), prominent germinal center (**c**) and Hurthle cell/follicular cells with reactive atypia (**d**)

- Normal thyroid function; sometimes hyper- or hypothyroidism
- Goiter with multiple nodules

Cytological Features

- Abundant colloid and small amount of follicular cells (Figs. 3.16, 3.17, 3.18, 3.19, 3.20, and 3.21).
- Mixed population of follicular cells, Hurthle cells, and histiocytes.
- Pigment-laden histiocytes, foamy histiocytes, and stromal cells.
- Follicular cells are arranged in a honeycomb pattern with follicles of variable sizes.
- Focal reactive atypical follicular cells can be seen.

Histologic Features

- A wide spectrum of histologic changes can be seen (Fig. 3.22a–c).
- Multiple nodules, some surrounded by partial or even complete capsules.
- Huge follicles lined by flattened follicular epithelium, a mixture of follicles of variable sizes, cellular nodules with microfollicles, or cellular nodules with hyperplastic changes, including papillary formations.
- Focal or diffuse Hurthle cell changes.
- Secondary changes such as hemorrhage, cystic degeneration, fibrosis, calcification, or even ossification.
- Rupture of follicles with granulomatous reaction, foreign body-type multinucleated giant cells, and variable numbers of chronic inflammatory cells.

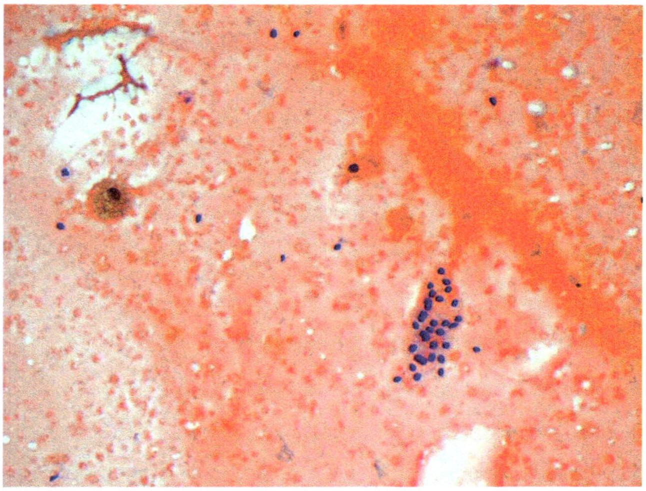

Fig. 3.16 Nodular goiter/hyperplasia with abundant watery colloid, benign follicular cells, and histiocytes (Pap stain)

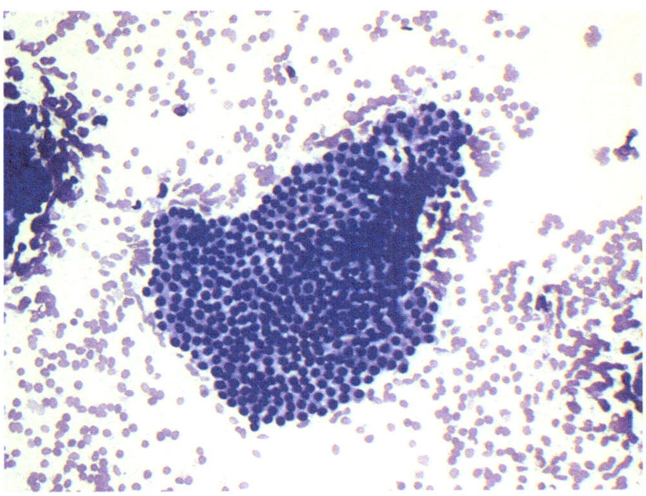

Fig. 3.17 Benign follicular cells in a nodular goiter/hyperplasia (DQ stain)

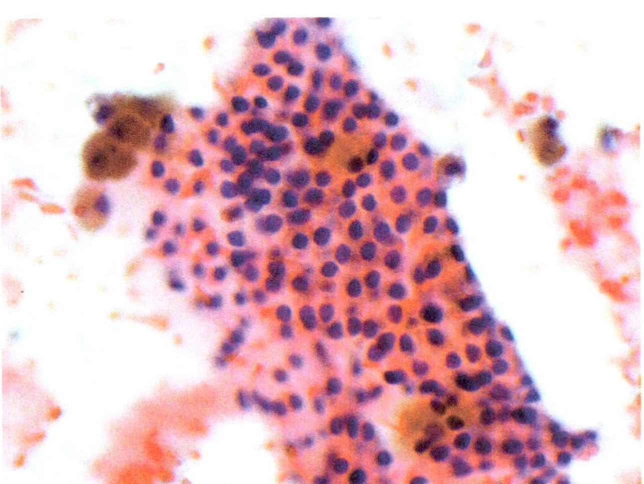

Fig. 3.18 Hurthle cells in a nodular goiter/hyperplasia (Pap stain)

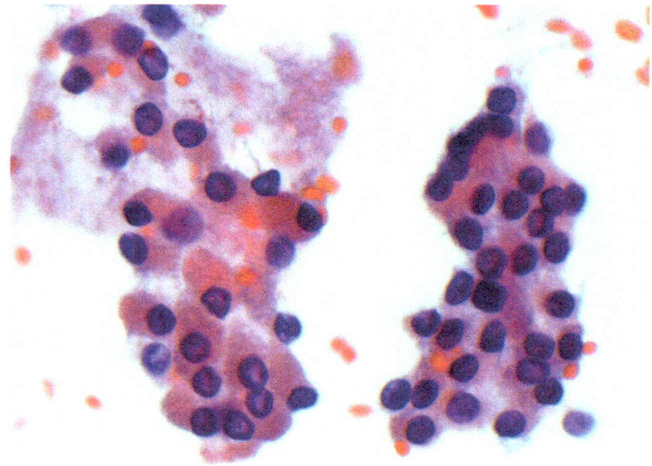

Fig. 3.19 Hurthle cells in a nodular goiter (Pap stain)

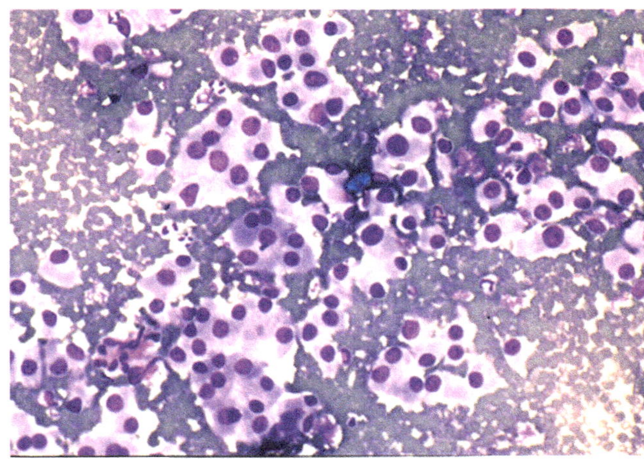

Fig. 3.20 Hurthle cells in a nodular goiter/hyperplasia (DQ stain)

Differential Diagnosis

- Follicular neoplasm
- Hurthle cell neoplasm
- Papillary carcinoma

Neoplastic Thyroid Lesions

Follicular Neoplasm

- Including follicular adenoma and follicular carcinoma

Follicular Adenoma

Clinical Features

- Common benign neoplasm
- More common in women
- Usually present with a solitary, well-circumscribed, mass

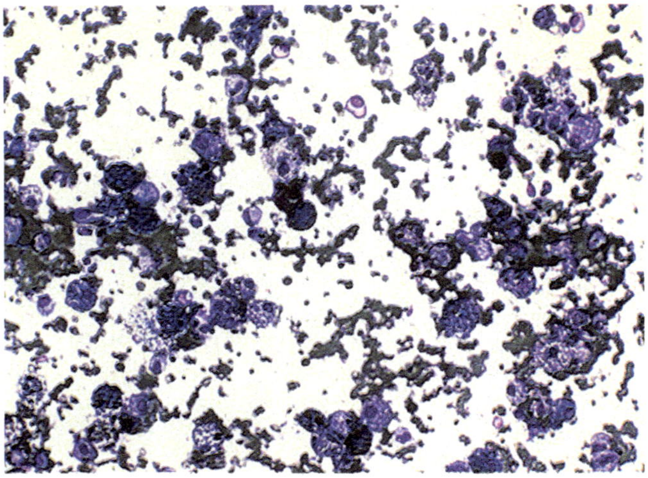

Fig. 3.21 Histiocytes in a nodular goiter/hyperplasia with degenerative change (DQ stain)

Cytological Features

- Hypercellular specimen with numerous groups of follicular cells and little or no colloid (Figs. 3.23 and 3.24).
- Microfollicular growth pattern (defined as 6–12 crowded follicular cells in a ring or rosette-like structure, with or without colloid in the center).
- Relatively uniform population of follicular cells without other types of cells, such as Hurthle cells and histiocytes.
- Follicular cells are enlarged in size with round nuclei.
- Focal nuclear atypia can be present.

Histologic Features

- A follicular nodule enclosed by a fibrous capsule of variable thickness (Fig. 3.25a).
- Absence of capsular or vascular invasion.

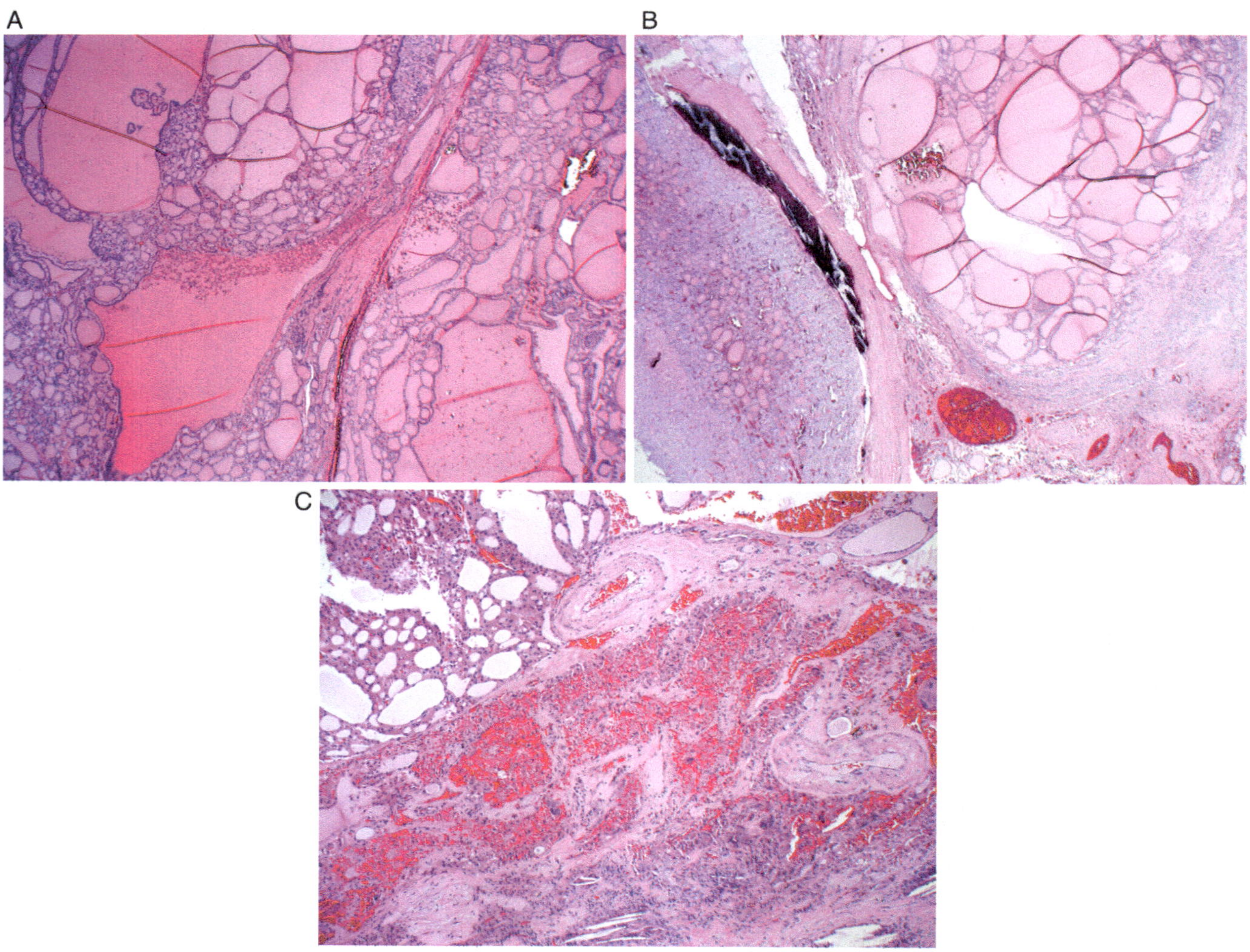

Fig. 3.22 Histologic sections of nodular goiter with Hurthle cells changes, calcification, and degenerative and regenerative changes

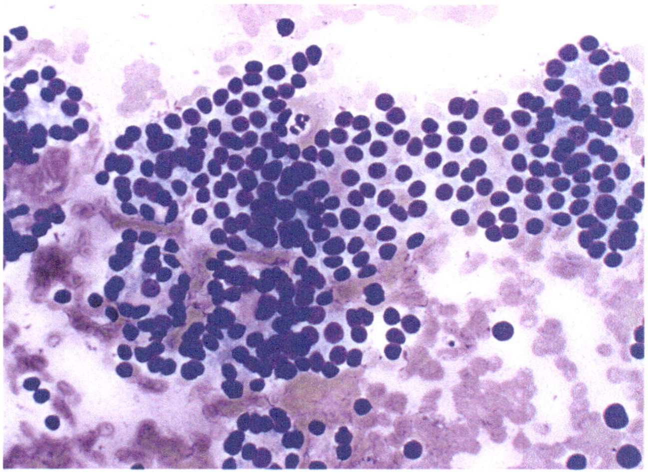

Fig. 3.23 Follicular neoplasm (DQ stain) with microfollicular growth pattern and lack of colloid in the background

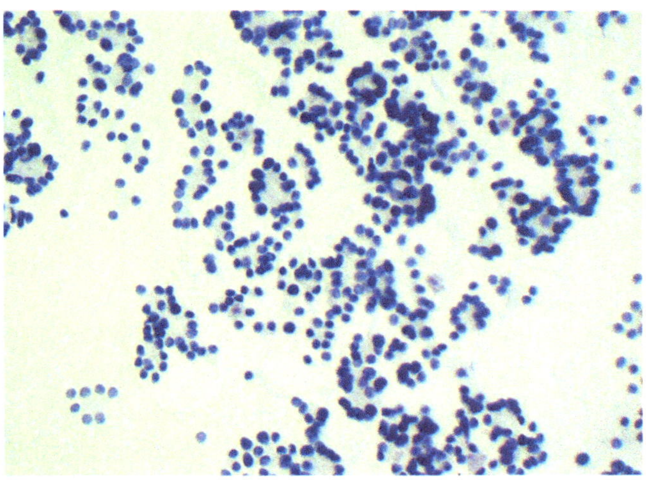

Fig. 3.24 Follicular neoplasm (DQ stain) with microfollicular growth pattern, nuclear enlargement, and nuclear crowding

- The architectural patterns may include microfollicular and solid (Fig. 3.25b), trabecular (Fig. 3.25c), normofollicular, and macrofollicular architectures (Fig. 3.25d).
- The tumor cells are cuboidal, columnar or polygonal, and frequently with uniform, dark, round nuclei.
- Foci of large nuclei or atypical nuclei with degenerative changes can be seen.
- Mitotic figures are rare.
- Many histologic variants have been described, such as clear cell follicular adenoma (Fig. 3.25e), oncocytic follicular adenoma, signet-ring cell follicular adenoma, lipoadenoma, mucinous follicular adenoma, follicular adenoma with bizarre nuclei (Fig. 3.25f), follicular adenoma with papillary hyperplasia, and hyperfunctioning follicular adenoma.
- Secondary changes, such as myxoid change, cyst formation, fibrosis, hyalinization, hemorrhage, cartilaginous metaplasia, ossification, and calcifications, can be seen.

Immunohistochemistry

- Positive for TTF1, PAX8, and thyroglobulin
- Negative for calcitonin and neuroendocrine markers
- Can be positive for HBME-1 and galectin-3; usually negative for CK19 and TROP2

Differential Diagnosis

- Cellular nodular goiter
- AUS/FLUS
- Follicular variant of papillary carcinoma

Follicular Carcinoma

Clinical Features

- More common in 40- to 60-year-old women.
- Accounts for 10% of thyroid carcinomas.
- A slow-growing neoplasm.
- Can be divided into two types: minimally invasive type which is rarely going for distant metastasis; another type is widely invasive type which is frequently goes for a distant metastasis and has a worse prognosis than papillary carcinoma of the thyroid.

Cytological Features (Figs. 3.26, 3.27, and 3.28)

- In general, there are no definitive criteria to separate follicular adenoma from follicular carcinoma on an FNA sample.
- Crowded and three-dimensional follicular structures.
- Microfollicles with irregular shapes and many single cells.
- Nuclear pleomorphism.
- Nuclear enlargement (three to four times that of normal follicular cells).
- Coarse and irregular nuclear chromatin.
- High nuclear-to-cytoplasmic ratio.
- Prominent and multiple nucleoli.
- Mitoses can be seen.

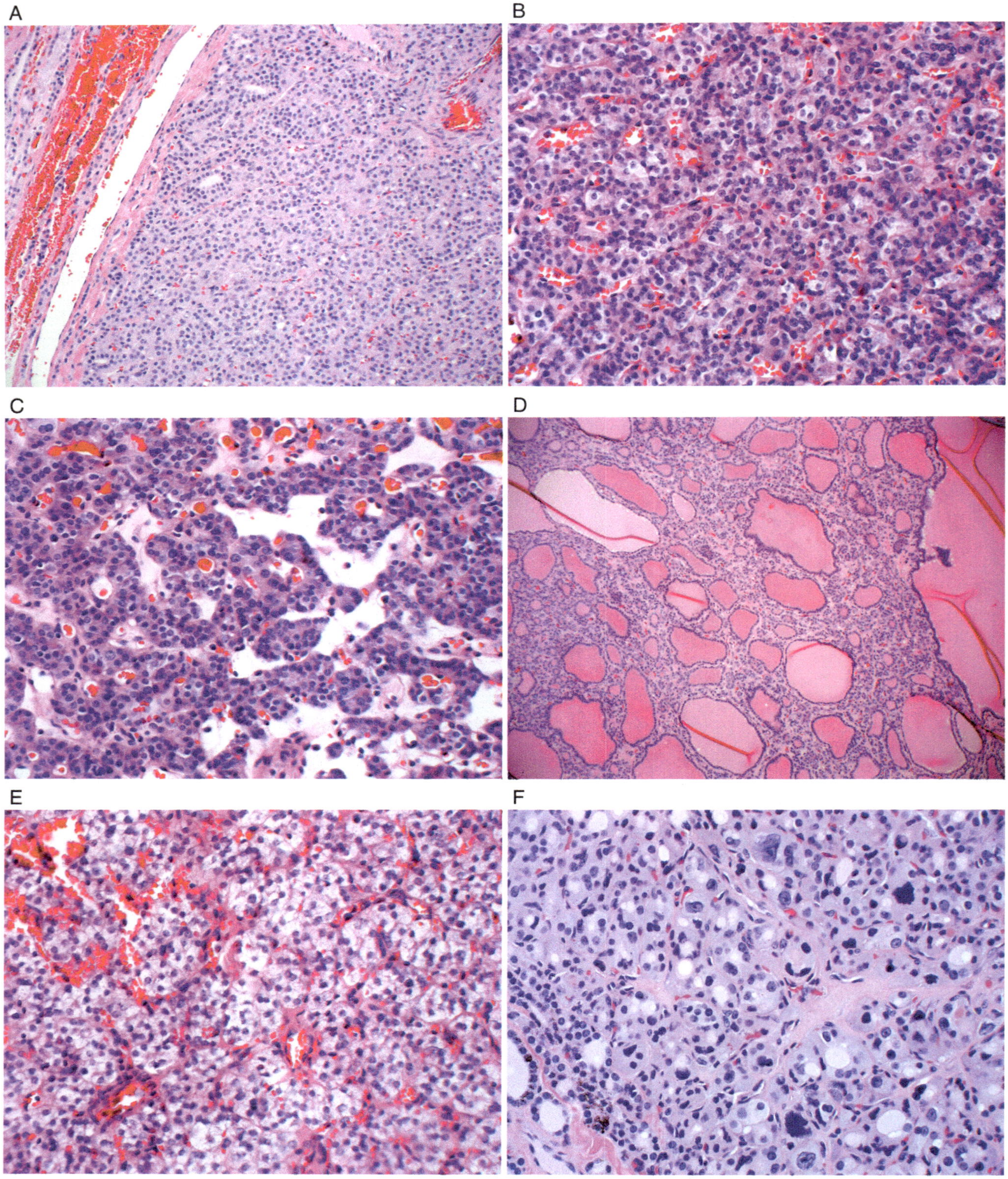

Fig. 3.25 Histologic sections of follicular adenoma with thin fibrous capsule (**a**), microfollicular and solid pattern (**b**), trabecular pattern (**c**), macrofollicular (**d**), clear cell changes (**e**), and bizarre nuclei (**f**)

Histologic Features

- A follicular nodule enclosed by a thick fibrous capsule showing definite capsular and/or vascular invasion.
- Lack of diagnostic nuclear features of PTC.
- Can have variable architectural patterns and cytological features.
- Classically, it can be divided into two categories: (1) minimally invasive follicular carcinoma with limited capsular invasive and vascular invasion (less than four vessels) and (2) widely invasive follicular carcinoma with widespread capsular and vascular invasion (greater than four vessels).

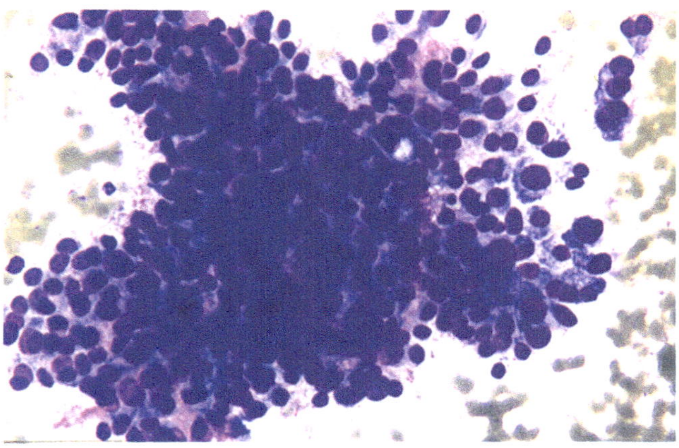

Fig. 3.26 Nuclear enlargement, crowding, and pleomorphism, suggestive of follicular carcinoma

- Fig. 3.29a–g shows some examples of capsular and vascular invasion.
- Oncocytic variant and clear cell variant have been described.

Immunohistochemistry

- Similar to follicular adenoma
- Can be positive for HBME-1 and galectin-3; usually negative for CK19 and TROP2

Differential Diagnosis

- Follicular adenoma
- Follicular variant of papillary carcinoma

Hurthle Cell Neoplasm (Figs. 3.30, 3.31, 3.32, and 3.33a–c)

- May be considered a subtype of follicular neoplasm
- Uniform population of Hurthle cells in small clusters and single cells
- Little or no colloid
- Prominent or small nucleoli
- Three-dimensional or crowded structures
- Features suggestive for Hurthle cell carcinoma, including nuclear pleomorphism, multiple and prominent nucleoli, high nuclear-to-cytoplasmic ratio, nuclear crowding, and mitoses

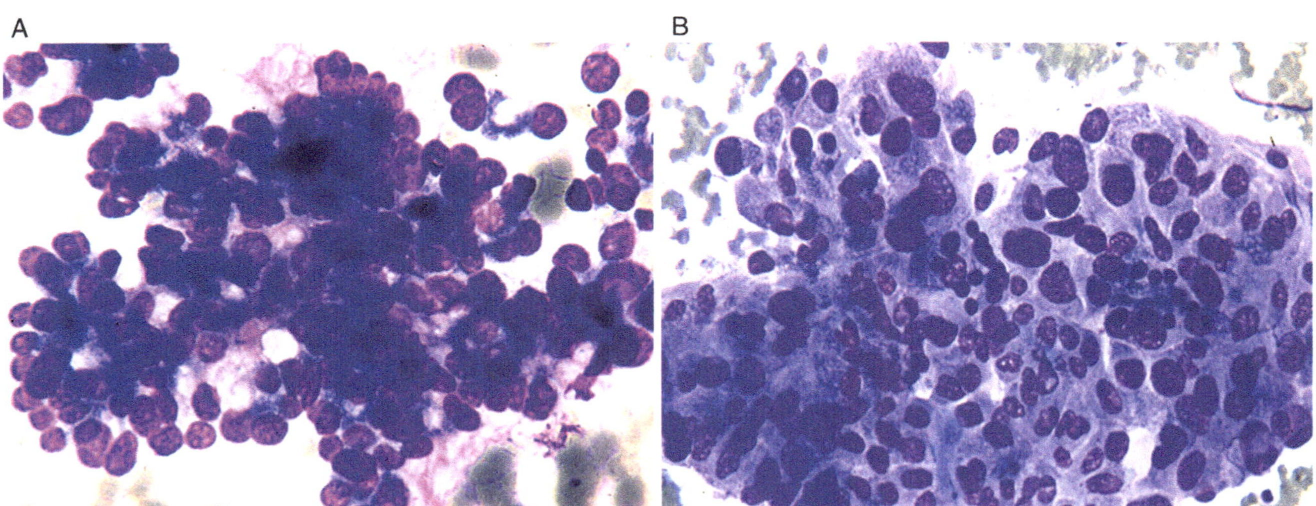

Fig. 3.27 Marked nuclear atypia, suggestive of follicular carcinoma (DQ stain)

Hyalinizing Trabecular Neoplasm

Clinical Features

- A rare tumor of follicular cell origin.
- The nuclear features of the tumor suggest that it may be related to PTC.
- Rearranged during transfection (RET)/PTC rearrangements have been reported in some tumors.
- Much more common in middle-aged women.

Cytological Features (Fig. 3.34a–d)

- Similar cytological features to papillary carcinoma.
- Hyalinizing material may be present between tumor cells.
- Tumor cells may be more elongated or even spindle.
- Nuclear grooves and intranuclear inclusions are frequent findings.
- Psammoma bodies can be seen.

Histologic Features

- A solid neoplasm with or without thin fibrous capsule.
- Trabecular or alveolar growth pattern.

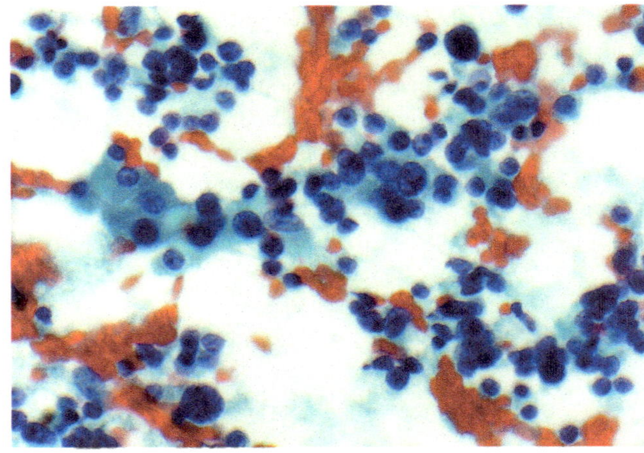

Fig. 3.28 Follicular carcinoma on Pap stain

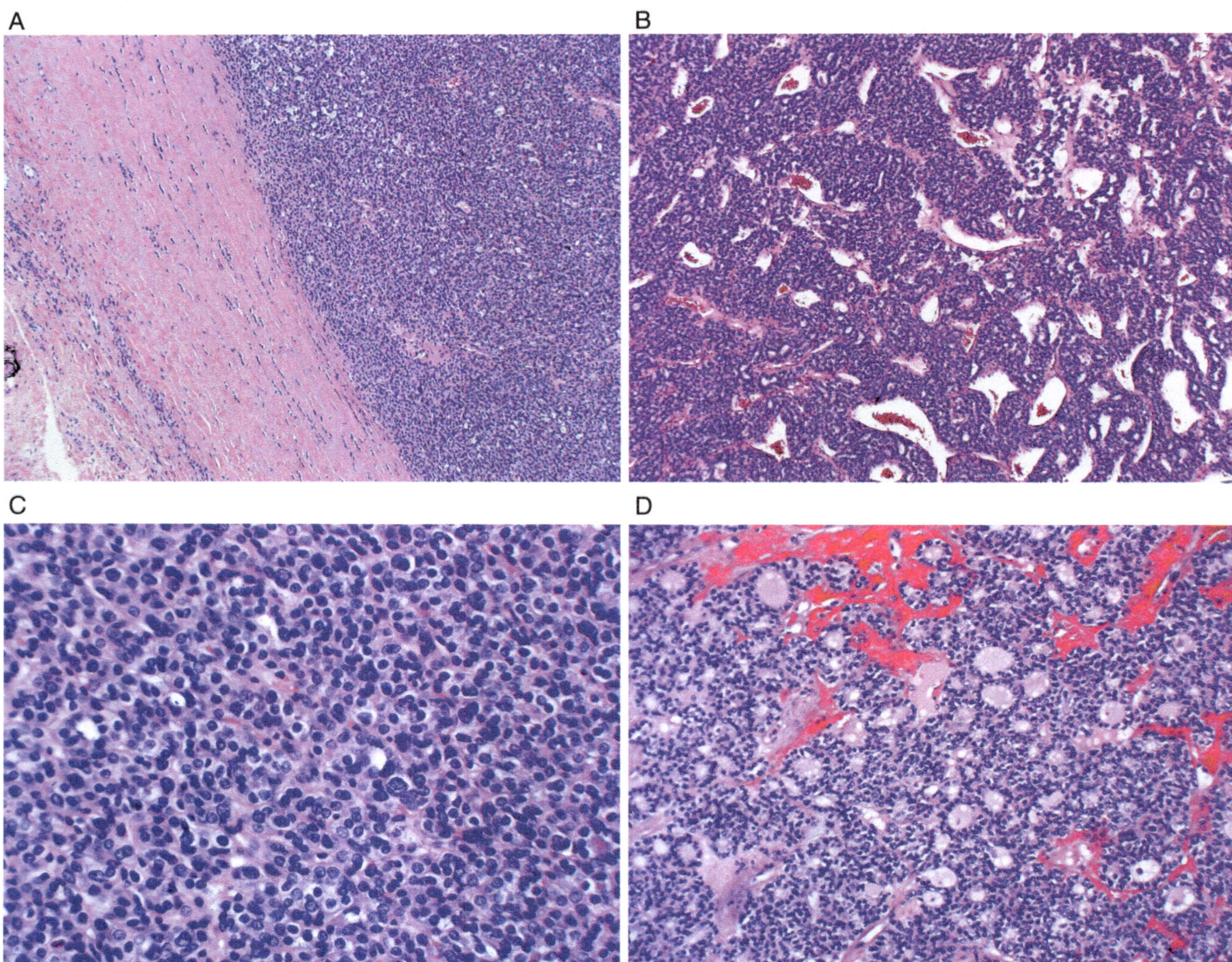

Fig. 3.29 Histology section of follicular carcinoma with capsular invasion (**e**) and vascular invasion (**f**, **g**)

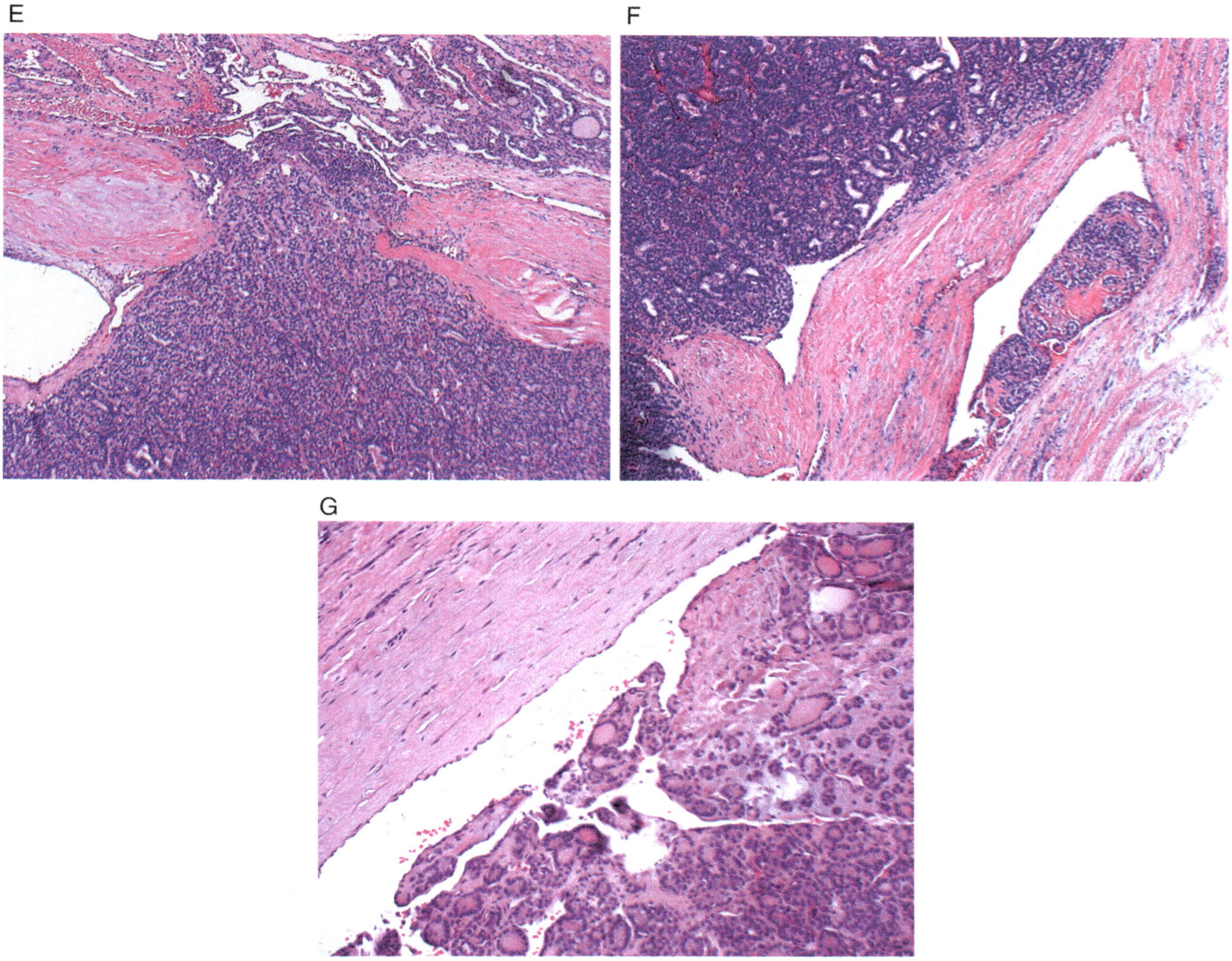

Fig. 3.29 (continued)

- Polygonal or spindle tumor cells, with granular to clear cytoplasm, with a prominent hyaline stroma between nests or trabeculae of tumors.
- Elongated nuclei, centrally located, with nuclear grooves and intranuclear pseudoinclusion (Fig. 3.35a, b).
- Mitotic figures are rarely seen; psammoma bodies may be present.
- Usually absence of colloid.

Immunohistochemistry

- MIB-1 (a specific clone for Ki-67) staining showing distinctive membranous staining pattern in the majority of cases (Fig. 3.35c)
- Frequently positive for galectin-3; can be positive for CK19
- Positive for TTF1 and PAX8 and negative for calcitonin and neuroendocrine markers

Differential Diagnosis

- Papillary carcinoma
- Medullary carcinoma
- Table 3.2 below summarizes useful markers for the distinction among these three tumors.

PTC (Papillary Thyroid Carcinoma)

Clinical Features

- Accounts for about 70% of malignant thyroid neoplasms.
- More common in young females, with female-to-male ratio of 4:1, especially under age 40.
- Slow growing; patient may survive for many years even after local lymph node metastasis.

- Papillary microcarcinoma is defined as a tumor 1 cm or less in diameter.
- Tall cell variant, columnar cell variant, diffuse sclerosing variant, and solid variant tend to show a more aggressive clinical behavior than a conventional PTC.

Cytological Features of Conventional PTC (Figs. 3.36, 3.37, 3.38, 3.39, 3.40, 3.41, 3.42, 3.43, 3.44, 3.45, 3.46, 3.47, and 3.48)

- Hypercellular specimen with three-dimensional or two-dimensional papillary structures
- Nuclear enlargement, overlapping, open nuclear chromatin, small and marginated nucleoli, nuclear grooves, and intranuclear cytoplasmic inclusions

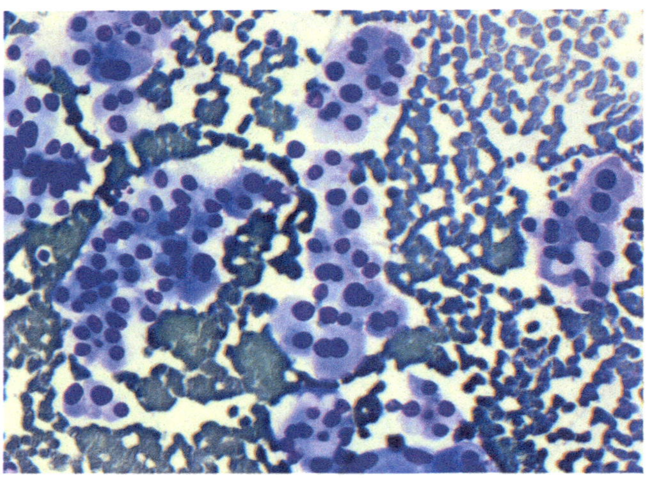

Fig. 3.30 Hurthle cell neoplasm with groups of Hurthle cells and absence of colloid in the background (DQ)

- Squamoid cytoplasm, oncocytic cytoplasm, or cytoplasm with small vacuoles
- Thick colloid or gummy colloid
- Multinucleated giant cells
- Psammoma bodies

Cytologic Features for Variants of PTC

Follicular Variant
- Resembles an FNA smear of follicular neoplasm.
- Tumor cells mostly arranged in microfollicles with absence or near absence of papillary structures.
- Nuclear features for PTC tend to be subtle when comparing to a classical PTC.
- Less intranuclear pseudoinclusions.
- Multinucleated giant cells, psammoma bodies, and cystic changes are usually absent.
- Follicular neoplasm and parathyroid neoplasm are included in the diagnostic consideration.

Tall Cell Variant
- Resembles a classic PTC.
- The tumor cells have an elongated shape, with a height-to-width ratio of 3:1 or greater (Fig. 3.49a, b).
- Classic nuclear features are needed to render a definitive diagnosis.

Columnar Cell Variant
- The neoplastic cells are arranged in papillae, groups, and sheets.
- The nuclei are elongated and stratified.
- The nuclear chromatin tends to be more hyperchromatic than open chromatin.
- The intranuclear inclusions are less prominent.
- Definitive nuclear changes for PTC are required to render a diagnosis.

A B

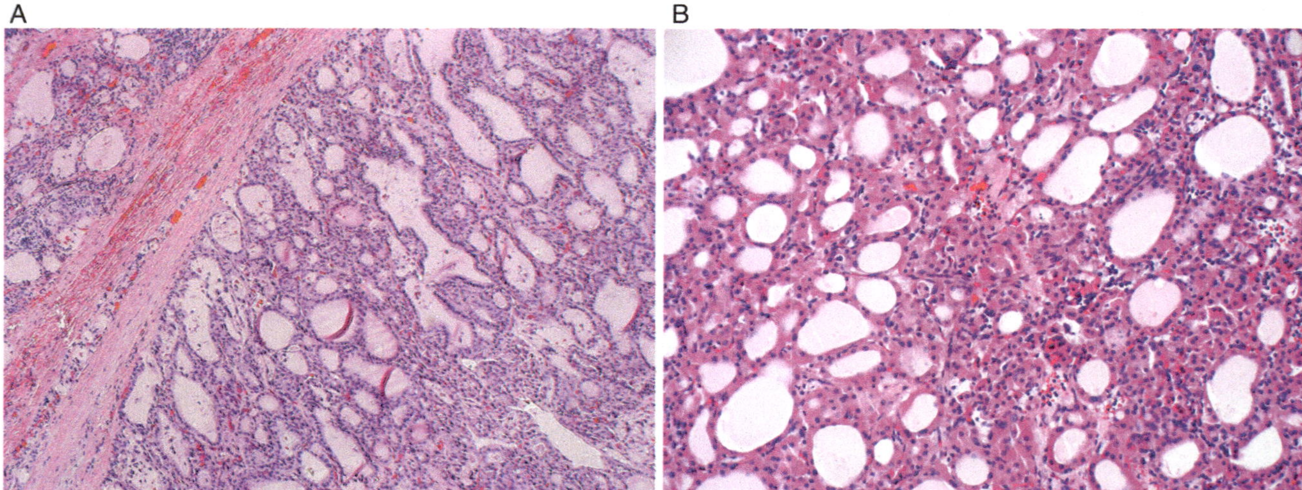

Fig. 3.31 Histology section of Hurthle cell adenoma

Macrofollicular Variant

- Resembles a benign colloid nodule on a low-power view with a mixture of sheets of follicular cells, some with microfollicular patterns, and abundant colloid.

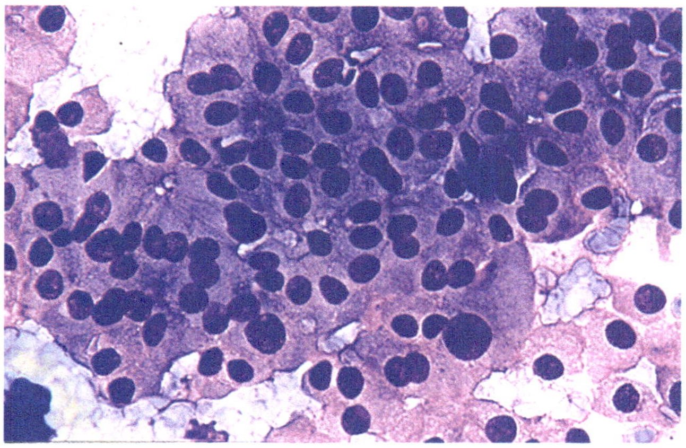

Fig. 3.32 Hurthle cell carcinoma on FNA smear (DQ)

- Diagnosis is based on the observation of nuclear changes for PTC at higher magnification. In general, these tend to be subtle.

Oncocytic Variant

- Resembles Hurthle cell proliferation, including Hurthle cell neoplasm.
- The majority of tumor cells contain abundant oncocytic cytoplasm and are isolated or arranged in sheets or papillae.
- Classic nuclear changes for PTC, including intranuclear inclusions.
- Absence of lymphoid cells.
- Nucleoli tend to be more conspicuous than in a conventional PTC; however, prominent nucleoli, frequently seen in a Hurthle cell neoplasm, are not typical features for an oncocytic variant of PTC.

Cystic Variant

- Resembles a colloid cyst with very low cellularity or mainly hemosiderin-laden histiocytes and clear background.

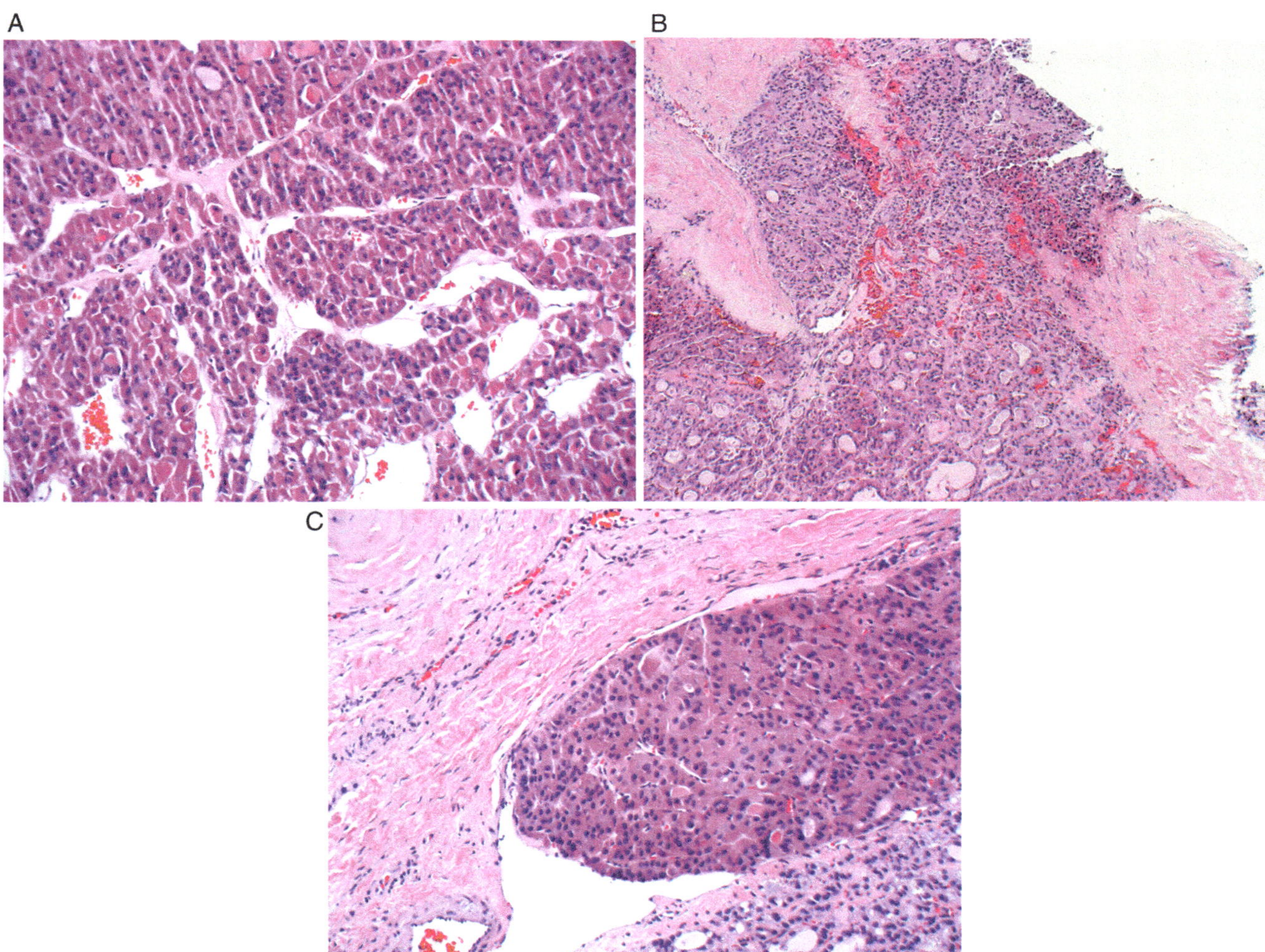

Fig. 3.33 Histologic sections of Hurthle cell carcinoma (a) with capsular (b) and vascular invasion (c)

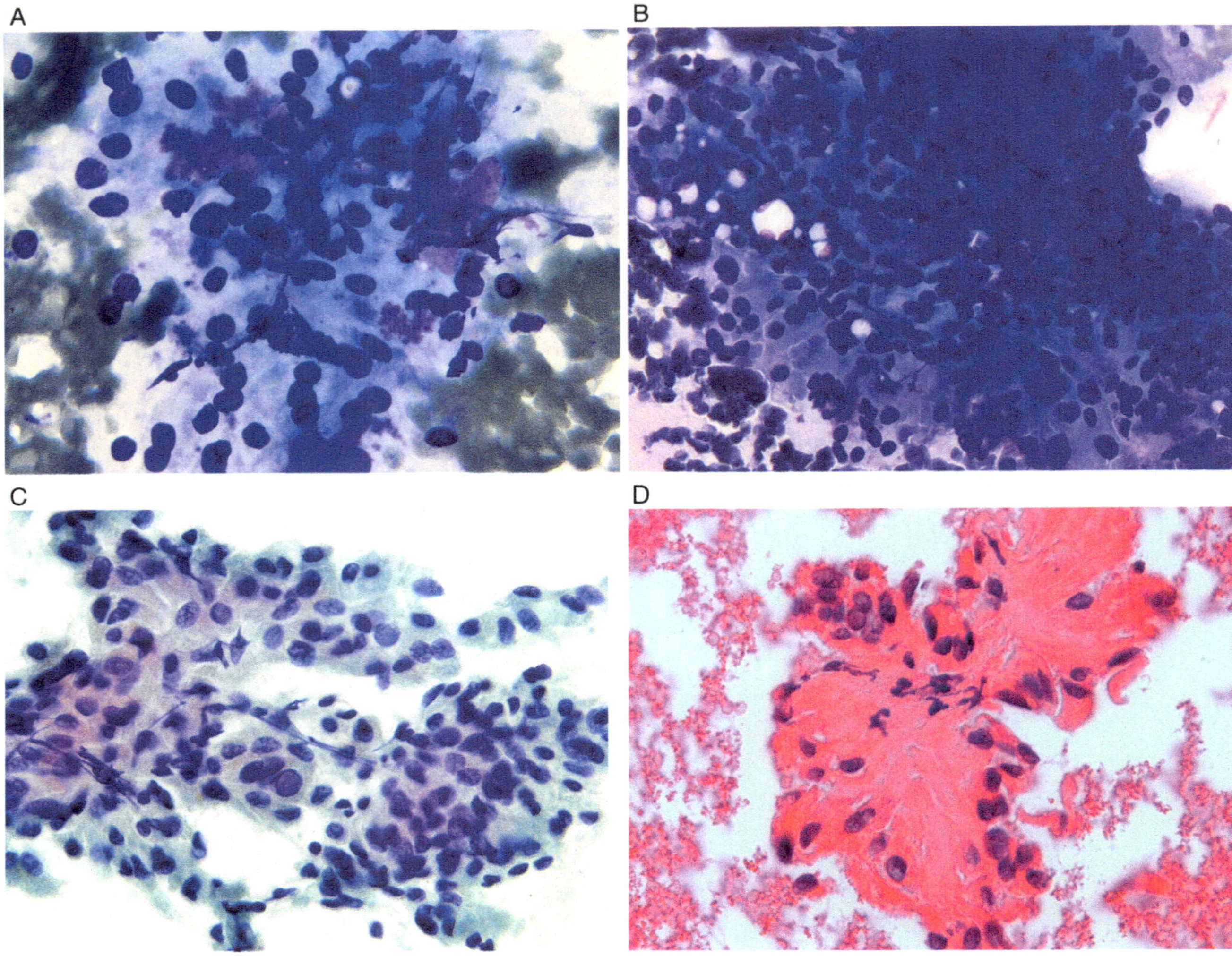

Fig. 3.34 Hyalinizing trabecular adenoma with many cytological features of PTC, including intranuclear inclusion. Note that eosinophilic hyalinizing material between cells (**a**, DQ) and cellblock (**d**)

- Only a few groups of neoplastic follicular cells are present, and they are usually arranged in a small groups, sheets, papillae, or follicles (Fig. 3.49c).
- The tumor cells may show "histiocytoid" features with cytoplasmic vacuoles.
- Identification of diagnostic nuclear features for PTC, including intranuclear inclusions, is required to render a diagnosis.

Warthin-Like Variant

- Resembles Hashimoto's thyroiditis.
- Oncocytic tumor cells arranged in sheets, groups, and papillary and follicular structures.
- Lymphoplasmacytic background with lymphoid cells and plasma cells intimately associated with tumor cells (Fig. 3.49d).
- Classic nuclear features for PTC are required to render a diagnosis.

Histologic Features

- The characteristic nuclear features mentioned above are the key to making a diagnosis.
- Complex papillary architectures with branching and squamous metaplasia are commonly seen.
- The papillae may have markedly edematous changes.
- Cystic changes are frequent.
- Psammoma is frequently present.
- Many histologic variants are present: (1) follicular variant (Fig. 3.50a), (2) oncocytic variant, (3) tall cell variant (Fig. 3.50b, c), (4) columnar cell variant, (5) diffuse sclerosing variant, (6) clear cell variant, (7) solid variant, (8) cystic variant (Fig. 3.50d, e), (9) cribriform variant (Fig. 3.50f, g), (10) macrofollicular variant, and (11) Warthin-like variant (Fig. 3.50h).

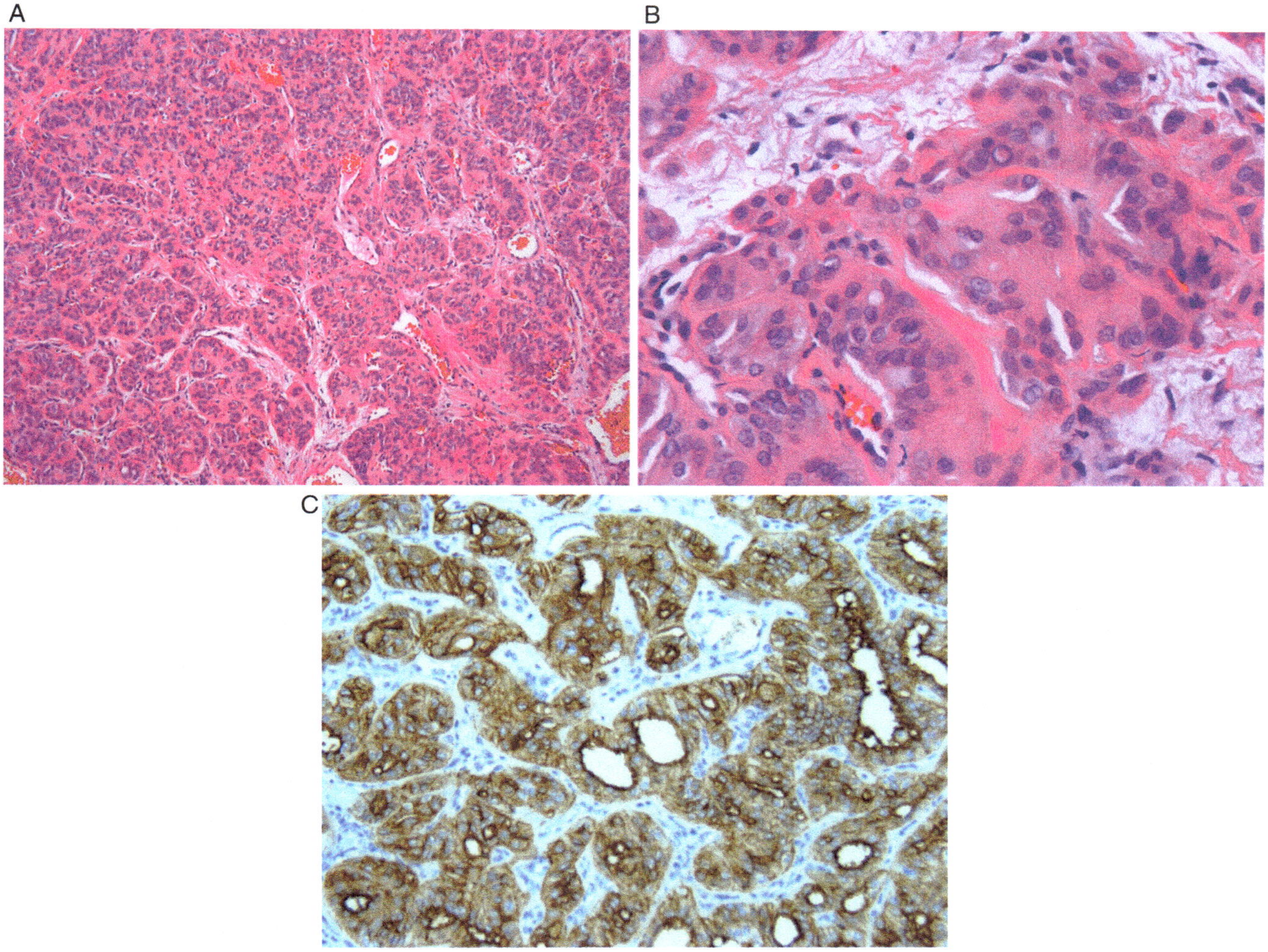

Fig. 3.35 Hyalinizing trabecular adenoma. Histologic sections showing elongated nuclei, centrally located with nuclear grooves and intranuclear pseudoinclusion (**a**, **b**). Note that MIB-1 (Ki-67) immunostain on histology section showing distinct membranous staining pattern (**c**)

Table 3.2 Differentiation of hyalinizing trabecular neoplasm, papillary carcinoma, and medullary carcinoma by immunostains

Marker	Hyalinizing trabecular neoplasm	Papillary carcinoma	Medullary carcinoma
Thyroglobulin	+	+	−
Calcitonin	−	−	+
MIB-1 (Ki-67)	Membranous	Nuclear	Nuclear

- A small proportion of papillary carcinomas may show a combination of histologic variants, with focus/foci of (1) insular carcinoma, (2) squamous cell carcinoma, (3) mucoepidermoid carcinoma, (4) spindle cell and giant cell carcinoma, (5) and medullary carcinoma.

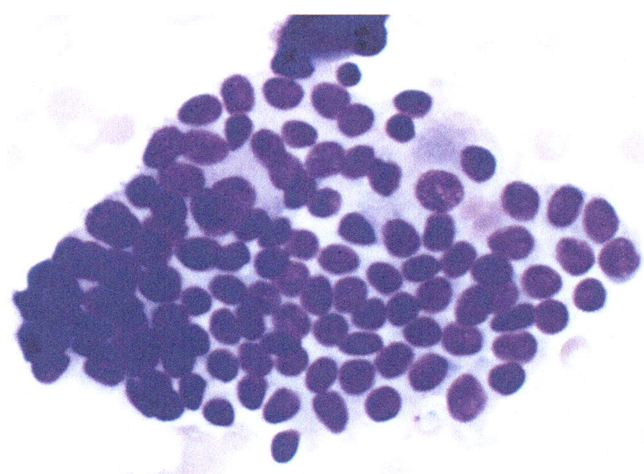

Fig. 3.36 Papillary carcinoma with two-dimensional papillary structure (DQ stain)

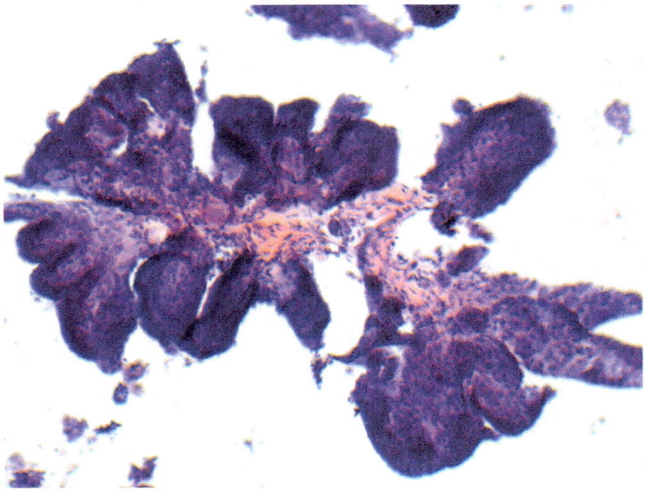

Fig. 3.37 Papillary carcinoma with three-dimensional papillary fronds (DQ stain)

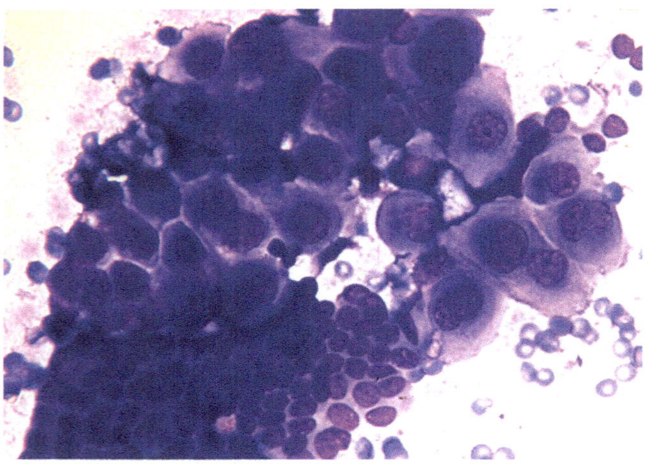

Fig. 3.38 Papillary carcinoma with nuclear enlargement and squamoid cytoplasm (DQ stain)

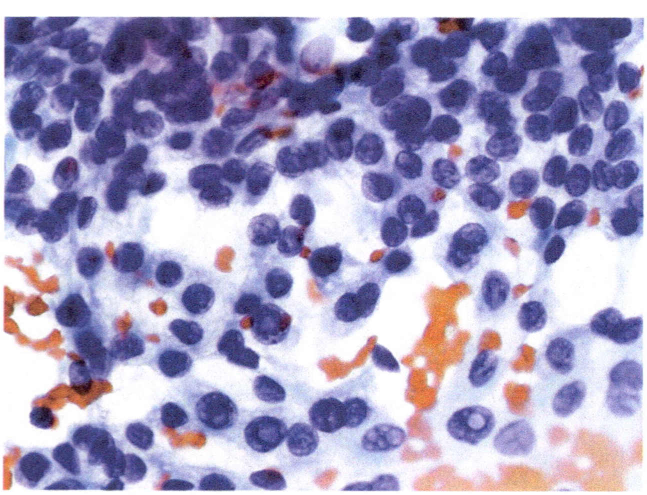

Fig. 3.39 Papillary carcinoma with nuclear enlargement, overlapping, nuclear grooves, and intranuclear inclusions (Pap stain)

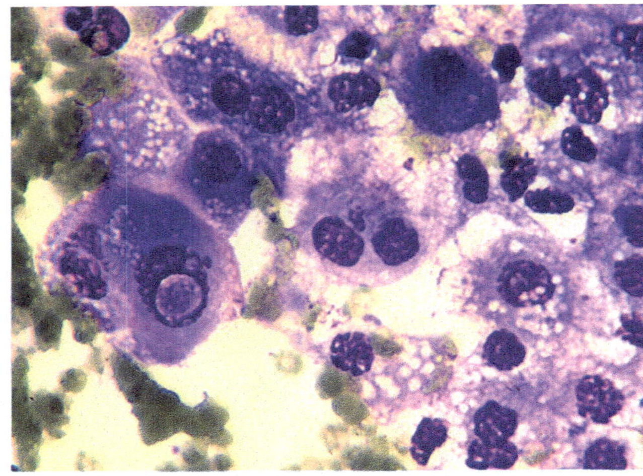

Fig. 3.40 Papillary carcinoma with squamoid cytoplasm and septated cytoplasmic vacuoles and intranuclear cytoplasmic inclusion (DQ stain)

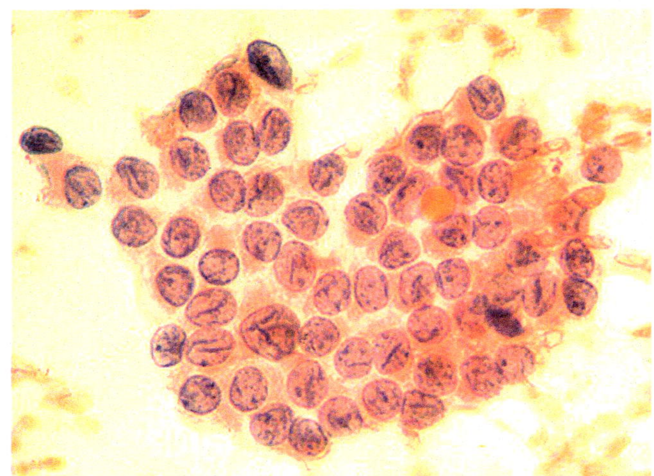

Fig. 3.41 Papillary carcinoma with open nuclear chromatin, grooves, and intranuclear cytoplasmic inclusions (Pap stain)

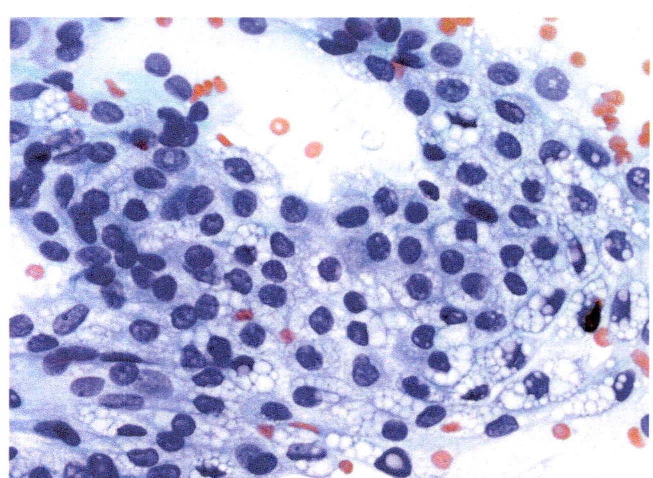

Fig. 3.42 Papillary carcinoma. Cytoplasmic vacuoles (Pap stain)

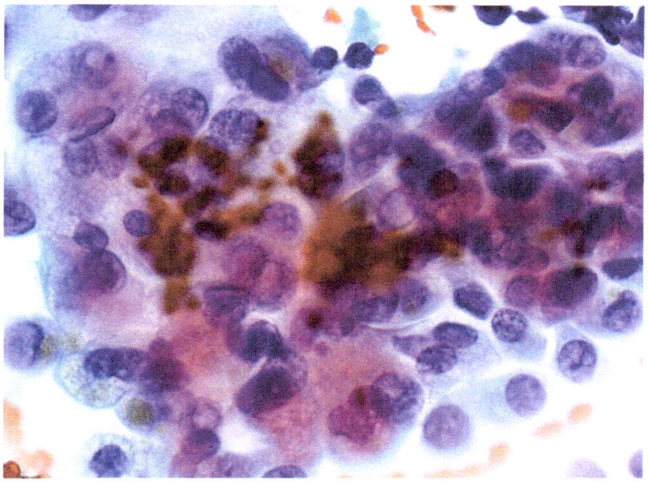

Fig. 3.43 Papillary carcinoma. Squamoid cytoplasm (Pap stain)

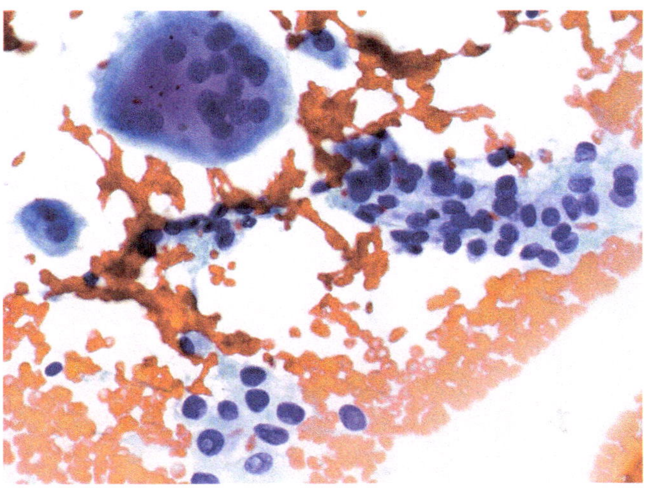

Fig. 3.44 Papillary carcinoma. Multinucleated giant cells (Pap stain)

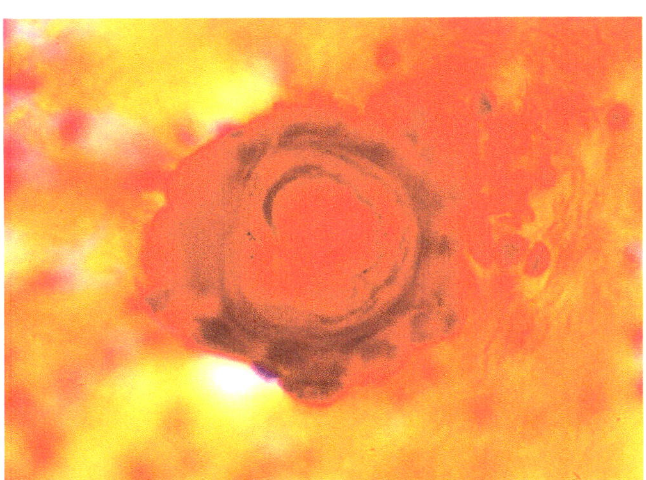

Fig. 3.45 Papillary carcinoma. Psammoma body (Pap stain)

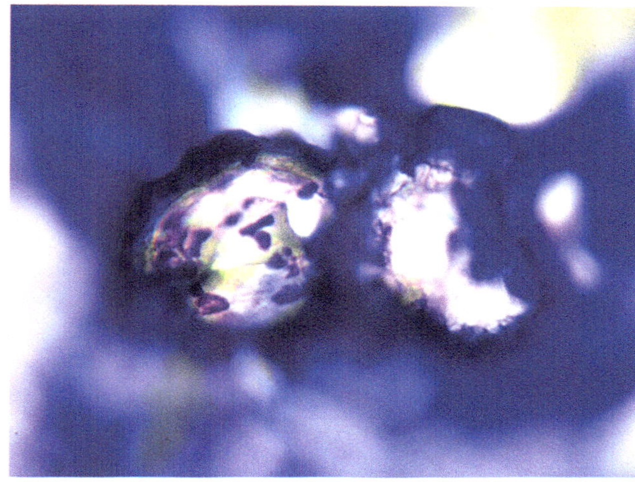

Fig. 3.46 Papillary carcinoma. Psammoma body (DQ stain)

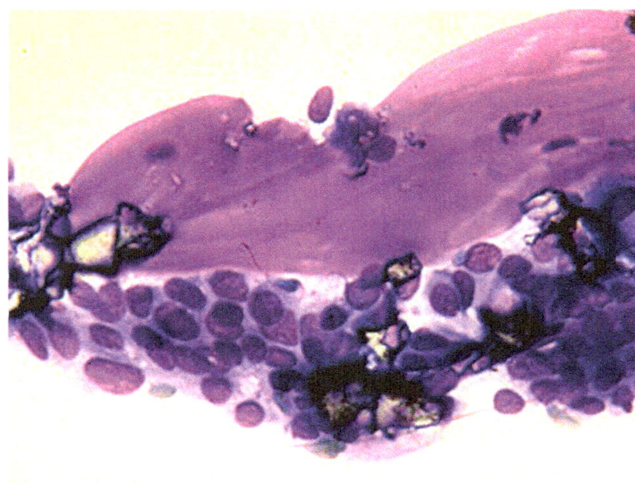

Fig. 3.47 Papillary carcinoma. Gummy/sticky colloid (DQ stain)

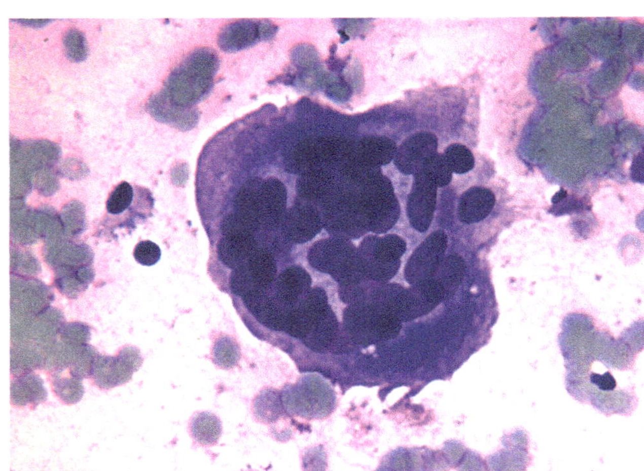

Fig. 3.48 Papillary carcinoma. Multinucleated giant cells (DQ stain)

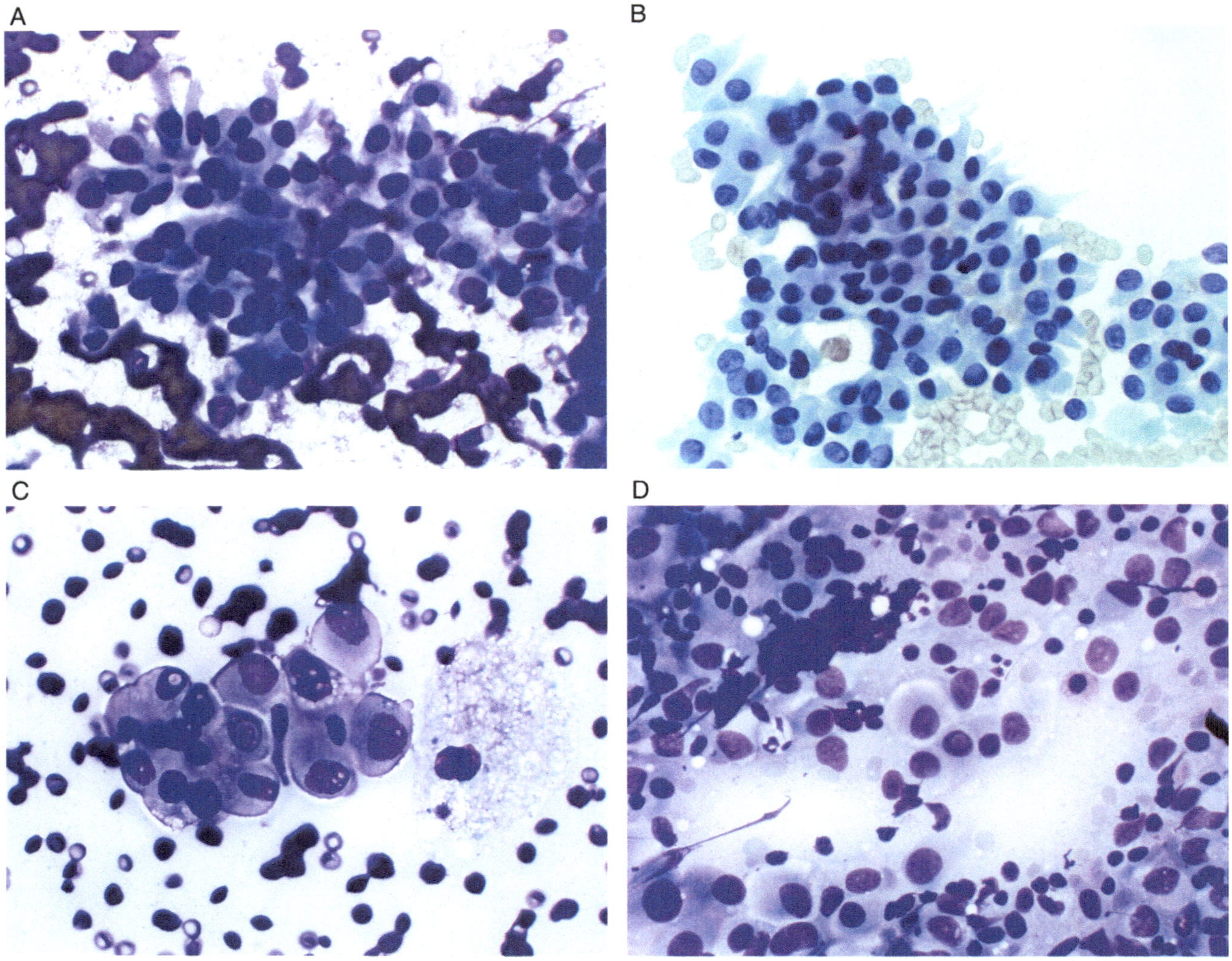

Fig. 3.49 Cytologic features of some variants, tall cell variant (**a**, **b**), cystic variant (**c**), and Warthin-like variant (**d**)

Immunohistochemistry

- Positive for thyroglobulin, TTF1, vimentin, and PAX8; negative for neuroendocrine markers and calcitonin.
- Calectin-3, CK19, HBME-1, and TROP2 are a useful panel of markers for the diagnosis of papillary carcinoma as summarized in Table 3.3. However, no single marker in this panel is entirely sensitive or specific for papillary carcinoma.
- Antibodies to RET/PTC rearrangement and BRAF mutation can be useful as well.
- An example of micropapillary PTC on FNA smear, CB, and positive for CK19, HBME-1, and TROP2 was shown in Fig. 3.51a–e. The histologic section was shown in Fig. 3.51f, g.

Molecular Alterations of Thyroid Tumors of Follicular Cell Origin

Table 3.4 summarizes the common genetic alterations reported in thyroid tumors of follicular cell origin.

Differential Diagnosis

- Atypical follicular cells in nodular goiter or Hashimoto's thyroiditis
- Hyalinizing trabecular neoplasm
- Medullary carcinoma
- Follicular carcinoma

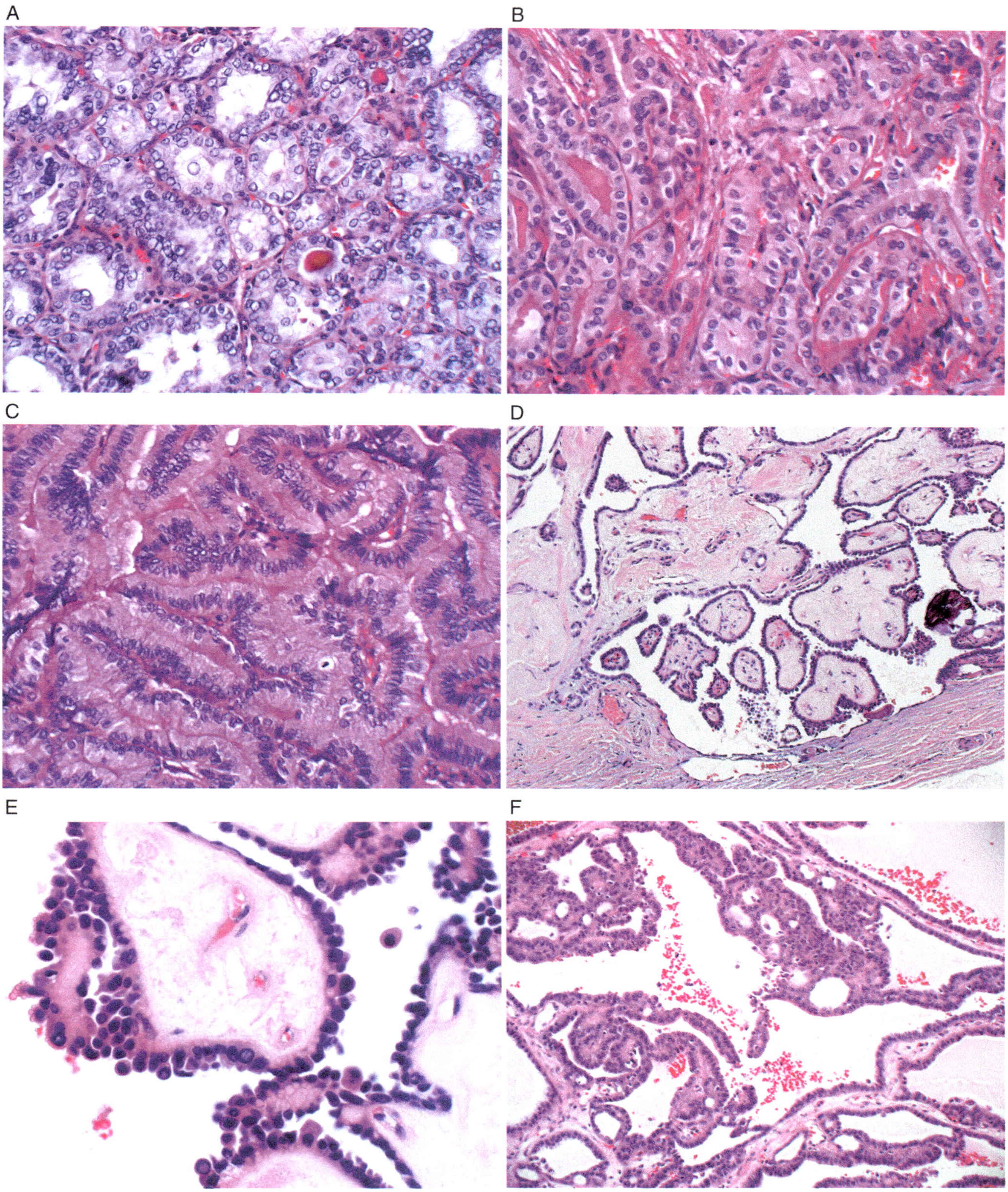

Fig. 3.50 Histologic sections of follicular variant (**a**), tall cell variant (**b**, **c**), cystic variant (**d**, **e**), cribriform variant (**f**, **g**), and Warthin-like variant (**h**)

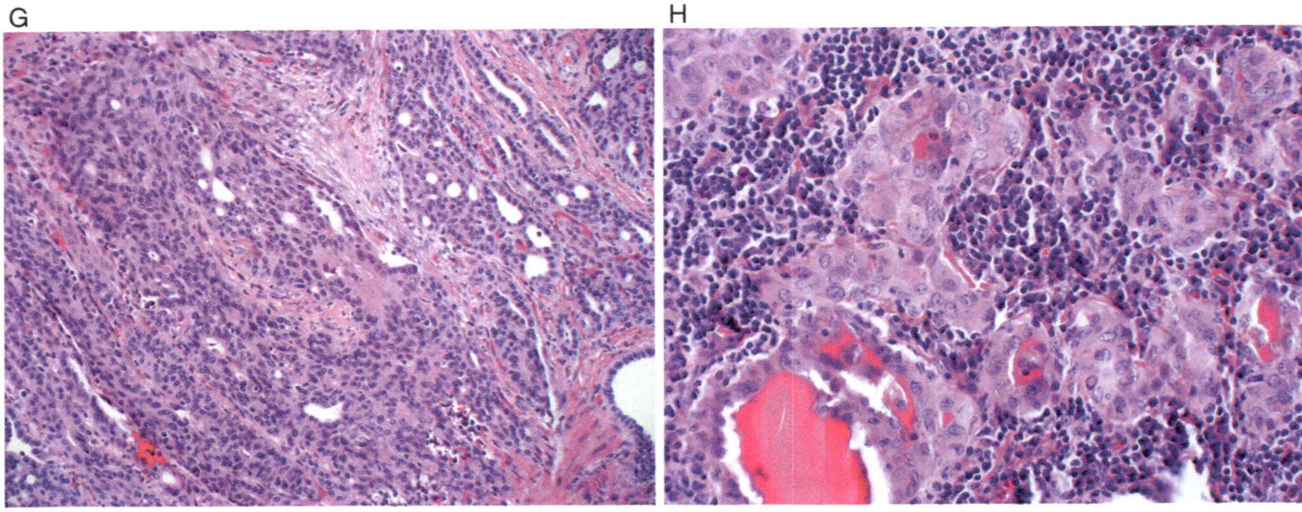

Fig. 3.50 (continued)

Table 3.3 Differentiation of PTC, follicular variant PTC, follicular adenoma, and reactive atypia by immunostains

Marker	PTC	Follicular variant PTC	Follicular adenoma	Reactive atypia
Galectin-3	+	+	−/+	−/+
CK19	+	+/−	−	−
HBME-1	+	+	−/+	−
TROP2	+	+/−	−	−

Medullary Carcinoma

Clinical Features

- Accounts for 5–10% of malignant thyroid neoplasms.
- More common in ages 40–60, male-to-female ratio is 2:3.
- Most cases are associated with RET oncogene in chromosome 10 q11.2.
- Associated with autosomal dominant trait in some patients.
- Over 90% of tumors secrete calcitonin.
- Painless thyroid mass.
- C-cell hyperplasia is the precursor of heritable medullary carcinoma.

Cytological Features (Fig. 3.52a–i)

- Mixed population of epithelioid and spindle neoplastic cells.
- The tumor cells can be predominately single or in clusters, including sheets, follicles, microfollicles, rosettes, cords, or papillae.
- Plasmacytoid cells with binucleation or multinucleation or bizarre cells.
- Small to inconspicuous nucleoli.
- Salt-and-pepper nuclear chromatin.
- Intranuclear cytoplasmic inclusions.
- Intracytoplasmic inclusions can be seen.
- Amyloid in the background.

Histologic Features (Fig. 3.53a–d)

- Variable histologic growth patterns and architectures, including sheets, nests, trabeculae, pseudopapillary, follicular, and solid.
- Polygonal, epithelioid, oncocytic, clear, spindle, melanotic, and small tumor cells or a mixture of different types of cells.
- Salt-and-pepper chromatin, granular cytoplasm, and small nucleoli are common.
- Prominent nucleoli are observed in oncocytic variant.
- Intranuclear inclusions are frequently seen.
- Intracytoplasmic lumen and mucin production have been reported.
- Amyloid stroma has been reported in 80% of cases; giant cell reaction and calcification may be present.
- Tumor necrosis and hemorrhage are uncommon.
- Focal nuclear pleomorphism may be present but does not indicate a more clinical aggressiveness.

Immunohistochemistry

- 95% of cases positive for calcitonin.
- Over 95% of cases positive for carcinoembryonic antigen (CEA).

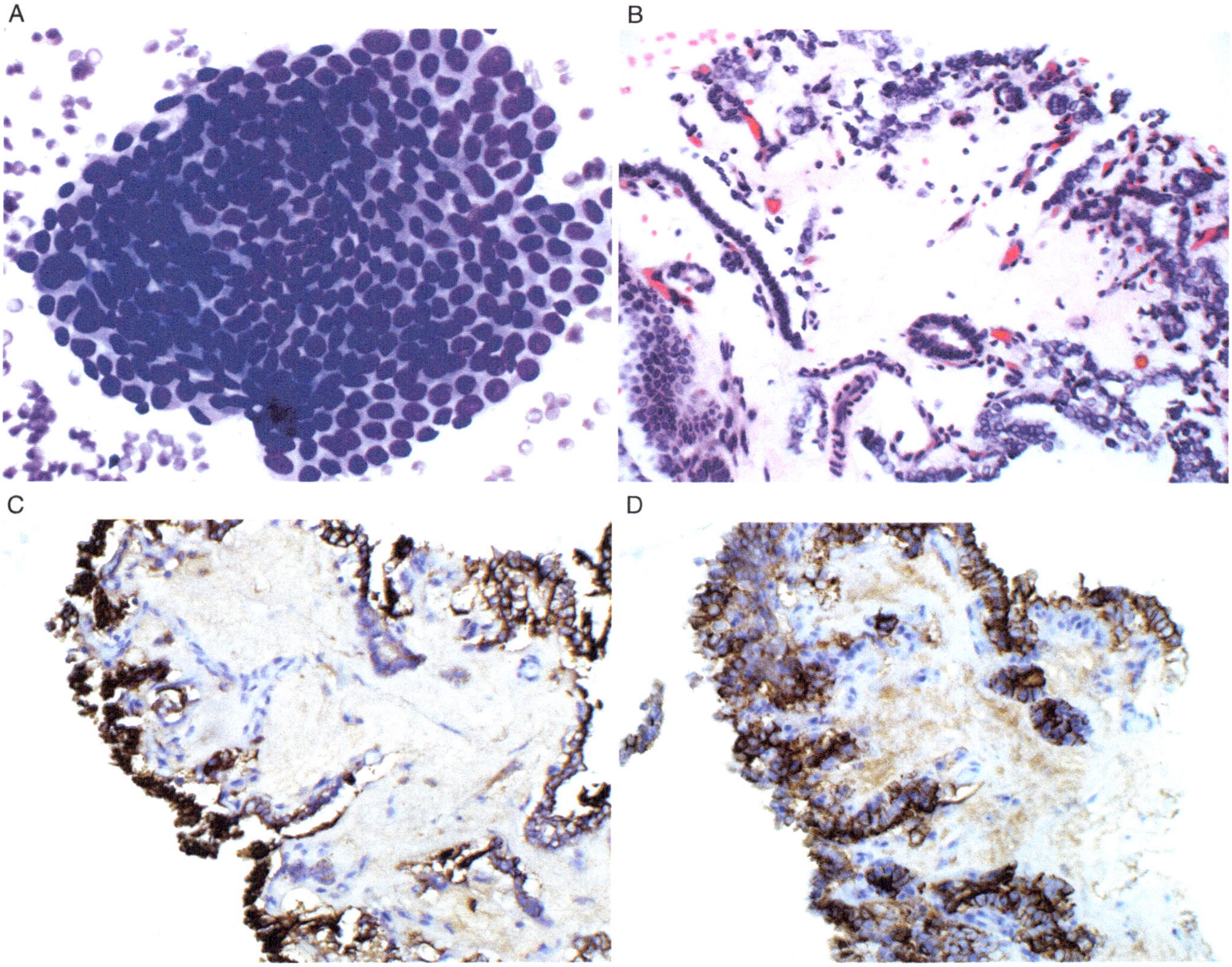

Fig. 3.51 Example of micropapillary carcinoma on FNA smear (**a**), cellblock (**b**), positive for CK19 (**c**), HBME-1 (**d**), and TROP2 (**e**), and the histologic section (**f**, **g**)

- Usually weakly positive for TTF1.
- Positive for chromogranin and synaptophysin.
- Negative for thyroglobulin and PAX8.
- An example of IHC is shown in Fig. 3.54a–c.

Differential Diagnosis

- Insular carcinoma/poorly differentiated carcinoma of the thyroid
- Anaplastic carcinoma of the thyroid
- Hyalinizing trabecular neoplasm
- Metastasis

Poorly Differentiated (Insular) Carcinoma

Clinical Features

- More common in elderly patients
- Prognosis better than anaplastic carcinoma but worse than papillary and follicular carcinoma

Cytological Features (Fig. 3.55a–c)

- Relatively uniform population of neoplastic cells.
- Single or small clusters of neoplastic cells.

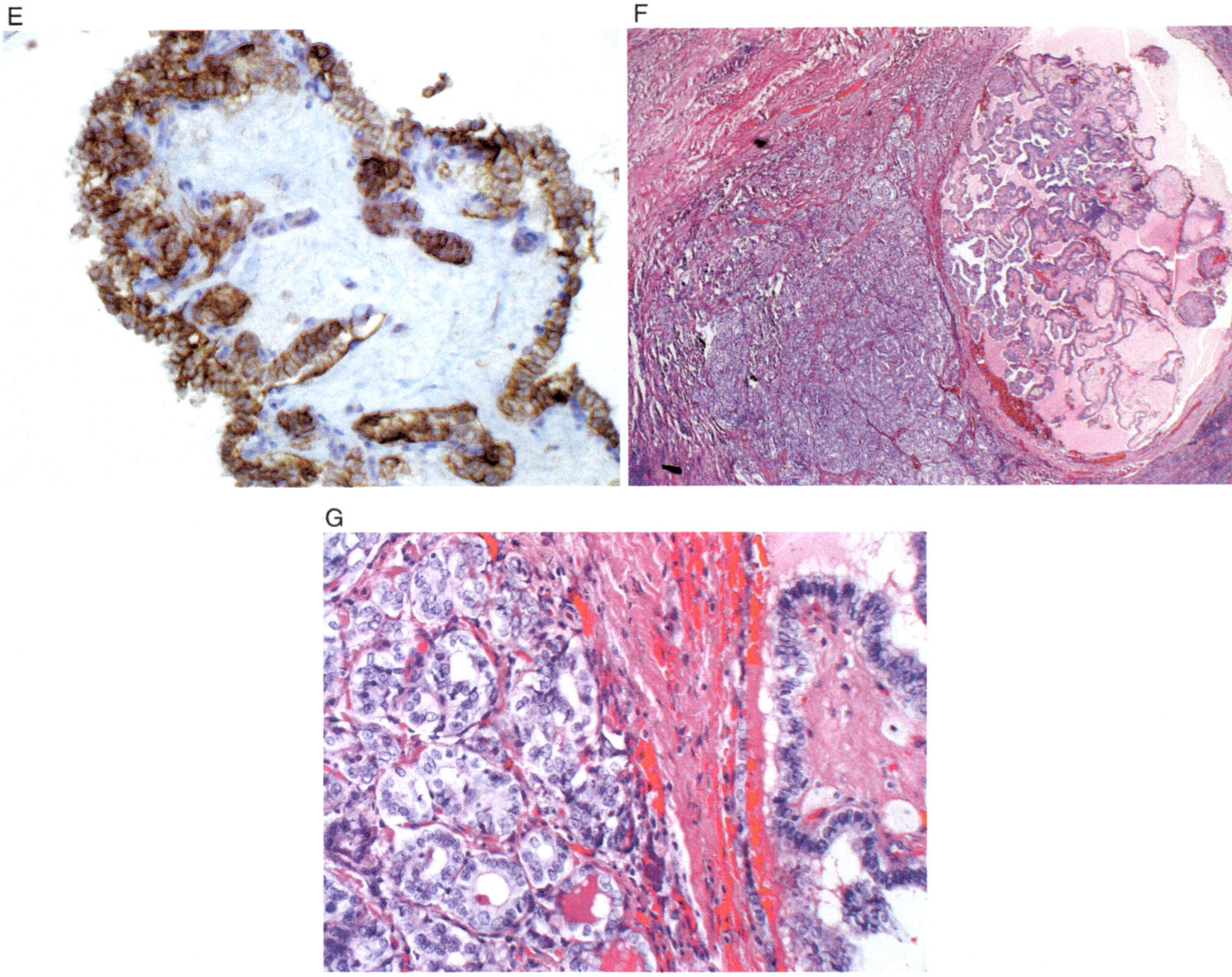

Fig. 3.51 (continued)

Table 3.4 Common molecular alterations in thyroid tumors of follicular cells

Diagnosis	Molecular alterations							
	BRAF	RET/PTC	RAS	PAX8-PARr	PIK3CA	B-catenin (CTNNB1)	TP53	PTEN
Papillary carcinoma	30–70%	20%	10%	–	–	–	–	–
Papillary carcinoma-encapsulated follicular variant	5–10%	5–10%	25–45%	0–30%	–	–	–	–
Follicular adenoma	–	–	20–40%	5–20%	–	–	–	–
Follicular carcinoma	–	–	45%	35%	<10%	–	–	<10%
Poorly differentiated (insular) carcinoma	5–15%	–	35%	–	–	20%	20%	–
Undifferentiated (anaplastic) carcinoma	25%	–	55%	–	5–25%	65%	70%	5–20%

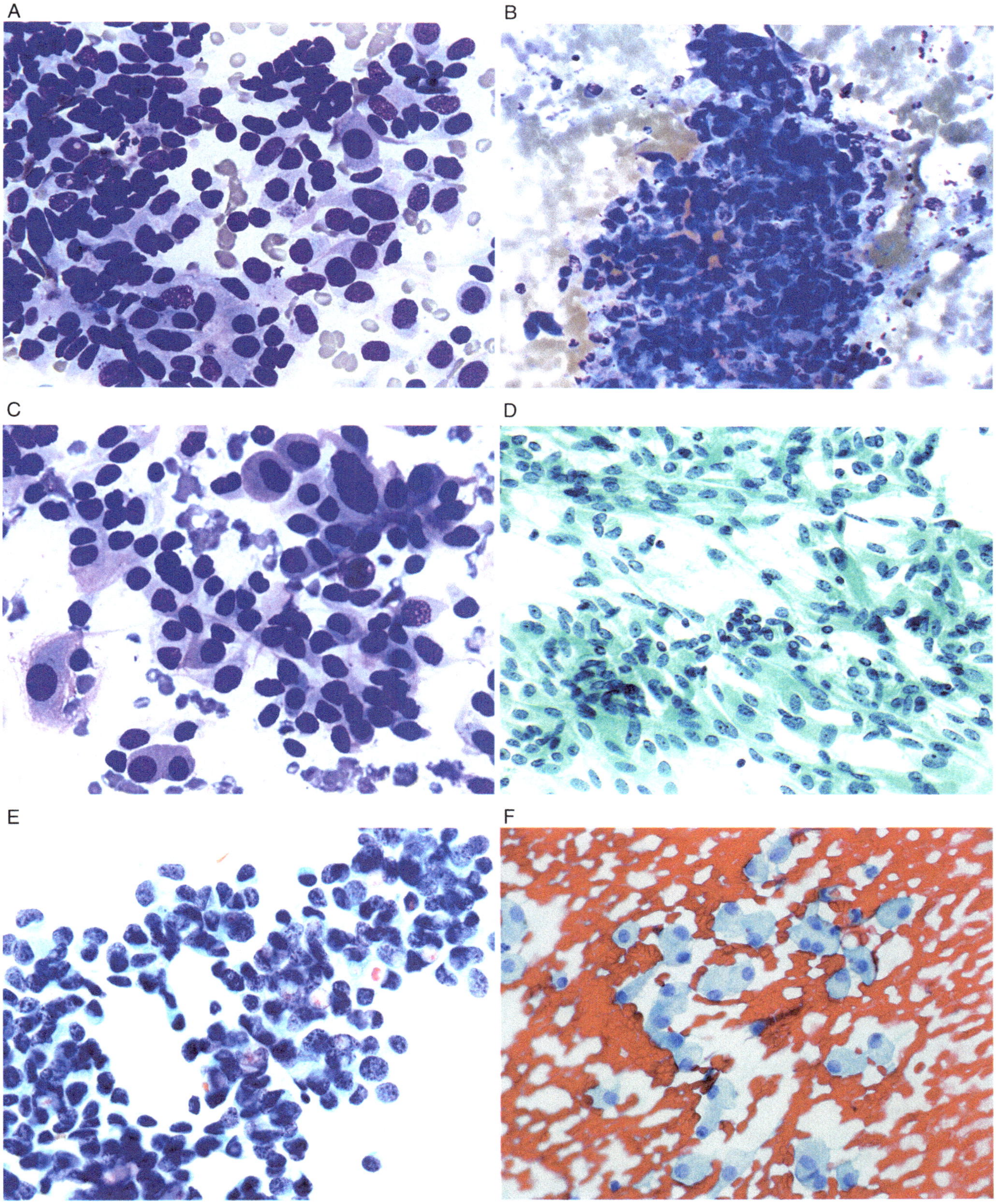

Fig. 3.52 Cytologic features of medullary carcinoma with epithelioid and spindle cells (**a**, **b**), plasmacytoid cells and binucleation (**c**), spindle cells (**d**), intracytoplasmic inclusion (**e**), foamy cytoplasm (**f**), amyloid stroma (**g**), amyloid on Congo-red stain (**h**), and positive for calcitonin on cellblock (**i**)

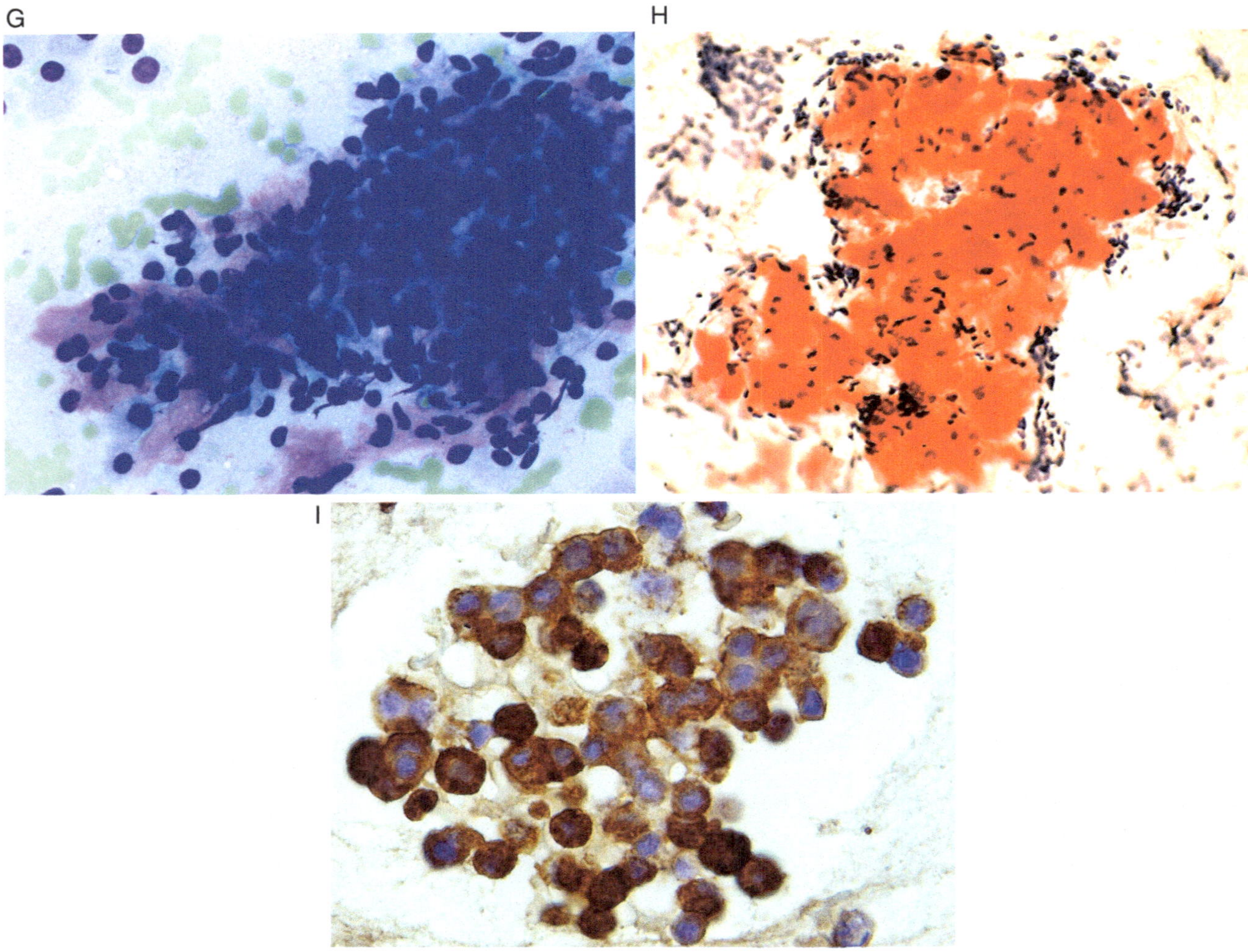

Fig. 3.52 (continued)

- Round to oval nuclei with hyperchromatic chromatin and high nuclear cytoplasmic ratio.
- Little or absence of colloid.
- Tumor necrosis can be seen.

Histologic Features

- Variable histologic growth patterns and insular, trabecular, solid, peritheliomatous, and infiltrating growth (Fig. 3.56a–c).
- Small uniform tumor cells with round, hyperchromatic to vesicular nuclear chromatin and small nucleoli.
- Mitotic figures, vascular invasion, and tumor necrosis are common.
- A small proportion of papillary carcinoma or follicular carcinoma may be present.
- Regardless of the percentage, the presence of undifferentiated carcinoma component should be reported.

Immunohistochemistry

- Positive for TTF1, PAX8, and thyroglobulin
- Focal p53 positivity
- Increased MIB-1 proliferative index
- Negative for calcitonin and neuroendocrine markers

Differential Diagnosis

- Medullary carcinoma
- Follicular carcinoma
- Metastasis

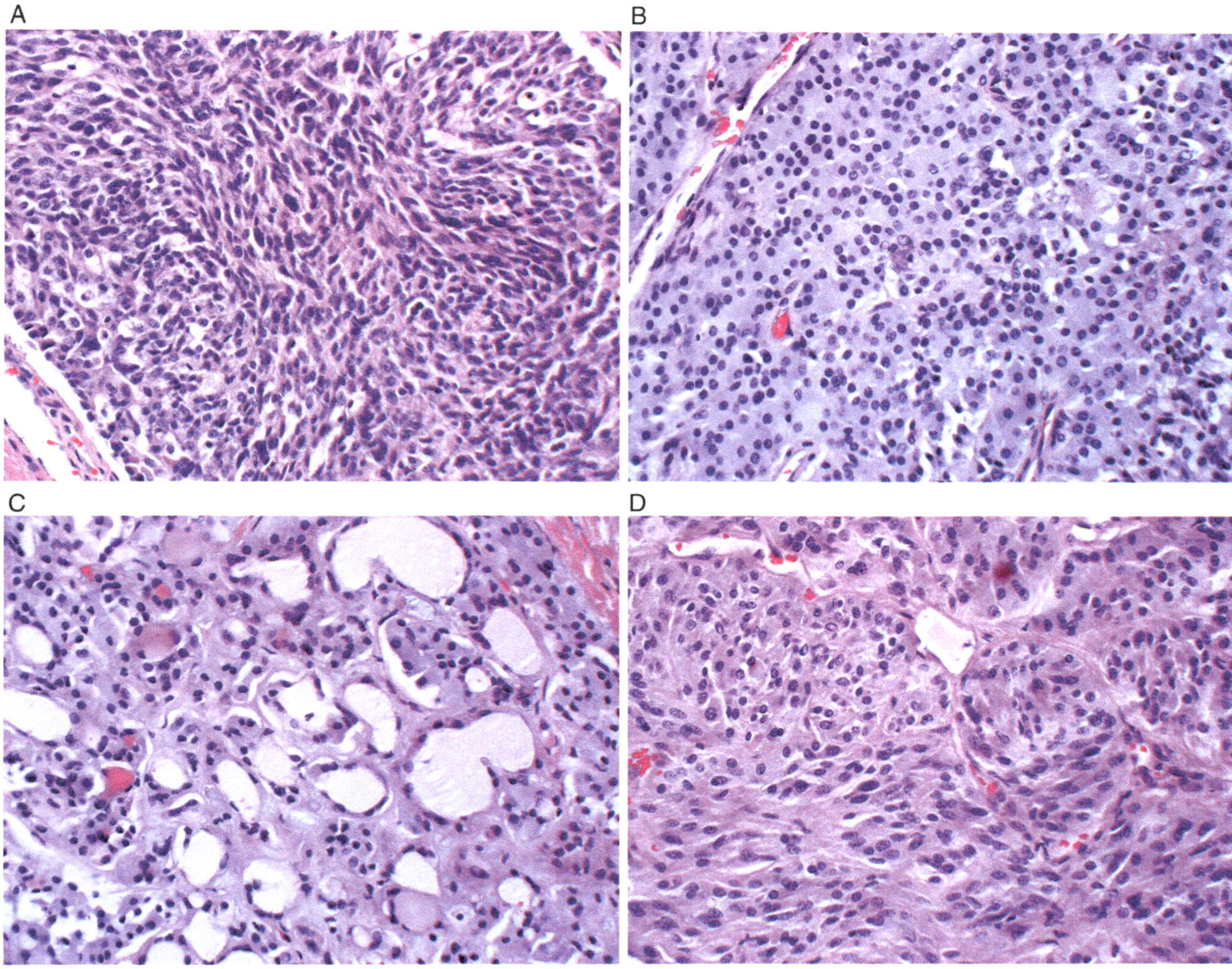

Fig. 3.53 Histologic pattern of medullary carcinoma

Undifferentiated (Anaplastic) Carcinoma

Clinical Features

- Rare, accounting for 5% of malignant thyroid neoplasms
- Usually occur after age 50, more common in women
- Rapid growth in months
- Diffuse enlargement of the thyroid with firm nodules and masses
- Can be a painful or painless mass

Cytological Features (Fig. 3.57a–d)

- Epithelioid, spindle, or giant neoplastic cells, singly or in small clusters
- Marked nuclear pleomorphism, bizarre nuclei, with single or multiple prominent nucleoli
- Frequent mitotic figures with abnormal mitoses
- Extensive tumor necrosis and acute inflammatory cells in the background

Histologic Features

- Admixture of spindle cells, pleomorphic giant cells, and epithelioid cells (Fig. 3.58a–d).
- Tumor may show predominately or exclusively spindle cells with a sarcomatoid appearance.
- Squamoid changes are common.
- Prominent neutrophilic infiltrate can be seen.
- Vascular invasion may be present.
- Several histologic variants have been described: osteoclastic variant, paucicellular variant, and lymphoepithelioma-like variant.

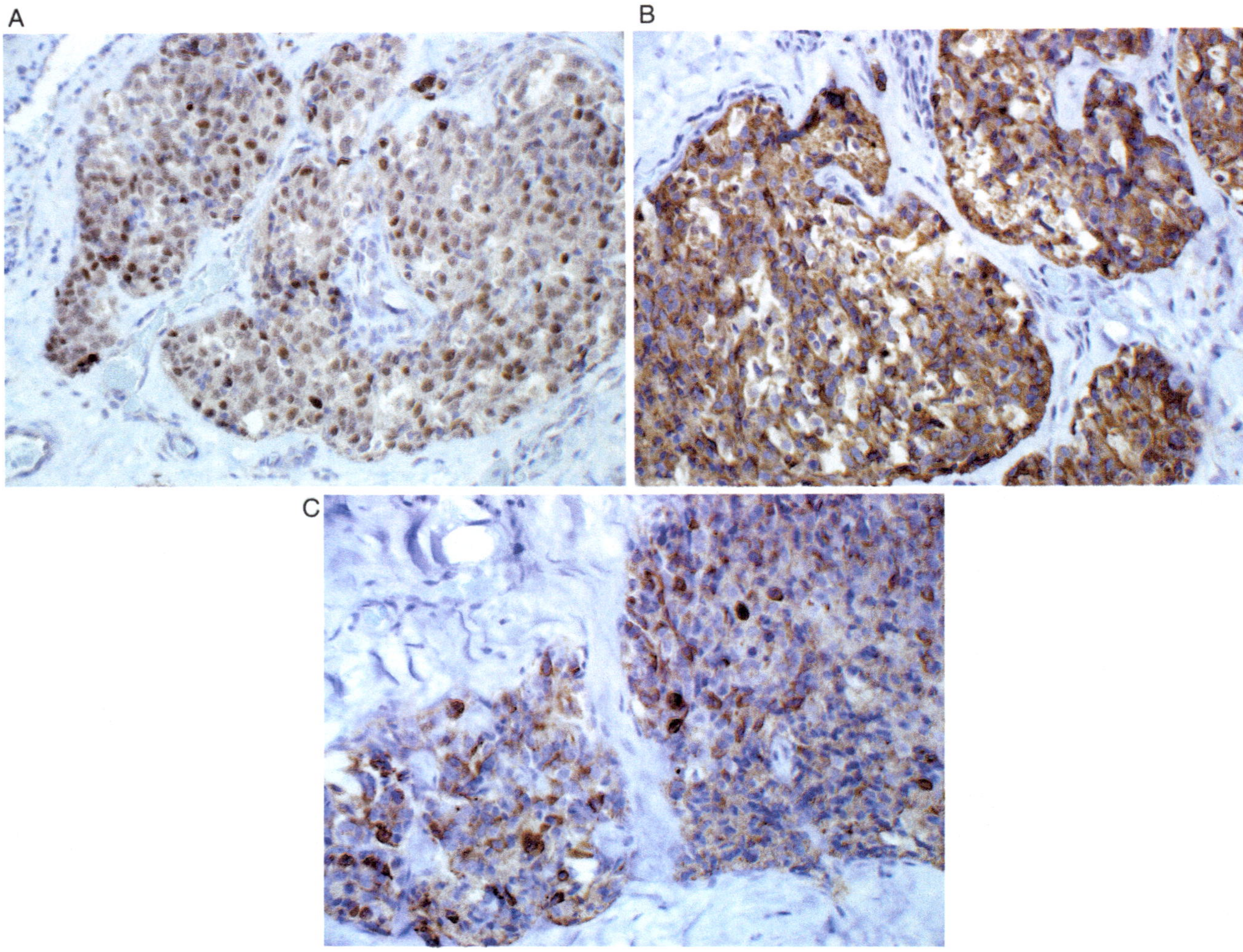

Fig. 3.54 Example of medullary carcinoma weakly positive for TTF1 (**a**) and positive for calcitonin (**b**) and chromogranin (**c**)

- A focus of well-differentiated or poorly differentiated thyroid carcinoma may be identified following an extensive sampling.

Immunohistochemistry

- Most cases are negative for TTF1 and thyroglobulin.
- About 50% of cases are positive for PAX8 (Fig. 3.59d) as shown in a needle core biopsy case (Fig. 3.59a–d).
- Strong p53 positivity is common.
- Over 80% of cases are positive for one of the cytokeratins (AE1/3, CAM5.2, CK5/6, and 34betaE12).
- Epithelial membrane antigen (EMA) is positive in less than 50% cases.

Differential Diagnosis

- Medullary carcinoma
- Soft tissue sarcomas
- Metastasis, especially from the lung and pancreas

Uncommon and Rare Thyroid Lesions

Lymphoma and Plasmacytoma

- Most cases are non-Hodgkin's lymphoma with secondary involvement of the thyroid (Fig. 3.60a, b).
- Approximately 15–20% of lymphomas may involve the thyroid.

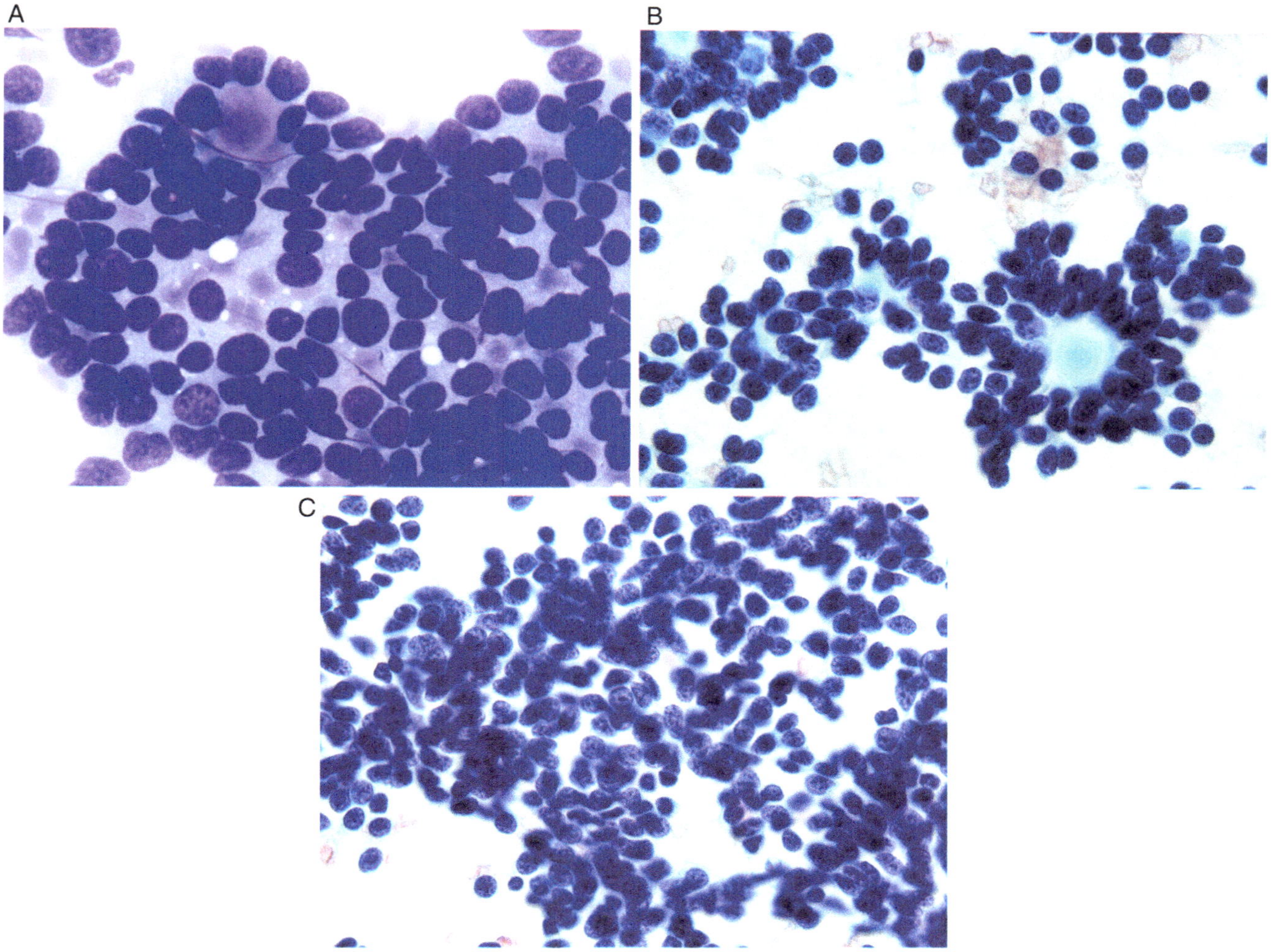

Fig. 3.55 Poorly differentiated (insular) carcinoma showing relatively uniform population of neoplastic cells with round to oval nuclei with hyperchromatic chromatin and high nuclear cytoplasmic ratio (**a**, DQ stain) and (**b**, **c**, Pap stain)

- Account for 1–3% of all malignant neoplasms of the thyroid
- Plasmacytoma/multiple myeloma as a primary presentation in the thyroid (Fig. 3.61a, b).

Squamous Cell Carcinoma

- Primary squamous cell carcinoma of the thyroid accounts for less than 1% of the malignant neoplasms of the thyroid. A metastasis especially from the head and neck, lung, and esophagus should be excluded.

Many other rare primary thyroid neoplasms have been recognized and reported in the literature. Table 3.5 summarizes the clinical, cytologic, and histologic features of these neoplasms and any ancillary tests which are potentially useful in making a diagnosis.

Metastases

- The most common metastases are from the kidney, skin (melanoma), lung, breast, stomach, and head and neck. Lymphomas and leukemias account for 15% of the cases.
- Can be a solitary mass or multiple nodules; 80% of cases involve a single lobe.
- Table 3.6 summarizes the useful IHC markers for the most common differential diagnosis.

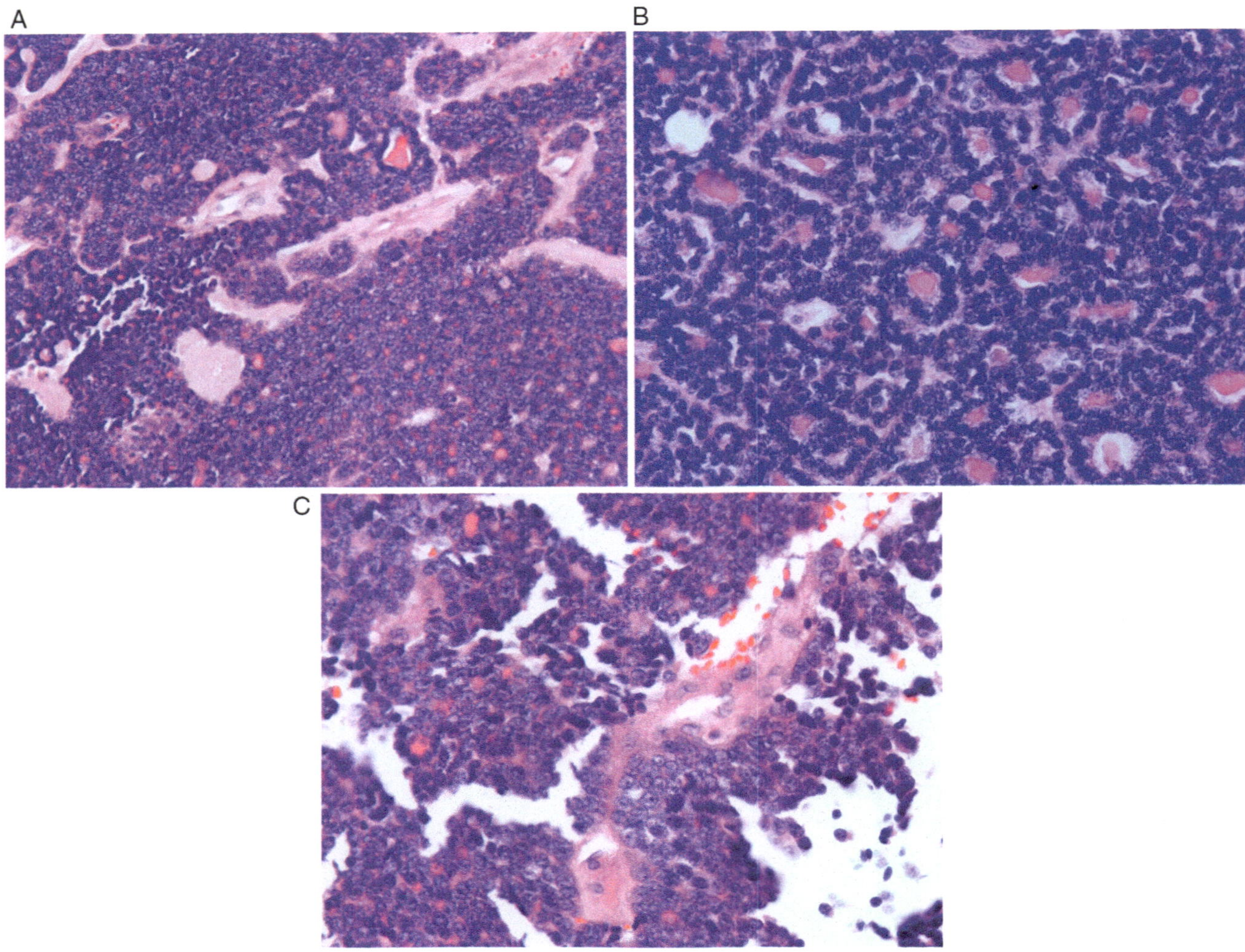

Fig. 3.56 Histologic sections showing insular and trabecular growth and follicular patterns

- Several examples of secondary tumors including metastatic renal cell carcinoma (Fig. 3.62a), breast carcinoma (Fig. 3.62b), and lung squamous cell carcinoma (Fig. 3.62c) are shown.

Parathyroid Adenoma/Neoplasm and Carcinoma

Parathyroid Adenoma/Neoplasm

Clinical Features

- Clinical hypercalcemia is very helpful.
- Usually involve a single parathyroid gland.
- More common in patients 50–60 years of age.
- Female-to-male ratio of approximately 3:1.

Cytologic Features (Fig. 3.63a–g)

- Hypercellular specimen with similar features to follicular neoplasm.
- Neoplastic cells tend to be smaller than follicular cells.
- Numerous naked nuclei in the background.
- Vascular-rich stroma.
- Neuroendocrine nuclear chromatin.
- Fine cytoplasmic vacuoles.
- Oncocytic cytoplasm resembling Hurthle cell neoplasm.
- Clear cell change is a frequent finding.
- Focal marked nuclear pleomorphism may be present.

Histologic Feature (Fig. 3.64a–g)

- With or without a well-defined fibrous capsule.
- Proliferation of chief cells, oncocytic cells, or a mixture of different cell types.

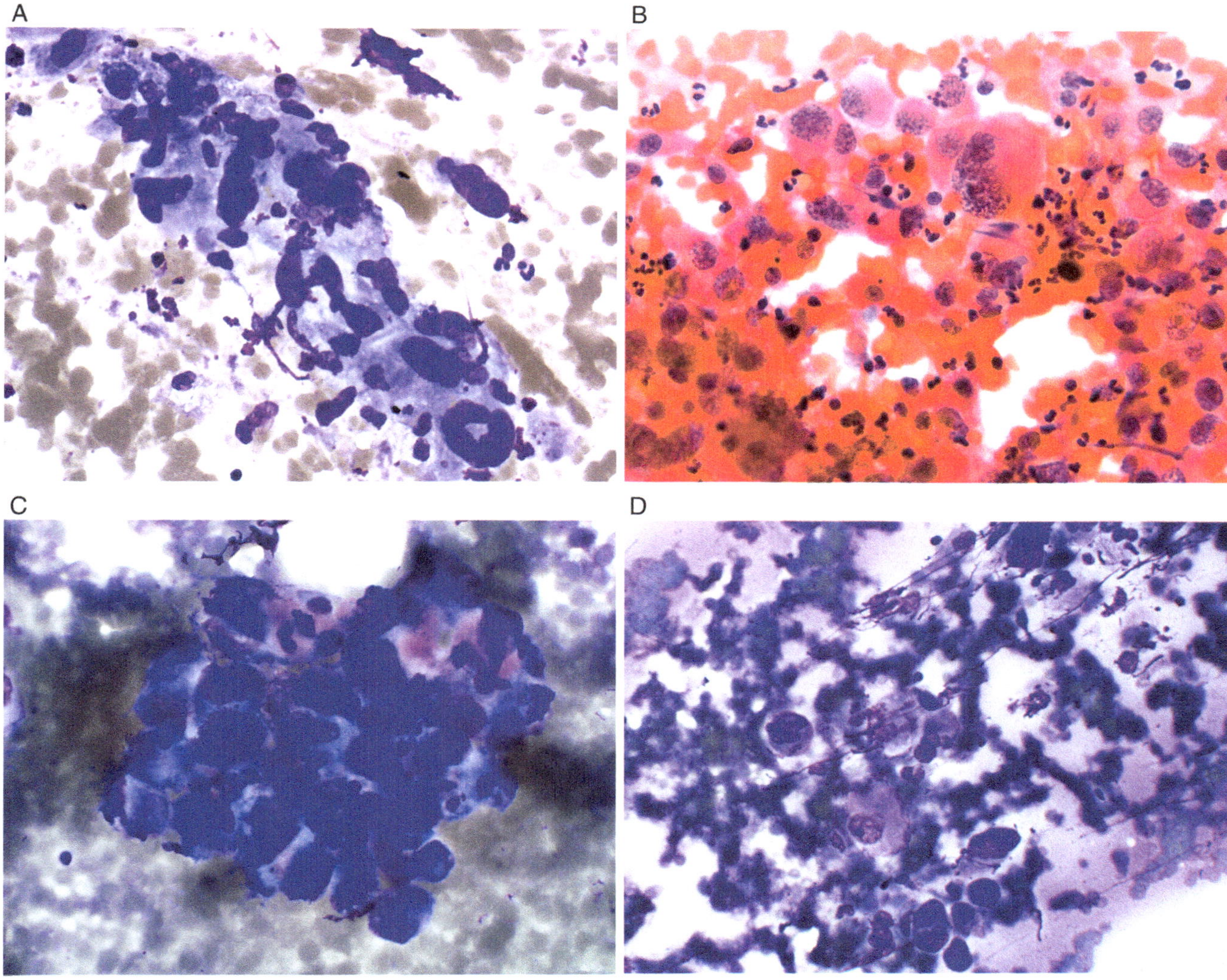

Fig. 3.57 Cytologic features of undifferentiated (anaplastic) carcinoma with a mixture of epithelioid, spindle, or giant neoplastic cells (**a**), numerous acute inflammatory cells (**b**, **c**), and abnormal mitosis (**d**)

- Many growth patterns such as solid sheets, nodular, trabecular, follicular, and acinar patterns; a mixture of growth patterns is common.
- Cystic degeneration may be present.
- Richly vascular stroma with limited fibrotic areas or fibrous bands.
- Calcification or even ossification can occur.
- The neoplastic chief cells show round nuclei, neuroendocrine chromatin, and small nucleoli.
- Focal nuclear pleomorphism with giant hyperchromatic and multilobar nuclei may be seen.
- A thin rim of normal parathyroid tissue at the periphery.
- Mitotic figures are generally absent.
- Massive infarction following an FNA can occur, but tumor necrosis is absent.
- Three histologic variants have been described: oncocytic adenoma, water-clear cell adenoma, and lipoadenoma.
- Absence or marked reduction of intracellular and extracellular neutral lipid by oil red O stain.
- Atypical parathyroid adenoma has been used to describe an adenoma with broad fibrous bands and lack of other malignant features, such as vascular invasion, capsular invasion, increased mitoses, and tumor necrosis.

Immunohistochemistry

- Table 3.7 summarizes a panel of useful IHC markers in the differential diagnosis.

Differential Diagnosis

- Follicular neoplasm
- Hurthle cell neoplasm
- Medullary carcinoma
- Papillary carcinoma

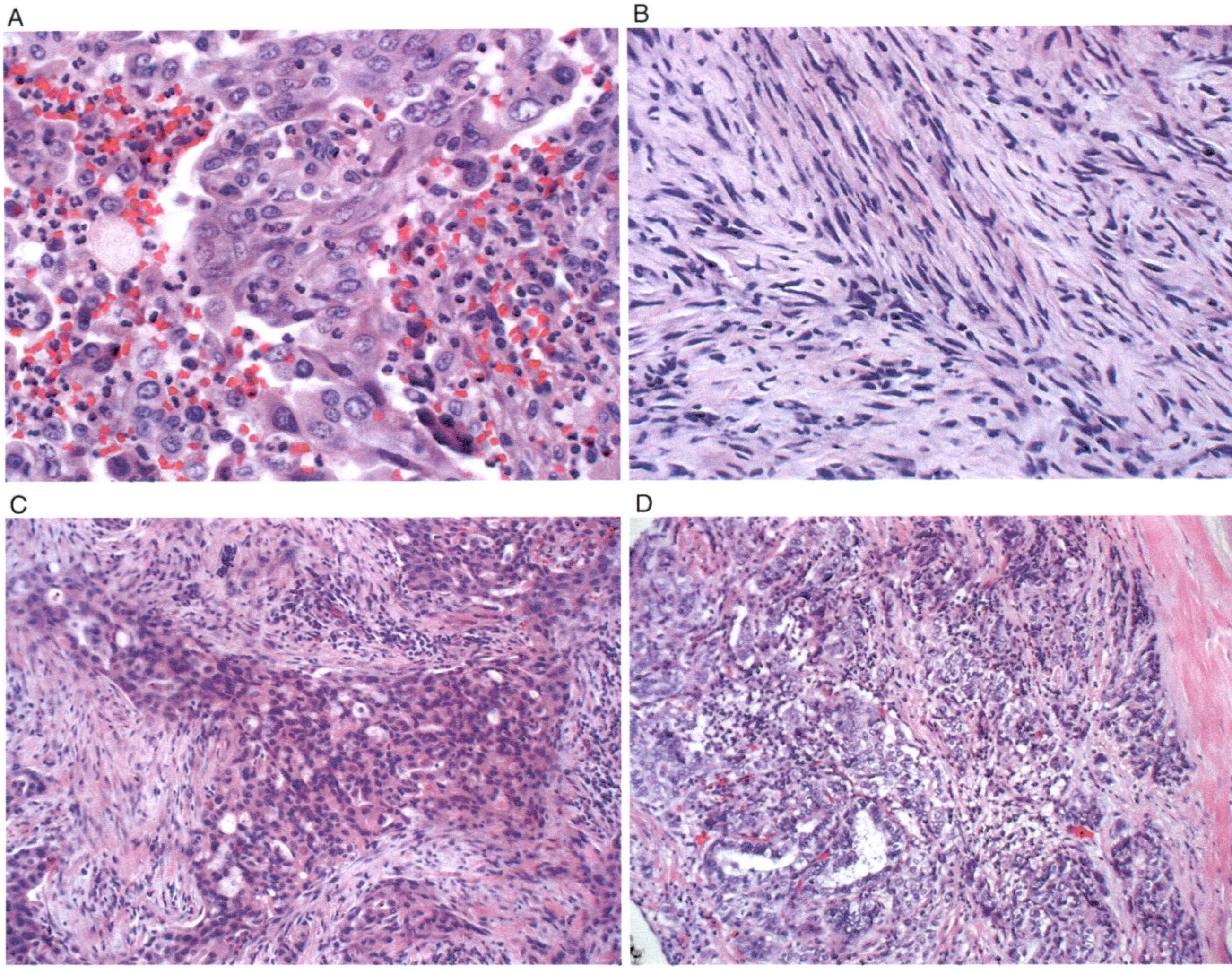

Fig. 3.58 Undifferentiated (anaplastic) carcinoma showing histologic sections with pleomorphic giant cells, and epithelioid cells (**a**), exclusively spindle cells (**b**), squamoid changes (**c**), and transformation from PTC (**d**)

Parathyroid Carcinoma

Clinical Features

- Rare; accounting for less than 1% of patients with primary hyperparathyroidism
- Male-to-female ratio of approximately 1:1
- High serum PTH and hypercalcemia

Cytologic Features

- Tumor cells with large nuclei and prominent nucleoli, diffuse nuclear atypia, tumor necrosis, and increased mitoses are suggestive of malignancy.

Histologic Features (Fig. 3.65a–c)

- Usually solid sheets, trabecular, follicular, rosette-like, and spindle cell growth patterns.
- Can be chief cells, oncocytic cells, clear cells, or a mixture.
- Broad fibrous bands and focal coagulative necrosis are commonly seen.
- Enlarged nuclei with prominent nucleoli may be present.
- Mitotic activity is extremely variable but often more than 5 per 50 high-power fields.
- For a definitive malignancy, one of these features must be seen: (1) vascular invasion in the fibrous capsule or the surrounding soft tissue, (2) capsular penetration with invasion into the adjacent tissues, or (3) metastasis.

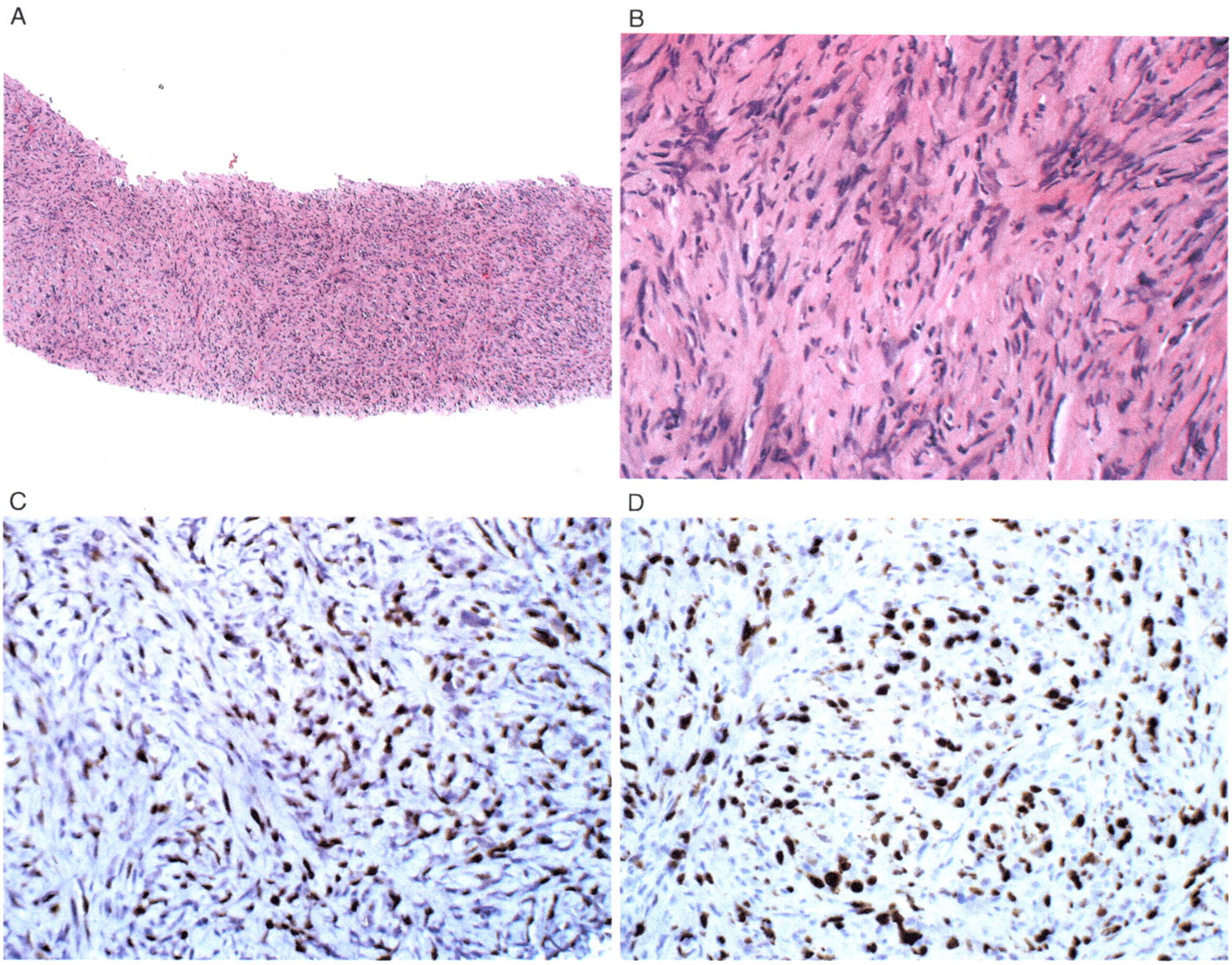

Fig. 3.59 An example of anaplastic carcinoma with spindle cell morphology on needle core biopsy specimen (**a** and **b**). Note tumor cell is positive for PAX8 (**c**) and high MIB1 proliferative index (**d**)

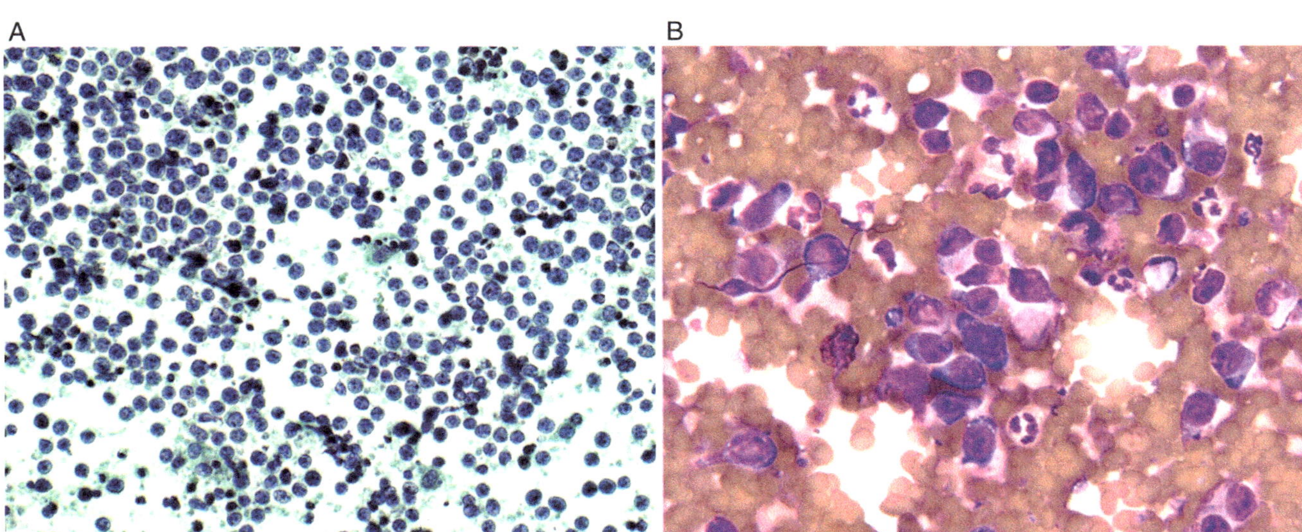

Fig. 3.60 A diffuse large B-cell lymphoma on FNA smear

A B

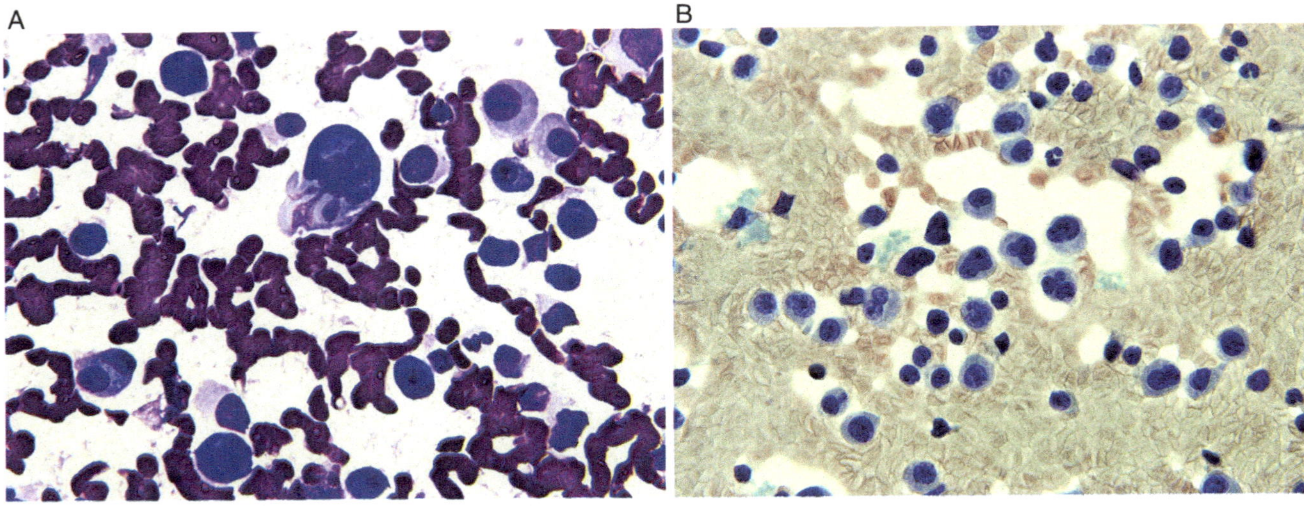

Fig. 3.61 A plasmacytoma involving the thyroid as a primary presentation

Table 3.5 Summary of uncommon and rare thyroid neoplasms/lesions

Diagnosis	Clinical features	Cytologic features	Histologic features	Ancillary tests
Mucoepidermoid carcinoma	Rare, more common in female adults	Epidermoid cells and mucin-containing cells in the background of mucin	Similar histologic features of the salivary gland	Mucicarmine stain for intracellular mucin positive, focally positive for TTF1 and thyroglobulin,
SMECE	Rare, nearly always in adult women	Bland-looking epithelial cells and mucin-containing cells	Sclerotic stroma with infiltrating epithelial tumor cells, mucin-containing cells, and numerous eosinophils and plasma cells, squamous metaplasia commonly seen	May be focally positive for TTF1 and CEA, usually negative for thyroglobulin
Mucinous carcinoma	Very rare	Groups of epithelial cells in a background of mucin	Clusters of tumor cells in pools of mucin	Focally positive for TTF1, thyroglobulin, and MUC2
SETTLE	Adolescents or young adults, male-to-female ratio about 1.5:1		Lobulated tumor growth in fibrous stroma, usually biphasic with both spindle cells and glandular or tubulopapillary structures, similar to synovial sarcoma	Both spindle cells and glands are positive for cytokeratin, spindle cells can be positive for myoepithelial markers, negative for calcitonin, CEA, S100, CD5, and S100
CASTLE	Very rare, middle-aged adults	Atypical epithelial cells in groups	Anastomosing epithelial tumor islands in a desmoplastic stroma, tumor cells with squamoid or syncytial appearance	IHC profile is similar to thymic carcinoma including positive for CD5, can be positive for PAX8 and p63
Angiosarcoma	Iodine deficiency has been suggested to be a possible etiologic factor, elderly, male-to-female ratio of 1.2:1	Large pleomorphic epithelioid tumor cells with large vesicular nuclei, prominent central nucleoli, and abundant eosinophilic cytoplasm in the background of necrosis	Anastomosing vascular channels lined by atypical endothelial cells, discrete cytoplasmic vacuoles, or sheets of atypical epithelioid cells	Positive for ERG, CD31, and CD34, focal or diffusely positive for cytokeratin, can be seen in epithelioid angiosarcoma, a metastasis must be excluded.

(continued)

Table 3.5 (continued)

Diagnosis	Clinical features	Cytologic features	Histologic features	Ancillary tests
PNST	Very rare	Spindle cells	Spindle cells with variable degree of atypia	Focal and weak positive for S100 in MPNST, diffusely and strongly positive for S100 in Schwannoma
SFT	Adults	Bland-looking spindles	Alternating hypercellular and hypocellular areas, with haphazardly distributed bland spindle or stellate cells in fibrous stroma of thick collagen fibers	Positive for STAT6, CD99, CD34, and Bcl2, negative for cytokeratin and S100
SMT	Very rare, more often malignant	Spindle cells with variable degree of atypia	Fascicles of mitotically active atypical spindle cells, with necrosis, hemorrhage, and invasive growth pattern in a leiomyosarcoma	Positive for SMA and desmin
FDCT	Rare, may be associated with Epstein-Barr virus	Spindle to epithelioid cells with vesicular chromatin, distinct nucleoli, and moderate amount of eosinophilic cytoplasm	Sheets of spindle to epithelioid cells with vesicular chromatin, distinct nucleoli, and moderate amount of eosinophilic cytoplasm, small lymphocytes are present, mitotic rate is variable from 0 to 10 per high-power field	Positive for vimentin, CD21, CD23, and CD35, may be focally positive for S100, CD68, CD45, and CD20
LCH	Rare, most patients are younger than 20	Histiocyte-like cells with prominent nuclear grooves, mixed with abundant eosinophils and lymphocytes in a hemorrhagic background	Sheets of large histiocyte-like cells with vesicular chromatin, prominent nuclear folds ("coffee-bean"), and small nucleoli, multinucleated cells may be present, abundant eosinophils and lymphocytes	Positive for CD1a and S100, can be positive or CD68, negative for cytokeratin, CD21, and CD35
RDD	Rare, reported in adult women	Large histiocytes with foamy cytoplasm containing intact lymphocytes	Nodules of histiocyte-like cells with emperipolesis and lymphoid cells in the background	Positive for S100 and CD68
Paraganglioma	Rare, female predilection, 40–60 years	Single cells or loose clusters of large cells with ovoid nuclei and focally discrete nucleoli	Lobules of ovoid cells with finely granular cytoplasm in the vascular-rich networks, scattered tumor cell nuclei can be enlarged, hyperchromatic, or bizarre	Positive for synaptophysin and chromogranin, S100 highlighting sustentacular cells
Ectopic thymoma	Very rare, most common in middle-aged women	Spindle cells, epithelioid cells, and lymphoid cells in a various proportions depending on the histologic type	Similar to the histologic types of mediastinal thymoma	Positive for PAX8 and p63
Teratoma	Very rare, about 75% in the neonates and infants and 25% in children and adults, >90% of the tumors are benign in the neonatal group, >50% of the tumors are malignant in the adult group	Various cellular components from a mixture of benign elements to small round cells from the immature elements	A wide range of tissue types and growth patterns as seen in other teratomas, the maturation of the neural-type tissue determines the grade, immature teratomas with prominent primitive neuroectodermal tissues (grade 3 or malignant)	Some IHC markers such as S100, myogenin, NSE, and GFAP are useful to further determine the immature components

Bcl2 B-cell CLL/lymphoma 2, *CASTLE* carcinoma showing thymus-like differentiation, *CD5* cluster of differentiation 5, *ERG* ETS-related gene, *FDCT* follicular dendritic cell tumor, *GFAP* glial fibrillary acidic protein, *IHC* immunohistochemical, *LCH* Langerhans cell histiocytosis, *MPNST* malignant peripheral nerve sheath tumor, *MUC2* mucin 2, *NSE* neuron-specific enolase, *PNST* peripheral nerve sheath tumor, *RDD* Rosai-Dorfman disease, *SETTLE* spindle epithelial tumor with thymus-like differentiation, *SFT* solitary fibrous tumor, *SMA* smooth muscle actin, *SMECE* sclerosing mucoepidermoid carcinoma with eosinophils, *SMT* smooth muscle tumor, *STAT6* signal transducer and activator of transcription 6

Table 3.6 Summary of useful IHC markers for the common differential diagnoses

Diagnosis/markers	Thyroid	CRCC	Lung	Breast	Stomach	SCC
CK7	+	−	+	+	+	−/+
CK20	−	−	−	−	−/+	−
Vimentin	+	+	−	−	−	−
TTF1	+	−	+	−	−	−
PAX8	+	+	−	−	−	−
Thyroglobulin	+	−	−	−	−	−
pVHL	−	+	−	−	−	−
RCCma	−	+/−	−	−	−	−
CD10	−	+	−/+	−	−	−
GATA3	−	−	−	+	−	−/+
ER	−/+	−	−	+	−	−
CDX2	−	−	−	−	+/−	−
p40	−	−	−	−	−	+

Breast breast carcinoma, *CDX2* caudal type homeobox 2, *CRCC* clear cell renal cell carcinoma, *GATA3* GATA-binding protein 3, *Lung* lung adenocarcinoma, *stomach* gastric and upper gastrointestinal adenocarcinoma, *pVHL* von Hippel-Lindau tumor suppressor gene protein, *RCCma* renal cell carcinoma marker, *SCC* squamous cell carcinoma, *Thyroid* thyroid carcinoma of follicular cell origin

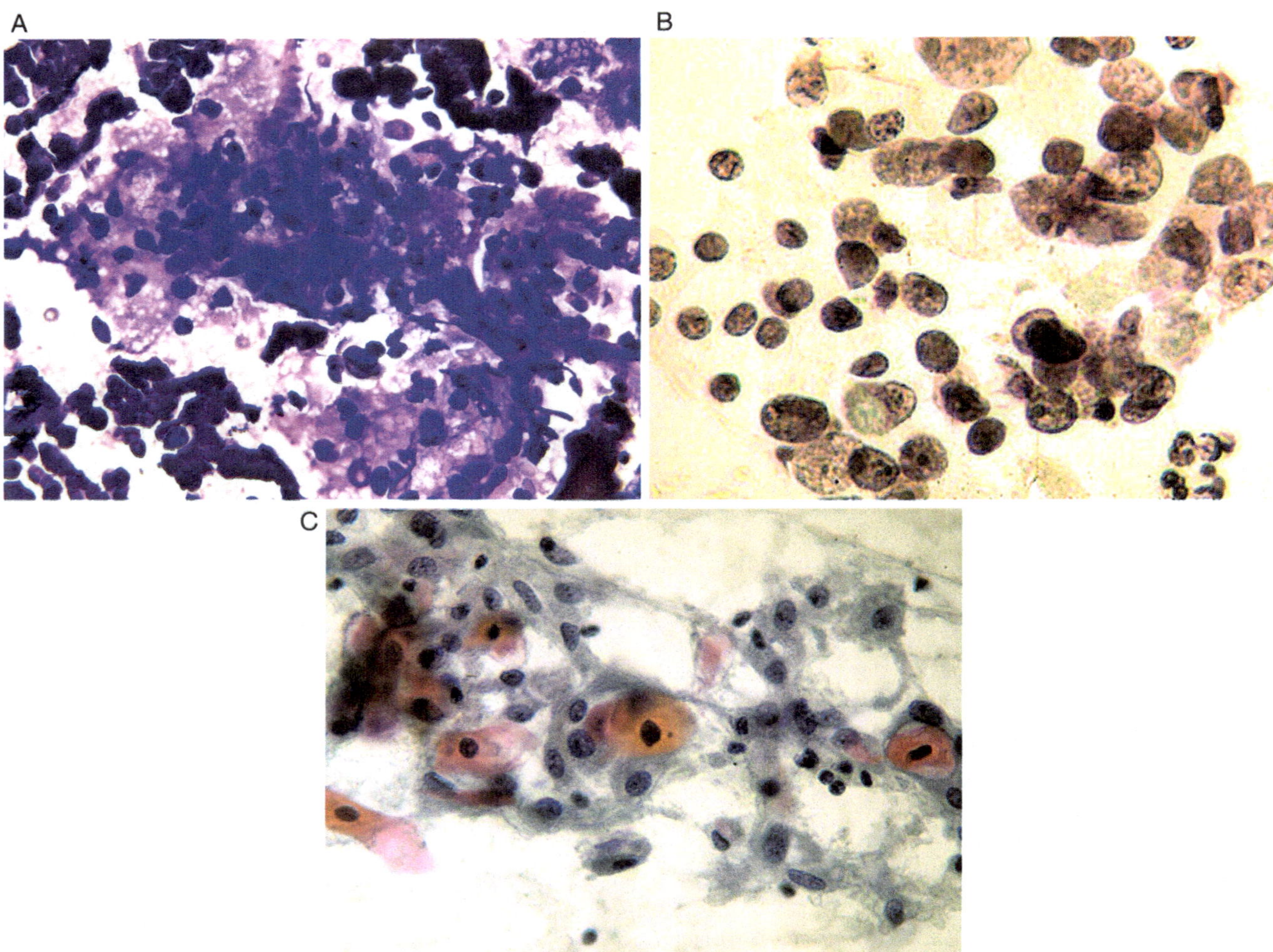

Fig. 3.62 Examples of secondary tumors with metastatic renal cell carcinoma (**a**), breast carcinoma (**b**), and squamous cell carcinoma (**c**)

Immunohistochemistry

- Positive for PTH, chromogranin, and GATA3.
- Negative for calcitonin, TTF1, PAX8, and thyroglobulin.
- Table 3.8 summarizes a panel of useful IHC markers in distinction of parathyroid carcinoma from parathyroid adenoma.

Differential Diagnosis

- Thyroid carcinoma
- Medullary carcinoma
- Metastasis

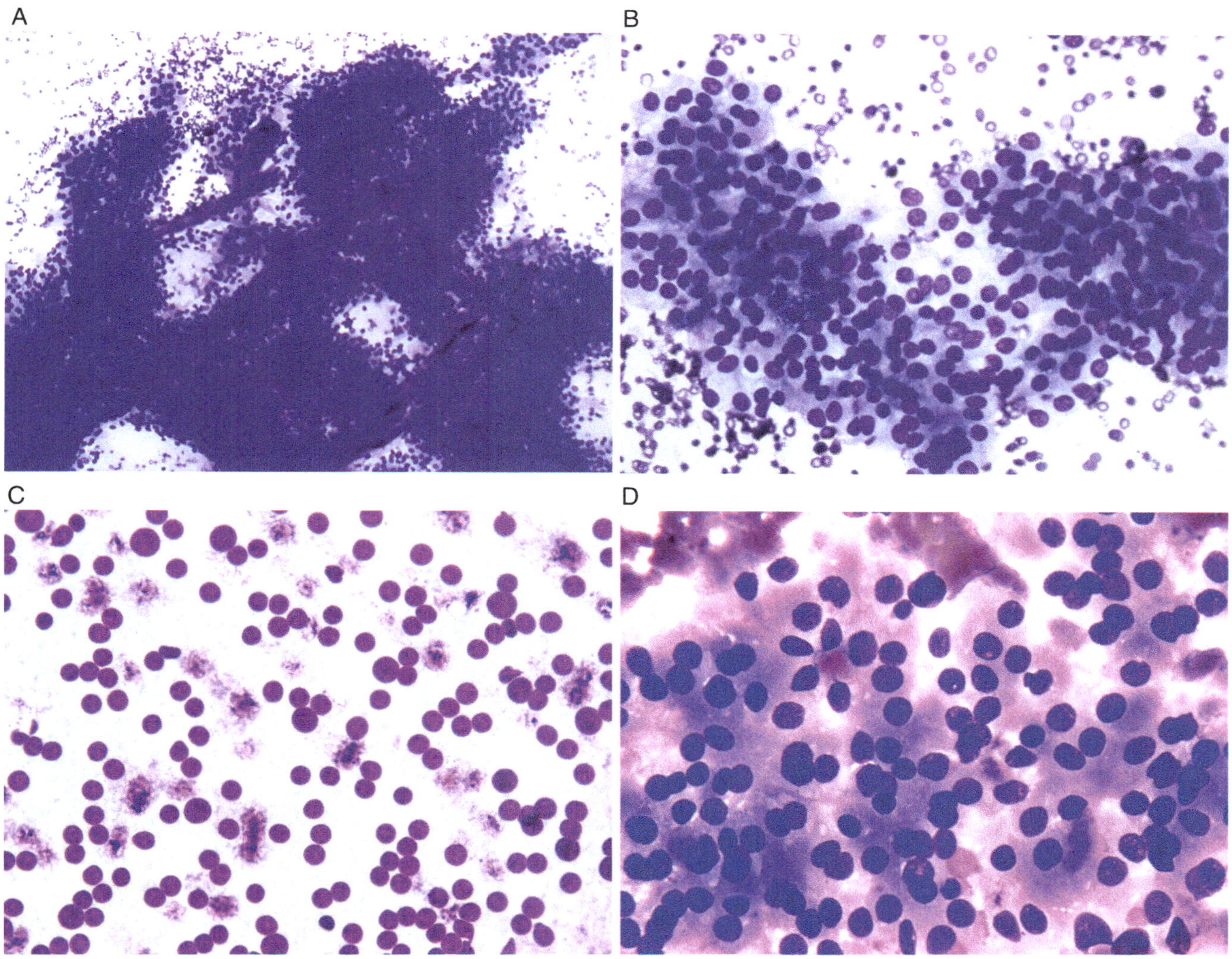

Fig. 3.63 Cytologic features of parathyroid neoplasm are similar to follicular neoplasm with neoplastic cells smaller than follicular cells, numerous naked nuclei in the background, vascular-rich stroma, and oncocytic changes (**a**–**e**). Note the cellblock section (**f**) and positive for PTH (**g**)

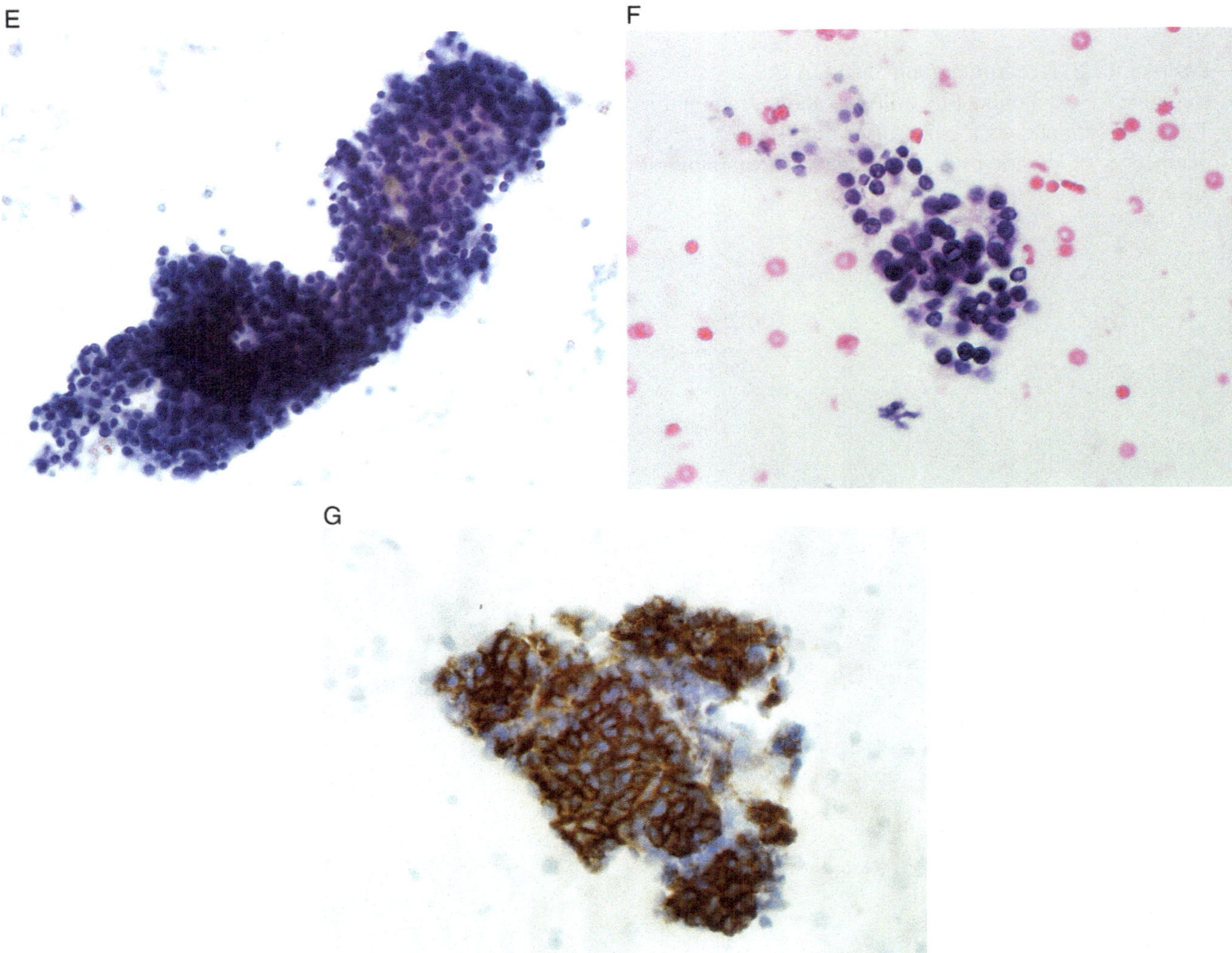

Fig. 3.63 (continued)

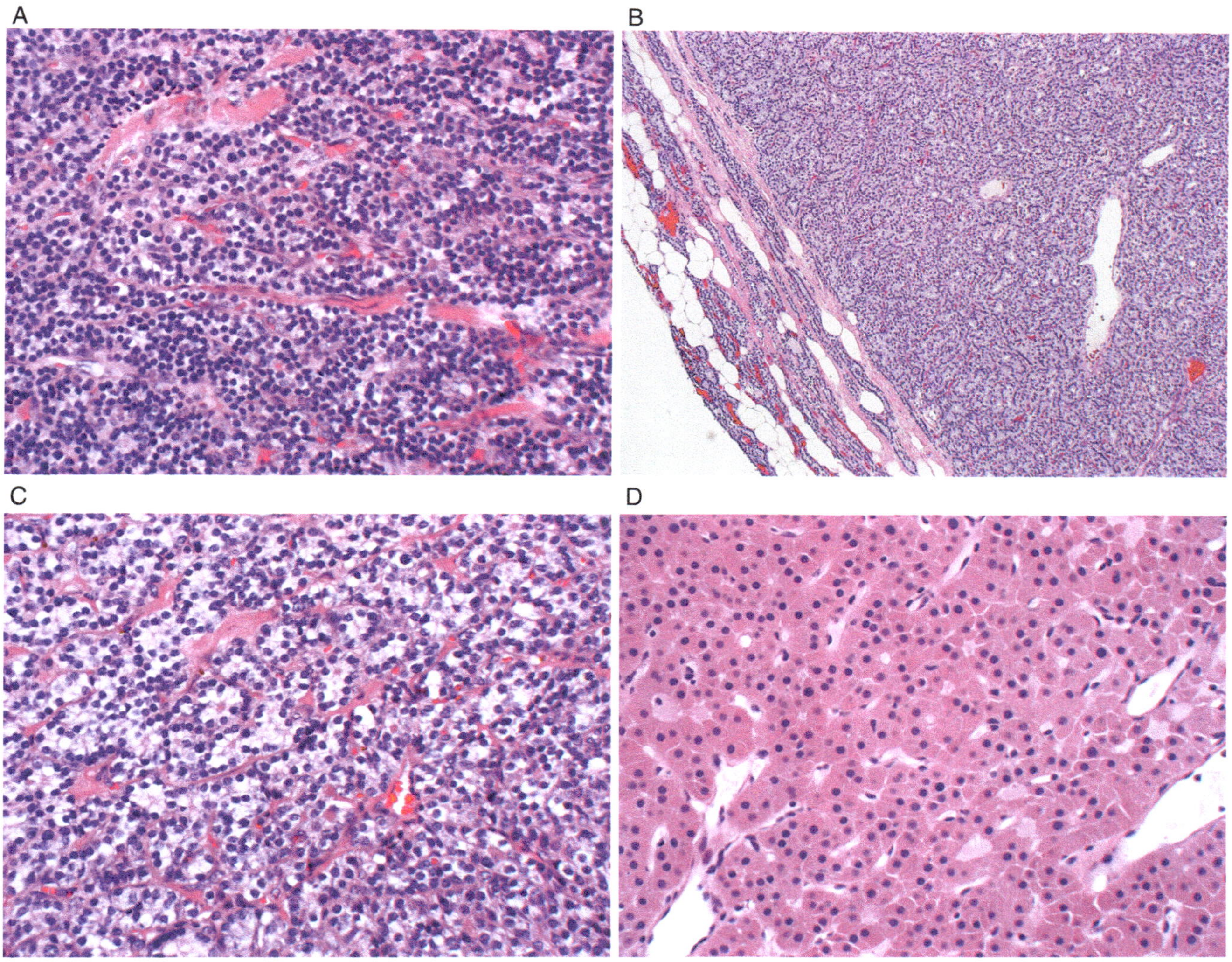

Fig. 3.64 Histologic sections of parathyroid adenoma with different growth patterns and cell changes. Note that a rim of normal parathyroid tissue (**b**), clear cell changes (**c**), oncocytic changes (**d**), cystic changes (**e**), follicular-like structures (**f**), and positive for PTH (**g**)

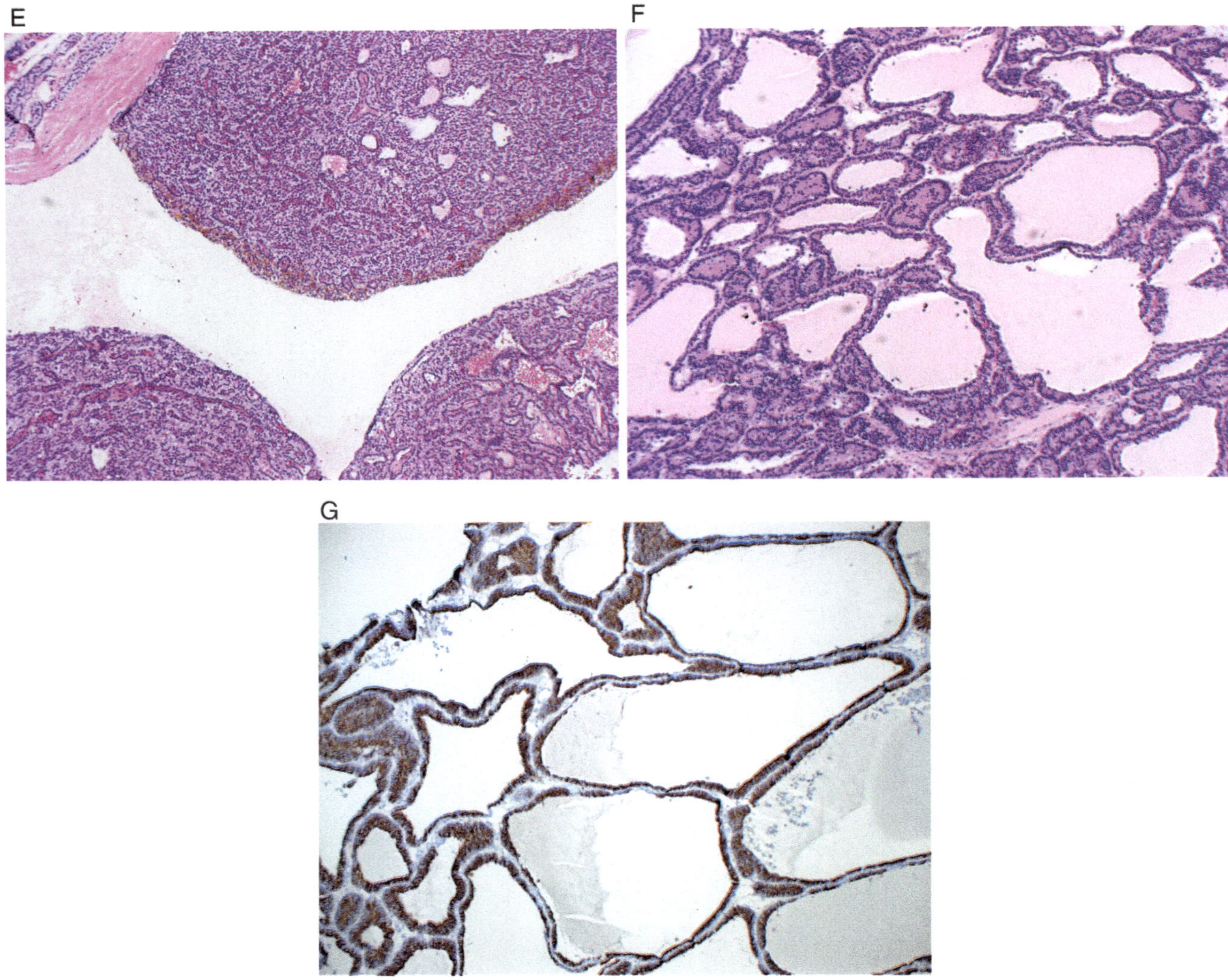

Fig. 3.64 (continued)

Table 3.7 Summary of useful IHC markers for differential diagnosis of follicular neoplasm/Hurthle cell neoplasm, parathyroid adenoma, and medullary carcinoma

Marker	Follicular neoplasm/ Hurthle cell neoplasm	Parathyroid adenoma	Medullary carcinoma
TTF1	+	−	Weak +
Thyroglobulin	+	−	−
PAX8	+	−	−
PTH	−	+	−
GATA3	−	+	−
Calcitonin	−	−	+

PTH parathyroid hormone

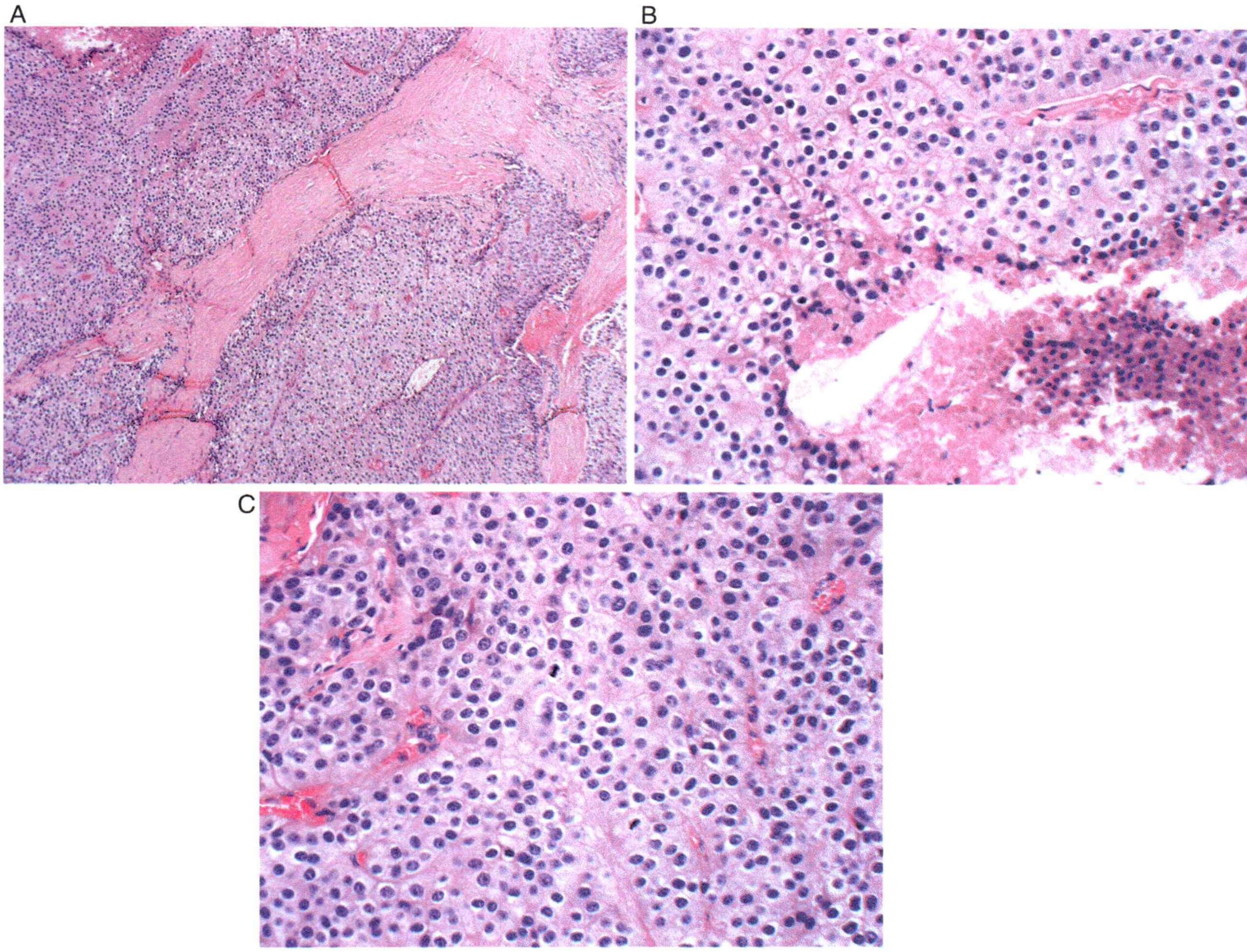

Fig. 3.65 Histologic sections of parathyroid carcinoma with thick fibrous bands (**a**), trabecular growth pattern, nuclear atypia, tumor necrosis (**b**), and many mitoses (**c**)

Table 3.8 Summary of IHC markers in distinction between parathyroid carcinoma from adenoma

Markers	Parathyroid carcinoma	Parathyroid adenoma
Parafibromin (HRPT2)	−/weak	+
Galectin-3	±	−
MIB-1 (Ki-67)	High or mildly increased	Low
PTH	+	+
GATA3	+	+

Case Presentations

Diagnosis of a common thyroid lesion such as nodular goiter, lymphocytic thyroiditis, papillary carcinoma, and follicular/Hurthle cell neoplasm in an adequately cellular FNA specimen is usually straightforward. There are three challenging scenarios sometimes encountered when evaluating an FNA biopsy of a mass lesion of the thyroid with or without a cellblock preparation. Case scenario 1 is how to identify a medullary carcinoma and its variants; case scenarios 2 and 3 are how to make a diagnosis of variants of papillary carcinoma; case scenario 4 is how to deal with an overt malignancy or neoplastic process in which an undifferentiated carcinoma, a rare primary tumor, and a secondary tumor are included in the diagnostic consideration.

Case Scenario 1

Learning Objectives

1. Reiterate the diagnostic criteria for medullary carcinoma of the thyroid.
2. Review the most effective panel of immunomarkers for diagnosis of medullary carcinoma and its mimics.

Case

A 22-year-old woman presented with a 1.0 × 0.8 cm nodule at the left lobe of the thyroid. She has no known history of a prior malignancy and no significant family history for cancer. An ultrasound-guided FNA was performed. The FNA smear showed a cellular specimen with cytologically bland histiocyte-like cells singly, in small groups, or follicular or acinar patterns. No colloid was seen. The cellular components showed small- to medium-sized nuclei with fine nuclear chromatin and abundant fine granular to foamy cytoplasm as shown in Fig. 3.66a–c. Occasional binucleation was noted. Significant nuclear atypia, nuclear grooves, intranuclear inclusions, or diagnostic nuclear features for papillary carcinoma were not observed. Spindle cells and inflammatory cells were not seen. The cellblock preparation was nearly acellular with occasional histiocyte-like cells as shown in Fig. 3.66d.

Based on the cytologic features, the diagnostic consideration included (1) medullary carcinoma, (2) follicular/Hurthle cell neoplasm, (3) histiocytic lesion, and (4) a secondary tumor. The presence of a mixture of cytologically bland small groups and single cells without colloid in the background was highly suspicious for medullary carcinoma. Follicular neoplasm can have clear cell changes, but it is unusual to have many single cells with intact cytoplasm. In addition, extensive microfollicular patterns were not seen. The presence of small cohesive clusters and binucleated cells made them less likely to be histiocytes. Lack of nuclear grooves and inflammatory cells, including eosinophils, excluded Langerhans cell histiocytosis. The absence of a vascular pattern, in addition to the patient's age and no known history of renal cell carcinoma, largely excluded a metastatic renal cell carcinoma.

As mentioned earlier, rare single cells were noted in the cellblock preparation. A small panel of IHC including calcitonin and CEA was attempted on the cellblock sections; the results showed that rare single cells were strongly positive for calcitonin and CEA (Fig. 3.66e, f), supporting the diagnosis of medullary carcinoma of the thyroid. A typical medullary carcinoma of the thyroid usually demonstrates a strong immunoreactivity for CEA, calcitonin, chromogranin, and other neuroendocrine markers, is weakly positive for TTF1, and is negative for PAX8, thyroglobulin, PTH, and GATA3. A thyroid tumor of follicular cell origin tends to be strongly positive for TTF1, PAX8, and thyroglobulin. In contrast, parathyroid neoplasm is positive for PTH, neuroendocrine markers, and GATA3 and negative for calcitonin, TTF1, and thyroglobulin. Thyroglobulin tends to show some background staining or a low staining sensitivity. Therefore, it is not a very useful marker in a daily practice.

Subsequently, a total thyroidectomy was performed. The histologic features of the tumor were similar to the cytologic findings, with predominately histiocyte-like tumor cells (Fig. 3.66g) and small foci of the tumor with spindle cell morphology as shown in Fig. 3.66h. Foci of C-cell hyperplasia were present. An incidental papillary thyroid microcarcinoma (3.0 mm) with a classic papillary growth pattern and typical nuclear features was also found.

Final Diagnosis on FNA Specimen

Medullary carcinoma of the thyroid

Final Diagnoses on Surgical Specimen

Medullary carcinoma of the thyroid

C-cell hyperplasia

Papillary microcarcinoma (3.0 mm)

What Are the Learning Points from This Case?

1. Regardless of the degree of cytologic atypia, a diagnosis of medullary carcinoma should be considered when many single cells with intact cytoplasm and absence of colloid were seen.

(continued)

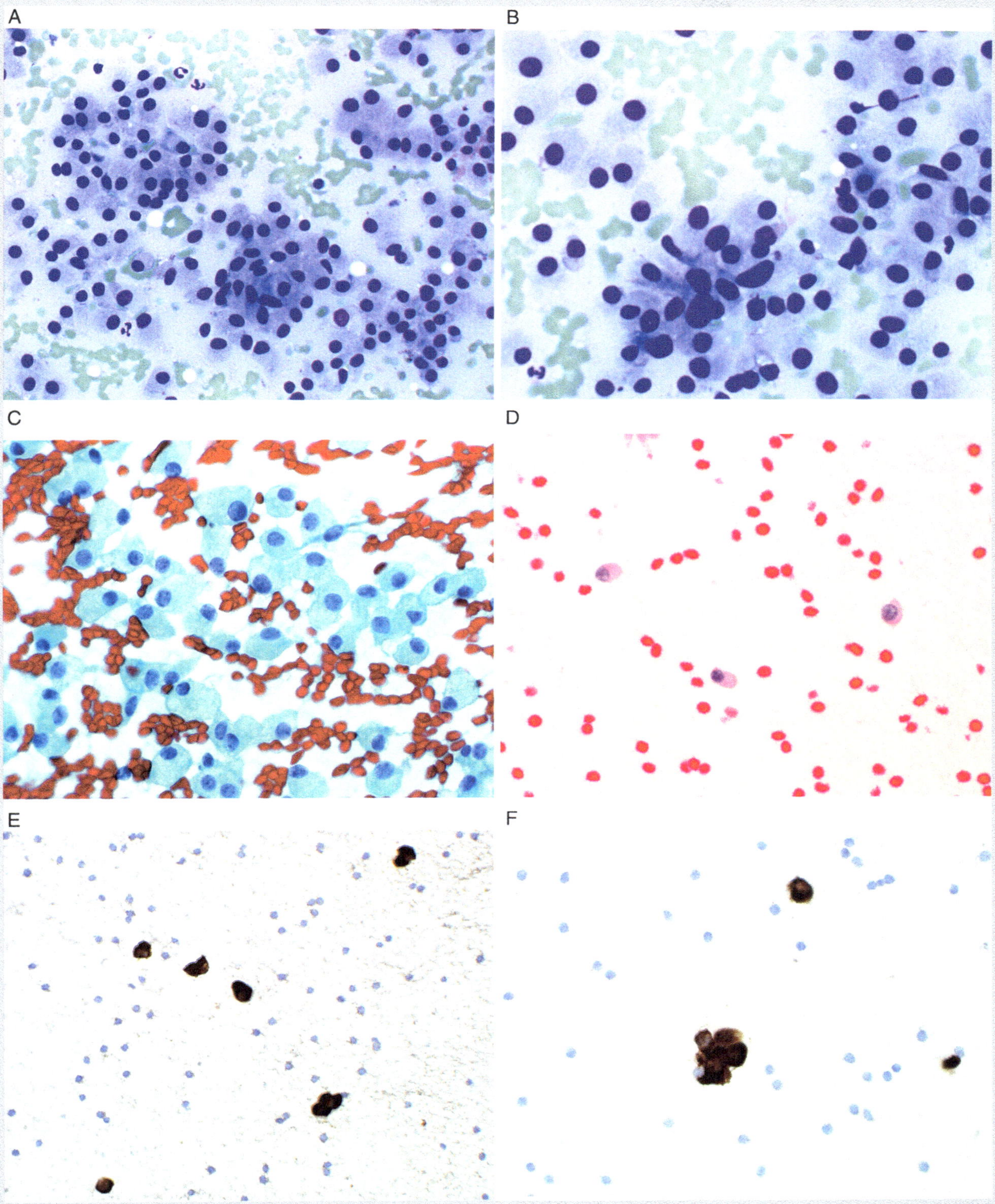

Fig. 3.66 A case of medullary carcinoma. Note that histiocyte-like cells, singly, in small groups, or follicular or acinar patterns (**a–c**). Cellblock (**d**), positive for CEA (**e**) and calcitonin (**f**), histologic sections (**g, h**)

(continued)

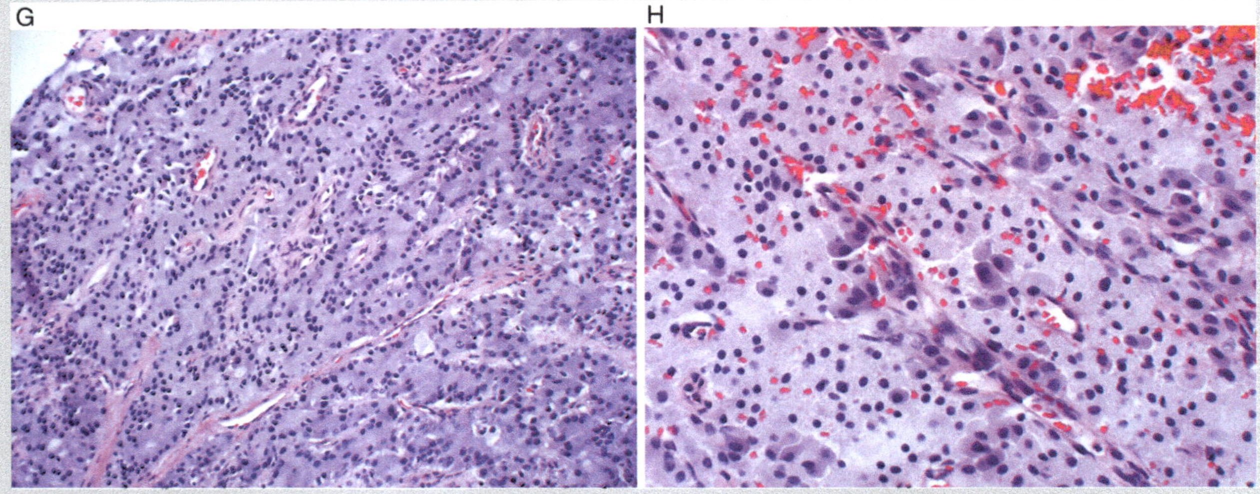

Fig. 3.66 (continued)

2. If a medullary carcinoma was suspected at time of an immediate assessment, additional passes of FNA for a cellblock should be obtained.
3. A small panel of immunostains including calcitonin and CEA should be attempted even if a cellblock preparation was essentially acellular on the hematoxylin and eosin (H&E)-stained slide as shown in the case.

Case Scenario 2

Learning Objectives

1. Reiterate the diagnostic criteria for this variant of PTC.
2. Review the differential diagnosis.

Case

A 23-year-old woman presented with a 0.9-cm-hypoechoic nodule with an irregular margin at the left lobe of the thyroid by ultrasound examination. An FNA was performed. The FNA smears were hypercellular with numerous oncocytic epithelial cells, singly or loosely in groups and small clusters, in the background of lymphoid cells. The epithelial cells contained moderate to abundant granular cytoplasm with round to ovoid nuclei, small to inconspicuous nucleoli, and scattered intranuclear pseudoinclusions as shown in Fig. 3.67a–c. Scattered spindle cells and atypical follicular cells with larger nuclei and small nucleoli were also noted. No colloid was seen. Neither distinct papillary structures nor a microfollicular pattern was observed. A cellblock preparation was obtained with essentially no cells identified.

Based on the cytologic findings above, the diagnostic consideration included (1) oncocytic variant of papillary carcinoma in the background of lymphocytic/ Hashimoto's thyroiditis, (2) oncocytic variant of medullary carcinoma, (3) Hurthle cell neoplasm and lymphocytic thyroiditis, (4) Hashimoto's thyroiditis with atypia, (5) metastatic PTC in a lymph node adjacent to the thyroid, and (6) less likely, hyalinizing trabecular neoplasm. A small panel of IHC including CEA and calcitonin was attempted on the cellblock sections. The results were negative for both markers in the rare cellular components. A diagnosis of suspicious for PTC was issued.

Subsequently, a left lobectomy was performed. The histologic sections showed an oncocytic tumor with diagnostic nuclear changes for papillary carcinoma and the presence of a dense lymphoplasmacytic infiltration as shown in Fig. 3.67d–f. The adjacent nonneoplastic thyroid tissue showed lymphocytic/Hashimoto's thyroiditis. A final diagnosis of Warthin-like variant of PTC was rendered.

Final Diagnosis on the FNA Specimen

Suspicious for papillary thyroid carcinoma

Final Diagnoses on the Surgical Specimen

Papillary thyroid carcinoma, Warthin-like variant
Lymphocytic thyroiditis

(continued)

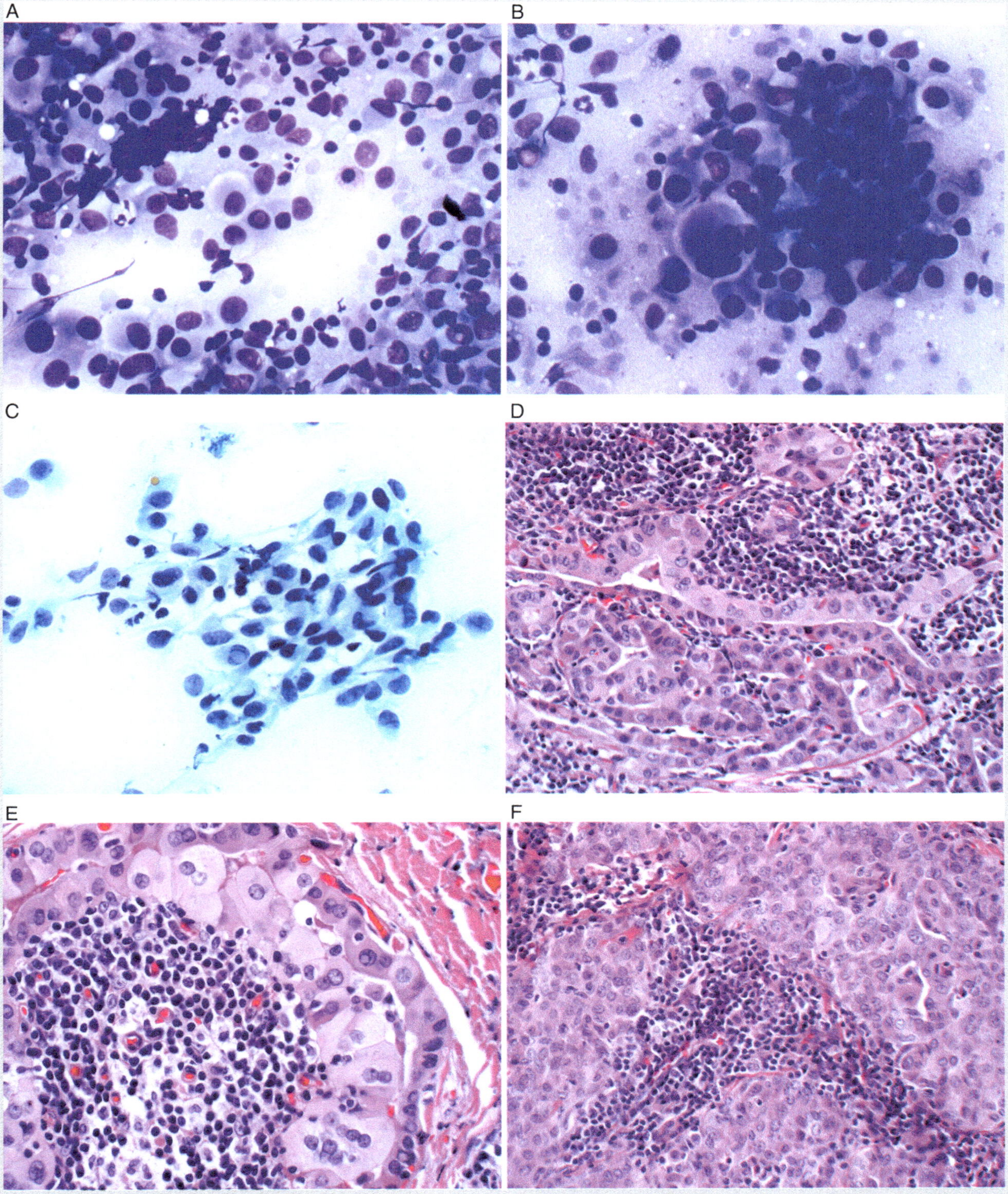

Fig. 3.67 A case of Warthin-like variant of PTC. Note that oncocytic follicular cells with nuclear changes of PTC (**a**–**c**) and histologic sections (**d**–**f**)

(continued)

What Are the Learning Points from This Case?

1. When an FNA sample demonstrates an oncocytic lesion with nuclear changes suspicious for PTC in the background of lymphoid cells, a Warthin-like variant PTC needs to be included in the differential diagnosis.
2. A Warthin-like PTC often coexists with a lymphocytic thyroiditis.
3. A small IHC panel including CEA and calcitonin can be useful in excluding a medullary carcinoma, even in a hypocellular cellblock preparation.

Case Scenario 3

Learning Objectives

1. Reiterate the diagnostic criteria for this variant of papillary carcinoma and its mimics.
2. Review the most effective panel of immunomarkers for diagnosis of this specific variant.

Case

A 60-year-old woman presented with a 3.0 cm mass at the right thyroid. Her previous medical history was significant for adenomatous colon polyps and nodular goiter which was confirmed by FNA 20 years ago. An ultrasound-guided FNA of the right lobe mass was performed. The FNA smears were hypercellular with numerous sheets and groups of atypical follicular cells with nuclear changes such as nuclear overlapping, grooves, and intranuclear inclusions for papillary carcinoma as shown in Fig. 3.68a, b. In addition to the characteristic nuclear features for a PTC, many epithelial groups/sheets showed (1) punched-out spaces resembling ductal carcinoma in situ of the breast (Fig. 3.68c), (2) large blunt papillary configuration without fibrovascular cores (Fig. 3.68d), (3) follicular cells highly cohesive and extremely overcrowded, and (4) foci of spindle cell morphology suggestive of squamous differentiation. Microfollicular pattern, colloid, and psammoma bodies were absent.

Based on the classic nuclear changes for PTC, the FNA diagnosis of PTC was issued.

Subsequently, a total thyroidectomy was performed. Histologic sections demonstrated a mixture of growth patterns, including cribriform, tubular/follicular, solid areas with spindled cells and squamoid changes, and large papillary fronds without distinct fibrovascular cores (Fig. 3.68e–h). Tumor cells exhibited definitive nuclear features for PTC and a moderate amount of granular cytoplasm. No colloid was seen throughout the tumor sections. The histologic findings raised a concern for cribriform variant of PTC. A panel of IHC including beta-catenin, CK19, HBME-1, p53, and galectin-3 was performed. The tumor cells demonstrated diffuse and strong nuclear and cytoplasmic positivity for beta-catenin and were positive for CK19, p53, and galectin-3, but negative for HBME-1 as shown in Fig. 3.68i–l. This immunostaining profile supported the morphologic impression of cribriform variant of PTC. Some investigators preferred to consider this as a distinct entity. It has been well documented that this tumor typically occurs in young patients with familial adenomatous polyposis (FAP) or Gardner syndrome. In this setting, the tumor tends to be multiple foci. A solitary sporadic tumor also has been reported as well. This particular patient most likely fit into a sporadic category since she was 60 at the time of this diagnosis and did not have a documented history of FAP.

Final Diagnosis on FNA Specimen

Papillary thyroid carcinoma

Final Diagnosis on Surgical Specimen

Papillary thyroid carcinoma, cribriform variant

What Are the Learning Points from This Case?

1. On an FNA smear, a cribriform variant of PTC should be excluded if one sees the following cytologic features: punched-out spaces resembling ductal carcinoma in situ of the breast, large blunt papillary configuration without fibrovascular cores, and foci of spindle cell morphology suggestive of squamous differentiation.
2. When this entity is suspected, additional sample should be requested for a cellblock preparation, and immunostains for beta-catenin and other useful diagnostic markers as mentioned earlier should be performed.
3. In a patient with this diagnosis, additional studies to exclude FAP in the patient and the family members are warranted.

Case Scenario 4

Learning Objectives

1. Review the differential diagnosis for an undifferentiated thyroid neoplasm.
2. Reiterate the diagnostic clues for an angiosarcoma.
3. Review the most effective panel of immunomarkers for diagnosis of this specific entity.

(continued)

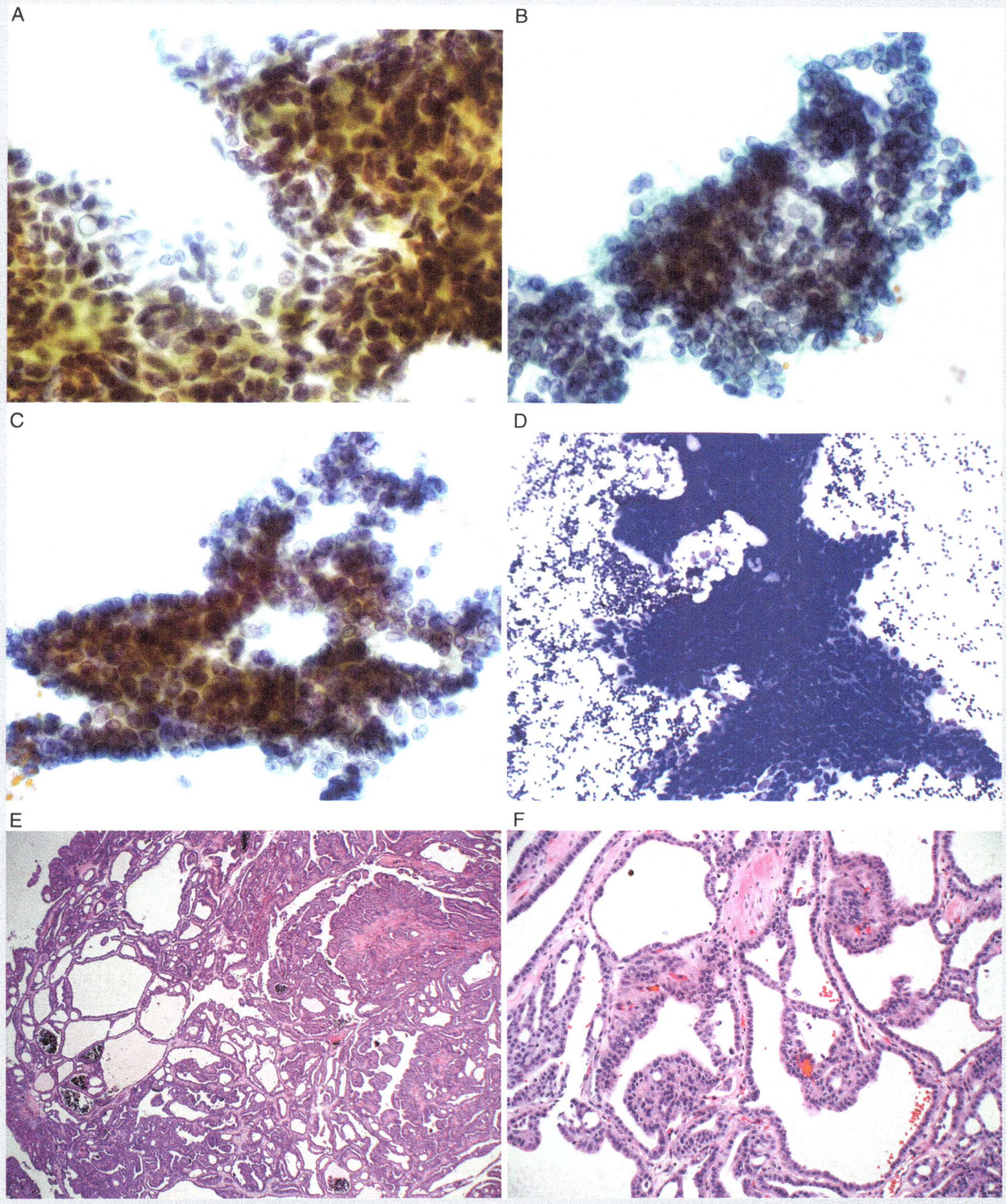

Fig. 3.68 A case of cribriform variant of PTC. Note that atypical follicular cells with nuclear changes such as nuclear overlapping, grooves, and intranuclear inclusions for papillary carcinoma (**a**, **b**), punched-out spaces resembling ductal carcinoma in situ of the breast (**c**), large blunt papillary configuration without fibrovascular cores (**d**), histologic sections (**e**–**h**), and positive stain for beta-catenin (both nuclear and cytoplasmic staining) (**i**), CK19 (**j**), and p53 (**k**) and negative for HBNE1 (**l**)

(continued)

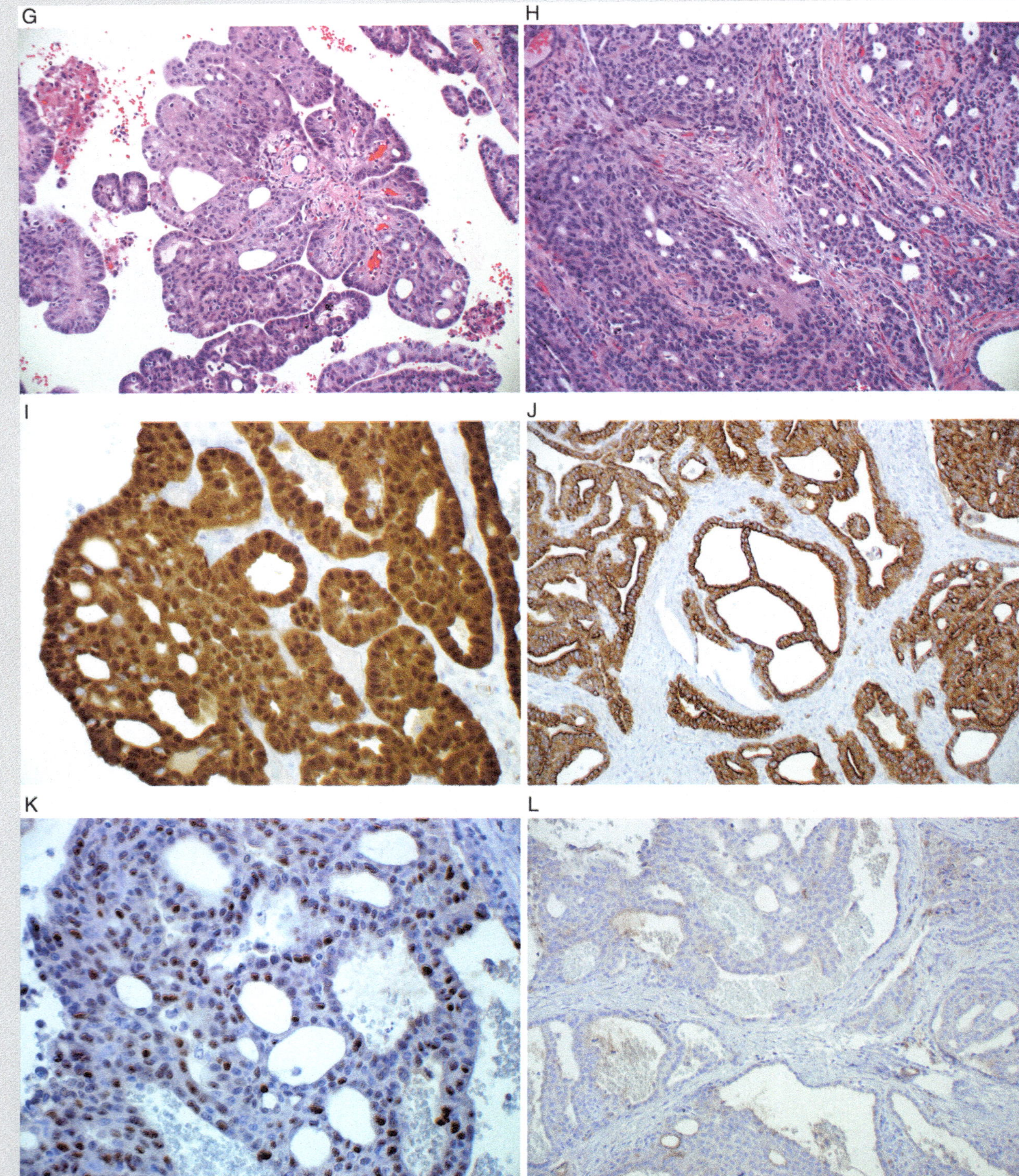

Fig. 3.68 (continued)

(continued)

Case

A 70-year-old man with a history of high-grade prostatic adenocarcinoma presented with a 4.0 cm mass at the left lobe of the thyroid. An ultrasound-guided FNA was performed. The FNA smears demonstrated low cellularity with large discohesive cells with enlarged nuclei, prominent nucleoli, some with a plasmacytoid appearance, and some with clear cytoplasm and cytoplasmic vacuoles containing red blood cells as shown in Fig. 3.69a–c. Necrosis and/or fibrin-like material were present in a bloody background. Fibrin and fibromuscular-like tissue were noted in the cellblock preparation as shown in Fig. 3.69d. Based on the cytologic features seen above, a diagnosis of positive for malignant cells, which favors poorly differentiated carcinoma, was rendered. It was recommended to obtain additional tissue for immunostains to further classify this malignant tumor.

Subsequently, a hemithyroidectomy was performed. Multiple sections contained a hemorrhagic and necrotic mass within the parenchyma of the thyroid gland. The mass expanded the thyroid lobe and infiltrated into the benign thyroid tissue. The tumor was composed of anastomosing vascular channels lined by pleomorphic, malignant endothelial cells with pleomorphic nuclei and prominent nucleoli as shown in Fig. 3.69e–g. Mitoses were frequent. Many of the vascular channels were necrotic and thrombosed. A panel of immunostains revealed that the atypical lining cells were positive for ERG, CD31, and CD34 as shown in Fig. 3.69h, i, and negative for cytokeratin and TTF1, which confirmed the diagnosis of angiosarcoma of the thyroid.

Final Diagnoses on the FNA Specimen

Positive for malignant cells
Favor poorly differentiated carcinoma
Recommend additional tissue for immunostains

Final Diagnosis on the Surgical Specimen

Angiosarcoma of the thyroid

What Are the Learning Points from This Case?

1. When the cytologic features of the atypical/malignant cells do not resemble a common thyroid tumor, such as papillary carcinoma, follicular/Hurthle cell neoplasm, and medullary carcinoma, an undifferentiated thyroid carcinoma, a rare primary thyroid tumor including angiosarcoma especially in an elderly man, and a secondary tumor should be included in the diagnostic consideration.
2. Atypical epithelioid cells with prominent nucleoli and cytoplasmic vacuoles containing red blood cells in a bloody background and the presence of fibrin-like material can be the clues for a diagnosis of angiosarcoma.
3. If an angiosarcoma is suspected, a panel of IHC markers including ERG and CD31 should be performed, even in a hypocellular cellblock. In the current case, if IHC would have done on the cellblock sections, a definitive diagnosis would have been reached. In retrospect, ERG and CD31 were performed on the cellblock sections, which showed that the "fibromuscular-like tissue" as shown in Fig. 3.69d was fibrin material, and the cellular components were positive for both ERG and CD31.

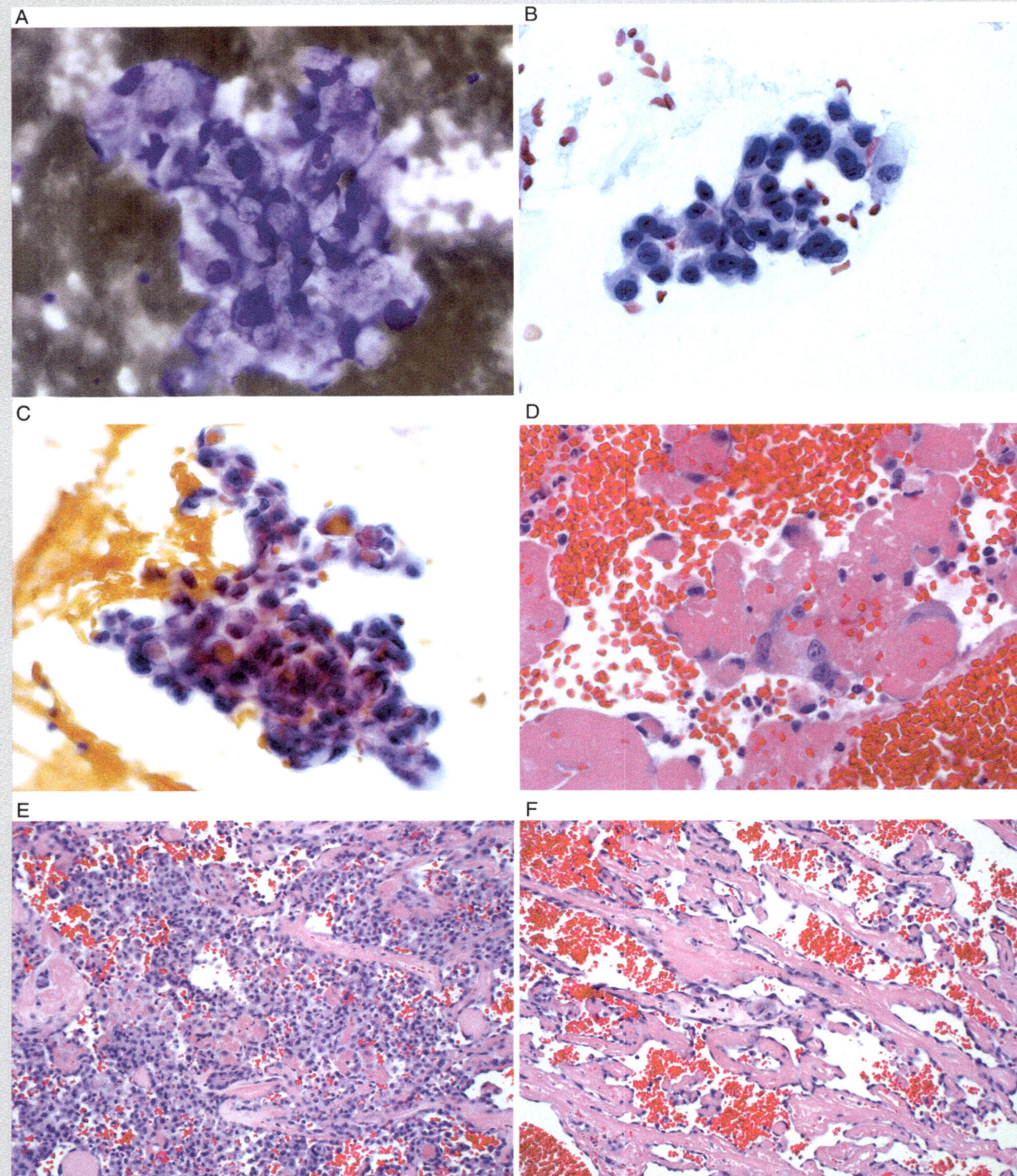

Fig. 3.69 A case of angiosarcoma of the thyroid. Note that large discohesive cells with enlarged nuclei, prominent nucleoli, some with plasmacytoid appearance, some with clear cytoplasm and cytoplasmic vacuoles containing red blood cells (**a–c**), cellblock (**d**), histologic sections of anastomosing vascular channels lined by pleomorphic, malignant endothelial cells (**e–g**) and positive for ERG (**h**) and CD31 (**i**) and negative or for cytokeratin and TTF1 (not shown)

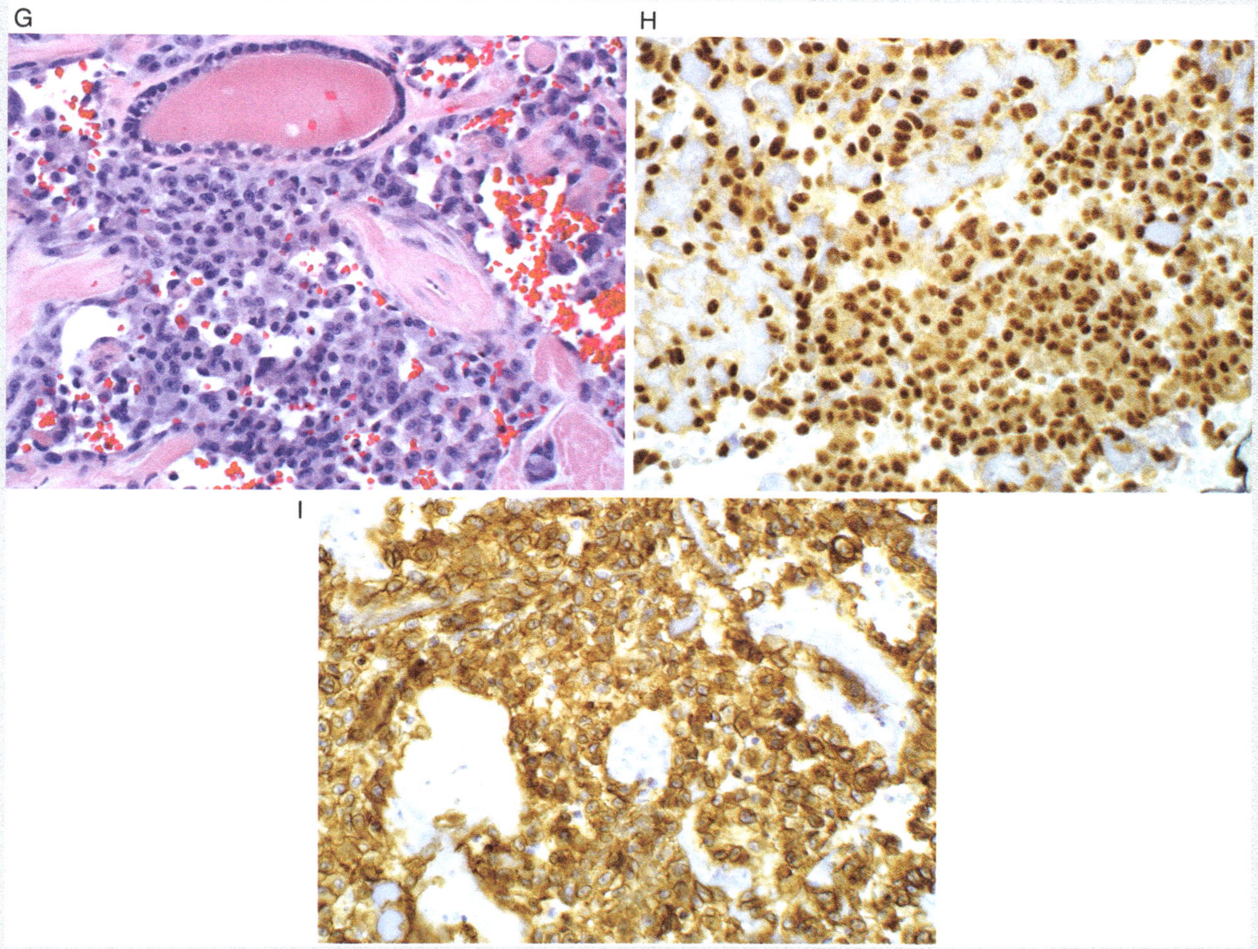

Fig. 3.69 (continued)

Abbreviation List

Abbreviation	Full text
AUS/FLUS	Atypia of Undetermined Significance/Follicular Lesion of Undetermined Significance
Bcl2	B-cell CLL/lymphoma 2
CASTLE	Carcinoma showing thymus-like differentiation
CD	Cluster of differentiation
CDX2	Caudal type homeobox 2
CEA	Carcinoembryonic antigen
CK	Cytokeratin
CRCC	Clear cell renal cell carcinoma
DQ	Diff-Quik
EMA	Epithelial membrane antigen
ERG	ETS-related gene
FDCT	Follicular dendritic cell tumor
FNA	Fine-needle aspiration
GATA3	GATA-binding protein 3
GFAP	Glial fibrillary acidic protein
GMS	Grocott's methenamine silver
HBME-1	Hector Battifora mesothelial epitope-1
IHC	Immunohistochemical
LCH	Langerhans cell histiocytosis
MIB-1	Mindbomb E3 ubiquitin protein ligase 1
MPNST	Malignant peripheral nerve sheath tumor
MUC2	Mucin 2
NSE	Neuron-specific enolase
Pap	Papanicolaou
PAX8	Paired box gene 8
PNST	Peripheral nerve sheath tumor

Abbreviation	Full text
PTC	Papillary thyroid carcinoma
PTH	Parathyroid hormone
pVHL	von Hippel-Lindau tumor suppressor gene protein
RCCma	Renal cell carcinoma marker
RDD	Rosai-Dorfman disease
RET	Rearranged during transfection
SCC	Squamous cell carcinoma
SETTLE	Spindle epithelial tumor with thymus-like differentiation
SFT	Solitary fibrous tumor
SMA	Smooth muscle actin
SMECE	Sclerosing mucoepidermoid carcinoma with eosinophils
SMT	Smooth muscle tumor
STAT6	Signal transducer and activator of transcription 6
TROP2	Tumor-associated calcium signal transducer 2
TTF1	Thyroid transcription factor 1
WHO	World Health Organization

Suggested Reading

Cytology/Fine-Needle Aspiration

Aggarwal SK, Jayaram G, Kakar A, Goel GD, Prakash R, Pant CS. Fine needle aspiration cytologic diagnosis of the solitary cold thyroid nodule. Comparison with ultrasonography, radionuclide perfusion study and xeroradiography. Acta Cytol. 1989;33(1):41–7.

Ali SZ, Cibas ES, editors. The bethesda system for reporting thyroid cytopathology. New York: Springer Science+Business Media; 2010.

Baloch ZW, LiVolsi VA. Cytologic and architectural mimics of papillary thyroid carcinoma. Diagnostic challenges in fine-needle aspiration and surgical pathology specimens. Am J Clin Pathol. 2006a;125(Suppl):S135–44.

Baloch ZW, LiVolsi VA. Warthin-like papillary carcinoma of the thyroid. Arch Pathol Lab Med. 2000a;124(8):1192–5.

Baloch ZW, LiVolsi VA, Asa SL, Rosai J, Merino MJ, Randolph G, et al. Diagnostic terminology and morphologic criteria for cytologic diagnosis of thyroid lesions: a synopsis of the National Cancer Institute thyroid fine-needle aspiration state of the science conference. Diagn Cytopathol. 2008;36(6):425–37.

Barroeta JE, Baloch ZW, Lal P, Pasha TL, Zhang PJ, LiVolsi VA. Diagnostic value of differential expression of CK19, galectin-3, HBME-1, ERK, RET, and p16 in benign and malignant follicular-derived lesions of the thyroid: an immunohistochemical tissue microarray analysis. Endocr Pathol. 2006a;17(3):225–34.

Bhatia A, Rajwanshi A, Dash RJ, Mittal BR, Saxena AK. Lymphocytic thyroiditis--is cytological grading significant? A correlation of grades with clinical, biochemical, ultrasonographic and radionuclide parameters. Cytojournal. 2007;4:10.

Bongiovanni M, Bloom L, Krane JF, Baloch ZW, Powers CN, Hintermann S, et al. Cytomorphologic features of poorly differentiated thyroid carcinoma: a multi-institutional analysis of 40 cases. Cancer. 2009a;117(3):185–94.

Bongiovanni M, Crippa S, Baloch Z, Piana S, Spitale A, Pagni F, et al. Comparison of 5-tiered and 6-tiered diagnostic systems for the reporting of thyroid cytopathology: a multi-institutional study. Cancer Cytopathol. 2012;120(2):117–25.

Bongiovanni M, Triponez F, McKee TA, Kumar N, Matthes T, Meyer P. Fine-needle aspiration of the diffuse sclerosing variant of papillary thyroid carcinoma masked by florid lymphocytic thyroiditis; a potential pitfall: a case report and review of the literature. Diagn Cytopathol. 2009b;37(9):671–5.

Bose S, Kapila K, Verma K. Medullary carcinoma of the thyroid: a cytological, immunocytochemical, and ultrastructural study. Diagn Cytopathol. 1992;8(1):28–32.

Cameselle-Teijeiro J, Chan JK. Cribriform-morular variant of papillary carcinoma: a distinctive variant representing the sporadic counterpart of familial adenomatous polyposis-associated thyroid carcinoma? Mod Pathol. 1999;12(4):400–11.

Casey MB, Sebo TJ, Carney JA. Hyalinizing trabecular adenoma of the thyroid gland identification through MIB-1 staining of fine-needle aspiration biopsy smears. Am J Clin Pathol. 2004;122(4):506–10.

Cersosimo E, Gharib H, Suman VJ, Goellner JR. "Suspicious" thyroid cytologic findings: outcome in patients without immediate surgical treatment. Mayo Clin Proc. 1993;68(4):343–8.

Chan JK, Saw D. The grooved nucleus. A useful diagnostic criterion of papillary carcinoma of the thyroid. Am J Surg Pathol. 1986;10(10):672–9.

Chang TC, Lai SM, Wen CY, Hsiao YL. Three-dimensional cytomorphology in fine needle aspiration biopsy of subacute thyroiditis. Acta Cytol. 2004;48(2):155–60.

Collins BT, Cramer HM, Tabatowski K, Hearn S, Raminhos A, Lampe H. Fine needle aspiration of medullary carcinoma of the thyroid. Cytomorphology, immunocytochemistry and electron microscopy. Acta Cytol. 1995;39(5):920–30.

DeLellis RA. Orphan Annie eye nuclei: a historical note. Am J Surg Pathol. 1993;17(10):1067–8.

DeMay RM. Thyroid. In:The art and science of cytopathology. 2nd ed. Chicago: ASCP Press; 2010. p. 841–95.

Deveci MS, Deveci G, LiVolsi VA, Baloch ZW. Fine-needle aspiration of follicular lesions of the thyroid. Diagnosis and follow-up. Cytojournal. 2006;3:9.

Dugan JM, Atkinson BF, Avitabile A, Schimmel M, LiVolsi VA. Psammoma bodies in fine needle aspirate of the thyroid in lymphocytic thyroiditis. Acta Cytol. 1987;31:330–4.

Gamboa-Domínguez A, Candanedo-González F, Uribe-Uribe NO, Angeles-Angeles A. Tall cell variant of papillary thyroid carcinoma. A cytohistologic correlation. Acta Cytol. 1997;41(3):672–6.

Gharib H, Goellner JR, Johnson DA. Fine-needle aspiration cytology of the thyroid. A 12-year experience with 11,000 biopsies. Clin Lab Med. 1993;13(3):699–709.

Giorgadze T, Rossi ED, Fadda G, Gupta PK, Livolsi VA, Baloch Z. Does the fine-needle aspiration diagnosis of "Hurthle-cell neoplasm/follicular neoplasm with oncocytic features" denote increased risk of malignancy? Diagn Cytopathol. 2004;31:307–12.

Goellner JR. Problems and pitfalls in thyroid cytology. Monogr Pathol. 1997;39:75–93.

Guarda LA, Peterson CE, Hall W, Baskin HJ. Anaplastic thyroid carcinoma: cytomorphology and clinical implications of fine-needle aspiration. Diagn Cytopathol. 1991;7(1):63–7.

Gutman PD, Henry M. Fine needle aspiration cytology of the thyroid. Clin Lab Med. 1998;18(3):461–82.

Jayaram G. Fine needle aspiration cytologic study of the solitary thyroid nodule. Profile of 308 cases with histologic correlation. Acta Cytol. 1985;29(6):967–73.

Kini SR, Miller JM, Hamburger JI. Cytopathology of Hürthle cell lesions of the thyroid gland by fine needle aspiration. Acta Cytol. 1981;25(6):647–52.

Kumarasinghe MP, De Silva S. Pitfalls in cytological diagnosis of autoimmune thyroiditis. Pathology. 1999;31(1):1–7.

Luze T, Tötsch M, Bangerl I, Hittmair A, Sandbichler P, Ladurner D, et al. Fine needle aspiration cytodiagnosis of anaplastic carcinoma and malignant haemangioendothelioma of the thyroid in an endemic goitre area. Cytopathology. 1990;1(5):305–10.

Oertel YC. Fine-needle aspiration and the diagnosis of thyroid cancer. Endocrinol Metab Clin North Am. 1996;25(1):69–91.

Oertel YC, Miyahara-Felipe L, Mendoza MG, Yu K. Value of repeated fine needle aspirations of the thyroid: an analysis of over ten thousand FNAs. Thyroid. 2007;17(11):1061–6.

Oertel YC, Oertel JE. Diagnosis of malignant epithelial thyroid lesions: fine needle aspiration and histopathologic correlation. Ann Diagn Pathol. 1998;2(6):377–400.

Papaparaskeva K, Nagel H, Droese M. Cytologic diagnosis of medullary carcinoma of the thyroid gland. Diagn Cytopathol. 2000;22(6):351–8.

Pérez F, Llobet M, Garijo G, Barceló C, Castro P, Bernadó L. Fine-needle aspiration cytology of columnar-cell carcinoma of the thyroid: report of two cases with cytohistologic correlation. Diagn Cytopathol. 1998;18(5):352–6.

Renshaw AA, Wang E, Haja J, Wilbur D, Henry MR, Hughes JH, Cytopathology Committee, College of American Pathologists. Fine-needle aspiration of papillary thyroid carcinoma: distinguishing between cases that performed well and those that performed poorly in the College of American Pathologists Nongynecologic Cytology Program. Arch Pathol Lab Med. 2006a;130(4):452–5.

Renshaw AA, Wang E, Wilbur D, Hughes JH, Haja J, Henry MR, College of American Pathologists Cytopathology Committee. Interobserver agreement on microfollicles in thyroid fine-needle aspirates. Arch Pathol Lab Med. 2006b;130(2):148–52.

Söderström N, Biörklund A. Intranuclear cytoplasmic inclusions in some types of thyroid cancer. Acta Cytol. 1973;17(3):191–7.

Wong LQ, LiVolsi VA, Baloch ZW. Diagnosis of atypia/follicular lesion of undetermined significance: an institutional experience. Cytojournal. 2014;11:23.

Yang GC, LiVolsi VA, Baloch ZW. Thyroid microcarcinoma: fine-needle aspiration diagnosis and histologic follow-up. Int J Surg Pathol. 2002;10:133–9.

Histology

Ahuja AT, Chan ES, Allen PW, Lau KY, King W, Metreweli C. Carcinoma showing thymiclike differentiation (CASTLE tumor). AJNR Am J Neuroradiol. 1998;19(7):1225–8.

Albores-Saavedra J, Gould E, Vardaman C, Vuitch F. The macrofollicular variant of papillary thyroid carcinoma: a study of 17 cases. Hum Pathol. 1991;22(12):1195–205.

Albores-Saavedra J, LiVolsi VA, Williams ED. Medullary carcinoma. Semin Diagn Pathol. 1985;2(2):137–46.

Aldinger KA, Samaan NA, Ibanez M, Hill CS Jr. Anaplastic carcinoma of the thyroid: a review of 84 cases of spindle and giant cell carcinoma of the thyroid. Cancer. 1978;41(6):2267–75.

Apel RL, Asa SL, LiVolsi VA. Papillary Hürthle cell carcinoma with lymphocytic stroma. "Warthin-like tumor" of the thyroid. Am J Surg Pathol. 1995;19(7):810–4.

Asa SL. My approach to oncocytic tumours of the thyroid. J Clin Pathol. 2004;57(3):225–32.

Baloch ZW, LiVolsi VA. Microcarcinoma of the thyroid. Adv Anat Pathol. 2006b;13(2):69–75.

Baloch ZW, LiVolsi VA. Our approach to follicular-patterned lesions of the thyroid. J Clin Pathol. 2007;60(3):244–50.

Baloch ZW, LiVolsi VA. Warthin-like papillary carcinoma of the thyroid. Arch Pathol Lab Med. 2000b;124(8):1192–5.

Baloch ZW, Solomon AC, LiVolsi VA. Primary mucoepidermoid carcinoma and sclerosing mucoepidermoid carcinoma with eosinophilia of the thyroid gland: a report of nine cases. Mod Pathol. 2000;13(7):802–7.

Ben Romdhane K, Khattech R, Ben Othman M, Gamoudi A, Ammar A, Cammoun M. Melanin production in medullary thyroid carcinoma. Histopathology. 1995;27(6):569–71.

Berho M, Suster S. The oncocytic variant of papillary carcinoma of the thyroid: a clinicopathologic study of 15 cases. Hum Pathol. 1997;28(1):47–53.

Bronner MP, LiVolsi VA. Spindle cell squamous carcinoma of the thyroid: an unusual anaplastic tumor associated with tall cell papillary cancer. Mod Pathol. 1991;4(5):637–43.

Cameselle-Teijeiro J. Mucoepidermoid carcinoma and solid cell nests of the thyroid. Hum Pathol. 1996;27(8):861–3.

Cameselle-Teijeiro J, Varela-Duran J, Fonseca E, Villanueva JP, Sobrinho-Simoes M. Solitary fibrous tumor of the thyroid. Am J Clin Pathol. 1994;101(4):535–8.

Carcangiu ML, Bianchi S. Diffuse sclerosing variant of papillary thyroid carcinoma. Clinicopathologic study of 15 cases. Am J Surg Pathol. 1989;13(12):1041–9.

Carcangiu ML, Steeper T, Zampi G, Rosai J. Anaplastic thyroid carcinoma. A study of 70 cases. Am J Clin Pathol. 1985;83(2):135–58.

Carcangiu ML, Zampi G, Rosai J. Poorly differentiated ("insular") thyroid carcinoma. A reinterpretation of Langhans' "wuchernde Struma". Am J Surg Pathol. 1984;8(9):655–68.

Carney JA, Ryan J, Goellner JR. Hyalinizing trabecular adenoma of the thyroid gland. Am J Surg Pathol. 1987;11(8):583–91.

Chan JK, Albores-Saavedra J, Battifora H, Carcangiu ML, Rosai J. Sclerosing mucoepidermoid thyroid carcinoma with eosinophilia. A distinctive low-grade malignancy arising from the metaplastic follicles of Hashimoto's thyroiditis. Am J Surg Pathol. 1991;15(5):438–48.

JKC C. Tumors of thyroid and parathyroid glands. In: Fletcher CDM, editor. Diagnostic histopathology of tumors. 4th ed. London: Churchill Livingstone; 2013. p. 1177–293.

Chem KT, Rosai J. Follicular variant of thyroid papillary carcinoma: a clinicopathologic study of six cases. Am J Surg Pathol. 1977;1(2):123–30.

Chetty R, Clark SP, Dowling JP. Leiomyosarcoma of the thyroid: immunohistochemical and ultrastructural study. Pathology. 1993;25(2):203–5.

Cheung CC, Boerner SL, MacMillan CM, Ramyar L, Asa SL. Hyalinizing trabecular tumor of the thyroid: a variant of papillary carcinoma proved by molecular genetics. Am J Surg Pathol. 2000;24(12):1622–6.

Chow SM, Law SC, Chan JK, Au SK, Yau S, Lau WH. Papillary microcarcinoma of the thyroid-prognostic significance of lymph node metastasis and multifocality. Cancer. 2003;98(1):31–40.

DeLellis RA, Williams ED. Tumors of the thyroid and parathyroid. In: DeLellis RA, Lloyd RV, Heitz PU, Eng C, editors. WHO classification of tumours. Pathology and genetics tumours of endocrine organs. Lyon: IARC Press; 2004. p. 49–136.

Dotto J, Nose V. Familial thyroid carcinoma: a diagnostic algorithm. Adv Anat Pathol. 2008;15(6):332–49.

Evans HL. Columnar-cell carcinoma of the thyroid. A report of two cases of an aggressive variant of thyroid carcinoma. Am J Clin Pathol. 1986;85(1):77–80.

Fenton PA, Clarke SE, Owen W, Hibbert J, Hodgson SV. Cribriform variant papillary thyroid cancer: a characteristic of familial adenomatous polyposis. Thyroid. 2001;11(2):193–7.

Flynn SD, Forman BH, Stewart AF, Kinder BK. Poorly differentiated ("insular") carcinoma of the thyroid gland: an aggressive subset of differentiated thyroid neoplasms. Surgery. 1988;104(6):963–70.

Franssila KO, Ackerman LV, Brown CL, Hedinger CE. Follicular carcinoma. Semin Diagn Pathol. 1985;2(2):101–22.

Ghossein R. Problems and controversies in the histopathology of thyroid carcinomas of follicular cell origin. Arch Pathol Lab Med. 2009;133(5):683–91.

Hazard JB, Kenyon R. Atypical adenoma of the thyroid. AMA Arch Pathol. 1954a;58(6):554–63.

Hazard JB, Kenyon R. Encapsulated angioinvasive carcinoma (angioinvasive adenoma) of the thyroid gland. Am J Clin Pathol. 1954b;24(7):755–66.

Hiltzik D, Carlson DL, Tuttle RM, Chuai S, Ishill N, Shaha A, et al. Poorly differentiated thyroid carcinomas defined on the basis of mitosis and necrosis: a clinicopathologic study of 58 patients. Cancer. 2006;106(6):1286–95.

Hunt JL, Barnes EL. Non-tumor-associated psammoma bodies in the thyroid. Am J Clin Pathol. 2003;119(1):90–4.

Iwasa K, Imai MA, Noguchi M, Tanaka S, Sasaki T, Katsuda S, et al. Spindle epithelial tumor with thymus-like differentiation (SETTLE) of the thyroid. Head Neck. 2002;24(9):888–93.

Kirby PA, Ellison WA, Thomas PA. Spindle epithelial tumor with thymus-like differentiation (SETTLE) of the thyroid with prominent mitotic activity and focal necrosis. Am J Surg Pathol. 1999;23(6):712–6.

Landon G, Ordonez NG. Clear cell variant of medullary carcinoma of the thyroid. Hum Pathol. 1985;16(8):844–7.

Lang W, Georgii G. Minimal invasive cancer in the thyroid. Clin Oncol. 1982;1:527–37.

Mendelsohn G, Baylin SB, Bigner SH, Wells SA Jr, Eggleston JC. Anaplastic variants of medullary thyroid carcinoma: a light-microscopic and immunohistochemical study. Am J Surg Pathol. 1980;4(4):333–41.

Mills SE, Gaffey MJ, Watts JC, Swanson PE, Wick MR, LiVolsi VA. Angiomatoid carcinoma and "angiosarcoma" of the thyroid gland. A spectrum of endothelial differentiation. Am J Clin Pathol. 1994;102(3):322–30.

Montone KT, Baloch ZW, LiVolsi VA. The thyroid Hurthle (oncocytic) cell and its associated pathologic conditions: a surgical pathology and cytopathology review. Arch Pathol Lab Med. 2008;132(8):1241–50.

Nikiforov YE, Erickson LA, Nikiforova MN, Caudill CM, Lloyd RV. Solid variant of papillary thyroid carcinoma: incidence, clinical-pathologic characteristics, molecular analysis, and biologic behavior. Am J Surg Pathol. 2001;25(12):1478–84.

Ostrowski M, Merino MJ. Tall cell variant of papillary thyroid carcinoma: a reassessment and immunohistochemical study with comparison to usual type of papillary carcinoma of the thyroid. Am J Surg Pathol. 1996;20(8):964–74.

Rosai J, Saxén EA, Woolner L. Undifferentiated and poorly differentiated carcinoma. Semin Diagn Pathol. 1985;2(2):123–36.

Rosai J, Tallini G. Thyroid gland. In: Rosai J, editor. Rosai and Ackerman's surgical pathology. 10th ed. London: Mosby Elsevier; 2011. p. 487–564.

Sambade C, Baldaque-Faria A, Cardoso-Oliveira M, Sobrinho-Simões M. Follicular and papillary variants of medullary carcinoma of the thyroid. Pathol Res Pract. 1988;184(1):98–107.

Schmid KW, Mesewinkel F, Böcker W. Hyalinizing trabecular adenoma of the thyroid--morphology and differential diagnosis. Acta Med Austriaca. 1996;23(1–2):65–8.

Schmidt RJ, Wang CA. Encapsulated follicular carcinoma of the thyroid: diagnosis, treatment, and results. Surgery. 1986;100(6):1068–77.

Sobrinho-Simoes M, Sambade C, Nesland JM, Johannessen JV. Tall cell papillary carcinoma. Am J Surg Pathol. 1989;13(1):79–80.

Thieblemont C, Mayer A, Dumontet C, Barbier Y, Callet-Bauchu E, Felman P. Primary thyroid lymphoma is a heterogeneous disease. J Clin Endocrinol Metab. 2002;87(1):105–11.

Volante M, Collini P, Nikiforov YE, Sakamoto A, Kakudo K, Katoh R, et al. Poorly differentiated thyroid carcinoma: the Turin proposal for the use of uniform diagnostic criteria and an algorithmic diagnostic approach. Am J Surg Pathol. 2007;31(8):1256–64.

Wang SA, Rahemtullah A, Faquin WC, Roepke J, Harris NL, Hasserjian RP. Hodgkin's lymphoma of the thyroid: a clinicopathologic study of five cases and review of the literature. Mod Pathol. 2005;18(12):1577–84.

Wenig BM, Adair CF, Heffess CS. Primary mucoepidermoid carcinoma of the thyroid gland: a report of six cases and a review of the literature of a follicular epithelial-derived tumor. Hum Pathol. 1995;26(10):1099–108.

Wenig BM, Thompson LD, Adair CF, Shmookler B, Heffess CS. Thyroid papillary carcinoma of columnar cell type. A clinicopathologic study of 16 cases. Cancer. 1998;82(4):740–53.

Zaatari GS, Saigo PE, Huvos AG. Mucin production in medullary carcinoma of the thyroid. Arch Pathol Lab Med. 1983;107(2):70–4.

Ancillary Tests: Immunohistochemistry

Abrosimov A. Histologic and immunohistochemical characterization of medullary thyroid carcinoma. Arkh Patol. 1996;58(4):43–8. Russian.

Barroeta JE, Baloch ZW, Lal P, Pasha TL, Zhang PJ, LiVolsi VA. Diagnostic value of differential expression of CK19, galectin-3, HBME-1, ERK, RET, and p16 in benign and malignant follicular-derived lesions of the thyroid: an immunohistochemical tissue microarray analysis. Endocr Pathol. 2006b;17(3):225–34.

Cheung CC, Ezzat S, Freeman JL, Rosen IB, Asa SL. Immunohistochemical diagnosis of papillary thyroid carcinoma. Mod Pathol. 2001;14(4):338–42.

DeLilles RA, Rule AH, Spiler I, Nathanson L, Tashjian AH Jr, Wolfe HJ. Calcitonin and carcinoembryonic antigen as tumor markers in medullary thyroid carcinoma. Am J Clin Pathol. 1978;70(4): 587–94.

Hirokawa M, Carney JA, Ohtsuki Y. Hyalinizing trabecular adenoma and papillary carcinoma of the thyroid gland express different cytokeratin patterns. Am J Surg Pathol. 2000;24(6):877–81.

Lin F, Liu H. Immunohistochemistry in undifferentiated neoplasm/tumor of uncertain origin. Arch Pathol Lab Med. 2014;138(12):1583–610.

Liu H, Lin F. Application of immunohistochemistry in thyroid pathology. Arch Pathol Lab Med. 2015;139(1):67–82.

Liu H, Shi J, Lin F. The potential diagnostic utility of TROP-2 in thyroid neoplasms. Appl Immunohistochem Mol Morphol. 2016. Epub 2016 Feb 9.

Liu H, Wilkerson M, Lin F. Thyroid, parathyroid and adrenal glands. In: Lin F, Prichard JW, Liu H, Wilkerson M, Chen ZE, editors. Handbook of practical immunohistochemistry – frequently asked questions. 2nd ed. New York: Springer Science+Business Media; 2015. p. 255–86.

LiVolsi VA, Brooks JJ, Arendash-Durand B. Anaplastic thyroid tumors. Immunohistology. Am J Clin Pathol. 1987;87(4):434–42.

Nonaka D, Tang Y, Chiriboga L, Rivera M, Ghossein R. Diagnostic utility of thyroid transcription factors Pax8 and TTF-2 (FoxE1) in thyroid epithelial neoplasms. Mod Pathol. 2008;21(2):192–200.

Ordóñez NG, El-Naggar AK, Hickey RC, Samaan NA. Anaplastic thyroid carcinoma. Immunohistochemical study of 32 cases. Am J Clin Pathol. 1991;96(1):15–24.

Rosai J. Immunohistochemical markers of thyroid tumors: significance and diagnostic applications. Tumori. 2003;89(5):517–9.

Williams ED, Ponder BJ, Craig RK. Immunohistochemical study of calcitonin gene-related peptide in human medullary carcinoma and C cell hyperplasia. Clin Endocrinol (Oxf). 1987;27(1):107–14.

Ancillary Tests: Molecular Testing

Barzon L, et al. Characterization of a novel complex BRAF mutation in a follicular variant papillary thyroid carcinoma. Eur J Endocrinol. 2008;159:77–80.

Capella G, Matias-Guiu X, Ampudia X, de Leiva A, Perucho M, Prat J. Ras oncogene mutations in thyroid tumors: polymerase chain reaction-restriction-fragment-length polymorphism analysis from paraffin-embedded tissues. Diagn Mol Pathol. 1996;5(1): 45–52.

Cohen Y, Xing M, Mambo E, Guo Z, Wu G, Trink B, et al. BRAF mutation in papillary thyroid carcinoma. J Natl Cancer Inst. 2003;95(8):625–7.

Elisei R, Romei C, Vorontsova T, Cosci B, Veremeychik V, Kuchinskaya E, et al. RET/PTC rearrangements in thyroid nodules: studies in irradiated and not irradiated, malignant and benign thyroid lesions in children and adults. J Clin Endocrinol Metab. 2001;86(7):3211–6.

Eng C, Mulligan LM, Smith DP, Healey CS, Frilling A, et al. Mutation of the RET protooncogene in sporadic medullary thyroid carcinoma. Genes Chromosomes Cancer. 1995;12(3):209–12.

Esapa CT, Johnson SJ, Kendall-Taylor P, Lennard TW, Harris PE. Prevalence of Ras mutations in thyroid neoplasia. Clin Endocrinol (Oxf). 1999;50(4):529–35.

Fabien N, Paulin C, Santoro M, Berger N, Grieco M, Galvain D. Detection of RET oncogene activation in human papillary thyroid carcinomas by in situ hybridisation. Br J Cancer. 1992;66(6):1094–8.

Frank-Raue K, Rondot S, Raue F. Molecular genetics and phenomics of RET mutations: impact on prognosis of MTC. Mol Cell Endocrinol. 2010;322(1–2):2–7.

Giordano TJ, Kuick R, Thomas DG, Misek DE, Vinco M, Sanders D, et al. Molecular classification of papillary thyroid carcinoma: distinct BRAF, RAS, and RET/PTC mutation-specific gene expression profiles discovered by DNA microarray analysis. Oncogene. 2005;24(44):6646–56.

Inaba M, Umemura S, Satoh H, Abe Y, Kurokawa K, Sakai H, et al. Expression of RET in follicular cell-derived tumors of the thyroid gland: prevalence and implication of morphological type. Pathol Int. 2003;53(3):146–53.

Jhiang SM, Fithian L, Weghorst CM, Clark OH, Falko JM, O'Dorisio TM, et al. RET mutation screening in MEN2 patients and discovery of a novel mutation in a sporadic medullary thyroid carcinoma. Thyroid. 1996;6(2):115–21.

Kimura ET, Nikiforova MN, Zhu Z, Knauf JA, Nikiforov YE, Fagin JA. High prevalence of BRAF mutations in thyroid cancer: genetic evidence for constitutive activation of the RET/PTC-RAS-BRAF signaling pathway in papillary thyroid carcinoma. Cancer Res. 2003;63(7):1454–7.

Kroll TG. Molecular events in follicular thyroid tumors. Cancer Treat Res. 2004;122:85–105.

Marques AR, Espadinha C, Catarino AL, Moniz S, Pereira T, Sobrinho LG, et al. Expression of PAX8-PPAR gamma 1 rearrangements in both follicular thyroid carcinomas and adenomas. J Clin Endocrinol Metab. 2002;87(8):3947–52.

Motomura T, Nikiforov YE, Namba H, Ashizawa K, Nagataki S, Yamashita S, et al. Ret rearrangements in Japanese pediatric and adult papillary thyroid cancers. Thyroid. 1998;8(6):485–9.

Mulligan LM, Eng C, Healey CS, Clayton D, Kwok JB, Gardner E, et al. Specific mutations of the RET proto-oncogene are related to disease phenotype in MEN 2A and FMTC. Nat Genet. 1994;6(1):70–4.

Nikiforov M, Biddinger PW, Caudill CM, Kroll TG, Nikiforov YE. PAX8-PPAR g rearrangement in thyroid tumors: RT-PCR and immunohistochemical analysis. Am J Surg Pathol. 2002;26(8):1016–23.

Nikiforov YE. Molecular analysis of thyroid tumors. Mod Pathol. 2011;24(Suppl 2):S34–43.

Nikiforov YE. RET/PTC rearrangement in thyroid tumors. Endocr Pathol. 2002;13(1):3–16.

Nikiforov YE. Thyroid carcinoma: molecular pathways and therapeutic targets. Mod Pathol. 2008;21(Suppl 2):S37–43.

Nikiforov YE, Steward DL, Robinson-Smith TM, Haugen BR, Klopper JP, Zhu Z, et al. Molecular testing for mutations in improving the fine-needle aspiration diagnosis of thyroid nodules. J Clin Endocrinol Metab. 2009;94(6):2092–8.

Nikiforova MN, Caudill CM, Biddinger P, Nikiforov YE. Prevalence of RET/PTC rearrangements in Hashimoto's thyroiditis and papillary thyroid carcinomas. Int J Surg Pathol. 2002;10(1):15–22.

Papotti M, Volante M, Giuliano A, Fassina A, Fusco A, Bussolati G, et al. RET/PTC activation in hyalinizing trabecular tumors of the thyroid. Am J Surg Pathol. 2000;24(12):1615–21.

Williams GH, Rooney S, Thomas GA, Cummins G, Williams ED. RET activation in adult and childhood papillary thyroid carcinoma using a reverse transcriptase-n-polymerase chain reaction approach on archival-nested material. Br J Cancer. 1996;74(4):585–9.

Wirtschafter A, et al. Expression of the RET/PTC fusion gene as a marker for papillary carcinoma in Hashimoto's thyroiditis. Laryngoscope. 1997;107(1):95–100.

Xing M. BRAF mutation in thyroid cancer. Endocr Relat Cancer. 2005;12(2):245–62.

Xing M, Tufano RP, Tufaro AP, Basaria S, Ewertz M, Rosenbaum E, et al. Detection of BRAF mutation on fine needle aspiration biopsy specimens: a new diagnostic tool for papillary thyroid cancer. J Clin Endocrinol Metab. 2004;89(6):2867–72.

Lymph Nodes

4

Xiaohong (Mary) Zhang and Fan Lin

Summary of Pearls and Pitfalls

- Always attempt to get sufficient sample for flow cytometric study, molecular analysis, and cellblock preparation if a lymphoma is suspected.
- A final diagnosis of lymphoma should not be based on cytomorphology alone. Ancillary tests such as flow cytometric study, immunohistochemistry (IHC), and cytogenetic analysis/fluorescence in situ hybridization (FISH) should be performed.
- Cell block preparation for immunostains is highly recommended if large B-cell lymphoma (LBCL) is suspected, since a significant number of cases have an inconclusive diagnosis from flow cytometric analysis due to the breakdown of the cytoplasm of lymphoid cells.
- Incisional or excisional biopsy is recommended for all cases suspicious for Hodgkin lymphoma, T-cell lymphoma, T-cell-rich B-cell lymphoma, transformation from a low-grade lymphoma into a high-grade non-Hodgkin lymphoma and unusual types of lymphoma.
- Culture should be considered when acute inflammation and necrosis are present.
- Mycobacterial infection should be considered when a granulomatous process and necrosis are present.
- Cohesive sheets and groups of lymphoid cells are frequently seen in an LBCL that might be mistaken for metastatic carcinoma.
- Noncaseating granulomas are frequently seen in Hodgkin lymphoma and T-cell lymphoma, in addition to benign conditions and metastatic tumors, such as seminoma.
- In addition to Burkitt lymphoma (BL), cytoplasmic vacuoles can be seen in other high-grade lymphomas, rhabdomyosarcoma, seminoma, and carcinomas.
- Lymphoglandular bodies are less frequently present in plasmacytoma or myeloid sarcoma.
- HIV-associated follicular hyperplasia and mononucleosis are more likely to mimic a high-grade lymphoma.
- Collision tumors, such as metastatic small cell carcinoma or melanoma in the background of small lymphocytic lymphoma (SLL), are infrequent, but can be seen.
- Most low-grade lymphomas have a mindbomb homolog 1 (MIB-1, Ki-67) proliferative index less than 26%; in contrast, high-grade lymphoma usually has a MIB-1 proliferative index greater than 26%.

2017 WHO Classification of Mature Lymphoid, Histiocytic, and Dendritic Neoplasms[1]

Mature B-Cell Neoplasms

Chronic lymphocytic leukemia/small lymphocytic lymphoma (CLL/SLL)
Monoclonal B-cell lymphocytosis[2]
B-cell prolymphocytic leukemia
Splenic marginal zone lymphoma (MZL)
Hairy cell leukemia
Splenic B-cell lymphoma/leukemia, unclassifiable
Splenic diffuse red pulp small B-cell lymphoma

[1]Used with permission from Arber et al. (Arber et al. 2016); and from Swerdlow et al. (Swerdlow et al. 2016a).

[2]Changes from the 2008 classification.

Provisional entities are listed in italics.

© Springer International Publishing AG 2018
F. Lin et al., *Handbook of Practical Fine Needle Aspiration and Small Tissue Biopsies*, DOI 10.1007/978-3-319-57386-1_4

Hairy cell leukemia variant
Lymphoplasmacytic lymphoma (LPL)
Waldenström macroglobulinemia
Monoclonal gammopathy of undetermined significance (MGUS), IgM[2]
Mu heavy chain disease
Gamma heavy chain disease
Alpha heavy chain disease
MGUS, IgG/A[3]
Plasma cell myeloma
Solitary plasmacytoma of the bone
Extraosseous plasmacytoma
Monoclonal immunoglobulin deposition diseases[3]
Extranodal MZL of mucosa-associated lymphoid tissue (MALT lymphoma)
Nodal MZL
Pediatric nodal MZL
Follicular lymphoma
In situ follicular neoplasia[3]
Duodenal-type follicular lymphoma[3]
Pediatric-type follicular lymphoma[3]
LBCL with interferon regulatory factor 4 (IRF4) rearrangement[3]
Primary cutaneous follicle center lymphoma
Mantle cell lymphoma (MCL)
In situ mantle cell neoplasia[3]
Diffuse large B-cell lymphoma (DLBCL), not otherwise specified (NOS)
Germinal center B-cell type[3]
Activated B-cell (ABC) type[3]
T-cell/histiocyte-rich LBCL
Primary DLBCL of the central nervous system (CNS)
Primary cutaneous DLBCL, leg type
Epstein-Barr virus (EBV)-positive DLBCL, NOS[4]
EBV+ mucocutaneous ulcer[4]
DLBCL associated with chronic inflammation
Lymphomatoid granulomatosis
Primary mediastinal (thymic) LBCL
Intravascular LBCL
ALK-positive LBCL
Plasmablastic lymphoma
Primary effusion lymphoma
Human herpes virus 8 (HHV8)-positive DLBCL, NOS[4]
Burkitt lymphoma
Burkitt-like lymphoma with 11q aberration[4]
High-grade B-cell lymphoma (HGBCL), with *MYC* and *BCL2* and/or *BCL6* rearrangements[4]
HGBCL, NOS[4]
B-cell lymphoma, unclassifiable, with features intermediate between DLBCL and CHL

[3] See footnote 2.
[4] See footnote 2.

Mature T- and Natural Killer (NK)-Cell Neoplasms

T-cell prolymphocytic leukemia
T-cell large granular lymphocytic leukemia
Chronic lymphoproliferative disorder of NK cells
Aggressive NK-cell leukemia
Systemic EBV+ T-cell lymphoma of childhood[5]
Hydroa vacciniforme-like lymphoproliferative disorder[5]
Adult T-cell leukemia/lymphoma
Extranodal NK/T-cell lymphoma, nasal type
Enteropathy-associated T-cell lymphoma
Monomorphic epitheliotropic intestinal T-cell lymphoma[5]
Indolent T-cell lymphoproliferative disorder of the gastrointestinal (GI) tract [5]
Hepatosplenic T-cell lymphoma
Subcutaneous panniculitis-like T-cell lymphoma
Mycosis fungoides
Sézary syndrome
Primary cutaneous CD30-positive T-cell lymphoproliferative disorders
Lymphomatoid papulosis
Primary cutaneous anaplastic large cell lymphoma
Primary cutaneous gamma-delta T-cell lymphoma
Primary cutaneous CD8-positive aggressive epidermotropic cytotoxic T-cell lymphoma
Primary cutaneous acral CD8-positive T-cell lymphoma[5]
Primary cutaneous CD4-positive small/medium T-cell lymphoproliferative disorder[5]
Peripheral T-cell lymphoma, NOS
Angioimmunoblastic T-cell lymphoma
Follicular T-cell lymphoma[6]
Nodal peripheral T-cell lymphoma with T follicular helper (TFH) phenotype[6]
Anaplastic large cell lymphoma, ALK positive
Anaplastic large cell lymphoma, ALK negative[6]
Breast implant-associated ALCL[6]

Hodgkin Lymphoma

Nodular lymphocyte-predominant Hodgkin lymphoma
Classical Hodgkin lymphoma (CHL)
Nodular sclerosis CHL
Lymphocyte-rich CHL
Mixed cellularity CHL
Lymphocyte-depleted CHL

[5] See footnote 2.
[6] See footnote 2.

Posttransplant Lymphoproliferative Disorders (PTLD)

Plasmacytic hyperplasia PTLD
Infectious mononucleosis PTLD
Florid follicular hyperplasia PTLD[6]
Polymorphic PTLD
Monomorphic PTLD (B- and T-/NK-cell types)
CHL PTLD

Histiocytic and Dendritic Cell Neoplasms

Histiocytic sarcoma
Langerhans cell histiocytosis (LCH)
Langerhans cell sarcoma
Indeterminate dendritic cell tumor
Interdigitating dendritic cell sarcoma
Follicular dendritic cell sarcoma
Fibroblastic reticular cell tumor
Disseminated juvenile xanthogranuloma
Erdheim-Chester disease[7]

B Lymphoblastic Leukemia/Lymphoma

B lymphoblastic leukemia/lymphoma, NOS
B lymphoblastic leukemia/lymphoma with recurrent genetic abnormalities
B lymphoblastic leukemia/lymphoma with t(9;22)(q34.1;q11.2); *BCR-ABL1*
B lymphoblastic leukemia/lymphoma with t(v;11q23.3); *KMT2A* rearranged
B lymphoblastic leukemia/lymphoma with t(12;21)(p13.2;q22.1); *ETV6-RUNX1*
B lymphoblastic leukemia/lymphoma with hyperdiploidy
B lymphoblastic leukemia/lymphoma with hypodiploidy
B lymphoblastic leukemia/lymphoma with t(5;14)(q31.1;q32.3) *IL3-IGH*
B lymphoblastic leukemia/lymphoma with t(1;19)(q23;p13.3); *TCF3-PBX1*
Provisional entity: B lymphoblastic leukemia/lymphoma, *BCR-ABL1-like*
Provisional entity: B lymphoblastic leukemia/lymphoma with *iAMP21*

T Lymphoblastic Leukemia/Lymphoma

Provisional entity: early T-cell precursor lymphoblastic leukemia
Provisional entity: NK-cell lymphoblastic leukemia/lymphoma

Nonneoplastic Lymph Nodes

Cytological Features (Fig. 4.1a, b)

- High cellularity
- Mixed population of lymphoid cells with small lymphocytes predominant
- Plasma cells, plasmacytoid cells, and immunoblasts
- Histiocytes and tingible-body macrophages

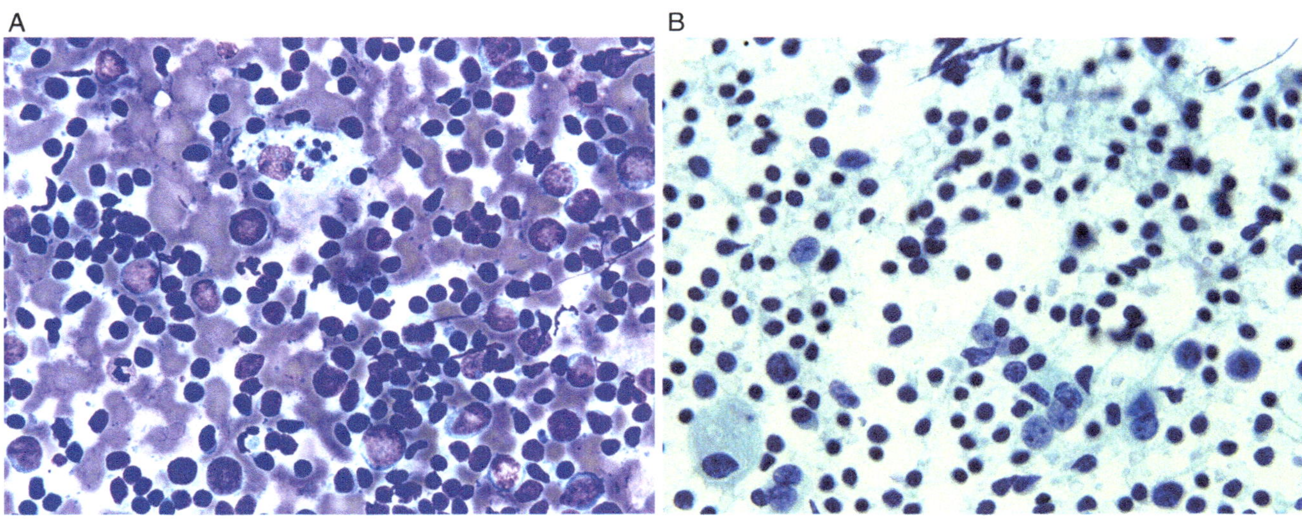

Fig. 4.1 (**a**, **b**) Reactive lymph node with a mixed population of lymphoid cells with small lymphocytes predominant on Diff-Quik (**a**) and Pap stain (**b**)

[7] See footnote 2.

Suppurative Lymphadenitis

Cytological Features (Fig. 4.2a, b)

- Mixed population of lymphoid cells with a variable number of neutrophils.
- Degenerated lymphoid cells, histiocytes, neutrophils, and necrotic debris.
- Bacteria or fungus may be seen.
- Etiologies could include cat-scratch disease, bacterial infection, lupus, and less commonly Hodgkin lymphoma and metastatic carcinomas.

Histologic Features

- Preserved nodal architecture with lymphoid follicular hyperplasia (Fig. 4.3).
- Hyperplastic lymphoid follicles show polarity with tingible-body macrophages (Fig. 4.4).
- Increased neutrophilic infiltrate, abscess formation, and perilymphadenitis (Fig. 4.5).

Infectious Mononucleosis

Cytological Features

- Highly cellular specimen
- Mixed population of lymphoid cells with many immunoblasts and plasmacytoid cells.
- Large atypical lymphoid cells are frequently present; some may mimic Hodgkin cells.
- Flow cytometry reveals an abundance of CD8-positive T cells and only a small population of B cells.

Histologic Features

- Preserved nodal architecture with paracortical expansion composed of mixed mature lymphocytes, plasma cells, immunoblasts, and histiocytes in a mottled pattern (Figs. 4.6 and 4.7)
- Lymphoid follicular hyperplasia
- EBV-positive by in situ hybridization stain (Fig. 4.8)

Differential Diagnosis

- HGBCL
- Hodgkin lymphoma

Rosai-Dorfman Disease

Cytological Features

- Mixed population of lymphoid cells.
- A large number of histiocytes with pale cytoplasm.
- Many histiocytes contain lymphoid cells or red blood cells.
- These histiocytes are positive for S100, but negative for CD1a.
- Tissue biopsy should be recommended for a final diagnosis.

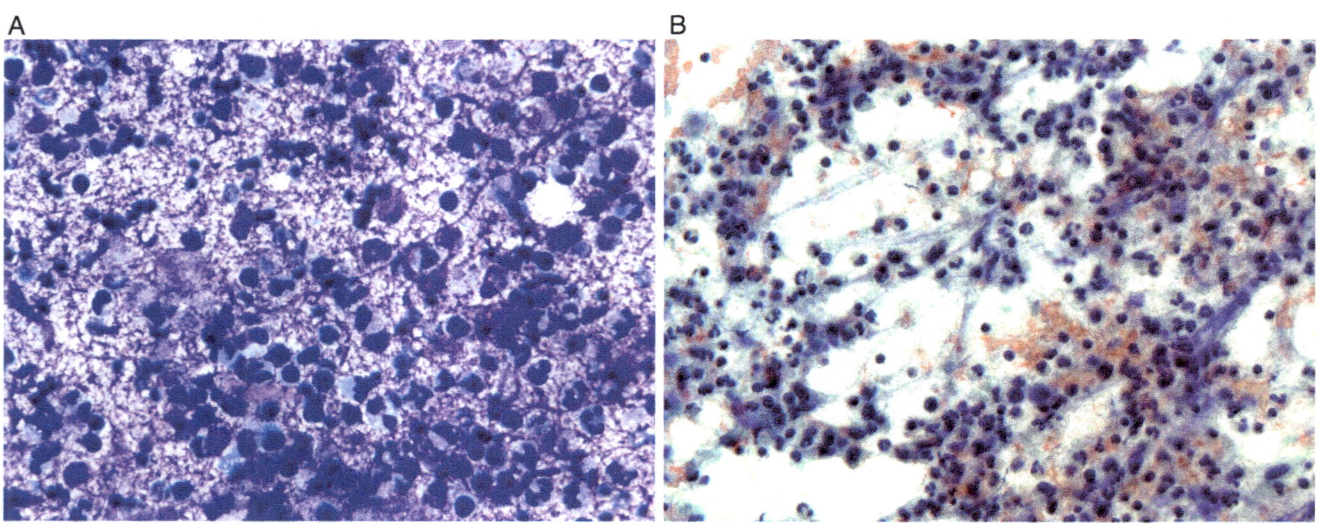

Fig. 4.2 (**a**, **b**) Suppurative lymphadenitis with degenerated lymphoid cells, histiocytes, neutrophils, and necrotic debris on Diff-Quik (**a**) and Pap stain (**b**)

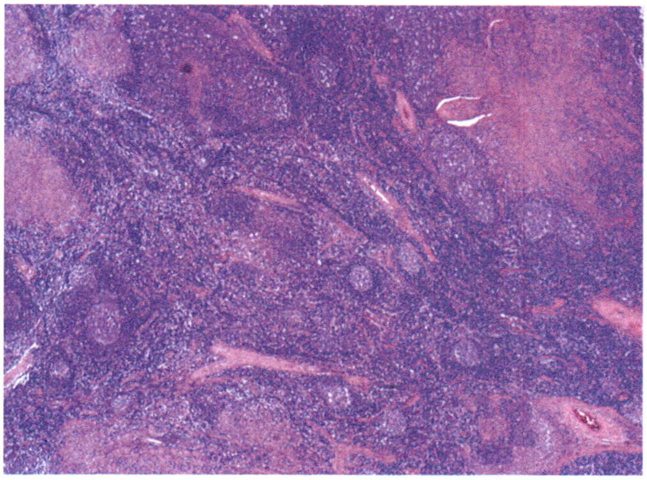

Fig. 4.3 Suppurative lymphadenitis showing preserved nodal architecture with reactive lymphoid follicles and focal abscess formation

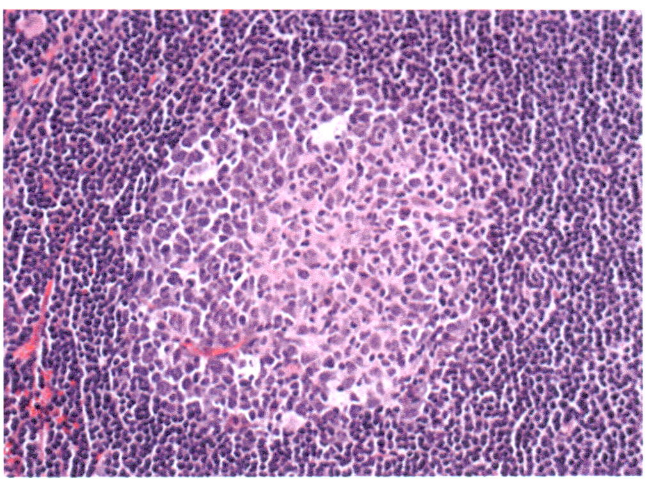

Fig. 4.4 Reactive lymphoid follicles with polarity and tingible-body macrophages

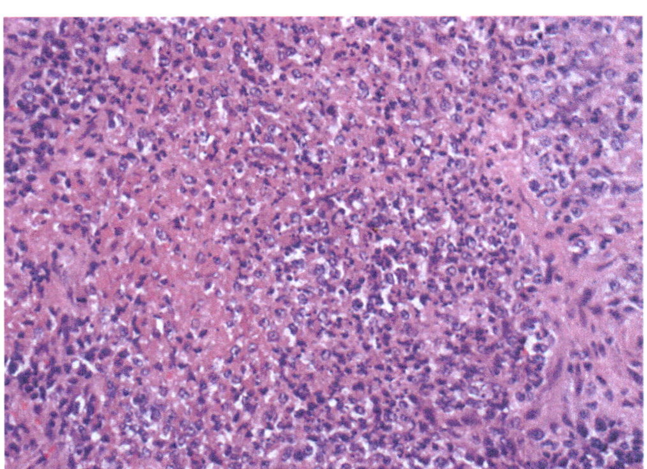

Fig. 4.5 Suppurative lymphadenitis with focal abscess formation and necrosis

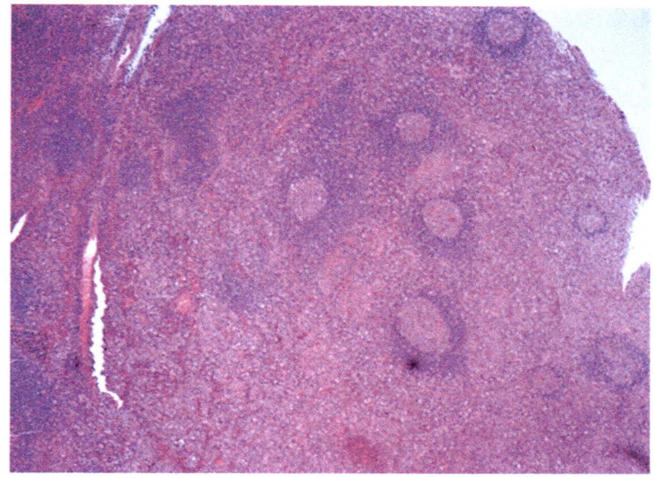

Fig. 4.6 Infectious mononucleosis with reactive lymphoid follicles and perifollicular expansion

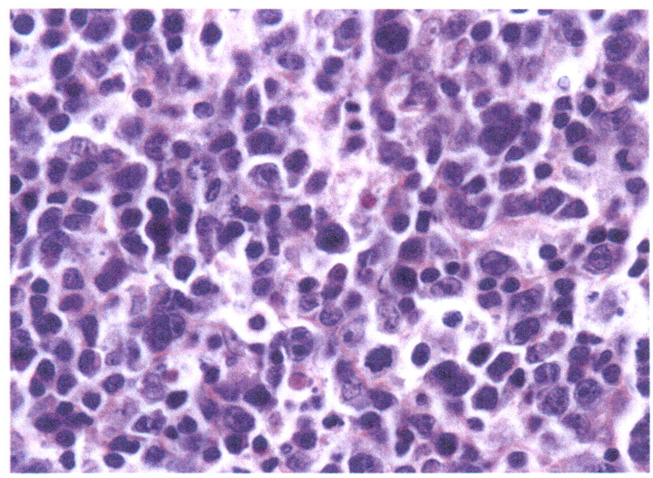

Fig. 4.7 Infectious mononucleosis with lymphoblasts and immunoblasts showing prominent nucleoli

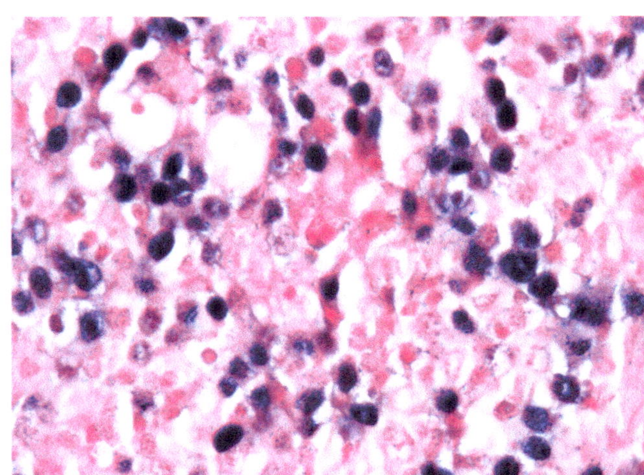

Fig. 4.8 Infectious mononucleosis with positive EBV by in situ hybridization stain

Histologic Features

- Marked sinus dilatation with sheets of foamy histiocytes (Figs. 4.9 and 4.10).
- Some histiocytes may contain lymphocytes, plasma cells, or red blood cells.

Granulomatous Lymphadenitis

Cytological Features (Fig. 4.11a–c)

- Mixed population of lymphoid cells.
- Epithelioid histiocytes in aggregates with or without multinucleated giant cells.
- Necrotic debris and acute inflammatory cells may or may not be present.
- Etiologies could include foreign body reaction, sarcoidosis, fungus, mycobacteria, and toxoplasmic lymphadenitis.
- Culture should be submitted.

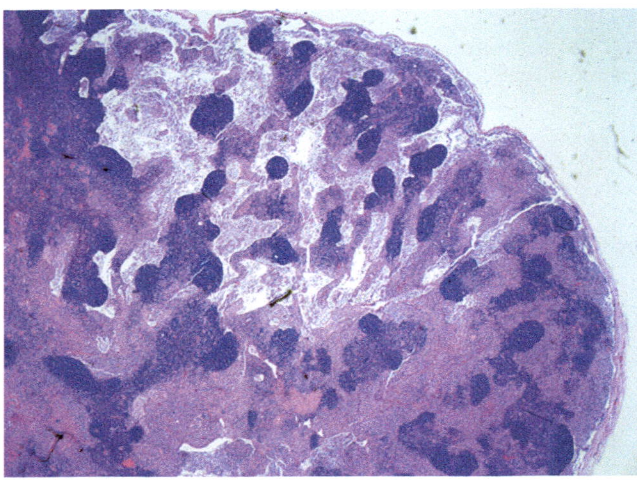

Fig. 4.9 Lymph node with Rosai-Dorfman disease shows marked sinus dilation

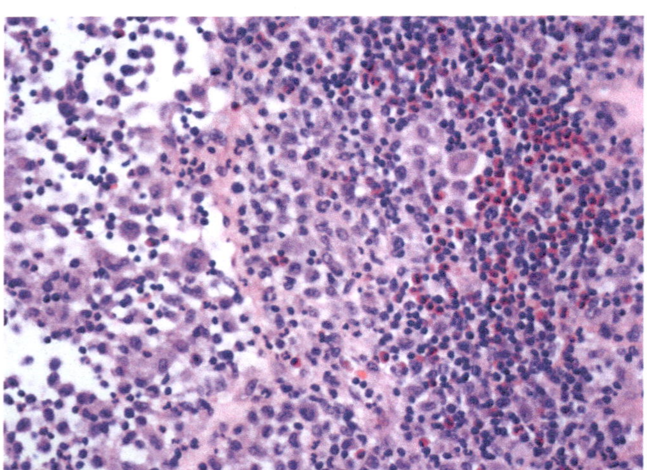

Fig. 4.10 Lymph node with Rosai-Dorfman disease shows sheets of histiocytes

Histologic Features

- Granulomas with necrosis in infection of mycobacteria (Figs. 4.12, 4.13, and 4.14)
- Granulomas surrounded by few or no lymphocytes (naked granuloma) in sarcoidosis (Figs. 4.15, 4.16, 4.17, and 4.18)
- Epithelioid granuloma and sheets of monocytoid lymphocytes in infection of Toxoplasma (Figs. 4.19 and 4.20)
- Multinucleated cells with foreign body in foreign body granuloma (Fig. 4.21)

Non-Hodgkin Lymphomas

Cytological Features

- Hypercellular specimen
- A relatively uniform population of lymphoid cells
- Can be divided into three groups
- Group 1 – small lymphoid cells (smaller than histiocytes), such as small lymphocytic lymphoma (SLL), grade I follicular lymphoma, MZL, LPL
- Group 2 –intermediate lymphoid cells (same size as histiocytes), such as MCL, grade II follicular lymphoma, BL, lymphoblastic lymphoma
- Group 3 – large lymphoid cells (larger than histiocytes), such as LBCL, grade III follicular lymphoma, ALCL, some T-cell lymphomas
- Immunophenotypes of B-cell lymphoma (Table 4.1) and frequent chromosomal translocations and gene mutations (Tables 4.2 and 4.3)

Small Lymphocytic Lymphoma (SLL)

Clinical Features

- Rare before 40 years of age
- General lymphadenopathy
- Bone marrow involvement

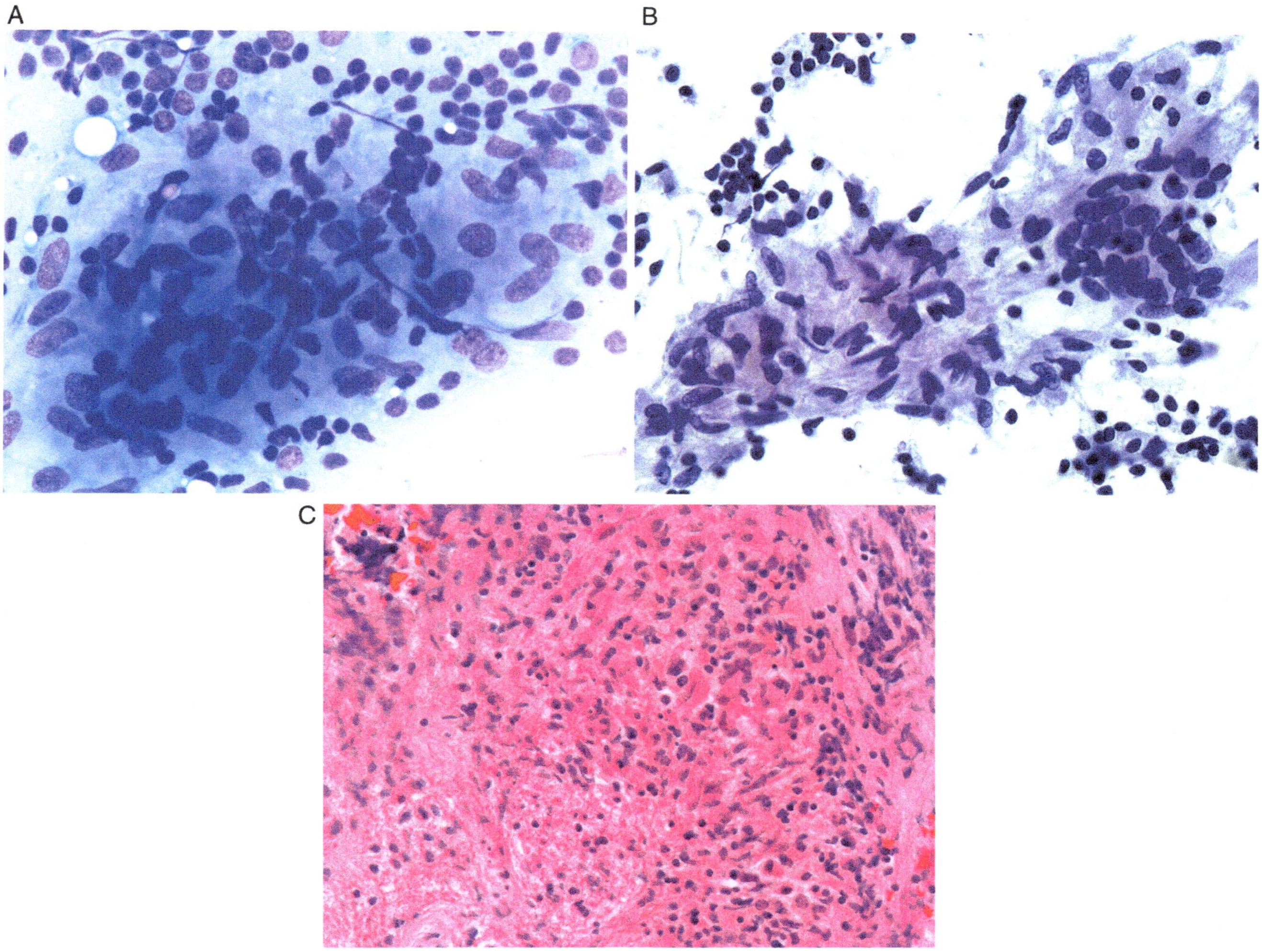

Fig. 4.11 (**a**–**c**) Granulomatous lymphadenitis with epithelioid histiocytes in aggregates with or without multinucleated giant cells and a mixed population of lymphoid cells on Diff-Quik (**a**), Pap stain (**b**), and cellblock preparation (**c**)

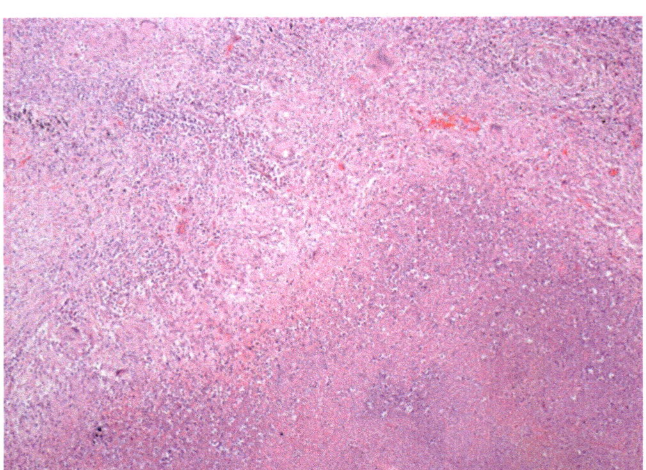

Fig. 4.12 Lymph node with caseating granulomas in tuberculosis

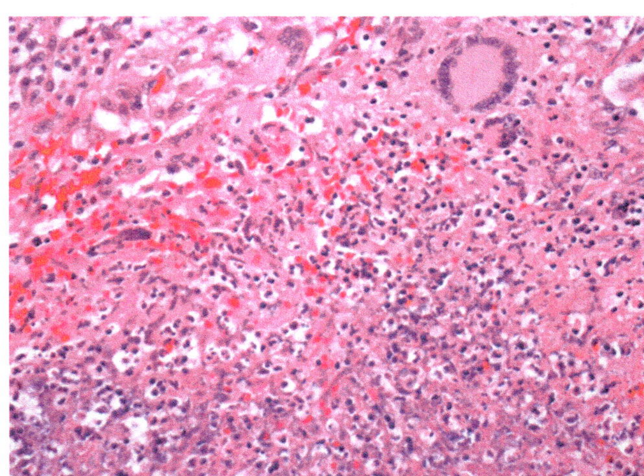

Fig. 4.13 Lymph node with caseating granulomas showing necrosis and giant cells

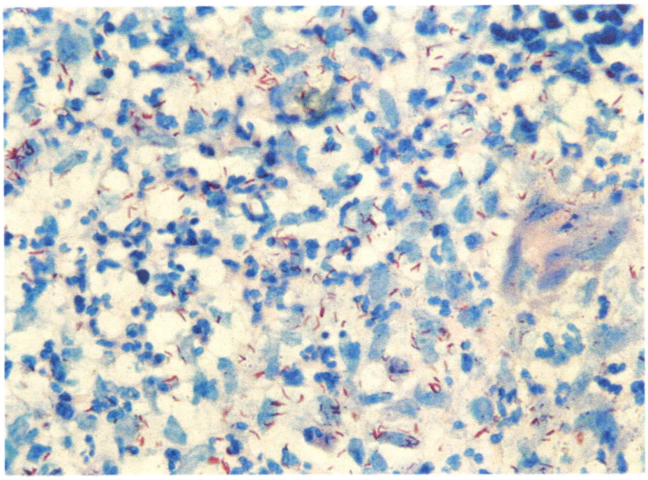

Fig. 4.14 Special stain (acid-fast bacilli [AFB], acid-fast Fite) reveals mycobacteria in caseating granulomas

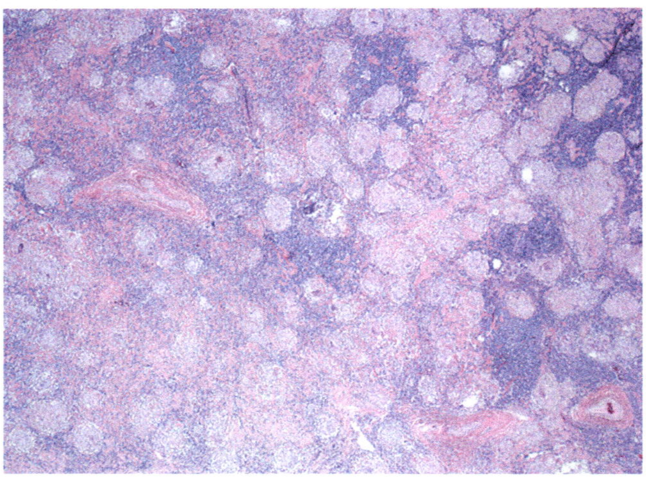

Fig. 4.15 Sarcoidosis in lymph node with noncaseating granulomas

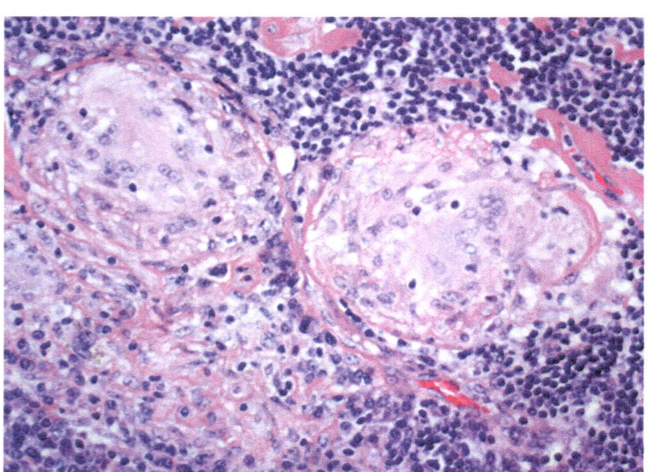

Fig. 4.16 Sarcoidosis in lymph node with "naked" noncaseating granulomas

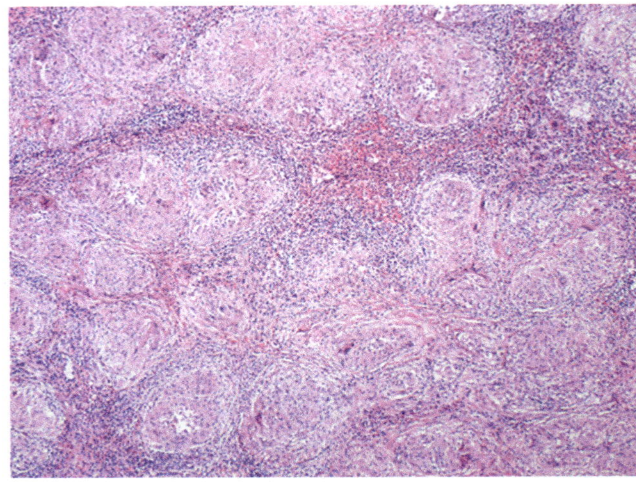

Fig. 4.17 Sarcoidosis in the spleen with noncaseating granulomas

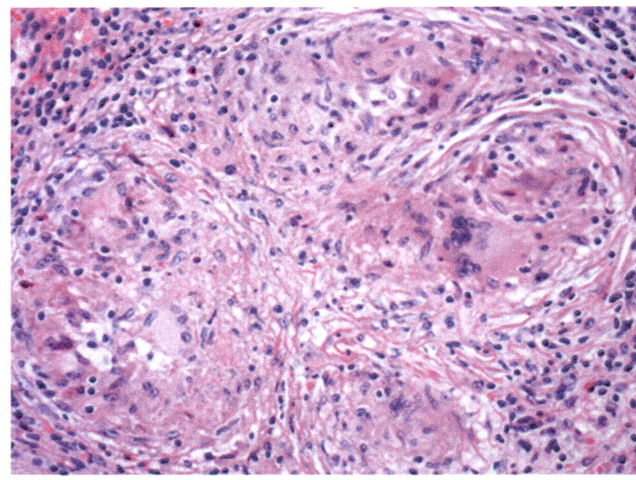

Fig. 4.18 Sarcoidosis in the spleen with "naked" noncaseating granulomas

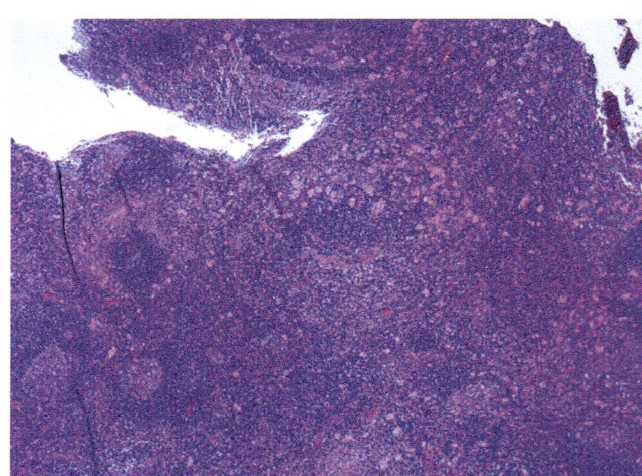

Fig. 4.19 Lymph node with toxoplasma shows reactive lymphoid follicles and expanded perifollicular area in a "mottled" appearance

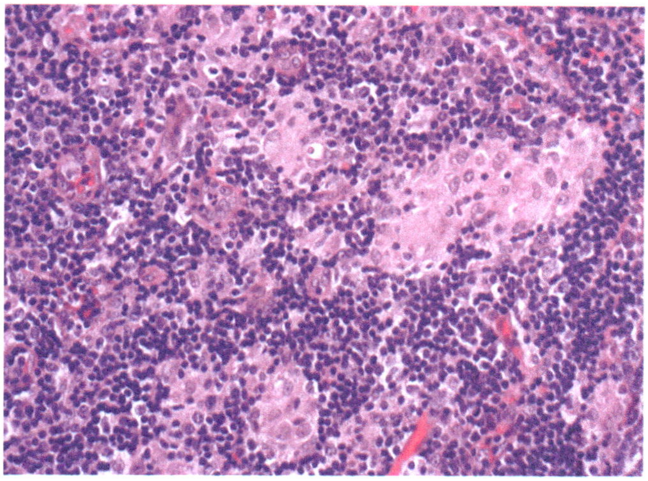

Fig. 4.20 Lymph node with toxoplasma shows cluster of epithelioid histiocytes and monocytoid lymphocytes

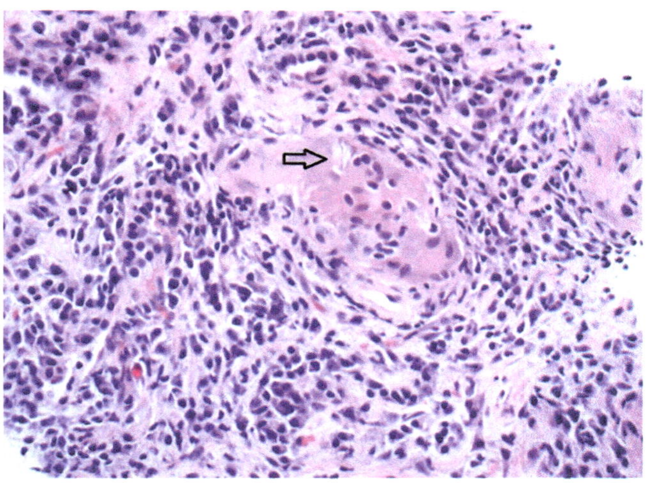

Fig. 4.21 Foreign body granuloma with giant cells containing foreign body (arrow)

Cytological Features (Fig. 4.22a, b)

- Highly cellular
- Monotonous population of small lymphocytes
- Smooth nuclear membrane, "clock face" nuclear chromatin, small to invisible nucleoli, and scant cytoplasm

Histologic Features

- Effaced nodal architecture in a vaguely nodular (pseudofollicular) pattern (Fig. 4.23).
- Sheets of neoplastic lymphocytes with hypercondensed chromatin and round to slightly irregular nuclear contour (Fig. 4.24).
- Admixed with prolymphocytes.
- Adenopathy <1.5 cm by computed tomography (CT) scan is called tissue-based monoclonal B-cell lymphocytosis.

Immunohistochemistry and Ancillary Studies

- Flow cytometry studies: CD19+, CD20+ (low intensity), CD5+, CD23+, CD43+, FMC7- (Fig. 4.25a–d); CD38 and zeta-chain-associated protein kinase 70 (ZAP-70) to evaluate the prognosis: both negative, most favorable; one positive and one negative, intermediate; and both positive, least favorable prognosis
- IHC: CD20+, PAX5+ (especially important after Rituxan treatment that cause CD20 negativity on IHC), CD5+, CD23+, lymphoid enhancer-binding factor 1 (LEF1)+ (Fig. 4.26)
- FISH: deletion of 13q14 in 50% of cases, trisomy 12 in 20% of cases (Figs. 4.27 and 4.28)

Differential Diagnosis

- Reactive lymph node
- Other low-grade lymphoma

Table 4.1 Immunophenotype of B-cell lymphomas

Category	CD20	CD5	CD10	CD23	BCL1	BCL2	BCL6	LEF1	LMO2	SOX11
SLL	+	+	−	+	−	+	−	+	−	−
FL	+	−	+	−	−	+	+	−	+	−
MZL	+	−	−	−	−	+	−	−	−	−
MCL	+	+	−	−	+	+	−	−	−	+

CD cluster of differentiation, *BCL* B-cell lymphoma, *LEF1* lymphoid enhancer-binding factor 1, *LMO2* LIM-only transcription factor 2, *SOX 11* sex-determining region Y box 11, *SLL* small lymphocytic lymphoma, *FL* follicular lymphoma, *MZL* marginal zone lymphoma, *MCL* mantle cell lymphoma

Table 4.2 Summary of chromosomal translocation-associated lymphomas and the affected genes

Chromosome	Lymphoma	Affected genes
t(8;14)(q24;q32)	BL	*c-MYC* and *IgH*
t(11;14)(q13;q32)	MCL	*Cyclin D1* and *IgH*
t(14;18)(q32;q21)	FL	*BCL2* and *IgH*
t(2;5)(p23;q35)	ALCL	*ALK* and *NPM*

BL Burkitt lymphoma, *IgH* immunoglobulin heavy, *MCL* mantle cell lymphoma, *FL* follicular lymphoma, *BCL2* B-cell CLL lymphoma 2, *ALCL* anaplastic large cell lymphoma, *ALK* anaplastic lymphoma kinase, *NPM* nucleophosmin

Table 4.3 Most common gene mutations in non-Hodgkin lymphomas

Lymphoma	Affected genes
Hairy cell leukemia	*BRAF V600E*
LPL Waldenström macroglobulinemia	*MYD88 L256P*
DLBCL, GC type	*EZH2, BCL2, GNA13*
DLBCL, ABC type	*MYD88, CD79A, CARD11, TNFAIP3*
Large granular lymphocyte leukemia	*STAT3*

BRAF v-raf murine sarcoma viral oncogene homolog B1, *LPL* lymphoplasmacytic lymphoma, *MYD88* myeloid differentiation primary response gene 88, *L256P* leucine to proline mutation at amino acid position 256, *DLBCL* diffuse large B-cell lymphoma, *GC* germinal center, *EZH2* enhancer of zeste homolog 2, *BCL2* B-cell lymphoma 2, *GNA13* guanine nucleotide-binding protein subunit alpha-13, *ABC* activated B-cell, *CD79A* cluster of differentiation 79A, *CARD11* caspase recruitment domain-containing protein 11, *TNFAIP3* tumor necrosis factor, alpha-induced protein 3, *STAT3* signal transducer and activator of transcription 3

Follicular Lymphoma

Clinical Features

- Accounts for 35% of adult non-Hodgkin lymphomas in the USA and 22% worldwide.
- Accounts for 70% of "low-grade" lymphomas in the USA.
- Affecting mainly adults, median age of 59 years, rarely occurs before age 20 years.
- 40% of patients have bone marrow involvement at the initial diagnosis.

Cytological Features (Fig. 4.29a–d)

- Usually cellular.
- Small lymphocytes with cleaved nuclei.
- Papanicolaou (Pap) stain better shows nuclear membrane irregularities.
- Small to inconspicuous nucleoli and scant cytoplasm.
- Increased numbers of large atypical lymphoid cells (centroblasts) in grade 2 and grade 3 follicular lymphoma.
- Grading of follicular lymphoma in a fine needle aspiration (FNA) specimen is similar to that of a histological specimen by counting the number of centroblasts at 40x high-power field (HPF); i.e., grade 1, 0–5 centroblasts/HPF; grade 2, 6–15 centroblasts/HPF; and grade 3, >15 centroblasts/HPF.

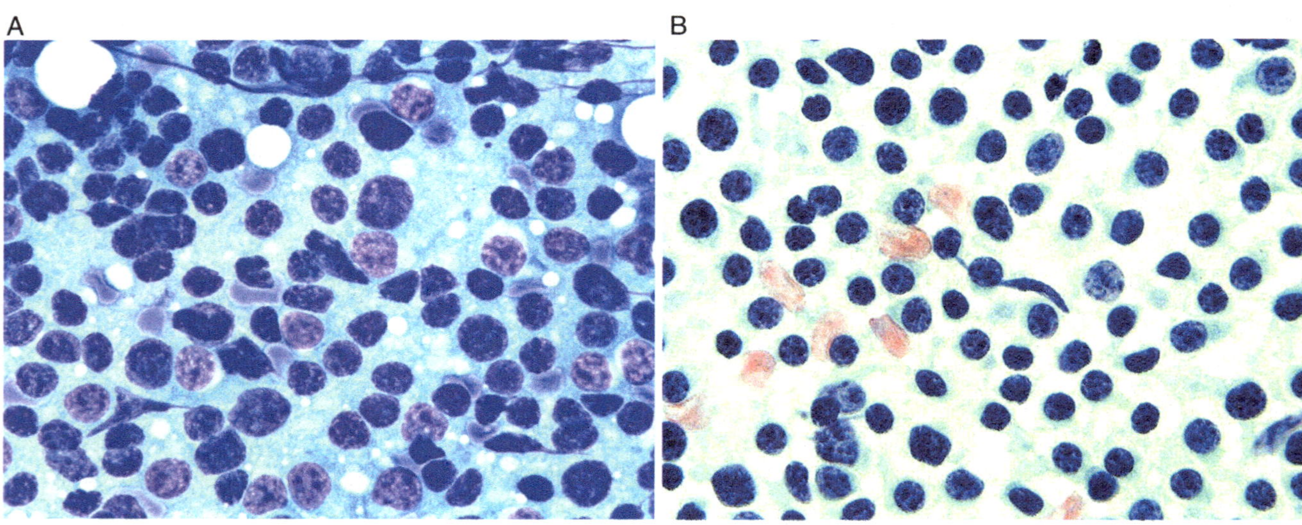

Fig. 4.22 (**a**, **b**) Small lymphocytic lymphoma with monotonous population of small lymphocytes on Diff-Quik (**a**) and Pap stain (**b**)

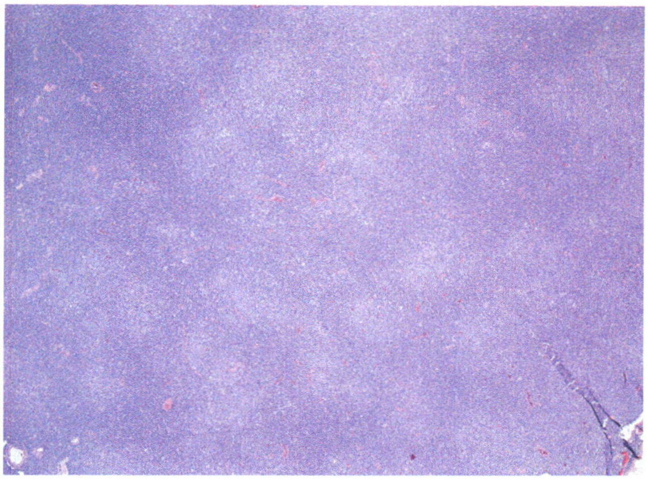

Fig. 4.23 Small lymphocytic lymphoma with effaced nodal architecture in a vaguely nodular (pseudofollicular) pattern

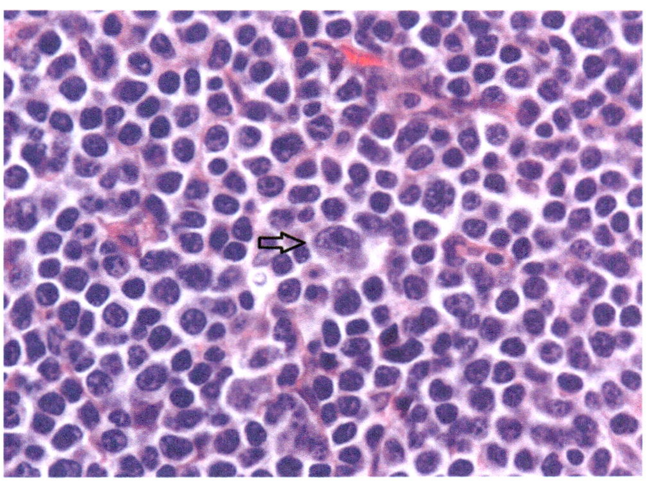

Fig. 4.24 Small lymphocytic lymphoma cells with hypercondensed chromatin and round nuclear contour; admixed prolymphocytes (*arrow*) with nucleolus and larger in size

- MIB-1 (Ki-67) is a useful marker to differentiate most grade 1 and grade 2 from grade 3.
- In situ follicular neoplasia with a low rate of progression can be detected by flow cytometry studies in half of the cases. Careful interpretation of FNA specimens is recommended.

Histologic Features

- Effaced nodal architecture in follicular pattern, follicles >75% (Fig. 4.30); in follicular and diffuse pattern, follicles 25–75%; in focally follicular pattern, follicles <25%; and in diffuse pattern, follicles 0%.
- Neoplastic follicles are usually round, surrounded by decreased mantle zone and composed of centrocytes and centroblasts without tingible-body macrophages.
- Centrocytes have mature chromatin and folded nuclear membrane; centroblasts show prominent nucleolus and round nuclear contour (Fig. 4.31).
- Grades 1–2 (low grade) with similar clinical prognosis
  - Grade 1: <5 centroblasts/HPF
  - Grade 2: 6–15 centroblasts/HPF
- Grade 3 (high grade): >15 centroblasts/HPF
  - Grade 3A: centroblasts separated by centrocytes
  - Grade 3B: sheets of centroblasts

Immunohistochemistry and Ancillary Studies

- Flow cytometry: CD19+, CD20+, CD10+ (Fig. 4.32a–d)
- IHC: CD20+, CD10+, BCL2+, BCL6+ and LIM-only transcription factor-2 (LMO2)+ (Fig. 4.33)
- FISH: positive for t(14;18)(q32;q21) (IGH;BCL2) (Fig. 4.34)

Differential Diagnosis

- Reactive lymph node
- Other low-grade lymphoma

Marginal Zone Lymphoma (MZL)

Clinical Features

- Involving nodal and extranodal sites
- Commonly in women
- Usually in the elderly

Cytological Features (Fig. 4.35a–f)

- Cellular smear
- A heterogeneous population of cells, including plasmacytoid cells, plasma cells, scattered immunoblasts, centrocyte-like cells
- Monocytoid B cells

Histologic Features

- Expanded marginal zone (Fig. 4.36)
- Neoplastic cells may appear as monocytoid, plasmacytoid, or centrocyte-like cells (Fig. 4.37).

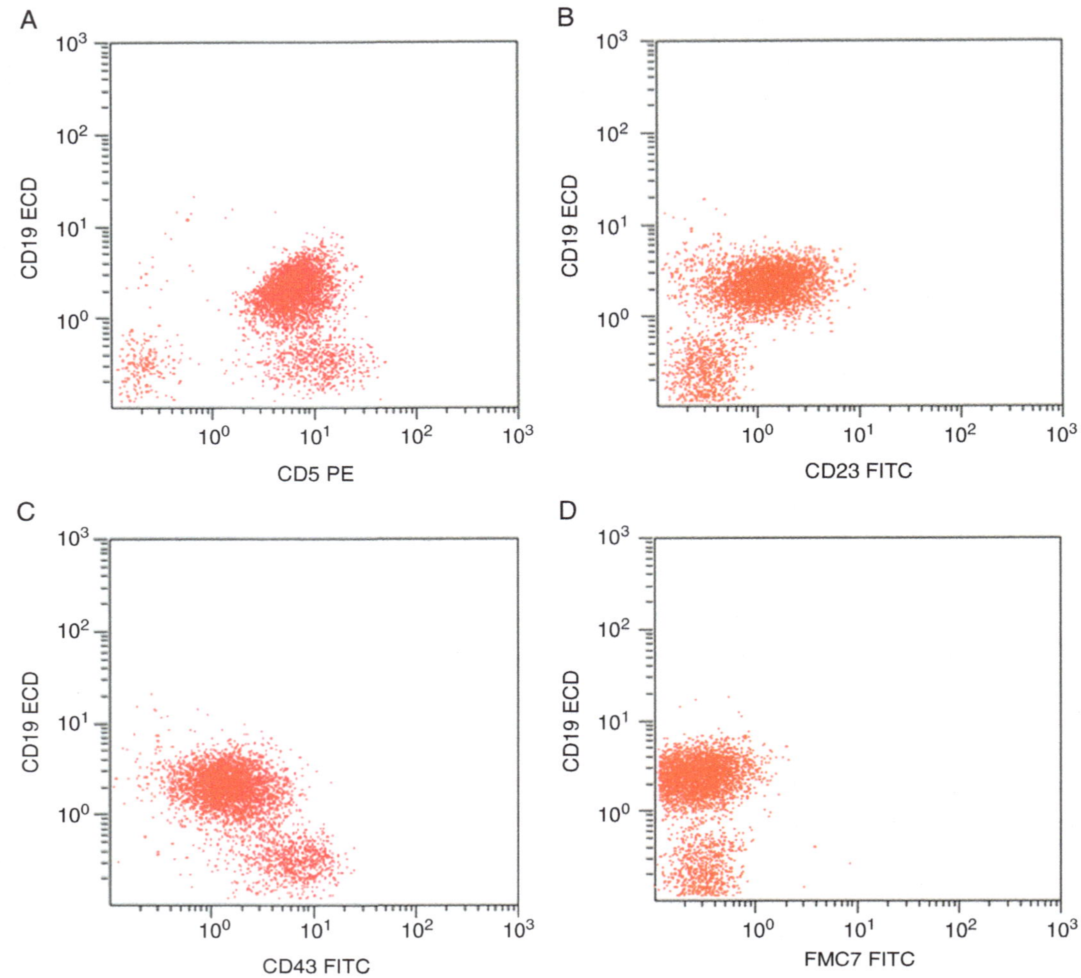

Fig. 4.25 (**a**–**d**) Flow cytometry studies in small lymphocytic lymphoma shows CD19+ lymphoma cells with coexpression of CD5 and CD23, positive for CD43 and negative for FMC7

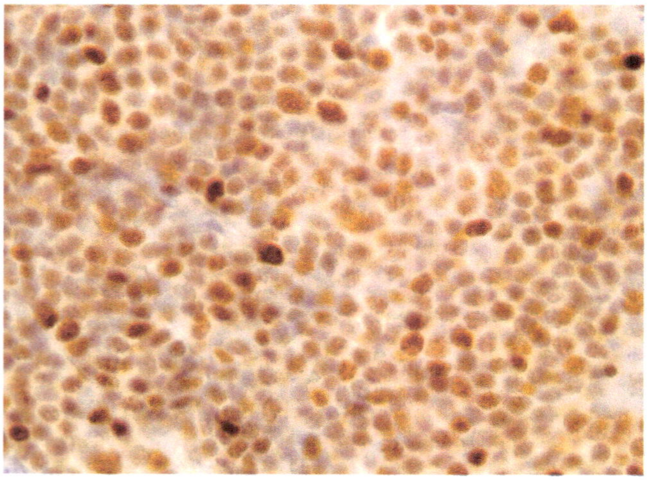

Fig. 4.26 Small lymphocytic lymphoma positive for LEF1

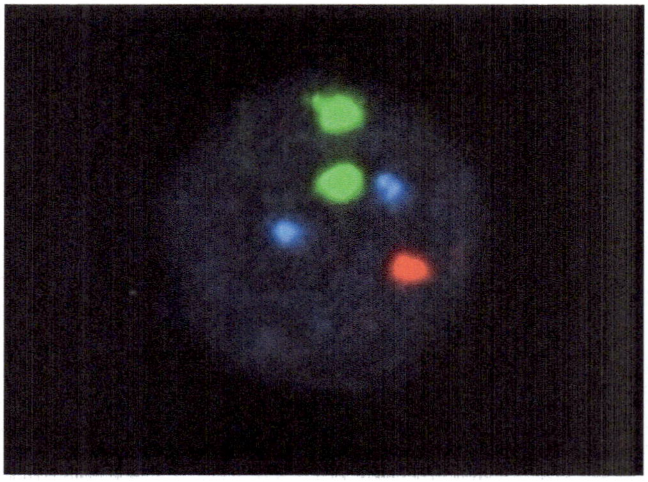

Fig. 4.27 FISH in small lymphocytic lymphoma with deletion of 13q14 (IR2G2A) in 50% of cases

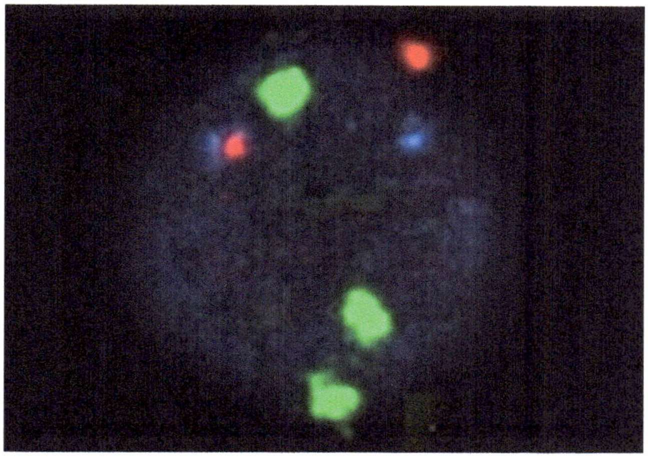

Fig. 4.28 FISH in small lymphocytic lymphoma with trisomy 12 (2R3G2A) in 20% of cases

Immunohistochemistry and Ancillary Studies

- Flow cytometry: CD19+, CD20+, CD5-, CD10-, CD23-
- IHC: CD20+, CD43+ (50% of cases), immunoglobulin superfamily receptor translocation associated 1(IRTA1)+ (Fig. 4.38)

Differential Diagnosis

- Reactive lymph node
- Other low-grade lymphoma

Mantle Cell Lymphoma (MCL)

Clinical Features

- 3–10% of non-Hodgkin lymphomas.
- Median age of 60 and male predominance.

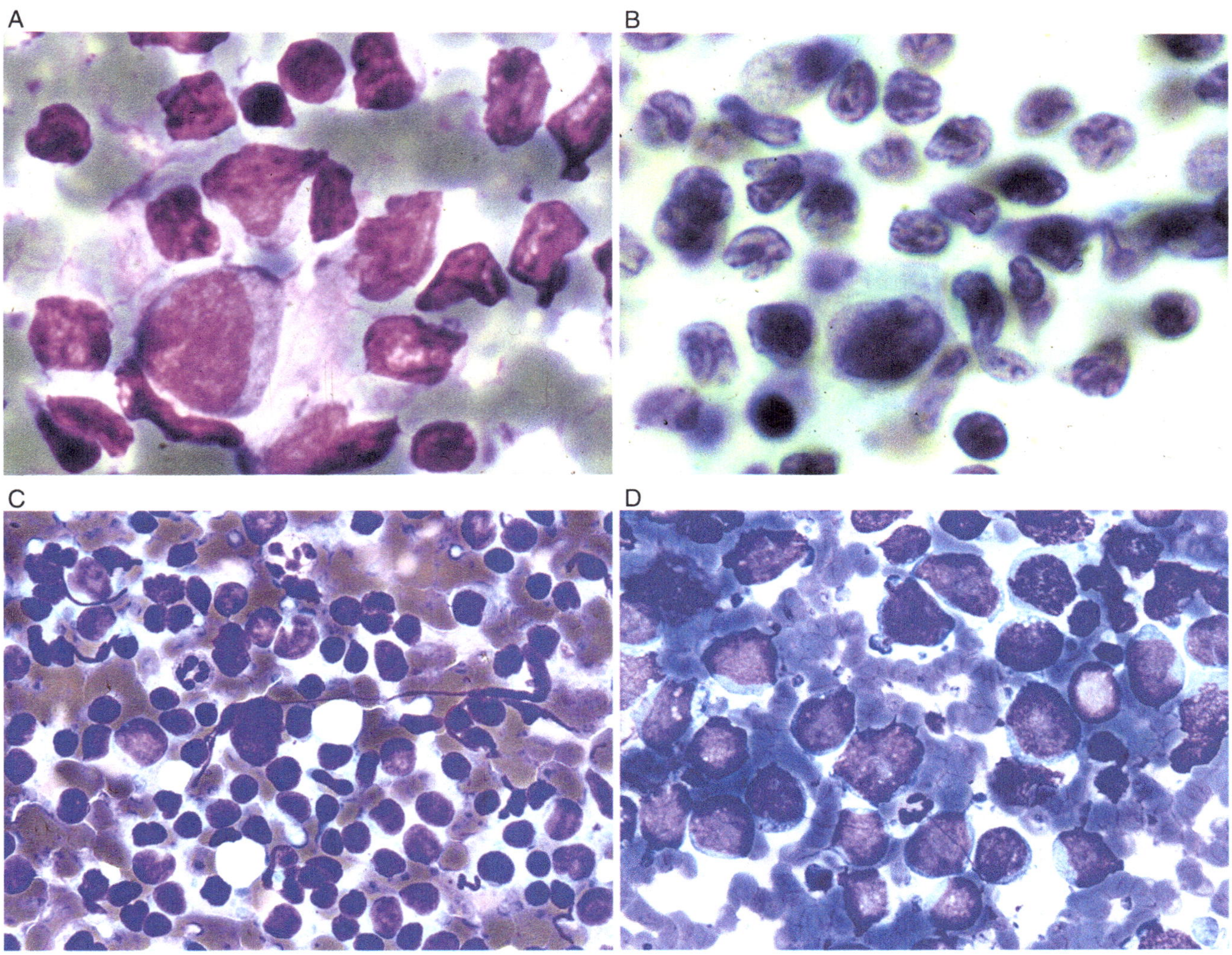

Fig. 4.29 (**a**–**d**) Follicular lymphoma with increased numbers of large atypical lymphoid cells (centroblasts) in grade 1 (**a**, **b**), grade 2 (**c**), and grade 3 (**d**) follicular lymphoma

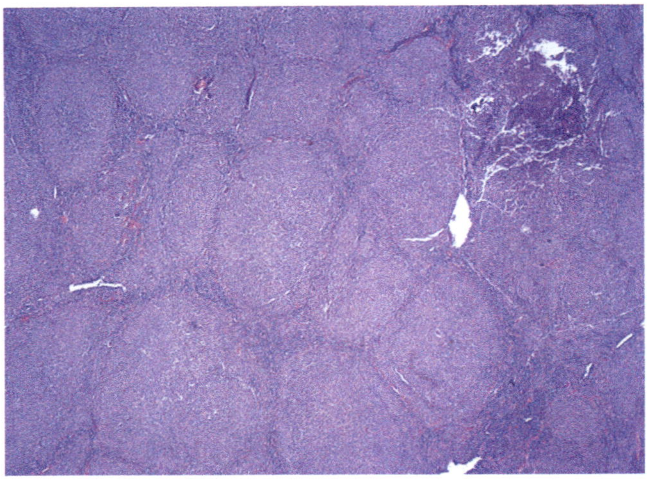

Fig. 4.30 Follicular lymphoma with effaced nodal architecture in a follicular pattern as "balls in a bag"

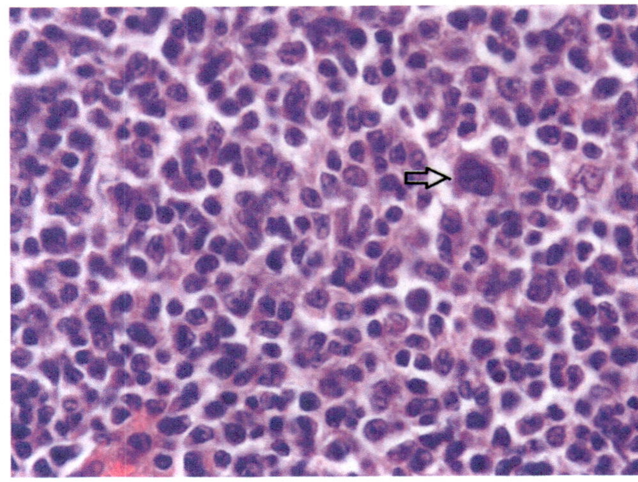

Fig. 4.31 Neoplastic cells (centrocytes) with folded nuclear contour and mature chromatin; admixed centroblasts (*arrow*) with smooth nuclear membrane and vesicular chromatin

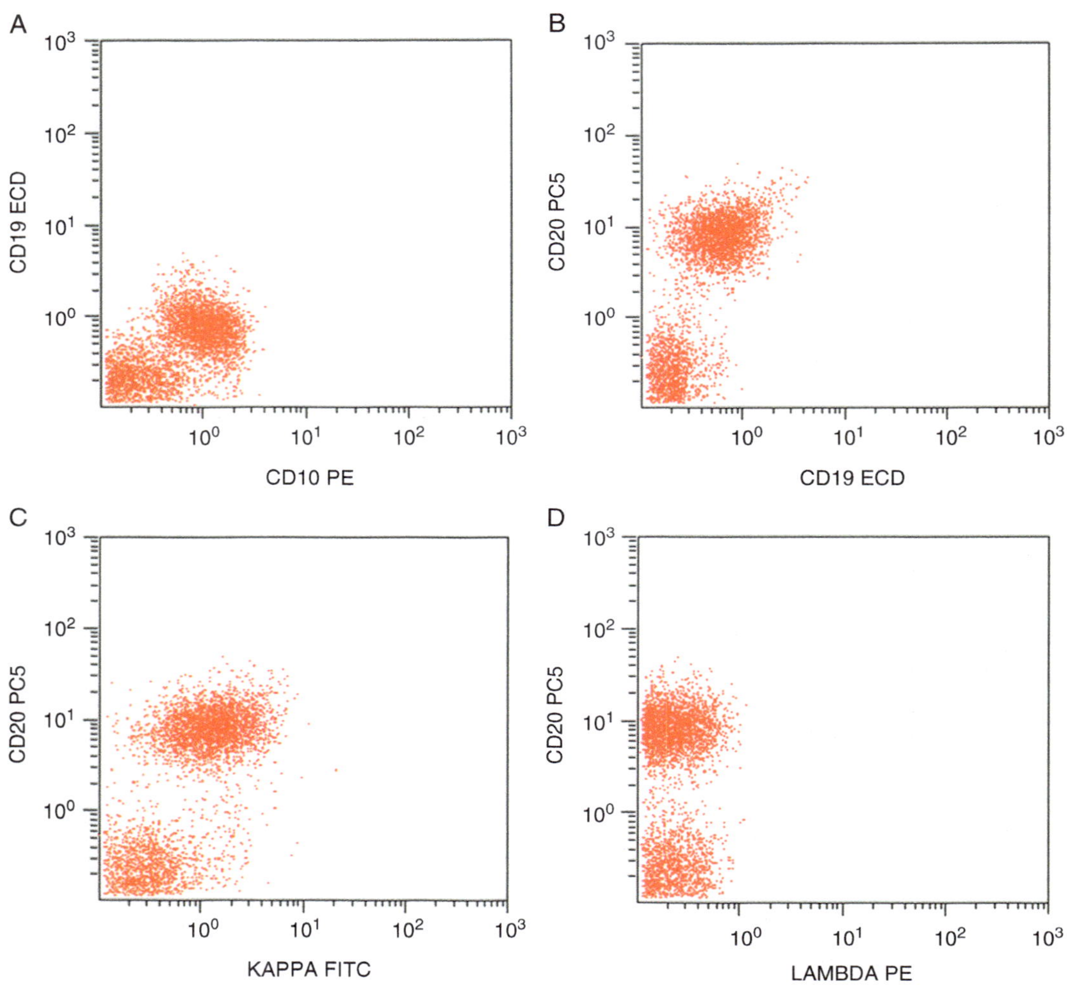

Fig. 4.32 (**a–d**) Flow cytometry studies of follicular lymphoma with coexpression of CD10, high intensity of CD20, and immunoglobulin light chain restriction

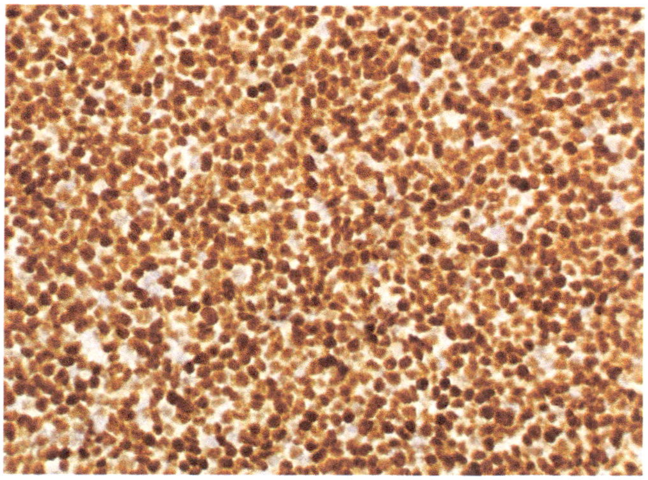

Fig. 4.33 Follicular lymphoma with LMO2 positivity

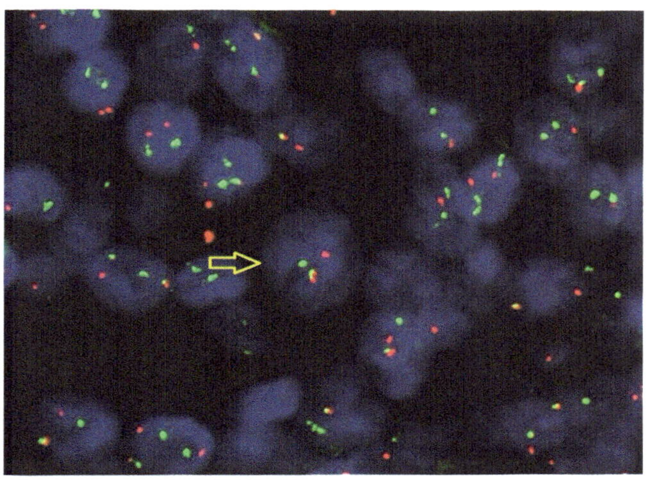

Fig. 4.34 FISH in follicular lymphoma with t(14;18) (*IGH; BCL2*) (1R1G2A, arrow)

- Involvement of the lymph nodes, spleen, and bone marrow.
- Up to 30% with GI involvement.
- Up to 25% with peripheral blood involvement.
- Two types: sex-determining region Y box (SOX)11-positive/immunoglobulin heavy chain variable *(IGHV)*-unmutated MCL typically involves lymph nodes and other extranodal sites with an aggressive clinical behavior; SOX11-negative/*IGHV*-mutated MCL usually involves the peripheral blood, bone marrow, and spleen with an indolent clinical course.

Cytological Features (Fig. 4.39a, b)

- Cellular smear.
- Homogeneous population of small- to intermediate-size lymphocytes
- Slightly cleft nuclear membrane.
- Condensed chromatin.
- Inconspicuous nucleoli.
- Many large cells are seen in a blastoid variant (resembling lymphoblasts) with a high mitotic index (>10/10 HPF).
- Positive for CD20, CD5, and negative for CD23 and CD10.
- FISH showing nearly 100% of cases with the t(11;14) translocation.
- Cyclin D1 overexpression by immunostain.

Histologic Features

- Nodular pattern with expanded mantle zone and may show a diffuse pattern (Fig. 4.40).
- Neoplastic cells with mature chromatin and irregular nuclear contour (Fig. 4.41).
- Capillary proliferation (Fig. 4.42).
- Aggressive variants:
  - Blastoid variant with lymphoblasts
  - Pleomorphic variant with oval to irregular nuclear contour and prominent nucleolus
- Other variants:
  - Small cell variant mimicking SLL
  - Marginal zone-like variant with monocytoid cells
- In situ mantle cell neoplasia with a low rate of progression and indolent clinical course. Careful interpretation of FNA specimen is recommended.

Immunohistochemistry and Ancillary Studies

- Flow cytometry: CD19+, CD20+, CD5+, FMC7+, CD43- (Fig. 4.43a–d)
- IHC: CD20+, CD5+, BCL1+, SOX11+ (Figs. 4.44 and 4.45)
- FISH: t(11;14) (CCND1;IGH) (Fig. 4.46)

Differential Diagnosis

- Reactive lymph node
- Other low-grade lymphoma

Plasmacytoma/Multiple Myeloma

Cytological Features (Fig. 4.47a, b)

- Mature or immature plasma cells.
- Binucleation or multinucleation.
- Intranuclear bodies (Dutcher body) or intracytoplasmic bodies (Russell body).
- Positive for CD38 and CD138 and negative for CD20.
- May be positive for epithelial membrane antigen (EMA), but negative for cytokeratin.
- IgM MGUS is more closely related to LPL.

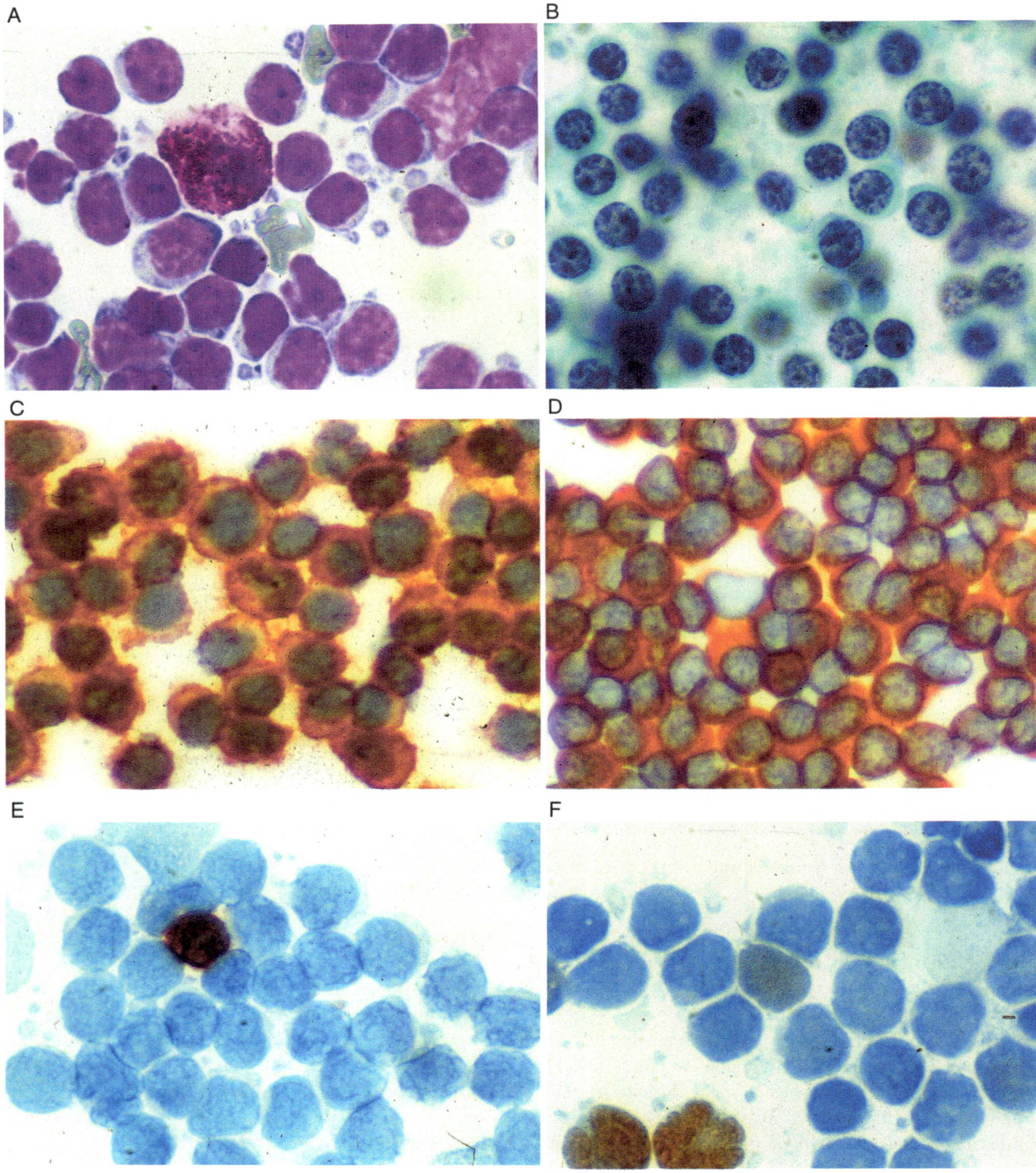

Fig. 4.35 (**a–f**) Marginal zone lymphoma with a heterogeneous population of cells, including plasmacytoid cells, plasma cells, scattered immunoblasts, centrocyte-like cells on Diff-Quik (S), and Pap stain (**b**). Note that immunostain performed on the direct FNA smears showed CD20 positivity (**c**), Kappa light chain restriction (**d**), lack of Lambda light chain (**e**), and low Ki-67 proliferative index (**f**)

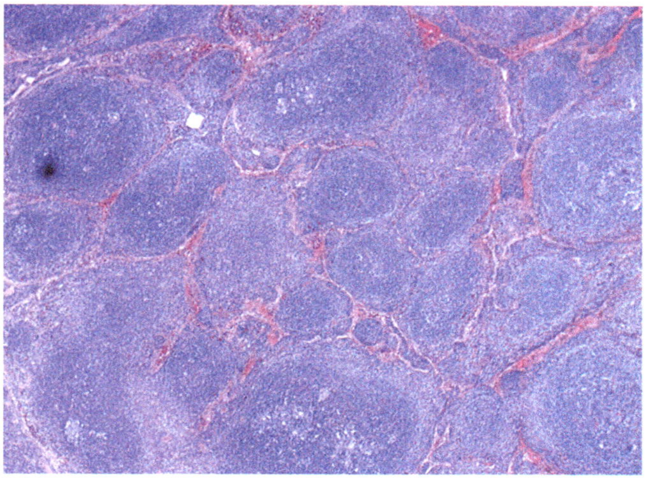

Fig. 4.36 Marginal zone lymphoma with effaced nodal architecture and marked marginal zone expansion

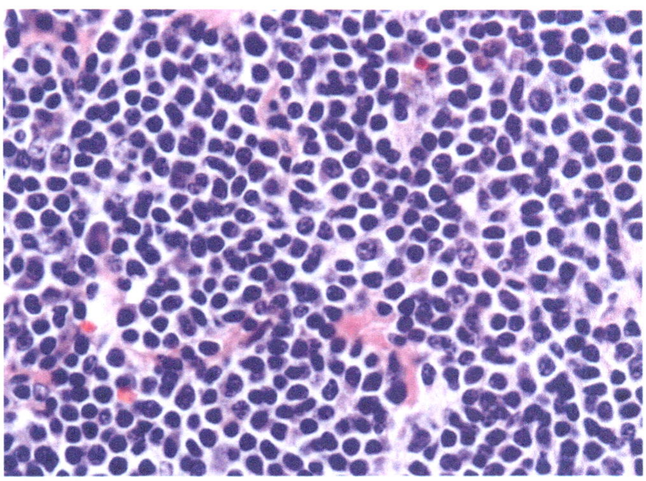

Fig. 4.37 Neoplastic marginal zone cells show round nuclear contour and mature chromatin with monocytoid or plasmacytoid appearance

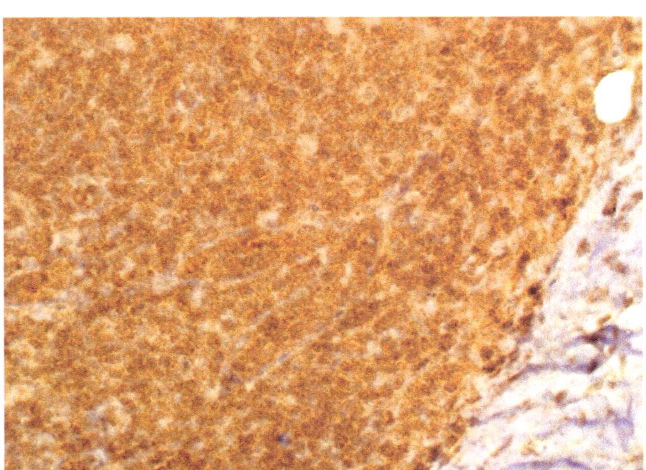

Fig. 4.38 Neoplastic marginal zone cells positive for IRTA1

Histologic Features

- Sheets of plasma cells in tissue or lymph node (Figs. 4.48 and 4.49).
- Multiple myeloma in bone marrow biopsy: monotypic plasma cells represent >30% of marrow cellularity.

Immunohistochemistry and Ancillary Studies

- IHC: CD138+ (Fig. 4.50) used to evaluate volume of plasma cells and kappa and lambda for clonality; some neoplastic plasma cells show aberrant expression of CD56, BCL1, and CD117.

Large B-Cell Lymphoma (LBCL)

Clinical Features

- Accounts for 30%–40% of adult non-Hodgkin lymphomas in western countries.
- Nodal or extranodal disease.
- Forty percent with initial extranodal presentation, GI tract most common.
- HIV or other immunodeficiency is a risk factor.
- Many morphologic variants, including centroblastic, immunoblastic, and anaplastic, and subtypes, such as T-cell/histiocytes-rich, primary DLBCL of the CNS, primary cutaneous DLBCL leg type and EBV-positive DLBCL, NOS, et al.
- t(14;18) chromosomal translocation in 30% of cases.
- Two major patterns of gene expression in DLBCL: germinal center (GC)-B cell type DLBCL and activated B-cell (ABC)-type DLBCL. GC-type DLBCL has a much better prognosis than ABC-type DLBCL.

Cytological Features (Fig. 4.51a–g)

- Highly cellular specimen.
- Dispersed large uniform to variable-size lymphoid cells.
- Numerous lymphoglandular bodies in the background.
- Large pleomorphic nuclei, irregular nuclear contour, and prominent nucleoli.
- Multinucleated giant cells can be seen.
- Variable nuclear-to-cytoplasmic ratio.
- Cohesive groups of large atypical lymphoid cells may mimic other malignant tumors, such as carcinoma, melanoma, and sarcoma.
- Tumor necrosis and mitosis are usually present.

Histologic Features

- Effaced nodal architecture in a diffuse pattern by medium to large neoplastic lymphocytes

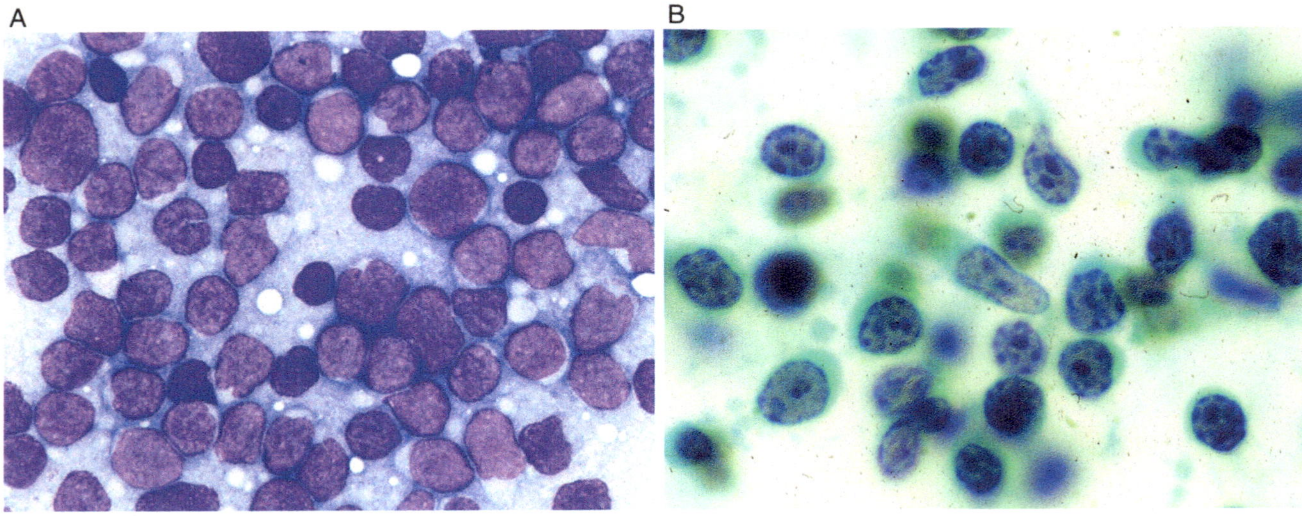

Fig. 4.39 (**a**, **b**) Mantle cell lymphoma with a homogeneous population of small to intermediate-size lymphocytes with slightly cleft nuclear membranes on Diff-Quik (**a**) and Pap stain (**b**)

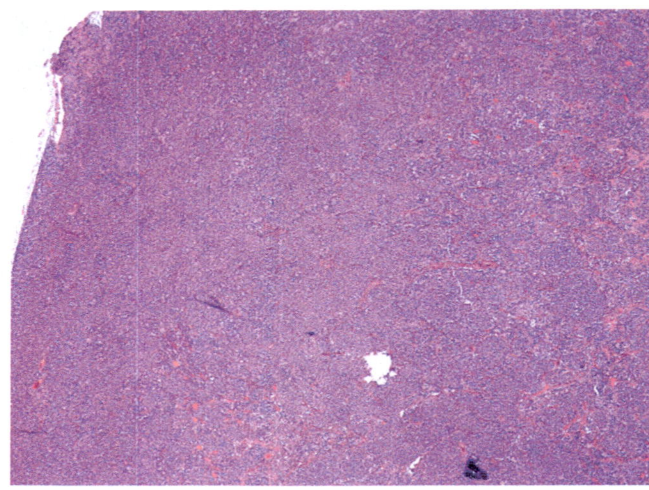

Fig. 4.40 Mantle cell lymphoma with effaced nodal architecture and mantle zone expansion in a vaguely nodular pattern

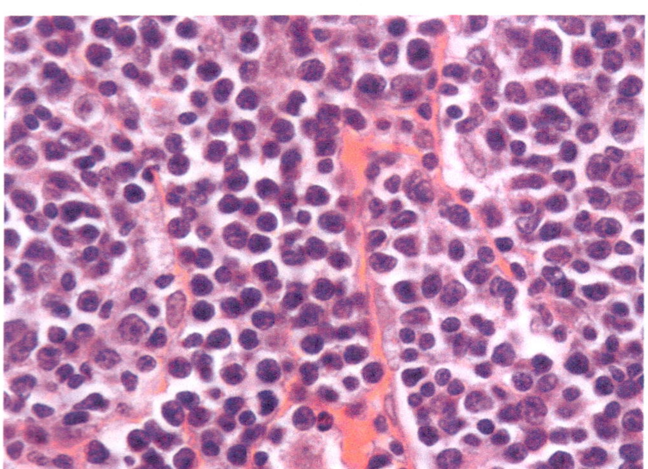

Fig. 4.41 Neoplastic mantle cells with irregular nuclear contour and mature chromatin

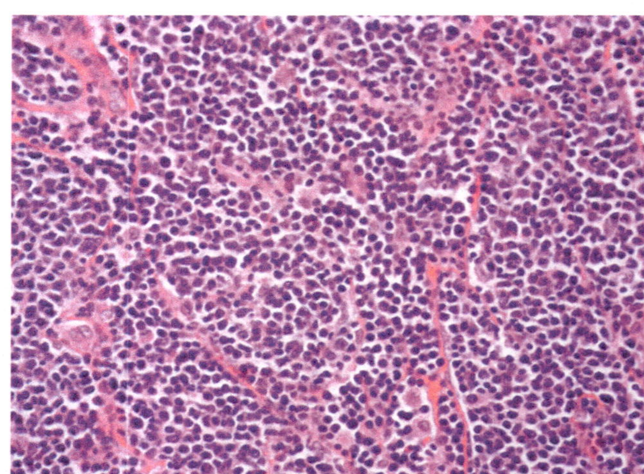

Fig. 4.42 Mantle cell lymphoma with capillary proliferation

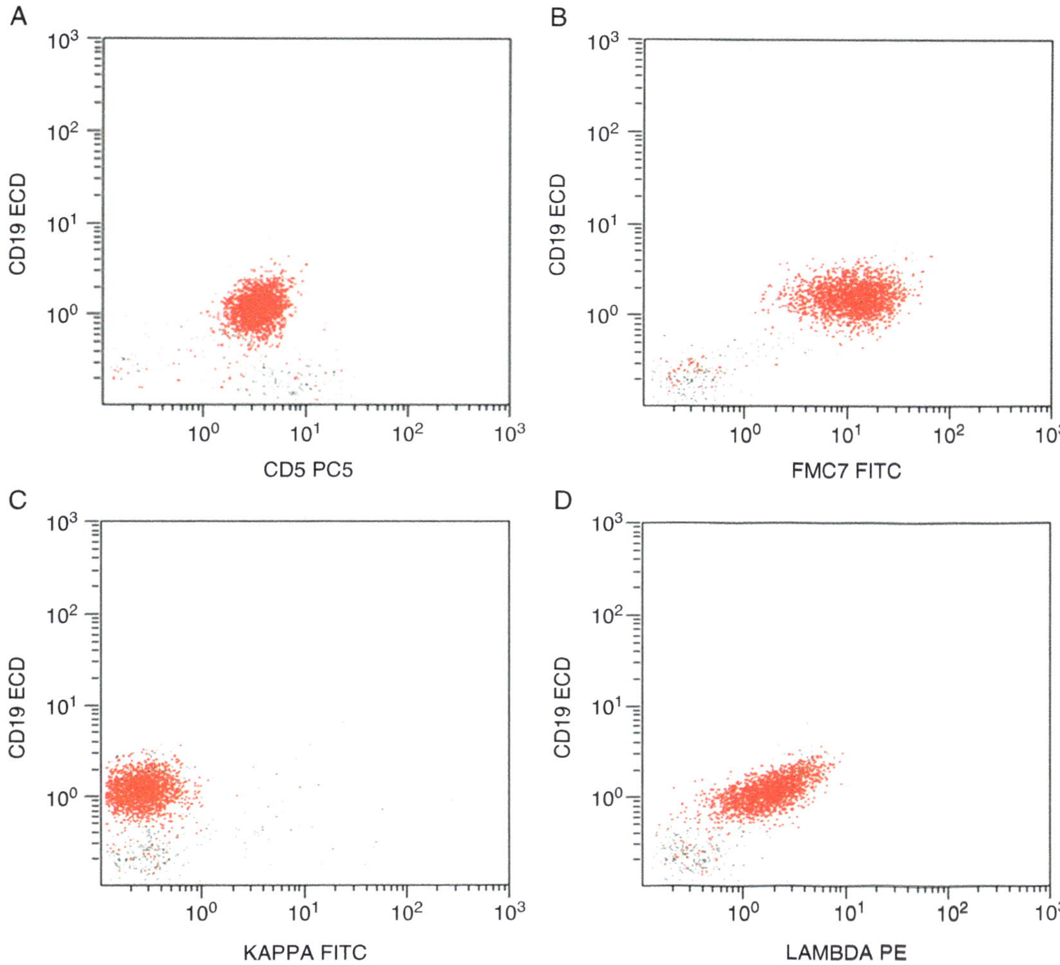

Fig. 4.43 (**a–d**) Flow cytometry studies of mantle cell lymphoma with coexpression of CD5, positivity of FMC7, and immunoglobulin light chain restriction

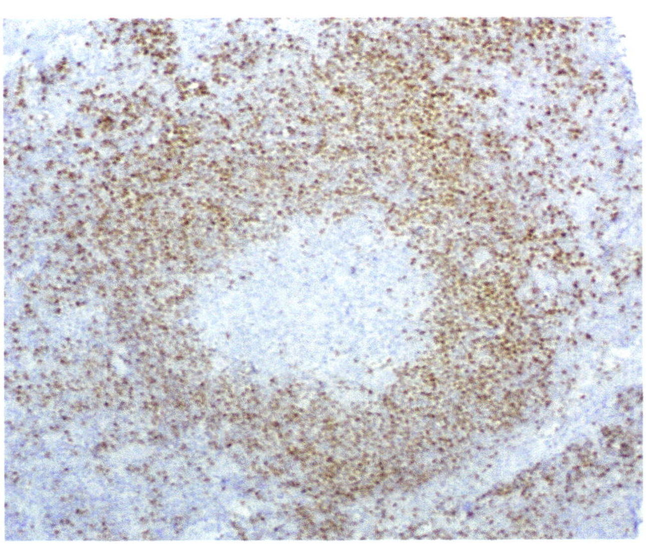

Fig. 4.44 Immunohistochemical study of SOX11 in mantle cell lymphoma shows mantle zone expansion

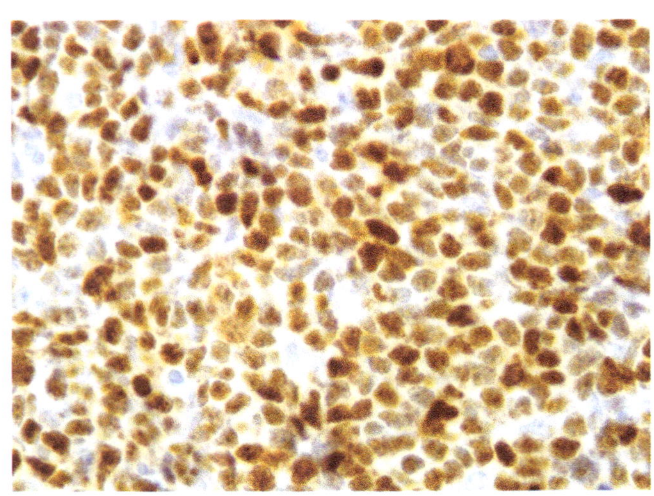

Fig. 4.45 Immunohistochemical study in mantle cell lymphoma shows mantle cells positive for SOX11

- Neoplastic cells in sheets or a scattered pattern, depending on the subtype (Figs. 4.52 and 4.55)

Immunohistochemistry and Ancillary Studies

- IHC: positive for the B-cell markers CD20 (Figs. 4.53 and 4.56), paired box gene (PAX)5 (Fig. 4.54), B-cell Oct binding protein 1 (BOB1), octamer-binding transcription factor 2 (Oct2); MIB evaluates the proliferation rate.
- Subclassification:
  - GCB-type DLBCL: CD10+, BCL6+, multiple myeloma 1 (MUM1)-
  - ABC-type DLBCL: CD10-, BCL6-, MUM1+

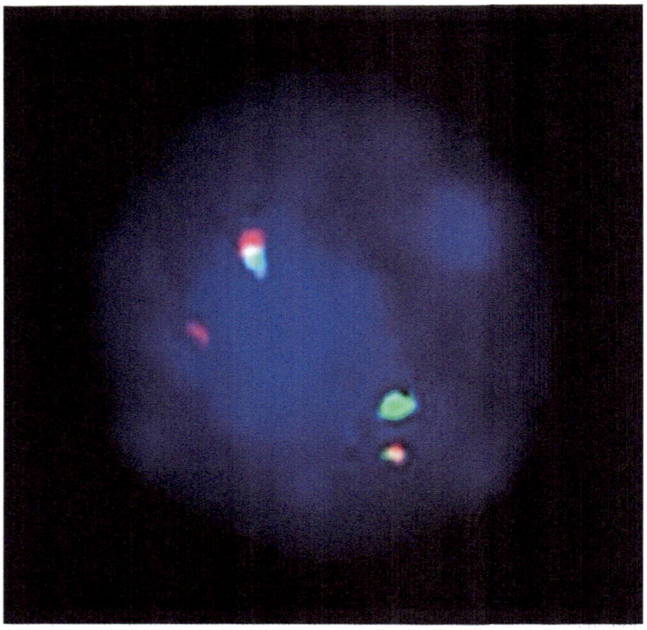

Fig. 4.46 FISH in mantle cell lymphoma with t(14;18) (*CCND1;IGH*) (1R1G2F)

- Other types include double-hit or triple-hit HGBCL with rearrangements of *MYC* and *BCL2* and/or *BCL6*, and double-expresser HGBCL with immunostain of MYC (>40%) and BCL2 (>50%) but lack *MYC* and *BCL2* chromosomal alteration.

Differential Diagnosis

- Reactive lymph node
- High-grade lymphoma and Hodgkin lymphoma
- Melanoma
- Carcinoma
- Sarcoma

Burkitt Lymphoma (BL)

Clinical Features

- Endemic BL, sporadic BL, and immunodeficiency-related BL.
- Extranodal involvement frequent in the jaw, facial bone, abdominal organs, and breast.
- EBV plays an important role in endemic BL.
- Transcription factor 3 (*TCF3*) mutation in 40% of endemic BLs and 70% of sporadic BLs and immunodeficiency-related BLs.

Cytological Features (Fig. 4.57)

- Cellular smear.
- Monotonous population of medium-size lymphoid cells.
- Usually smooth nuclear membrane, small notched or indented, may be seen.
- Finely stippled nuclear chromatin.

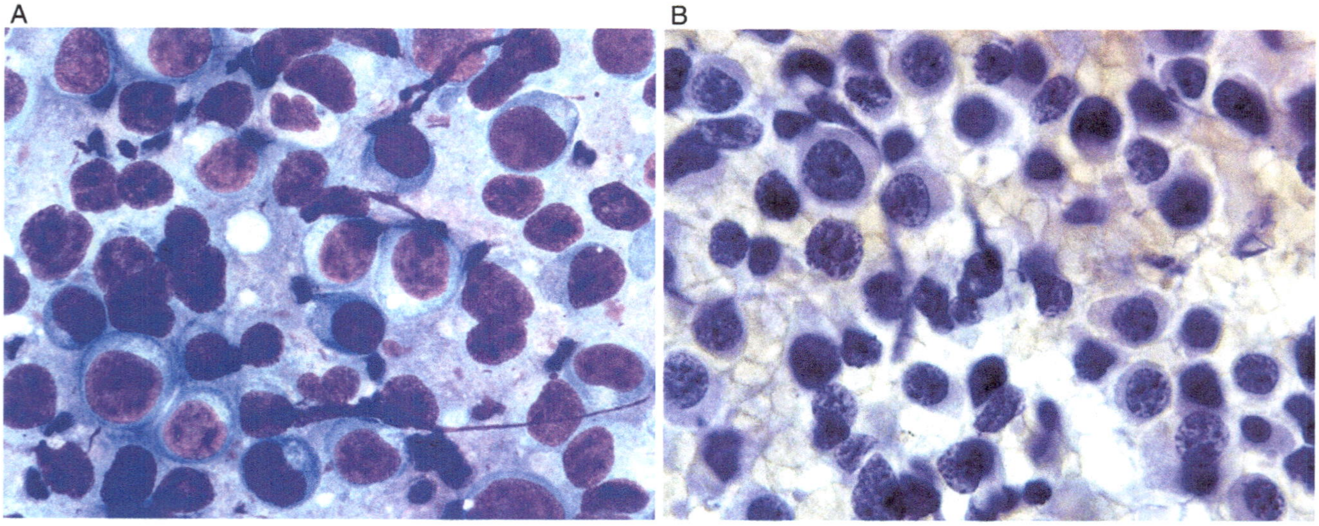

Fig. 4.47 (**a**, **b**) Plasmacytoma on Diff-Quik (**a**) and Pap stain (**b**)

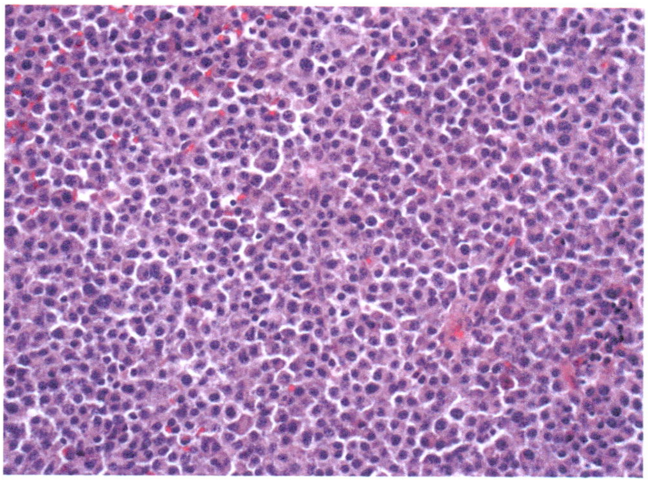

Fig. 4.48 Plasmacytoma with sheets of plasma cells

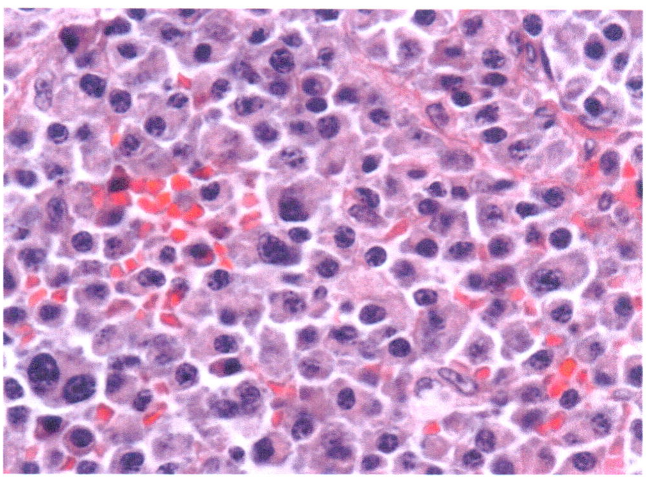

Fig. 4.49 Neoplastic plasma cells with less mature chromatin, nucleolus, and scattered binucleation

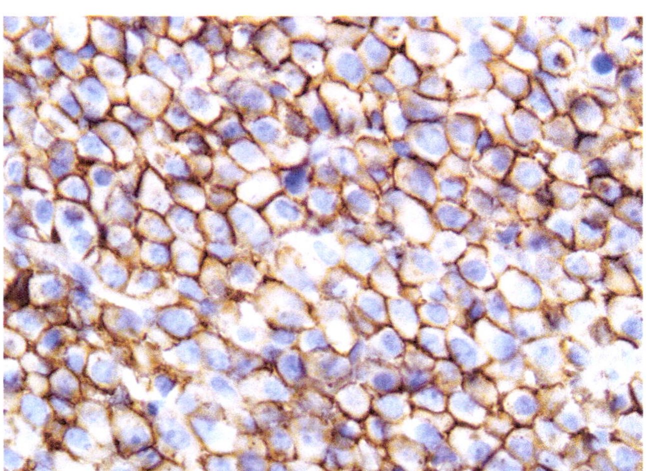

Fig. 4.50 Plasmacytoma with sheets of CD138 positive plasma cells

- Multiple conspicuous nucleoli.
- Moderate amount, deeply basophilic cytoplasm with tiny vacuoles.
- CD20, CD10, BCL6 positive.
- All cases positive for the t(8;14) translocation, involving *MYC*.

Histologic Features

- Effaced nodal architecture with a "starry sky" pattern and composed of sheets of neoplastic lymphocytes and scattered tingible-body histiocytes (Fig. 4.58)
- Neoplastic lymphocytes are medium in size with a round to slightly irregular nuclear contour and small nucleoli with a "snake head" appearance (Fig. 4.59).

Immunohistochemistry and Ancillary Studies

- IHC: strongly positive for CD20, CD10, BCL6, c-MYC and negative for BCL2 with proliferation rate of 100% by MIB-1 stain (Fig. 4.60)
- FISH: MYC translocation (Fig. 4.61)
- A subset lacking *MYC* rearrangement called "Burkitt-like lymphoma with 11q aberration" shows the same morphology and similar clinical course.

Differential Diagnosis

- LBCL
- Viral infection with reactive change
- Lymphoblastic lymphoma

T-Cell Lymphoma

Clinical Features

- Relatively uncommon lymphoid neoplasm, accounting for less than 12% of non-Hodgkin lymphomas, including peripheral T-cell lymphoma (PTCL), unspecified T-cell lymphoma, NK-cell lymphoma, ALCL, and nodal T-cell lymphoma with TFH phenotype
- More common in Asia

Cytological Features (Fig. 4.62a, b)

- Polymorphous population of a spectrum of small, medium, and large lymphocytes.
- Convoluted nuclear membranes, vesicular or coarse chromatin, and prominent nucleoli.
- Binucleation and multinucleation can be seen.
- Cytoplasm ranging from scant to abundant, pale to basophilic.

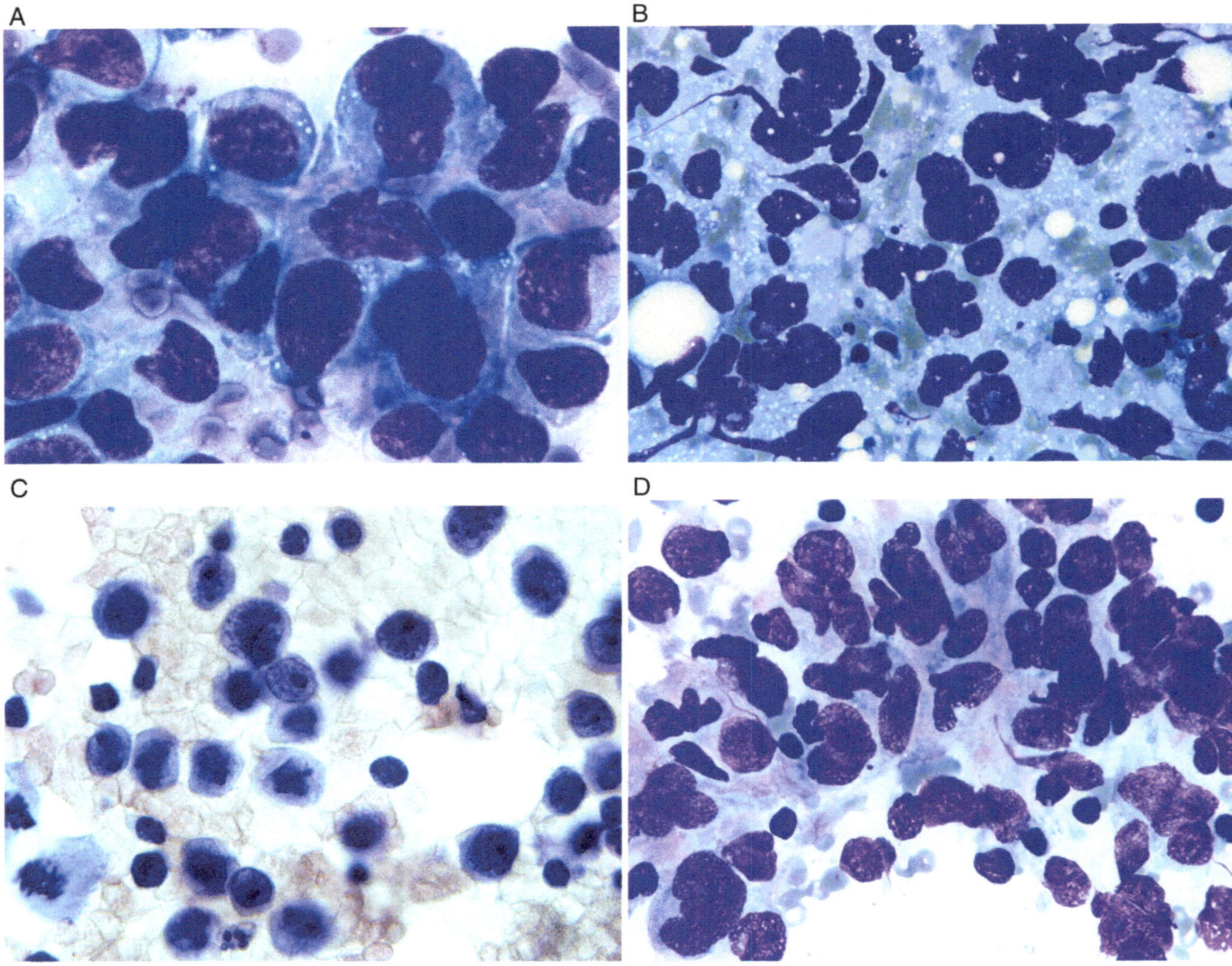

Fig. 4.51 (**a**–**g**) Large B-cell lymphoma with large uniform to variable-size lymphoid cells on Diff-Quik (**a**, **b**) and Pap stain (**c**). Note that LBCL may mimic other malignant tumors, such as carcinoma, as shown in (**d**), on cellblock preparation (**e**), positive for CD20 (**f**) and increased Ki-67 proliferative index (**g**)

- Histiocytes, eosinophils, plasma cells and neutrophils can be seen.
- Granulomas can be seen.

Histologic Features

- Effaced nodal architecture with perifollicular (T-cell zone) expansion (Fig. 4.63).
- Neoplastic lymphocytes are medium in size with irregular nuclear contour, vesicular chromatin, and prominent nucleoli; they form sheets or a scattered pattern (Fig. 4.64).

Immunohistochemistry and Ancillary Studies

- Positive for, but often loss of one or more of, the T-cell markers CD2, CD3, CD5 and CD7 with either CD4 or CD8.
- Angioimmunoblastic T-cell lymphoma (Fig. 4.65) and two new subtypes – follicular center T-cell lymphoma and nodal PTCL with TFH type – show the follicular center markers CD279/programmed death 1 (PD1), CD10, BCL6, chemokine (C-X-C motif) ligand 13 (CXCL13), inducible T-cell co-stimulator (ICOS), serum amyloid P (SAP), and chemokine receptor type 5 (CCR5).

Anaplastic Large Cell Lymphoma (ALCL)

Clinical Features

- Three percent of adult non-Hodgkin lymphomas.
- ALK+ ALCL represents 10–20% of childhood lymphomas; ALK- ALCL peaks in adults (40–65 years).
- CD30-positve T-cell lymphoma.

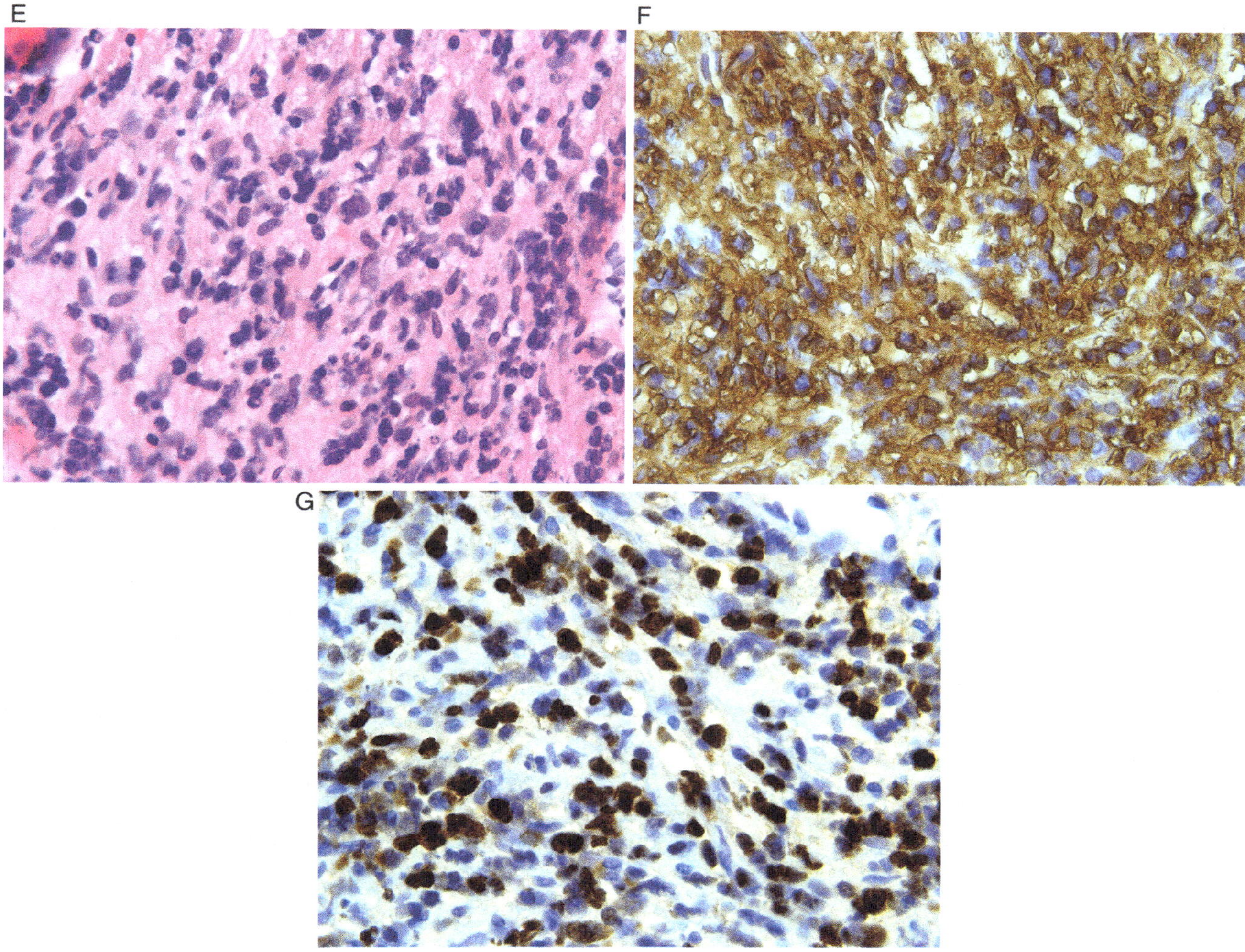

Fig. 4.51 (continued)

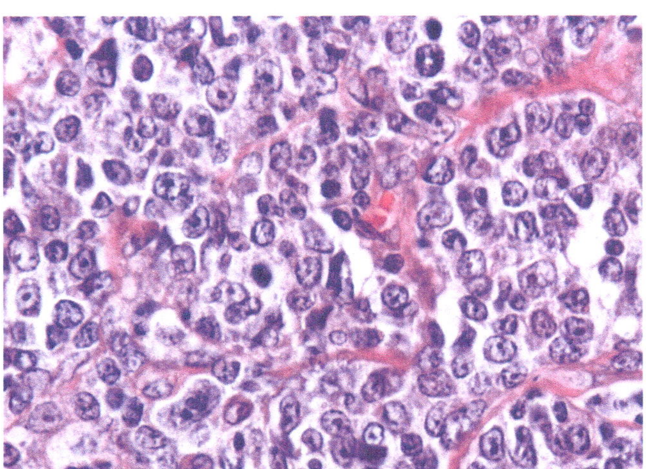

Fig. 4.52 Diffuse large B-cell lymphoma with effaced nodal architecture in a diffuse pattern by sheets of large cells showing vesicular chromatin and prominent nucleolus

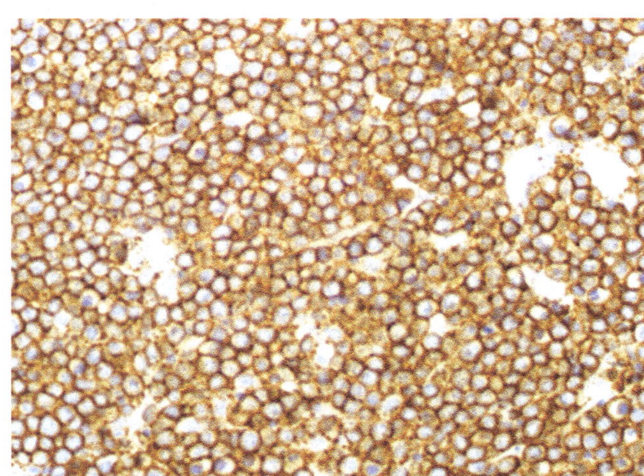

Fig. 4.53 Diffuse large B-cell lymphoma with sheets of CD20-positive neoplastic cells

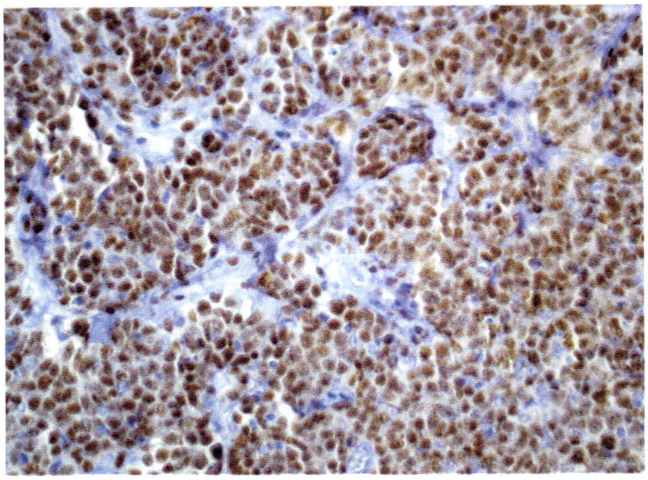

Fig. 4.54 Diffuse large B-cell lymphoma with sheets of PAX5-positive neoplastic cells

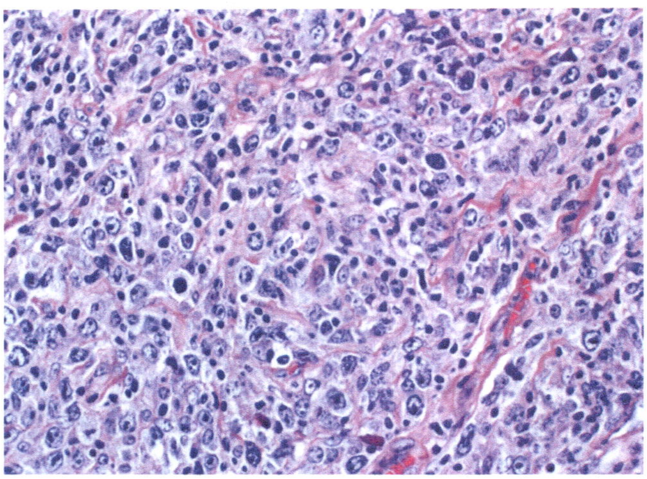

Fig. 4.55 Diffuse large B-cell lymphoma with effaced nodal architecture in a diffuse pattern by scattered large cells showing pleomorphism

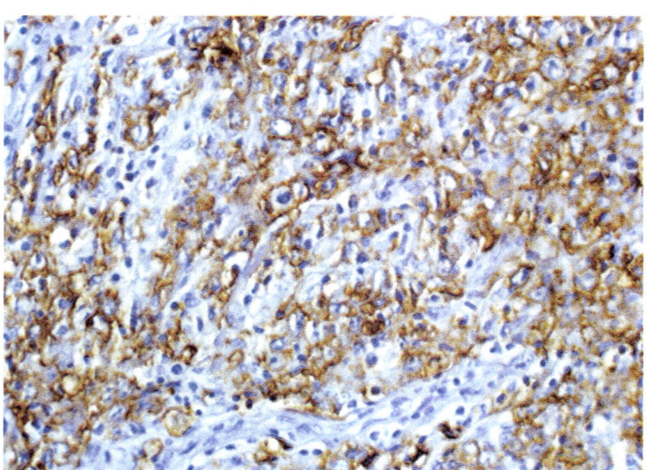

Fig. 4.56 The large pleomorphic cells in diffuse large B-cell lymphoma with CD20 positivity

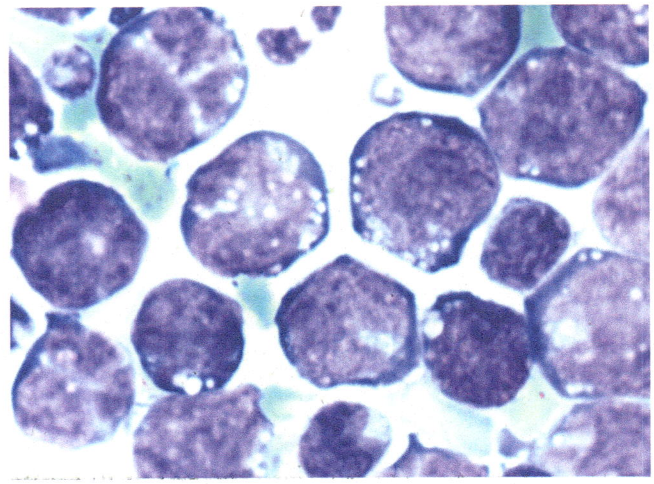

Fig. 4.57 Burkitt lymphoma with a monotonous population of medium-size lymphoid cells. Note the deeply basophilic cytoplasm with tiny vacuoles

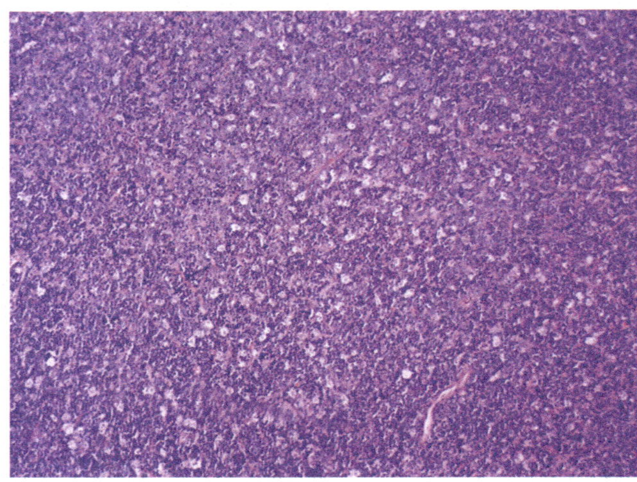

Fig. 4.58 Burkitt lymphoma with sheets of lymphoma cells admixed with histiocytes as a "starry sky" pattern

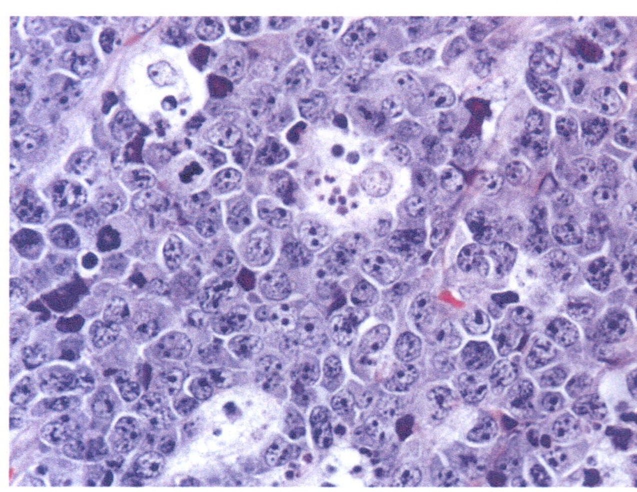

Fig. 4.59 Burkitt lymphoma cells with round nuclear contour and small nucleoli as a "snake head" appearance

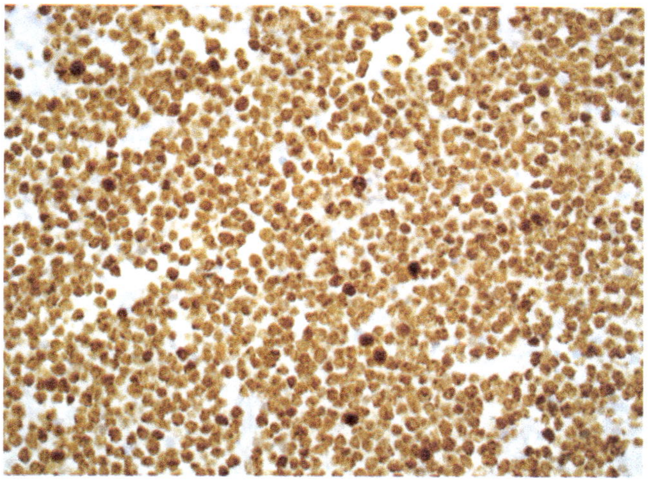

Fig. 4.60 Burkitt lymphoma cells with 100% of proliferation rate by Ki67 (MIB) immunohistochemical stain

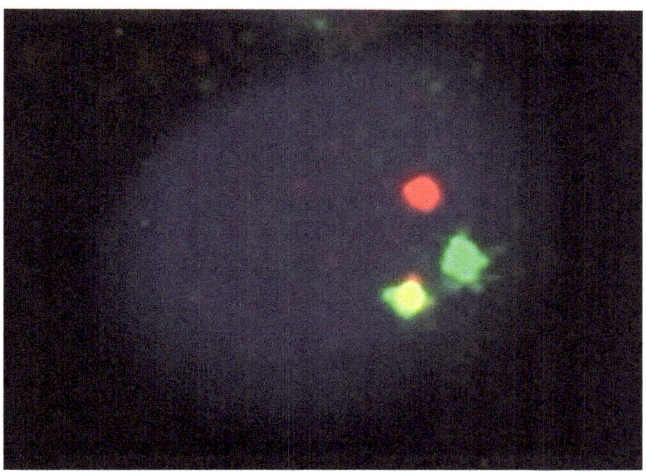

Fig. 4.61 FISH in Burkitt lymphoma with *MYC* rearrangement (break-apart, 1R1G1F)

- 70–80% with t(2;5) translocation and ALK expression.
- ALK-positive cases frequently involve both nodal and extranodal sites and have a better prognosis.

Cytological Features (Fig. 4.66a–d)

- Cellular smear.
- Pleomorphic cells with variable sizes.
- Binucleation or multinucleation or bizarre cells can be seen.
- Large nuclei with indentation and lobulation.
- Variable amount of cytoplasm.
- Heterogeneous population in the background, including small lymphoid cells, histiocytes, and plasma cells.
- CD2 and CD4 are the more sensitive markers.
- More than 75% of cases are negative for CD3.
- CD30 positive in all cases, usually in large lymphoid cells; most cases are positive for EMA.
- Seventy percent of cases show ALK expression (either nuclear or cytoplasmic staining).
- EBV is negative.

Histologic Features

- Effaced nodal architecture with expanded perifollicular areas (Fig. 4.67).
- Neoplastic cells are pleomorphic and hallmark cells with horseshoe-like nucleus (Fig. 4.68).

Immunohistochemistry and Ancillary Studies

- Positive for T-cell markers, CD30 (Fig. 4.69), and ALK1 (Fig. 4.70) and negative for CD15
- ALK1+ and ALK1- types share a similar molecular Janus kinase/signal transducer and activator of transcription 3 (JAK/STAT3) pathway.

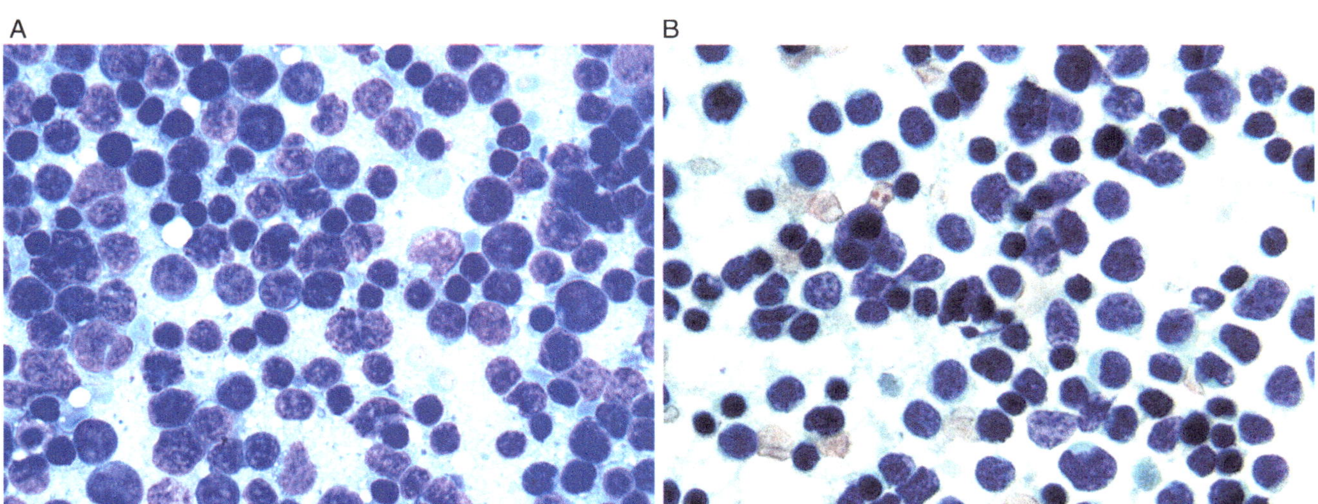

Fig. 4.62 (**a**, **b**) T-cell lymphoma with a polymorphous population of a spectrum of small, medium, and large lymphocytes on Diff-Quik (**a**) and Pap stain (**b**)

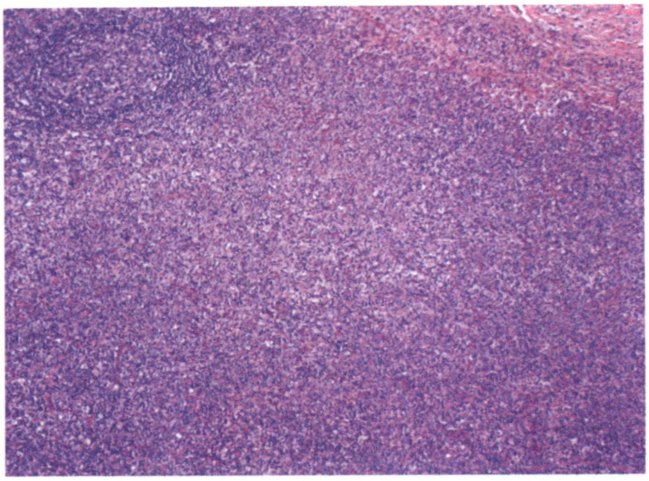

Fig. 4.63 Peripheral T-cell lymphoma with effaced nodal architecture and perifollicular expansion

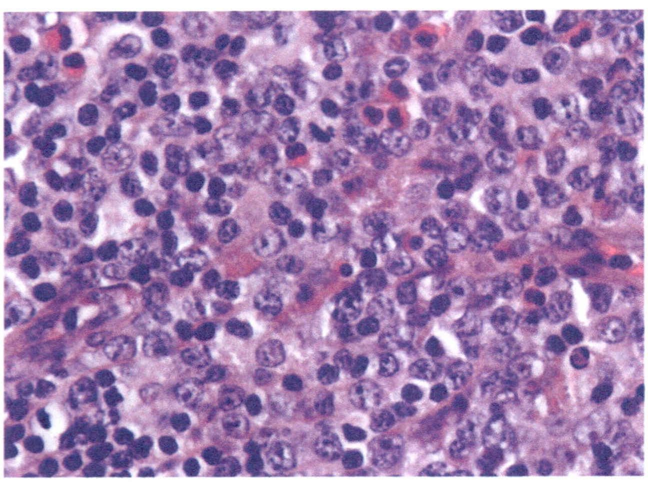

Fig. 4.64 Neoplastic T cells are medium in size with vesicular chromatin and nucleolus; there is a background of mature lymphocyte and scattered eosinophils

- New type: ALK-negative ALCL arising in association with breast implants shows similar morphological features, but neoplastic cells are confined to the seroma fluid without invasion of the capsule. Treatment is removal of the implant and capsule.

Differential Diagnosis

- Hodgkin lymphoma
- Other high-grade lymphoma
- Carcinoma
- Melanoma
- Sarcoma

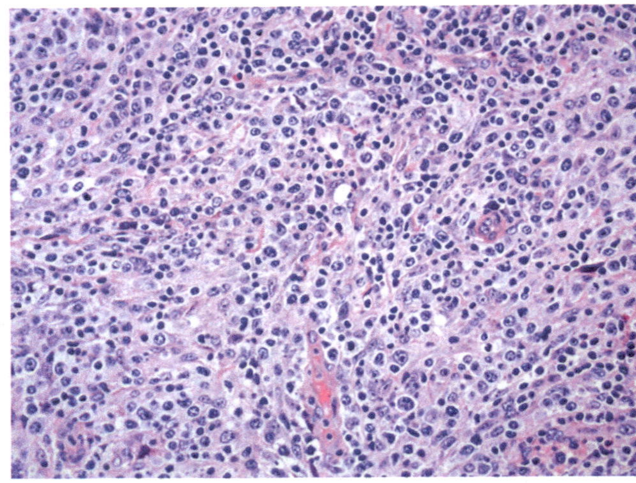

Fig. 4.65 Angioimmunoblastic T-cell lymphoma with effaced nodal architecture and perifollicular expansion by monocytoid lymphocytes and capillary proliferation

Hodgkin Lymphoma

Clinical Features

- Cervical, mediastinal, or axillary mass
- Bimodal age curve with a peak in young adults (15–35 years) and a second in the elderly

Cytological Features (Fig. 4.71a–h)

- Low to moderate cellularity.
- Polymorphous population of small lymphoid cells, plasma cells, histiocytes, and eosinophils.
- Classic multinucleated Reed-Sternberg cells and mononuclear Hodgkin cells.
- Fibrosis and crushed cellular components are frequently seen.
- Excisional biopsy should be suggested for further classification.

Histologic Features

- Effaced nodal architecture in a nodular or diffuse pattern with two types: CHL (nodular sclerosis, mixed cellularity, lymphocyte rich, and lymphocyte depleted) (Figs. 4.72a–d and 4.73a–c) and nodular lymphocyte-predominant Hodgkin lymphoma (NLPHL) (Figs. 4.74 and 4.75a–d)
- Large neoplastic cells including Reed-Sternberg cells, Hodgkin cells, lacunar cells, and popcorn cells (Fig. 4.76a–d)

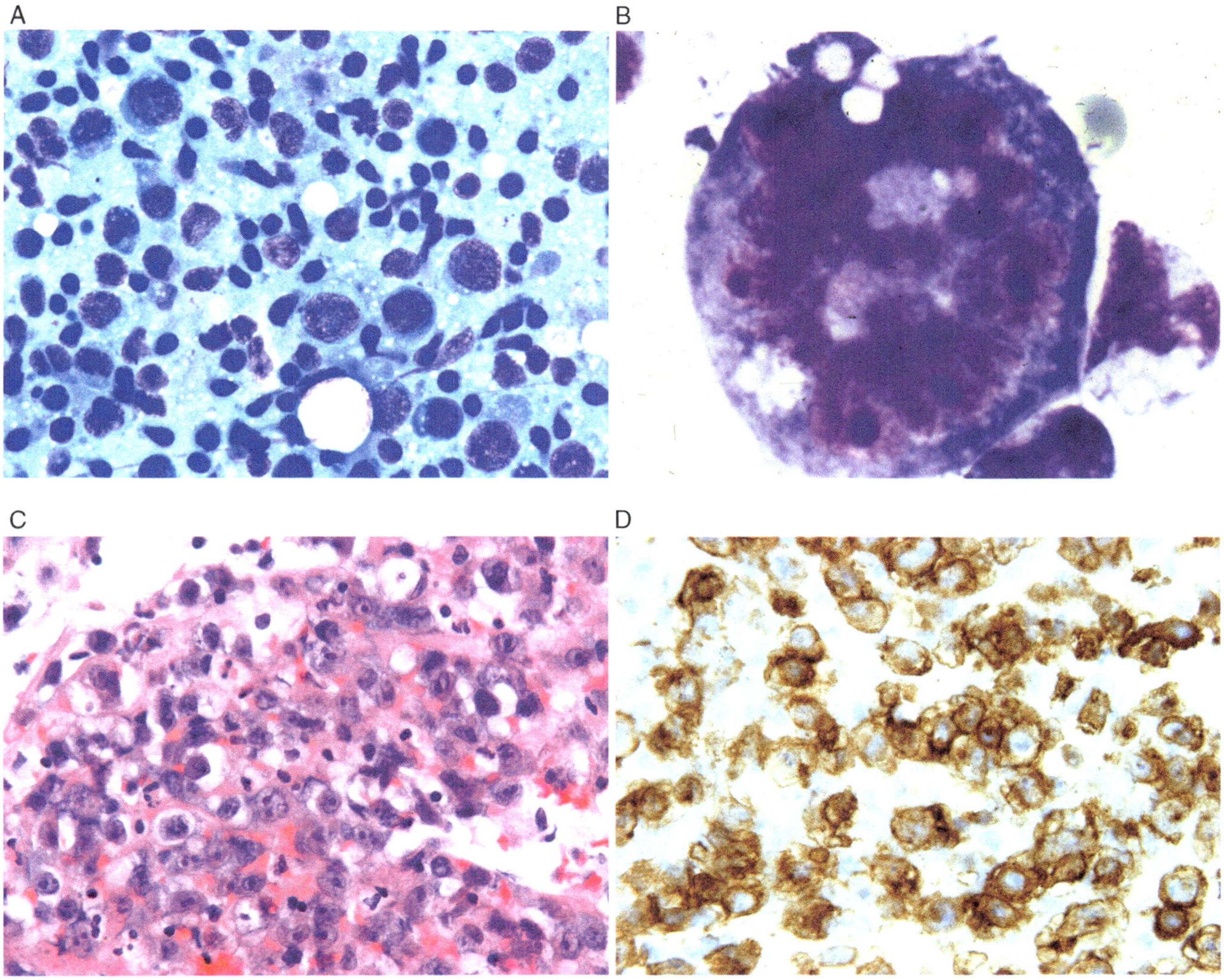

Fig. 4.66 (**a**–**d**) Anaplastic large cell lymphoma with pleomorphic cells with variable sizes on Diff-Quik (**a**, **b**), cellblock (**c**), positive for CD30 (**d**)

Immunohistochemistry and Ancillary Studies

- Reed-Sternberg cells in CHL are positive for CD15, CD30, and K homology domain-containing protein over-expressed in cancer 1 (KOC1) (Fig. 4.77a–c) and negative for CD3 and CD20.
- NLPHL is a monoclonal B-cell neoplasm that is CD45 positive, CD20 positive, PAX5 positive, CD15 negative, and CD30 negative (Fig. 4.78a–e).
- Lymphocyte-rich CHL has features intermediate between CHL and NLPHL.

Differential Diagnosis

- Poorly differentiated carcinoma
- Melanoma
- Sarcoma
- Reactive lymph node with many immunoblasts

Others

Langerhans Cell Histiocytosis (LCH)

Cytological Features (Fig. 4.79a–e)

- Langerhans histiocytes and eosinophils.
- Nuclear grooves or linear folds are seen in Langerhans cells.
- Immunostain shows positivity for both S100 and CD1a.
- Multinucleated giant cells may be present.
- Some of these neoplasms may have transdifferentiation to follicular lymphoma, CLL, B- or T-lymphoblastic

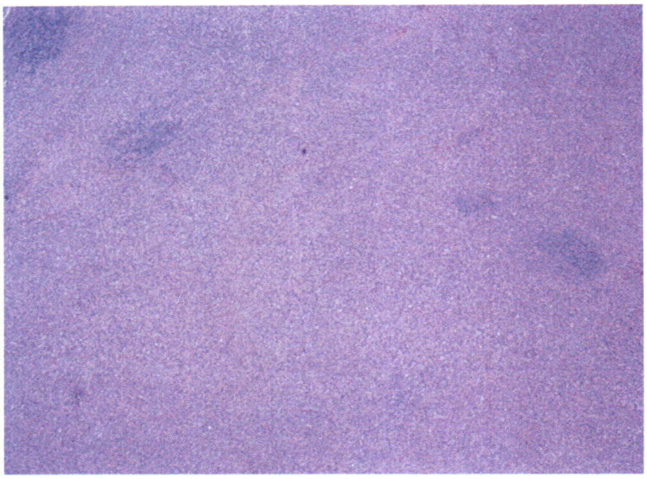

Fig. 4.67 Anaplastic large cell lymphoma with effaced nodal architecture and perifollicular expansion

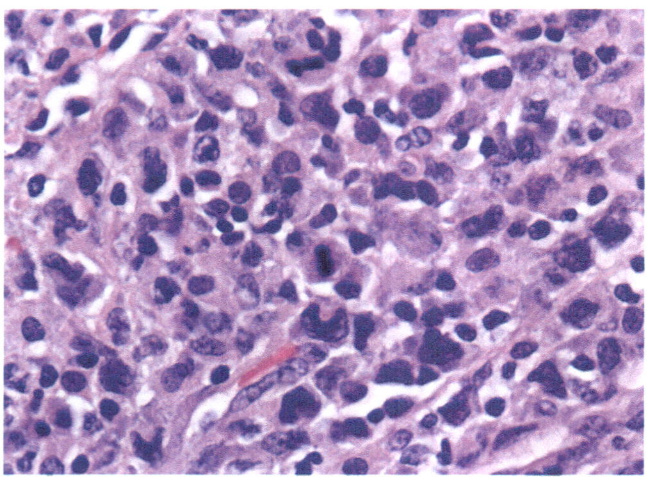

Fig. 4.68 Neoplastic T cells are pleomorphic and some with horseshoe-like nucleus – hallmark cells

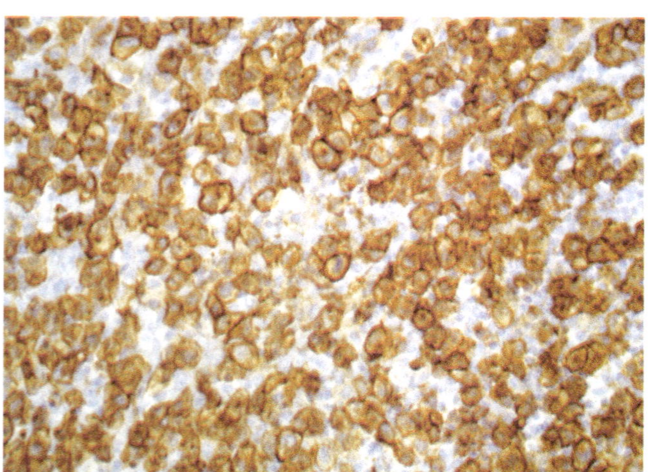

Fig. 4.69 Neoplastic T cells positive for CD30

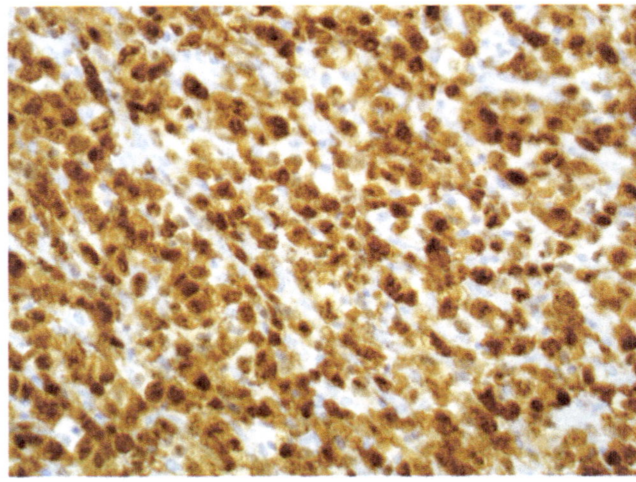

Fig. 4.70 Neoplastic T cells positive for ALK1

neoplasms carrying the same *IGHV*, or T-cell receptor (*TCR*) gene rearrangement.

Histologic Features

- Effaced nodal architecture with expanded sinus and pericortex by large neoplastic Langerhans cells
- In early stage, Langerhans cells prominent admixed with eosinophils and neutrophils; in late stage, the number of Langerhans cells is decreased with fibrosis and increased foamy macrophages.

Myeloid Sarcoma

Cytological Features (Fig. 4.80a–e)

- Myeloid cells in various stages of differentiation
- Can be mainly blasts or a mixed population of myeloid cells in different stages
- Eosinophilic myelocytes may be seen.

Histologic Features

- Effaced nodal or tissue architecture with sheets of myeloblasts (Figs. 4.81 and 4.82), rarely, of erythroid precursors or megakaryoblasts
- May present de novo, with peripheral and bone marrow involvement, relapse of acute myeloid leukemia (AML) or progression of a prior myelodysplastic syndrome (MDS), myeloproliferative neoplasm (MPN), or MDS/MPN. Recommend clinical correlation.

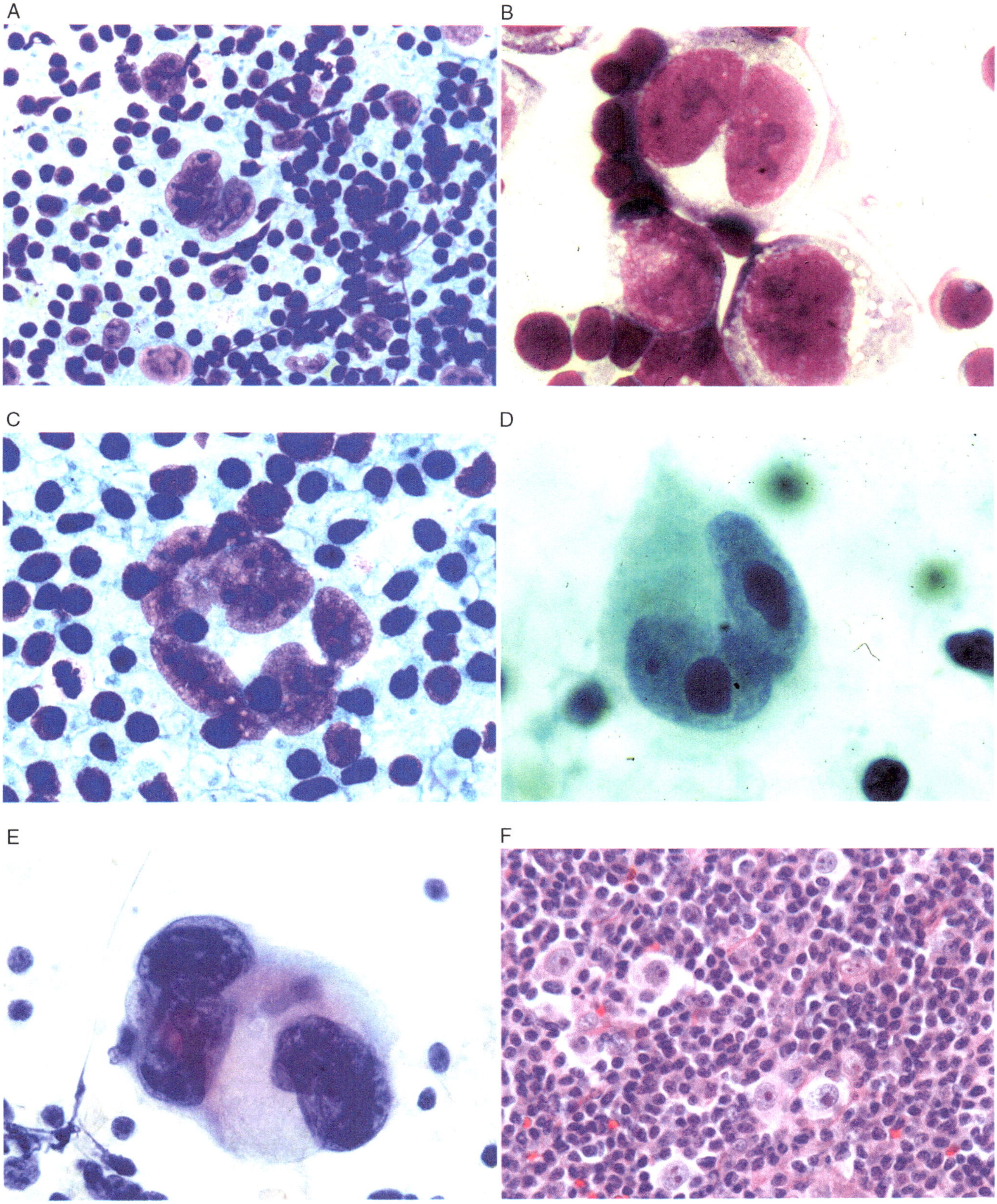

Fig. 4.71 (**a–h**) Hodgkin lymphoma with classic Reed-Sternberg cells and mononuclear or multinucleated Hodgkin cells in the background of a polymorphous population of small lymphoid cells, plasma cells, histiocytes, and eosinophils (**a–e**), and small tissue section (**f**), Hodgkin cells positive for CD15 (**g**), and CD30 (**h**)

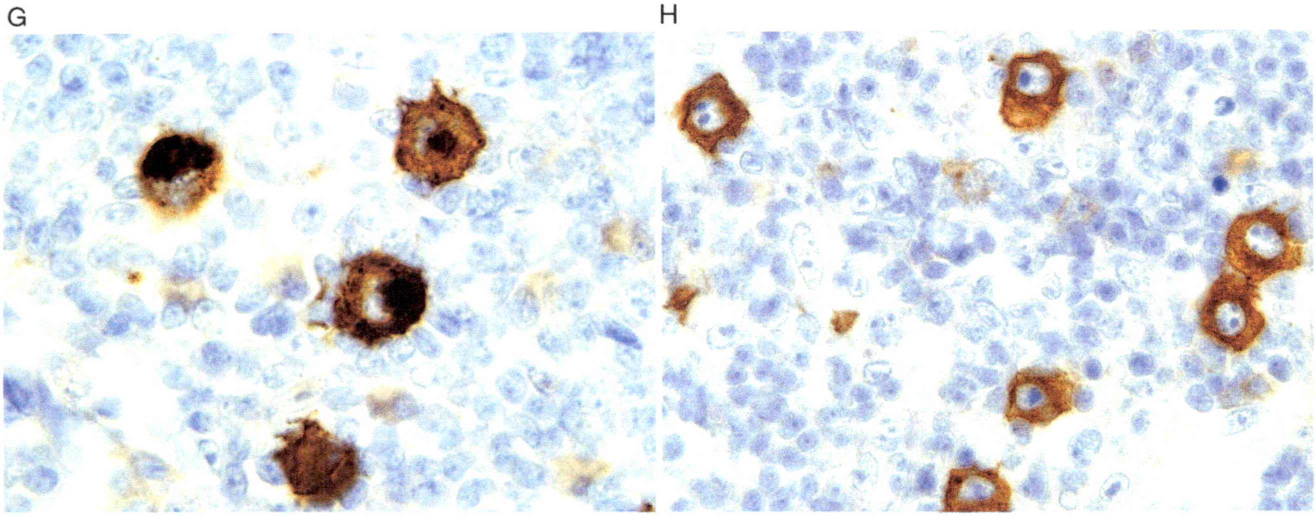

Fig. 4.71 (continued)

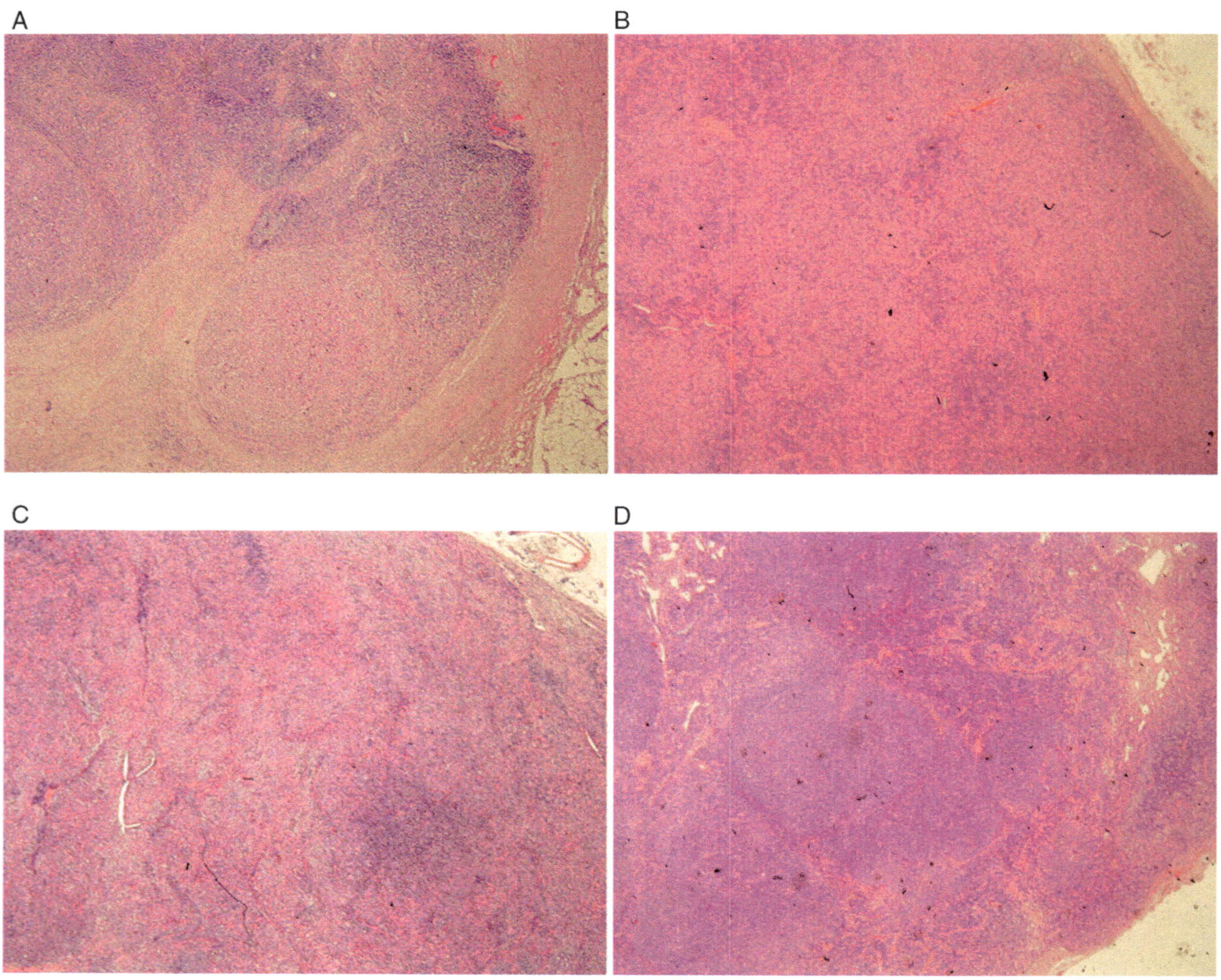

Fig. 4.72 (**a**–**d**) Classical Hodgkin lymphoma with nodular sclerosis (**a**), mixed cellularity (**b**), lymphocyte rich (**c**), and lymphocyte depleted (**d**)

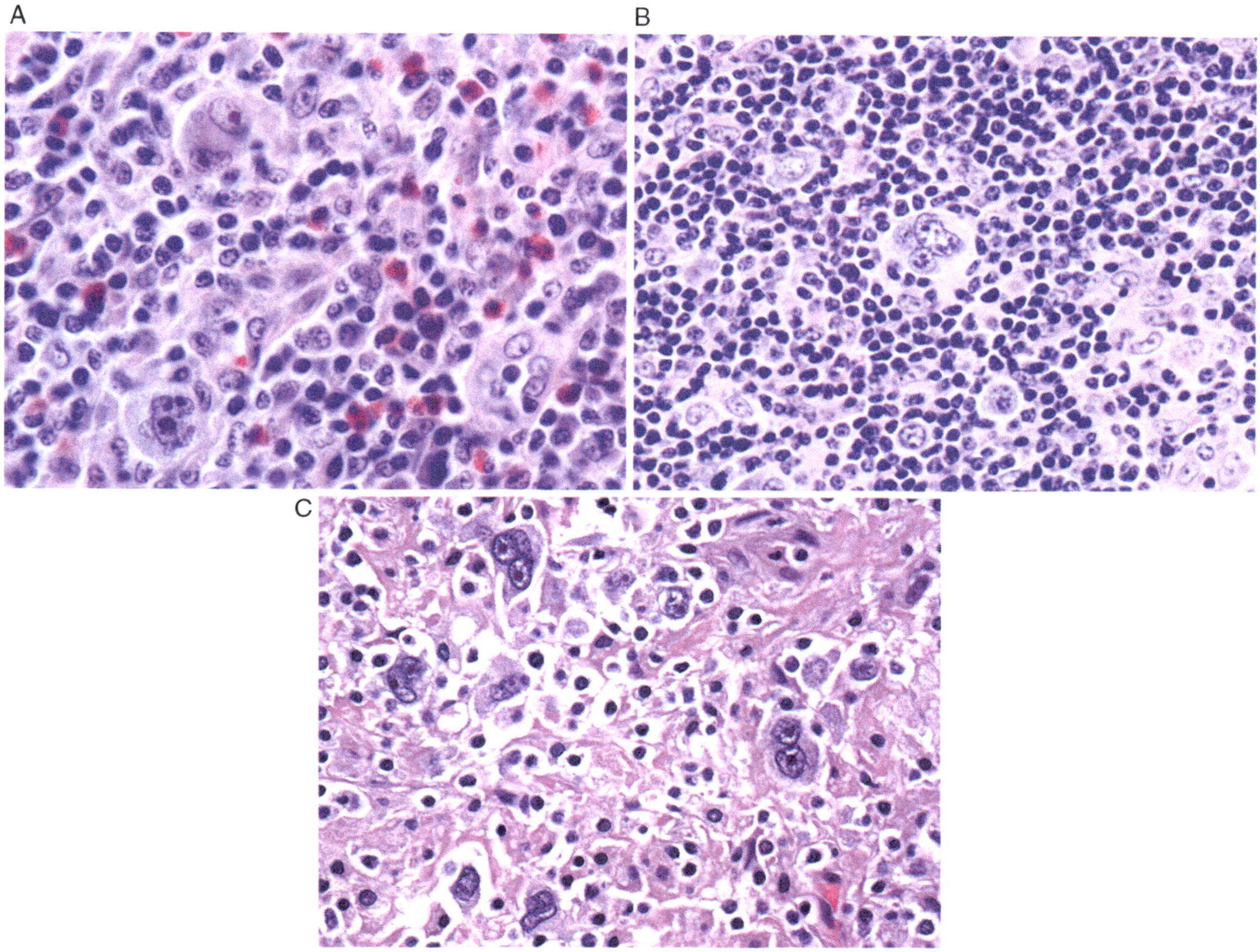

Fig. 4.73 (**a–c**) High-power view of classical Hodgkin lymphoma with Reed-Stenberg cells in a background of mixed lymphocytes, plasma cells, and eosinophils in nodular sclerosis and mixed cellularity (**a**), neoplastic cells with background of lymphocytes in lymphocyte-rich (**b**) and neoplastic cells with background of hypocellularity in lymphocyte depleted (**c**)

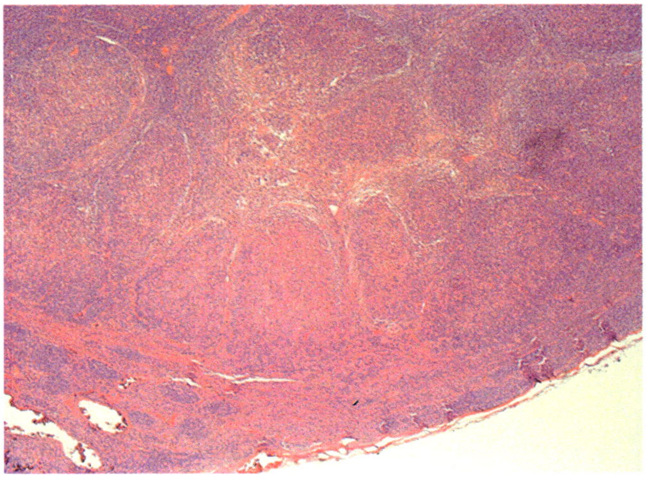

Fig. 4.74 Nodular lymphocytic-predominant Hodgkin lymphoma with large nodular pattern

Immunohistochemistry and Ancillary Studies

- Myeloblasts positive for myeloperoxidase (MPO, Fig. 4.83), CD117, lysozyme (Fig. 4.84), CD68, CD99, and CD34

Lymphoblastic Lymphoma

Clinical Features

- A childhood disease
- 90% precursor T-lymphoblastic cells and 10% precursor B lymphoblastic cells.
- A designation of lymphoma is given when a patient presents as a mass lesion and less than 25% blasts in bone marrow.
- T-lymphoblastic lymphoma frequently present with a mediastinal mass.

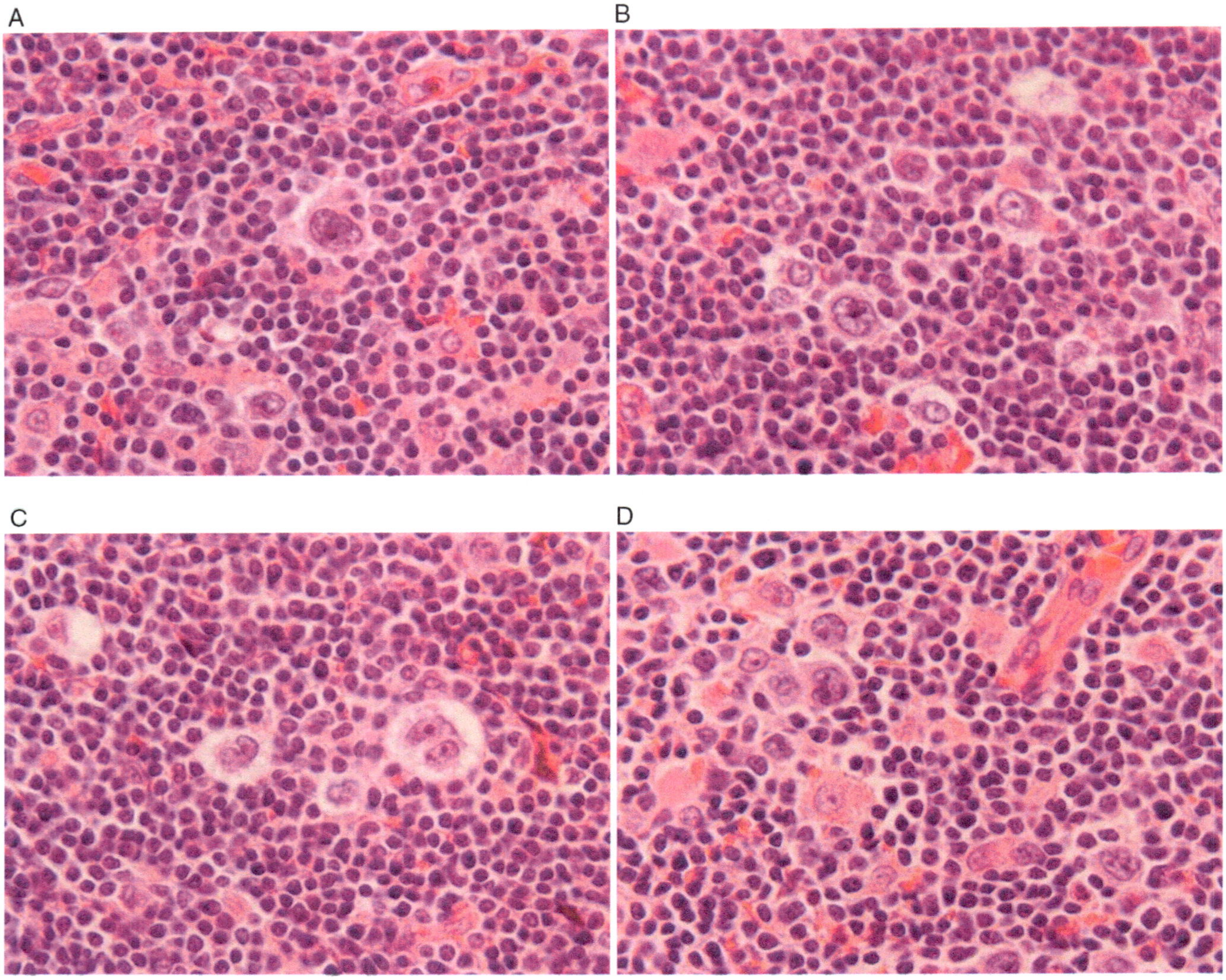

Fig. 4.75 (**a–d**) Nodular lymphocytic-predominant Hodgkin lymphoma with scattered lymphocyte-predominant cells in a background of mature lymphocytes

- Indolent T-lymphoblastic proliferation may mimic T-lymphoblastic lymphoma. It typically involves lymphoid tissue of the upper aerodigestive tract without systemic dissemination and also no clonality detected.

Cytological Features (Fig. 4.85a–c)

- Cellular smear
- Relatively uniform population of medium-size lymphoid cells
- Fine, delicate, and powdery nuclear chromatin
- Small to conspicuous nucleoli
- Nuclear membrane variable from smooth to convoluted
- Scant to small amount of cytoplasm
- Cytoplasmic vacuoles can be seen

Histologic Features

- Effaced nodal architecture with sheets of blasts (Fig. 4.86) and may have a "starry sky" pattern.
- Neoplastic cells are medium in size with vesicular chromatin and small nucleolus (Fig. 4.87).
- New type: Early T-precursor (ETP) lymphoblastic leukemia shows blasts positive for CD2, CD7, cytoplasmic CD3, and CD4 and negative for CD1a, CD5 (or weak expression) and CD8 with one or more of the myeloid/stem cell markers CD34, CD117, CD13, CD33, CD11b, or CD65 (Figs. 4.88 and 4.89a, b). It has a very poor outcome.
- New provisional entity: Indolent T-lymphoblastic proliferation belongs to nonneoplastic entity and may mimic

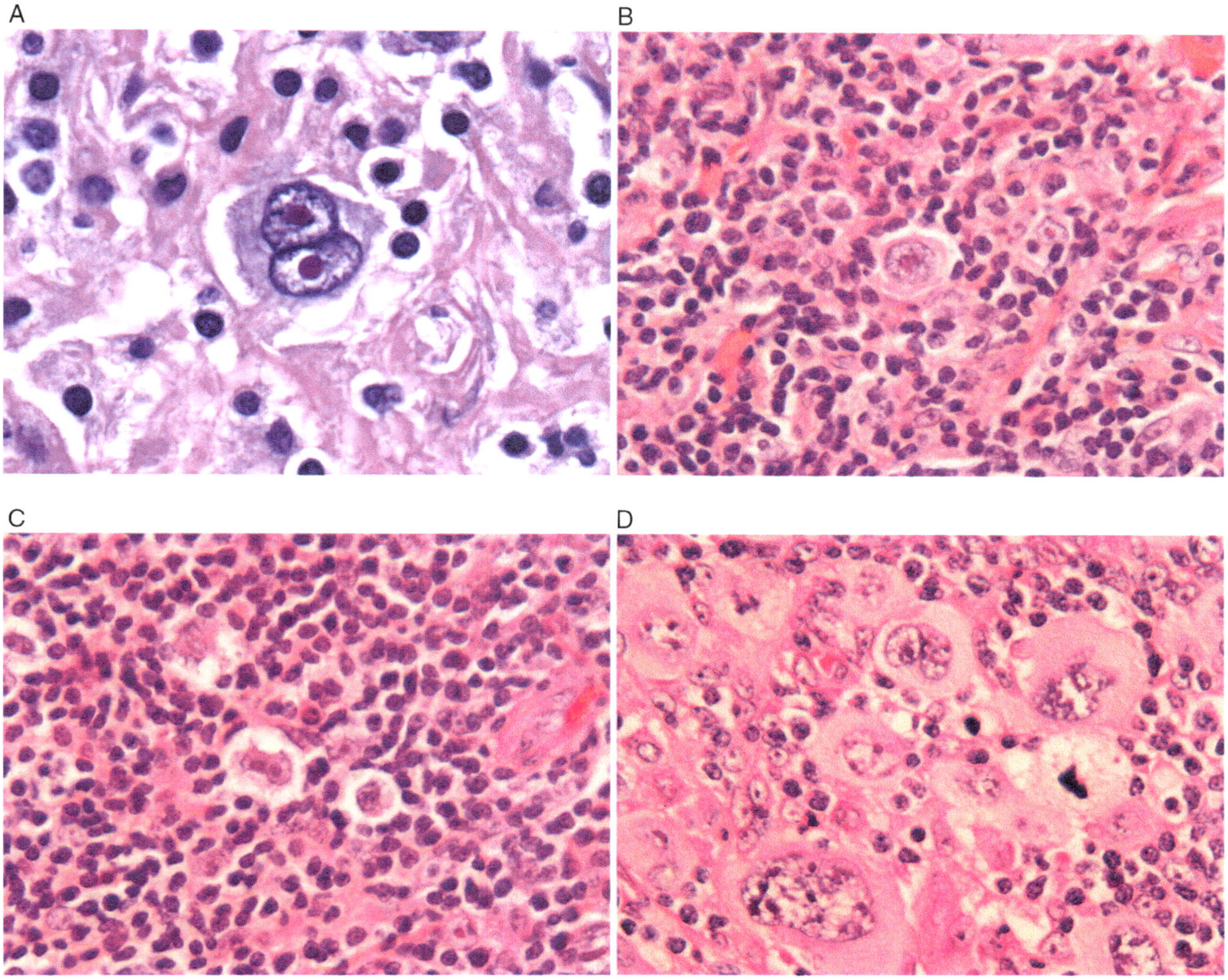

Fig. 4.76 (**a**–**d**) Hodgkin lymphoma with Reed-Sternberg cells (**a**), Hodgkin cells (**b**), lacunar cells (**c**), and popcorn cells (**d**)

T-lymphoblastic lymphoma. IHC: TdT+, no aberrant phenotype, and not clonal. It mostly occurs in lymphoid tissue of upper aerodigestive tract with good prognosis.

Immunohistochemistry and Ancillary Studies

- Terminal deoxynucleotidyl transferase (TdT)-positive in both T and B lymphoblasts.
- T lymphoblasts are positive for CD7 and cytoplasmic CD3 with coexpression of CD4 and CD8 and also positive for other T-cell markers, such as CD1a and CD2.
- B lymphoblasts are positive for CD19, CD79a, CD10, and CD34.

Tumors Mimicking Lymphomas

Melanoma

Cytological Features

- Loosely cohesive groups and single cells
- Binucleation and multinucleation
- Intranuclear inclusions
- Plasmacytoid cells with abundant cytoplasm
- Prominent nucleoli
- Dusty pigments

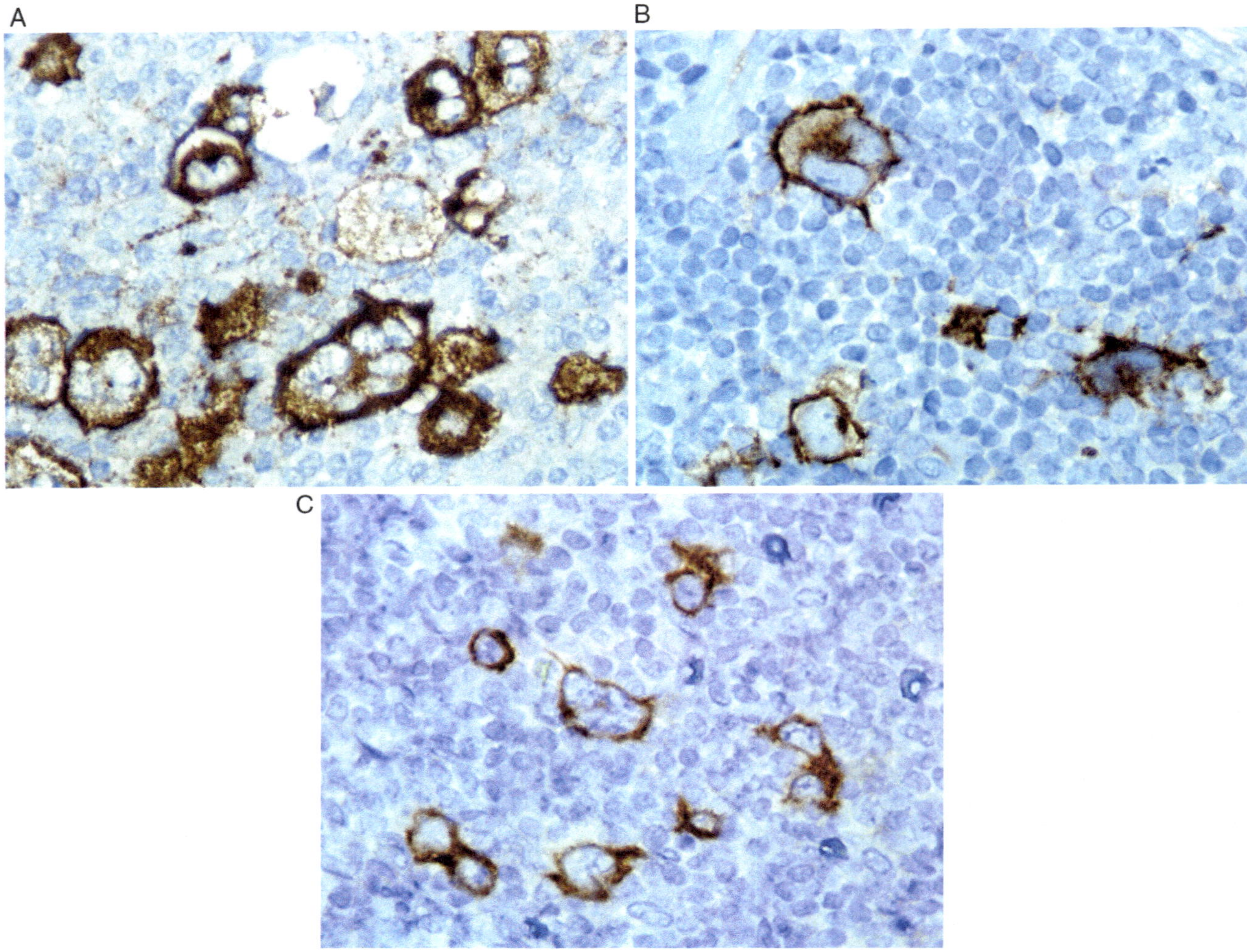

Fig. 4.77 (**a**–**c**) Reed-Sternberg cells in classical Hodgkin lymphoma with positive CD15 (**a**), positive CD30 (**b**), and positive KOC1 (**c**)

Small Cell Undifferentiated Carcinoma

Cytological Features

- Cohesive and single neoplastic cells.
- Very high nuclear-to-cytoplasmic ratio.
- Neuroendocrine chromatin.
- Inconspicuous nucleoli.
- Single cell necrosis and many mitosis.
- Blue bodies in the background may resemble lymphoglandular bodies.

Undifferentiated Carcinoma

- Nasopharyngeal carcinoma
- Poorly differentiated squamous cell carcinoma
- Basaloid squamous cell carcinoma
- Merkel cell carcinoma

Small Round Cell Tumors

- Rhabdomyosarcoma
- Ewing's sarcoma/primitive neuroectodermal tumor (PNET)
- Neuroblastoma
- Desmoplastic small round cell tumor

Seminoma

Cytological Features

- Two populations of cells: large neoplastic tumor cells and small benign lymphoid cells.
- The neoplastic cells are large and relatively uniform in size.
- Single prominent nucleoli.
- Cytoplasmic vacuoles can be seen.

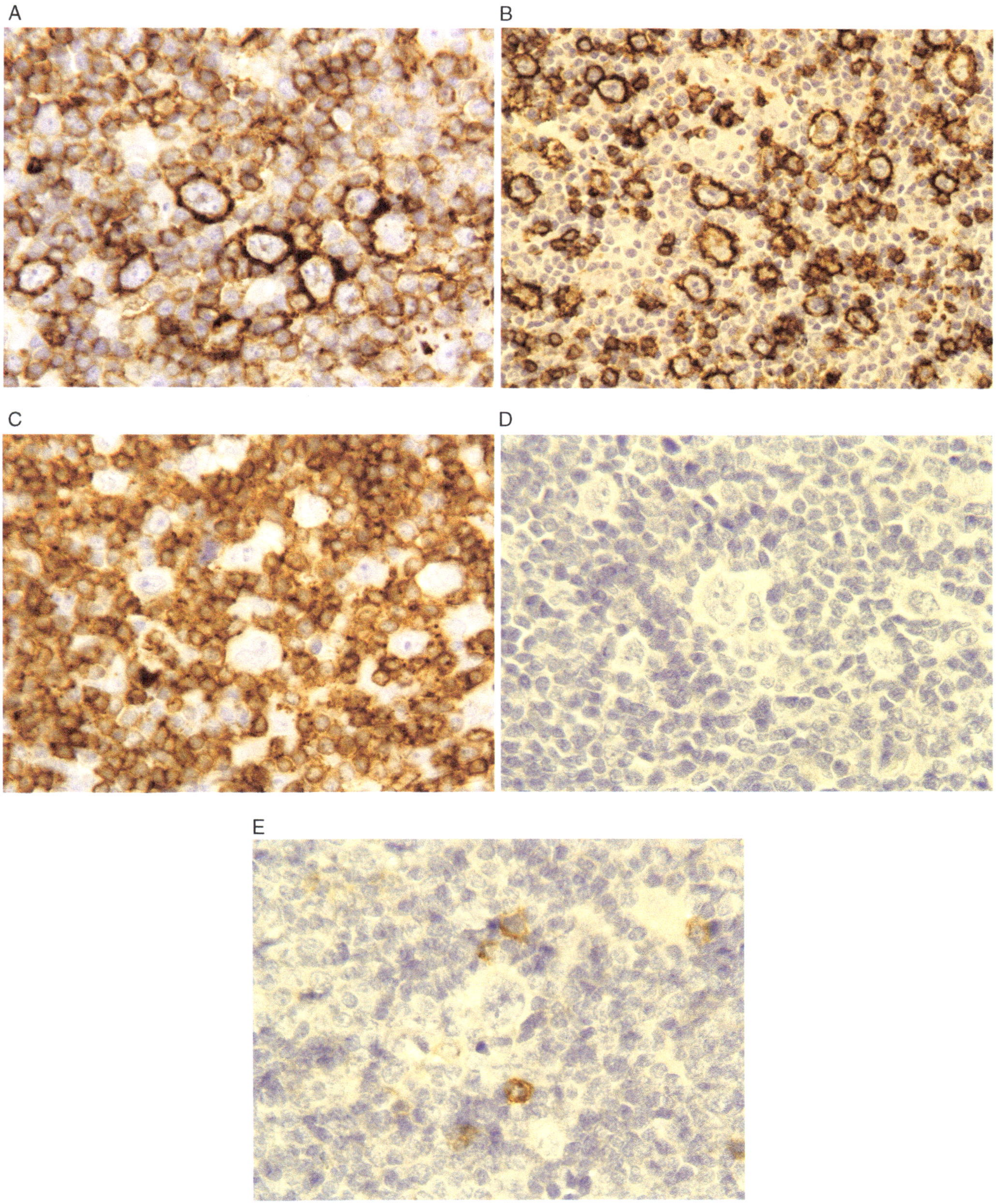

Fig. 4.78 (**a–e**) Lymphocyte-predominant cells in nodular lymphocytic-predominant Hodgkin lymphoma with positive CD45 (**a**), positive CD20 (**b**), negative CD3 (**c**), negative CD15 (**d**), and negative CD30 (**e**)

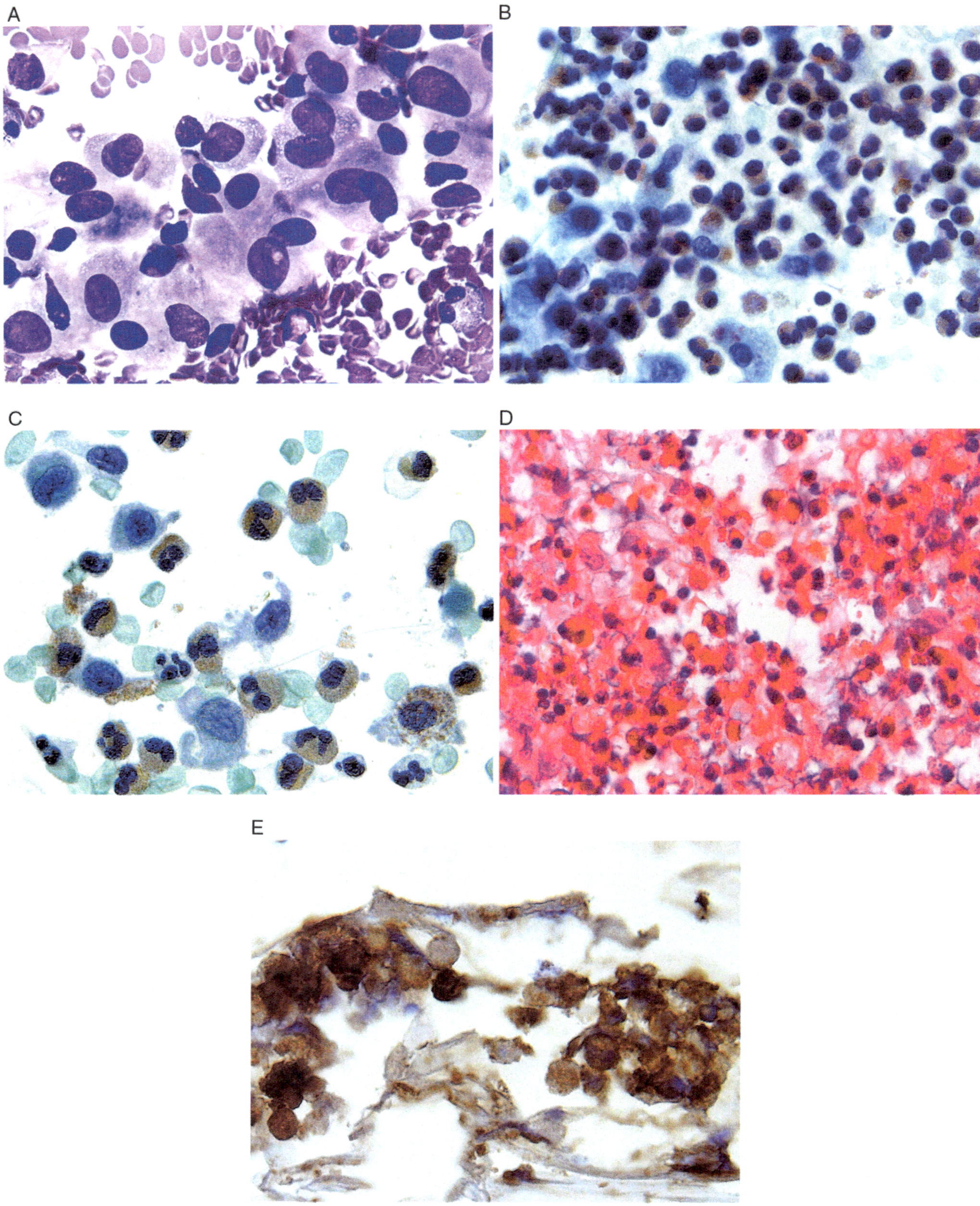

Fig. 4.79 (**a**–**e**) Langerhans cell histiocytosis with Langerhans histiocytes and eosinophils in (**a**) and (**b**), prominent nuclear grooves or linear folds seen in Langerhans histiocytes (**c**), on cellblock (**d**) and positive for CD1a (**e**)

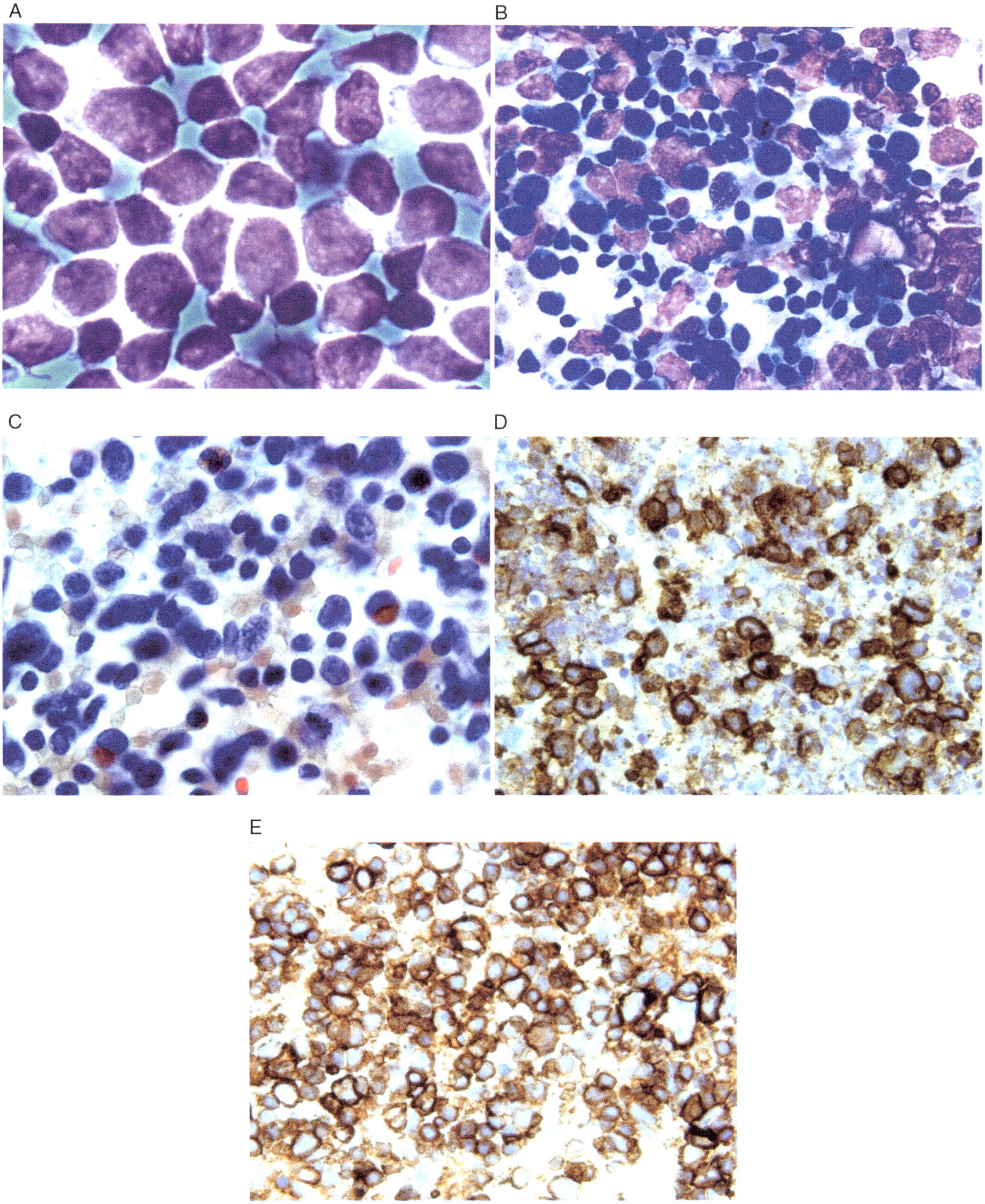

Fig. 4.80 (**a**–**e**) Myeloid sarcoma on Diff-Quik (**a**, **b**), Pap stain (**c**), positive for CD34 (**d**) and CD43 (**e**) on cellblock sections

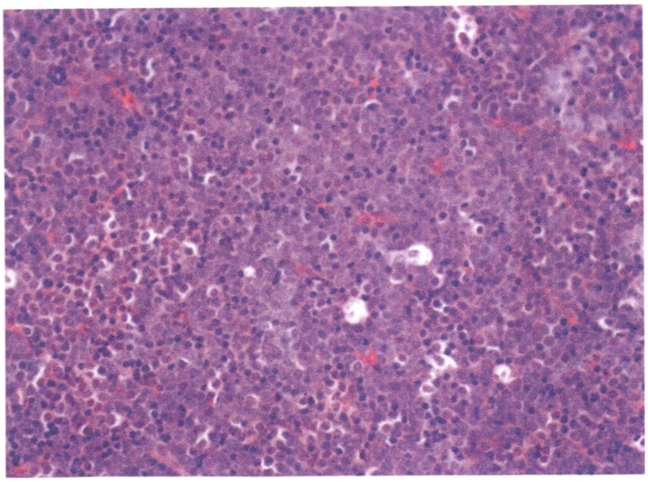

Fig. 4.81 Myeloid sarcoma with sheets of blasts

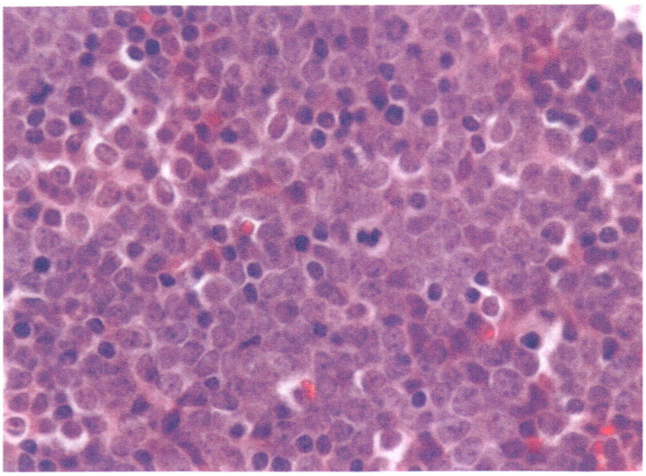

Fig. 4.82 Myeloblasts with fine chromatin, round nuclear contour, and frequent mitotic figures

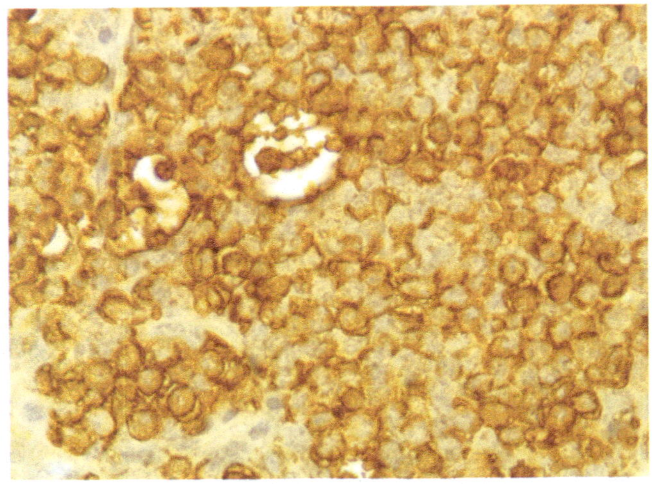

Fig. 4.83 Myeloblasts with positive myeloperoxidase

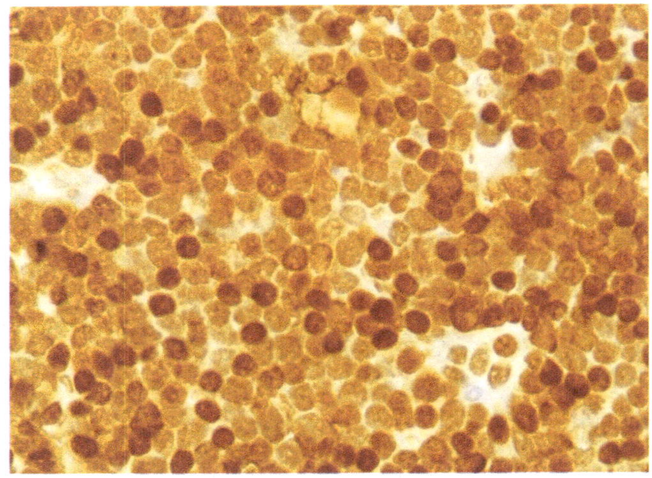

Fig. 4.84 Myeloblasts with positive lysozyme

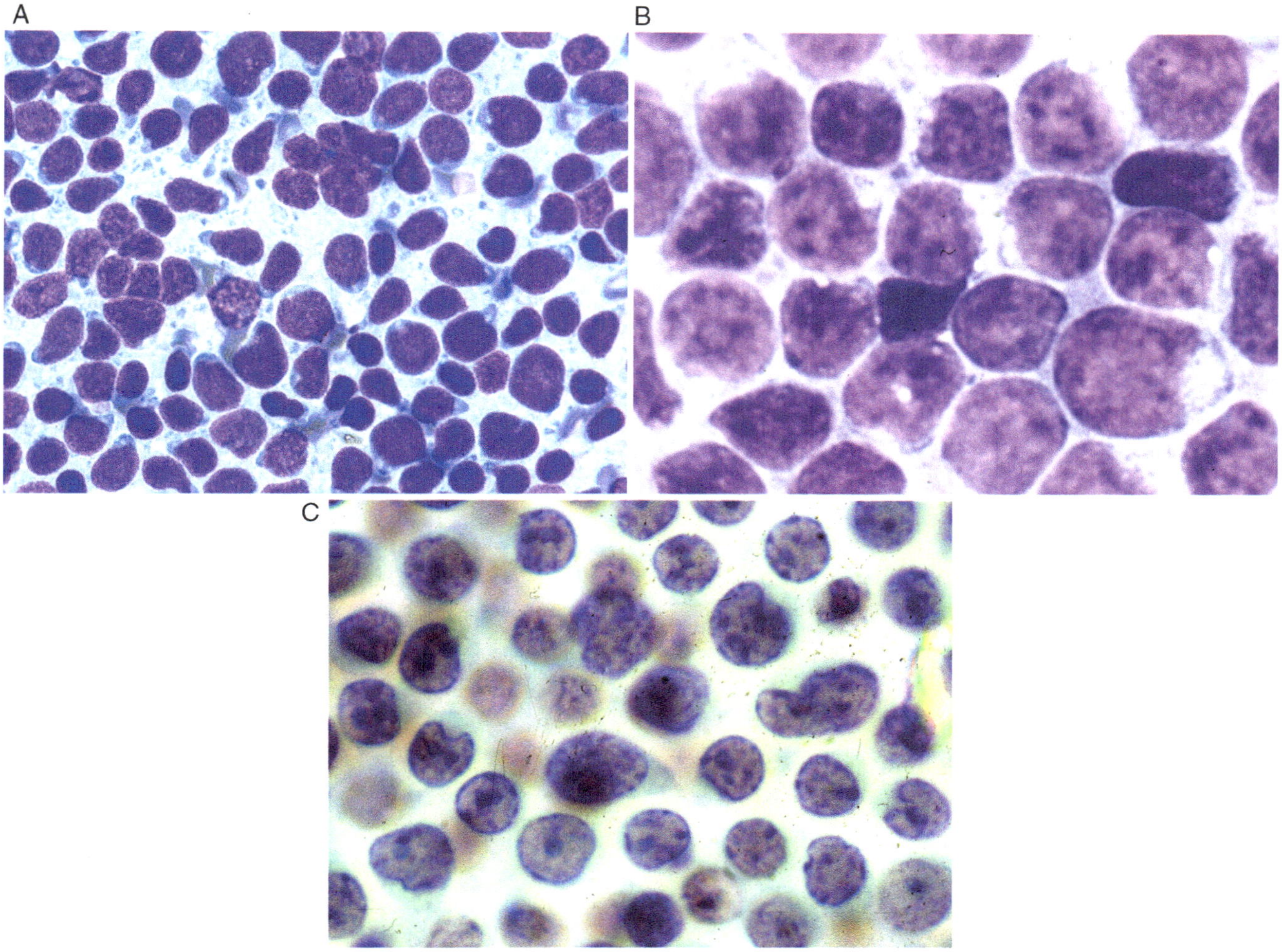

Fig. 4.85 (**a**–**c**) Lymphoblastic lymphoma with relatively uniform population of medium-size lymphoid cells, with fine, delicate, and powdery nuclear chromatin on Diff-Quik (**a**, **b**) and Pap stain (**c**)

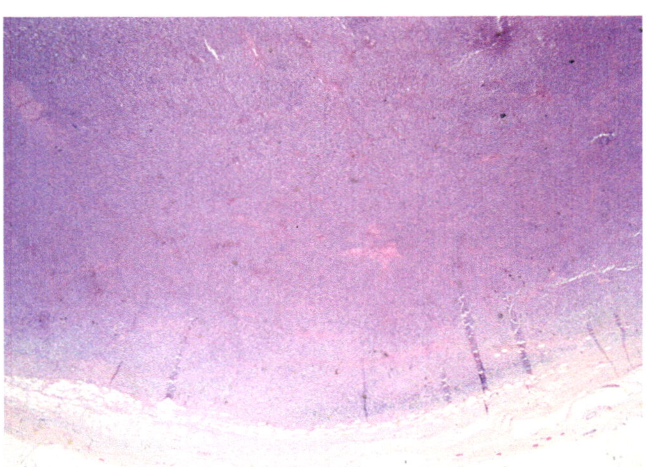

Fig. 4.86 Lymphoblastic lymphoma with effaced nodal architecture in a diffuse pattern by sheets of neoplastic cells

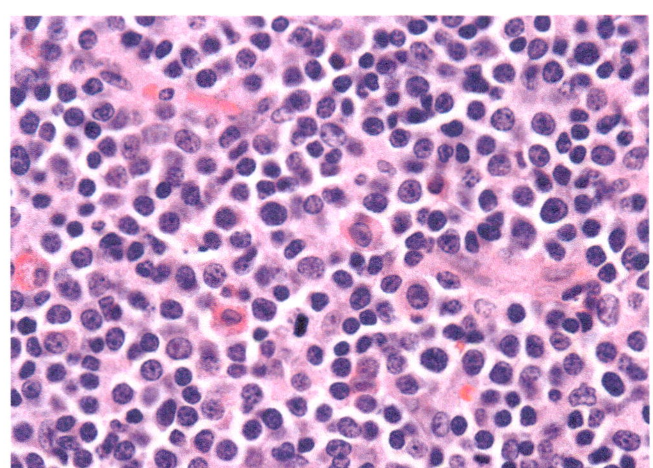

Fig. 4.87 Neoplastic cells with round nuclear contour, vesicular chromatin, and small nucleoli; in a background of mature lymphocytes and eosinophils

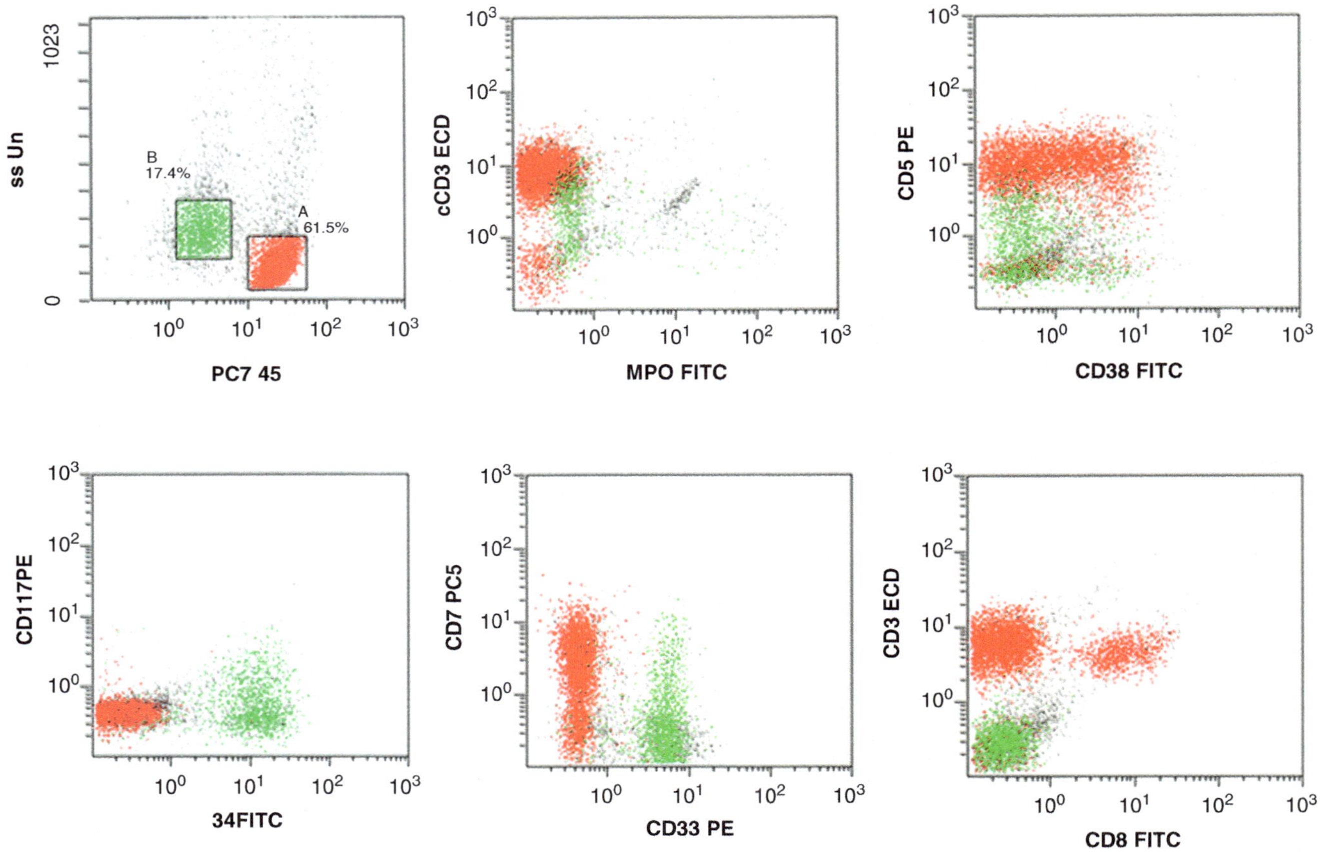

Fig. 4.88 Flow cytometry studies of lymphoblast positive for cCD3 and CD34, and low intensity of CD5 and negative for sCD3, CD8, and MPO (a few blasts expressing MPO in low intensity) with aberrant expression of CD33

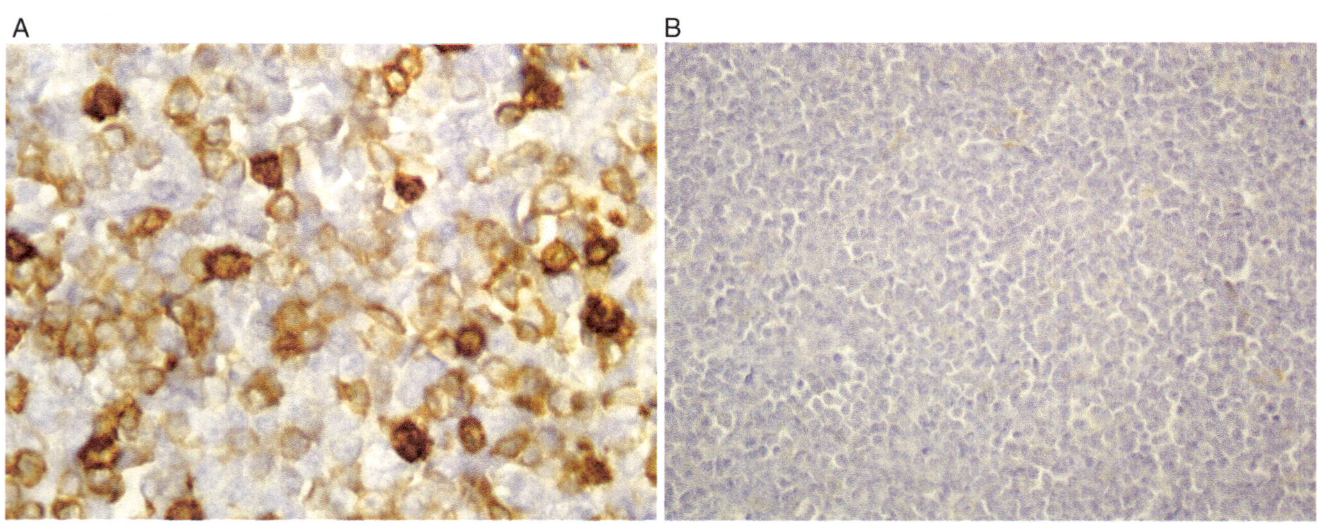

Fig. 4.89 Neoplastic cells positive for cCD3 (**a**) and negative for CD1a (**b**)

Thymoma

Cytological Features

- Two populations of cells: epithelial cells and lymphoid cells.
- Can be predominately lymphoid cells.
- Lymphoid cells are CD3-positve and TdT-positive cortical thymocytes.
- Epithelial cells are positive for p63.

Case Presentations

There are three scenarios encountered in practice when evaluating an enlarged lymph node. Case Scenario 1 is how to make a diagnosis and classification of low-grade B-cell lymphoma based on morphology, flow cytometry, and molecular studies; Case Scenario 2 is how to work on a blast-looking lymphoma in a young patient and what immunophenotypic and molecular tests should be ordered; and Case Scenario 3 is how to deal with a T-cell lymphoma in an elderly patient and what immunophenotypic features need to be paid attention to.

Case Scenario 1

Learning Objective

1. To reiterate the diagnostic criteria for low-grade B-cell lymphomas on morphological, immunophenotypic, and molecular features (Table 4.4)

Case

A 67-year-old female presented with a 2 x 1 cm left neck mass located in zone 5. She first noticed it 6 months ago and was not treated. She was otherwise healthy with no significant past medical history, no symptoms, and no weight loss. CT scan revealed a few tiny lymph nodes other than the enlarged lymph node mentioned above. Excisional biopsy was performed. The morphological features are shown in Figs. 4.90 and 4.91. Flow cytometry studies revealed a population of monotypic B cells positive for CD19 and CD20 and negative for CD5, CD10, and CD23 (Fig. 4.92a–d).

At this point, it is a low-grade B-cell lymphoma. Based on immunophenotypes, the differential diagnosis includes MZL, LPL, and other atypical B-cell lymphomas. Typically B-cell SLL coexpresses CD5 and CD23; MCL is positive for CD5 and FMC7; and follicular lymphoma is positive for CD10, but all the B-cell lymphomas can show an atypical immunophenotype with loss of one or more immunophenotypic marker(s). The morphological pattern showed perifollicular expansion by monotonous monocytoid/plasmacytoid cells, favoring LPL. Now the molecular test will be helpful to make the right classification of this low-grade B-cell lymphoma. Molecular testing showed MYD88 mutation (Fig. 4.93).

Final Diagnosis

Lymphoplasmacytic lymphoma (LPL).

What Are the Learning Points from This Case?

The learning points from this case include:

1. It is important to evaluate the pattern of effaced nodal architecture and cytological features of neoplastic cells, although there is overlapping in different low-grade B-cell lymphomas.
2. Every low-grade B-cell lymphoma has its typical immunophenotypic features, but it should be noted that any lymphomas could have atypical immunophenotypic features.
3. FISH and molecular tests, including specific translocation or mutation, would be helpful to make an accurate classification when immunophenotypic features are equivocal.

Case Scenario 2

Learning Objectives

1. To identify high-grade lymphomas, especially in young patients
2. To review the clinical, morphological, immunophenotypic, and molecular features of high-grade hematopoietic tumors (Table 4.5)

Case

A previously heathy 14-year-old boy presented with new-onset dysphagia and snoring, followed by a change in his voice. Symptom started around the time when he and his family had upper respiratory infections. He visited his family doctor, who found him with right tonsillar hypertrophy and positive for *Streptococcus*. The boy was treated with multiple courses of antibiotics with minimal improvement in symptoms. A tonsillectomy was performed. The right tonsil was 4.0 x 3.5 x 1.5 cm and left tonsil 3.2 x 2.0 x 1.2 cm. Morphologically, the left tonsil showed lymphoid follicular hyperplasia; the right tonsil revealed focal effacement by sheets of blasts in a "starry sky" pattern (Fig. 4.58). High-power view showed neoplastic cells with round nuclear contour, small nucleoli, and frequent mitotic figures (Fig. 4.59).

At this point, a diagnosis of high-grade hematolymphoid tumor can be made. Differential diagnosis includes lymphoblastic lymphoma, DLBCL, BL, or myeloid sarcoma. A definite diagnosis cannot be rendered without immunophenotypic study.

(continued)

Table 4.4 Summary of most common low-grade B-cell lymphomas

Diagnosis	Clinical features	Cytological features	Histological features	IHC features	Molecular features
CLL/SLL	-Most common leukemia/ lymphoma in west countries -Mostly occurs in adults >40 years -M:F ratio - 1.5–2:1 -Involving PB, BM, and LN	Round nuclear contour and hypercondensed chromatin	-Vaguely nodular pattern -Small lymphoma cells admixed with prolymphocytes	CD20+, CD5+, CD23+, LEF1+, CD38, and ZAP-70 to evaluate prognosis	50%: del 13q, 20%:+12 Less common: del 11, del 17q, del 6q
FL	-20% of all lymphomas with highest incidence in the USA and Western Europe -M:F – 1:1.7 -Involving LN, also BM, PB, and GI tract	Centrocytes with folded nuclear contour and mature chromatin Centroblasts with round nuclear membrane, vesicular chromatin, and small nucleoli	Neoplastic follicles with neither polarity nor tingible-body macrophages Pattern with follicular, diffuse and follicular, focally follicular, and diffuse Grade with centroblasts: 1–2: <15/HPF 3:>15/HPF 3A: scattered centroblasts; 3B: sheets of centroblasts	CD20+ CD10+ BCL2+ BCL6+ LMO2+	80% with t(14;18) 20% with +7, +18 15% with abnormal 3q27–28, 6q23–26, 17p
MCL	–3–10% of non-Hodgkin lymphomas -Adults of middle age to older -M:F – > 2:1 -Involving the LN, spleen, BM, and GI	Irregular nuclear contour and mature chromatin	Mantle zone expansion to diffuse pattern Vascular proliferation In situ mantle cell neoplasia: limited to mantle zone	CD20+ CD5+ BCL1 (cyclinD1)+ SOX11+	t(11;14) (*CCND1;IGH*) Rare with *cyclinD2* or *D3* translocation
MZL	-10% of B-cell lymphomas -Involving the GI, LN, spleen	Mature chromatin with monocytoid, plasmacytoid, or centrocytoid appearance	Expanded marginal zone	CD20+ CD5- CD10- CD23- IRTA1+	In GI MALT lymphoma: t(11;18) (*API2;MALT1*)

CLL/SLL chronic lymphocytic leukemia/small lymphocytic lymphoma, *M:F* male to female ratio, *PB* peripheral blood, *BM* bone marrow, *LN* lymph node, *CD* cluster of differentiation, *LEF1* lymphoid enhancer-binding factor 1, *ZAP-70* zeta-chain-associated protein kinase 70, *FL* follicular lymphoma, *GI* gastrointestinal, *HPF* high-power field, *BCL* B-cell lymphoma, *LMO2* LIM-only transcription factor-2, *MCL* mantle cell lymphoma, *SOX11* sex-determining region Y box 11, *CCND1* cyclin D1, *IGH* immunoglobulin heavy, *MZL* marginal zone lymphoma, *IRTA1* immunoglobulin superfamily receptor translocation associated 1, *MALT* mucosa-associated lymphoid tissue, *API2* apoptosis inhibitor 2, *MALT1* mucosa-associated lymphoid tissue lymphoma translocation 1

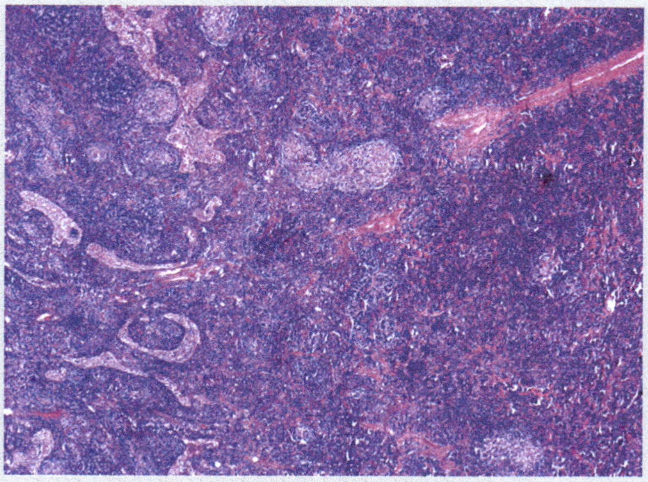

Fig. 4.90 Lymphoplasmacytic lymphoma with effaced nodal architecture and perifollicular expansion

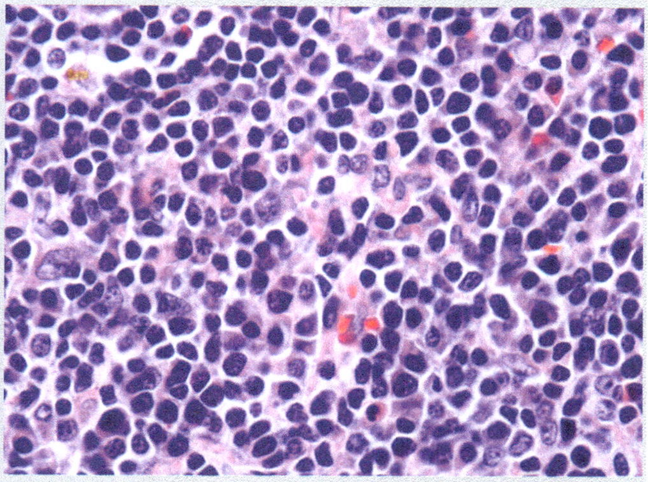

Fig. 4.91 Neoplastic cells in lymphoplasmacytic lymphoma show round nuclear contour and mature chromatin with plasmacytoid appearance

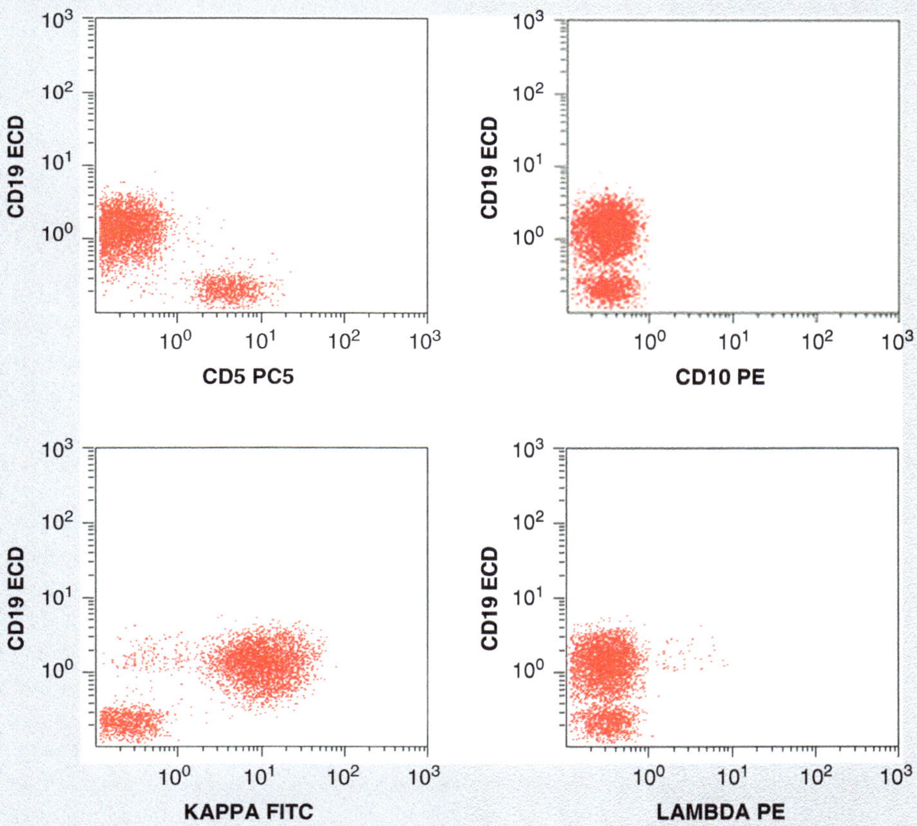

Fig. 4.92 (**a–d**) Flow cytometry studies of lymphoplasmacytic lymphoma show lymphoma cells negative for CD5 (**a**) and CD10 (**b**) with immunoglobulin light chain restriction (**c**, **d**)

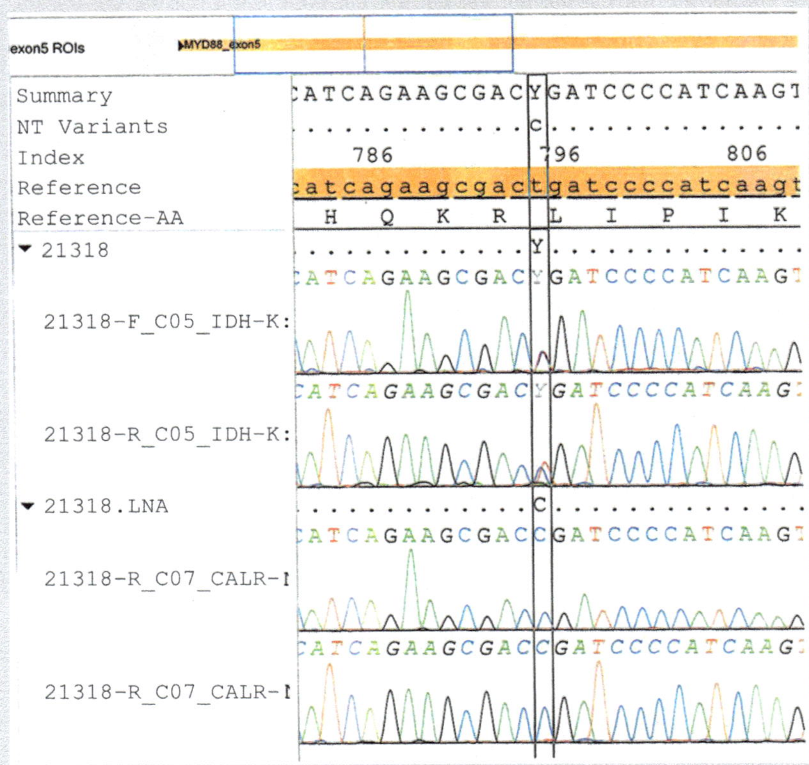

Fig. 4.93 Molecular study of lymphoplasmacytic lymphoma with *MYD88 L265P* mutation: a mutation in chromosome 3p22 in a single nucleotide change, T to C (*inside frame*), in MYD88, resulting a switch of leucine to proline at amino acid position 265 (L265P)

Flow cytometry studies showed a population of monotypic B cells with coexpression of CD10 and negative for the blast markers of CD34 and TdT and T-cell or myelomonocytic markers. Immunohistochemical stains revealed the neoplastic cells to be positive for CD20, BCL6, and MYC and negative for BCL2 with a proliferation rate of 100% by Ki67 stain (Fig. 4.37). EBV was negative by in situ hybridization. FISH study was positive for MYC (8q24.1) rearrangement (Fig. 4.61).

Final Diagnosis
Burkitt lymphoma (BL)

What Are the Learning Points from This Case?
The learning points from the case include:

1. High-grade hematolymphoid tumor can partially involve lymphoid tissue in the early stage.
2. Immunophenotypic features by flow cytometry and immunohistochemical studies are useful to classify the tumor.
3. FISH or molecular studies are the gold standard to further confirm the diagnosis.

Case Scenario 3

Learning Objectives

1. To review the T-cell leukemia/lymphomas
2. To pay attention to immunophenotypic features for classification and guided treatment

Case
A 60-year-old male presented with a rapidly progressive left axillary mass. He had night sweats and a 15-pound weight loss over the previous one to two months. His laboratory tests showed WBC of 7.3, hemoglobin of 11.9, and platelets of 248,000. CT scan revealed lymphadenopathy, including a left axillary lymph node of 3.0 x 3.4 cm with necrosis; periportal, retroperitoneal, bilateral iliac chain, and extensive mesenteric adenopathy, up to 2.4 cm; the enlarged spleen was 15 cm. There was no mediastinal or hilar mass. An excisional biopsy from left axillary lymph node was performed and showed an effaced nodal architecture in a diffuse pattern (Fig. 4.86). Neoplastic cells were medium in size with round nuclear contour, vesicular chromatin, and small nucleolus; there was a background of mature lymphocytes and eosinophils (Fig. 4.87).

(continued)

Table 4.5 Summary of most common high-grade hematolymphoid tumors

Diagnosis	Clinical features	Cytological features	Histological features	IHC features	Molecular features
DLBCL	-30% of adult non-Hodgkin lymphomas -More in elderly adult -Involving LN or extranodal areas -May occur de novo or transform from any low-grade B-cell lymphomas	Medium to large in size with pleomorphic nuclei and vesicular chromatin	Effaced nodal architecture with a diffuse pattern	CD20+ PAX5+ ABC-type: CD10-, BCL6-, MUM1+ GCB type: CD10+, BCL6+, MUM1-. BCL2, BCL6, and MYC to evaluate aggressive behavior	FISH for BCL2, BCL6, MYC for double-hit or triple-hit lymphoma that has worse prognosis and needs more intensive treatment
BL	Three clinical variants -Endemic: mostly in Africa, in children, peak at 4–7 years, M:F – 2:1 -Sporadic: mainly in children and young adults, 30%–50% of all childhood lymphoma, M:F – 2–3:1 -Immunodeficiency-associated: occurs in HIV infection, transplant, or other immunodeficient patients	Medium in size with round nuclear contour, vesicular chromatin, and small nucleoli (snake head appearance)	Sheets of tumor cells with scattered tingible-body macrophages (starry sky pattern)	CD20+ CD10+ BCL6+ BCL2- MYC+ EBV may+, mostly in endemic BL	*MYC* gene rearrangement TCF3 mutation in up to 70% of cases
ALL	-Mostly in children -B-ALL: 80–85% of all lymphoblastic leukemia -T-ALL: 85–90% of all lymphoblastic lymphoma	Medium in size with round nuclear contour and blast-looking chromatin Same in both B- or T-ALL	Same as BL	B-ALL: CD19+, CD10+ CD22+ CD79a+ T-ALL: CD1a+ CD2+ cCD3+ CD4 or/and CD8+ CD5+ CD7+ ALL: CD34+, TdT+	B-ALL: clonal *IGH* gene rearrangement t(9;22) (*BCR-ABL*) with worse prognosis: p190kd-in childhood ALL; p210kd in adult T-ALL: clonal *TCR* gene rearrangement
ALCL	-3% of adult non-Hodgkin lymphomas and 10–20% of childhood lymphomas -M:F – 1.5:1 -Involving the LN, skin, bone, soft tissue, lung, and liver	Neoplastic cells are pleomorphic. Hallmark cells with horseshoe-like or kidney-like nucleus and eosinophilic cytoplasm	-Lymphohistiocytic pattern: hallmark cells and reactive histiocytes -Small cell pattern: small to medium-size neoplastic cells admixed with hallmark cells; -Hodgkin-like pattern: mimic CHL	CD30+ ALK+/- CD2+ CD5+ CD4+ CD3+ in 25% of cases TIA+ Granzyme+ EBV-	T(2;5) (*ALK;NPM*) or *ALK* translocation to other chromosomes 1, 2, 3, 17, 19, 2, and X

(continued)

Table 4.5 (continued)

Diagnosis	Clinical features	Cytological features	Histological features	IHC features	Molecular features
Myeloid sarcoma	-mostly in adults -M:F – 1.2:1 -involving any site -may occur de novo, or proceed or coincide with AML or transformation of MDS and/or MPN	Myeloblasts with fine chromatin and high N/C ratio. Rare case with erythroid precursors or megakaryoblasts	Sheets of blasts with frequent mitotic figures	MPO+ CD117+ Lysozyme+ CD68/KP1+ CD34+ TdT may +	55% of cases: +7, +8, *MLL*-rearrangement, inv.(16), +4, −16, 16q-, 5q-, 20q-, +1p

DLBCL diffuse large B-cell lymphoma, *CD* cluster of differentiation, *PAX5* paired box gene 5, *ABC* activated B-cell, *BCL* B-cell lymphoma, *MUM1* multiple myeloma 1, *GC* germinal center, *FISH* fluorescence in situ hybridization, *BL* Burkitt lymphoma, *M:F* male to female ratio, *EBV* Epstein-Barr virus, *ALL* acute lymphoblastic leukemia, *B-ALL* B-cell acute lymphoblastic leukemia, *IGH* immunoglobulin heavy chain, *T-ALL* T-cell acute lymphoblastic leukemia, *TdT* terminal deoxynucleotidyl transferase, *BCR* breakpoint cluster region, *ABL* Abelson murine leukemia viral oncogene homolog 1, *TCR* T-cell receptor, *ALCL* anaplastic large cell lymphoma, *LN* lymph node, *CHL* classical Hodgkin lymphoma, *ALK* anaplastic lymphoma kinase, *TIA* T-cell intracellular antibody, *NPM* nucleophosmin, *AML* acute myeloid leukemia, *MDS* myelodysplastic syndrome, *MPN* myeloproliferative neoplasm, *N/C* nuclear to cytoplasmic, *MPO* myeloperoxidase, *TdT* terminal deoxynucleotidyl transferase, *MLL* mixed-lineage leukemia, *TCF3* transcription factor 3

At this point, a diagnosis of high-grade hematolymphoid tumor can be made. Differential diagnosis includes lymphoblastic lymphoma, myeloid sarcoma, or acute hematolymphoid tumor with bi-phenotypic features. A definite diagnosis cannot be rendered without immunophenotypic study.

Flow cytometry studies showed a population of blasts positive for cytoplasmic CD3 (cCD3) and CD34 and low intensity of CD5 and negative for surface CD3, CD8, and MPO (a few of blasts expressing MPO in low intensity) with aberrant expression of CD33 (Fig. 4.88). Immunohistochemical studies revealed neoplastic cells positive for cCD3 and negative for CD1a (Fig. 4.89a, b). Molecular test showed clonal TCR gene rearrangement.

Final Diagnosis

Early T-cell precursor lymphoma

What Are the Learning Points from This Case?

The learning points from the case include:

1. Lymphoblastic leukemia/lymphoma shares the same morphological features in B-cell acute lymphoblastic leukemia (B-ALL) and T-cell acute lymphoblastic leukemia (T-ALL).
2. Immunophenotype by flow cytometry and immunohistochemical studies are helpful to make a right diagnosis.
3. The aberrant immunophenotypes that would indicate the prognosis and guide the treatment should be carefully evaluated and mentioned.

Abbreviations List

Abbreviation	Full text
ABC	Activated B-cell
ABL	Abelson murine leukemia viral oncogene homolog 1
ALCL	Anaplastic large cell lymphoma
ALK	Anaplastic lymphoma kinase
ALL	Acute lymphoblastic leukemia
AML	Acute myeloid leukemia
B-ALL	B-cell acute lymphoblastic leukemia
BCL	B-cell lymphoma (BCL1, BCL2, BCL6)
BCR	Breakpoint cluster region
BL	Burkitt lymphoma
BM	Bone marrow

Abbreviation	Full text
BOB1	B-cell Oct binding protein 1
BRAF	v-raf murine sarcoma viral oncogene homolog B1
CARD11	Caspase recruitment domain-containing protein 11
cCD3	Cytoplasmic CD3
CCND1	Cyclin D1
CCR5	Chemokine receptor type 5
CD	Cluster of differentiation
CHL	Classical Hodgkin lymphoma
CLL	Chronic lymphocytic leukemia
CNS	Central nervous system
CT	Computed tomography
CXCL13	Chemokine (C-X-C motif) ligand 13
DLBCL	Diffuse large B-cell lymphoma
EBV	Epstein-Barr virus
EMA	Epithelial membrane antigen
ETP	Early T precursor
ETV6	ETS variant 6
EZH2	Enhancer of zeste homolog 2
FISH	Fluorescence in situ hybridization
FL	Follicular lymphoma
FMC7	A monoclonal antibody and an epitope of CD20
FNA	Fine needle aspiration
GC	Germinal center
GI	Gastrointestinal
GNA13	Guanine nucleotide-binding protein subunit alpha-13
HGBCL	High-grade B-cell lymphoma
HHV8	Human herpes virus 8
HPF	High-power field
iAMP2	Intrachromosomal amplification of chromosome 21
ICOS	Inducible T-Cell co-stimulator
IgG/A	Immunoglobulin G/A
IGH	Immunoglobulin heavy chain
IGHV	Immunoglobulin heavy-chain variable
IgM	Immunoglobulin M
IHC	Immunohistochemistry
IL3	Interleukin 3
IRF4	Interferon regulatory factor 4
IRTA1	Immunoglobulin superfamily receptor translocation associated 1
JAK/STAT3	Janus kinase/signal transducer and activator of transcription
KMT2A	Lysine methyltransferase 2A
KOC1	K homology domain-containing protein overexpressed in cancer
L256P	Leucine to proline mutation at amino acid position 256
LBCL	Large B-cell lymphoma
LCH	Langerhans cell histiocytosis
LEF1	Lymphoid enhancer-binding factor 1
LMO2	LIM-only transcription factor-2

Abbreviation	Full text
LN	Lymph node
LPL	Lymphoplasmacytic lymphoma
MALT	Mucosa-associated lymphoid tissue
MCL	Mantle cell lymphoma
MDS	Myelodysplastic syndrome
MGUS	Monoclonal gammopathy of undetermined significance
MIB-1	Mindbomb homolog 1
MLL	Mixed-lineage leukemia
MPN	Myeloproliferative neoplasm
MPO	Myeloperoxidase
MUM1	Multiple myeloma 1
MYC/c-MYC	A regulator gene that codes for a transcription factor
MYD88	Myeloid differentiation primary response gene 88
MZL	Marginal zone lymphoma
N/C	Nuclear to cytoplasmic
NK	Natural killer
NOS	Not otherwise specified
NPM	Nucleophosmin
Oct2	Octamer-binding transcription factors
Pap	Papanicolaou
PAX	Paired box gene
PB	Peripheral blood
PBX1	Pre-B-cell leukemia homeobox 1
PD1	Programmed death 1
PNET	Primitive neuroectodermal tumor
PTCL	Peripheral T-cell lymphoma
PTLD	Posttransplant lymphoproliferative disorders
RUNX1	Rnt-related transcription factor 1
SAP	Serum amyloid P
sCD3	Surface CD3
SLL	Small lymphocytic lymphoma
SOX	Sex-determining region Y box
STAT3	Signal transducer and activator of transcription 3
T-ALL	T-cell acute lymphoblastic leukemia
TCF3	Transcription factor 3
TCR	T-cell receptor
TdT	Terminal deoxynucleotidyl transferase
TFH	T follicular helper
TIA	T-cell intracellular antibody
TNFAIP3	Tumor necrosis factor, alpha-induced protein 3
US, USA	United States (not spelled out in chapter)
WHO	World Health Organization
ZAP-70	Zeta-chain-associated protein kinase 70

References

Alikhan M, Song JY, Sohani AR, Moroch J, Plonquet A, Duffield AS, et al. Peripheral T-cell lymphomas of follicular helper T-cell type frequently display an aberrant CD3−/dimCD4+ population by flow cytometry: an important clue to the diagnosis of a Hodgkin lymphoma mimic. Mod Pathol. 2016;29:1173–82.

Arber DA, Orazi A, Hasserjian R, Thiele J, Borowitz MJ, Le Beau MM, et al. The 2016 revision to the World Health Organization classification of myeloid neoplasms and acute leukemia. Blood. 2016;127(20):2391–405.

Arcaini L, Rossi D, Paulli M. Splenic marginal zone lymphoma: from genetics to management. Blood. 2016;127(17):2072–81.

Berndt SI, Skibola CF, Joseph V, Camp NJ, Nieters A, Wang Z, et al. Genome-wide association study identifies multiple risk loci for chronic lymphocytic leukemia. Nat Genet. 2013;45(8):868–76.

Bigras G, Dong WF, Canil S, Lai R, Morel D, Swanson PE, et al. New MYC IHC classifier integrating quantitative architecture parameters to predict MYC gene translocation in diffuse large B-cell lymphoma. Appl Immunohistochem Mol Morphol. 2016.; Epub 2016 May 20.

Bob R, Falini B, Marafioti T, Paterson JC, Pileri S, Stein H. Nodal reactive and neoplastic proliferation of monocytoid and marginal zone B cells: an immunoarchitectural and molecular study highlighting the relevance of IRTA1 and T-bet as positive markers. Histopathology. 2013;63(4):482–98.

Bogusz AM, Bagg A. Genetic aberrations in small B-cell lymphomas and leukemias: molecular pathology, clinical relevance and therapeutic targets. Leuk Lymphoma. 2016;27:1–23.

Burotto M, Berkovits A, Dunleavy K. Double hit lymphoma: from biology to therapeutic implications. Expert Rev Hematol. 2016:1–10.

de Jonge AV, Roosma TJ, Houtenbos I, Vasmel WL, van de Hem K, de Boer JP, et al. Diffuse large B-cell lymphoma with MYC gene rearrangements: current perspective on treatment of diffuse large B-cell lymphoma with MYC gene rearrangements; case series and review of the literature. Eur J Cancer. 2016;55:140–6.

DeMay RM. Lymph node. In:The art and science of cytopathology. 2nd ed. Chicago: ASCP Press; 2010. p. 966–1028.

Dunleavy K. Aggressive B cell lymphoma: optimal therapy for MYC-positive, double-hit, and triple-hit DLBCL. Curr Treat Options in Oncol. 2015;16(12):58.

Dyhdalo KS, Lanigan C, Tubbs RR, Cook JR. Immunoarchitectural patterns of germinal center antigens including LMO2 assist in the differential diagnosis of marginal zone lymphoma vs follicular lymphoma. Am J Clin Pathol. 2013;140(2):149–54.

Falini B, Agostinelli C, Bigerna B, Pucciarini A, Pacini R, Tabarrini A, et al. IRTA1 is selectively expressed in nodal and extranodal marginal zone lymphomas. Histopathology. 2012;61(5):930–41.

Freedman A. Follicular lymphoma: 2015 update on diagnosis and management. Am J Hematol. 2015;90(12):1171–8.

Ioachim HL, Medeiros LJ, editors. Ioachim's lymph node pathology. 4th ed. Philadelphia: Lippincott William & Wilkins; 2009. p. 1–291.

Jain N, Lamb AV, O'Brien S, Ravandi F, Konopleva M, Jabbour E, et al. Early T-cell precursor acute lymphoblastic leukemia/lymphoma (ETP-ALL/LBL) in adolescents and adults: a high-risk subtype. Blood. 2016;127(15):1863–9.

Karnik T, Ozawa MG, Lefterova M, Luna-Fineman S, Alvarez E, Link M, et al. The utility of IgM, CD21, HGAL and LMO2 in the diagnosis of pediatric follicular lymphoma. Hum Pathol. 2015;46(4):629–33.

Menter T, Dirnhofer S, Tzankov A. LEF1: a highly specific marker for the diagnosis of chronic lymphocytic B cell leukaemia/small lymphocytic B cell lymphoma. J Clin Pathol. 2015a Jun;68(6):473–8.

Menter T, Gasser A, Juskevicius D, Dirnhofer S, Tzankov A. Diagnostic utility of the germinal center-associated markers GCET1, HGAL, and LMO2 in hematolymphoid neoplasms. Appl Immunohistochem Mol Morphol. 2015b;23(7):491–8.

Nakashima MO, Durkin L, Bodo J, Lin J, Quintanilla-Martinez L, Fu K, et al. Utility and diagnostic pitfalls of SOX11 monoclonal antibodies in mantle cell lymphoma and other lymphoproliferative disorders. Appl Immunohistochem Mol Morphol. 2014;22(10):720–7.

Swerdlow SH. Diagnosis of 'double hit' diffuse large B-cell lymphoma and B-cell lymphoma, unclassifiable, with features intermediate between DLBCL and Burkitt lymphoma: when and how, FISH versus IHC. Hematology Am Soc Hematol Educ Program. 2014;2014(1):90–9.

Swerdlow SH, Campo E, Pileri SA, Harris NL, Stein H, Siebert R, et al. The 2016 revision of the World Health Organization classification of lymphoid neoplasms. Blood. 2016a;127(20):2375–90.

Swerdlow SH, Campo E, Pileri SA, Harris NL, Stein H, Siebert R, et al. WHO classification of tumours of hematopoietic and lymphoid tissues. 4th ed. Lyon: IARC; in press; expected Spring 2017.

Swerdlow SH, Kuzu I, Dogan A, Dirnhofer S, Chan JK, Sander B, et al. The many faces of small B cell lymphomas with plasmacytic differentiation and the contribution of MYD88 testing. Virchows Arch. 2016b;468(3):259–75.

Tandon B, Peterson L, Gao J, Nelson B, Ma S, Rosen S, et al. Nuclear overexpression of lymphoid-enhancer-binding factor 1 identifies chronic lymphocytic leukemia/small lymphocytic lymphoma in small B-cell lymphomas. Mod Pathol. 2011;24(11):1433–43.

Vose JM. Mantle cell lymphoma: 2015 update on diagnosis, risk-stratification, and clinical management. Am J Hematol. 2015;90(8):739–45.

Zhang YH, Liu J, Dawlett M, Guo M, Sun X, Gong Y. The role of SOX11 immunostaining in confirming the diagnosis of mantle cell lymphoma on fine-needle aspiration samples. Cancer Cytopathol. 2014;122(12):892–7.

Zucca E, Bertoni F. The spectrum of MALT lymphoma at different sites: biological and therapeutic relevance. Blood. 2016;127(17):2082–92.

5 Breast

Haiyan Liu, Fan Lin, and Jun Zhang

Summary of Pearls and Pitfalls

- Fine needle aspiration (FNA) cytology and core needle biopsy (CNB) of breast lesions are the key components of the triple test for detecting breast malignancies.
- The advantages of FNA cytology are its rapid, cost-effective and, in experienced hands, highly sensitive and specific as well.
- The major limitations of FNA of breast lesions are the need for expertise in cytology for the interpretation of FNA material, inability to differentiate atypical ductal hyperplasia (ADH) from ductal carcinoma in situ (DCIS), limited ability to diagnose invasion, and often inadequate sample (and/or inadequate preparation of the material) for hormonal analyses in cases of carcinomas.
- For nonpalpable breast lesions, CNB has become the standard procedure for pathologic diagnosis.
- For palpable lesions, FNA is still utilized but has rapidly declined in popularity in recent years.
- At the current time, the common indications for FNA of breast lesions are as follows: (a) an expected benign cyst by ultrasound; (b) a sonographic lesion in a pregnant or postpartum patient or a patient with contraindications for CNB; (c) a sonographic lesion in a location unsuitable for CNB, such as behind the nipple or close to the chest wall; (d) to confirm an inoperable and locally advanced malignancy; (e) a suspected recurrence or metastasis; and (f) preoperative staging of axillary lymph nodes.
- Complications are rare, with the most common being bleeding.

Normal Cytology of Breast

- The female mammary gland is composed of 15–20 (or 25) lobes or segments that converge on the nipple in a radial pattern.
- Each lobe consists of a lactiferous duct, lactiferous sinus, segmental collecting duct, subsegmental duct, ductule (terminal duct), and acini (terminal ductules).
- The terminal duct lobular units (TDLUs) are comprised of ductile and acini, as shown in Fig. 5.1a, b, which is the most hormone-sensitive, therefore, the major site of origin of breast pathology.
- The smears of benign non-neoplastic glandular tissue are usually low cellularity, arranged in tight small, large or branching clusters, as well as monolayer sheets.
- The cells are cohesive; uniform; with small, round-to-oval, hyperchromatic nuclei; inconspicuous or very small nucleoli, and scant cytoplasm without distinct cell borders.
- The nuclei are irregularly distributed within the clusters to impart a crowded, overlapping appearance, as shown in Fig. 5.2a.
- Myoepithelial cells or stromal cells are appreciated at the periphery or admixed within the clusters.
- Naked bipolar nuclei (myoepithelial cells) may be seen in the background.
- Figure 5.2b illustrates a sample of benign glandular epithelial cells in a monolayer sheet.

Nipple Discharge Cytology

A spontaneous nipple discharge in a non-lactating or pregnant woman is abnormal and may suggest an underlying breast lesion (such as papilloma/papillomatosis or carcinoma) or

© Springer International Publishing AG 2018
F. Lin et al., *Handbook of Practical Fine Needle Aspiration and Small Tissue Biopsies*, DOI 10.1007/978-3-319-57386-1_5

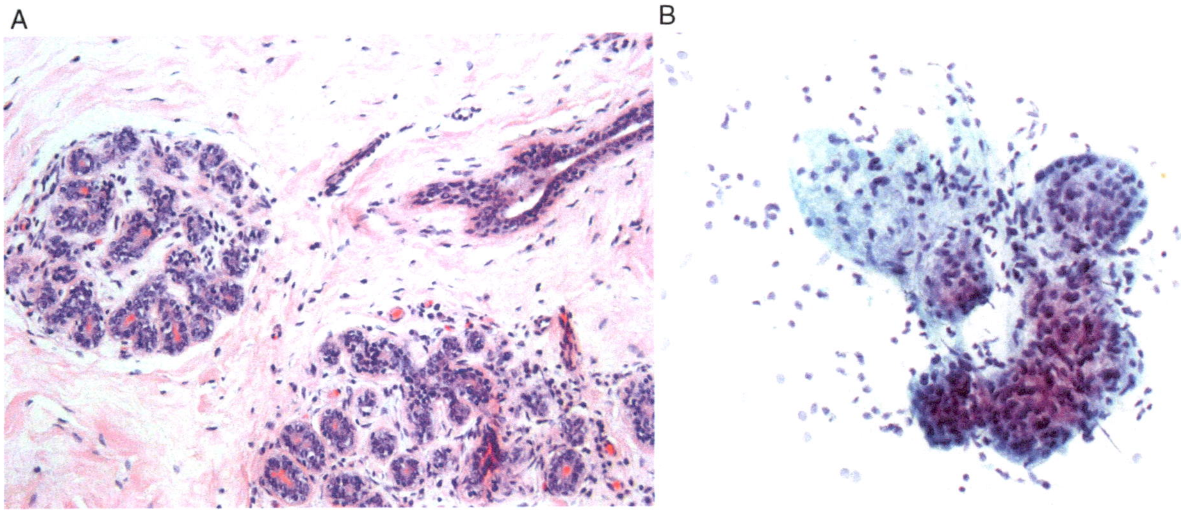

Fig. 5.1 (**a**, **b**) Normal terminal duct lobular unit (TDLU). (**a**) Histology, H&E; (**b**) cytology, Pap stain

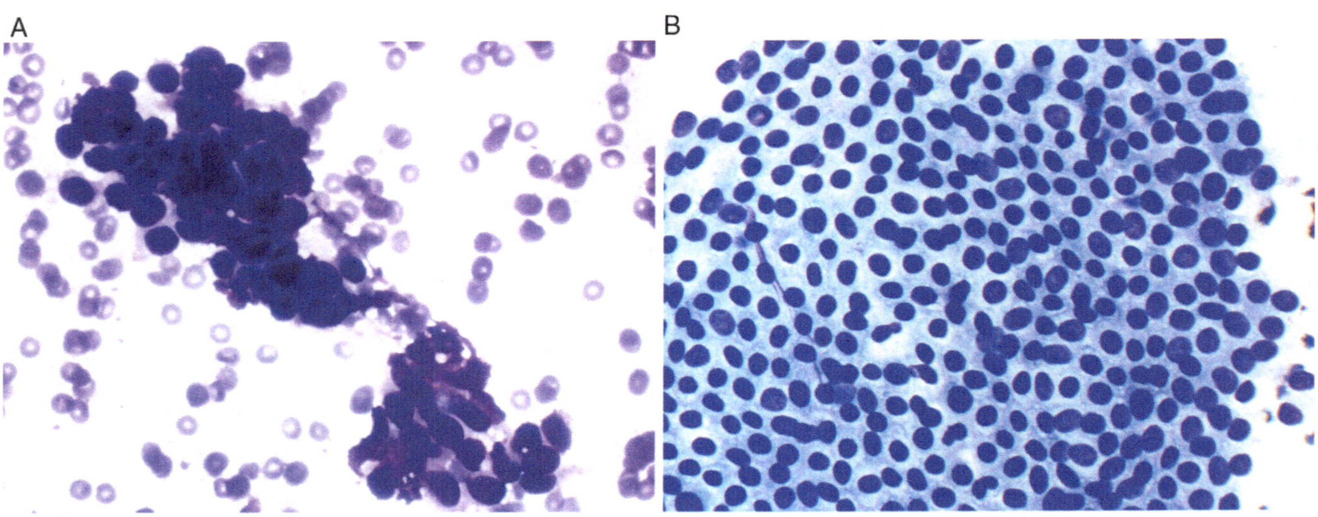

Fig. 5.2 (**a**, **b**) Benign ductal and lobular epithelial cells. (**a**) Benign ductal cells in crowded cluster, Diff-Quik; (**b**) benign ductal cells in monolayer sheet, Pap stain

hormonal abnormalities. However, nipple discharge cytology has a low sensitivity for detecting an underlying malignancy. Cases with unilateral, serous, bloody nipple discharge from a single duct are pathological and frequently associated with papillary lesions. In addition, the probability of detecting an underlying malignancy is increased in those specimens.

Cytological Features

Benign Nipple Discharge

- Usually sparsely cellular.
- Scattered foamy histiocytes.
- Rare benign ductal cells in small clusters.
- Inflammatory cells may be present.
- Proteinaceous debris in background.
- Figure 5.3a, b.

Atypical or Malignant Nipple Discharge

- Significant increase of cellularity.
- Clusters or isolated ductal cells with enlarged and pleomorphic nuclei displaying nucleoli.
- Stripped nuclei.
- Papillary groups may be seen.
- Necrosis may present.

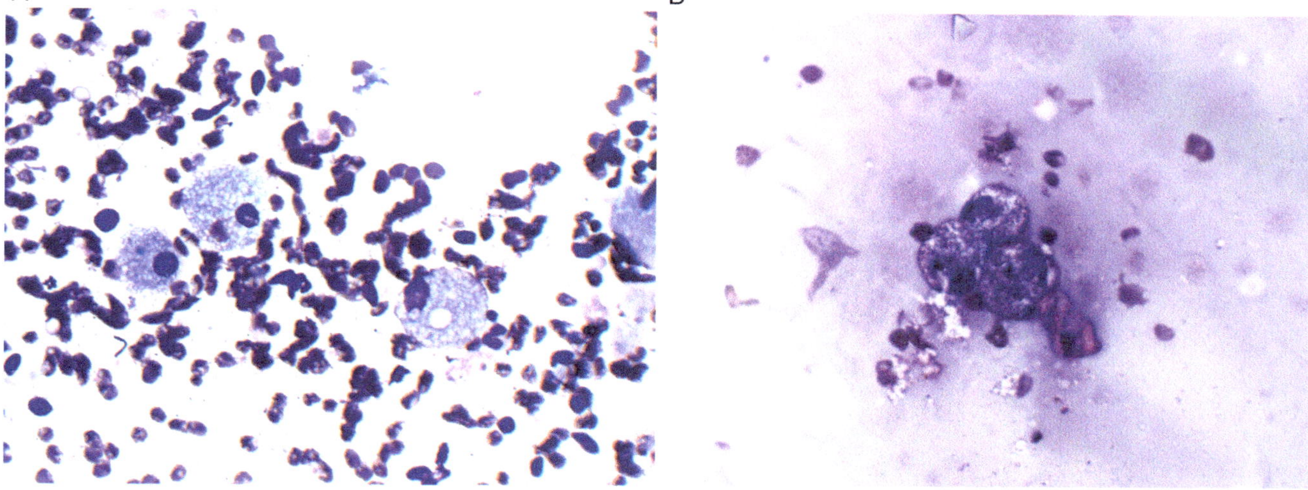

Fig. 5.3 (**a**, **b**) Contents of benign nipple discharge. Sparsely cellular smear contains few foam histiocytes and proteinaceous debris. (**a**) histiocytes, Diff-Quik; (**b**) degenerated histiocytes and rare crystals in a background of proteinaceous debris, Diff-Quik

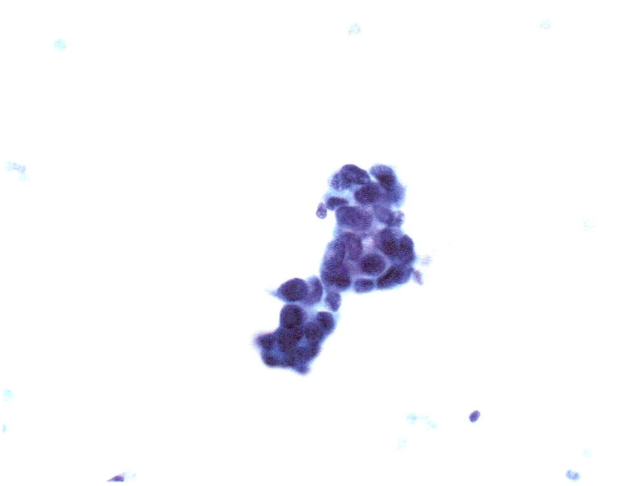

Fig. 5.4 Contents of atypical nipple discharge, showing a tight cluster of atypical ductal epithelial cells with enlarged nuclei, hyperchromatic chromatin, and moderate nuclear pleomorphism, Pap stain

- Acute inflammation and bloody background.
- Figure 5.4.

Fat Necrosis

Key Clinical Features

- The result of various injuries, such as trauma, previous procedure, chemoradiation therapy, and rupture of cyst
- Mimics breast carcinoma clinically, such as a firm mass, skin retraction, or thickening

Key Radiological Features

- Variable, may mimic breast carcinomas radiographically

Cytological Features

- Degenerated adipose tissue, giant cells, and foamy histiocytes
- Dirty background with amorphous or granular debris, fat droplets, and normal or degenerating adipose tissue
- Reactive stromal cells and occasional inflammatory cells
- Paucity of epithelial cells
- Figure 5.5a, b

Differential Diagnosis

- Infectious panniculitis
- Invasive lobular carcinoma

Histology

- Usually a well-demarcated area of vacuolated fat admixed with infiltrates of foamy histiocytes, multinucleated giant cells, lymphocytes, and plasma cells.
- Hemosiderin-laden macrophages and occasional cholesterol clefts are present.
- Granulation tissue with fibrosis and reactive ductal epithelial cells are occasionally identified.
- Representative image is illustrated in Fig. 5.5c, d.

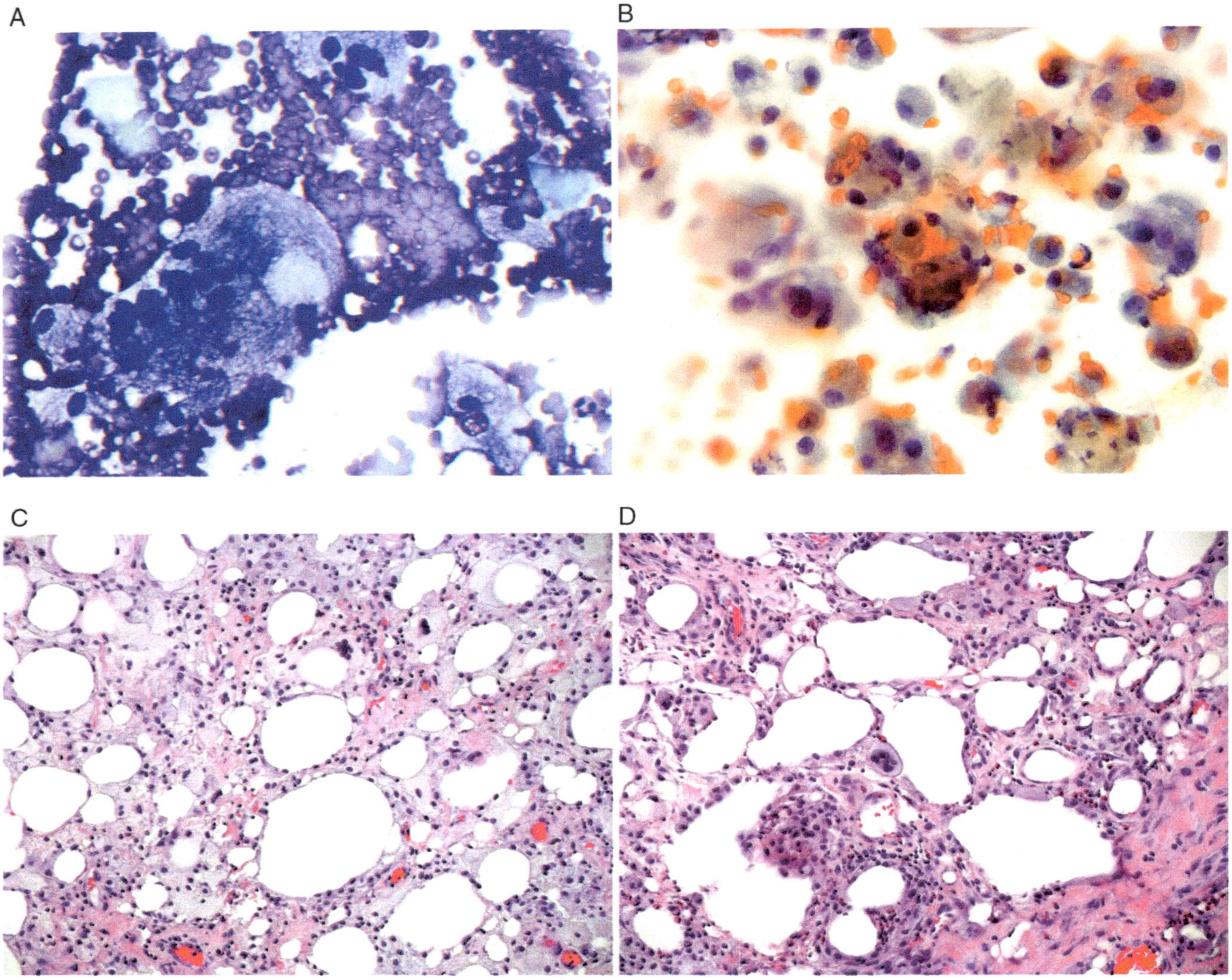

Fig. 5.5 (**a–d**) Fat necrosis. (**a**, **b**) Cytology, showing foamy histiocytes including multinucleated forms and debris (**a**, Diff-Quik; **b**, Papanicolaou [Pap] stain); (**c**, **d**) histology, abundant foam histiocytes including multinucleated forms, fat and fibrous tissue, hematoxylin, and eosin (H&E)

Immunohistochemistry

- Fat necrosis is mainly a histological diagnosis.
- Immunohistochemistry (IHC) is rarely applied on post-procedural specimens from breast carcinoma patients when the histiocytes show significant atypia; cluster of differentiation 68 (CD68) decorates histiocytes, while cytokeratin (CK) AE1/3 is nonreactive.

Subareolar Abscess

Key Clinical Features

- Also called "recurrent subareolar abscess"
- In the subareolar region, starts as a localized inflammation to form abscess, with subsequent healing and squamous metaplasia of the lactiferous ducts, then keratin plugging, dilatation and rupture of the ducts, as well as sinus tract formation

Cytological Features

- Abundant anucleated squames and neutrophils (Fig. 5.6a–d).
- Keratin debris, cholesterol crystals, and strips of squamous epithelial cells may be present.
- Rare ductal cells.
- Reactive stromal cells and giant cells.

Differential Diagnosis

- Epidermal inclusion cyst: peripheral and periareolar location

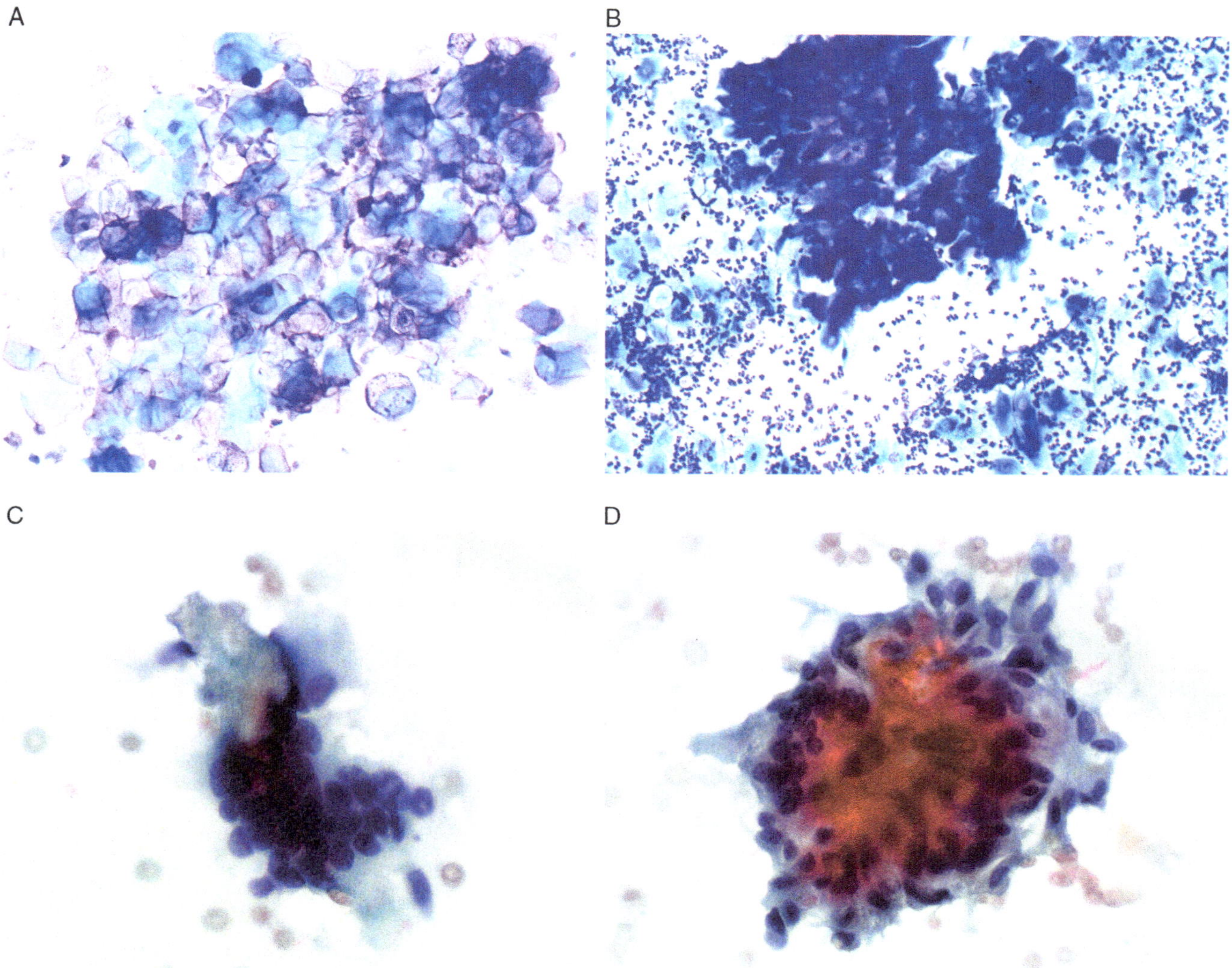

Fig. 5.6 (**a–d**) Subareolar abscess, cytology. There are abundant anucleated squamous epithelial cells, neutrophils, and dirty debris (**a**, **b**, Diff-Quik). Occasional multinucleated giant cells with adjacent keratin debris are seen (**c**, Pap stain), may form granulomatous aggregate (**d**, Pap stain)

Histology

- Breast tissue is displaced by chronic active inflammation with numerous neutrophils and a scant mixture of plasma cells and histiocytes.
- In recurrent cases, dilated duct with inflamed wall, granulation tissue, and intraluminal debris is present; may form a fistula.
- Representative images are shown in Fig. 5.7a, b.

Immunohistochemistry

- Immunohistochemistry is usually not applied for the diagnosis of subareolar abscess.

Fibrocystic Change

Fibrocystic change is the most common breast disorder, characterized by any combination of small/large cysts, apocrine metaplasia, fibrosis, adenosis, and duct hyperplasia.

Key Clinical Features

- Usually palpable nodularity in women of 20–50 years of age.
- The nodules are not well-defined, usually tender or even painful, changing with menstrual cycle.
- Generally multifocal, may be bilateral.

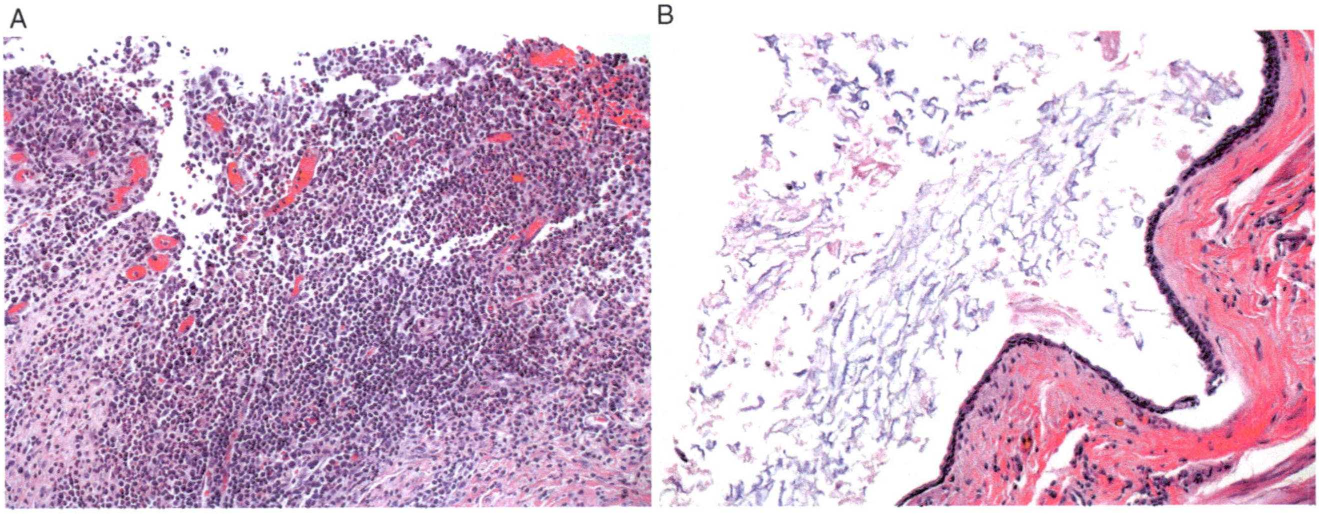

Fig. 5.7 (**a**, **b**) Subareolar abscess, histology. (**a**) Breast tissue with chronic active inflammation with numerous neutrophils and a scant mixture of plasma cells and histiocytes, H&E; (**b**) dilated duct with inflamed wall, granulation tissue, and intraluminal debris, including abundant anucleated squamous epithelial cells, H&E

- May be more localized to produce a palpable mass: the most common mass-producing lesion in women older than 30 years.
- May come to attention due to calcifications on mammogram.

Radiological Features

- Nodular densities or solitary, round or ovoid, and/or well-circumscribed masses of low-to-intermediate density on mammogram; may have microcalcifications.
- Simple cysts show lack of internal echoes and increased echogenicity of the posterior tissue on ultrasound.

Cytological Features

Nonproliferative Fibrocystic Changes

- Low-to-moderate cellularity
- A mixture of cellular components: cohesive groups or sheets of bland ductal cells, myoepithelial cells, apocrine cells, and histiocytes
- Scattered naked bipolar nuclei, fat, stromal tissue, and proteinaceous fluid in the background
- Figure 5.8a–d

Proliferative Fibrocystic Change

Ductal Proliferative Lesion Without Atypia

- Sheets and tight clusters of cells without significant nuclear overlap
- Finely granular chromatin pattern
- Inconspicuous to small nucleoli

Ductal Proliferative Lesion with Atypia

- Sheets and tight clusters of cells with significant nuclear overlap, loss of polarity, punched-out spaces, and mitosis
- Finely to coarsely granular chromatin
- Prominent to multiple nucleoli
- Figure 5.9a, b

Differential Diagnosis

Ductal Proliferative Lesion Without Atypia

- Intraductal papilloma
- Fibroadenoma

Ductal Proliferative Lesion with Atypia

- ADH and/or DCIS
- Ductal carcinoma

Histology

- Fibrocystic change refers to a complex of lesions, including dilated ducts/cysts, stromal fibrosis, apocrine metaplasia, blunt duct adenosis, mild sclerosing adenosis, and usual ductal hyperplasia (UDH).
- Atypical ductal proliferative lesions show ADH or DCIS.

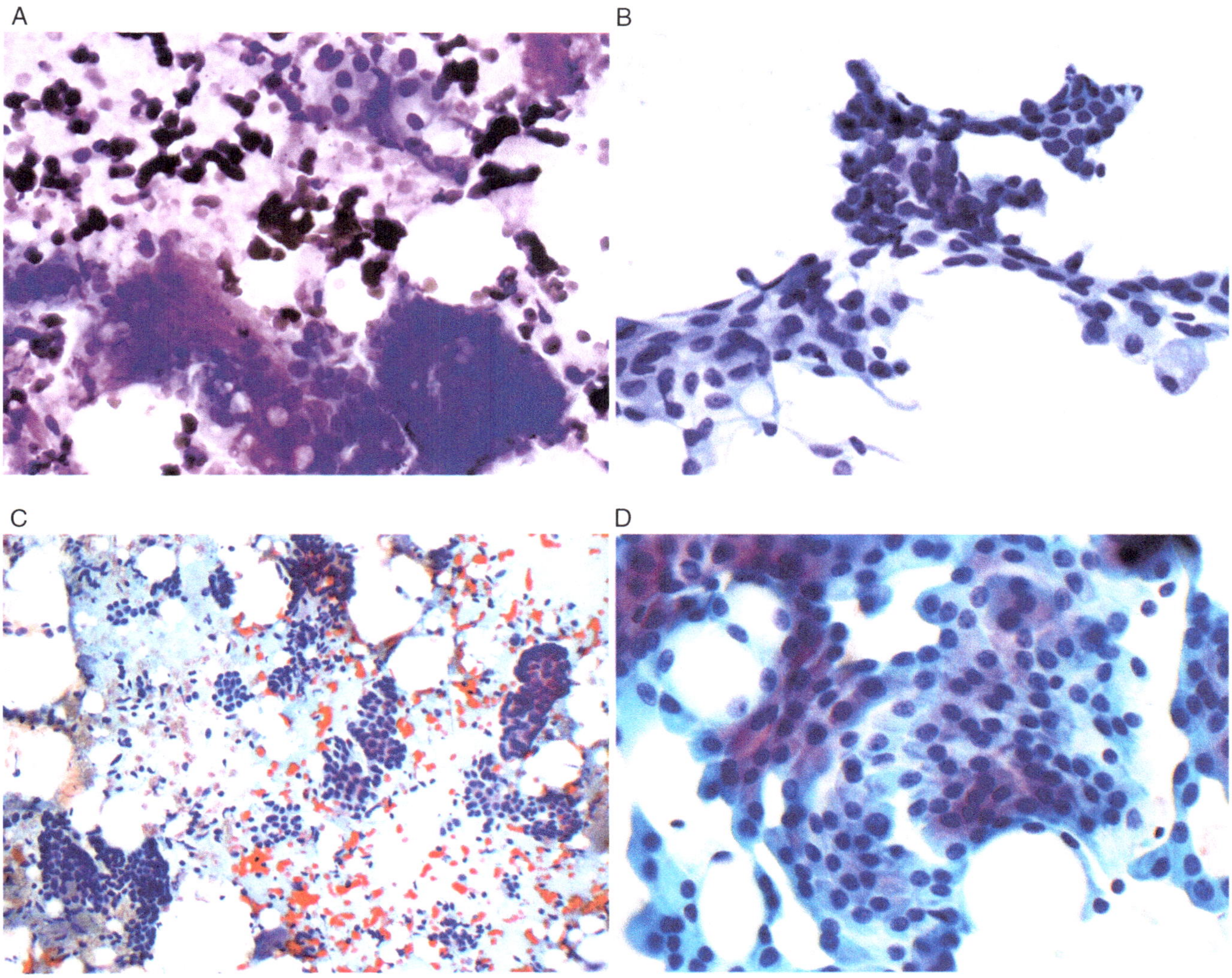

Fig. 5.8 (**a**–**d**) Nonproliferative fibrocystic changes. (**a**) Benign ductal cells in cohesive cluster with appreciable myoepithelial cells and stromal fragment, Diff-Quik; (**b**) myoepithelial cells are easily identified, in addition, few macrophages are seen, Pap stain; (**c**) Cohesive groups and sheet of benign ductal epithelial cells in a background of many bipolar naked stromal nuclei, Pap stain; (**d**) cluster of bland-looking ductal epithelial cells admixed with adipocytes and myoepithelial cells, Pap stain

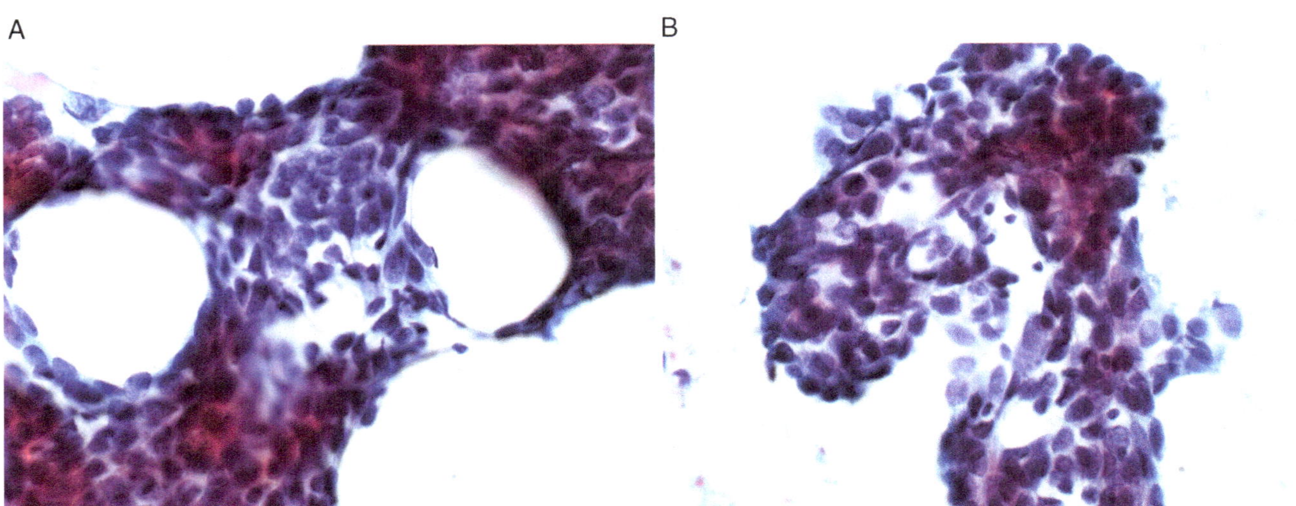

Fig. 5.9 (**a**, **b**) Ductal proliferative lesion with atypia. (**a**) Cluster of atypical ductal epithelial cells with monotonous enlarged nuclei, coarsely granular chromatin pattern, nucleoli, and punched-out spaces, suggesting ductal carcinoma in situ. Myoepithelial cells are identified at the periphery, Pap stain; (**b**) group of atypical ductal cells with appreciable punched-out spaces, myoepithelial cells identified focally, Pap stain

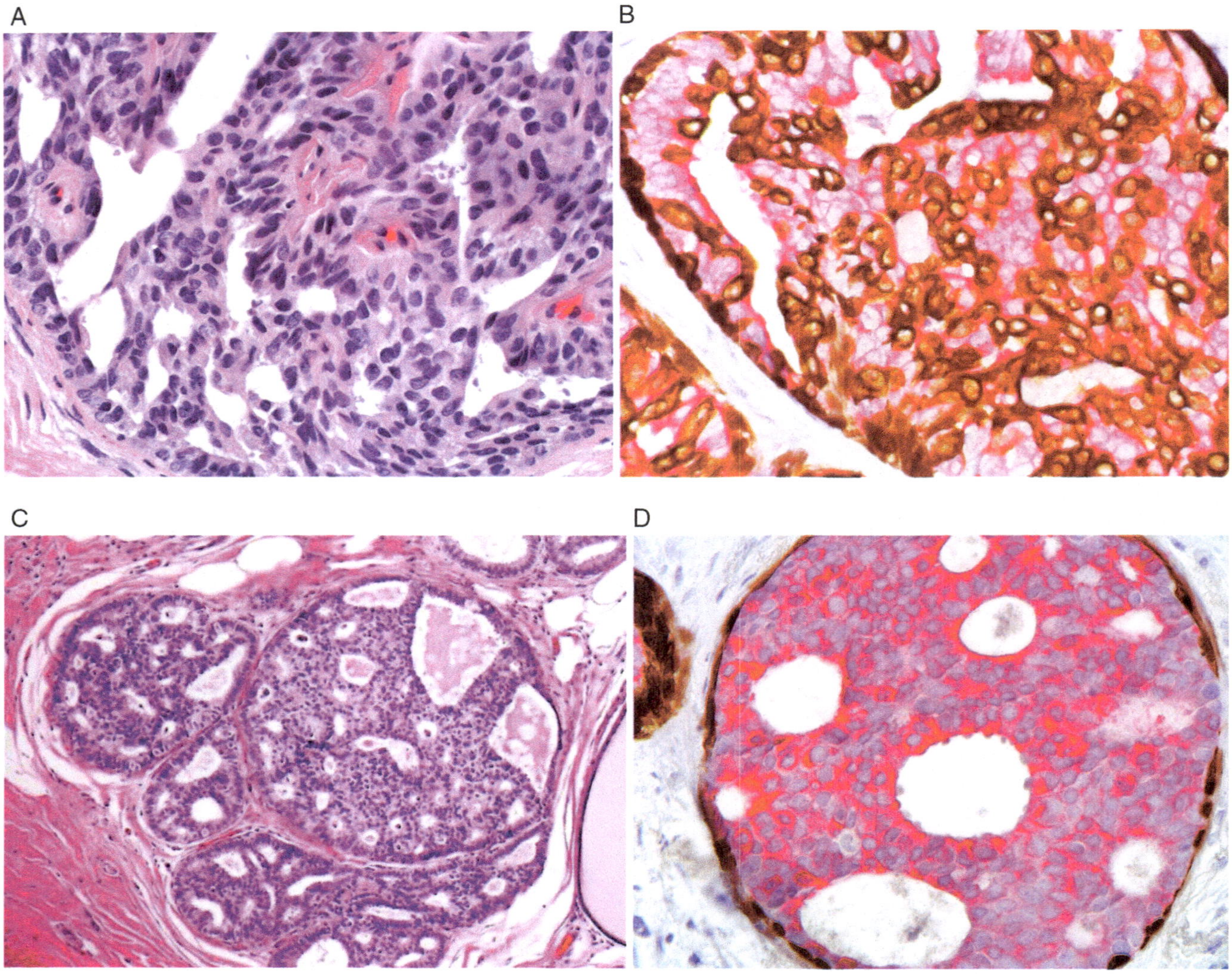

Fig. 5.10 (**a**–**d**) Differential immunophenotype of atypical ductal hyperplasia (ADH)/ductal carcinoma in situ (DCIS) vs usual ductal hyperplasia (UDH). (**a**) UDH, H&E; (**b**) UDH, ADH5 shows a mosaic pattern, both CK903 and luminal cytokeratin staining pattern, IHC; (**c**) ADH, H&E; (**d**) ADH, loss of expression for HMWCK, CK903, ADH5 staining, IHC

Immunohistochemistry

- Nonproliferative fibrocystic change is mainly a histomorphological diagnosis.
- IHC comes to play a role only when a ductal hyperplasia is present and the morphological features border on UDH and ADH.
- UDH is a hyperplastic process, with high expression of basal cell-type keratin or high molecular weight cytokeratin (HMWCK) and scattered ER expression.
- ADH/DCIS is neoplastic with a clonal proliferation of luminal epithelial cells, showing loss or focal weak expression of basal cell-type keratin or HMWCK and diffuse ER positivity.
- By application of ADH5, a breast marker cocktail consisting of CK5, CK14, p63, CK7, and CK18, UDH exhibits a mosaic staining pattern, and ADH/DCIS shows a clonal proliferation of luminal epithelial cells with negative HMWCK (basal cell type) staining, as shown in Fig. 5.10a–d, respectively.

Tumors of the Breast

The World Health Organization (WHO) classifications of tumors of the breast are summarized in Table 5.1.

Table 5.1 WHO Classification of Tumors of the Breast, 2012

Epithelial tumors
Microinvasive carcinoma
Invasive breast carcinoma
Invasive carcinoma of no special type (NST)
Pleomorphic carcinoma
Carcinoma with osteoclast-like stromal giant cells
Carcinoma with choriocarcinomatous features
Carcinoma with melanotic features
Invasive lobular carcinoma
Classic, solid, alveolar, pleomorphic, tubulolobular, mixed lobular carcinomas
Tubular carcinoma
Cribriform carcinoma
Mucinous carcinoma
Carcinoma with medullary features
Medullary carcinoma
Atypical medullary carcinoma
Invasive carcinoma NST with medullary features
Carcinoma with apocrine differentiation
Carcinoma with signet-ring-cell differentiation
Invasive micropapillary carcinoma
Metaplastic carcinoma NST
Low-grade adenosquamous carcinoma
Fibromatosis-like metaplastic carcinoma
Squamous cell carcinoma
Spindle cell carcinoma
Metaplastic carcinoma with mesenchymal differentiation
Chondroid, osseous, other types of mesenchymal differentiations
Mixed metaplastic carcinoma
Myoepithelial carcinoma
Rare types
Carcinoma with neuroendocrine features
Neuroendocrine tumor, well-differentiated
Neuroendocrine carcinoma, poorly differentiated (small cell carcinoma)
Carcinoma with neuroendocrine differentiation
Secretory carcinoma
Invasive papillary carcinoma
Acinic cell carcinoma
Mucoepidermoid carcinoma
Polymorphous carcinoma
Oncocytic carcinoma
Lipid-rich carcinoma
Glycogen-rich clear cell carcinoma
Sebaceous carcinoma
Salivary gland/skin adnexal-type tumors
Cylindroma, clear cell hidradenoma
Epithelial-myoepithelial tumors
Pleomorphic adenoma
Adenomyoepithelioma
Adenomyoepithelioma with carcinoma
Adenoid cystic carcinoma
Precursor lesions
DCIS
Lobular neoplasia
Lobular carcinoma in situ
Classic or pleomorphic lobular carcinoma in situ
Atypical lobular hyperplasia
Intraductal proliferative lesions
UDH
Columnar cell lesions, including flat epithelial atypia
ADH
Papillary lesions
Intraductal papilloma
Intraductal papillomas with ADH, or DCIS, or LCIS
Intraductal papillary carcinoma
Encapsulated papillary carcinoma
Encapsulated papillary carcinoma with invasion
Solid papillary carcinoma
In situ, invasive
Benign epithelial proliferations
Sclerosing adenosis
Apocrine adenosis
Microglandular adenosis
Radial scar/complex sclerosing lesion
Adenomas
Tubular, lactating, apocrine, ductal adenomas
Mesenchymal tumors
Nodular fasciitis
Myofibroblastoma
Desmoid-type fibromatosis
Inflammatory myofibroblastic tumor
Benign vascular lesions
Haemangioma, angiomatosis, atypical vascular lesions
Pseudoangiomatous stromal hyperplasia
Granular cell tumor
Benign peripheral nerve sheath tumors
Neurofibroma, schwannoma
Lipoma
Angiolipoma
Liposarcoma
Angiosarcoma
Rhabdomyosarcoma
Osteosarcoma
Leiomyoma
Leiomyosarcoma
Fibroepithelial tumors
Fibroadenoma
Phyllodes tumor
Benign, borderline, malignant, periductal stromal sarcoma, low grade
Hamartoma
Tumors of the nipple
Nipple adenoma
Syringomatous tumor
Paget disease of the nipple

(continued)

Table 5.1 (continued)

Malignant lymphoma	
Diffuse large B-cell lymphoma	
Burkitt lymphoma	
T-cell lymphoma	
	Anaplastic large cell lymphoma, anaplastic lymphoma kinase (ALK) negative
Extranodal marginal-zone B-cell lymphoma of mucosa-associated lymphoid tissue (MALT) type	
Follicular lymphoma	
Metastatic tumors	
Tumors of the male breast	
Gynecomastia	
Carcinoma	
	Invasive carcinoma, in situ carcinoma
Clinical patterns	
	Inflammatory carcinoma
	Bilateral breast carcinoma

Used with permission from WHO Classification of Tumours of the Breast. Edited by Lakhani SR et al. Lyon: IARC Press; 2012

Fibroepithelial Tumors

Fibroadenoma

Key Clinical Features

- Most common benign tumor
- Asymptomatic or a mobile, painless, well-defined breast nodule/mass
- In premenopausal women, usually in their second or third decades
- Usually solitary
- Occasionally multifocal and bilateral, reported in Afro-Caribbean women

Key Radiological Features

- Well-defined mass, with or without microcalcifications
- Homogeneous, hypoechoic, and well-circumscribed mass on ultrasound

Cytological Features

- Cohesive benign ductal epithelial cells arranged in a branching antler-horn configuration in a background of many naked bipolar or spindled nuclei
- Myoepithelial cells at periphery
- Hypocellular myxoid stroma
- Focal ductal cells with apocrine changes
- Figure 5.11a–d

Differential Diagnosis

- Benign proliferative fibrocystic changes
- Phyllodes tumor
- Mammary hamartoma
- Tubular adenoma

Histology

- Fibroadenomas are composed of both epithelium and stroma with a well-demarcated, lobulated, or smooth border.
- The epithelium shows two growth patterns: pericanalicular and intracanalicular, as illustrated in Fig. 5.11e, f.
- The stroma is variable in morphology and cellularity, however homogeneous throughout in individual cases.

Immunohistochemistry

- Immunohistochemistry is usually not applied for the diagnosis of fibroadenoma.

Phyllodes Tumor

Key Clinical Features

- 0.3–1% of all breast neoplasms
- In peri- and postmenopausal women, usually their fifth decade
- Presents with a palpable breast mass, usually painless, mobile, multinodular and firm, or presents with an abnormal mammography

Key Radiological Features

- Well-circumscribed, lobulated mass on mammography
- Solid, hypoechoic, well-circumscribed mass on ultrasound

Cytological Features

- Cellular specimen
- Mixed epithelial and stromal fragments
- Hypercellular stromal fragments, comprised of spindle-shaped cells singly or enmeshed in stroma; significant atypia of the spindle cells with mitotic activity suggesting malignant phyllodes tumor
- Many naked bipolar or spindle nuclei in the background
- Occasional ductal hyperplasia with or without atypia
- Figure 5.12a–c

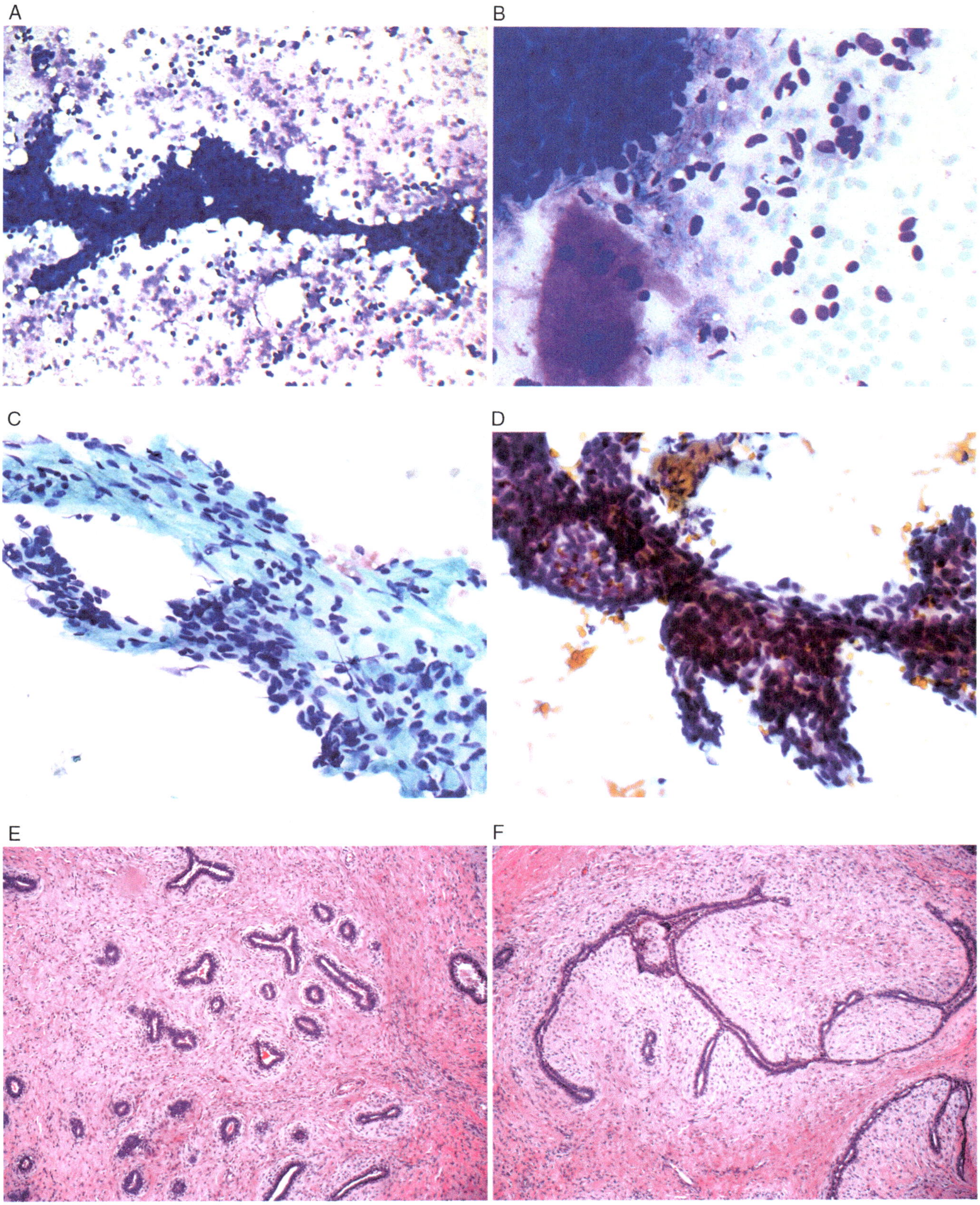

Fig. 5.11 (**a**–**f**) Fibroadenoma, cytology and histology. (**a**, **b**) Branching antler-horn benign ductal cells in a background of many bipolar or spindled naked nuclei and rare stromal tissue, Diff-Quik; (**c**) benign ductal epithelial cells and stromal tissue, Pap stain; (**d**) Antler-horn fragment of benign ductal epithelial cells and scant stroma. Myoepithelial cells are present, Pap stain; (**e**) pericanalicular pattern, H&E; (**f**) Intracanalicular pattern, H&E

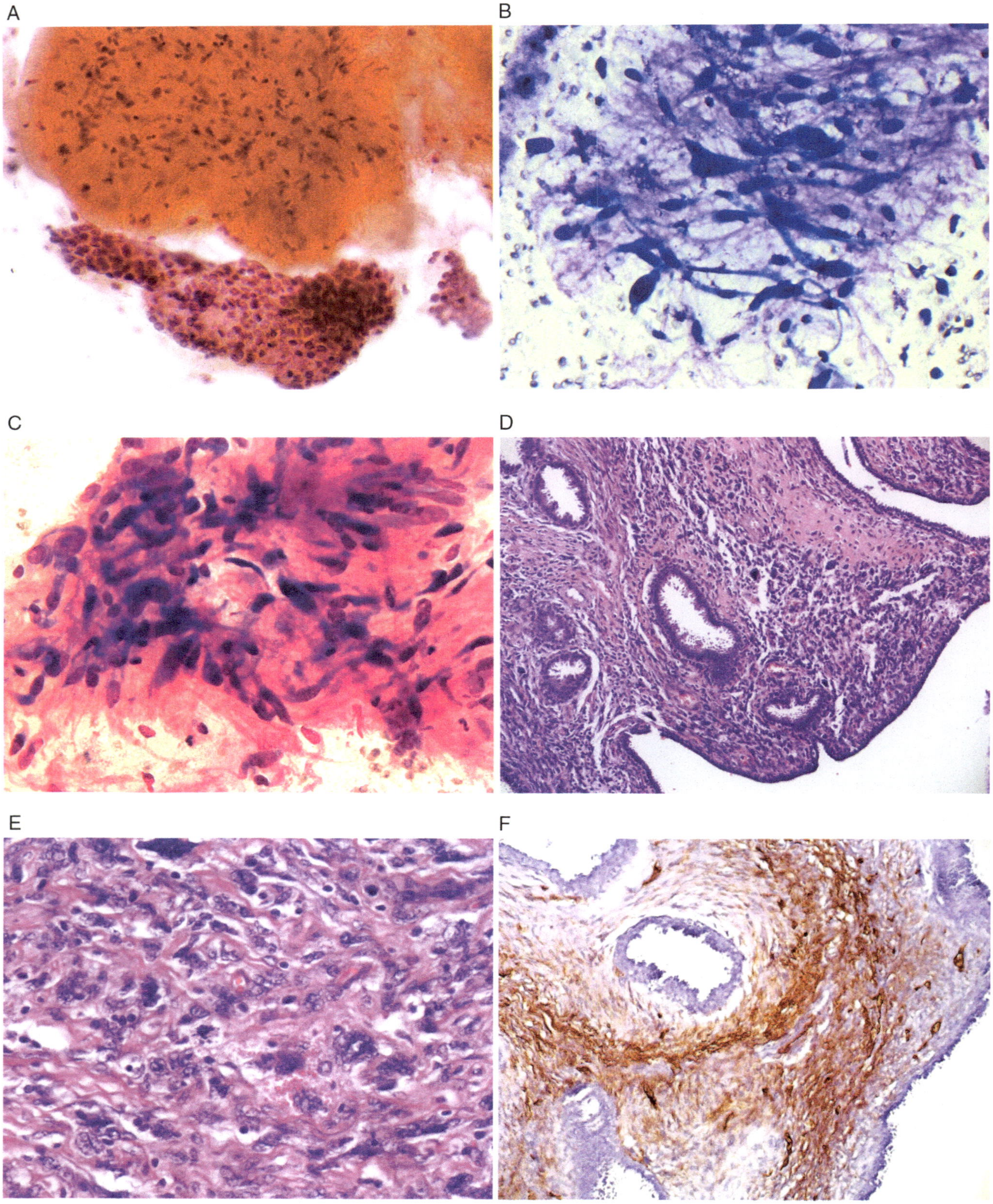

Fig. 5.12 (**a**–**h**) Phyllodes tumor, cytology, histology, and immunophenotype. (**a**) Cohesive cluster of ductal epithelial cells with mild atypia and fragment of stroma, Pap stain; (**b**) the stromal cells are spindled with atypia and a rare mitotic figure, Diff-Quik; (**c**) stroma with increased cellularity and atypia, Pap stain; (**d**, **e**) leaflike pattern, highly cellular and atypical stroma with mitotic figures, H&E; (**f**) positive CD34 staining, IHC; (**g**) high expression of p53, IHC; (**h**) high proliferative index (MIB-1), IHC

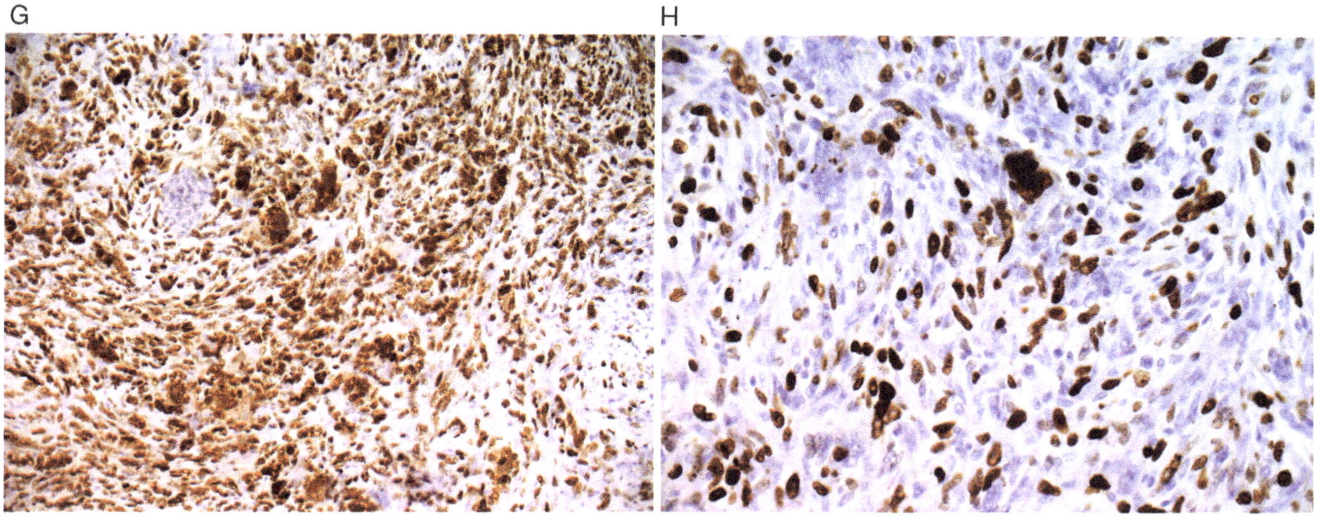

Fig. 5.12 (continued)

Differential Diagnosis

- Fibroadenoma
- Metaplastic carcinoma
- Primary sarcoma
- Sclerosing adenosis

Histology

- A biphasic tumor contains epithelial and stromal components, usually with a prominent intracanalicular growth pattern to form leaf-like structures.
- The stroma is usually heterogeneous in cellularity with mitotic activity.
- Representative images are illustrated in Fig. 5.12d, e.

Immunohistochemistry

- Immunohistochemistry does not usually contribute to the diagnosis of phyllodes tumor. However, the expression of Ki-67 and p53 correlates with tumor grade.
- CD34 and B-cell CLL/lymphoma-2 (Bcl2) were reported to be positive and can be used to differentiate a malignant phyllodes tumor from metaplastic (spindle cell) carcinoma.
- Representative images are illustrated in Fig. 5.12e–h.

Hamartomas

Key Clinical Features

- Less than 1% of benign breast masses
- Common in pre- and perimenopausal women
- Presents as a mobile, painless, soft-to-firm, well-defined palpable mass

Key Radiological Features

- Well-circumscribed, round-to-oval inhomogeneous mass on mammogram; characteristically, the mass is centrally dense with a radiolucent rim.
- Sonographic features are variable; difficult to delineate the margins due to the resemblance to normal breast tissue; and may appear as a well-defined, solid lesion with mixed internal echotextures and without any lesional microcalcifications.

Cytological Features

- Low-to-moderate cellularity specimen
- Scattered sheets of benign ductal epithelial cells, some showing irregular branching
- Lobular cells forming acini, presenting as an intact lobular units
- Minimal-to-absent cellular discohesion or atypia
- Adipose tissue in various amounts and occasional stromal fragments, may have attached epithelial cells
- Frequent bipolar stromal nuclei, occasional apocrine cells, foam cells, and myoepithelial cells

Differential Diagnosis

- Fibrocystic changes
- Fibroadenoma

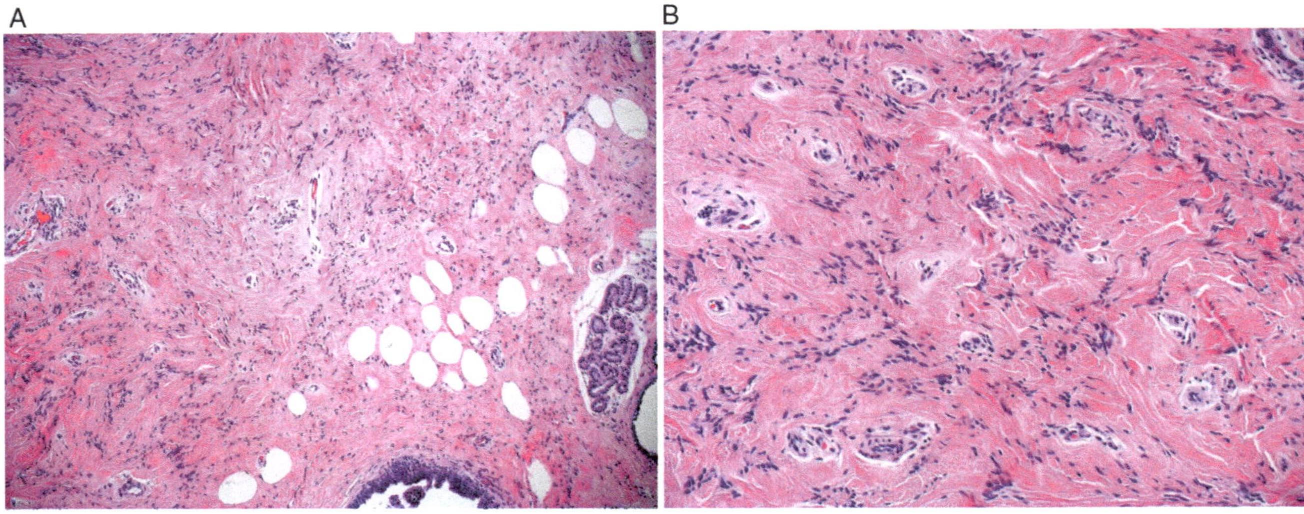

Fig. 5.13 (**a**, **b**) Mammary hamartoma, histology. (**a**) Disorganized growth of fat, fibrous connective tissue forming nodule, H&E; (**b**) disorganized growth of fibrous connective tissue, H&E

Histology

- A disproportionate and disorganized growth of mature mammary tissues, including ducts, lobules, fat, fibrous connective tissue, and smooth muscle, forming well-defined nodules.
- The presence of fibrous tissue within the lobules (interlobular fibrosis) or fibrous tissue and fat in the stroma should alert the pathologist to the possibility of a hamartoma.
- Representative images are shown in Fig. 5.13a, b.

Immunohistochemistry

- Immunohistochemistry plays no role in the diagnosis of a mammary hamartoma.

Epithelial Tumors

Benign Epithelial Proliferation

Lactating Adenoma
Lactating adenoma is a term used for a fibroadenoma with superimposed changes of lactation.

Key Clinical Features

- Typically a breast mass in a young pregnant or postpartum woman
- Occasionally can be large and painful

Key Radiological Features

- Similar to fibroadenoma; occasionally shows atypical features on ultrasound, such as irregular margins, heterogeneous echogenicity, and posterior shadowing

Cytological Features

- Cellular specimen with a milky or lipid background
- Ductal epithelial cells with nuclear enlargement and conspicuous nucleoli
- Ductal cells with smooth nuclear contour and evenly distributed chromatin
- Many naked nuclei with small-to-prominent nucleoli
- Figure 5.14a, b

Differential Diagnosis

- Carcinoma, ductal, or lobular
- Non-Hodgkin's lymphoma

Histology

- Lactating adenoma is composed of a compact aggregate of lobules exhibiting secretory hyperplasia during pregnancy or postpartum.
- The glandular elements are diffusely distributed in a sparsely cellular stroma; the glandular cells show vacuolated cytoplasm.
- A representative image is shown in Fig. 5.14c, d.

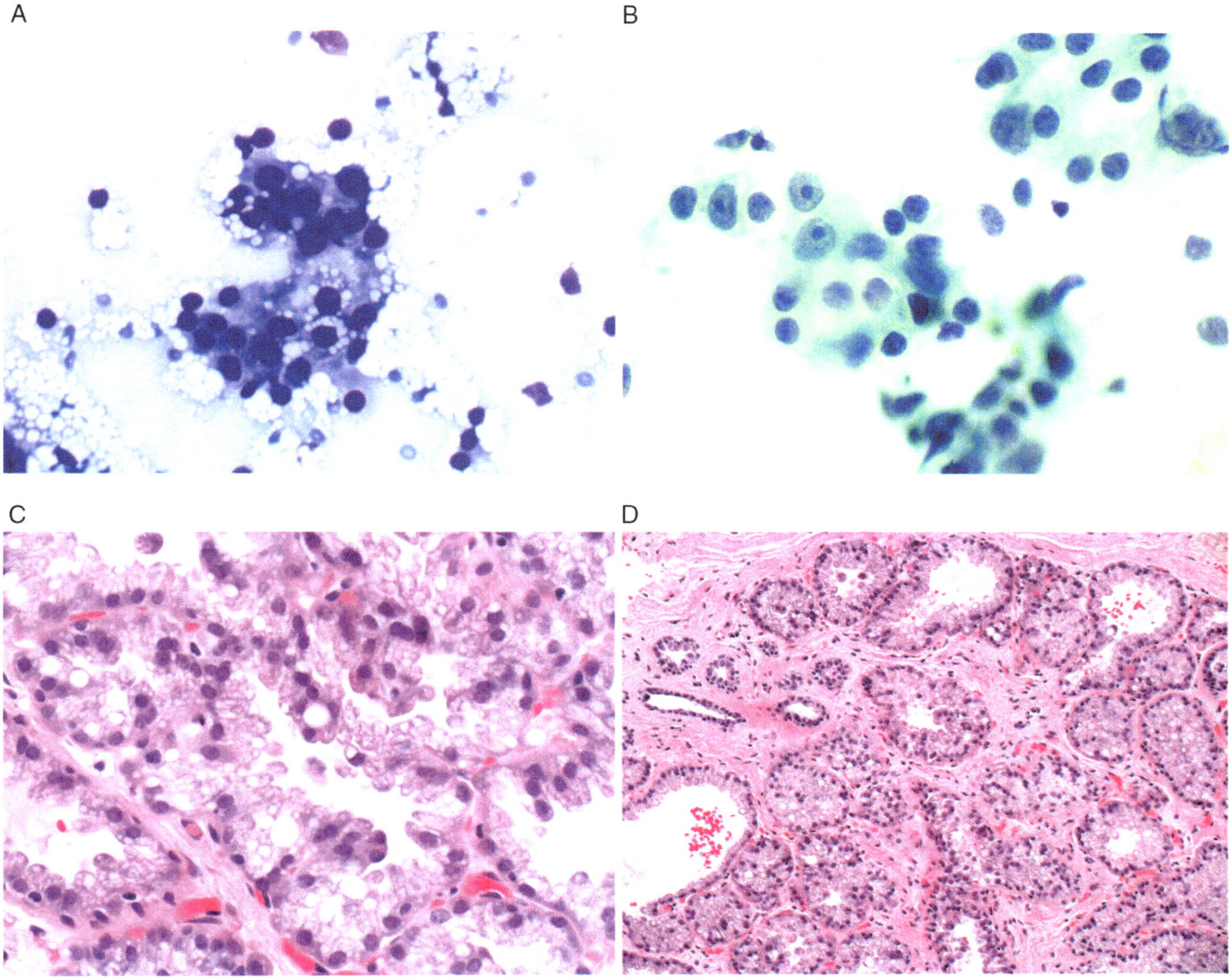

Fig. 5.14 (**a–d**) Lactating adenoma. (**a, b**) Cellular smear contains loosely cohesive clusters of ductal epithelial cells with enlarged nuclei, small to prominent nucleoli, and vacuolated cytoplasm in a milky or lipid background with naked nuclei, (**a**) Diff-Quik; (**b**) Pap stain; (**c, d**) Hiatology, H&E; well-circumscribed, compact aggregate of lobules exhibiting secretory hyperplasia (**d**); the glandular cells show vacuolated cytoplasm, diffusely distributed in a sparsely cellular stroma (**c**)

Immunohistochemistry

- Immunohistochemistry is usually not applied for the diagnosis of lactating adenoma.

Papillary Lesions

Key Clinical Features

- Intraductal papilloma: solitary, usually centrally located tumor in peri- and postmenopausal women, often presents as bloody nipple discharge; can be peripheral and multiple, may present as mass lesions
- Papillary carcinoma: 1–2% of breast cancers; usually in postmenopausal women; can present as a mass; one-third of patients present with bloody nipple discharge; favorable prognosis.

Key Radiological Features

- Central papillary lesions may present as a circumscribed subareolar mass with well-defined borders, without stromal distortion on mammography; an intraductal mass with associated dilated duct or a complex cystic lesion on ultrasonography. Peripheral papillary lesions present as mammographic abnormalities or may be radiographically occult.

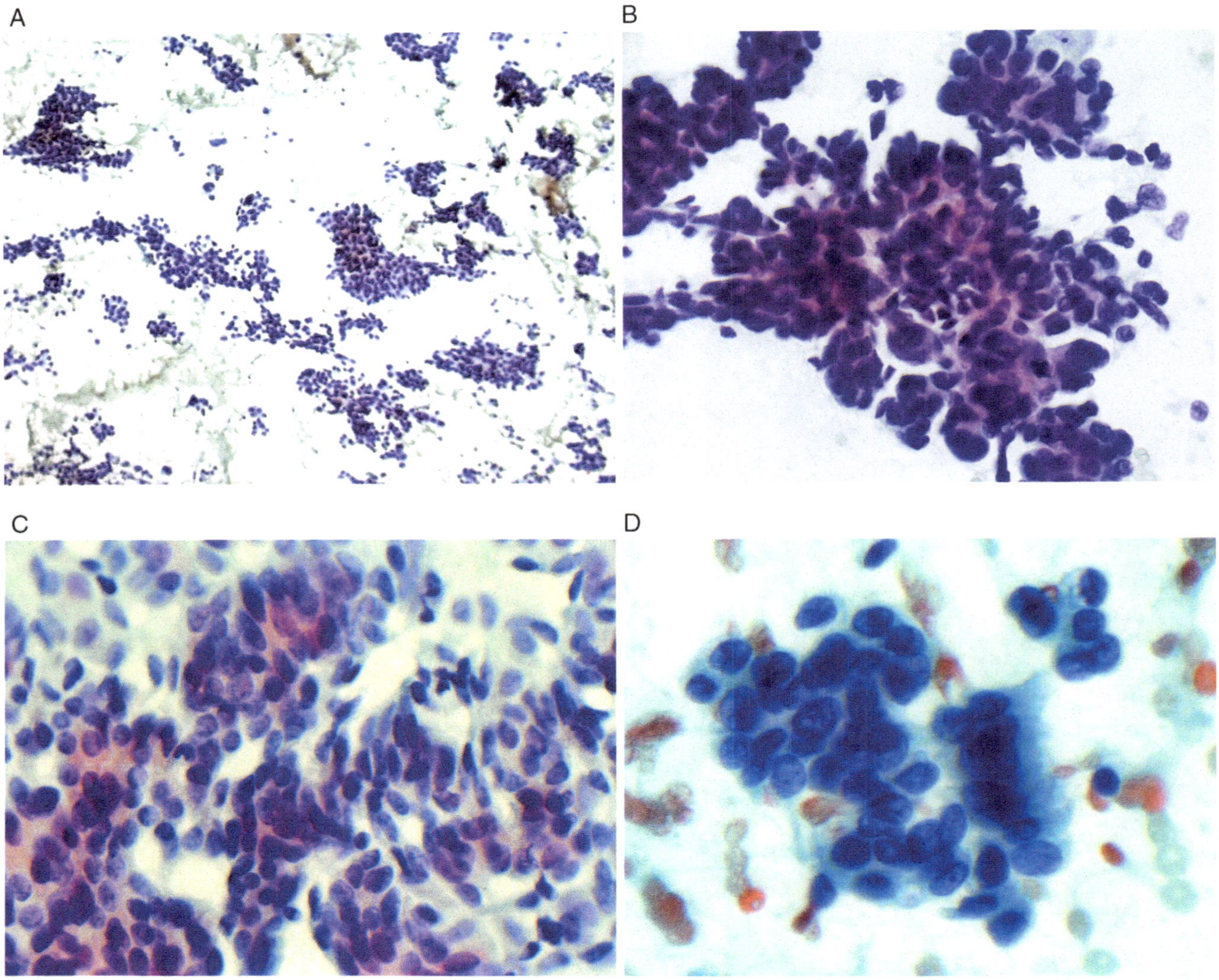

Fig. 5.15 (**a**–**d**) Papillary lesions, cytology, histology, and immunophenotype. (**a**) numerous papillary groups, Pap stain; (**b**) Papillary groups with the overlying epithelial cells showing columnar morphology; (**c**, **d**) loosely cohesive and single columnar cells with intact cytoplasm in background, Diff-Quik and Pap stain

Cytological Features

- Highly cellular sample
- Many groups and sheets of ductal cells with papillary fronds (Fig. 5.15a, b)
- Cells usually columnar shaped with many single or loosely cohesive cells with tall columnar-shaped and intact cytoplasm (Fig. 5.15c, d)
- Nuclear atypia and mitosis indicating atypical hyperplasia or more severe lesion
- A mixture of cellular components such as ductal cells, apocrine cells, and histiocytes indicating a papilloma

Differential Diagnosis

- Intraductal hyperplasia
- Fibroadenoma
- Ductal carcinoma

Histology

- Papillary lesions include a heterogeneous group of epithelial proliferations ranging from benign to malignant.
- Benign intraductal papilloma is composed of a few broad fronds with well-defined fibrovascular cores lined by two

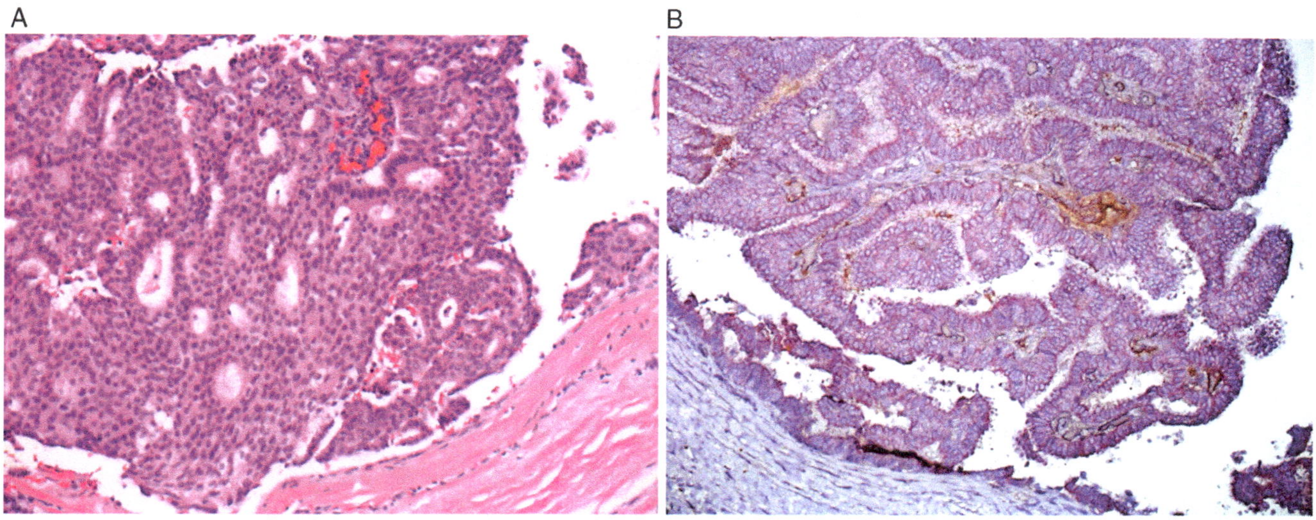

Fig. 5.16 (**a**, **b**) Intracystic papillary carcinoma, histology, and immunophenotype. (**a**) Cystically dilated duct with a fibrotic wall encircling an arborizing, complex papillary network lined by one or more layers of uniform epithelial cells, H&E; (**b**) ADH5 staining reveals loss of basal cells at periphery and over fibrous vascular core, with loss of CK903 staining, IHC

layers of cells: the ductal epithelial cells and myoepithelial cells. The ductal epithelial cells may undergo hyperplasia, atypical hyperplasia, or metaplasia. There may be sclerosis in the stroma.
- Papillary DCIS is a DCIS with a papillary growth pattern. The papillary stalks are usually thin and inconspicuous with frequent epithelial hyperplasia and atypia without myoepithelial cells, except at the periphery. The epithelial cells are monotonous.
- Encapsulated (intracystic) papillary carcinoma is traditionally considered a variant of DCIS, although this has been challenged recently. Histologically, the tumor is composed of a cystically dilated duct with a fibrotic wall encircling an arborizing, complex papillary network lined by one or more layers of uniform epithelial cells. Myoepithelial cells are absent within and at the periphery of the tumor.
- Representative images are shown in Fig. 5.16a, b.

Immunohistochemistry

- IHC plays an important role in the diagnosis of papillary lesions, especially in small biopsy specimens.
- Myoepithelial cell (MEC) markers (p63, calponin, smooth muscle myosin heavy chain [SM-MHC]), in conjunction with HMWCK (CK903, CK5/6, CK14) and ER, are most useful in the differential diagnosis of papillary lesions.
- The loss of myoepithelial cells (at the periphery and over the fibrovascular core) classifies a papillary lesion as malignant (encapsulated papillary carcinoma or solid papillary carcinoma).
- When a papillary lesion with intact myoepithelial cells (at the periphery, may or may not be over the fibrovascular core), immunoassays for HMWCK (CK903, CK5/6, CK14) and ER should be utilized; benign papilloma expresses HMWCK with a mosaic staining pattern and ER with focal weak staining pattern in the area of proliferation, while atypical papilloma or papillary DCIS shows loss of expression for HMWCK and strong diffuse reactivity to ER. However, caution should be exercised when interpreting ER results because papilloma is usually diffusely reactive to ER.
- In addition, neuroendocrine markers (synaptophysin and chromogranin) are positive in the majority of solid papillary carcinomas but negative in benign and atypical papillary lesions.
- Representative images are illustrated in Fig. 5.17a–d.

Invasive Ductal Carcinoma (NST)

Key Clinical Features

- Accounts for about 55–80% of invasive breast carcinomas.
- Symptomatic, presents as a breast lump with or without pain; asymptomatic, with mammographic abnormalities.
- Nipple abnormalities or skin dimpling/changes may present.

Key Radiological Features

- Mammography: variable, including well-defined, ill-defined, and spiculated masses, parenchymal deformity, and calcifications with or without mass lesions.

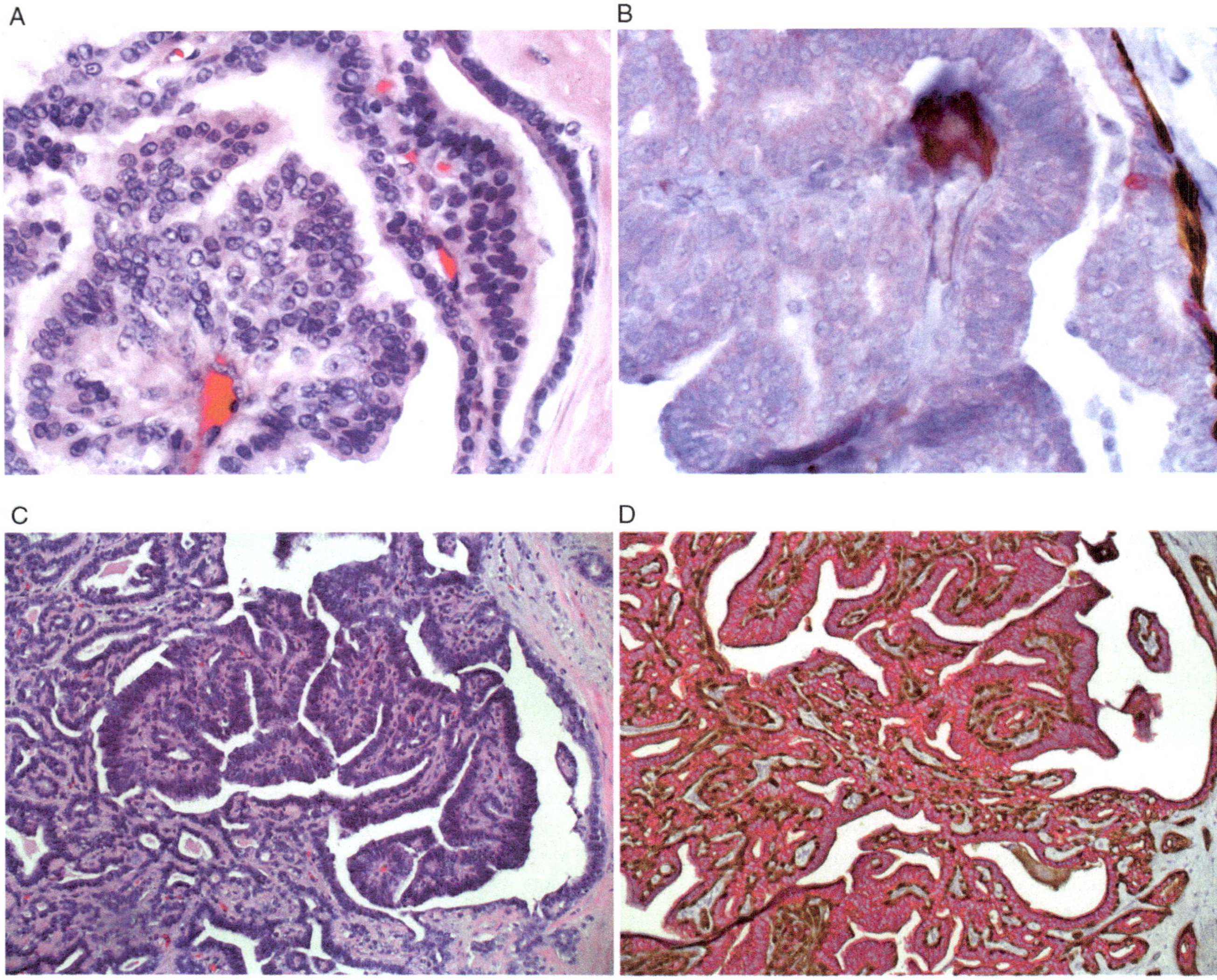

Fig. 5.17 (**a**–**d**) Differential immunophenotypes of papillary ductal carcinoma in situ and papilloma. (**a**) Papillary DCIS, H&E; (**b**) papillary DCIS, ADH5 showing intact basal cells at the periphery (nuclear decoration by p63 and cytoplasmic brown staining for CK903) and loss of expression for CK903 with luminal cytokeratin decoration, IHC; (**c**) benign papilloma, H&E; (**d**) papilloma, ADH5 showing intact basal cells at the periphery and in the stalks (nuclear decoration by p63 and cytoplasmic brown staining for CK903) and mosaic staining pattern for CK903 (brown; pink staining for luminal cytokeratins)

- Sonography: an irregular mass with ill-defined margins and an inhomogeneous echo texture with acoustic shadowing. The anteroposterior diameter is greater than the transverse diameter.

Cytological Features

- Moderate-to-high cellularity specimen
- Many loosely cohesive groups and singles
- Nuclear enlargement >2–3 times the size of a red blood cell (RBC)
- Single cells with intact cytoplasm
- Hyperchromasia, prominent nucleoli, nuclear membrane irregularity, and nuclear pleomorphism
- Mitosis and tumor necrosis
- Intracytoplasmic lumina
- Apocrine changes and cytoplasmic vacuoles
- Figure 5.18a–e

Differential Diagnosis

- DCIS
- Cytological atypia in benign lesions, such as fibroadenoma, papillary neoplasm, or epithelial hyperplasia
- Gynecomastia (male breast)
- Metastases

A B C D E F

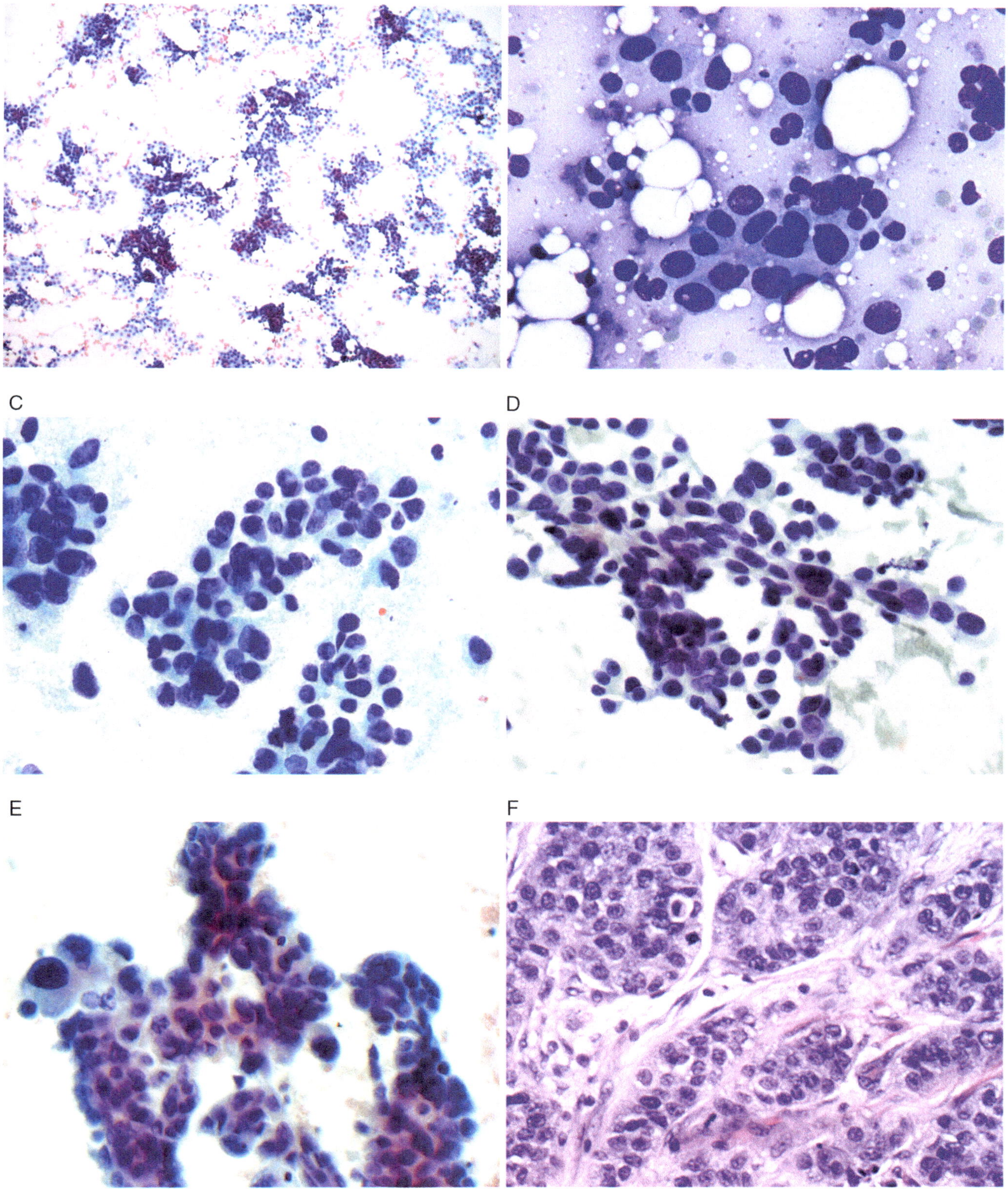

Fig. 5.18 (**a**–**f**) Invasive ductal carcinoma, NST. (**a**) Moderately to highly cellular smear comprised of loosely cohesive clusters and many single cells with intact cytoplasm, Pap stain; (**b**) Diff-Quik showing individual cells with pleomorphic nuclei, prominent nucleoli and intact cytoplasm; (**c**, **d**) Pap stain reveals the tumor cells with enlarged nuclei (at least 2–3× RBC), irregular nuclear membrane, nucleoli and coarse chromatin pattern; (**e**) Carcinoma cells show apocrine changes, Pap stain; (**f**) histology, H&E

Histology

- A non-specialized pattern comprises at least 50% of the tumor.
- Malignant cells arranged in cords, trabeculae, poorly formed tubular structures, or sheets infiltrate a desmoplastic or collagenous stroma.
- A representative image is shown in Fig. 5.18f.

Immunohistochemistry

- The loss of myoepithelial cells confirms its malignant nature.
- Intact membranous staining pattern for E-cadherin and p120 catenin.
- GATA3 positive in 94% of cases.
- 70–80% of invasive ductal carcinomas are ER positive.
- 15–25% of tumors overexpress human epidermal growth factor receptor-2 (Her-2/neu).

Invasive Lobular Carcinoma

Key Clinical Features

- Represents 5–15% of all invasive breast carcinomas.
- Usually presents as a palpable mass with irregular borders; may present as a poorly defined thickening or fine diffuse nodularity.
- Multifocal and bilateral lesions are more frequent, often in the central area.

Key Radiological Features

- Asymmetrical, ill-defined, or irregular masses or densities on mammography
- Usually presents as a hypoechoic mass with irregular or indistinct margins and posterior acoustic shadowing on sonography; about 10% invisible on ultrasonography

Cytological Features

- Low-to-moderate cellularity specimen
- Small loosely clusters and single lobular carcinoma cells, some lining up as a row
- The lobular carcinoma cells with mildly enlarged nuclei (1.5–2 times the size of an RBC), intact cytoplasm, and high nuclear-to-cytoplasmic ratio
- Hyperchromasia and nuclear membrane irregularity
- Intracytoplasmic lumina often seen
- Single atypical cells within adipose tissue
- Figure 5.19a–e

Differential Diagnosis

- Low-grade ductal carcinoma
- Neuroendocrine tumors
- Melanoma
- Lymphoma

Histology

- Invasive carcinomas showing lobular morphology in greater than 90% of the tumor are classified as invasive lobular carcinomas.
- For those with a 50–90% lobular morphology in addition to NST pattern, a mixed ductal and lobular carcinoma should be classified.
- The invasive lobular carcinoma cells are usually uniform, dyshesive, and round or oval cells with eccentrically placed nuclei containing small nucleoli and a scant amount of cytoplasm, classically in a single-file pattern. Intracytoplasmic lumina may be appreciated.
- There are subtypes, such as tubulolobular, solid, alveolar, and mixed patterns.
- Representative images are shown in Fig. 5.19f, g.

Immunohistochemistry

- A complete loss of expression of E-cadherin or aberrant localization of E-cadherin protein (cytoplasmic, as apical or perinuclear): due to loss of E-cadherin function or a dysfunctional cadherin-catenin complex or both caused by *cadherin 1 (CDH1)* gene aberrations at molecular genetic level. See Fig. 5.19h.
- Cytoplasmic staining pattern for p120 catenin, with loss of membranous staining.
- In morphologically challenging cases, E-cadherin and p120 catenin can be used to accurately classify a tumor as ductal or lobular type. Differential patterns of staining are illustrated in Fig. 5.20a–f.
- GATA3 positive in 100% of cases.
- 67–92% of lobular carcinomas are ER positive.
- Her-2/neu overexpression is uncommon.
- When lobular carcinoma metastasizes, especially to the gastrointestinal (GI) tract (e.g., stomach), a panel of immunomarkers consisting of ER, GATA binding protein 3 (GATA3), CK7, and caudal-type homeobox (CDX2) is most helpful in reaching a differential diagnosis.

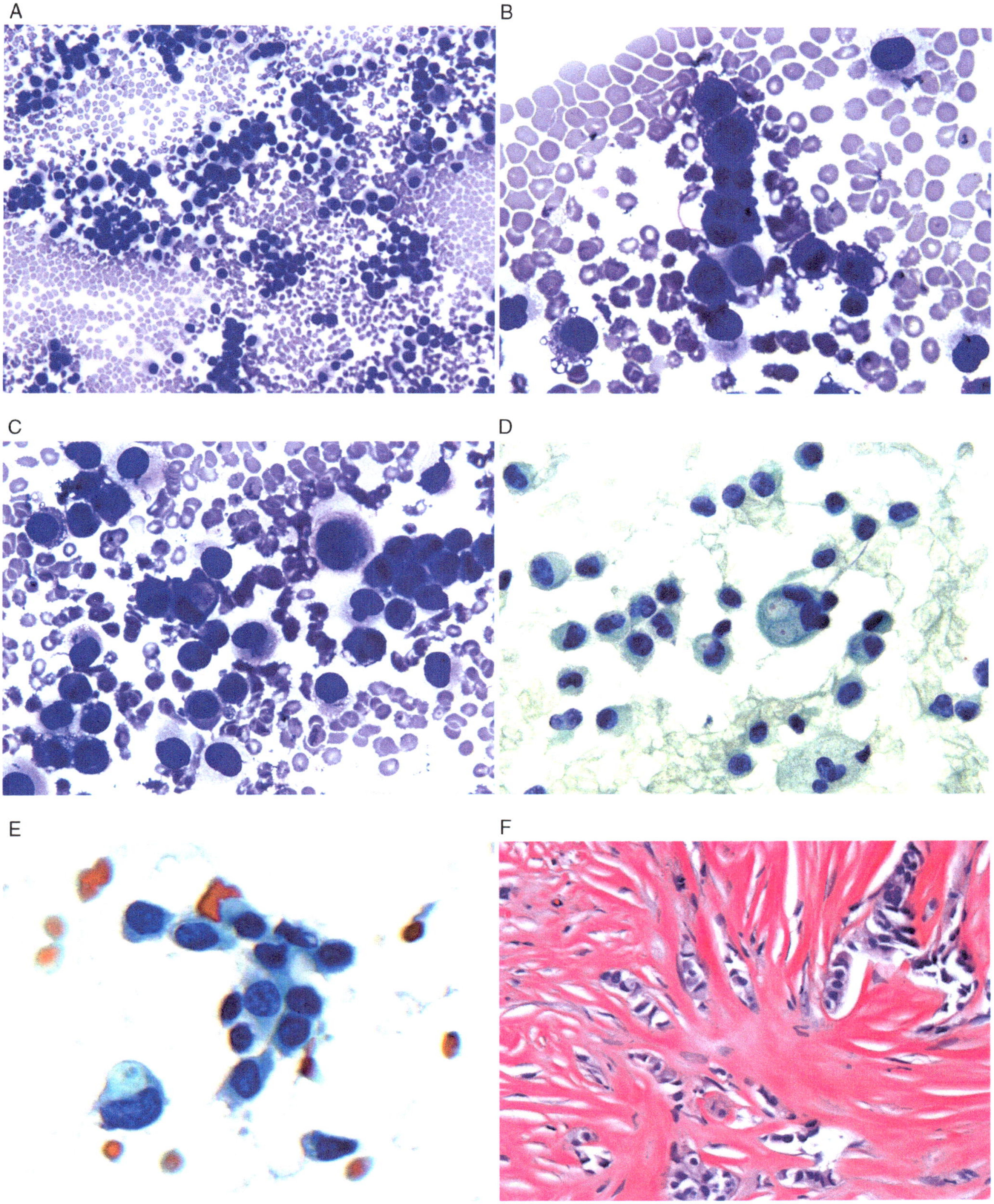

Fig. 5.19 (**a–h**) Invasive lobular carcinoma. (**a**, **b**) Low-to-moderate cellularity specimen contains small loose clusters and many single lobular carcinoma cells, some lining up as a row, Diff-Quik; (**c**) the lobular carcinoma cells are single, with mildly enlarged nuclei of 1.5–2 × RBC, some containing intracytoplasmic lumen, Diff-Quik; (**d**, **e**) intracytoplasmic lumen containing targetoid mucin noted, Pap stain; (**f**) classic lobular carcinoma, H&E; (**g**) pleomorphic lobular carcinoma, H&E; (**h**) pleomorphic lobular carcinoma, loss of E-cadherin expression

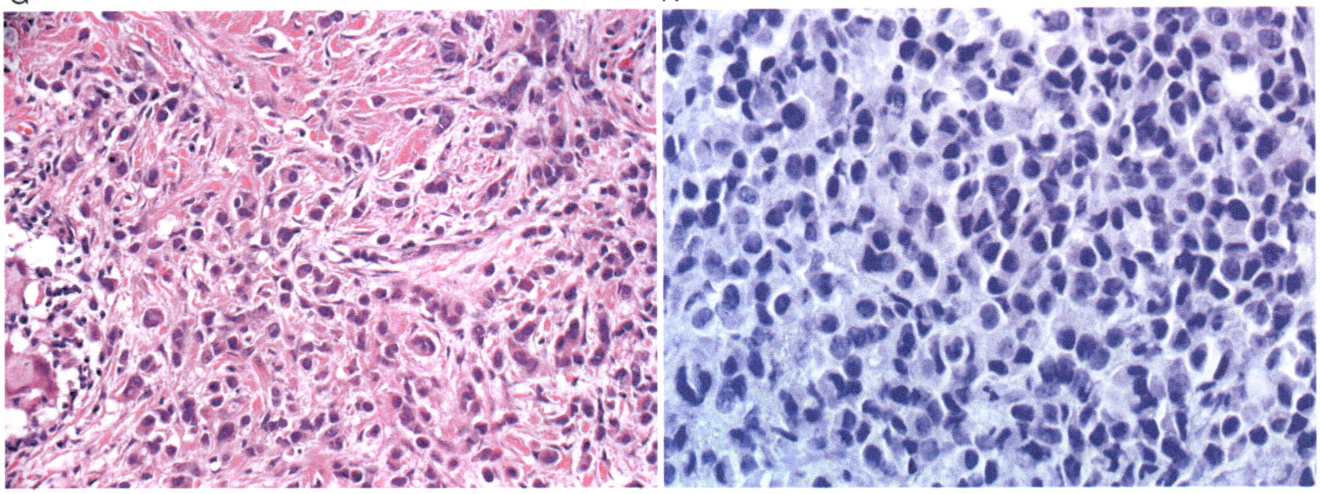

Fig. 5.19 (continued)

Tubular Carcinoma

Key Clinical Features

- Less than 2% of all invasive breast carcinomas
- More common in women in their late 50s and early 60s, rare in men
- Majority present with a palpable mass in the past; nonpalpable mammographic abnormalities at current time
- Excellent prognosis

Key Radiological Features

- A mass lesion, oval or round or lobulated, with irregular or spiculated margins, central density, and occasional microcalcifications on mammography
- Ill-defined hypoechoic masses with posterior acoustic shadowing on ultrasonography

Cytological Features

- Relatively low-cellularity specimen
- Angulated, pointed tubular/glandular structures
- Little or no nuclear atypia
- Few single cells with intact cytoplasm
- Lack of myoepithelial cells
- Bipolar naked stromal nuclei generally absent
- Figure 5.21a, b

Differential Diagnosis

- Sclerosing adenosis, tubular adenosis, and radial scars
- Fibroadenoma
- Invasive lobular carcinoma
- Invasive ductal carcinoma, not otherwise specified (NOS)

Histology

- Characterized by a haphazard proliferation of infiltrative tubules distributed in a stellate configuration.
- The tubules are angulated with a single layer of monotonous cuboidal to low columnar ductal epithelial cells, often showing apical "snouts" and open lumina.
- The stroma is desmoplastic, often with elastosis.
- Mitoses are rare.

Immunohistochemistry

- IHC is often applied in small biopsy specimens.
- The lack of myoepithelial cells confirms the diagnosis of tubular carcinoma, as illustrated in Fig. 5.21c, d.
- GATA3 positive.

Medullary Carcinoma

Key Clinical Features

- 1–10% of all invasive breast carcinomas
- Affects younger women, in their 30s and 40s, with a predominantly early-onset age distribution in which the incidence increases until age 50, then plateaus or decreases

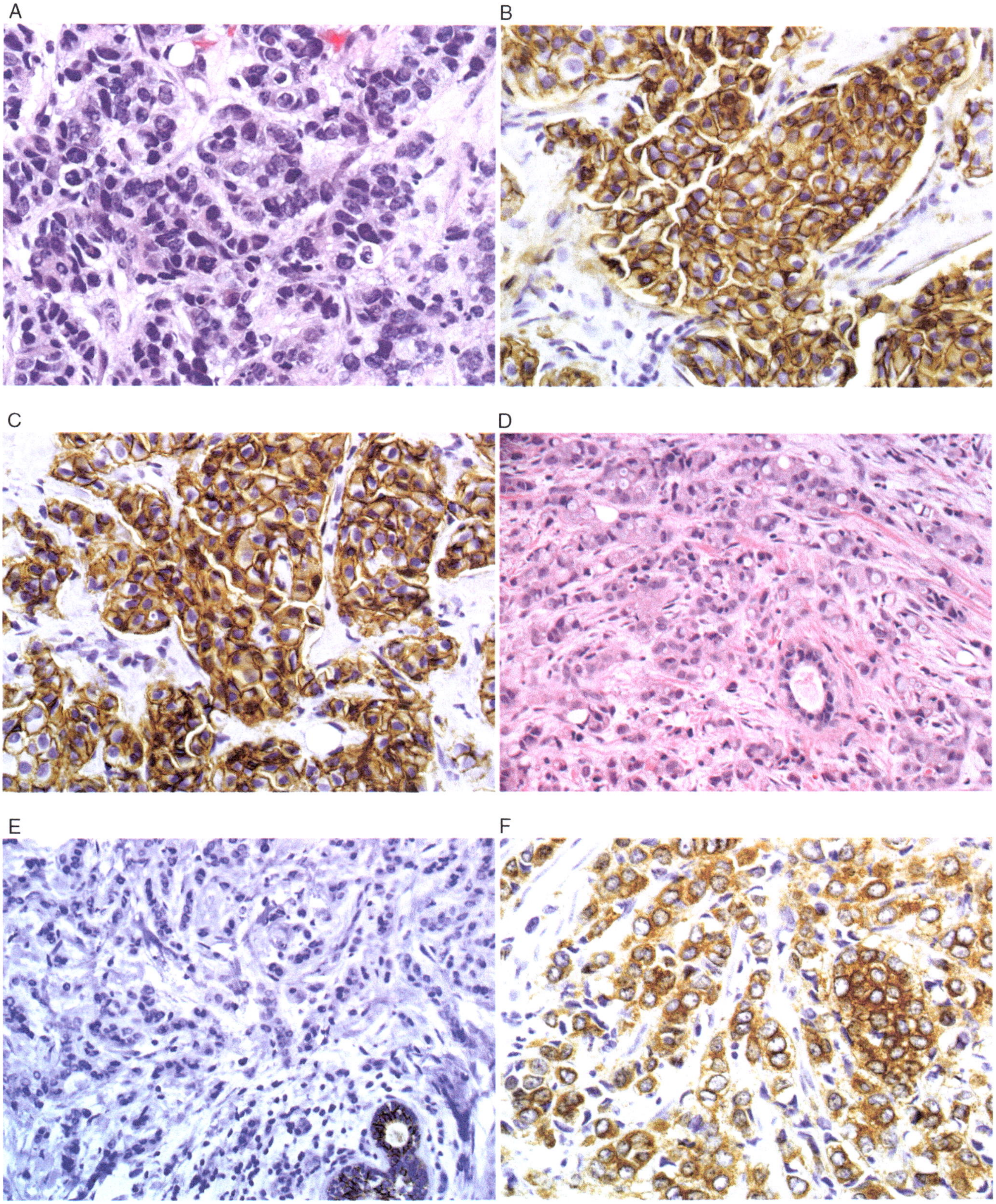

Fig. 5.20 (**a**–**f**) Differential immunophenotype for invasive ductal (IDC) and lobular carcinomas (ILC). (**a**) IDC, H&E; (**b**) IDC, membranous staining for E-Cadherin; (**c**) IDC, membranous staining for p120; (**d**) ILC, H&E; (**e**) ILC, loss E-Cadherin staining; (**f**) ILC, cytoplasmic staining for p120

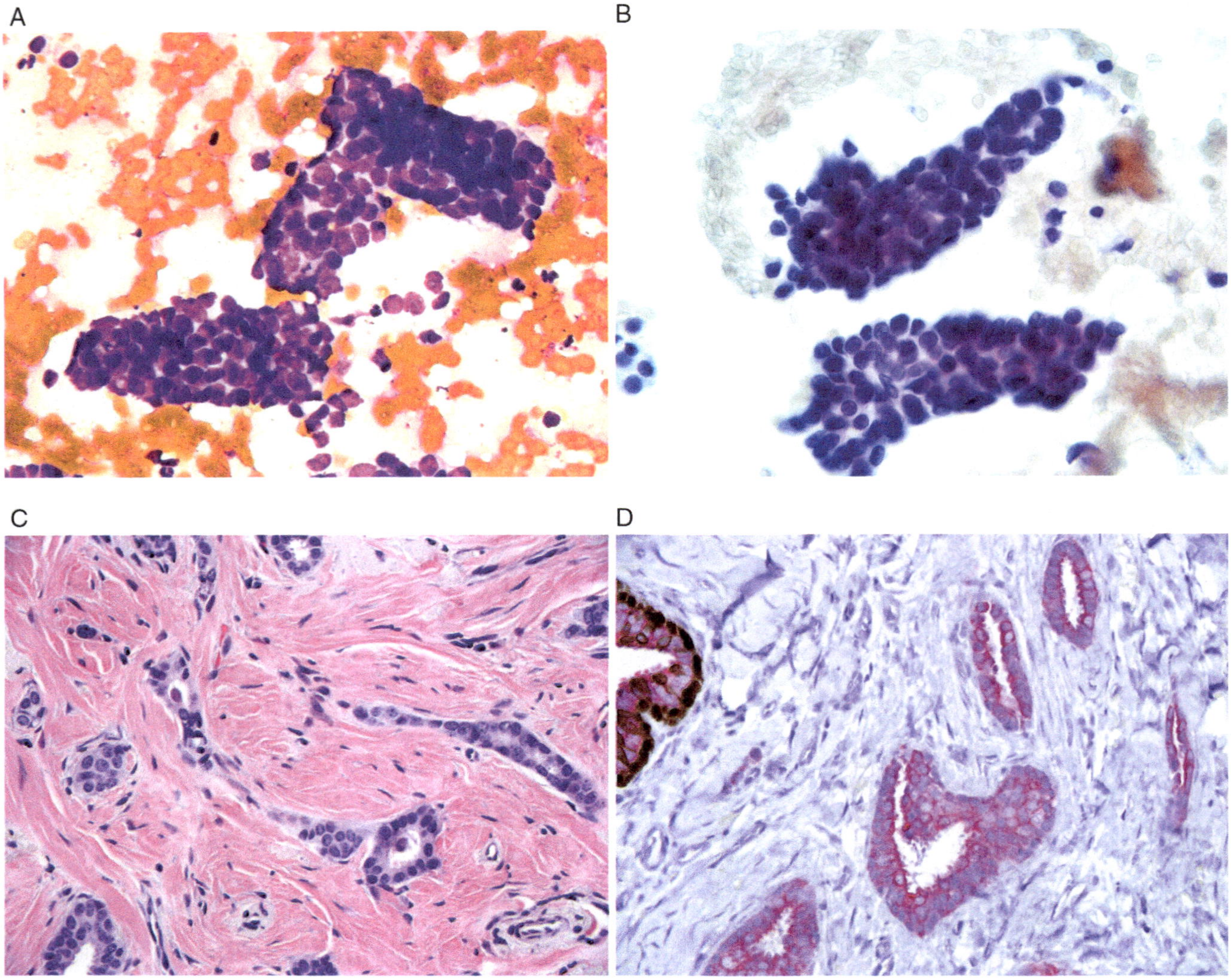

Fig. 5.21 (**a**–**d**) Invasive tubular carcinoma. (**a**) Angulated, pointed atypical ductal epithelial cells with low-grade morphology, Diff-Quik; (**b**) PAP; (**c**) tubular carcinoma, H&E; (**d**) ADH5 staining reveal loss of basal cells

- Usually a palpable soft mass, often in the upper outer quadrant
- Favorable prognosis
- Higher frequency in harboring *breast cancer 1* (*BRCA1*) mutations

Key Radiological Features

- A round, oval, lobulated noncalcified mass with well-defined borders on mammography
- A well-circumscribed, hypoechoic, round or oval, or lobulated mass on ultrasonography

Cytological Features

- Cohesive groups or sheets of ductal cells with marked nuclear atypia
- Many lymphoid cells including plasma cells in the background
- Fig. 5.22a–e

Differential Diagnosis

- Invasive ductal carcinoma, high grade
- High-grade DCIS (comedocarcinoma)
- Metastasis

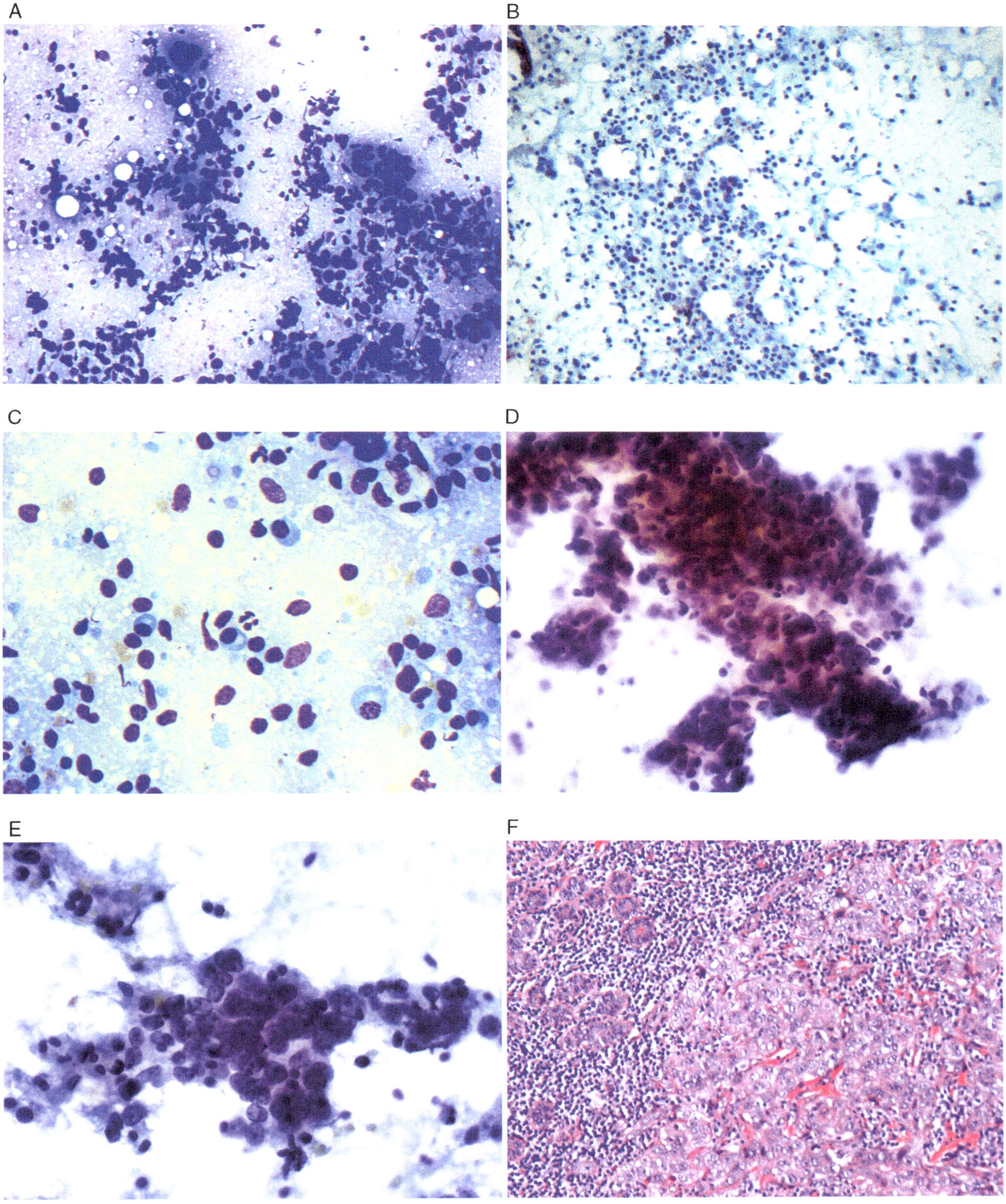

Fig. 5.22 (**a–h**) Medullary carcinoma. (**a**) Cellular smear contains clusters of atypical ductal cells in a background of lymphoid cells, Diff-Quik; (**b**) the same, Pap stain; (**c**) Background lymphocytes and plasma cells, Diff-Quik; (**d**) cohesive cluster of highly atypical ductal epithelial cells with prominent nucleoli admixed with lymphocytes, Diff-Quik; (**e**) the same, Pap stain; (**f**, **g**) histology, medullary carcinoma with syncytial growth pattern and lymphocytes, H&E; (**h**) CK5/6 decorates tumor cells, IHC

G H

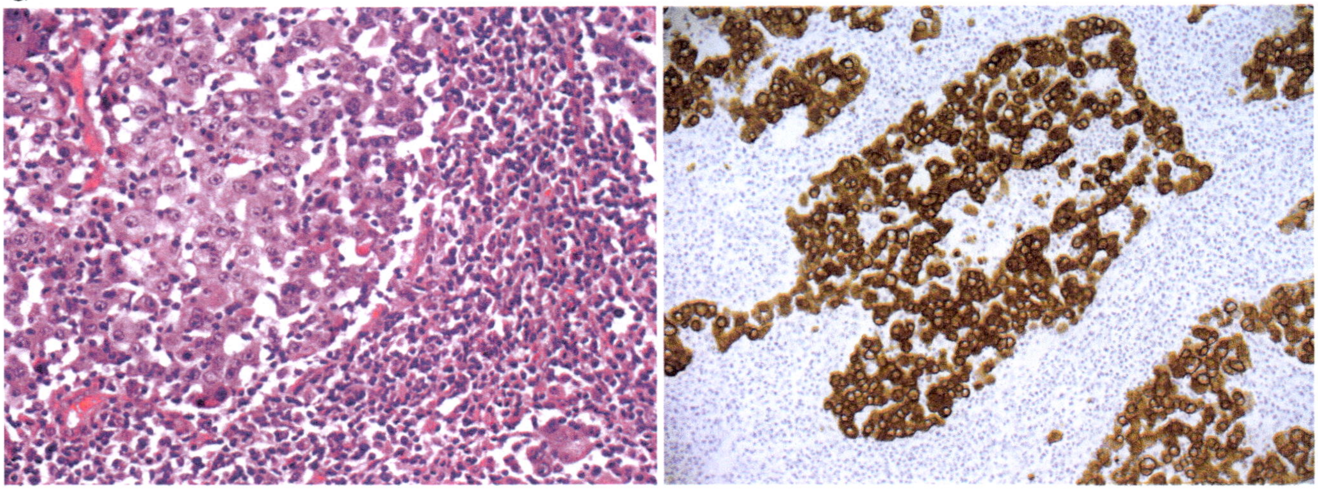

Fig. 5.22 (continued)

Histology

- The diagnostic criteria for medullary carcinoma include a predominantly syncytial growth pattern (>75%), absence of glandular differentiation, a diffuse moderate to marked lymphoplasmacytic infiltrate, high nuclear grade (grade 3), and microscopic circumscription.
- The tumor cells are usually poorly differentiated with high mitotic activity, showing pleomorphic nuclei, coarse chromatin pattern, and prominent nucleoli.
- Representative images are shown in Fig. 5.22f, g.

Immunohistochemistry

- Medullary carcinomas show a basal-like phenotype, expressing epithelial growth factor receptor (EGFR), HMWCK, and CD117 (Fig. 5.22h, CK5/6 staining).
- p53 is positive in a majority of medullary carcinomas.
- GATA3 positive in approximately 50% of cases, usually weak expression
- Typically triple negative (ER-, progesterone [PR]-, Her-2/neu-)

Mucinous Carcinoma

Key Clinical Features

- 1–2% of all invasive breast carcinomas
- More common in older women, with median age of 71 years
- Often presents as a palpable soft mass in the past; nonpalpable mammographic abnormalities at the current time
- Favorable prognosis

Key Radiological Features

- An oval or lobulated mass, well circumscribed, rarely associated with microcalcifications on mammography
- Ultrasonography: a mass with well-defined borders and isoechoic echo texture or hypoechoic with microlobulated margins

Cytological Features

- Cohesive groups or balls of mildly atypical ductal cells without myoepithelial cells
- Single cells with intact cytoplasm
- Mucinous background, which is more easily identifiable on Diff-Quik stain
- Figure 5.23a–d

Differential Diagnosis

- Benign or atypical mucocele-like lesions
- Micropapillary carcinoma

Histology

- The diagnosis of invasive mucinous carcinoma is reserved for tumors with at least a 90% mucinous component.
- The characteristic feature of invasive mucinous carcinoma is the presence of pools of extracellular mucin with nests, trabeculae, acini, or sheets of neoplastic cells.
- Representative images are shown in Fig. 5.23e, f.

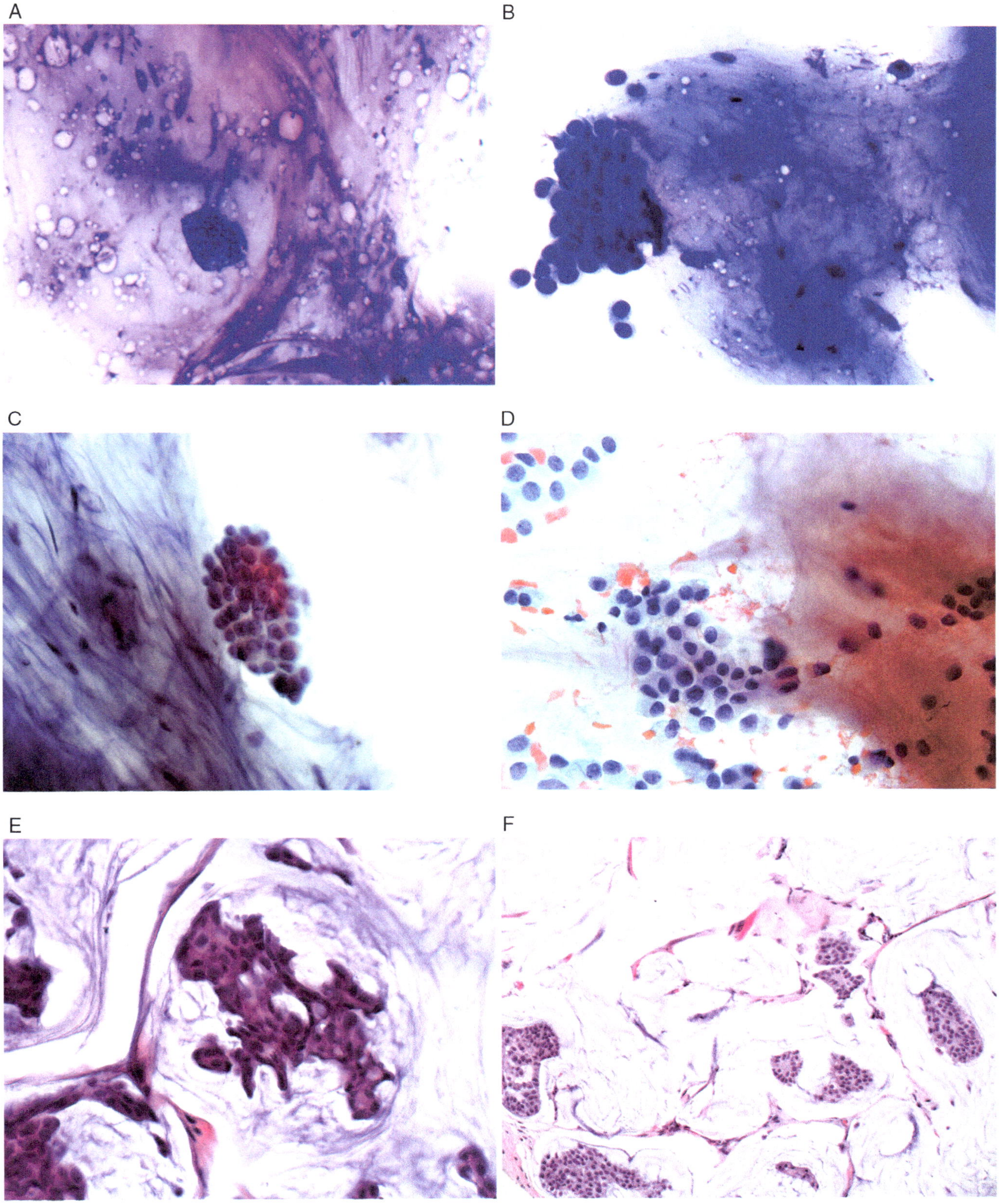

Fig. 5.23 (**a–h**) Mucinous carcinoma. (**a**) Cohesive cluster of mildly atypical ductal epithelial cells in a background of thick mucin, Diff-Quik; (**b**) high-power view shows low-grade morphology, Diff-Quik; (**c**, **d**) the same, Pap stain; (**e**, **f**) Small clusters of mildly atypical ductal epithelial cells with a cribriform pattern floating in a pool of mucin, H&E; (**g**) tumor cell strongly positive for ER, IHC; (**h**) MUC2 decorates tumor cells

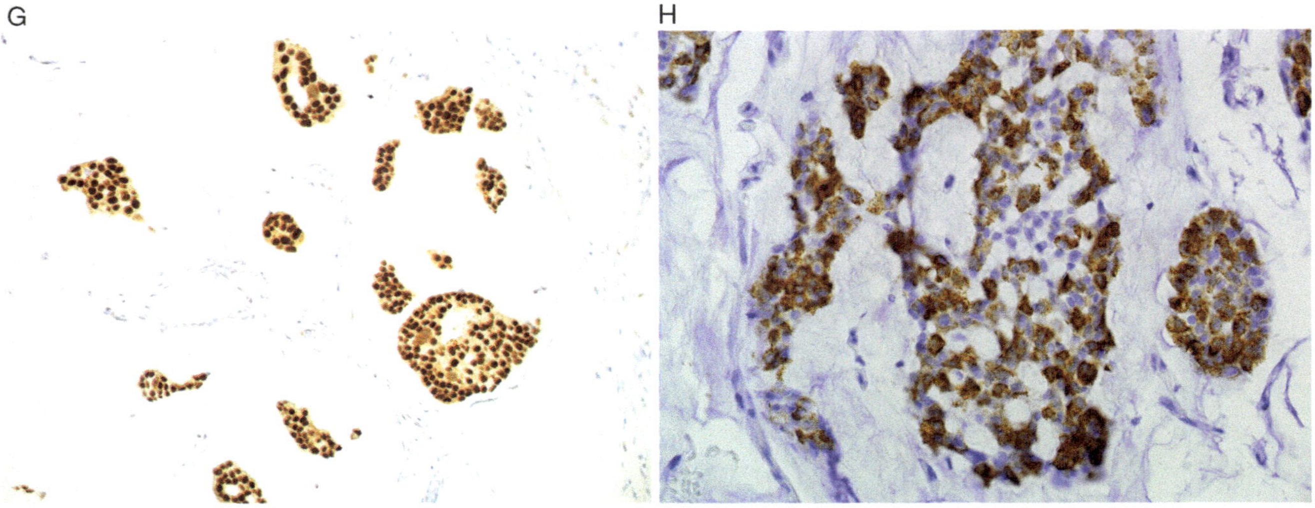

Fig. 5.23 (continued)

Immunohistochemistry

- MEC markers (p63, calponin and SMM-HC) are occasionally utilized to document the lack of myoepithelial cells in neoplastic clusters.
- Neuroendocrine differentiation in mammary mucinous carcinoma has been reported.
- GATA3 positive.
- Mucinous carcinomas are usually positive for ER and PR, negative for Her-2/neu.
- Representative images shown in Fig. 5.23g, h.

Carcinoma with Apocrine Differentiation

Key Clinical Features

- Less than 5% of all invasive breast carcinomas.
- Clinical presentation is no different from that of invasive ductal carcinoma, NOS.

Key Radiological Features

- No distinct imaging features, similar to that of invasive ductal carcinoma, NOS

Cytological Features

- Cellular specimen
- Syncytial fragments or individual atypical cells with large, pleomorphic nuclei, macronucleoli, and abundant basophilic to eosinophilic granular cytoplasm
- Figure 5.24a–c

Differential Diagnosis

- Lipid-rich carcinoma
- Secretory carcinoma
- Granular cell tumor
- Alveolar soft part sarcoma
- Carcinoma with squamous differentiation

Histology

- The overall growth pattern of apocrine carcinoma is no different from invasive ductal carcinoma, NST.
- The neoplastic cells with apocrine differentiation in >90% of the tumor (Rosen's strict definition is the entire tumor.).
- The cytological features of apocrine differentiation include abundant eosinophilic granular cytoplasm or foamy vacuolated cytoplasm and enlarged round vesicular nuclei with prominent eosinophilic (occasionally basophilic) nucleoli.
- Representative images are shown in Fig. 5.24d.

Immunohistochemistry

- Usually androgen receptor (AR) + and triple-negative (ER-, PR-, Her-2/neu-) or Her-2/neu overexpressed (ER-, PR-, Her-2/neu+) tumors.
- A higher rate of EGFR expression is reported in apocrine carcinoma than in conventional ductal carcinoma.
- Nearly all of the apocrine lesions are positive for gross cystic disease fluid protein-15 (GCDFP-15), however, which also decorates non-apocrine breast epithelial cells.
- Apocrine carcinoma is frequently positive for p53, especially in in situ carcinoma.

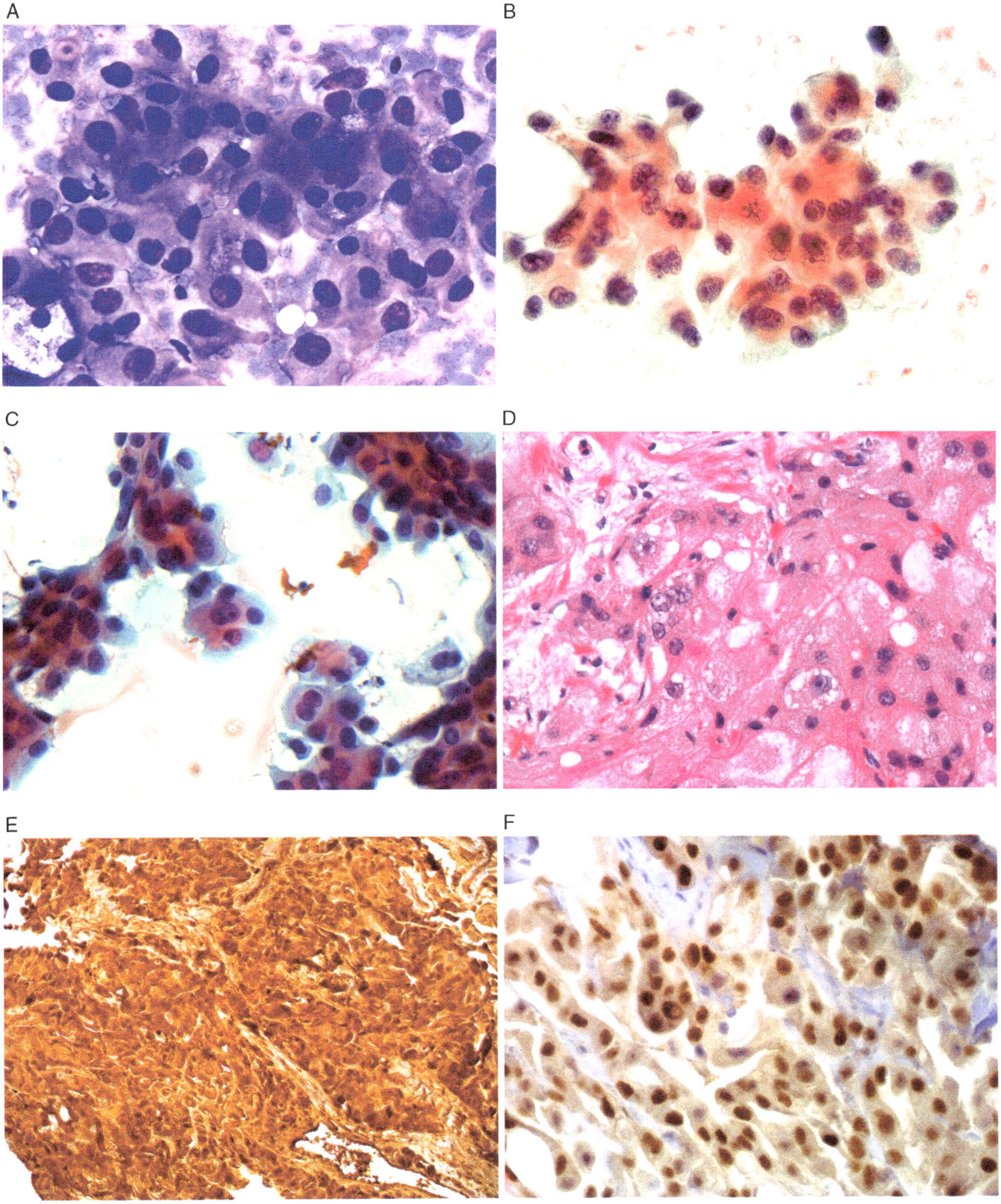

Fig. 5.24 (**a–f**) Apocrine carcinoma. (**a**) Apocrine carcinoma cells with large nuclei, prominent nucleoli and abundant granular cytoplasm, Diff-Quik; (**b**, **c**) the same, PAP; (**d**) histology, tumor cells contain enlarged, round, vesicular nuclei with prominent nucleoli, and abundant eosinophilic granular or foamy vacuolated cytoplasm, H&E; (**e**) strong GCDFP15 staining, IHC; (**f**) nuclear staining for AR, IHC

- GATA3 expression in apocrine carcinomas, in our experience, is variable, showing a heterogeneous staining pattern. Among the six apocrine carcinomas included in our study, two showed strong diffuse positivity, one weak diffuse, two weak focal, and one negative.
- Representative images are illustrated in Fig. 5.24e, f.

Metaplastic Carcinoma

Key Clinical Features

- Less than 1% of all invasive breast carcinomas
- Most common in older women, with a mean age of 68 years
- Presentation similar to that of invasive ductal carcinoma, NOS

Key Radiological Features

- Well-defined mass or densities on mammography or ultrasonography; may reveal microcalcifications or ossifications

Cytological Features

- Heterogeneous, with a mixture of atypical spindle cells and epithelial cells with a variety of differentiations
- Spindle cells and epithelial cells with squamous features
- Inflammatory cells and amorphous debris in the background
- Figure 5.25a–c

Differential Diagnosis

- Adenomyoepithelioma
- Myofibroblastoma
- High-grade ductal carcinoma
- High-grade sarcoma or malignant phyllodes tumor
- Metastasis

Histology

In 2012, WHO defined metaplastic carcinoma as "a group of neoplasms characterized by differentiation of the neoplastic epithelium into squamous cells and/or mesenchymal-looking elements, including but not restricted to spindle, chondroid, osseous, and rhabdomyoid cells." These neoplasms may be composed of either entirely metaplastic elements or a complex admixture of carcinoma and metaplastic areas. Histologically, metaplastic carcinoma has been further subclassified as the following types:

- Low-grade adenosquamous carcinoma (Fig. 5.25d)
- Fibromatosis-like metaplastic carcinoma (Fig. 5.25e)
- Squamous cell carcinoma (Fig. 5.25f)
- Spindle cell carcinoma (Fig. 5.25g)
- Metaplastic carcinoma with mesenchymal differentiation: chondroid differentiation, osseous differentiation, other types of mesenchymal differentiation
- Mixed metaplastic carcinoma (Fig. 5.25h)
- Myoepithelial carcinoma

Immunohistochemistry

- Typically triple-negative tumors (ER-, PR-, Her-2/neu-).
- A broad panel of low molecular weight cytokeratins (LMWCKs) (CAM 5.2, CK19), HMWCKs (CK5/6, CK14, CK17, and CK903), and pan-CK (MNF116) should be applied.
- CK7 was reported in the epithelial element only.
- HMWCKs and pan-CK are among the most sensitive markers to detect CK expression in this setting.
- MEC markers (p63, calponin, CD10, smooth muscle actin [SMA]) are often expressed in metaplastic carcinoma in the spindle cell element.
- The HMWCKs and p63 are most likely to be positive, as shown in Fig. 5.25i, j.

Adenoid Cystic Carcinoma

Key Clinical Features

- Only 0.1% of all invasive breast carcinomas.
- Usually in postmenopausal women, with a mean age of 66 years.
- Clinical presentation is no different from that of invasive ductal carcinoma, NOS.
- Better prognosis.

Key Radiological Features

- No distinct imaging features, similar to that of invasive ductal carcinoma, NOS

Cytological Features

- Hypercellular specimen.
- Cohesive groups of uniform, small basaloid cells with hyperchromatic, angulated nuclei with coarse chromatin pattern, small nucleolus and scant cytoplasm.
- Hyaline globules of basement membrane material are present, eosinophilic on Diff-Quik and pale green on Papanicolaou stain.
- Figure 5.26a–d.

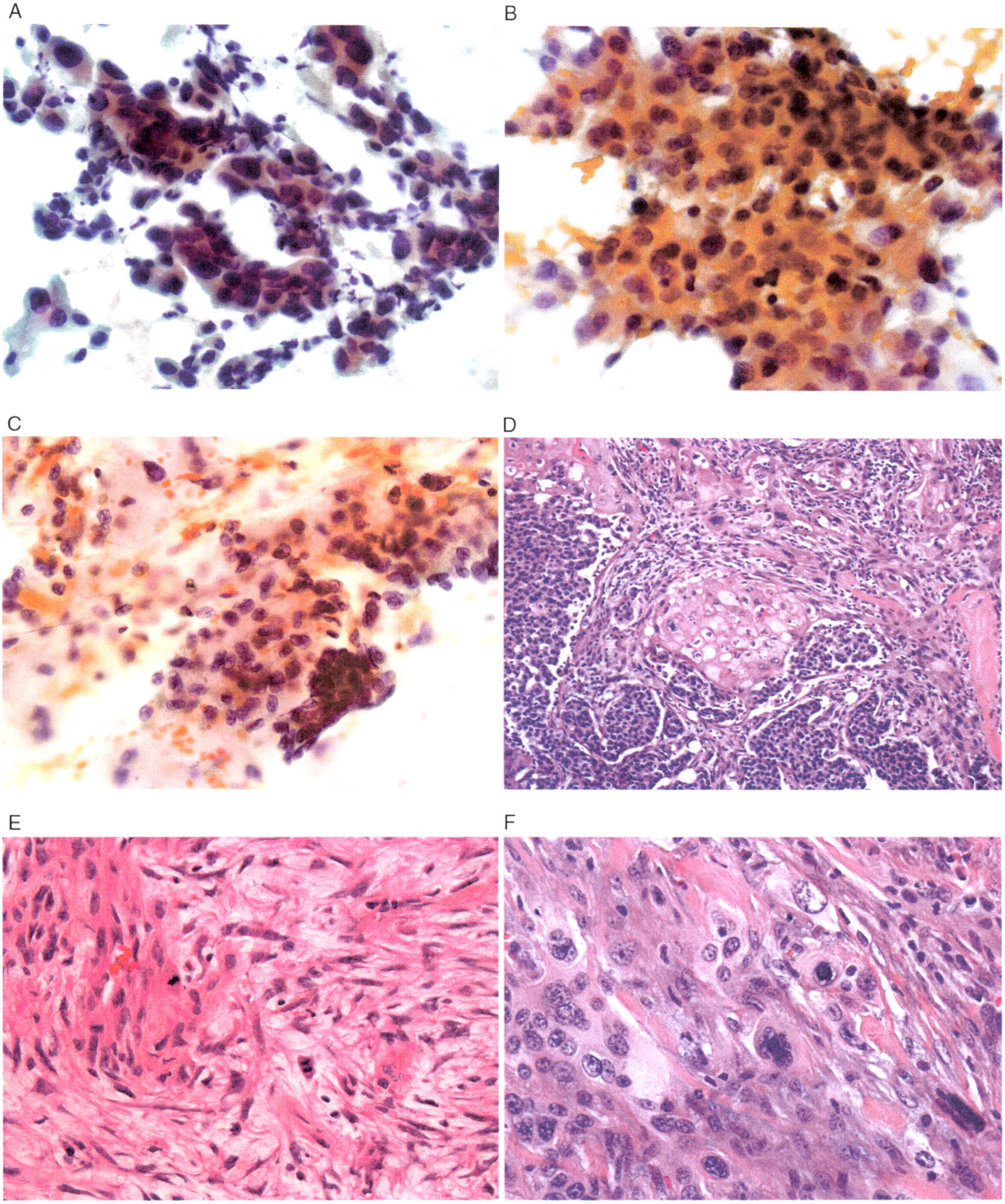

Fig. 5.25 (**a**–**j**) Metaplastic carcinoma, cytology and histology. (**a**, **b**) Spindle cells and epithelial cells with squamous features, Pap stain; (**c**) inflammatory cells and amorphous debris in the background, Pap stain; (**d**) low-grade adenosquamous carcinoma, H&E; (**e**) Fibromatosis-like metaplastic carcinoma, H&E; (**f**) squamous cell carcinoma, H&E; (**g**) spindle cell carcinoma, H&E; (**h**) mixed metaplastic carcinoma, H&E; (**i**) positive CK903 staining in area with squamoid morphology, IHC; (**j**) positive p63 staining in area with squamoid morphology, IHC

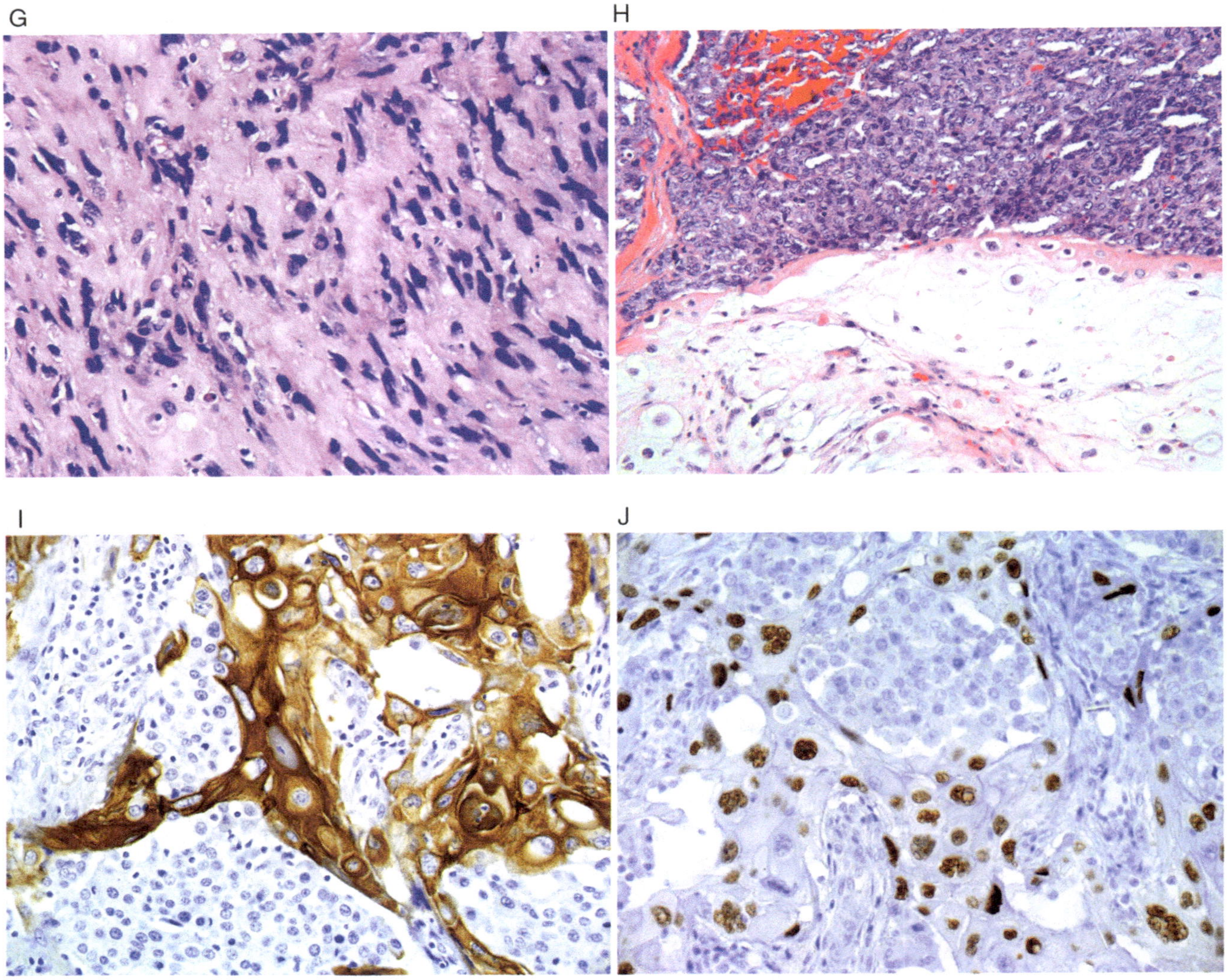

Fig. 5.25 (continued)

Differential Diagnosis

- Collagenous spherulosis
- Invasive cribriform carcinoma

Histology

- Composed of a dual-cell population of epithelial (luminal) and myoepithelial (basaloid) cells forming tubular, cribriform, and solid patterns.
- The neoplastic cells are polarized around glandular spaces or pseudolumina.
- The majority of tumor cells are small and hyperchromatic with scant cytoplasm.
- The glandular spaces are lined by epithelial cells, while the pseudolumina are surrounded by myoepithelial cells containing eosinophilic spherules or cylinders of hyaline material.
- Representative images are shown in Fig. 5.26e–g.

Immunohistochemistry

- Typically a triple-negative (ER-, PR-, and Her-2/neu-) and basal-like carcinoma.
- p63 is a specific myoepithelial marker labeling the myoepithelial (basaloid) cells at the periphery or in the solid area.
- c-kit (CD117) labels the epithelial (luminal) cells, not the myoepithelial cells; therefore, the solid area (which is composed of myoepithelial cells) is nonreactive.
- The eosinophilic hyaline material in the pseudolumens is periodic acid-Schiff (PAS) positive, diastase (D) resistant,

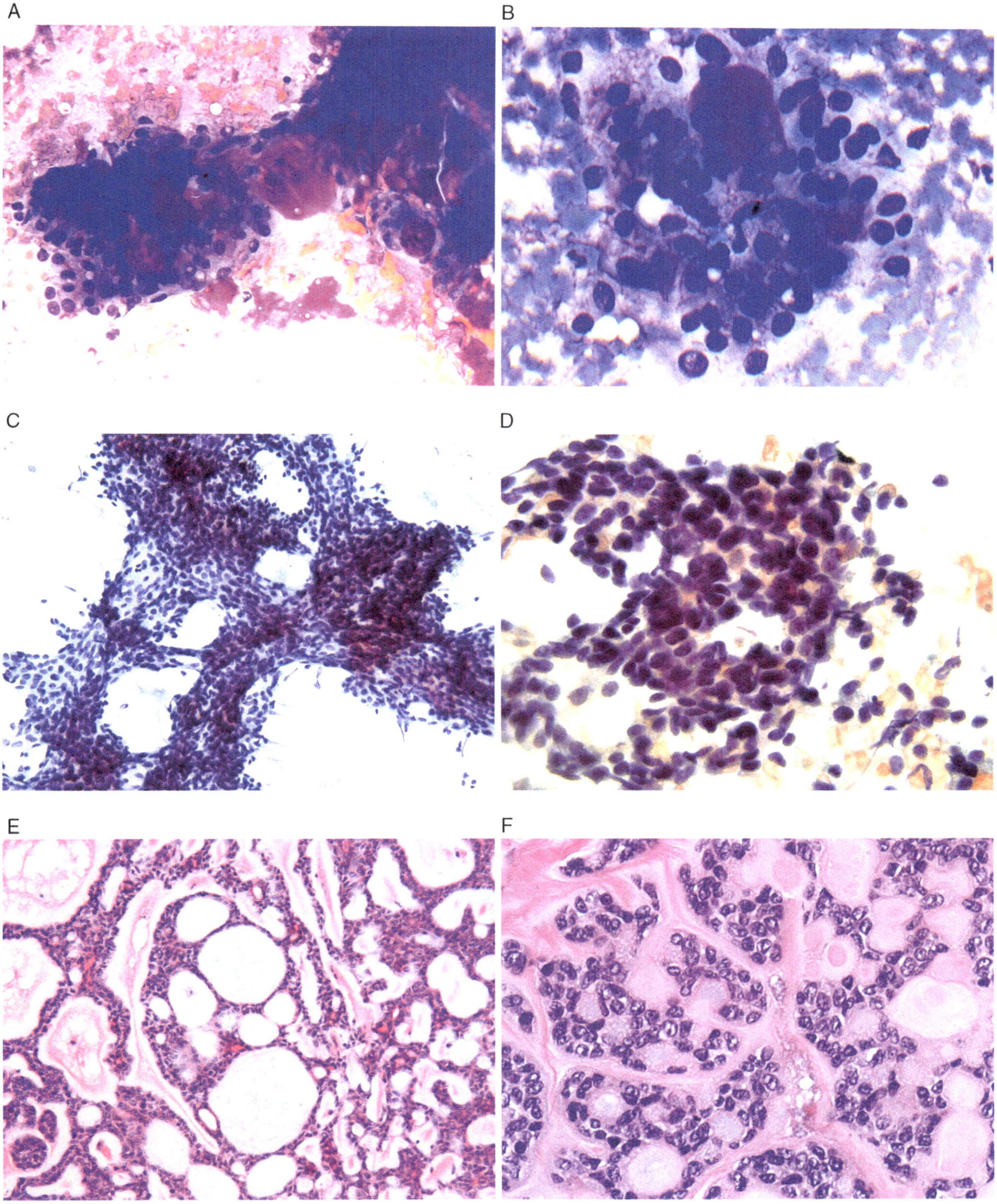

Fig. 5.26 (**a–h**) Adenoid cystic carcinoma, cytology, histology, and immunophenotype. (**a**, **b**) Cohesive groups of uniform, small basaloid cells surrounding eosinophilic hyaline globules, Diff-Quik; (**c**, **d**) the hyaline globules appear pale on Pap stain; the tumor cells are hyperchromatic with an angulated appearance, Pap stain; (**e**) cribriform pattern, H&E; (**f**) pseudolumina containing eosinophilic hyaline material, H&E; (**g**) solid pattern with hyperchromatic, basaloid cells, H&E; (**h**) cocktail p63 and CD117 staining, p63 decorating basal cells (brown, nuclei), while CD117 highlighting luminal cells (pink, cytoplasm), IHC

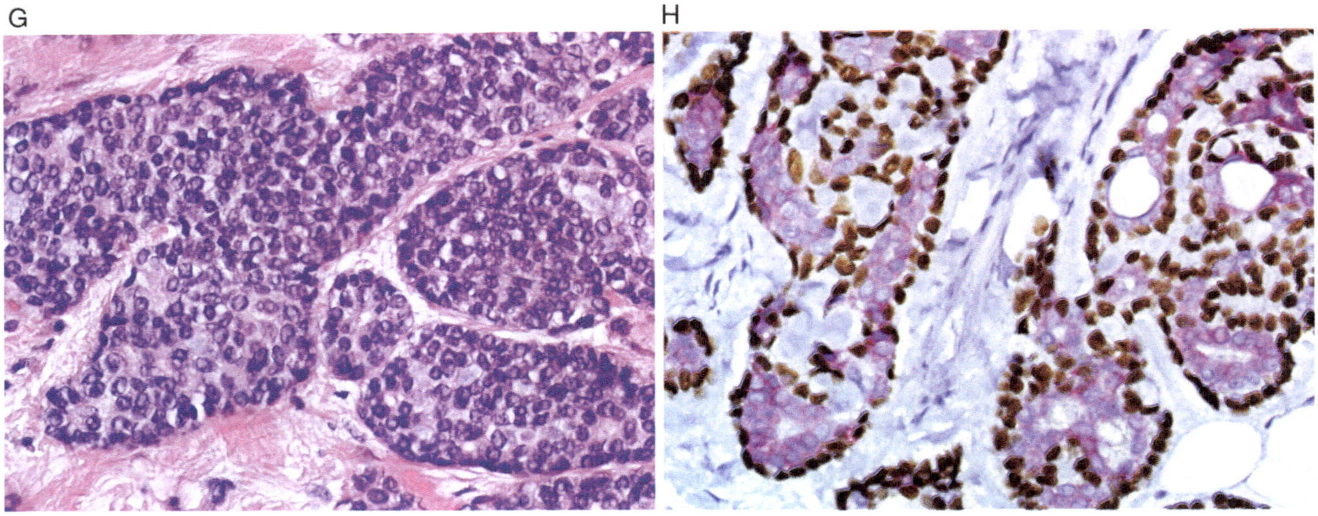

Fig. 5.26 (continued)

and immunohistochemically reactive to collagen IV and laminin; the lightly basophilic myxoid substance in glandular spaces is Alcian blue positive.

- Representative image is illustrated in Fig. 5.26h.

Mesenchymal Tumors

Myofibroblastoma

Key Clinical Features

- Most common in elderly men and women, occasionally associated with gynecomastia
- Usually presents as a slowgrowing, solitary nodule/mass, rarely bilateral and multifocal

Key Radiological Features

- Usually a well-circumscribed, homogeneous solid mass devoid of microcalcifications

Cytological Features

- Cellular smears containing single and clusters of mesenchymal cells with elongated or oval nuclei, a finely granular chromatin pattern, inconspicuous nucleoli, nuclear grooves, occasional intranuclear inclusions, and scant cytoplasm

Differential Diagnosis

- Nodular fasciitis
- Fibromatosis
- Spindle cell metaplastic carcinoma
- Leiomyoma
- Invasive lobular carcinoma: to differentiate from epithelioid cell myofibroblastoma

Histology

- Usually composed of uniform spindle to oval cells arranged in short, haphazardly intersecting fascicles interrupted by thick bands of brightly eosinophilic collagen.
- Adipocytes are present in variable amounts.
- Smooth muscle, cartilaginous, or osseous metaplasia occasionally may be observed.
- No necrosis and rare mitoses are evident.
- There is usually no entrapment of mammary ducts or lobules within the tumor.
- Representative images are shown in Fig. 5.27a–c.

Immunohistochemistry

- The neoplastic cells are positive for desmin, CD34, SMA, Bcl2, CD99, CD10, and hormone receptors (ER, PR, AR).
- H-caldesmon expression is reported in 2–10% of myofibroblastoma cells.
- Representative images are illustrated in Fig. 5.27d–f.

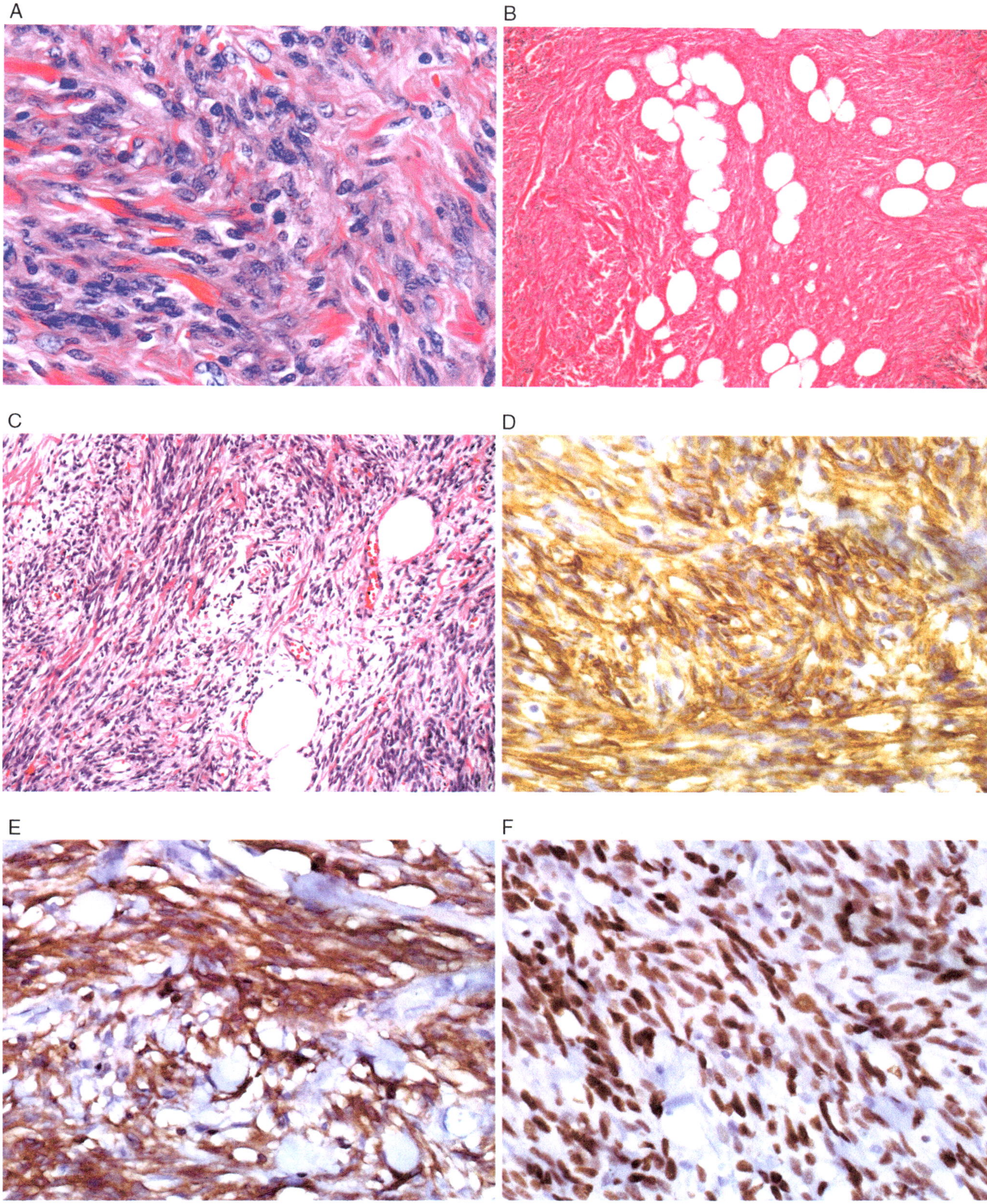

Fig. 5.27 (**a**–**f**) Myofibroblastoma, histology, and immunophenotype. (**a**) Uniform spindled to oval cells arranged in short, haphazardly intersecting fascicles interrupted by thick bands of brightly eosinophilic collagen, H&E; (**b**, **c**) adipocytes are present in variable amounts, H&E; (**d**) rumor cells are positive for CD34; (**e**) Bcl2 decorating tumor cells; (**f**) nuclear staining for AR

Desmoid-Type Fibromatosis

Key Clinical Features

- Most common in women in their second to fourth decades.
- Presents as a firm palpable mass; may be associated with dimpled skin.
- May be sporadic or associated with FAP.
- The sporadic cases may be associated with trauma or history of breast surgery, including implant surgery.

Key Radiological Features

- Mammography: a spiculated mass that simulates carcinoma
- Ultrasonography: a hypoechoic mass

Cytological Features

- Usually sparsely cellular, contains fibrohistiocytic cells, singly or in tissue fragments.
- The cells are spindled and bland; occasional small groups of benign ductal cells may be present.

Differential Diagnosis

- Spindle cell carcinoma
- Lipomatous myofibroblastoma
- Nodular fasciitis

Histology

- Cytologically bland spindle cells arranged in long, sweeping and intersecting fascicles in a collagenous or myxoid background.
- The margins are ill-defined and infiltrative, blending into adjacent normal breast stroma or deep skeletal muscle.
- There are often lymphoid aggregates at the edge.
- Representative images are shown in Fig. 5.28a, b.

Immunohistochemistry

- Aberrant nuclear expression of beta-catenin is reported in 67–100% of cases.
- Keratin, epithelial membrane antigen (EMA), CD31, Bcl-2, and CD34 are negative.
- Actin, desmin, and S100 may be expressed in occasional cases.
- Representative images shown in Fig. 5.28c, d.

Primary Sarcoma

Key Clinical Features

- A heterogeneous group of neoplasms, account for <1% of all breast neoplasms
- Any age of adults, women or men, average age in the sixth decade
- Presenting as a progressively enlarging, typically solitary breast mass, may be associated with pain or skin changes
- Coexisting lymphadenopathy in up to one-third of patients, however reactive by histology.

Key Radiological Features

- Mass lesion, usually lobulated

Cytological Features

- Smears usually contain fragments of cellular mesenchymal tissue and dispersed spindle cells with variable degree of nuclear atypia.
- Primary high-grade sarcomas of the breast are highly cellular, comprised of pleomorphic spindled to plump cells with hyperchromatic nuclei, a coarse chromatin pattern and prominent nucleoli; necrosis is common.
- High-grade angiosarcomas are moderately cellular, composed of clusters and single of atypical plump, spindled and oval cells with a moderate amount of cytoplasm in background of hemorrhage.
- The presence of a few single pleomorphic cells with intracytoplasmic hemosiderin deposits in a hemorrhagic background should raise the diagnostic possibility of angiosarcoma.
- The presence of small clusters of cells or vasoformative features, such as microacini, fragments of arborizing microtissue, and intracytoplasmic lumen in a bloody background, suggests vascular differentiation.

Differential Diagnosis

- Spindle cell carcinoma
- Malignant phyllodes tumor
- Fibromatosis
- Nodular fasciitis
- Spindle cell melanoma

Histology

- Depending on the specific tumor type, primary mammary sarcomas show histologic features similar to those arising from soft tissue.

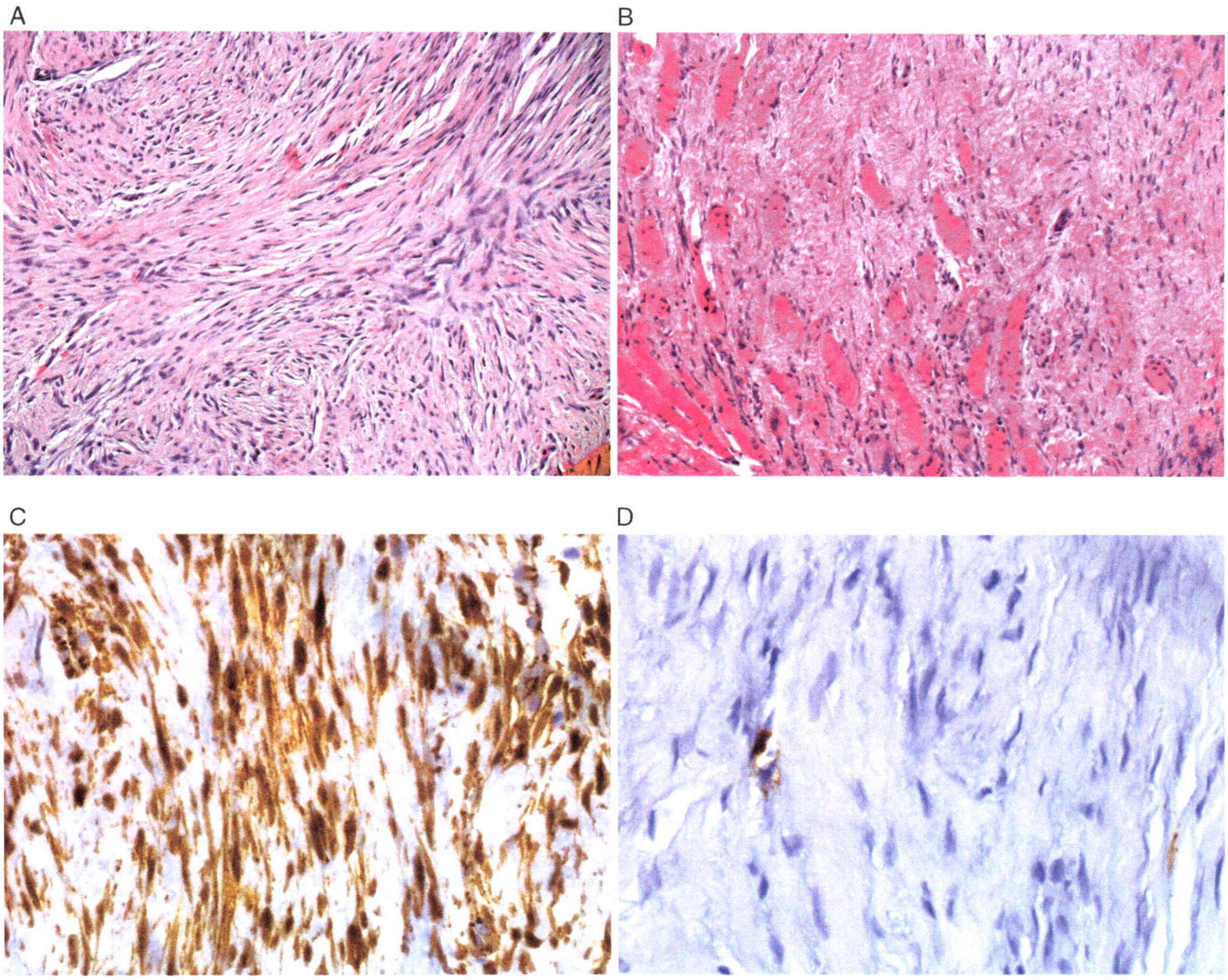

Fig. 5.28 (**a–d**) Desmoid-type fibromatosis, histology, and immunophenotype. (**a**, **b**) Cytologically bland spindle cells arranged in long, sweeping, and intersecting fascicles in a collagenous or myxoid background, focally infiltrating underlying skeletal muscle, H&E; (**c**) nuclear staining for β-catenin; (**d**) negative for CD34, rare capillary highlighted

- Angiosarcoma: the most common, composed of a broad spectrum of growth patterns (vasoformative, solid, papillary endothelial, and capillary-type patterns) and variable nuclear atypia; the neoplastic cells may be flat, plump, spindled, or epithelioid in shapes; can be classified as low (type I), intermediate (type II), and high (type III) grade based on histomorphology on resection specimens.
- Liposarcoma: includes well-differentiated, myxoid, pleomorphic, and dedifferentiated.
- Leiomyosarcoma is composed of fascicles of smooth muscle cells with nuclear atypia, mitosis, and necrosis; epithelioid morphology and heterogeneous elements have been reported.
- Representative images of angiosarcoma are shown in Fig. 5.29a–d.

Immunohistochemistry

- For liposarcoma, IHC or fluorescence in situ hybridization (FISH) for mouse double minute 2 homolog (MDM2) and cyclin-dependent kinase 4 (CDK4) may help to confirm the diagnosis and exclude other types of sarcoma or benign fatty tumors.
- Leiomyosarcoma is immunohistochemically positive for actin and desmin.
- Angiosarcoma is positive for vascular markers (CD31, CD34, Factor VIII) and ETS-related gene (ERG) and negative for cytokeratin and EMA; ER and PR are negative in the majority of angiosarcomas.
- An example of angiosarcoma is illustrated in Fig. 5.29e, f.

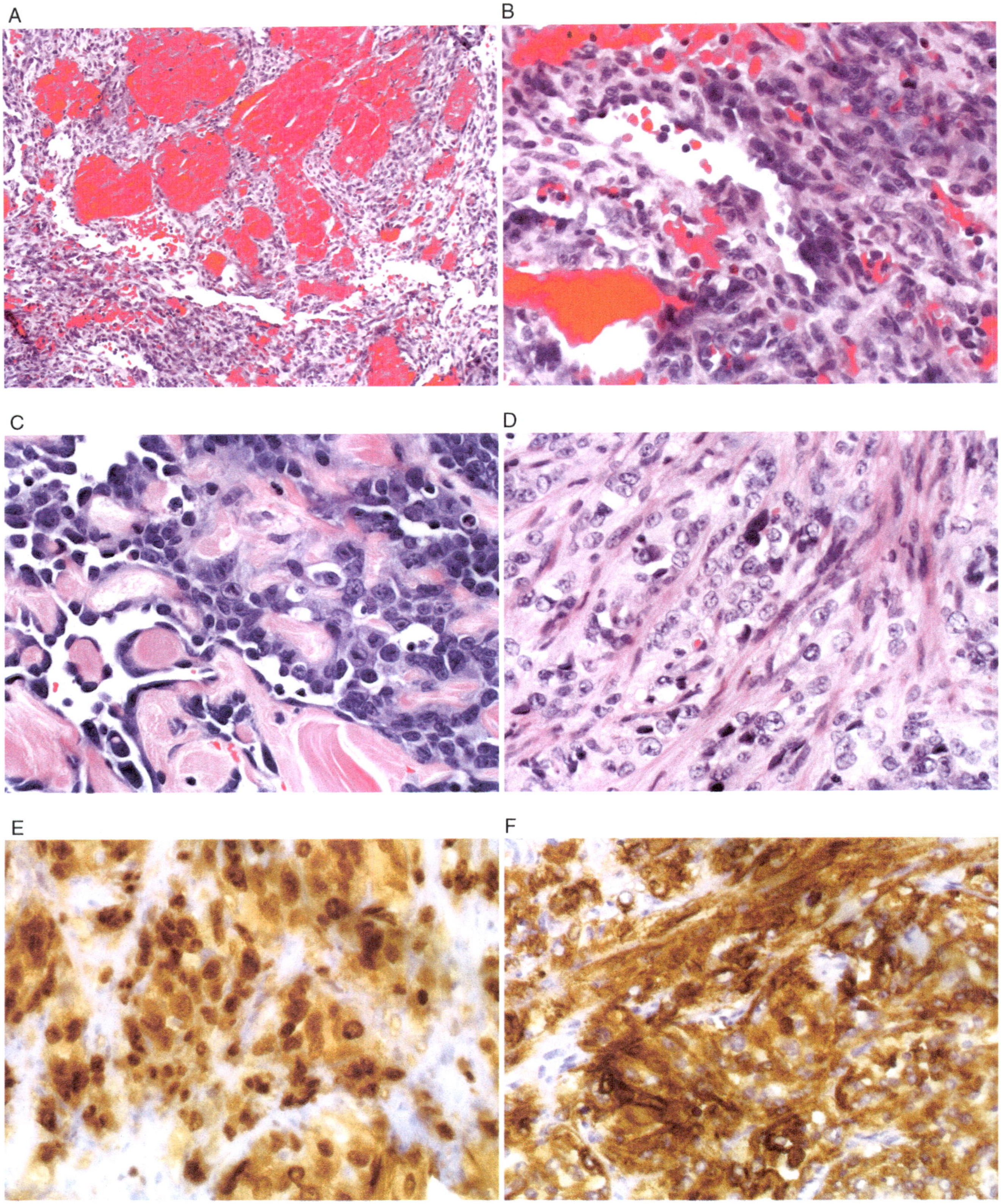

Fig. 5.29 (**a**–**f**) Angiosarcoma of the breast, histology and immunophenotype. (**a**–**d**) Vasoformative growth, with production of highly infiltrative, irregularly configured vascular channels, with intraluminal papillary projections, and variety of growth patterns that varies from sieve-like to solid, H&E; (**e**) ERG decorates tumor cells, nuclear staining pattern; (**f**) tumor cells are positive for CD31

Lymphoma

Clinical Features

- Rare, <0.5% of all breast malignancies.
- Often seen in postmenopausal women.
- The majority are non-Hodgkin's lymphomas, most common diffuse large B-cell lymphoma.
- Usually presents with a palpable, painless breast mass lesion.

Radiological Features

- Radiographic features are variable, indistinguishable from invasive carcinomas.

Cytological Features

- Hypercellular smears consist of a population of monomorphic atypical lymphocytes in a background of round basophilic cytoplasmic fragments (lymphoglandular bodies).
- Cytological features of the tumor cells are identical to those of lymphomas arising from lymph nodes, based on the type of lymphoma.
- Figure 5.30a, b.

Differential Diagnosis

- Poorly differentiated carcinomas
- Neuroendocrine tumors
- Granulocytic sarcoma
- Chronic mastitis

Histology

- The diagnosis of lymphomas of the breast requires integration of clinical, morphologic, immunophenotypic, genetic, and flow cytometric information.
- Lymphomas of the breast are commonly well-circumscribed tumors of varying size; however, histologically, the borders are infiltrative, with tumor cells permeating around lobules and ducts.
- The histomorphology is similar to those seen at other anatomic sites, depending on the tumor type. Diffuse large B-cell lymphoma is composed of sheets of large atypical lymphoid cells with irregular nuclear contours, a vesicular chromatin pattern, and prominent nucleoli. The tumor cells infiltrate and replace the underlying normal breast lobular structures.
- Representative image of a cell block section is shown in Fig. 5.30c.

Immunohistochemistry and Flow Cytometry Studies

- Depending on the tumor type, mammary lymphomas show identical phenotypes by IHC, flow cytometry studies, and/or cytogenetic evaluations.
- Diffuse large B-cell lymphomas express CD20, CD79a, and paired box gene 5 (PAX5) and variably express germinal center-associated and other B-cell subset markers, including CD10 (−/+), CD5 (−/+), Bcl6 (+/−), and interferon regulatory factor 4 protein/multiple myeloma 1 [IRF4/MUM-1] (+/−). Immunostains for CD3, cyclin D1, and cytokeratins are negative. Representative images shown in Fig. 5.30d–f.

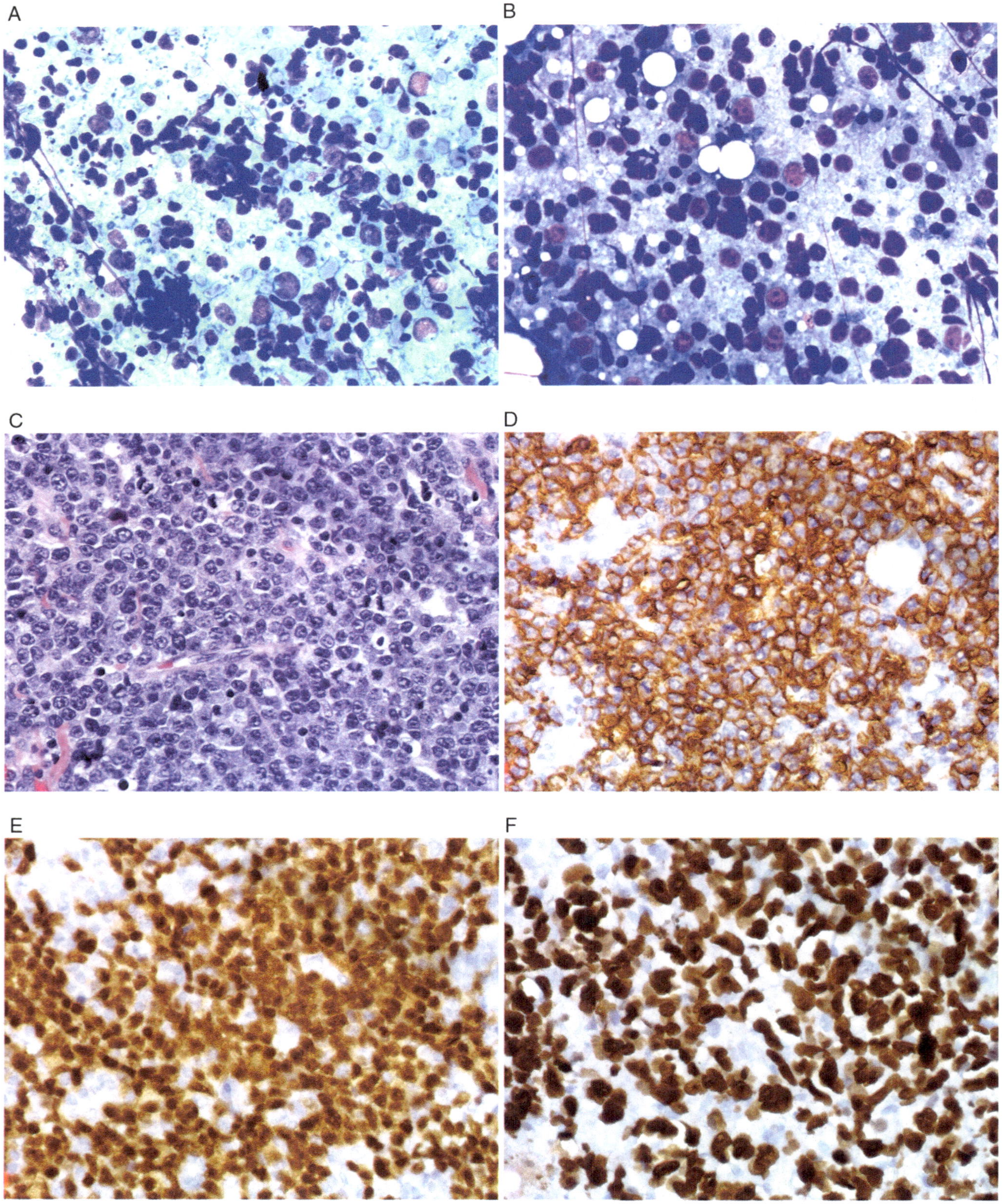

Fig. 5.30 (**a–f**) Diffuse large B-cell lymphoma of the breast. (**a**) Highly cellular smear comprised of individual blue cells, Diff-Quik; (**b**) tumor cells with large, vesicular nuclei, prominent nucleoli in background of lymphoglandular bodies, Diff-Quik; (**c**) core biopsy shows monotonous atypical lymphocytes with large nuclei, prominent nucleoli, and abundant mitotic activity, H&E; (**d**) positive for CD20, IHC; (**e**) nuclear decoration with PAX5, IHC; (**f**) high MIB-1 labeling, estimated at over 90%, IHC

Case Presentations

The following are three cases that are commonly encountered in daily practice. Case Scenario 1 is a case of intracystic (encapsulated) papillary carcinoma of the breast. The objective of this case presentation is to demonstrate an algorithmic approach for the workup of papillary lesions. Case Scenario 2 is a mammary spindle cell carcinoma. The objective is to illustrate the crucial role of IHC in the diagnosis of spindle cell lesions. Case Scenario 3 is a gastric metastasis of mammary lobular carcinoma. The objective is to illustrate the utility and pitfalls of breast organ-specific immunomarkers.

Case Scenario 1

Learning Objectives

1. To exercise histo- and cytomorphological diagnosis of papillary lesions
2. To illustrate an algorithmic approach for the diagnostic workup of papillary lesions
3. To suggest the effective panel of immunomarkers for the diagnosis of papillary lesions

Case

The diagnosis of papillary lesions of the breast is often challenging, especially in small biopsy specimens. IHC is commonly applied in this setting, using the algorithmic approach as provided in the previous section. The role of IHC workup on cytology cell block material is limited in the setting of papillary lesions.

A 69-year-old female presented with nipple discharge and a slow growing nodule/mass for a year. Mammogram revealed a multinodular increased density in upper right quadrant toward central region. An ultrasound-guided FNA and CNB were performed. The smears were cellular, comprised of papillary fragments and abundant single cells with a columnar or elongated appearance, as illustrated in Fig. 5.31a–e. The CNB revealed multiple cores of tissue comprised of vaguely papillary fragments containing a delicate fibrovascular stalk with overlying proliferation of monotonous neoplastic epithelial cells showing low-to-intermediate-grade nuclei. The neoplastic cells were focally arranged in solid or cribriform patterns. Focal surrounding thick fibrous capsule and cystic spaces were appreciated. No discernible myoepithelial cells were identified in the stalks and at periphery. Immunohistochemical studies including ADH5 and ER were performed and illustrated in Fig. 5.31f–h.

Papillary lesions encompass a spectrum of tumors from benign papilloma to invasive papillary carcinoma. The first step in the workup of a papillary lesion is to determine its benign vs malignant nature; this can be achieved by morphological assessment and, more accurately, the application of basal/myoepithelial markers, especially p63, calponin and HMWCKs (CK903, CK5/6, and CK14). The lack of basal/myoepithelial cells (both at the periphery and over fibrovascular stalks) identifies a malignancy, either intracystic (encapsulated) papillary carcinoma or invasive papillary carcinoma. The presence of basal/myoepithelial cells classifies the papillary lesion as benign or atypical. The latter includes ADH or DCIS involving papilloma and papillary carcinoma in situ. The next step is to separate benign from atypical, which is often achieved by the application of HMWCK (commonly CK903 or CK5/6) and ER. Studies well documented that ADH/DCIS is a neoplastic process with a clonal proliferation of luminal epithelial cells; by immunohistochemistry, these lesions show lack of or focal weak expression for HMWCK. In contrast, UDH is a hyperplastic process, exhibiting a mosaic staining pattern for ADH5, a cocktail consisting CK7, CK AE1/3, p63, CK903, and CK14. In addition, ER expression is scattered in UDH and diffuse in ADH/DCIS. However, papilloma itself is usually ER positive in a diffuse and strong fashion; therefore, caution should be exercised when interpreting the ER result. The loss of expression for HMWCK in conjunction with diffuse strong expression of ER in an area of proliferation suggests an atypical papillary lesion (ADH/DCIS involving papilloma or papillary DCIS), while a mosaic pattern of staining for HMWCK in conjunction with patchy weak expression for ER is in favor of a benign papilloma.

The current case reveals loss of myoepithelial cells (p63-, both at the periphery and over the stalks), loss of expression for HMWCK, and diffuse strong nuclear staining for ER; the phenotype supports the diagnosis of an encapsulated papillary carcinoma.

Case Scenario 2

Learning Objectives

1. To exercise histo- and cytomorphological diagnosis of spindle cell lesions
2. To illustrate the diagnostic workup of spindle cell lesions, especially metaplastic carcinoma
3. To suggest the effective panel of immunomarkers for the diagnosis of metaplastic carcinoma

(continued)

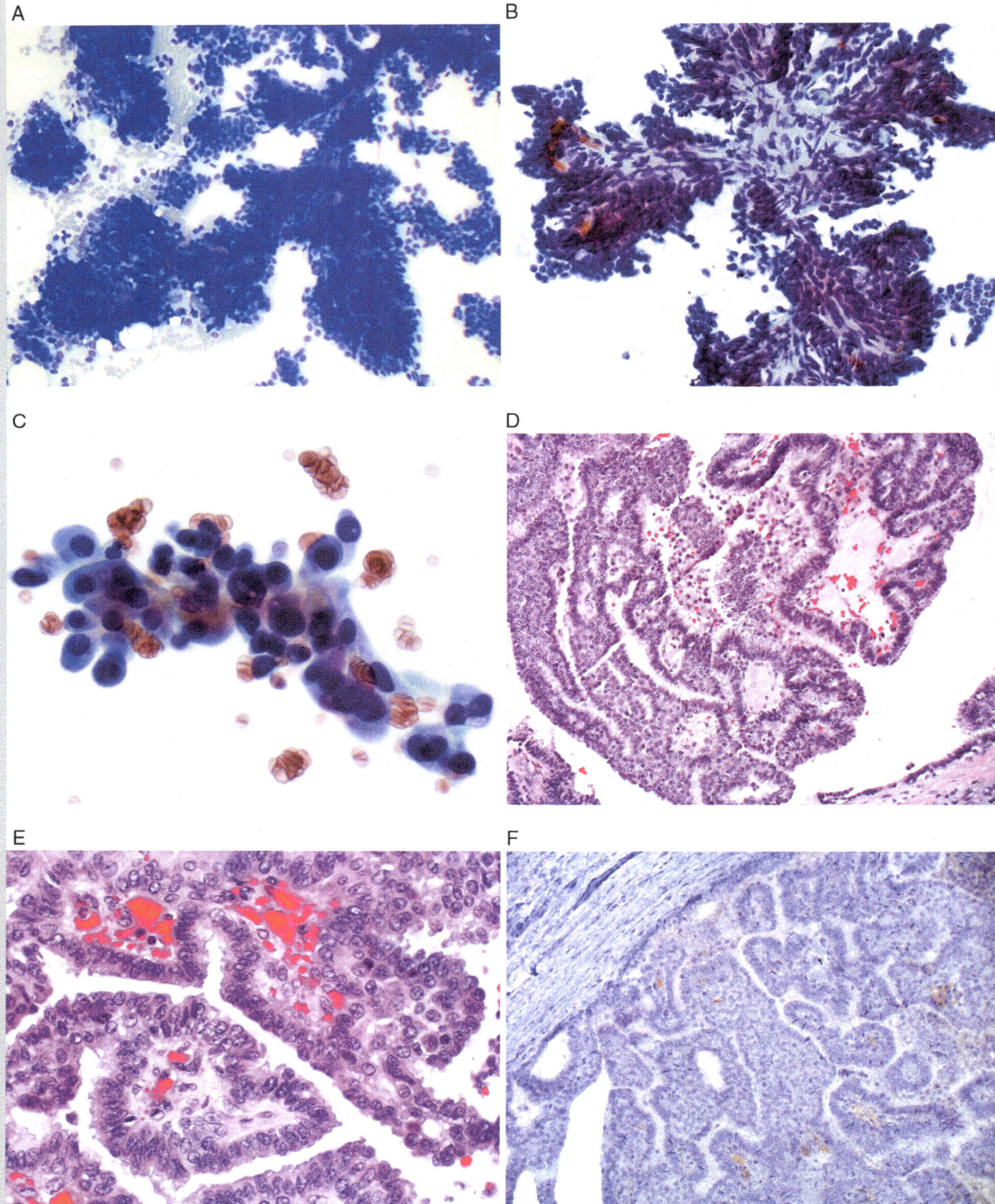

Fig. 5.31 (**a–h**) Encapsulated papillary carcinoma, cytology, histology, and immunophenotype. (**a**) Many papillary fragments of atypical ductal cells, Diff-Quik; (**b**) fibrovascular core with overlying monomorphic tumor cells, some with columnar morphology, Pap stain; (**c**) focally mild pleomorphic, with columnar morphology, Pap stain; (**d**) histology, papillary proliferation within cystic space, H&E; (**e**) high-power view of fibrovascular cores with overlying single or focally stratified ductal cells with columnar morphology, H&E; (**f**) p63 stain reveals lack of basal cells at the periphery and over vascular cores, IHC; (**g**) tumor cells show loss of expression for CK903, BNC5, IHC; (**h**) diffuse ER expression, IHC

(continued)

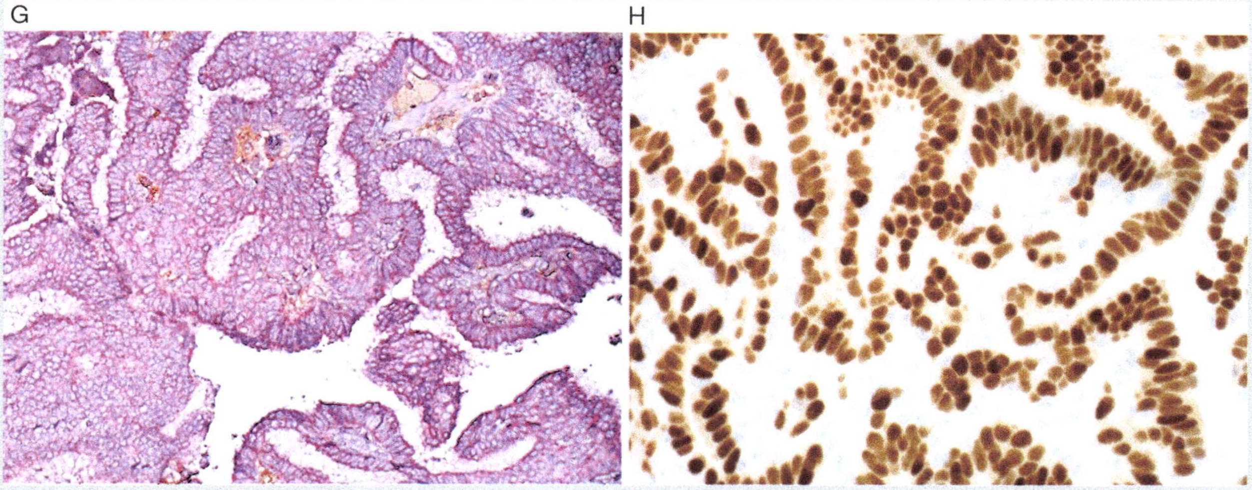

Fig. 5.31 (continued)

Case

The diagnostic approach for spindle cell lesion of the breast should focus on the exclusion of spindle cell carcinoma, due to the fact that primary spindle cell lesions of other types are rare. Therefore, is this a spindle cell carcinoma? That is always the first question to ask when encountering a spindle cell lesion of the breast. If the answer is yes, the case is done. If the answer is no, the next question is: is this a benign or malignant lesion? If it is malignant, the next question is: primary or secondary? Is it low grade or high grade? What is the lineage of the tumor? To answer those questions, IHC analysis plays an essential role. Here we propose an effective small panel of immunomarkers in the workup of a spindle cell lesion, particularly the metaplastic carcinoma of the mammary gland.

A 52-year-old female presented with a palpable breast mass of 2 cm. An ultrasound-guided FNA was performed, followed by CNB. The smears were moderately cellular, comprised of a mixture of mildly atypical spindle cells singly or in clusters, and occasional atypical epithelial cells with squamoid features. Neutrophils and amorphous debris were seen in the background, as illustrated in Fig. 5.32a, b. The CNB specimen revealed cores of tissue composed of a proliferation of mildly atypical spindle cells, rare multinucleated giant cells, and focal nests of epithelial cells with squamous differentiation. Focal necrosis and neutrophilic infiltrates were noted. Immunoassays were performed. Representative images are illustrated in Fig. 5.32c–h.

The World Health Organization Classification of Tumors of the Breast (2012) defines the metaplastic carcinoma of the mammary gland as "a group of neoplasms characterized by differentiation of the neoplastic epithelium into squamous cells and/or mesenchymal-looking elements, including but not restricted to spindle, chondroid, osseous, and rhabdomyoid cells." Histologically, there is a wide range of appearances. In 2012, WHO further classified metaplastic carcinoma into the following subtypes: (1) low-grade adenosquamous carcinoma, (2) fibromatosis-like metaplastic carcinoma, (3) squamous cell carcinoma, (4) spindle cell carcinoma, (5) metaplastic carcinoma with mesenchymal differentiation, and (6) mixed metaplastic carcinomas. The diagnosis of metaplastic carcinoma is challenging and often requires IHC studies with multiple immunomarkers, especially in small biopsy tissues. For tumors with spindled, low-grade morphology, the differential diagnosis usually includes malignant phyllodes tumor, fibromatosis, or even nodular fasciitis. For tumors with high-grade morphology,

(continued)

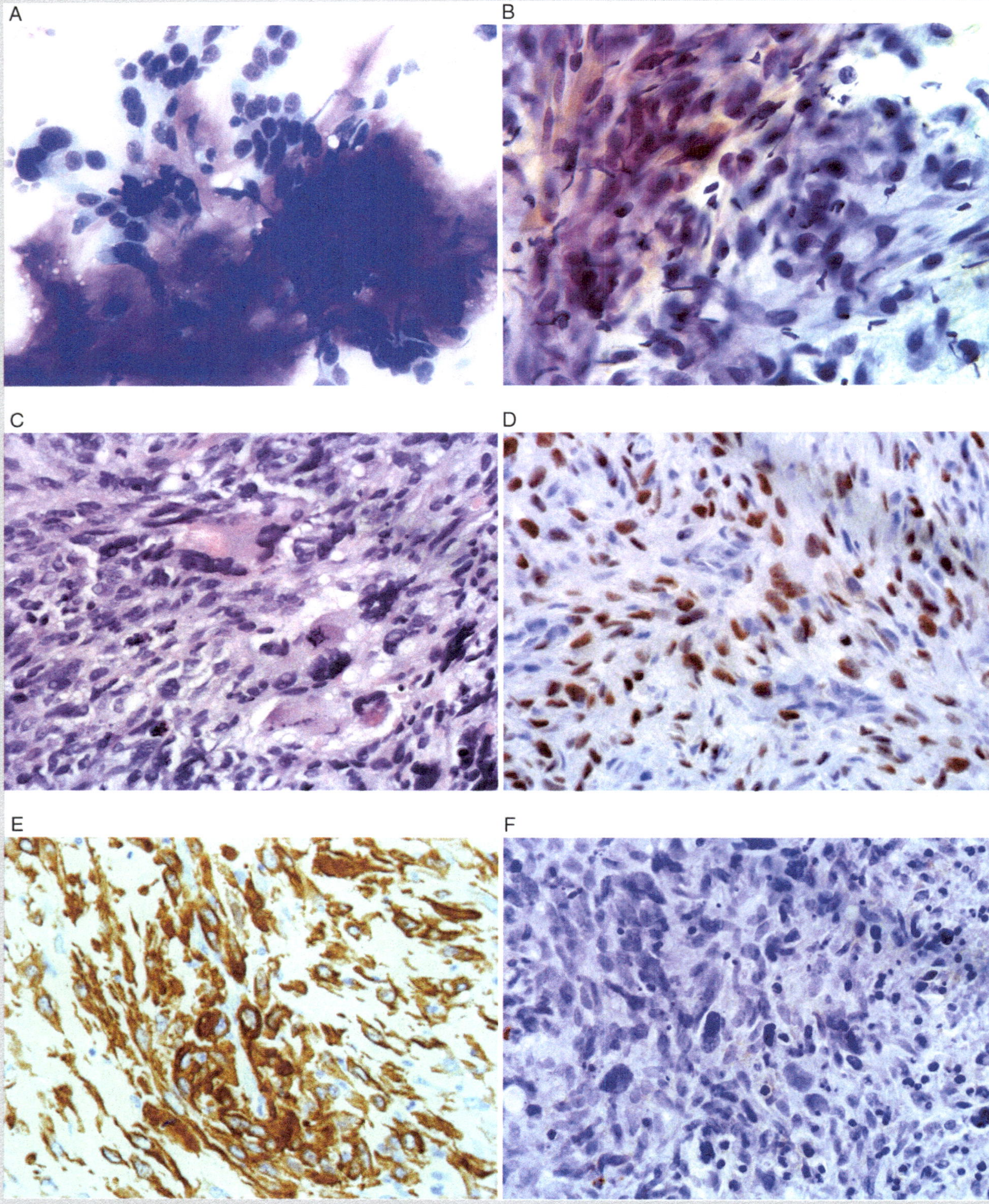

Fig. 5.32 (**a**–**h**) Metaplastic carcinoma. (**a**) Cluster of plump to spindled cells embedded in stromal tissue, Diff-Quik; (**b**) a typical spindled cells with scattered neutrophils, Pap stain; (**c**) H&E section revealing a metaplastic carcinoma comprised of highly atypical spindle cells with few multinucleated forms. Nests of malignant epithelial cells with squamoid features are noted but not shown in the photo; (**d**) p63 decorating scattered nuclei in spindle cell component as well as the epithelial nests (not shown); (**e**) CK903 decorating the epithelial cells and the spindle cell component; (**f**) CD34 is negative; (**g**) β-catenin stain shows a cytoplasmic granular pattern, no nuclear positivity; (**h**) EMA positive in spindle cell component

(continued)

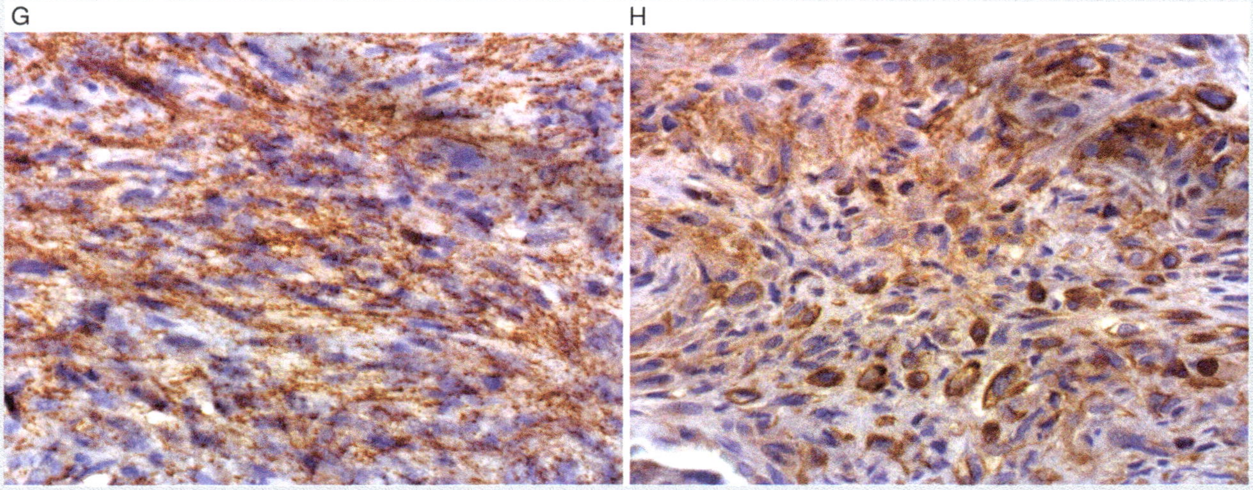

Fig. 5.32 (continued)

primary mammary sarcoma and metastasis should be considered in the differential diagnosis. The first step in establishing a diagnosis of metaplastic carcinoma is to confirm its epithelial differentiation; therefore, a broad panel of cytokeratins, especially HMWCK (CK903, CK5/6, and CK14) and pan-cytokeratin, such as AE1/AE3, is often applied. The majority of metaplastic carcinomas express cytokeratins in the spindle cell components, usually focally. Luminal cytokeratins, such as CK7 and CAM5.2, are commonly negative. No single cytokeratin is expressed in all metaplastic carcinomas; therefore, a panel of a variety of cytokeratins, including both basal and luminal types, is essential. However, not all spindle cell lesions with cytokeratin expression are metaplastic carcinomas. Metastatic spindle cell melanomas and leiomyosarcomas may express cytokeratin, usually CAM5.2. Therefore, one should interpret IHC results on the basis of histomorphology. In addition to the frequent expression of cytokeratins, especially basal keratins, metaplastic carcinomas often express other basal or myoepithelial markers. p63 is positive in >90% of cases and carries a higher specificity. p63 has not been reported in the entities in the differential diagnosis of metaplastic carcinomas, such as phyllodes tumors and

Table 5.2. Differential immunophenotypes of metaplastic carcinoma, phyllodes tumor, and fibromatosis

Tumor/marker	CK903	AE1/AE3	p63	β-catenin	CD34	Bcl2
MCA	+, focal	+, focal	+	−/+, N	−	−
PT	−	−	−	+, N	+	+
Fibromatosis	−	−	−	+, N	−	−

NOTE: The differential phenotype applies to the spindle cell component of the tumors
MCA metaplastic carcinoma, *N* nuclear, *PT* phyllodes tumor, + positive, − negative

fibromatosis. Therefore, the best panel of immunomarkers consists of CK903 or CK5/6, AE1/AE3, and p63. In addition, CD34 and Bcl2 should be included in the panel to differentiate metaplastic carcinoma from phyllodes tumor. When fibromatosis is in the differential consideration, the addition of β-catenin may be helpful. The differential IHC phenotypes are summarized in Table 5.2.

Metaplastic carcinomas are often triple-negative tumors with the expression of CK5/6 and/or EGFR, belonging to the basal-like tumor group.

The current case revealed patchy positivity for AE1/AE3, CK903, and p63, while negative for CD34 and Bcl2, supporting the diagnosis of a metaplastic

(continued)

carcinoma. Hormonal analyses reveal the tumor to be triple negative (ER-, PR-, Her-2/neu-).

Case Scenario 3

Learning Objectives

1. To illustrate the diagnostic workup for metastatic breast carcinomas
2. To suggest the effective panel of immunomarkers for the identification of breast primary
3. To discuss the applications and pitfalls of commonly used immunomarkers in breast pathology

Case

Gastric metastases are rare events. Breast carcinoma has been reported as the most common tumor to metastasize to the stomach. The histomorphology may suggest a possible primary site; however, IHC assays are essential for an accurate diagnosis in this context.

A 60-year-old female with no known past medical history of malignancy presented with dyspepsia and heartburn not responsive to medical treatment. An upper GI endoscopy was performed, revealing erythematous gastric mucosa with thickening of the folds. Biopsies were taken and consisted of fragments of gastric mucosa in which an abnormal population of cells is present in the lamina propria and submucosa, singly as well as focally, in a single-file pattern. The abnormal cells are plasmacytoid in appearance, relatively uniform, with small to prominent nucleoli. Occasional intracytoplasmic lumina are noted. Representative images are shown in Fig. 5.33a, b.

The histomorphology raises the differential diagnosis of metastatic lobular carcinoma of the breast, gastric signet-ring cell carcinoma, and, less likely, a metastatic urothelial carcinoma of plasmacytoid morphology. A panel of IHC markers was performed, including CK7, CK20, GATA3, ER, E-cadherin, and uroplakin II. Representative images are illustrated in Fig. 5.33c–f.

The relatively low-grade morphology of the tumor cells is in favor of a metastasis. Primary gastric carcinoma with signet-ring cell features tends to show a higher nuclear grade. CK7 expression is common for all three tumors included in the differential considerations. However, a positive CK7 stain can rule out other tumors with plasmacytoid morphology, such as plasmacytic neoplasia or malignant melanoma. CK20 can be positive in urothelial carcinoma and occasionally gastric carcinoma. Negative CK20 reaction in this case does not rule in or rule out a diagnosis. E-cadherin decorates epithelial cells in a membranous pattern; however, this pattern of expression for E-cadherin is characteristically lost in lobular carcinomas. A positive GATA3 stain suggests a breast or urothelial primary. However, ER expression favors the breast in this setting.

The vast majority of the breast carcinomas express CK7, of course. When working on a CK7-positive metastatic tumor with unknown primary, especially in a female patient, breast carcinoma should always be included in the differential considerations. The immunomarkers may serve as breast organ-specific, including GATA3, ER, mammaglobin (MGB), and GCDFP-15. In metastatic breast carcinomas, the ER-positive rate is about 50%. Both GCDFP-15 and MGB suffer low sensitivities, reported in the ranges of 35–55% and 65–70%, respectively. Our data on tissue microarrays (TMAs) of 250 cases of invasive breast carcinomas, including ductal, lobular, and other special types, is even lower: 30% for GCDFP-15 and 50% for MGB. GATA3, at the current time, is the most optimal breast organ-specific immunomarker. The expression of GATA3 in CK7+ tumors was reported mainly in breast carcinoma, urothelial carcinoma, benign Brunner tumor of the ovary, and salivary gland tumors. Our published data reveal that GATA3 is expressed in 94% (138/147) of breast carcinomas overall and 69% (66/96) of ER-negative breast carcinomas. When working up a metastatic tumor, if a breast primary is considered, a panel of immunomarkers including CK7,

(continued)

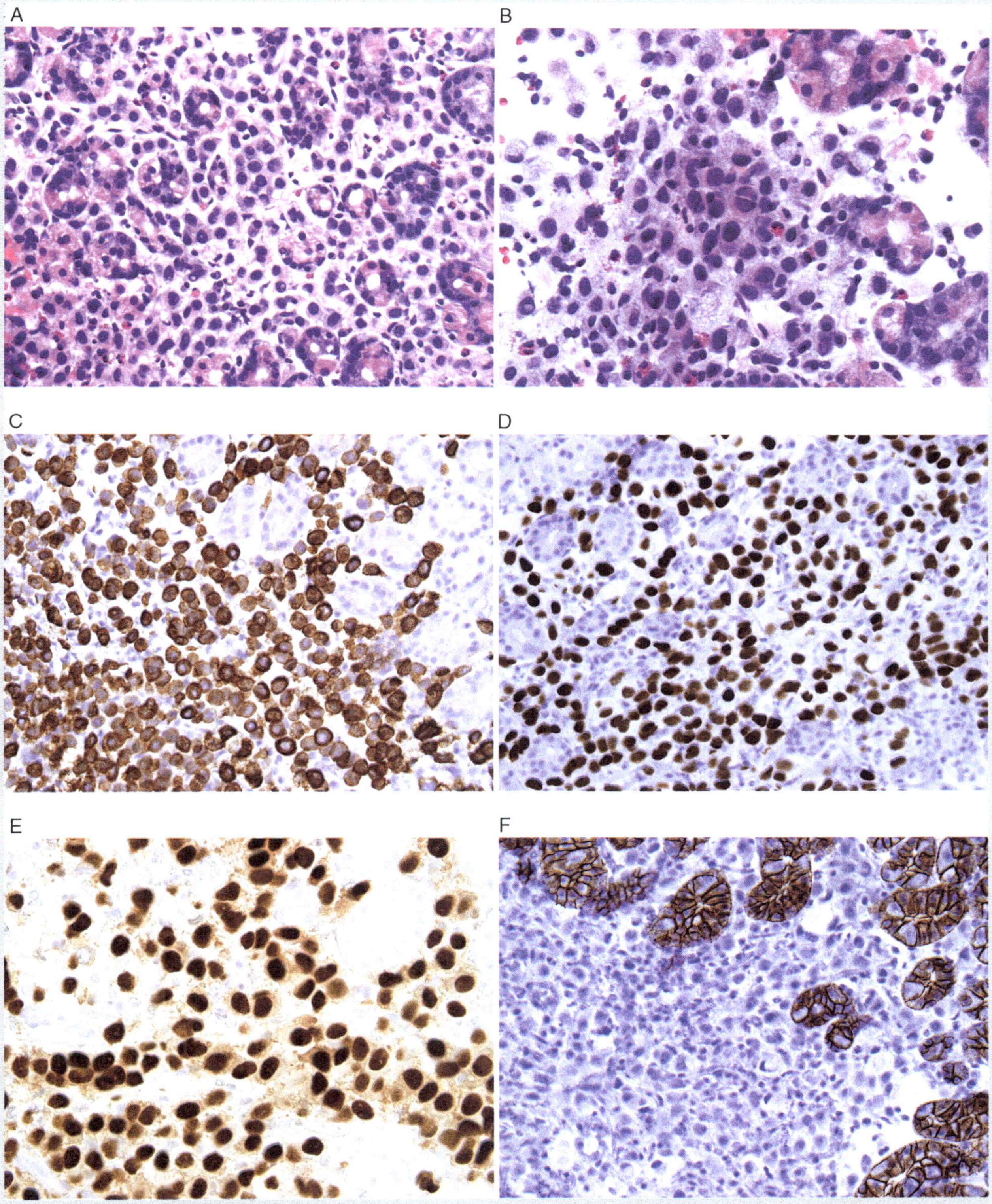

Fig. 5.33 (**a**–**f**) Metastatic lobular carcinoma of the breast to stomach. (**a**). An abnormal population of cells is present in the lamina propria and submucosa, singly as well as focally, in a single-file pattern, H&E; (**b**) the abnormal cells are plasmacytoid in appearance, relatively uniform, with small to prominent nucleoli. Occasional intracytoplasmic lumina are noted, H&E; (**c**) the tumor cells are positive for CK7; (**d**). Nuclear staining for GATA3; (**e**) positive for ER; (**f**) lack of membranous staining pattern for E-cadherin; note the gastric submucosal glands showing membranous staining for E-cadherin

Abbreviations List

Abbreviation	Full Text
ADH	Atypical ductal hyperplasia
ADH5	Breast marker cocktail consisting of CK5, CK14, p63, CK7, and CK18
ALK	Anaplastic lymphoma kinase
AR	Androgen receptor
Bcl (Bcl2, Bcl6)	B-cell CLL/lymphoma (2, 6)
Bcl2	B-cell CLL/lymphoma-2
BRCA1	Breast cancer 1
CDH1	Cadherin 1
CDK4	Cyclin-dependent kinase 4
CDX2	Caudal type homeobox 2
CK	Cytokeratin
c-kit	CD117
CNB	Core needle biopsy
D	Diastase
DCIS	Ductal carcinoma in situ
EGFR	Epithelial growth factor receptor
EMA	Epithelial membrane antigen
ER	Estrogen receptor
ERG	ETS-related gene
FISH	Fluorescence in situ hybridization
FNA	Fine needle aspiration
GATA3	GATA binding protein 3
GCDFP-15	Gross cystic disease fluid protein-15
GI	Gastrointestinal
Her-2/neu	Human epidermal growth factor receptor 2
HMWCK	High molecular weight cytokeratin
IHC	Immunohistochemistry
ILC	Invasive lobular carcinoma
IRF4/MUM1	Interferon regulatory factor 4/myeloma oncogene 1
IVD	Invasive ductal carcinoma
LMWCK	Low molecular weight cytokeratin
MALT	Mucosa-associated lymphoid tissue
MCA	Metaplastic carcinoma
MDM2	Mouse double minute 2 homolog
MEC	Myoepithelial cell
MGB	Mammaglobin
NOS	Not otherwise specified
NST	No special type
Pap	Papanicolaou stain
PAS	Periodic acid-Schiff
PAX	Paired box gene
PR	Progesterone receptor
PT	Phyllodes tumor
SMA	Smooth muscle actin
SMM-HC	Smooth muscle myosin heavy chain
TDLU	Terminal duct lobular unit
TMA	Tissue microarray
UDH	Usual ductal hyperplasia
WHO	World Health Organization

Suggested Reading

Cytology/Fine Needle Aspiration

Bibbo M, Wilbur DC. Comprehensive cytopathology. 4th ed. Philadelphia: Elsevier, Saunders; 2015.

Cibas ES, Ducatman BS. Cytology: diagnostic principles and clinical correlates. 2nd ed. Philadelphia: Saunders; 2003.

DeMay RM. The art & Science of cytopathology. 2nd ed. Chicago: American Society for Clinical Pathology (ASCP) PRESS; 2012.

Kiyozuka Y, Koyama H, Nakata M, Matsuyama T, Nikaido Y, Shimano N, et al. Diagnostic cytopathology in type II angiosarcoma of the breast: a case report. Acta Cytol. 2005;49(5):560–6.

Klijanienko J, Caillaud JM, Lagacé R, Vielh P. Cytohistologic correlations in angiosarcoma including classic and epithelioid variants: Institut Curie's experience. Diagn Cytopathol. 2003;29(3):140–5.

Martin HE, Ellis EB. Biopsy by needle puncture and aspiration. Ann Surg. 1930;92(2):169–81.

Ordi J, Riverola A, Solé M, Sentis M, Velasco M, Bernet M, et al. Fine needle aspiration of myofibroblastoma of the breast in a man. A report of two cases. Acta Cytol. 1992;36(2):194–8.

Pfeiffer DF, Bode-Lesniewska B. Fine needle aspiration biopsy diagnosis of angiosarcoma after breast-conserving therapy for carcinoma supported by use of a cell block and immunohistochemistry. Acta Cytol. 2006;50(5):553–6.

Simsir A, Cangiarella J, Boppana S, Waisman J. Aspiration cytology of the collagenized variant of mammary myofibroblastoma: a case report with review of the literature. Diagn Cytopathol. 2001;24(6):399–402.

Stewart FW. The diagnosis of tumors by aspiration. Am J Pathol. 1933;9(Suppl):801–812.3.

Histology

Al-Nafussi A. Spindle cell tumours of the breast: practical approach to diagnosis. Histopathology. 1999;35(1):1–13.

Brogi E. Benign and malignant spindle cell lesions of the breast. Semin Diagn Pathol. 2004;21(1):57–64.

Dabbs DJ. Breast pathology. Philadelphia: Elsevier, Saunders; 2012.

Lakhani SR, Ellis IO, Schnitt SJ, et al. WHO Classification of tumours of the breast. Lyon, France: IARC; 2012.

Lee AH. Recent developments in the histological diagnosis of spindle cell carcinoma, fibromatosis and phyllodes tumour of the breast. Histopathology. 2008;52(1):45–57.

Lee AH, Hodi Z, Ellis IO, Elston CW. Histological features useful in the distinction of phyllodes tumour and fibroadenoma on needle core biopsy of the breast. Histopathology. 2007;51(3):336–44.

O'Malley FP, Pinder SE, Mulligan AM. Breast pathology: a volume in the foundations in diagnostic pathology series. 2nd ed. Philadelphia: Elsevier, Saunders; 2011.

Rosen PP. Rosen's breast pathology. 3rd ed. Philadelphia: Lippincott, Williams & Wilkins; 2008.

Ancillary Tests

Abdel-Fatah TM, Powe DG, Hodi Z, Reis-Filho JS, Lee AH, Ellis IO. Morphologic and molecular evolutionary pathways of low nuclear grade invasive breast cancers and their putative precursor lesions: further evidence to support the concept of low nuclear grade breast neoplasia family. Am J Surg Pathol. 2008;32(4):513–23.
Aitken SJ, Thomas JS, Langdon SP, Harrison DJ, Faratian D. Quantitative analysis of changes in ER, PR and HER2 expression in primary breast cancer and paired nodal metastases. Ann Oncol. 2010;21(6):1254–61.
Asselin-Labat ML, Sutherland KD, Barker H, Thomas R, Shackleton M, Forrest NC, et al. Gata-3 is an essential regulator of mammary-gland morphogenesis and luminal-cell differentiation. Nat Cell Biol. 2007;9(2):201–9.
Bankfalvi A, Ludwig A, De-Hesselle B, Buerger H, Buchwalow IB, Boecker W. Different proliferative activity of the glandular and myoepithelial lineages in benign proliferative and early malignant breast diseases. Mod Pathol. 2004;17(9):1051–61.
Bhargava R, Dabbs DJ. Use of immunohistochemistry in diagnosis of breast epithelial lesions. Adv Anat Pathol. 2007;14(2):93–107.
Bhattacharya B, Dilworth HP, Iacobuzio-Donahue C, Ricci F, Weber K, Furlong MA, et al. Nuclear beta-catenin expression distinguishes deep fibromatosis from other benign and malignant fibroblastic and myofibroblastic lesions. Am J Surg Pathol. 2005;29(5):653–9.
Broom RJ, Tang PA, Simmons C, Bordeleau L, Mulligan AM, O'Malley FP, et al. Changes in estrogen receptor, progesterone receptor and her-2/neu status with time: discordance rates between primary and metastatic breast cancer. Anticancer Res. 2009;29(5):1557–62.
Buza N, Zekry N, Charpin C, Tavassoli FA. Myoepithelial carcinoma of the breast: a clinicopathological and immunohistochemical study of 15 diagnostically challenging cases. Virchows Arch. 2010;457(3):337–45.
Carlson JW, Fletcher CD. Immunohistochemistry for beta-catenin in the differential diagnosis of spindle cell lesions: analysis of a series and review of the literature. Histopathology. 2007;51(4):509–14.
Carter MR, Hornick JL, Lester S, Fletcher CD. Spindle cell (sarcomatoid) carcinoma of the breast: a clinicopathologic and immunohistochemical analysis of 29 cases. Am J Surg Pathol. 2006;30(3):300–9.
Chang HJ, Han SW, Oh DY, Im SA, Jeon YK, Park IA, et al. Discordant human epidermal growth factor receptor 2 and hormone receptor status in primary and metastatic breast cancer and response to trastuzumab. Jpn J Clin Oncol. 2011;41(5):593–9.
Chia Y, Thike AA, Cheok PY, Yong-Zheng Chong L, Man-Kit Tse G, Tan PH. Stromal keratin expression in phyllodes tumours of the breast: a comparison with other spindle cell breast lesions. J Clin Pathol. 2012;65(4):339–47.
Cimino-Mathews A, Sharma R, Illei PB, Vang R, Argani P. A subset of malignant phyllodes tumors express p63 and p40: a diagnostic pitfall in breast core needle biopsies. Am J Surg Pathol. 2014;38(12):1689–96.
D'Alfonso TM, Ross DS, Liu YF, Shin SJ. Expression of p40 and laminin 332 in metaplastic spindle cell carcinoma of the breast compared with other malignant spindle cell tumours. J Clin Pathol. 2015;68(7):516–21.
Dunne B, Lee AHS, Pinder SE, Bell JA, Ellis IO. An immunohistochemical study of metaplastic spindle cell carcinoma, phyllodes tumor and fibromatosis of the breast. Hum Pathol. 2003;34(10):1009–15.
Geyer FC, Lacroix-Triki M, Savage K, Arnedos M, Lambros MB, MacKay A, et al. β-catenin pathway activation in breast cancer is associated with triple-negative phenotype but not with CTNNB1 mutation. Mod Pathol. 2011;24:209–31.
Gomez-Fernandez C, Daneshbod Y, Nassiri M, Milikowski C, Alvarez C, Nadji M. Immunohistochemically determined estrogen receptor phenotype remains stable in recurrent and metastatic breast cancer. Am J Clin Pathol. 2008;130(6):879–82.
Higgins JP, Kaygusuz G, Wang L, Montgomery K, Mason V, Zhu SX, et al. Placental S100 (S100P) and GATA3: markers for transitional epithelium and urothelial carcinoma discovered by complementary DNA microarray. Am J Surg Pathol. 2007;31(5):673–80.
Koker MM, Kleer CG. p63 expression in breast cancer: a highly sensitive and specific marker of metaplastic carcinoma. Am J Surg Pathol. 2004;28(11):1506–12.
Lacroix-Triki M, Geyer FC, Lambros MB, Savage K, Ellis IO, Lee AH, et al. β-catenin/Wnt signalling pathway in fibromatosis, metaplastic carcinomas and phyllodes tumours of the breast. Mod Pathol. 2010;23(11):1438–48.
Lacroix-Triki M, Mery E, Voigt JJ, Istier L, Rochaix P. Value of cytokeratin 5/6 immunostaining using D5/16 B4 antibody in the spectrum of proliferative intraepithelial lesions of the breast. A comparative study with 34betaE12 antibody. Virchows Arch. 2003;442(6):548–54.
Lakhani SR, Collins N, Stratton MR, Sloane JP. Atypical ductal hyperplasia of the breast: clonal proliferation with loss of heterozygosity on chromosomes 16q and 17p. J Clin Pathol. 1995;48(7):611–5.
Lin F, Liu H. Unknown primary/undifferentiated neoplasm. In: Lin F, Prichard JW, Liu H, Wilkerson M, Chen ZE, editors. Handbook of practical immunohistochemistry: frequent asked questions. 2nd ed. New York: Springer Science+Business Media; 2015. p. 119–63.
Liu H. Application of immunohistochemistry in breast pathology: a review and update. Arch Pathol Lab Med. 2014;138(12):1629–42.
Liu H. Breast. In: Lin F, Prichard JW, Liu H, Wilkerson M, Chen ZE, editors. Handbook of practical immunohistochemistry: frequent asked questions. 2nd ed. New York: Springer Science+Business Media; 2015. p. 183–215.
Liu H, Shi J, Prichard J, Gung Y, Lin F. Immunohistochemical evaluation of GATA-3 expression in ER-negative breast carcinomas. Am J Clin Pathol. 2014;141(5):648–55.
Liu H, Shi J, Wilkerson ML, Lin F. Immunohistochemical evaluation of GATA3 expression in tumors and normal tissues: a useful immunomarker for breast and urothelial carcinomas. Am J Clin Pathol. 2012;138(1):57–64.
Miettinen M, Sarlomo-Rikala M, Kovatich AJ. Cell-type- and tumour-type-related patterns of bcl-2 reactivity in mesenchymal cells and soft tissue tumours. Virchows Arch. 1998;433(3):255–60.
Moinfar F, Man YG, Lininger RA, Bodian C, Tavassoli FA. Use of keratin 35betaE12 as an adjunct in the diagnosis of mammary intraepithelial neoplasia-ductal type--benign and malignant intraductal proliferations. Am J Surg Pathol. 1999;23(9):1048–58.
Moore T, Lee AH. Expression of CD34 and bcl-2 in phyllodes tumours, fibroadenomas and spindle cell lesions of the breast. Histopathology. 2001;38(1):62–7.
Namikawa T, Hanazaki K. Clinicopathological features and treatment outcomes of metastatic tumors in the stomach. Surg Today. 2014;44(8):1392–9.
Nonaka D, Wang BY, Edmondson D, Beckett E, Sun CC. A study of gata3 and phox2b expression in tumors of the autonomic nervous system. Am J Surg Pathol. 2013;37(8):1236–41.
Ordóñez NG. Value of GATA3 immunostaining in tumor diagnosis: a review. Adv Anat Pathol. 2013;20(5):352–60.
Pectasides D, Psyrri A, Pliarchopoulou K, Floros T, Papaxoinis G, Skondra M, et al. Gastric metastases originating from breast cancer: report of 8 cases and review of the literature. Anticancer Res. 2009;29(11):4759–63.
Perou CM, Sørlie T, Eisen MB, van de Rijn M, Jeffrey SS, Rees CA, et al. Molecular portraits of human breast tumours. Nature. 2000;406(6797):747–52.

Schmitt FC, AC Mera A. Fine needle aspiration cytology presentation of a cellular variant of breast myofibroblastoma. Report of a case with immunohistochemical studies. Acta Cytol. 1998;42(3):721–4.

Sneige N, Yaziji H, Mandavilli SR, Perez ER, Ordonez NG, Gown AM, et al. Low-grade (fibromatosis-like) spindle cell carcinoma of the breast. Am J Surg Pathol. 2001;25(8):1009–16.

Suster S, Fisher C, Moran CA. Expression of bcl-2 oncoprotein in benign and malignant spindle cell tumors of soft tissue, skin, serosal surfaces, and gastrointestinal tract. Am J Surg Pathol. 1998;22(7):863–72.

Tse GM, Tan PH, Chaiwun B, Putti TC, Lui PC, Tsang AK, Wong FC, Lo AW. p63 is useful in the diagnosis of mammary metaplastic carcinomas. Pathology. 2006;38(1):16–20.

Lung and Mediastinum

6

Haiyan Liu, Jun Zhang, and Fan Lin

Summary of Pearls and Pitfalls

- The concept of personalized medicine and the remarkable advances in lung cancer genetics and therapy in the past decade have changed lung pathology practice dramatically.
- The 2015 World Health Organization (WHO) classification of tumors of the lung specifies that immunohistochemistry is required for lung cancer diagnosis, not only for small biopsies and fine needle aspiration (FNA) specimens but also for certain resected specimens such as solid adenocarcinoma (ADC), nonkeratinizing squamous cell carcinoma, large cell carcinoma, neuroendocrine tumors, and sarcomatoid carcinomas.
- New criteria and terminology for the diagnosis of lung cancer based on small biopsies and cytology are proposed in the 2015 WHO classification and are summarized in Tables 6.1 and 6.2.
- The role of cytopathologists has expanded to not only making a specific diagnosis, including histopathological subtyping of tumors, but also to thoughtfully utilizing the limited material for necessary genetic studies to help personalize treatment strategies for advanced lung cancer patients.
- Thyroid transcription factor 1 (TTF1) and napsin A are accepted markers for ADC differentiation; p40 is reported to be the most specific and sensitive marker for squamous cell differentiation. A reasonable recommendation is that, when immunohistochemistry is deemed necessary, at least one antibody each for squamous and glandular differentiation, but no more than two antibodies, should be used for an initial workup (e.g., TTF1 and p40 or p63). Thus a limited panel of TTF1 and p40 (or p63) is suggested for subtyping the tumor to preserve tissue for molecular testing.
- Molecular testing for epithelial growth factor receptor (*EGFR*) mutation and anaplastic lymphoma kinase (*ALK*) rearrangement is recommended in tumors classified as ADC and in cases where an ADC component cannot be excluded.
- When evaluating a computed tomography (CT)-guided FNA of a lung lesion in the periphery, mesothelial cells are frequently seen on smears; reactive mesothelial cells may mimic carcinoma, and caution should be taken.
- Diagnosis of ADC with a lepidic growth pattern can be challenging in FNA specimens. Both quality (degree of atypia) and quantity (groups of atypical cells) need to be considered. In a typical case of ADC with a lepidic growth pattern, the smears tend to be very cellular, containing many groups of atypical epithelial cells. In contrast, in a reactive condition, such as pulmonary infarction, atypical reactive pneumocytes are usually less numerous.
- In mucinous ADC with a lepidic growth pattern, the neoplastic epithelial cells may mimic pulmonary macrophages. Features such as a mucinous background, cytoplasmic mucin/vacuoles, eccentrically located nuclei, and more abundant cytoplasm are helpful in reaching a correct diagnosis.
- Basaloid squamous cell carcinoma may mimic small cell carcinoma; therefore, cellblock preparation in conjunction with immunostains will be helpful.
- Infection such as aspergillosis may result in squamous cells with significant cytological atypia; therefore, infectious etiologies should be excluded before a diagnosis of well-differentiated squamous cell carcinoma is rendered.

© Springer International Publishing AG 2018

F. Lin et al., *Handbook of Practical Fine Needle Aspiration and Small Tissue Biopsies*, DOI 10.1007/978-3-319-57386-1_6

- A lesion from the mediastinum should be considered if cytological features do not fit the description of a typical "lung lesion."
- Thymoma is rare in young patients and children. In lymphocyte-dominant thymoma, the main component of the aspirate may contain cortical thymocytes with expression of terminal deoxynucleotidyl transferase (TdT) and cluster of differentiation (CD)99; therefore, caution should be taken to avoid misdiagnosing it as a lymphoblastic lymphoma.
- Thymic neuroendocrine neoplasm may mimic an epithelial-dominant thymoma; therefore, immunohistochemistry should be performed in cases with equivocal features.

Lung

Tables 6.1 and 6.2 summarize new criteria and terminology for the diagnosis of lung cancer based on small biopsies and cytology from the 2015 WHO classification.

Normal Cytology

Upper Respiratory Tract

- Ciliated columnar cells, see Fig. 6.1.
- Squamous cells, see Fig. 6.2.

Lower Respiratory Tract

- Trachea and bronchi
  - Ciliated columnar cells
  - Goblet cells, see Fig. 6.3.
  - Basal/reserve cells, see Fig. 6.4.
- Terminal bronchioles
  - Non-ciliated cuboidal/columnar cells (Clara cells)
  - Alveoli
  - Type I and II pneumocytes
  - Alveolar macrophages, see Fig. 6.5.

Respiratory Infections

Viral Infections

Specific viral infections, such as herpes simplex (Fig. 6.6) and cytomegalovirus (Fig. 6.7), can cause significant cyto-

Table 6.1 Terminology and criteria for adenocarcinoma, squamous cell carcinoma, and non-small cell carcinoma, not otherwise specified, in small biopsies and cytology specimens compared with those for resection specimens

Small biopsy/cytology terminology	Morphology/immunohistochemistry	2015 WHO classification of resection specimens
ADC (describe patterns)	Morphologic ADC patterns clearly present	ADC predominant pattern: lepidic, acinar, papillary, solid, and micropapillary
ADC with lepidic pattern (if pure, add note: an invasive component cannot be excluded)		Minimally invasive ADC, ADC in situ, or an invasive ADC with a lepidic component
Invasive mucinous ADC (describe patterns; use term mucinous ADC with lepidic pattern if pure)		Invasive mucinous ADC
ADC with colloid features		Colloid ADC
ADC with fetal features		Fetal ADC
ADC with enteric features		Enteric ADC
NSCC, favor ADC	Morphologic ADC patterns not present but supported by special stains (i.e., TTF1+)	ADC (solid pattern may be just one component of the tumor)
SqCC	Morphologic squamous cell pattern clearly present	SqCC
NSCC, favor SqCC	Morphologic squamous cell patterns not present but supported by stain (i.e., p40+)	SqCC (solid pattern may be just one component of the tumor)
NSCC NOS	No clear ADC, squamous or neuroendocrine morphology or staining pattern	Large cell carcinoma

Adapted with permission of Elsevier from Travis WD, Brambilla E, Nicholson AG, Yatabe Y, Austin JH, Beasley MB, et al.; WHO Panel. The 2015 World Health Organization classification of lung tumors: impact of genetic, clinical and radiologic advances since the 2004 classification. J Thorac Oncol. 2015;10(9):1243–60

ADC adenocarcinoma, *TTF1* thyroid transcription factor 1, *SqCC* squamous cell carcinoma, *NSCC* non-small cell carcinoma, *NOS* not otherwise specified, *WHO* World Health Organization

Table 6.2 Diagnostic terminology for small biopsy/cytology compared with that of the 2015 World Health Organization (WHO) in resection specimens with small cell carcinoma, LCNEC, adenosquamous carcinoma, and sarcomatoid carcinoma

Small biopsy/cytology terminology/criteria	2015 WHO classification of resections
Small cell carcinoma	Small cell carcinoma
NSCC with NE morphology and positive NE markers, possible LCNEC	LCNEC
NSCC with NE morphology. If negative NE markers comment: This is an NSCC where LCNEC is suspected, but stains fails to demonstrate NE differentiation	LCNEM
Morphologic squamous cell and ADC patterns present: NSCC, NOS. Comment that ADC and squamous components are present, and this could represent adenosquamous carcinoma	Adenosquamous carcinoma (if both components ≥10%)
No morphologic squamous cell or ADC patterns, but immunostains favor separate squamous and ADC components: NSCC, NOS. Specify the IHC results and the interpretation. Comment that this could represent adenosquamous carcinoma	ADC, SqCC, adenosquamous carcinoma, or large cell carcinoma with unclear IHC features
NSCC with spindle cell and/or giant cell carcinoma (mention if ADC or SqCC is present)	Pleomorphic, spindle cell, and/or giant cell carcinoma

Adapted with permission of Elsevier from Travis WD, Brambilla E, Nicholson AG, Yatabe Y, Austin JH, Beasley MB, et al.; WHO Panel. The 2015 World Health Organization classification of lung tumors: impact of genetic, clinical and radiologic advances since the 2004 classification. J Thorac Oncol. 2015;10(9):1243–60

WHO World Health Organization, *LCNEC* large cell neuroendocrine carcinoma, *NSCC* non-small cell carcinoma, *NE* neuroendocrine, *LCNEM* large cell carcinoma with neuroendocrine morphology, *ADC* adenocarcinoma, *NOS* not otherwise specified, *SqCC* squamous cell carcinoma, *IHC* immunohistochemistry

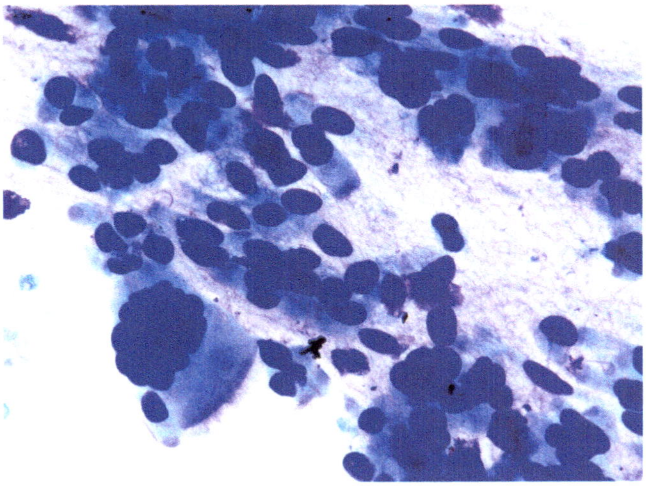

Fig. 6.1 Normal ciliated respiratory columnar cells, Diff-Quik stain

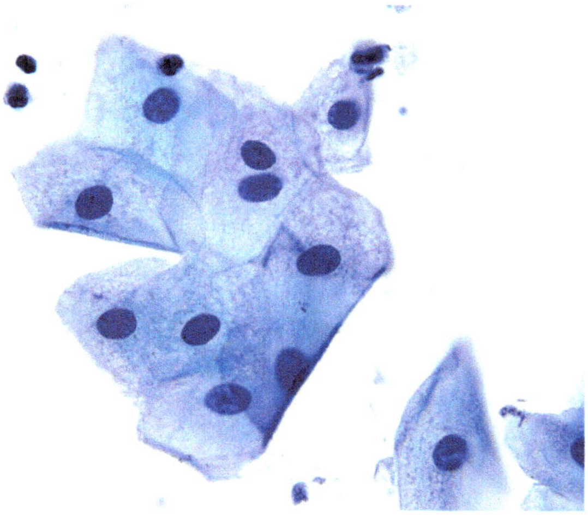

Fig. 6.2 Normal squamous cells, Pap stain

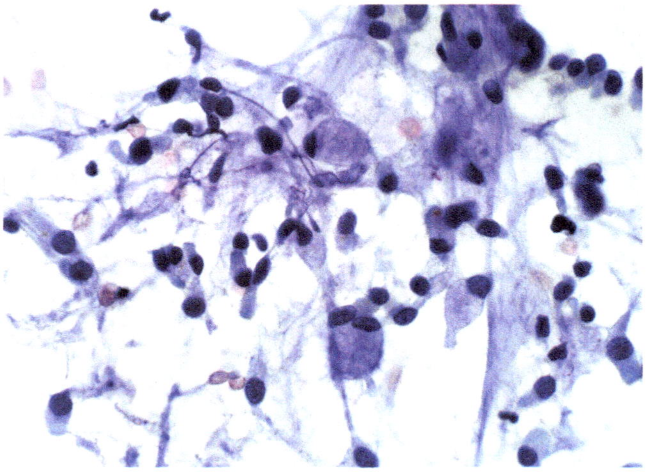

Fig. 6.3 Benign goblet cells, Pap stain

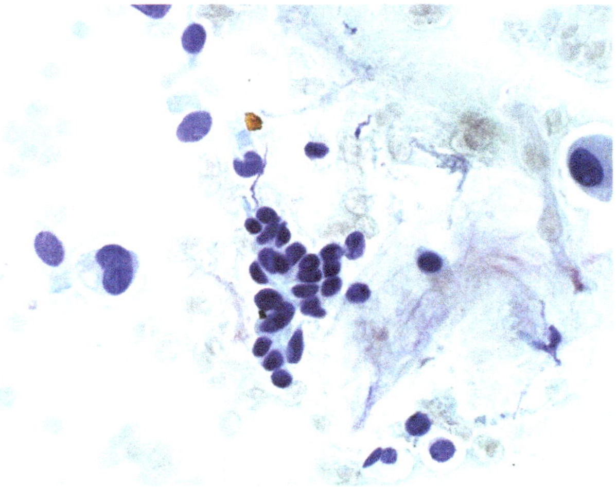

Fig. 6.4 Normal reserve cells, Pap stain

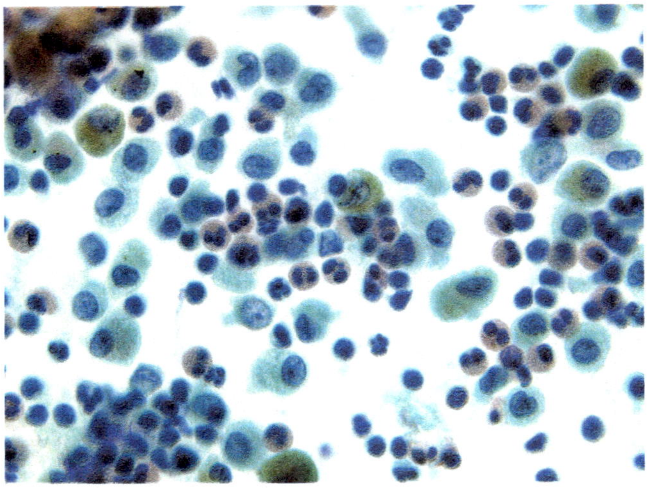

Fig. 6.5 Pulmonary macrophages, Pap stain

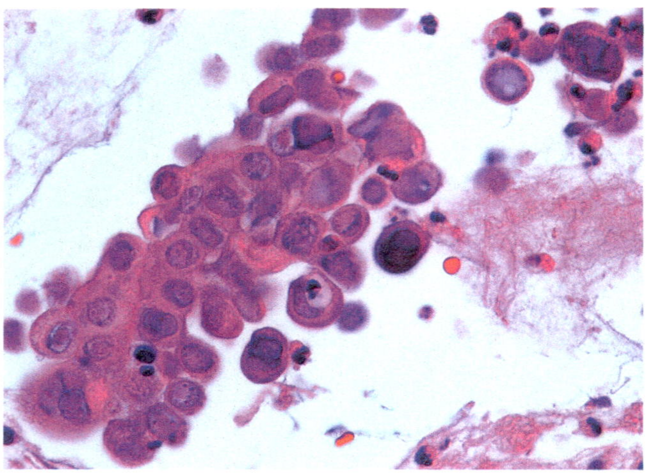

Fig. 6.6 Herpes simplex viral inclusions, H&E

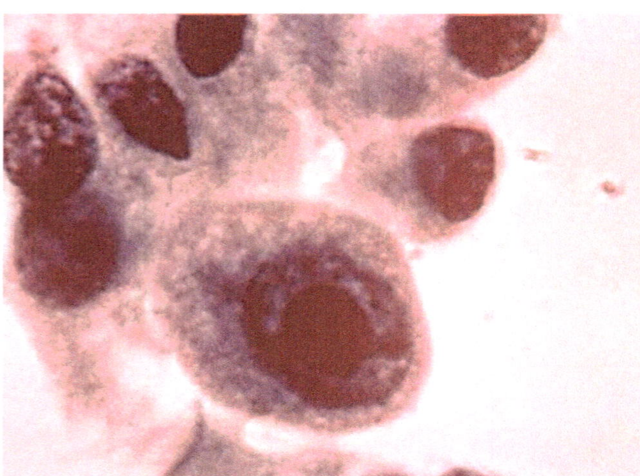

Fig. 6.7 Cytomegaloviral inclusion, Pap stain

logical changes that may mimic a malignant process. The diagnosis can be confirmed by immunoperoxidase studies.

Severe acute respiratory syndrome (SARS) caused by a novel coronavirus (SARS-CoV) became a worldwide outbreak in 2003, affecting more than 8000 patients, with a fatality rate of 9.2%. SARS-CoV belongs to a family of large, positive, single-stranded ribonucleic acid (RNA) viruses. The key pathologic finding is diffuse alveolar damage (DAD). Depending on different phases in the disease progression, the composition of inflammatory cells may vary; however, macrophages (including multinucleated forms) and lymphocytes usually predominate. Other pathologic findings, such as fibrosis, prominent vascular injury, hemophagocytosis, squamous metaplasia, apoptosis, and atypical pneumocytes, including multinucleated giant pneumocytes with irregularly distributed nuclei or pneumocytes with large atypical nuclei, prominent eosinophilic nucleoli, and granular amphophilic cytoplasm, were reported. Ancillary tests, such as in situ hybridization, immunohistochemistry, viral isolation, or reverse transcription polymerase chain reaction (RT-PCR), are necessary to confirm the diagnosis. Representative images are shown in Fig. 6.8a, b.

Fungal Infections

FNA is a useful means of diagnosing pulmonary fungal infection, which should be suspected whenever there is granulomatous inflammation. Silver or periodic acid-Schiff (PAS) stains are used on cellblock sections.

The common fungal infections include (1) *Candida* species; (2) *Aspergillus* species, Fig. 6.9; (3) phycomycosis (such as mucormycosis); (4) *Cryptococcus neoformans*, Fig. 6.10a–d; (5) *Histoplasma capsulatum*, Fig. 6.11a, b; (6) *Blastomyces dermatitidis*, Fig. 6.12a, b; (7) *Coccidioides immitis*, Fig. 6.13a, b; and (8) *Pneumocystis carinii*, Fig. 6.14a–c. The morphological features of these fungi are summarized in Table 6.3.

Strongyloidiasis

Pulmonary strongyloidiasis affects immunocompetent and, more commonly, immunosuppressed persons presenting with pneumonitis with hemoptysis. The etiological agent is the nematode. *Strongyloides stercoralis* in sputum is shown in Fig. 6.15.

Bacterial Infection

Infection by *Mycobacterium tuberculosis* is often a granulomatous inflammation containing clusters of epithelioid histiocytes, lymphocytes, and Langhans giant cells, with or without necrosis. In immunocompromised patients there may be abundant acid-fast organisms without obvious granulomatous inflammation.

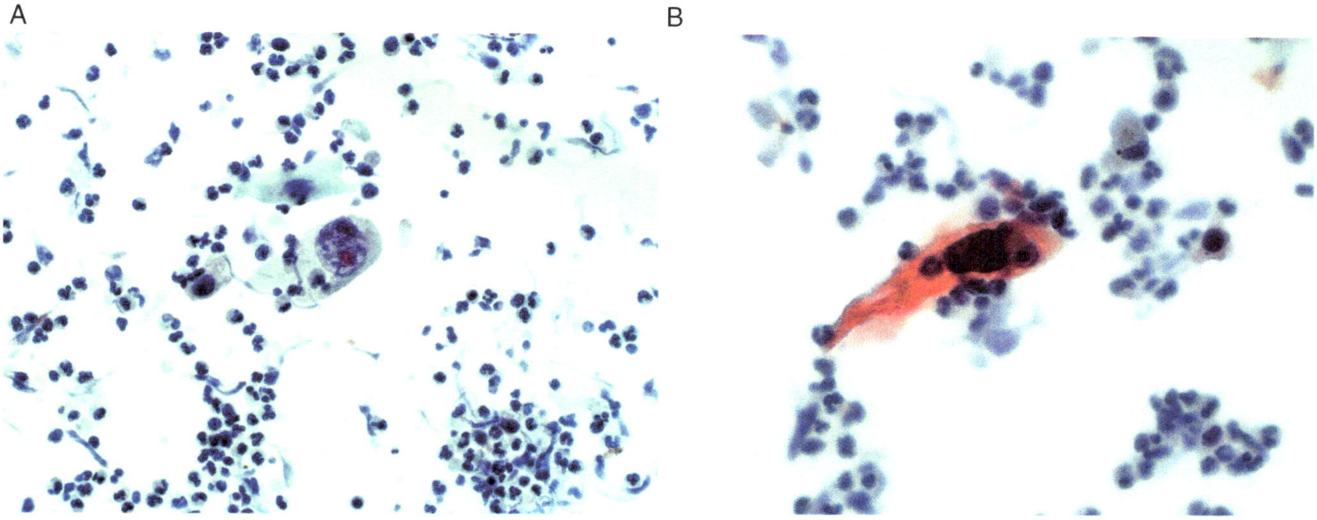

Fig. 6.8 Alveolar lavage from a patient with severe acute respiratory syndrome, with confirmed coronavirus infection. (**a**) Atypical pneumocytes with large nuclei, prominent eosinophilic nucleoli, and granular amphophilic cytoplasm in a background of marked acute inflammation, Pap stain; (**b**) typical metaplastic squamous cells with enlarged nuclei, hyperchromatic, smudged chromatin, Pap stain

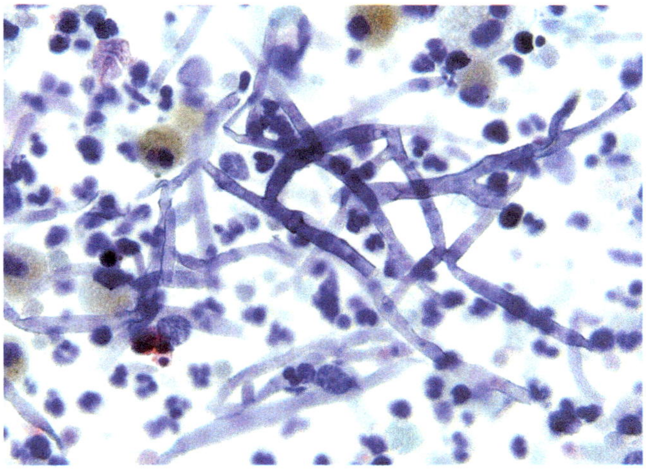

Fig. 6.9 *Aspergillus* species, alveolar lavage, Pap stain. The fungal hyphae exhibit septation, with dichotomous 45 degree angle branching. There are pulmonary macrophages and neutrophil-predominant mixed inflammatory cells in the background

Acquired immunodeficiency syndrome (AIDS) patients are especially susceptible to *Mycobacterium avium-intracellulare*, an acid-fast organism producing negative images on Romanowsky stain. Special stains on cellblock section are particularly helpful.

Nocardia, a weakly acid-fast filamentous organism, often infects immunocompromised patients, producing cavitary nodules on radiographs, which may mimic a neoplastic process.

Other Types of Granulomatous Inflammation

Sarcoidosis

Key Clinical Features

- Sarcoidosis is characterized by non-caseating granulomas in many organs, most commonly the lung.

Key Radiological Features

- Chest x-ray: bilateral hilar adenopathy is a classic finding; variable lung parenchyma changes, from normal, diffuse reticular, or ground glass opacities, nodular consolidation or cystic scarring.
- CT and positron emission tomography (PET) scan can also be used.

Cytological Features

- Aggregates of epithelioid histiocytes, with or without Schaumann and asteroid bodies
- Multinucleated giant cells and lymphocytes

Differential Diagnosis

An essential part of the diagnosis of sarcoidosis is the exclusion of alternative possibilities:

- Granulomas caused by infectious agents, such as mycobacterial infection and fungal infection
- Drug-induced, hypersensitivity pneumonitis, or foreign body granulomatosis

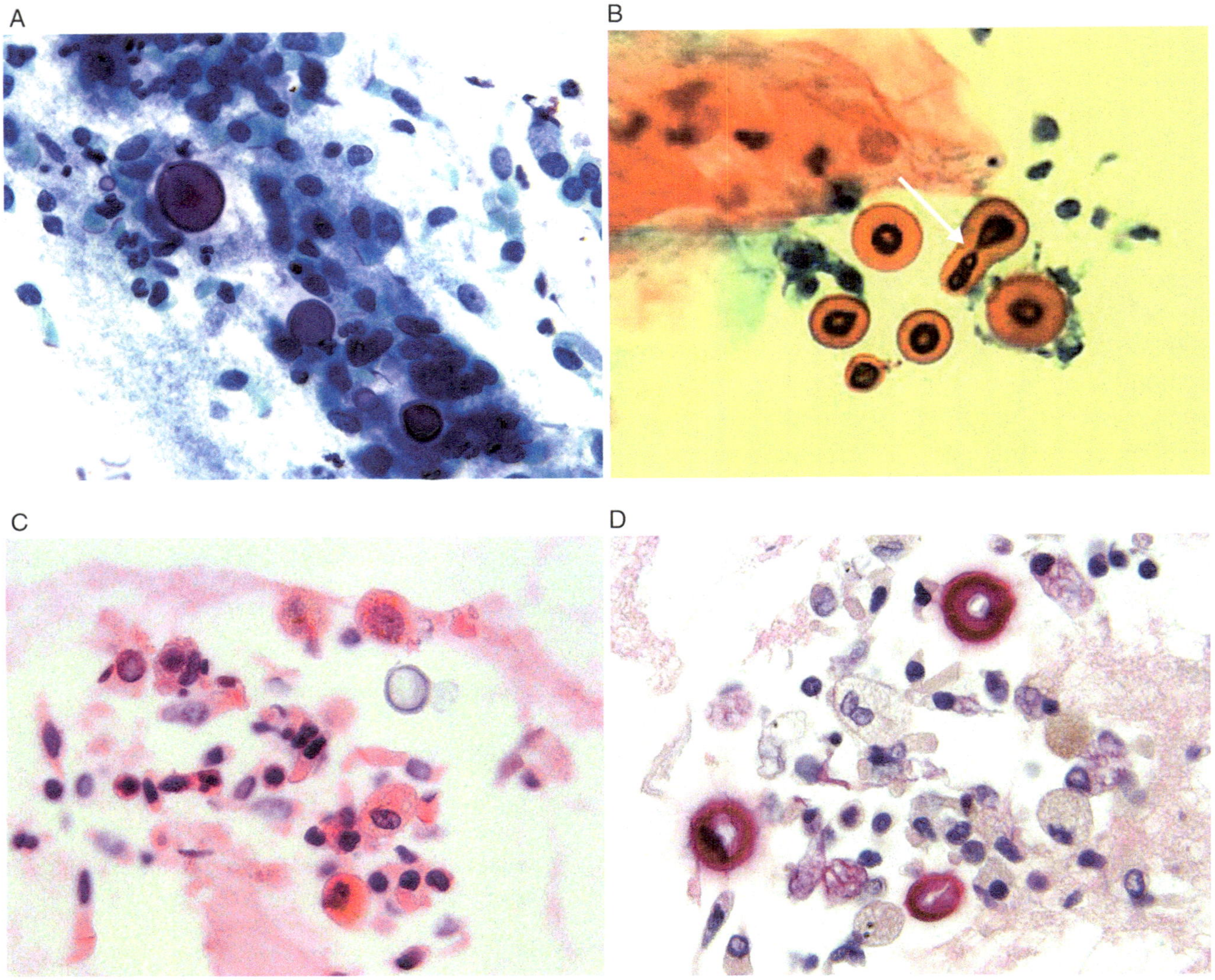

Fig. 6.10 *Cryptococcus neoformans*, bronchial brushing and alveolar lavage. (**a**) Round/oval, variable size yeast forms in background of respiratory epithelial cells, bronchial brushing, Pap stain; (**b**) alveolar lavage, showing slightly variable size, round/oval yeast forms with thick capsule and narrow-necked budding, H&E; (**c**) alveolar lavage, cellblock, H&E, showing round to oval yeast form; (**d**) alveolar lavage, the thick mucinous capsule showing bright red stain with mucicarmine, cellblock

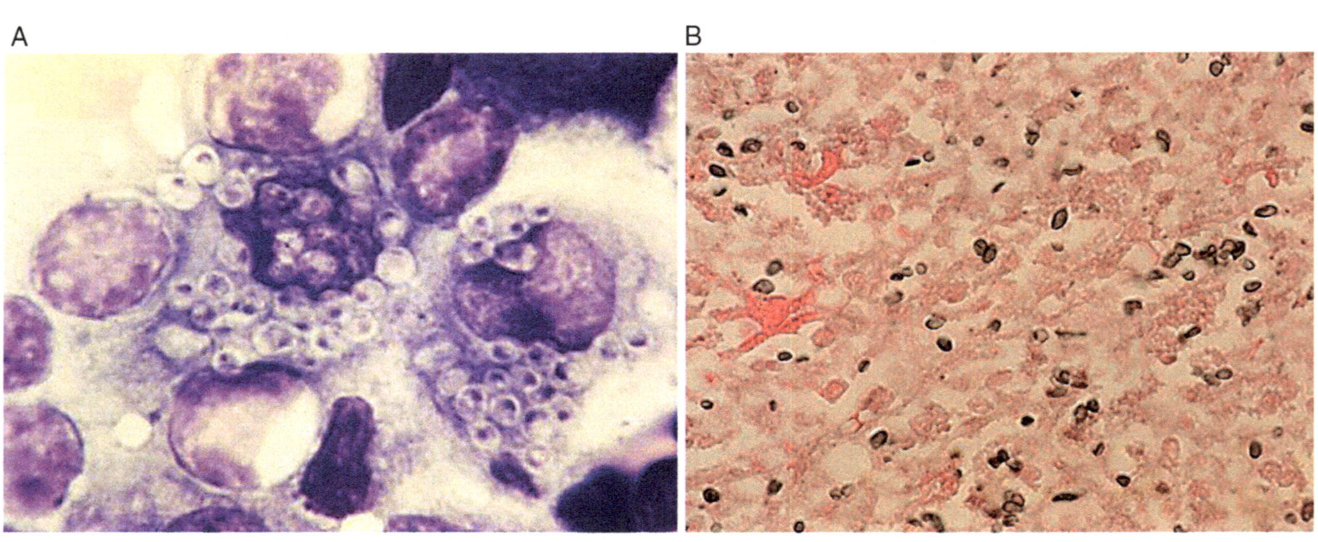

Fig. 6.11 *Histoplasma capsulatum*, lung lesion, fine needle aspiration. (**a**) Small, budding, intracellular yeast forms, 2–5 microns, Diff-Quick; (**b**) cellblock, Grocott's methenamine silver (GMS) stain, showing small yeast forms

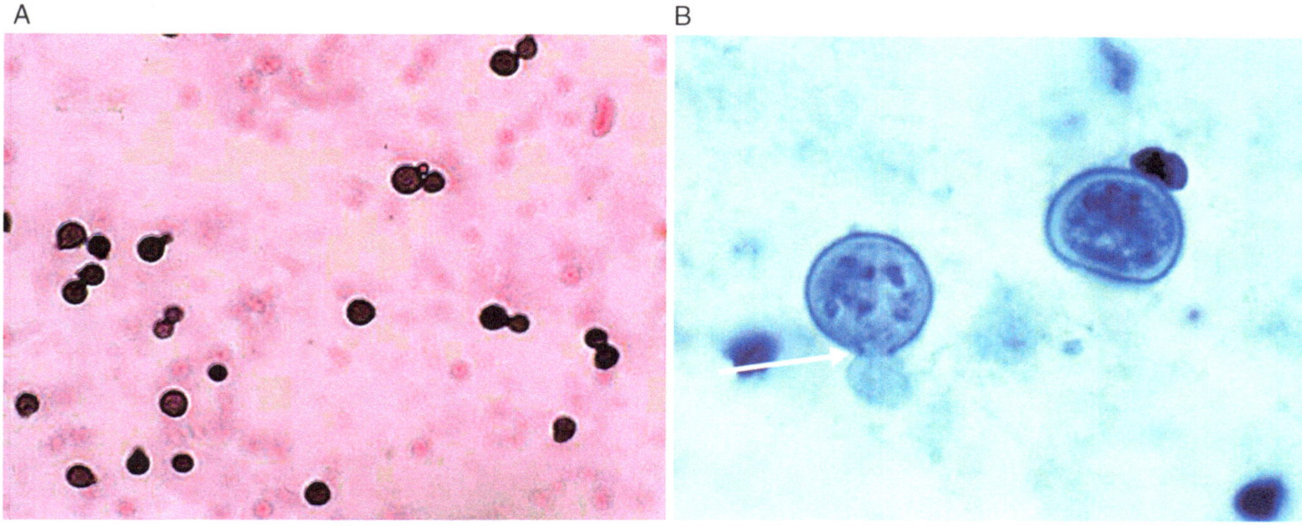

Fig. 6.12 *Blastomyces dermatitidis*, lung lesion, sputum. (**a**) Budding yeast form, broad base, cellblock, H&E; (**b**) sputum, broad-based budding yeast form, Pap stain

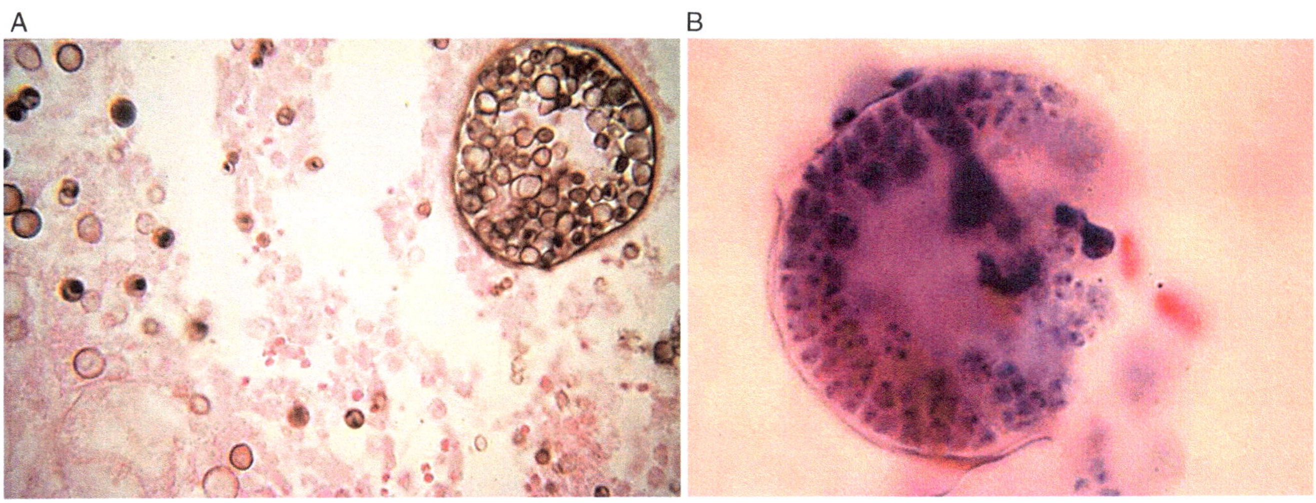

Fig. 6.13 *Coccidioides immitis*. (**a**) Cellblock, spherule form containing endospores, H&E; (**b**) spherule form containing endospores, Pap stain

- Pulmonary histiocytic disorders
- Granulomatous disorders associated with vascular inflammation such as Wegener granulomatosis and Churg-Strauss syndrome

Wegener Granulomatosis

Key Clinical Features

- Wegener granulomatosis is characterized by necrotizing vasculitis and may present as a lung mass with or without involvement of nasal passages and kidneys.

Key Radiological Features

- Multiple pulmonary nodules on imaging

Cytological Features

- Neutrophils, giant cells, necrotic collagen, and epithelioid histiocytes
- The findings are nonspecific; therefore, serologic studies are necessary.

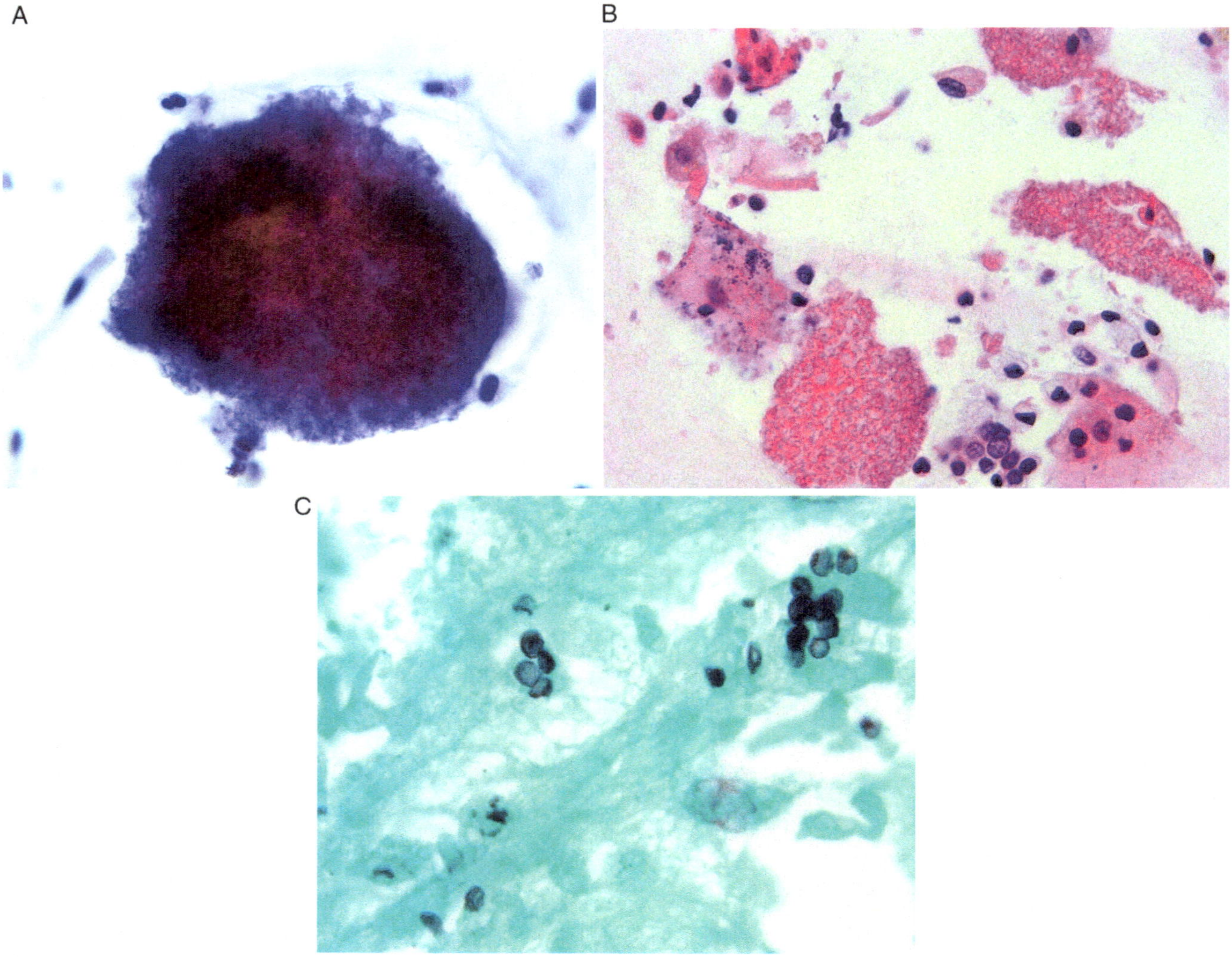

Fig. 6.14 *Pneumocystis carinii*, alveolar lavage. (**a**) Foamy proteinaceous spheres, Pap stain; (**b**) foamy proteinaceous spheres, cellblock, H&E; (**c**) GMS stain reveals small oval or cup-shaped yeast forms, cellblock

Table 6.3 Morphological features of fungi commonly seen in pulmonary cytological samples

Fungi	Forms	Hyphal branches	Average diameter (um)	Budding pattern
Candida spp.	Budding yeast Pseudohyphae	Not applicable	4	Constricted neck
Aspergillus spp.	Hyphae with 45-degree angle	45 degree	5–10	Not applicable
Mucormycosis	Hyphae with acute angle	90 degree	10–15	Not applicable
Histoplasma capsulatum	Budding yeast	Not applicable	2–4	Constricted neck
Cryptococcus neoformans	Yeast	Not applicable	5–8	Constricted neck
Blastomyces dermatitidis	Yeast	Not applicable	8–15	Broad-based
Coccidioides immitis	Endospores Spherules	Not applicable	Endospores 2–5 Spherules −100	Not applicable
[a]*Pneumocystis carinii*	Helmet-shaped cysts	Not applicable	6–8	Not applicable

[a]Genetic data suggest *Pneumocystis carinii* is more closely related to fungi
spp species (many)

Differential Diagnosis

- Granulomatous inflammations
- Metastatic diseases
- Non-Hodgkin lymphomas

Nodular Pulmonary Amyloidosis (Amyloid Tumor)

Key Clinical Features

- Amyloid deposits in the lung, forming discrete nodular masses

Key Radiological Features

- Discrete pulmonary nodules/masses (amyloidomas) on imaging

Cytological Features

- Irregular, waxy, amorphous, hypocellular material with a scalloped, occasionally cracked appearance, which is blue-green on Papanicolaou (Pap) stain and shows apple-green dichroism under polarized light after staining with Congo red

Differential Diagnosis

- Granulomatous inflammations
- Metastatic diseases
- Non-Hodgkin lymphomas

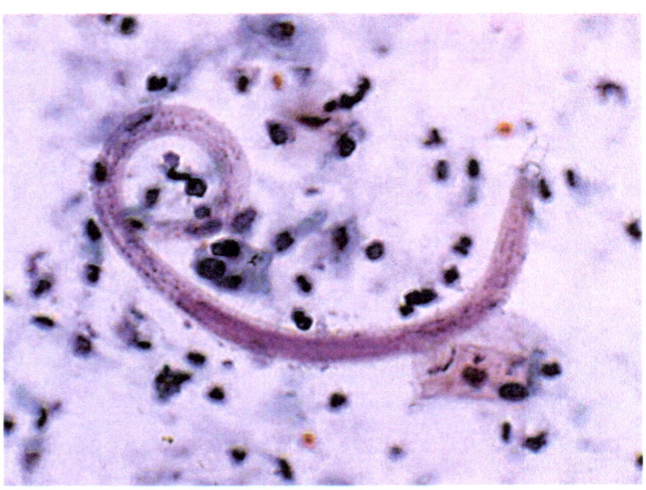

Fig. 6.15 Strongyloides stercoralis, sputum, Pap stain

Pulmonary Neoplasms

The 2015 *WHO Classification of Tumors of the Lung, Pleura, Thymus and Heart* has been published recently. There are numerous important changes in the classification of lung tumors, as summarized in Table 6.4.

Table 6.4 2015 World Health Organization (WHO) classification of lung tumors

Epithelial tumors	
Adenocarcinoma	Neuroendocrine tumors (continued)
Lepidic adenocarcinoma	Preinvasive lesion
Acinar adenocarcinoma	Diffuse idiopathic pulmonary neuroendocrine cell hyperplasia
Papillary adenocarcinoma	Large cell carcinoma
Micropapillary adenocarcinoma	Adenosquamous carcinoma
Solid adenocarcinoma	Sarcomatoid carcinomas
Invasive mucinous adenocarcinoma	Pleomorphic carcinoma
Mixed invasive mucinous and nonmucinous adenocarcinoma	Spindle cell carcinoma
Colloid adenocarcinoma	Giant cell carcinoma
Fetal adenocarcinoma	Carcinosarcoma
Enteric adenocarcinoma	Pulmonary blastoma
Minimally invasive adenocarcinoma	Other and Unclassified carcinomas
Nonmucinous	Lymphoepithelioma-like carcinoma
Mucinous	Nuclear protein in testis (NUT) carcinoma
Preinvasive lesions	Salivary gland-like tumors
Atypical adenomatous hyperplasia	Mucoepidermoid carcinoma
Adenocarcinoma in situ	Adenoid cystic carcinoma
Nonmucinous	Epithelial-myoepithelial carcinoma
Mucinous	Pleomorphic adenoma
Squamous cell carcinoma	Papillomas
Keratinizing squamous cell carcinoma	Squamous cell papilloma
Nonkeratinizing squamous cell carcinoma	Exophitic
Basaloid squamous cell carcinoma	Inverted
Preinvasive lesion	Glandular papilloma
Squamous cell carcinoma in situ	Mixed squamous and glandular papilloma
Neuroendocrine tumors	Adenomas
Small cell carcinoma	Sclerosing pneumocytoma
Combined small cell carcinoma	Alveolar adenoma
Large cell neuroendocrine carcinoma	Papillary adenoma
Combined large cell neuroendocrine carcinoma	Mucinous cystadenoma
Carcinoid tumors	Mucous gland adenoma
Typical carcinoid tumor	
Atypical carcinoid tumor	

(continued)

Table 6.4 (continued)

Mesenchymal tumors	
Pulmonary hamartoma	Epithelioid hemangioendothelioma
Chondroma	Pleuropulmonary blastoma
PEComatous tumors	Synovial sarcoma
Lymphangioleiomyomatosis	Pulmonary artery intimal sarcoma
PEComa, benign	Pulmonary myxoid sarcoma with *EWSR1-CREB1* translocation
Clear cell tumor	Myoepithelial tumors
PEComa, malignant	Myoepithelioma
Congenital peribronchial myofibroblastic tumor	Myoepithelial carcinoma
Diffuse pulmonary lymphangiomatosis	
Inflammatory myofibroblastic tumor	
Lymphohistiocytic tumors	
Extranodal marginal zone lymphoma of mucosa-associated lymphoid tissue (MALT lymphoma)	
Diffuse large cell lymphoma	
Lymphomatoid granulomatosis	
Intravascular large B-cell lymphoma	
Pulmonary Langerhans cell histiocytosis	
Erdheim-Chester disease	
Tumors of ectopic origin	
Germ cell tumors	
Teratoma, mature	
Teratoma, immature	
Intrapulmonary thymoma	
Melanoma	
Meningioma, not otherwise specified (NOS)	
Metastatic tumors	

Used with permission from Travis WD, Brambilla E, Burke AP, Marx A, Nicholson A. WHO classification of tumours of the lung, pleura, thymus and heart. Lyon, France: IARC; 2015

Representative Benign Neoplasms of the Lung

Pulmonary Hamartoma

Key Clinical Features

- The most common benign pulmonary neoplasm
- Usually asymptomatic, incidental finding
- Common in males, especially elderly men

Key Radiological Features

- Chest x-ray: solitary or multiple discrete, round, golf ball-like lesions ("coin lesions"), usually peripherally located, about 10% endobronchial

Cytological Features

- A mixture of mesenchymal and epithelial elements
- Immature fibromyxoid matrix
- Mature cartilage with chondrocytes in lacunae
- Benign glandular cells
- Adipocytes
- Representative images are shown in Fig. 6.16a, b.

Differential Diagnosis

- Epithelial malignancy

Histology

- Round to multilobulated, well-circumscribed tumor nodules composed of mesenchymal tissues, including chondroid or chondromyxoid tissue, fat, connective tissue, smooth muscle, and bone in various proportions, intermixed with clefts of respiratory epithelial cells
- Chondromyxoid tissue usually predominates.
- Representative images are shown in Fig. 6.16c, d.

Immunohistochemistry

- Immunohistochemistry is usually not necessary for diagnosis.
- Pulmonary hamartomas have a high frequency of translocation t(3;12)(q27–28;q14–15) leading to a gene fusion of the high mobility group protein gene AT-hook 2 (*HMGA2*) and the lipoma preferred partner (*LPP*) gene.

Inflammatory Myofibroblastic Tumor

Key Clinical Features

- Most often young patients, under the age of 40
- Male = female
- The most common endobronchial mesenchymal lesion in childhood

Key Radiological Features

- Chest x-ray: a peripheral, discrete, solitary nodule. If endobronchial location, post-obstructive pneumonia and atelectasis may be evident.

Cytological Features

- Spindle cells
- Storiform pattern
- Polymorphous inflammatory cells
- Minimal to no necrosis

Differential Diagnosis

- Sarcoma
- Mesothelioma
- Solitary fibrous tumor

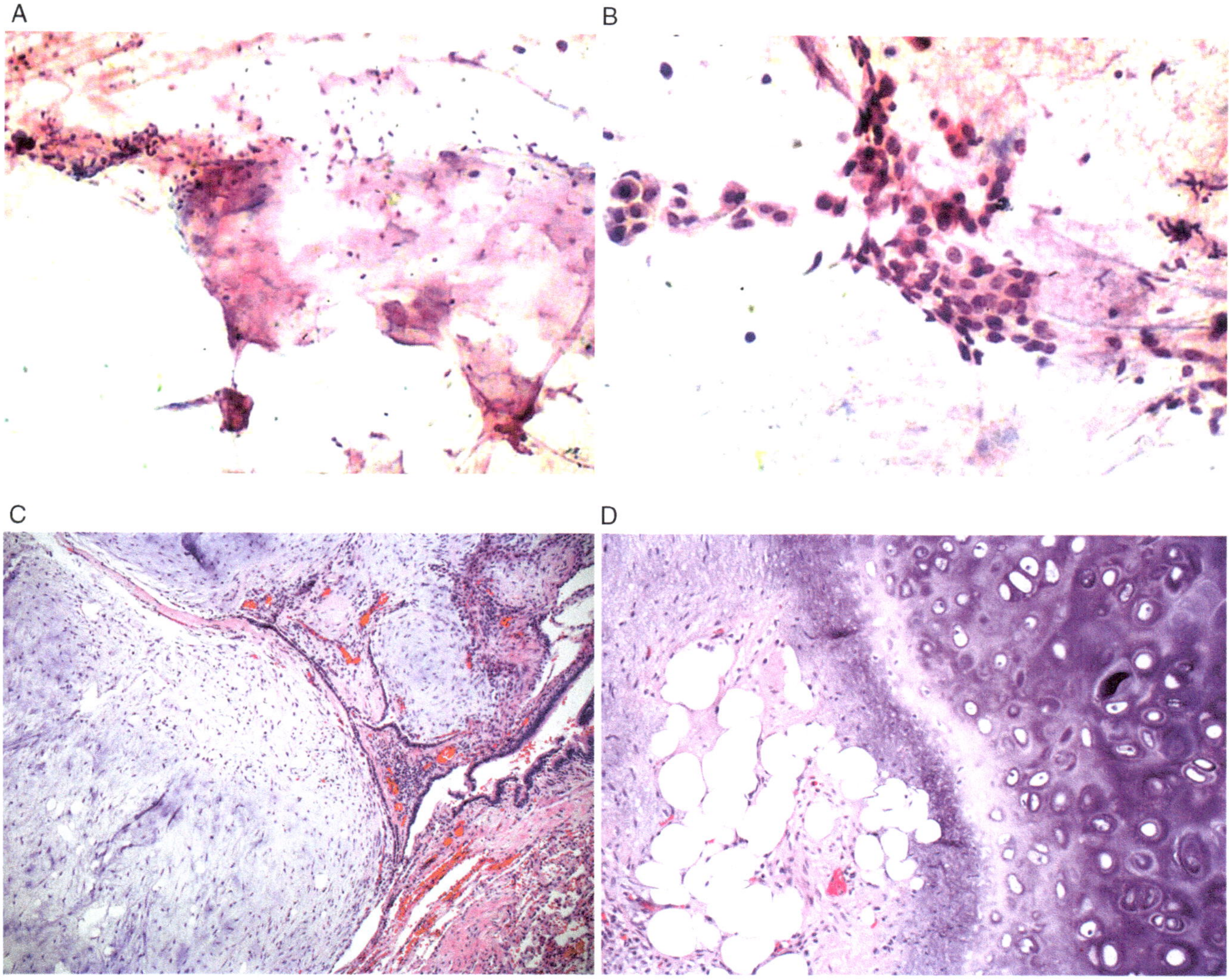

Fig. 6.16 Pulmonary hamartoma. (**a**) Sparsely cellular chondromyxoid matrix material containing scattered, benign, spindled, and stellate mesenchymal cells, Pap stain; (**b**) clusters of epithelial cells embedded in stromal, Pap stain; (**c**, **d**) histopathology, well-circumscribed, lobulated nodules of mesenchymal tissue including chondroid or chondromyxoid tissue, fat, and connective tissue intermixed with clefts of respiratory epithelial cells, H&E

Histology

- Composed of a mixture of spindle cells and obscuring inflammatory cell infiltrates, including lymphocytes, plasma cells, and histiocytes.
- Touton giant cells are often seen.
- The spindle cells contain oval nuclei with a fine chromatin pattern, inconspicuous nucleoli, and abundant bipolar lightly eosinophilic cytoplasm arranged in fascicles or a storiform architecture.
- Representative images are illustrated in Fig. 6.17a, b.

Immunohistochemistry

- Positive for vimentin, smooth muscle actin (SMA), and rarely to desmin
- Negative for myogenin, myoglobin, CD117, and S100 protein
- Focal cytokeratin (CK) positivity was reported in 1/3 of cases, likely due to alveolar entrapment.
- Anaplastic lymphoma kinase 1 (ALK1) expression was noted in 40% of cases.
- p53 is negative; however, positivity is associated with recurrence and malignant transformation.
- Representative images are illustrated in Fig. 6.17c, d.

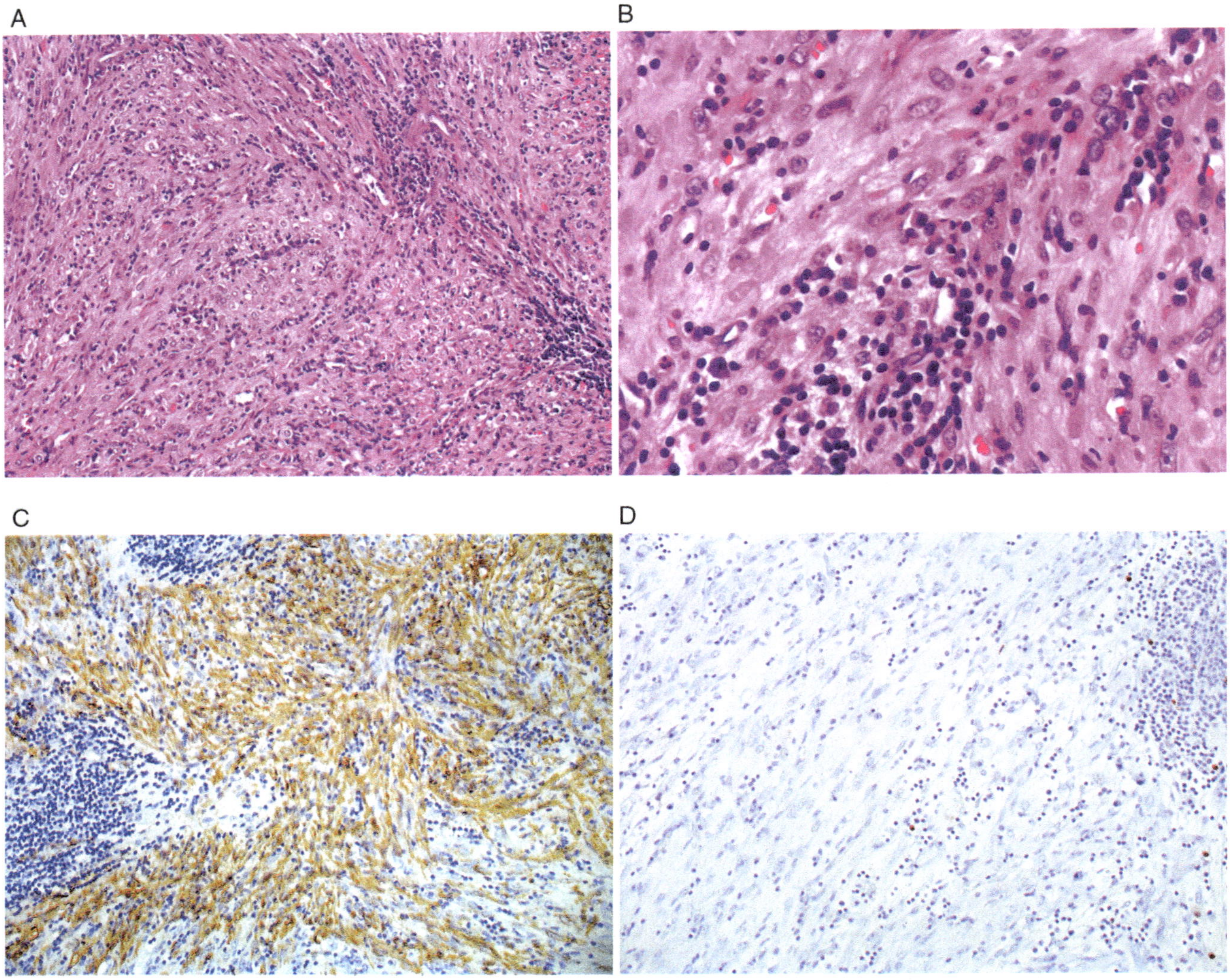

Fig. 6.17 Inflammatory myofibroblastic tumor. (**a**, **b**) Histopathology, a mixture of spindle cells and obscuring inflammatory cell infiltrates including lymphocytes, plasma cells, and histiocytes, H&E; (**c**) positive for SMA, IHC; (**d**) negative for S100, IHC

Representative Malignant Neoplasms of the Lung

Squamous Cell Carcinoma

Squamous cell carcinomas are malignant tumors that either morphologically show squamous cell differentiation (keratinization and/or intercellular bridges) or are morphologically undifferentiated non-small cell carcinomas but show squamous cell differentiation immunohistochemically. The 2015 WHO classifications of tumors of the lung reclassified squamous cell carcinomas into keratinizing, nonkeratinizing, and basaloid subtypes. The nonkeratinizing tumors require immunohistochemical proof of squamous differentiation.

Key Clinical Features

- About 20% of all pulmonary malignancies
- Clinical presentation is similar to other non-small cell carcinomas.

Key Radiological Features

- Usually a central mass with cavitation and post-obstructive pneumonia

Cytological Features

Keratinizing squamous cell carcinoma:

- Abundant dyshesive cells with dense cytoplasm, may be orangeophilic
- Polygonal, rounded, or elongated cells
- Tadpole or fiber-like cells
- Pleomorphic, pyknotic nuclei with obscured nucleoli and chromatin detail
- Anucleated cells and twisted keratin strands (Herxheimer spirals)
- Representative images are shown in Fig. 6.18a–d.

Nonkeratinizing or basaloid squamous cell carcinoma:

- Cohesive groups of cells with larger nuclei and coarsely granular chromatin
- Cyanophilic cytoplasm on Pap stain
- Rare or no keratinization
- Representative images are shown in Fig. 6.19a–f.

Differential Diagnosis

- Squamous metaplasia
- Cavitary infection
- Pemphigus vulgaris

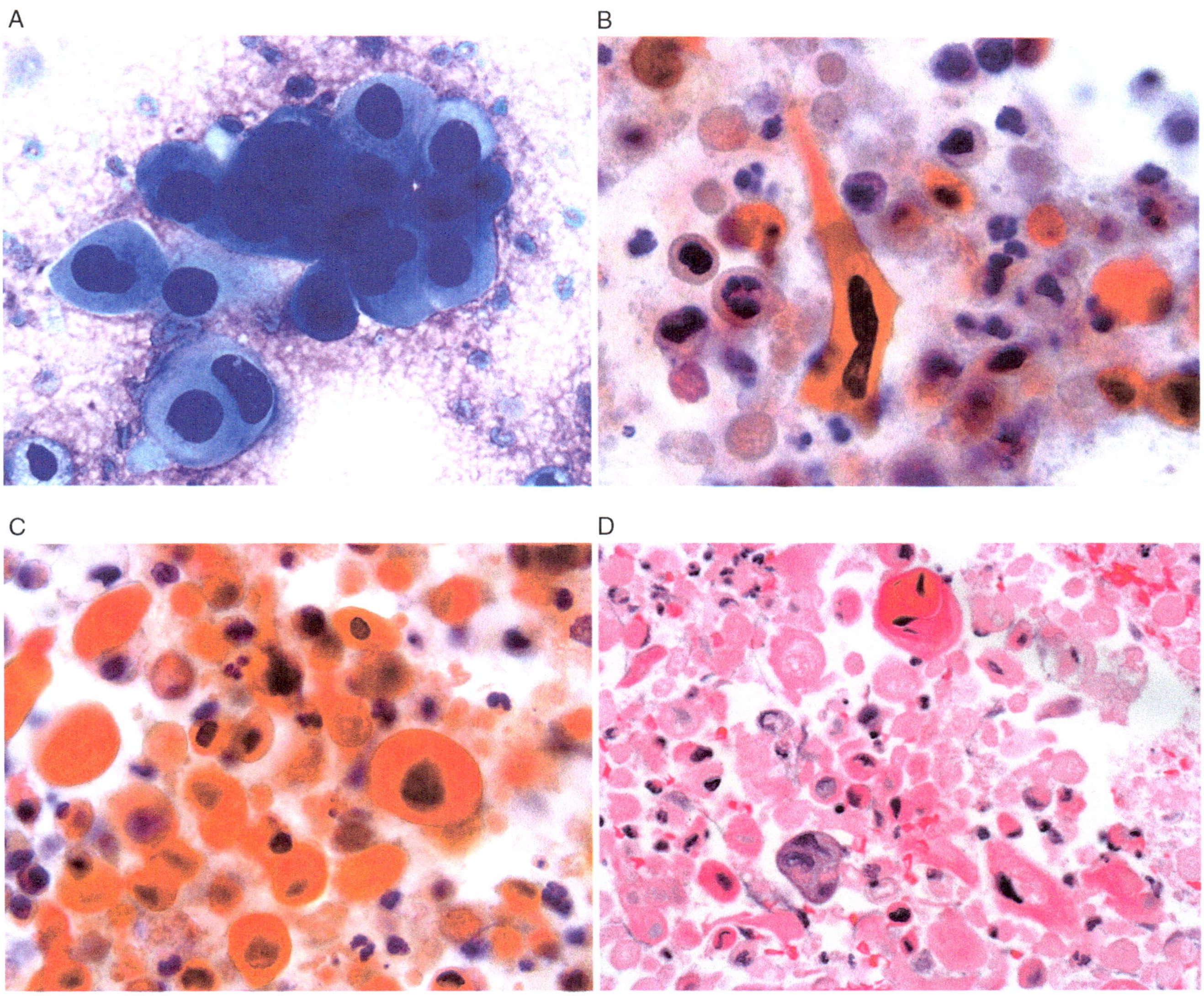

Fig. 6.18 Keratinizing squamous cell carcinoma, cytology. (**a**) Polygonal to round cells with hyperchromatic nuclei and hard cytoplasm, Diff-Quik; (**b**, **c**) polygonal or tadpole cells with pyknotic nuclei and dense, orangeophilic cytoplasm, Pap stain; (**d**) keratin pearls and debris, cell block, H&E

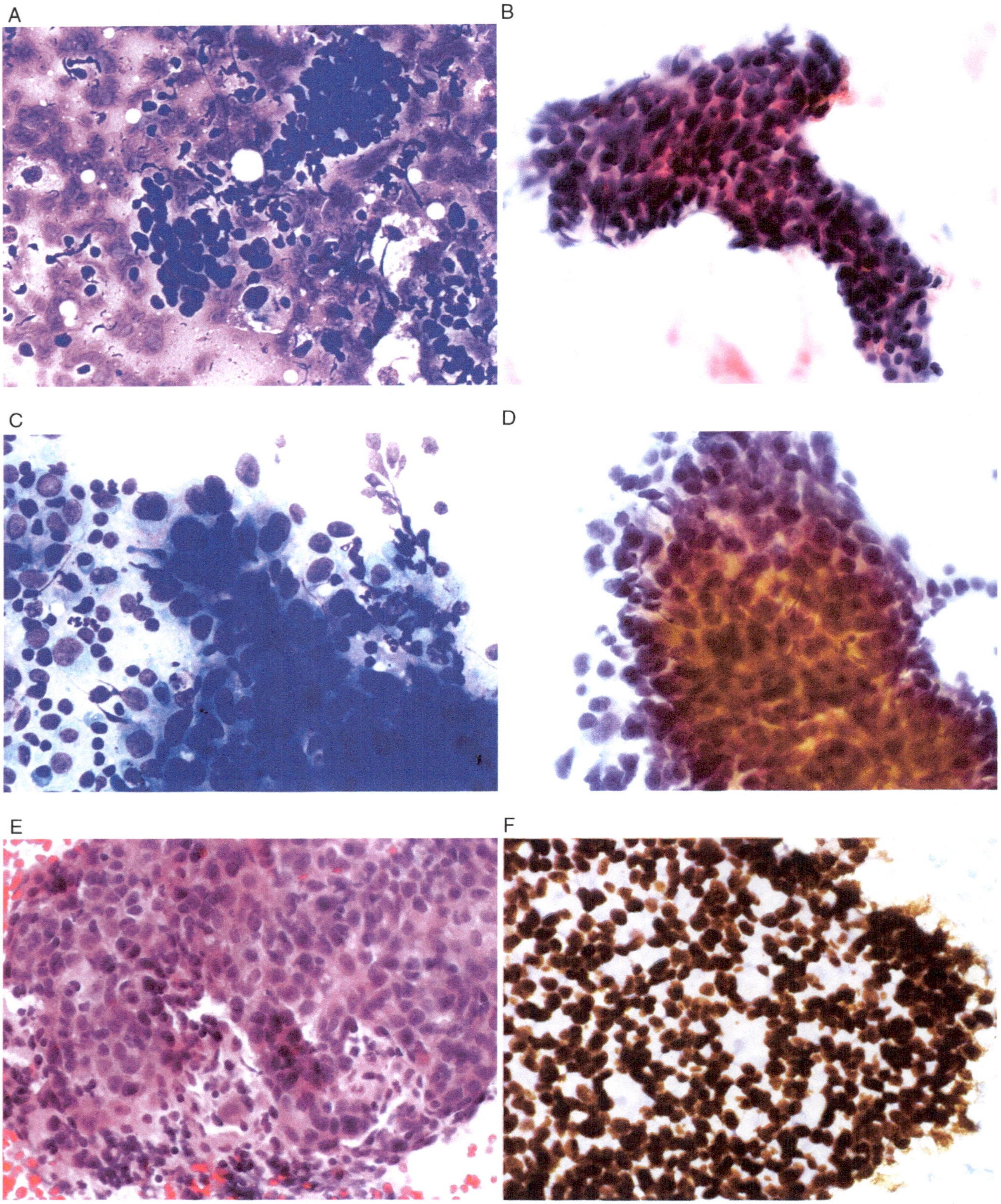

Fig. 6.19 Nonkeratinizing, basaloid squamous cell carcinoma, cytology. (**a**) Cohesive groups of atypical cells with hyperchromatic nuclei and coarse, granular chromatin texture, basaloid, Diff-Quik; (**b**) similar, basaloid, Pap stain; (**c**) cohesive cluster of atypical epithelial cells, no keratinization identified, Diff-Quik; (**d**) similar to C, Pap stain; (**e**) tumor cell cluster in cellblock, H&E; F. p40-decorated tumor nuclei, IHC

- Radiation/chemotherapy effect
- Other non-small cell carcinoma
- Small cell carcinoma
- Upper airway cancer contamination

Histology

- Three subtypes of squamous cell carcinoma in the 2015 WHO classification of tumors of the lung: keratinizing, nonkeratinizing, and basaloid subtypes:
  1. Keratinizing squamous cell carcinomas exhibit recognizable keratinization, keratin pearls, and/or intercellular bridges, as illustrated in Fig. 6.20a, b.
  2. Nonkeratinizing squamous cell carcinomas are without recognizable keratinization, keratin pearls, or intercellular bridges, as illustrated in Fig. 6.20c.
  3. Basaloid squamous cell carcinomas are tumors with a basaloid component in greater than 50% of the tumor, regardless of the presence of any keratinization, as illustrated in Fig. 6.20d.

Immunohistochemistry

- Immunohistochemistry is required for the diagnosis of nonkeratinizing squamous cell carcinomas.
- Squamous cell carcinomas express p40, p63, and CK5/6.
- TTF1 is usually negative in keratinizing squamous cell carcinomas, may be weakly focally positive in nonkeratinizing squamous cell carcinomas.
- Representative images are illustrated in Fig. 6.21a–d.
- Squamous cell carcinomas of lung are characterized by complex genomic alterations, frequently involving the following pathways:

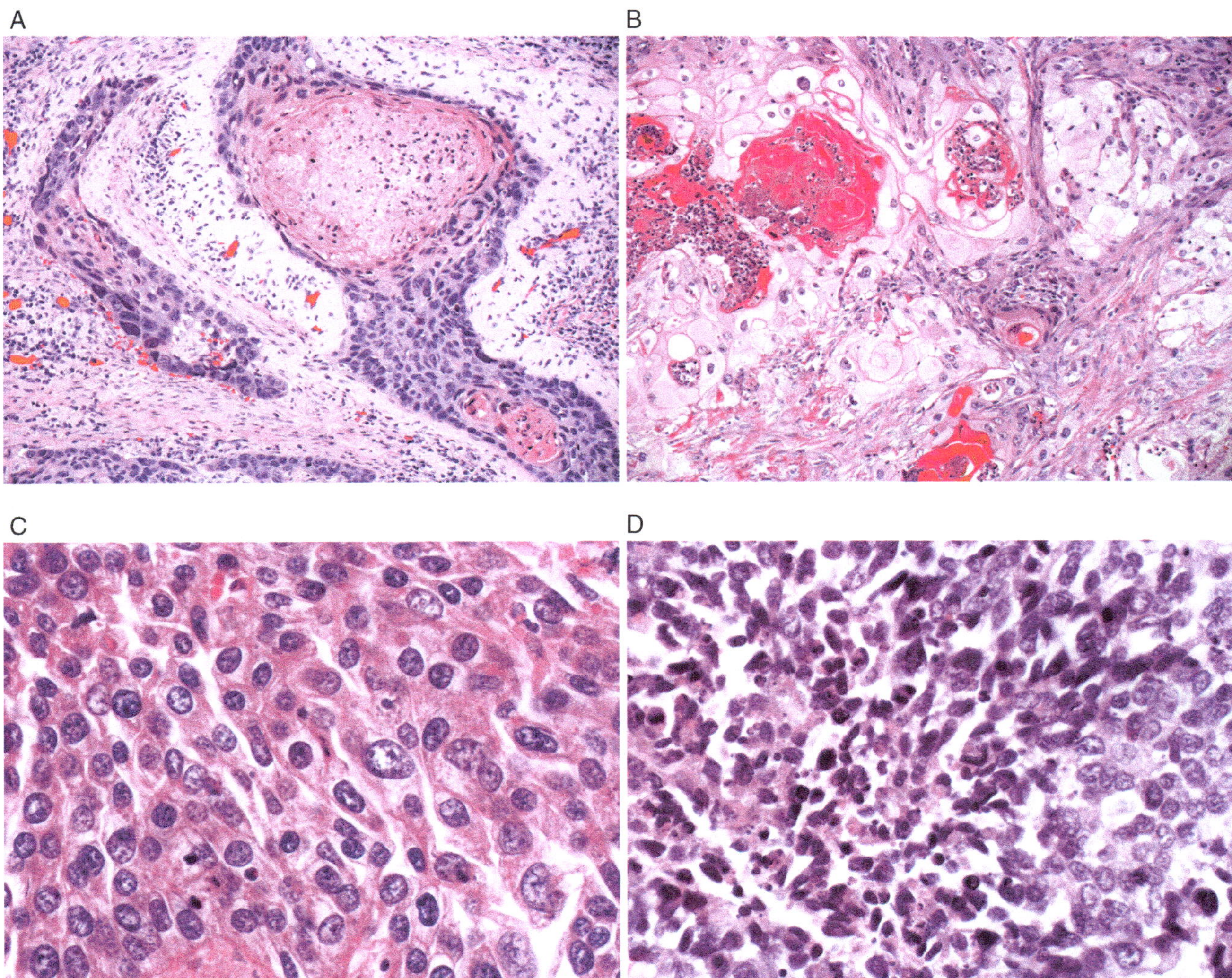

Fig. 6.20 Squamous cell carcinoma, histopathology. (**a**, **b**) Keratinizing squamous cell carcinoma, H&E; (**c**) nonkeratinizing squamous cell carcinoma, H&E; (**d**) basaloid squamous cell carcinoma exhibits solid islands of larger, hyperchromatic tumor cells with peripheral palisading, H&E

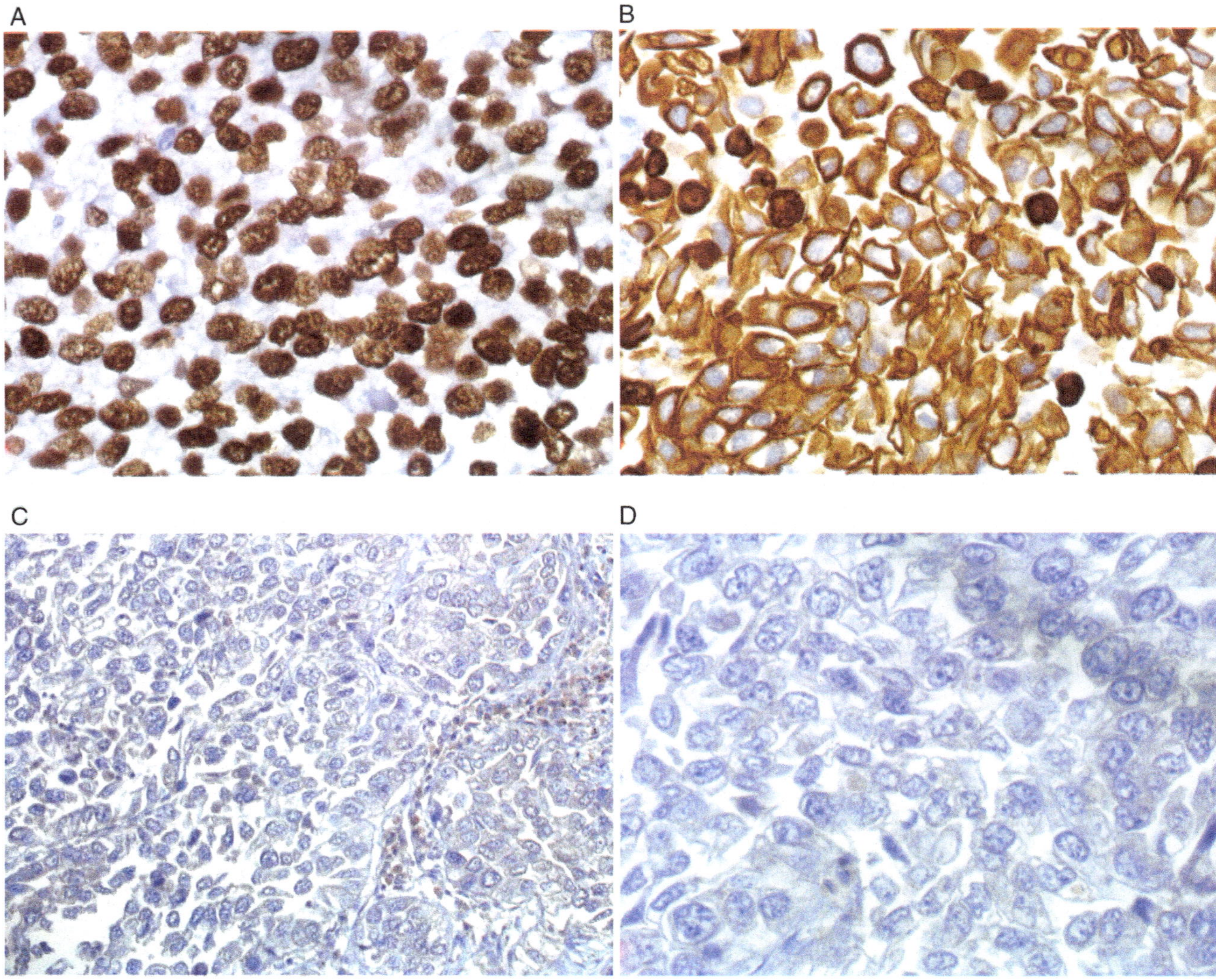

Fig. 6.21 Immunophenotype of squamous cell carcinoma. (**a**) Positive nuclear staining for p40, IHC; (**b**) positive CK5/6 staining, IHC; (**c**) negative TTF1 staining, IHC; (**d**) negative CK7 staining, IHC

1. Cyclin-dependent kinase inhibitor 2A/retinoblastoma 1/nuclear factor, erythroid 2 like 2/Kelch-like ECH-associated protein 1/cullin 3 (CDKN2A/RB1, NFE2L2/KEAP1/CUL3)
2. Phosphoinositide 3-kinase/protein kinase B (PI3K/AKT)
3. Sex-determining region Y box 2/tumor protein 63/Notch (Drosophila) homolog 1(*SOX2/TP63/NOTCH1)*

Gene copy number alterations involving chromosomes 3q (*SOX2, TP63*), 7p (*EGFR*), and 8p (fibroblast growth factor receptor 1 [*FGFR1*]) are characteristic. Almost all tumors display somatic mutation of tumor protein 53 (*TP53)*. Deletion of chromosome 9p (*CDKN2A*) was observed in 72% of cases.

Adenocarcinoma (ADC)

Key Clinical Features

- The most common primary pulmonary malignancy, accounting for about 40% of cases.
- Mortality and incidence rates have generally been highest in high-income countries but are now declining, especially in younger males and females.
- Has been more common in men than in women, but has begun to converge.

Key Radiological Features

- Usually a solitary peripheral nodule/mass

Cytological Features

- Cohesive, three-dimensional groups.
- Eccentric, irregular nuclei with granular chromatin, and prominent nucleoli.
- Transparent, foamy cytoplasm, may have secretory vacuoles.
- Invasive mucinous ADC: high cellularity, sheets and three-dimensional groups of relatively uniform cells, nuclear enlargement and irregular contour, and nucleoli. May have pseudoinclusions, psammoma bodies, and nuclear grooves/clearing.
- Poorly differentiated ADC: cohesive groups of overtly malignant cells with nuclear pleomorphism, nuclear membrane irregularity, and coarse chromatin pattern; cytoplasmic mucin is inconspicuous.
- Representative images are shown in Fig. 6.22a–h.

Differential Diagnosis

- Metastatic ADC
- Reactive/reparative changes
- Goblet cell hyperplasia
- Granulomatous inflammation
- Vegetable cells

Histology

- In 2011, the new International Association for the Study of Lung Cancer (IASLC)/American Thoracic Society (ATS)/European Respiratory Society (ERS) classification of lung ADC proposed significant changes to the 2004 WHO classification for resected tumors:
  1. Discontinuing the terms bronchioloalveolar carcinoma (BAC) and mixed subtype ADC
  2. Adding adenocarcinoma in situ (AIS) as a preinvasive lesion to join atypical adenomatous hyperplasia
  3. Adding minimally invasive adenocarcinoma (MIA)
  4. Classifying invasive ADCs according to the predominant subtype after comprehensive histologic subtyping in 5% increments
  5. Using of "lepidic" to describe a noninvasive component (previously BAC) as part of an invasive ADC
  6. Replacing mucinous BAC with invasive mucinous ADC excluding tumors that meet the criteria for AIS or MIA
  7. Discontinuing the subtypes of clear cell and signet ring ADC
  8. Discontinuing the term mucinous cystadenocarcinoma and including these under the category of colloid ADC
- In the 2015 WHO classification, large cell carcinomas with expression of TTF1 and/or napsin A are reclassified as solid ADCs even if mucin is absent. The solid ADC must be distinguished from squamous cell carcinomas and large cell carcinomas by the identification of at least two high-power fields with five or more cells showing intracytoplasmic mucin and/or the expression of TTF1 and/or napsin A.
- The diagnostic criteria for AIS:
  1. Solitary, small tumor ≤3 cm.
  2. Purely lepidic growth pattern.
  3. No invasion: stromal, vascular, or pleural.
  4. No pattern of invasive ADC: acinar, papillary, micropapillary, solid, colloid, enteric, fetal, or invasive mucinous ADC.
  5. No spread through air spaces.
  6. Mainly nonmucinous cell type, rare mucinous.
  7. No or inconspicuous nuclear atypia.
  8. Septal widening with sclerosis/elastosis is common.
- The diagnostic criteria for MIA:
  1. Solitary, small tumor ≤3 cm.
  2. Predominantly lepidic growth pattern.
  3. ≤0.5 cm invasive component in greatest dimension in any one focus.
  4. The invasive component to be measured includes any histologic subtype other than a lepidic pattern; tumor cells infiltrating myofibroblastic stroma.
  5. MIA diagnosis is excluded if the tumor invades lymphatics, blood vessels, air spaces, or pleura, contains tumor necrosis, and spreads through air spaces.
  6. The cell type is mostly nonmucinous, but rarely may be mucinous.
- The 2015 WHO classification of tumors of lung classifies ADC as lepidic, acinar, papillary, micropapillary, or solid according to the predominant pattern after a comprehensive histologic subtyping to identify all of the different histologic patterns in 5% increments.
- Other variants of ADCs include invasive mucinous ADC, colloid ADC, fetal ADC, and enteric ADC.
- Representative images are shown in Fig. 6.23a–d.

Immunohistochemistry

- Positive for TTF1 and napsin A: commonly used markers for pneumocytes, with comparable sensitivity, about 75%; much lower TTF1 expression in solid ADCs and mucinous ADCs
- Positive for CK7
- Negative for squamous cell markers; however, p63 positivity was reported in up to 30% of lung ADCs.

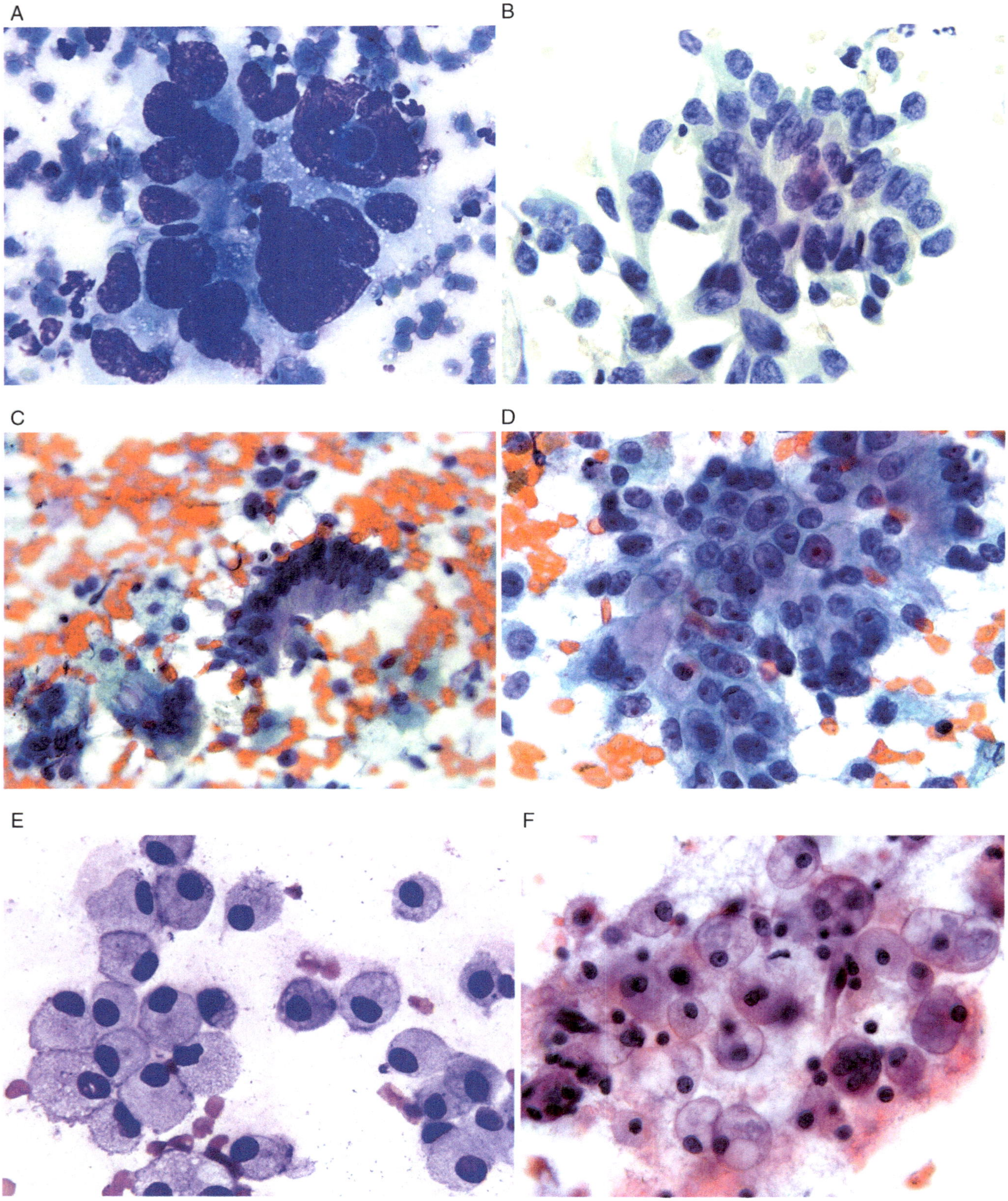

Fig. 6.22 Adenocarcinoma, cytology. (**a**) Cohesive groups of tumor cells with nuclear pleomorphism, nucleoli, and abundant foamy cytoplasm, forming acinar or ductal structure, Diff-Quik; (**b**) the same, Pap stain; (**c**, **d**) invasive mucinous adenocarcinoma, basally located nuclei with no atypia, Pap stain; (**e**) mucinous tumor cells mimic macrophages in background of mucin, Diff-Quik; Pap stain; (**f**) mucinous tumor cells mimic macrophages in background of mucin, Pap stain; (**g**) poorly differentiated adenocarcinoma showing pleomorphic tumor cells with no mucinous features identified, Diff-Quik; (**h**) poorly differentiated adenocarcinoma, Pap stain

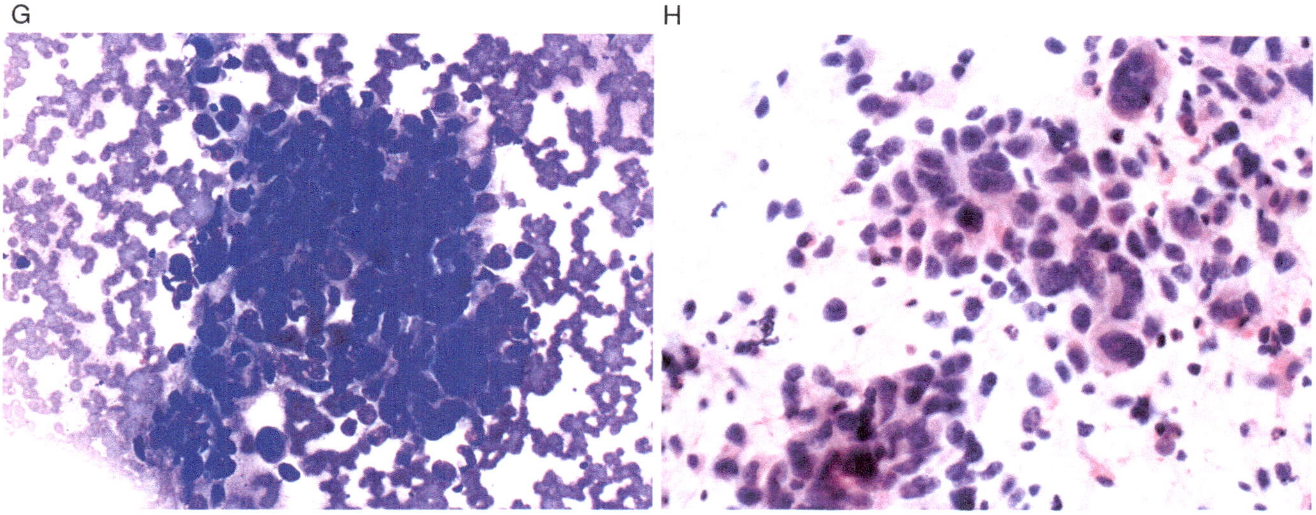

Fig. 6.22 (continued)

- Representative images are shown in Fig. 6.23e–h.
- EGFR, Kirsten rat sarcoma viral oncogene (KRAS), and ALK mutations are specific for lung ADCs. The ADCs with *EGFR* or *ALK* alteration are usually located in the periphery; in contrast, the ADCs with *KRAS* mutation are frequently located in hilar region. The prevalence for *KRAS* and *EGFR* mutations is 10–30%; the transforming fusion gene echinoderm microtubule-associated protein-like 4 (*EML4)-ALK* is found in 5% of lung ADCs. The characteristics of patients with *EGFR* mutation are Asians, never smokers, with nonmucinous tumors; for *ALK* mutation, patients are younger age, male gender, and never or light smokers; for *KRAS* mutation patients are non-Asians, smokers, with invasive mucinous ADCs usually negative for TTF1, and positive for mucin (MUC) 2,5,6 immunophenotypes.

Neuroendocrine Tumors

This group of tumor represents a morphologic and biologic spectrum of tumors that is classified by the 2015 WHO classification of tumors of the lung into four types: preinvasive lesion (including diffuse idiopathic pulmonary neuroendocrine cell hyperplasia), carcinoid tumors (including typical and atypical carcinoid tumors), large cell neuroendocrine carcinoma (LCNEC), including combined LCNEC, and small cell carcinoma (including combined small cell carcinoma).

Carcinoid Tumor

Carcinoid tumors are neuroendocrine epithelial malignancies, including typical carcinoids, defined as those with <2 mitoses/per 2 mm^2, lacking necrosis, ≥0.5 cm in size, and atypical carcinoids, which are those with 2–10 mitoses/per 2 mm^2 and/or foci of necrosis.

Key Clinical Features

- Account for <1% of all lung cancers.
- Majority (70–90%) are typical carcinoids.
- More common in female, white, and <60 years old.
- Clinical syndromes are uncommon, including carcinoid syndrome, Cushing syndrome, and acromegaly.

Key Radiographic Findings

- Chest x-ray: usually a centrally located, lobulated mass with a prominent endobronchial component; one third of tumors in periphery.
- CT using intravenous contrast medium shows considerable enhancement; calcification, especially in centrally located tumors; atelectasis; bronchiectasis; and hyperlucency for tumors with bronchial involvement.

Cytological Features

- Loosely cohesive groups and single uniform cells with granular nuclei and ample eosinophilic cytoplasm and naked nuclei.
- Round, columnar, or plasmacytoid cells, forming acinar or rosette-like structures.
- Branching capillaries.
- Clean background.

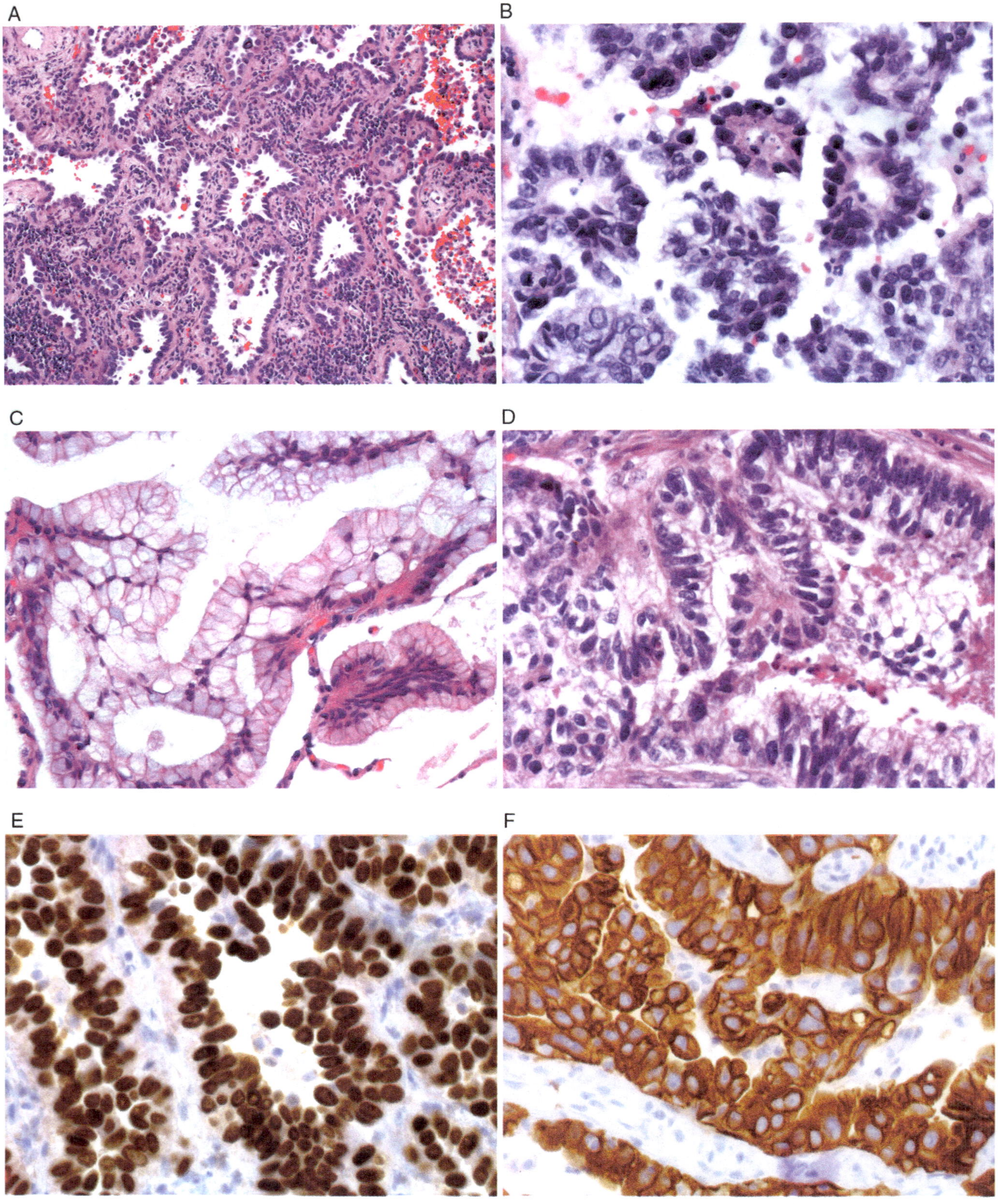

Fig. 6.23 Adenocarcinoma, histopathology and immunophenotype. (**a**) Lepidic growth pattern, H&E; (**b**) micropapillary pattern, H&E; (**c**) mucinous, H&E; (**d**) fetal adenocarcinoma, H&E; (**e**) nuclear staining for TTF1, IHC; (**f**) positive for CK7, IHC; (**g**) positive for napsin-A, IHC; (**h**) negative for p40, IHC

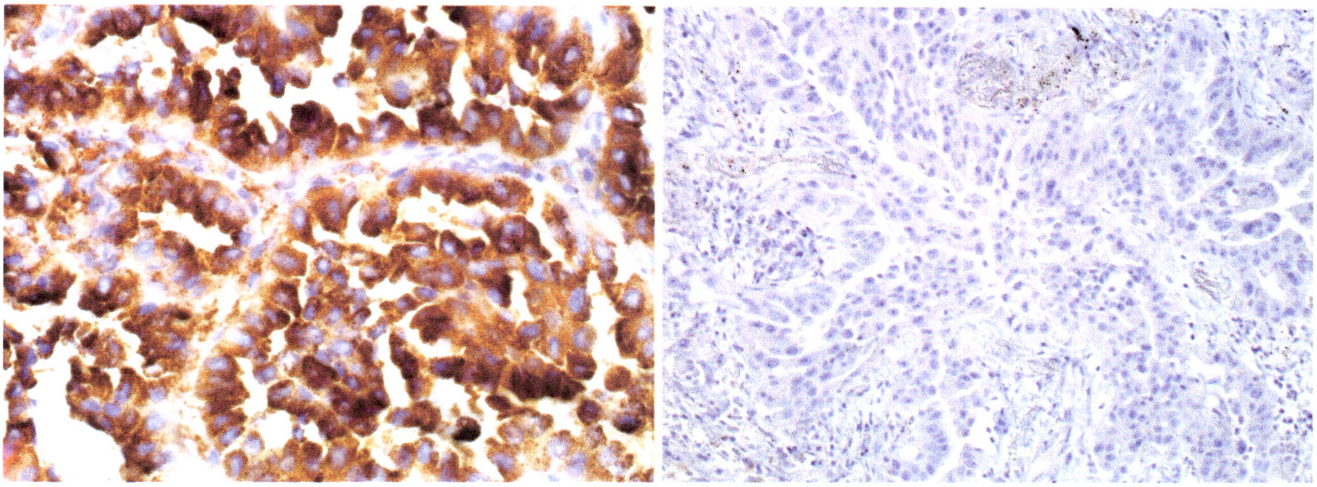

Fig. 6.23 (continued)

- May show pleomorphism and prominent nucleoli in atypical carcinoids.
- Mitoses uncommon, no necrosis in typical carcinoids; necrosis and mitosis seen in atypical carcinoids.
- Representative images are shown in Fig. 6.24a, b.

Differential Diagnosis

- Small cell carcinoma
- Lymphoma
- Benign bronchial epithelial cells
- Mesenchymal tumor (spindle cell carcinoid)
- ADC

Histology

- Usually uniform polygonal or spindled cells arranged in organoid or trabecular patterns.
- Other growth patterns also seen: rosette formation, papillary, pseudoglandular, or follicular patterns.
- Significant pleomorphism and prominent nucleoli may be seen in typical carcinoids.
- The differential features for atypical carcinoids are the presence of 2–10 mitoses per 2 mm^2 and/or necrosis. These changes may be focal.
- Representative images are shown in Fig. 6.24c–f.

Immunohistochemistry

- Immunohistochemistry is recommended for the diagnosis of neuroendocrine tumors, not only in small biopsy or cytology cases but also in resected specimens.
- The typical phenotype expresses neuroendocrine markers (CD56, synaptophysin, chromogranin); most are positive for panCK and negative for high molecular weight cytokeratins (HMWCKs) and TTF1. However, TTF-1 expression was reported in 43–53% of cases.
- The proliferative index (ki-67) is valuable in distinguishing carcinoids from high-grade neuroendocrine carcinomas, especially in small biopsies or cytology specimens with significant crush artifact. Small cell carcinomas have high proliferative index (>50%) in contrast to <10–20% in carcinoids.
- Ki-67 is not recommended for the distinction of typical from atypical carcinoids due to the lack of cutoff value.
- Representative images are shown in Fig. 6.25a–d.

Large Cell Neuroendocrine Carcinoma (LCNEC)

Key Clinical Features

- Heavy smokers in >90% of cases.
- Paraneoplastic syndrome is uncommon.

Key Radiological Findings

- Usually a periphery mass with irregular margin, with or without intratumoral calcification
- The tumors are usually large, showing central inhomogeneous enhancement on CT with contrast.
- Cavitation uncommon

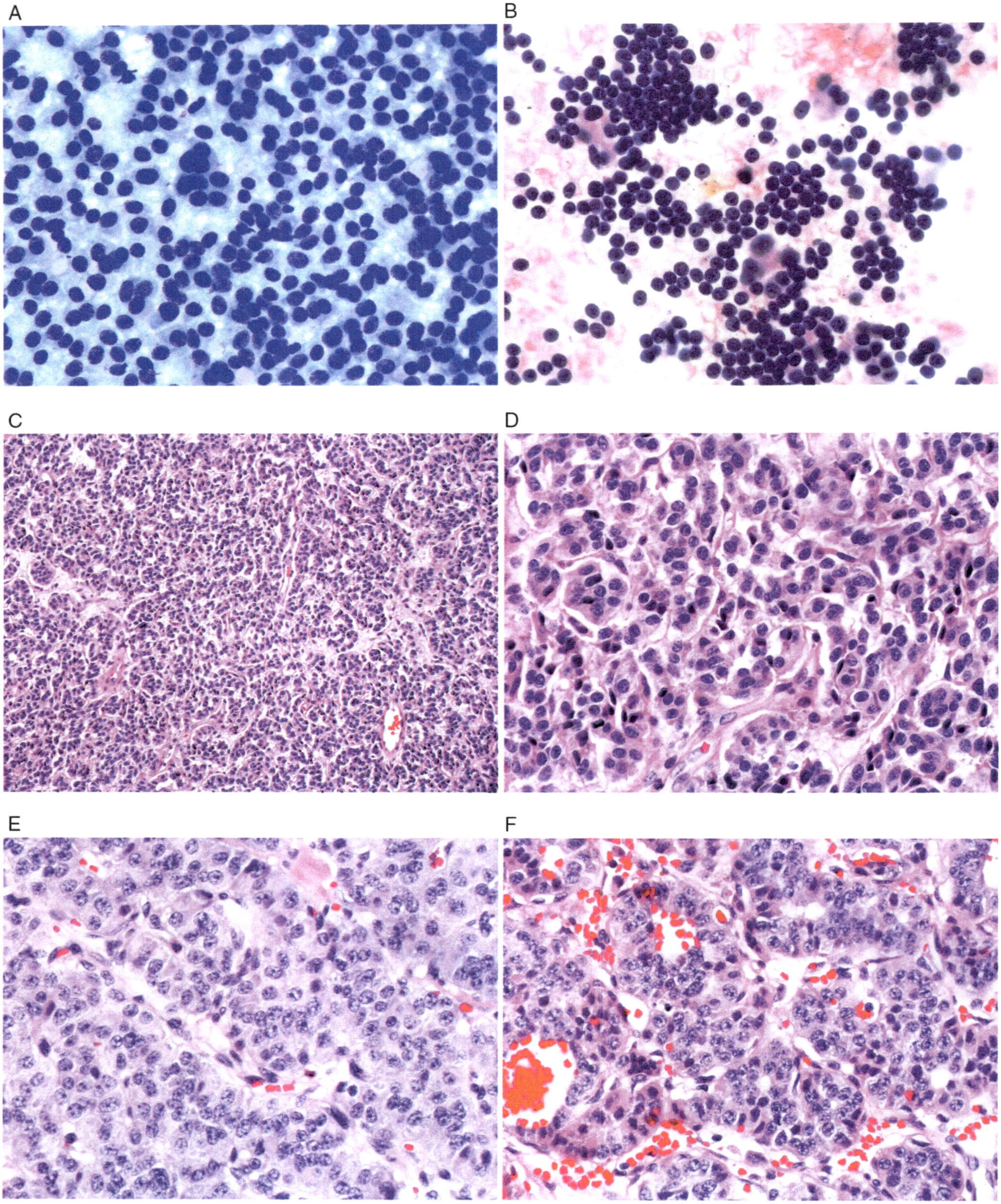

Fig. 6.24 Carcinoid tumors, cytology. (**a**) Loosely cohesive groups and single uniform round to oval cells with granular nuclei and ample eosinophilic cytoplasm, Diff-Quik stain; (**b**) same, Pap stain; (**c**, **d**) typical carcinoid, composed of uniform polygonal and spindled cells arranged in organoid and trabecular patterns, H&E; (**e**, **f**) atypical carcinoid, the cells are more atypical with focal prominent nucleoli, rare necrosis, and 2–10 mitoses/per 2 mm^2

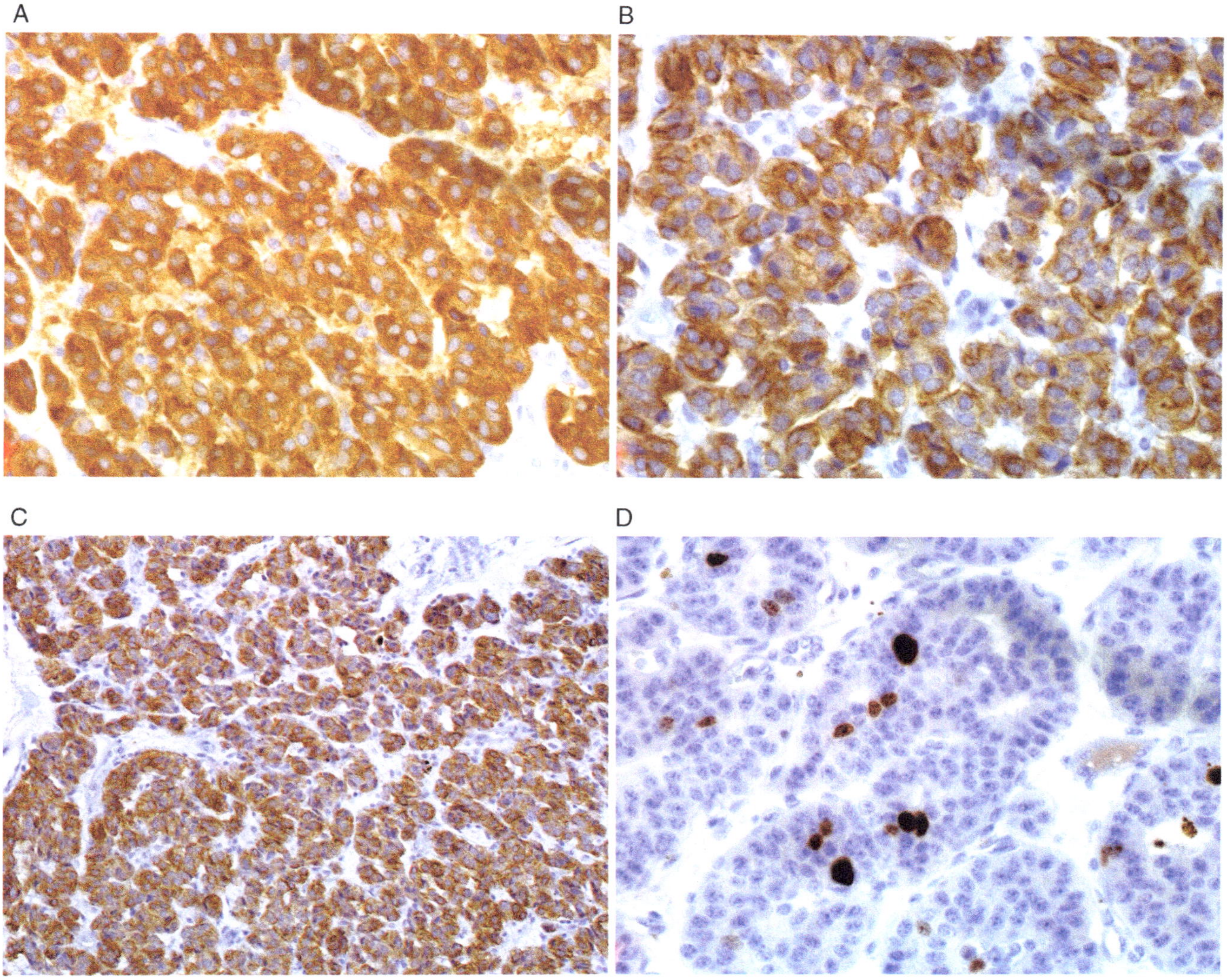

Fig. 6.25 Carcinoids, immunohistophenotype. (**a**) Positive for synaptophysin, IHC; (**b**) positive for chromogranin, IHC; (**c**) positive for AE1/3, IHC; (**d**) very low MIB-1, IHC

Cytological Features

- Overlapping with other neuroendocrine tumors and ADCs
- Loosely cohesive or single, monotonous tumor cells with a hyperchromatic nuclear chromatin pattern but easily appreciated nucleoli, nuclear membrane irregularity, and preserved moderate to abundant, delicate cytoplasm
- Necrosis or apoptotic debris may be seen.
- Representative images are shown in Fig. 6.26a, b.

Differential Diagnosis

- Other neuroendocrine tumors, including small cell carcinoma
- Other non-small cell carcinomas, such as ADC, basaloid squamous cell carcinoma, and large cell carcinoma
- Melanoma
- Metastasis

Histology

- Usually arranged in typical neuroendocrine tumor growth patterns, such as organoid, trabecular, rosette-like, peripheral palisading, or solid patterns.
- The tumor cells are often larger, with nucleoli (often prominent) and moderate to abundant cytoplasm.
- Mitotic figures >10/per 2 mm^2 (with an average of 75) of viable tumor; tumors with <30 mitoses/per 2 mm^2 are rare.

- The proliferative index (ki-67) is usually in the range of 40–80%.
- Necrosis is common.
- Representative images are shown in Fig. 6.26c, d.

Immunohistochemistry

- Immunohistochemical markers such as synaptophysin, chromogranin, and CD56 are required to confirm neuroendocrine differentiation of the tumor.
- CD56 was reported in 92–100% of cases, chromogranin in 80–85%, and synaptophysin in 50–60%.
- About 50% of cases are positive for TTF1.
- PanCK, low molecular weight cytokeratin (LMWCK), and CK7 are expressed in either dot-like or diffuse cytoplasmic patterns.
- CD117 positivity was reported in >70% of cases.

Small Cell Carcinoma

Key Clinical Features

- Thirteen percent of all newly diagnosed lung cancers are small cell carcinomas.
- Virtually all are heavy smokers, male predominant.

Key Radiological Findings

- Usually a centrally located lobulated mass, with occasional endobrochial involvement; 5% peripherally located
- A large hilar mass with bulky mediastinal lymph nodes is characteristic; invasion of hilar vessels and vena cava is common; cavitation is rare.

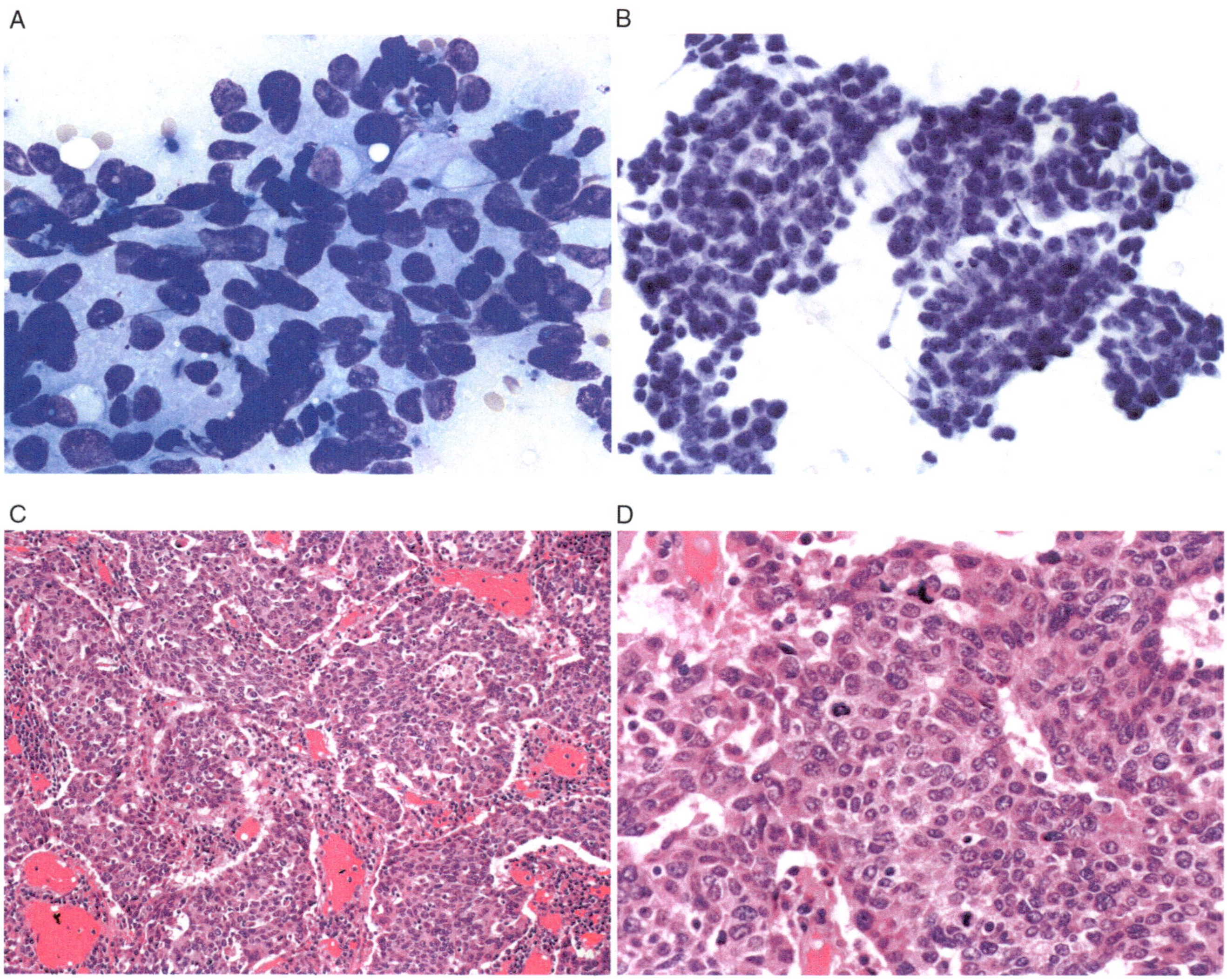

Fig. 6.26 Large cell neuroendocrine carcinoma. (**a**, **b**) Loosely cohesive cluster of mildly pleomorphic tumor cells with hyperchromatic nuclear chromatin pattern but easily appreciated nucleoli, nuclear membrane irregularity, and preserved moderate to abundant, delicate cytoplasm, Diff-Quik (**a**) and Pap (**b**) stains; (**c**) large tumor cells with prominent nucleoli and moderate to abundant cytoplasm, arranged in irregular nests, H&E; (**d**) mitotic figures are easily identified, H&E

Cytological Features

- Small cells with hyperchromatic nuclei, powdery chromatin texture, indistinct nucleoli, nuclear molding, and scant cytoplasm
- Marked mitosis and single cell necrosis
- Nuclear debris and crush artifact in the background
- Representative images are shown in Fig. 6.27a–d.

Differential Diagnosis

- Reserve cell hyperplasia
- Carcinoids
- Small blue cell tumors, such as lymphoma, Ewing sarcoma, and rhabdomyosarcoma
- Non-small cell carcinoma
- Pulmonary blastoma
- Merkel cell carcinoma

Histology

- The tumor usually presents in a sheetlike pattern.
- The tumor cells are small, containing round, oval, or spindled nuclei, with a fine granular chromatin pattern, inconspicuous nucleoli, and scant cytoplasm, without defined cell borders.
- Nuclear molding is frequent.
- High mitotic rate is seen, at least 10 mitoses/per 2 mm^2, with an average of 60 mitoses/per 2 mm^2. The proliferative index (ki-67) is >50%, with an average of >80%.
- May show extensive necrosis
- Representative image is shown in Fig. 6.27e.

Immunohistochemistry

- Immunohistochemical studies may be required to confirm neuroendocrine and epithelial differentiation of the tumor.
- CK AE1/3, CAM5.2, and MNF116 are positive in nearly 100% of cases, with either dot-like, paranuclear, or diffuse cytoplasmic staining patterns.
- Neuroendocrine markers (CD56, synaptophysin, and chromogranin) are reactive in the majority of cases; CD56 and synaptophysin are usually diffuse and strong, but chromogranin is often focal and weak.
- <10% of small cell carcinomas may lack or have only very focal expression of neuroendocrine markers.
- TTF1 is positive in up to 90–95% of cases.
- CD117 positivity was reported in 60% of cases.
- Representative images are shown in Fig. 6.27f–j.

The features of differential diagnosis for neuroendocrine tumors are summarized in Table 6.5.

Large Cell Carcinoma

Key Clinical Features

- About 2.3% of all pulmonary malignancies.
- Usually in the sixth decade, male predominant.
- Most patients are smokers.

Key Radiographic Features

- Chest x-ray: usually a peripheral mass, rarely may be cavitated

Cytological Features

- Single cells or loose clusters
- Vesicular, pleomorphic nuclei with irregular nuclear membrane, multiple nucleoli and high nuclear-to-cytoplasmic ratio
- Ill-defined, feathery cytoplasm

Differential Diagnosis

- Poorly differentiated non-small cell carcinoma
- Melanoma
- Metastatic carcinoma
- Radiation reaction
- Large cell non-Hodgkin lymphoma
- Anaplastic lymphoma
- Sarcoma

Histology

- Large cell carcinoma can only be diagnosed in a resected specimen, after ruling out the presence of squamous cell carcinoma, ADC, and small cell carcinoma morphologically, immunohistochemical evidence of squamous or ADC differentiation, and mucin stain.
- For small biopsy or cytology cases, large cell carcinomas can only be diagnosed as non-small cell lung carcinoma, not otherwise specified (NSCLC, NOS).
- Composed of sheets or nests of polygonal cells with vesicular nuclei, prominent nucleoli, and moderate amounts of cytoplasm.

Immunohistochemistry

- Immunohistochemical evaluation for TTF1, p40, and, if indicated, neuroendocrine markers (synaptophysin, chromogranin, and CD56) to exclude the presence of ADC, squamous cell carcinoma, and high-grade neuroendocrine carcinomas (small and large cell).

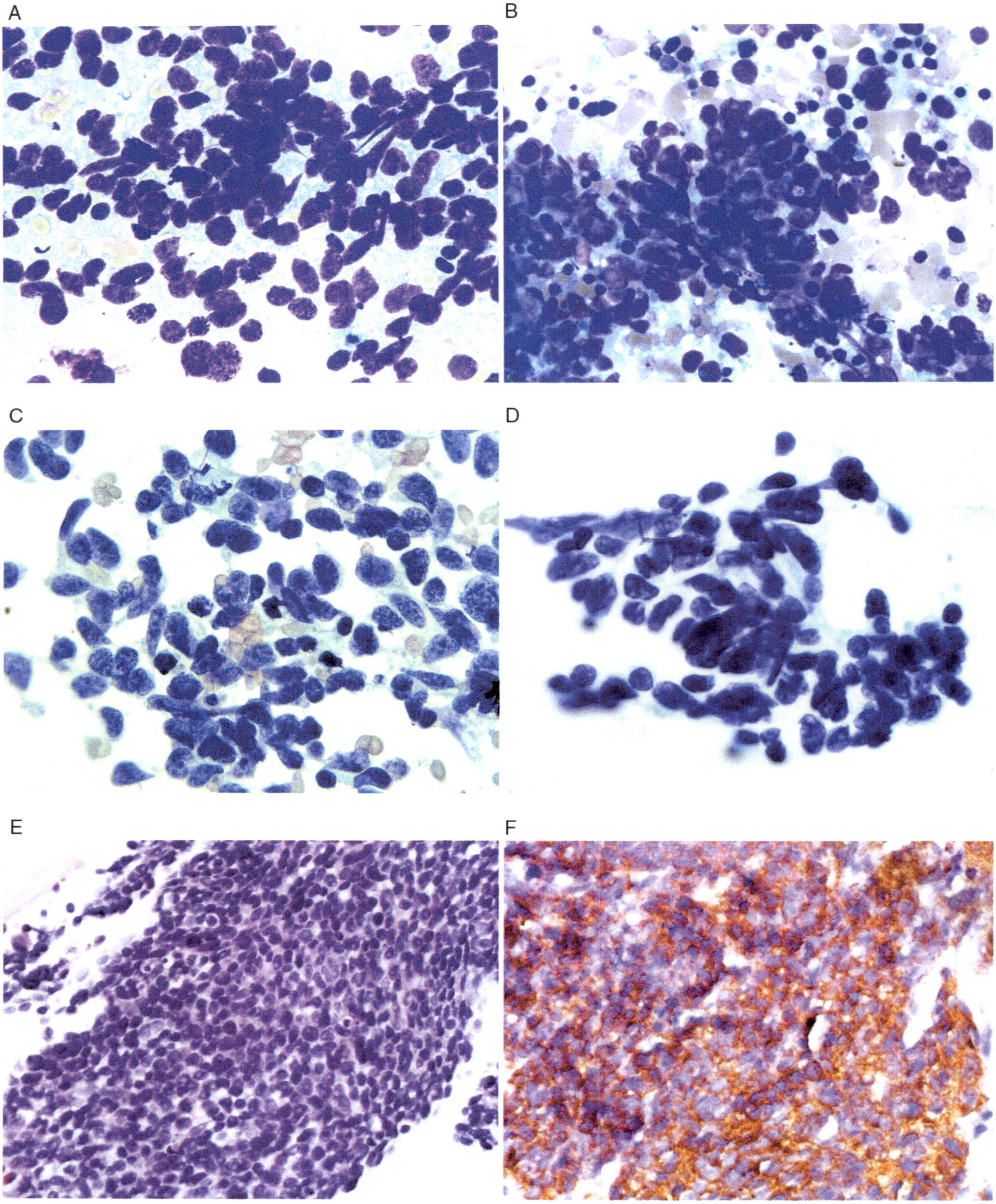

Fig. 6.27 Small cell carcinoma, cytology with immunophenotype. (**a**, **b**) Small uniform tumor cells with nuclear hyperchromasia, molding, powdery chromatin pattern, very scant cytoplasm, and abundant apoptotic cells, Diff-Quik; (**c**, **d**) lack of nucleoli, frequent mitoses, in clean background, Pap stain; (**e**) cellblock preparation shows thin cores of tumor tissue comprised of small, round to oval to spindled tumor nuclei with fine, granular chromatin pattern, inconspicuous nucleoli, and scant cytoplasm without defined cell borders, as well as abundant mitoses, H&E; (**f**) tumor cells are decorated by synaptophysin, IHC; (**g**) focal weak positivity with chromogranin, IHC; (**h**) diffuse nuclear staining for TTF-1, IHC; (**i**) positive CK7 staining, in a granular and dot-like pattern, IHC; (**j**) proliferative index (MIB-1) is estimated at 95%, IHC

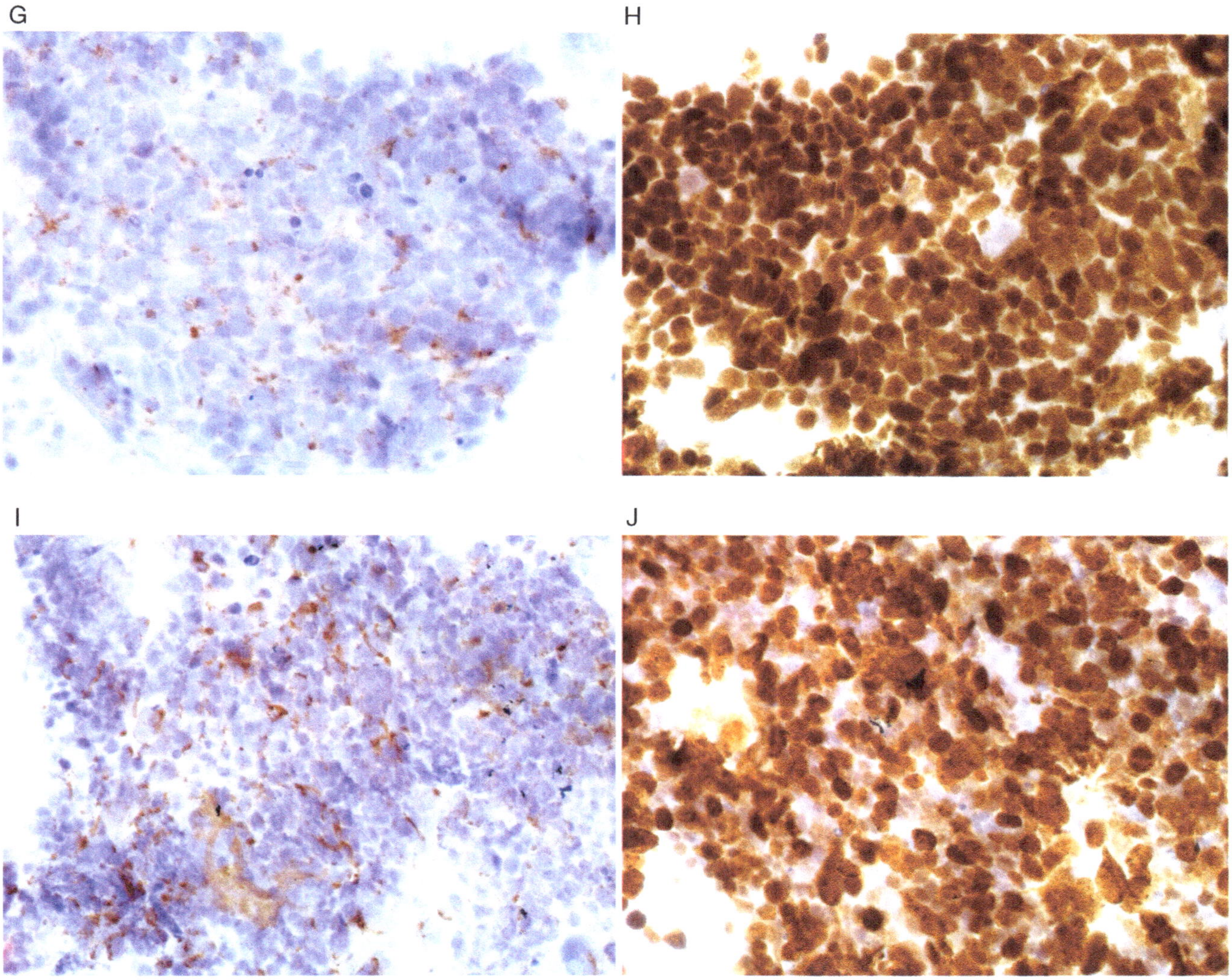

Fig. 6.27 (continued)

Table 6.5 Differential diagnosis of neuroendocrine tumors

	Typical carcinoid	Atypical carcinoid	LCNEC	SCNC
Clinical features				
Age	6th decade	6th decade	7th decade	7th decade
Gender	Female	Female	Male	Male
Smoker	No	Variable	Yes	Yes
Diagnostic criteria				
Mitosis per 2 mm²	0–1	2–10	> 10 (Med 70)	> 10 (Med 80)
Necrosis	No	Focal if any	Yes	Yes
Ki-67 index	Up to 5%	Up to 20%	40–80%	50–100%
IHC				
TTF1	Mostly –	Mostly –	+ in 50%	+ in 90–95%
SYN	+	+	+ in 80–90%	+ in 80–90%
CHR	+	+	+ in 80–90%	+ in 80–90%, F
CD56	+	+	+ in 80–90%	+ in 80–90%

LCNEC large cell neuroendocrine carcinoma, *SCNC* small cell neuroendocrine carcinoma, *Med* median, *IHC* immunohistochemistry, *TTF1* thyroid transcription factor 1, *SYN* synaptophysin, *CHR* chromogranin, *CD56* cluster of differentiation 56, *F* focal

- Only cases with negative phenotypes for those markers or cases with unclear patterns are classified as large cell carcinomas.
- Three subtypes of large cell carcinomas are based on immunophenotype:
  1. Large cell carcinoma with null immunohistochemical features: mucin –; cytokeratin +; TTF1 –; p63/p40/CK5/6 –
  2. Large cell carcinoma with unclear immunohistochemical features: mucin –; cytokeratin +; TTF1 –; p63/p40/CK5/6: any one of them showing focal +
  3. Large cell carcinoma with no additional stains: no immunohistochemical or mucin staining available
- Genomic data are limited to marker-null large cell carcinomas. The mutations found are those showing association with ADCs, such as *KRAS* and occasional *EGFR*. *TP53* mutations, *CDKN2A* deletions, and *MYC* as well as cyclin E1 (*CCNE1*) amplifications are also reported, with a similar frequency to that of other histological types. Therefore, molecular testing is recommended for large cell carcinomas.

Sarcomatoid Carcinoma

Sarcomatoid carcinoma is a general term that includes pleomorphic carcinoma, carcinosarcoma, and pulmonary blastoma, which are individual entities in the 2015 WHO classification. This group of tumors accounts for 2–3% of all cancer cases in a surgical series and <1% of all lung cancers. Definitive diagnosis of this group of tumors is very difficult or impossible in small biopsies and cytology specimens.

The characteristic features of individual tumors in this group are summarized in Table 6.6.

Representative images are illustrated in Fig. 6.28a–h.

Nuclear Protein in Testis (NUT) Carcinoma

This is a new entity in the 2015 WHO classification of tumors of lung. The group of carcinomas associated with

Table 6.6 Features of sarcomatoid carcinomas

	Pleomorphic, spindle cell, and giant cell CA	Carcinosarcoma	Pulmonary blastoma
Clinical features	Often smokers	Often heavy smokers Men > women, 7–8 times Median age of 65 years	Often smokers No sex predominance Common in the fifth decade
Radiographic features	A large peripheral mass, favoring the upper lobes; CT: low central attenuation, with frequent invading to adjacent pleura.	Usually centrally located mass with necrosis	Usually solitary, large, peripherally located mass
Cytologic features	1. Both malignant epithelial (ADC or SqCC) and mesenchymal-like elements 2. Discohesive, round to oval tumor giant cells with single or multiple large, irregular, lobulated nuclei, and abundant eosinophilic cytoplasm 3. Collagen or myxoid stroma, mitosis, necrosis, lymphocytes, and neutrophils	1. Both malignant epithelial and mesenchymal elements 2. The epithelial component is often SqCC with marked keratinization 3. The mesenchymal component can be heterologous differentiation	1. Biphasic tumor with fetal ADC (LG) and primitive mesenchymal stroma 2. Fetal ADC: uniform, small columnar cells with small nuclei, inconspicuous nucleoli and clear vacuolated cytoplasm 3. Stroma: loose aggregate or single dispersed small homogeneous cells with oval to elongated nuclei without nucleoli and high N/C ratio; may be embedded in myxoid tissue fragment 4. Reticulated, bubbly background
Histology	1. Pleomorphic CA: a mixture of giant and/or spindle cell elements (at least 10%) and epithelial elements, commonly ADC (31–72%), followed by undifferentiated NSCC (up to 43%) and SqCC (12–26%) 2. Spindle cell CA: composed of almost entirely malignant spindle cells in fascicular or storiform patterns 3. Giant cell CA: composed almost entirely pleomorphic giant tumor cells	1. Feature intimately admixed NSCC and sarcoma 2. The NSCLC component is often SqCC, followed by ADC, adenosquamous CA, and large cell CA 3. The sarcomatous components include, in descending order of frequency, rhabdomyosarcoma, chondrosarcoma, and osteosarcoma; often in combination	1. Areas of epithelial and mesenchymal differentiation in various proportions 2. Epithelial element: essentially LG fetal ADC, composed of branching tubules or glandular structures lined by pseudostratified columnar cells with bland morphology and clear to weakly eosinophilic cytoplasm 3. Mesenchymal element: tightly packed primitive cells with oval or elongated nuclei and high N/C ratio in myxoid or fibrous background; heterologous elements may be seen

(continued)

Table 6.6 (continued)

	Pleomorphic, spindle cell, and giant cell CA	Carcinosarcoma	Pulmonary blastoma
Immunohistochemistry	1. Positive for vimentin and fascin 2. Epithelial elements: positive for corresponding differentiation markers 3. Keratin expression is not required in giant or spindle cell elements	1. Helpful to highlight the epithelial and sarcomatous differentiation 2. The NSCLC component express markers of the conventional count parts 3. The sarcomatous component expresses corresponding linage markers	1. Epithelial element: positive for CK7, CK AE1/3, CEA, EMA, and TTF1; focally positive for CHR, SYN, and vimentin 2. Mesenchymal element: positive for vimentin, MSA, focal to CK AE1/3; heterologous elements: positive for linage specific markers 3. N/C accumulation of β-catenin: both epithelial and mesenchymal elements
Molecular Genetics	*KRAS* mutation in up to 38% of cases; *EGFR* mutation in up to 25% of cases; *TP53* mutation in spindle cell and pleomorphic CAs	Frequent for *TP53* mutation Less frequent for *KRAS* mutation Very uncommon for *EGFR* mutation	Frequent missense mutations in exon 3 of *CTNNB1* *TP53* mutation and both p53 and MDM2 protein accumulation occasionally detected

CA carcinoma, *CT* computed tomography, *ADC* adenocarcinoma, *SqCC* squamous cell carcinoma, *LG* low-grade, *N/C* nuclear to cytoplasmic ratio, *NSCC* non-small cell carcinoma, *NSCLC* non-small cell lung carcinoma, *CK* cytokeratin, *CEA* carcinoembryonic antigen, *EMA* epithelial membrane antigen, *TTF1* thyroid transcription factor 1, *CHR* chromogranin, *SYN* synaptophysin, *MSA* muscle-specific actin, *KRAS* Kirsten rat sarcoma oncogene, *EGFR* epithelial growth factor receptor, *TP53* tumor protein 53, *CTNNB1* catenin beta 1, *MDM2* mouse double minute 2 homolog

chromosomal rearrangement in the *NUT* gene is designated as NUT carcinoma.

Key Clinical Features

- Affects people of all ages, although, it was originally reported in children and younger adults
- Male equals female
- Fewer than 100 cases reported
- Usually presents at an advanced stage, with pleural effusion, chest pain, weight loss, and respiratory symptoms

Key Radiological Features

- Chest x-ray: extremely rapid-growing tumor, with complete opacification of the thorax within 2–8 weeks
- CT: a hypoattenuating, heterogeneously enhancing, often extensively necrotic mass with poorly defined, infiltrative borders. High fluorodeoxyglucose (FDG) uptake is characteristic.

Cytologic Findings

- Usually cellular smears
- Discohesive clusters and single of small to intermediate size, monomorphic cells with irregular nuclear membrane, granular to coarse chromatin pattern, and discrete nucleoli
- Mitoses, necrotic debris, and crush artifact are common.
- Representative image is shown in Fig. 6.29a.

Differential Diagnosis

- Poorly differentiated malignant neoplasms
- Basaloid squamous cell carcinoma
- Small cell carcinoma
- Ewing sarcoma
- Germ cell tumor
- Acute leukemia

Histology

- NUT carcinoma, also known as NUT midline carcinoma
- Usually composed of sheets and nests of small- to intermediate-size undifferentiated cells with a monomorphic appearance
- The tumor cells are primitive-appearing, with irregular nuclear membrane, distinct nucleoli, granular to coarse chromatin, and pale eosinophilic to basophilic cytoplasm.
- Neutrophil infiltration is a prominent feature.
- Foci of abrupt keratinization are characteristic.
- Representative image is shown in Fig. 6.29b.

Immunohistochemistry

- Speckled nuclear positivity in more than 50% of tumor cells with NUT antibody is a constant finding and is diagnostic.
- Broad-spectrum cytokeratins are positive in majority of cases.
- Other epithelial markers, such as epithelial membrane antigen (EMA), epithelial cell adhesion molecule (BerEP4), and carcinoembryonic (CEA) antigen showed variable results.
- Most of cases are positive for p63/p40 and CD34.
- Occasional reactivity to synaptophysin, chromogranin, and even TTF1 was observed.

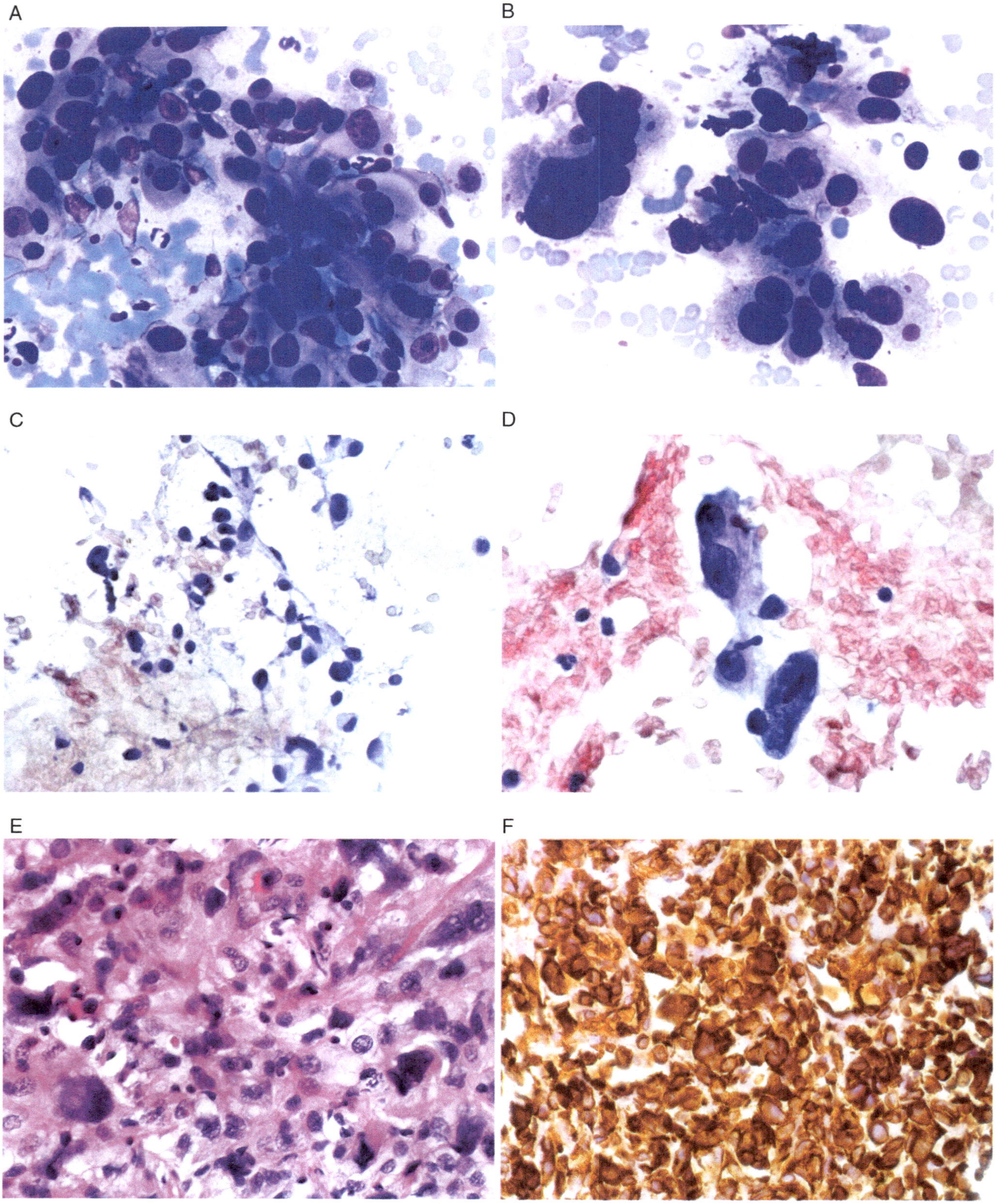

Fig. 6.28 Pleomorphic, spindle cell and giant cell carcinoma. (**a**, **b**) Discohesive, round to oval tumor giant cells with multiple large, irregular, lobulated nuclei and abundant eosinophilic cytoplasm, rare squamoid cells, and neutrophils are present, Diff-Quik; (**c**, **d**) spindled and giant tumor cells, Pap stain; (**e**) focal squamous differentiation is seen; spindled and giant tumor cells with abundant mitoses and necrosis (not shown), H&E; (**f**) vimentin positive, IHC; (**g**) AE1/3 positive, IHC; (**h**) focal CK5/6 positive, IHC

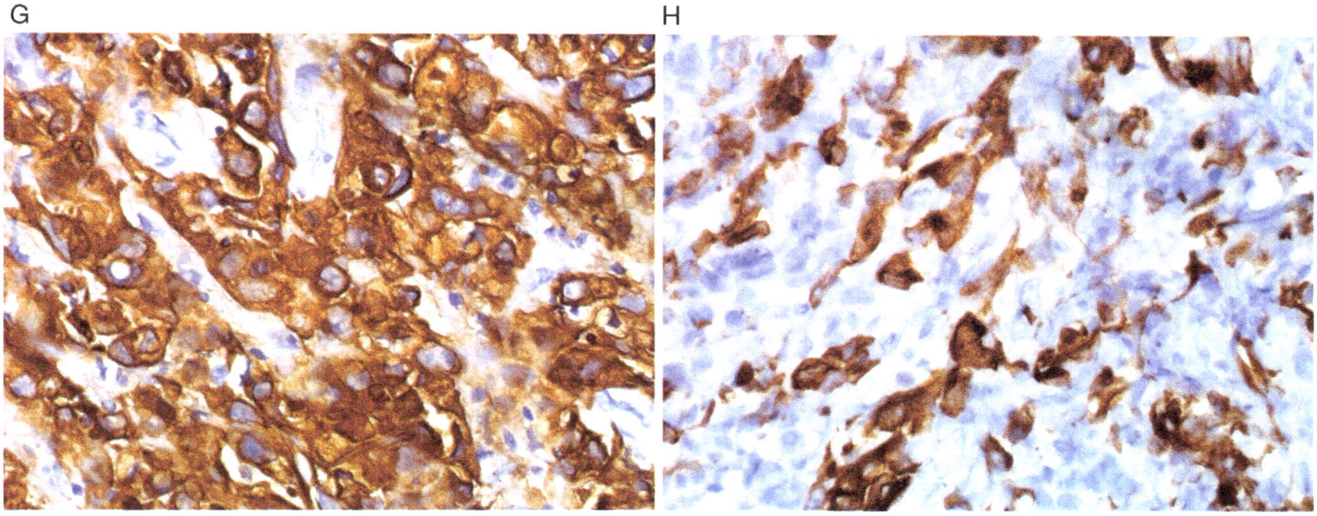

Fig. 6.28 (continued)

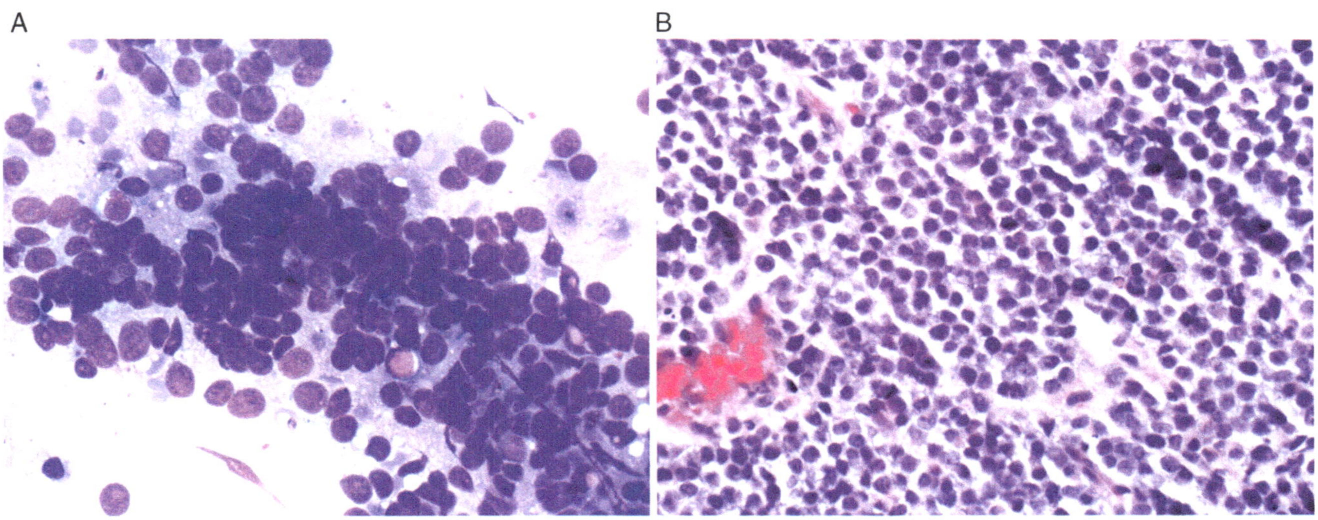

Fig. 6.29 NUT carcinoma. (**a**) Highly cellular smears contain discohesive clusters and single of small to intermediate sized, monomorphic cells, Diff-Quik; (**b**) sheets of small- to intermediate-sized, primitive-appearing cells with distinct nucleoli, granular to coarse chromatin, and pale eosinophilic to basophilic cytoplasm, H&E

- NUT carcinomas are defined by the presence of NUT gene rearrangement, which is a chromosomal translocation between the *NUT* gene (*NUTM1*) on chromosome 15q14 and other genes: Bromodomain containing *4* (*BRD4*) on chromosome 19p13.1 (70%), *BRD3* on chromosome 9q34.2 (6%), or an unknown partner gene (24%).

Metastasis to the Lung (See Chap. 7 on the Liver and Other Chapters)

The most common metastatic tumors are carcinomas, especially from the gastrointestinal tract, gynecological tract, breast, urothelial, head and neck, prostate, and other sites, followed by sarcomas, melanomas, and germ cell tumors. Sex and age distribution depend on tumor types, such as colorectal cancers in elderly patients of both sexes, breast cancer and melanoma in younger adults, and germ cell tumors and sarcomas in young adults or children. Metastases can be single or multiple, usually involving the lung parenchyma and the pleura. However, bilateral, multiple, peripherally located round, variable-size nodules (hematogenous metastases), or diffuse thickening of the interstitium (lymphangitic carcinomatosis) are typical.

Cytological features, histological findings, and immunoprofile are the same as the primary tumors. The differential immunophenotypes for the most common metastatic carcinomas are summarized in Table 6.7.

Table 6.7 Typical immunophenotypes of the common metastatic carcinomas

Antibody	Upper GI	Lower GI	Breast	GYN	Thyroid	Prostate	Urinary Bladder
CK7	+	−	+	+	+	−	+
CK20	+/−	+	−	−/+	−	−	+/−
TTF1	−	−	−	−	+	−	−
PAX8	−	−	−	+	+	−	−
GATA3	−	−	+	−	−	−	+
ER	−	−	+/−	+	−	−	−
SATB2	−	+	−	−	−	−	−
NKX3.1	−	−	−	−	−	+	−
Thyroglobulin	−	−	−	−	+	−	−
p63	−	−	−	−	−	−	+/−
CK5/6	−	−	−/+, F	−	−	−	+

− positive in <5% of cells, + positive in >70% of cells, +/− positive in 50–70% of cells, −/+ positive in <50% of cells
GI gastrointestinal tract, *GYN* gynecologic, *CK* cytokeratin, *TTF1* thyroid transcription factor-1, *PAX8* paired box gene 8, *GATA3* GATA binding protein 3, *ER* estrogen receptor, *SATB2* special AT-rich sequence-binding protein 2, *NKX3.1* NK3 homeobox 1, *F* focal

Table 6.8 2015 World Health Organization (WHO) classification of tumors of the pleura

Mesothelial tumors	*Mesenchymal tumors*
Diffuse malignant mesothelioma	Epithelioid hemangioendothelioma
Epithelioid mesothelioma	Angiosarcoma
Sarcomatoid mesothelioma	Synovial sarcoma
Desmoplastic mesothelioma	Solitary fibrous tumor
Biphasic mesothelioma	Malignant solitary fibrous tumor
Localized malignant mesothelioma	Desmoid-type fibromatosis
Epithelioid mesothelioma	Calcifying fibrous tumor
Sarcomatoid mesothelioma	Desmoplastic round cell tumor
Biphasic mesothelioma	
Well-differentiated papillary mesothelioma	
Adenomatoid tumor	
Lymphoproliferative disorders	
Primary effusion lymphoma	
Diffuse large B-cell lymphoma associated with chronic inflammation	

Used with permission from Travis WD, Brambilla E, Burke AP, Marx A, Nicholson A. WHO classification of tumors of the lung, pleura, thymus, and heart. Lyon, France: IARC; 2015

Pleura

The WHO classifications of tumors of the pleura, 2015, are summarized in Table 6.8.

Mesothelioma

Key Clinical Features

- Usually occurs in older adults, ≥60 years
- More often in men
- A strong association with asbestos exposure
- Pleural effusion is very common.

Key Radiological Features

- Variety of presentations, classically exhibiting a diffuse circumferential ring of nodular pleura associated with ipsilateral effusion
- Less commonly presents with pleural effusion without obvious pleural nodularity
- Pleural plaques, especially associated with calcifications, are suggestive of asbestos exposure.

Cytological Features

- Hypercellular specimen with mixed epithelial and spindle cells.
- Can be epithelial or spindle cell dominate.
- Resemble ordinary mesothelial cells.
- Tumor giant cells, granulomas, and psammoma can be seen.
- Representative images are shown in Fig. 6.30a–c.

Differential Diagnosis

- Pulmonary ADC (Table 6.9)
- Metastatic carcinoma
- Reactive mesothelial cells (Table 6.10)

Histology

Epithelioid Mesotheliomas

- Account for 60–80% of malignant mesotheliomas
- Variety of histological patterns. Most common patterns: solid, tubulopapillary, and trabecular; less common patterns: micropapillary, adenomatoid (microcystic), clear cell, transitional, deciduoid, and small cell

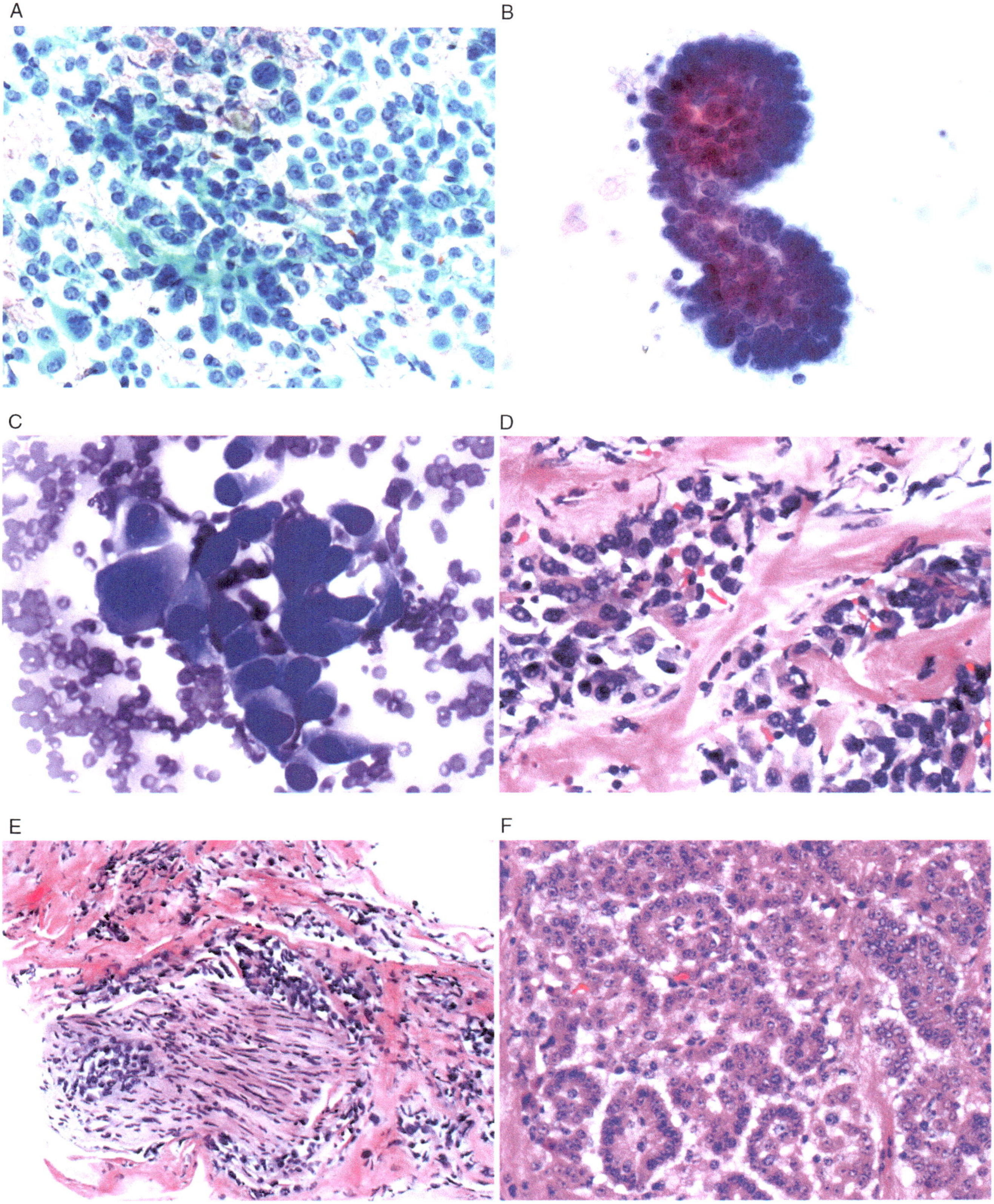

Fig. 6.30 Mesothelioma cytology and histopathology. (**a**) Cellular smears contain single and loosely clusters of plump and spindled cells, Pap stain; (**b**) epithelioid cells in papillary configuration, Diff-Quik; (**c**) atypical epithelioid cells, Diff-Quik; (**d**) histopathology, mesothelioma in nested pattern infiltrating dense fibrous tissue, H&E; (**e**) histopathology, perineural invasion, H&E; (**f**) histopathology, mesothelioma with papillary pattern, H&E

Table 6.9 Distinction of lung adenocarcinoma from mesothelioma

Markers	Mesothelioma	Adenocarcinoma
Calretinin	+	–
Cytokeratin 5/6	+	–
WT1	+	–
D2–40	+	–
MOC-31	–	+
CEA	–	+
TTF1	–	+
LeuM1	–	+
BerEP4	–	+
B72.3	–	+

"+" positive in majority of cases, "-" negative in majority of cases
Note: Two positive markers and two negative markers are usually needed to make a diagnosis of mesothelioma: (1) Two positive markers: calretinin and cytokeratin 5/6 (or Wilms tumor 1[WT1]); (2) two negative markers: CEA and MOC-31 (or B72.3)
WT1 Wilms tumor 1, *D2–40* podoplanin, *MOC-31* epithelial-related antigen, *CEA* carcinoembryonic antigen, *TTF1* thyroid transcription factor 1, *LeuM1* cluster of differentiation (CD)15, *BerEP4* epithelial cell adhesion molecule, *B72.3* tumor-associated glycopotein (TAG)72

Table 6.10 Benign mesothelial cells vs. mesothelioma

Markers	Benign mesothelial cells	Mesothelioma
GLUT1	–/+	+
CD146	–	+
IMP3	–/+	+
E-Cadherin	–	+
EMA	+/–	+
p53	–/+	+
Desmin	+	–/+
p16	+/–	–/+

– positive in <5% of cells, + positive in >70% of cells, +/– positive in 50–70% of cells, –/+ positive in <50% of cells
GLUT1 glucose transporter 1, *CD146* cluster of differentiation 146, *IMP3* insulin-like growth factor II messenger RNA binding protein-3, *EMA* epithelial membrane antigen

- The tumor cells are usually bland, with eosinophilic cytoplasm and a bland vesicular chromatin pattern. Occasional anaplastic forms may be observed.
- The fibrous stroma can vary from scant to prominent, showing varying degree of cellularity from hyalinized acellular to highly cellular stroma. Myxoid changes may be seen in 5–10% of cases, with nests of bland-looking, vacuolated epithelioid cells floating in the matrix.
- Representative images are shown in Fig. 6.30d–f.

Sarcomatoid Mesotheliomas

- Characterized by a proliferation of spindle cells arranged in fascicles or with a haphazard pattern and involves the adipose tissue of the parietal pleura or the adjacent lung parenchyma.
- The tumor cells show variety of morphology, from plump to thin, elongated cells with scant cytoplasm.
- The degree of nuclear atypia, mitotic activity, and necrosis vary from minimal to moderate to marked.

Desmoplastic Mesotheliomas

- Characterized by areas of atypical spindle cells arranged in a so-called patternless pattern within a dense, hyalinized, fibrous stroma constituting at least 50% of the tumor
- Invasion of adipose tissue is the most reliable criterion to distinguish desmoplastic mesothelioma from organizing pleuritis.

Biphasic Mesotheliomas

- Show any combination of the patterns described above constituting at least 10% of the tumor

Immunohistochemistry

- Positive for CK AE1/3, calretinin, CK5/6, WT1, and D2–40.
- Negative for BerEP4, MOC-31, B72.3, and CEA.
- See Tables 6.8 and 6.9 for differential diagnosis.
- Multiple chromosomal alterations, more common with chromosomal losses, especially on chromosomal arms 1p, 3p, 4q, 6q, 9p, 13q, 14q, and 22q; alterations in several tumor suppressor genes, including neurofibromin 2 (NF2), CDKN2A (p16INK4a), CDKN2B (p15INK4b), and BRCA1-associated protein 1 (BAP1).
- Representative images are shown in Fig. 6.31a–f.

Mesenchymal Tumors

Solitary Fibrous Tumor

Key Clinical Features

- Most common in sixth to seventh decades
- No sex predisposition
- Accounting for <5% of primary pleural tumors
- Unknown etiology
- Slow-growing, relatively benign tumors, up to 10% malignant
- Usually asymptomatic, incidental finding

Key Radiological Features

- Usually solitary, well-circumscribed mass arising from visceral pleura
- Can be multiple and distributed throughout the pleural cavity

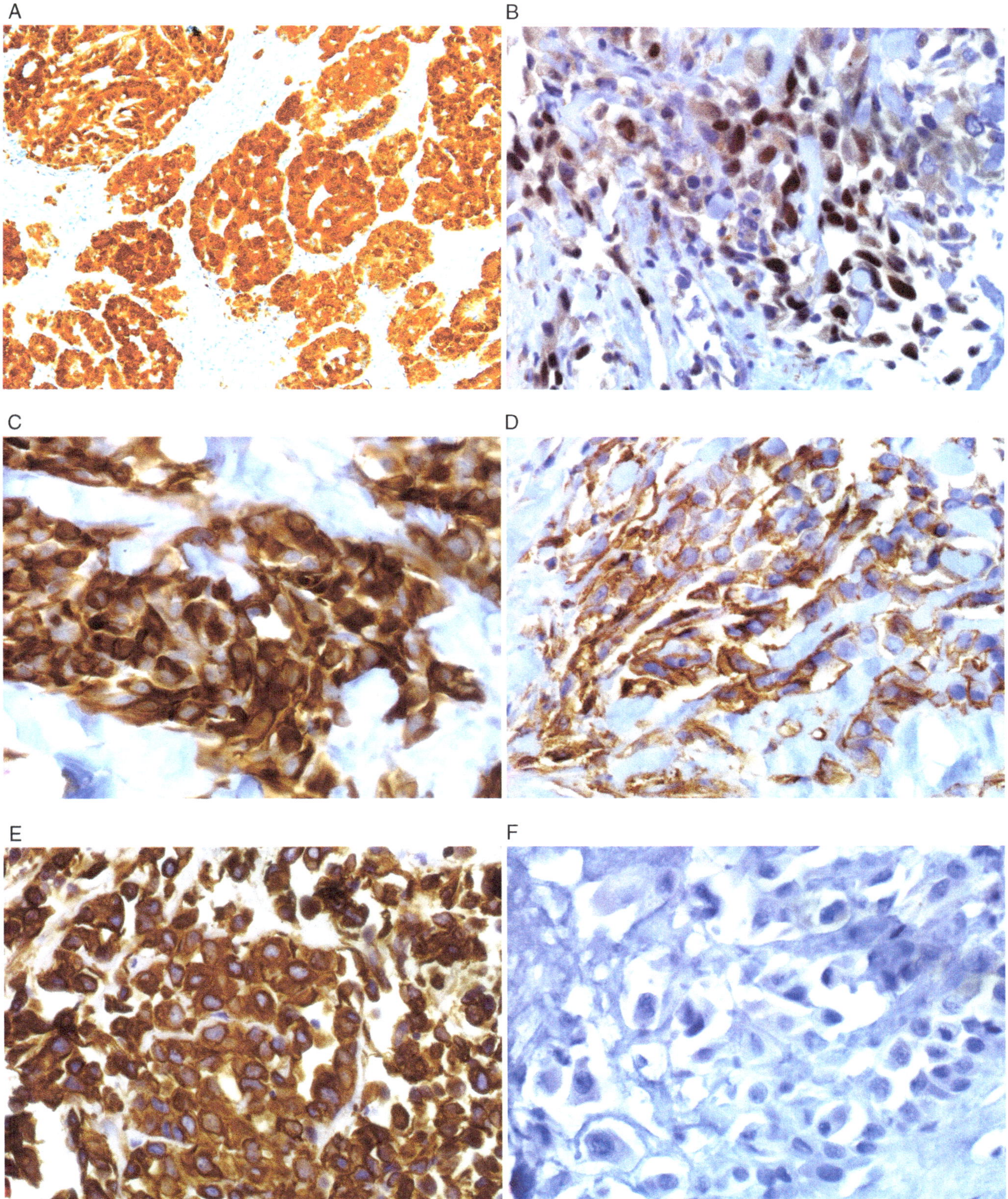

Fig. 6.31 Mesothelioma, immunophenotype. (**a**) Calretinin decorates tumor cells, IHC; (**b**) positive for WT-1, IHC; (**c**) CK5/6 positive, IHC; (**d**) positive for GLUT1, IHC; (**e**) positive for AE1/3, IHC; (**f**) MOC31 negative, IHC

Cytological Features

- Cellular smear with bland-appearing, small, oval to spindled cells
- No mitosis or necrosis
- Representative images are shown in Fig. 6.32a, b.

Differential Diagnosis

- Neuroendocrine tumors
- Synovial sarcoma
- Sarcomatoid mesothelioma
- Nerve sheath tumor
- Type A thymoma

Histology

- Uniform fibroblastic spindle cells with tapering nuclei, scant, pale, indistinct cytoplasm, variable cellularity, and patternless architecture.
- Focal storiform or fascicular growth pattern may be seen.
- Prominent stromal and perivascular hyalinization.
- Branching hemangiopericytoma-like vessels of varying size and number.
- Usually <3 mitoses/per 2 mm^2; malignant: > 4 mitoses/per 2 mm^2, rarely showing dedifferentiation.
- Representative images are shown in Fig. 6.32c, d.

Immunohistochemistry

- Positive for signal transducer and activator of transcription 6 (STAT6): > 95% of cases, specific.
- Positive for CD34, B-cell CLL/lymphoma 2 (Bcl2), and CD99: nonspecific.
- Occasionally may be positive for SMA, epithelial membrane antigen (EMA), keratin, S100, or desmin.
- Representative images are shown in Fig. 6.32e, f.
- The tumor harbors characteristic gene fusion NGFI-A binding protein 2 (*NAB2*)-*STAT6*.

Mediastinum

Overview

The mediastinum can be divided into four hypothetical compartments: superior, anterior, middle, and posterior. The distribution of organs and tumors of the mediastinum is summarized in Table 6.11.

In adults, the distribution of tumors is as follows: 46% thymic epithelial tumors, 23% lymphomas, 16% endocrine tumors, and 15% germ cell tumors. In children, the frequency of tumors is 47% neurogenic neoplasms, 19% germ cell tumors, 12% lymphomas, 10% thymic epithelial tumors, 6% cysts, and 6% mesenchymal tumors. The 2015 WHO classification of tumors of the thymus is summarized in Table 6.12.

Selected entities will be discussed in the section below.

Cysts

Key Clinical Features

- Bronchogenic cyst –any part of the mediastinum
- Enteric cyst – posterior mediastinum
- Thymic cyst – anterior mediastinum
- Pericardial cyst –middle mediastinum

Cytological Features

- Hypocellular smear
- Dependent upon the type of the cyst

Epithelial Tumors

Thymoma

Key Clinical Features

- Rare malignancy overall, but the most common mediastinal tumors in adults
- Median age of 50 years, rare in children
- May present as a mass lesion or an incidental finding
- May be associated with myasthenia gravis, pure red cell aplasia, hypogammaglobulinemia (Good syndrome), and/or other autoimmune disorders

Key Radiological Features

- Usually a mass lesion, well-circumscribed or invasive borders, depending on the subtypes of thymoma

Cytological Features

- Usually moderate to hypercellular smear
- Two populations of relatively bland neoplastic epithelial cells and lymphocytes
- The proportion of epithelial cells and lymphocytes is dependent upon subtype.
- In epithelial subtype, epithelial cells are dominant; in lymphocyte-predominant subtype, small mature lymphocytes are dominant; and in spindle cell type, spindle epithelial cells are predominant.
- Neoplastic epithelial cells tend to be cohesive and have a delicate nuclear membrane, fine nuclear chromatin, and small nucleoli.
- Few or no mitoses are present.
- Representative images are shown in Fig. 6.33a–f.

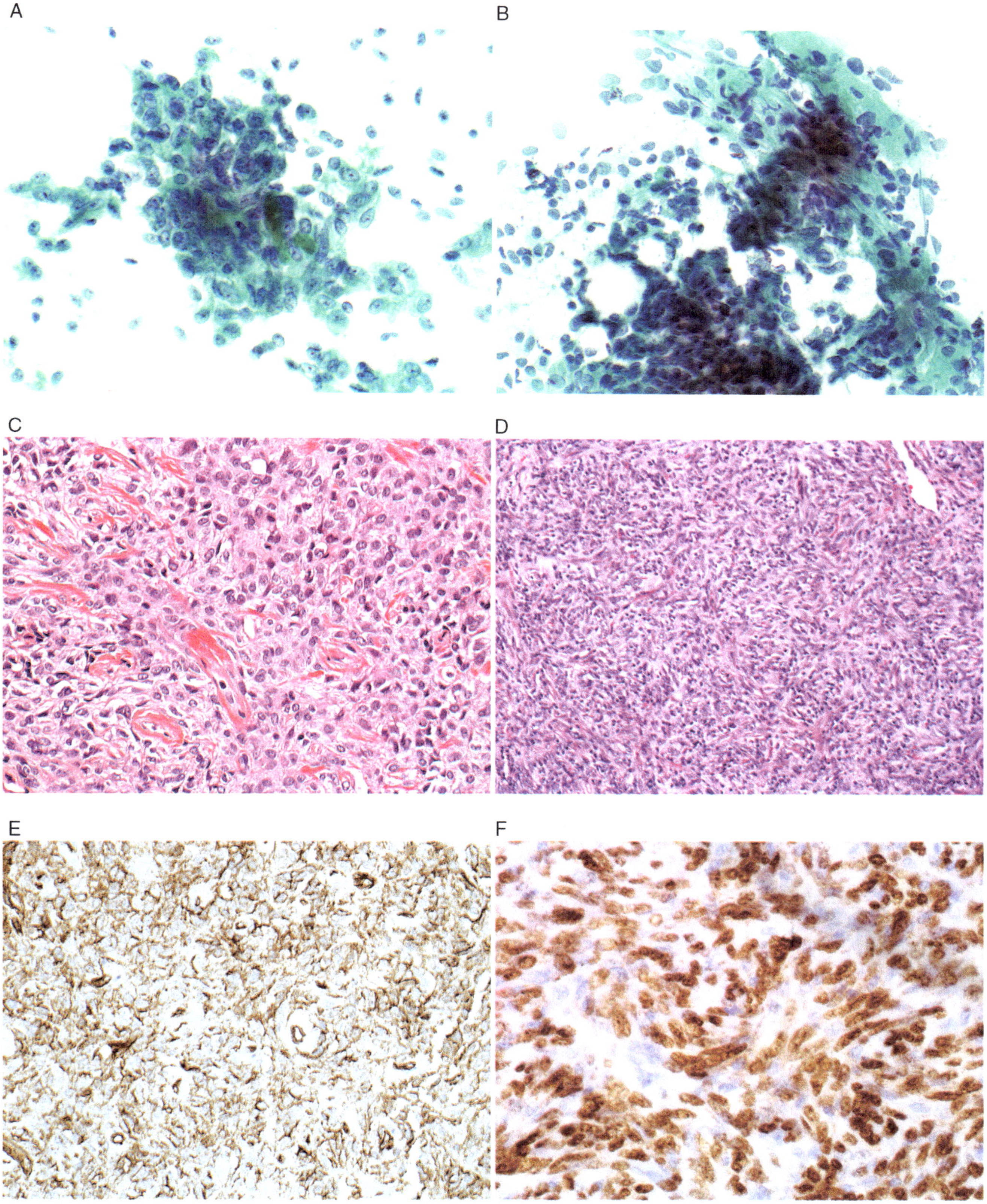

Fig. 6.32 Solitary fibrous tumor. (**a**, **b**) Cellular smear with bland-appearing, small, oval to spindled cells, Pap stain; (**c**, **d**) surgical resection tissue showing patternless spindle cells with significant hyalinized stroma, H&E; (**e**) diffuse CD34 positivity, IHC; (**f**) positive for STAT6, IHC

Table 6.11 Distribution of organs and tumors of the mediastinum

Superior					
Thymus (thymoma, cyst, carcinoid, lymphoma) *Lymph node* (metastases, lymphoma, inflammation) *Thyroid* (goiter, neoplasm) *Parathyroid* (adenoma, cyst) *Other* (cysts, aneurysm)					
Anterior	*Thymus* (thymoma, cyst, carcinoid, lymphoma) *Germ cell tumors* *Lymph node* (metastases, lymphoma, inflammation) *Thyroid* (goiter, neoplasm) *Parathyroid* (adenoma, cyst) *Paraganglia tumors* *Other* (angioma, lipoma, other mesenchymal tumors	Middle	*Cysts* (pericardial, bronchogenic) *Lymph node* (metastases, lymphoma, inflammation) *Other* (atrial myxoma, mediastinal fibrosis)	Posterior	*Neurogenic* (nerve sheath and sympathetic, paraganglioma) *Lymph node* (metastases, lymphoma, inflammation) *Cyst* (gastroenteric) *Other* (esophageal lesions, abscess, aneurysm, meningocele)

Table 6.12 2015 World Health Organization (WHO) classification of tumors of the thymus

Epithelial tumors	
Thymoma Type A thymoma, including atypical variant Type AB thymoma Type B1 thymoma Type B2 thymoma Type B3 thymoma Micronodular thymoma with lymphoid stroma Metaplastic thymoma Other rare thymoma Microscopic thymoma Sclerosing thymoma Lipofibroadenoma Thymic carcinoma Squamous cell carcinoma Basaloid carcinoma Mucoepidermoid carcinoma Lymphoepithelioma-like carcinoma Clear cell carcinoma Sarcomatoid carcinoma Adenocarcinomas Papillary adenocarcinoma Thymic carcinoma with adenoid cystic carcinoma-like features Mucinous adenocarcinoma Adenocarcinoma, not otherwise specified (NOS)	Thymic carcinoma (continued) NUT carcinoma Undifferentiated carcinoma Other rare thymic carcinomas Adenosquamous carcinoma Hepatoid carcinoma Thymic carcinoma, NOS Thymic neuroendocrine tumors Carcinoid tumors Typical carcinoid Atypical carcinoid Large cell neuroendocrine carcinoma Combined large cell neuroendocrine carcinoma Small cell carcinoma Combined small cell carcinoma Combined thymic carcinomas
Germ cell tumors of the mediastinum	
Seminoma Embryonal carcinoma Yolk sac tumor Choriocarcinoma Teratoma Teratoma, mature Teratoma, immature	Mixed germ cell tumors Germ cell tumors with somatic-type solid malignancy Germ cell tumors with associated hematological malignancy
Lymphomas of the mediastinum	
Primary mediastinal large B-cell lymphoma Extranodal marginal zone lymphoma of mucosa-associated lymphoid tissue (MALT lymphoma) Other mature B-cell lymphomas T lymphoblastic leukemia/lymphoma	Anaplastic large cell lymphoma (ALCL) and other rare mature T- and natural killer (NK)-cell lymphomas ALCL, ALK-positive (ALK+) ALCL, ALK-negative (ALK-) Hodgkin lymphoma B-cell lymphoma, unclassifiable, with features intermediate between diffuse large B-cell and classical Hodgkin lymphoma
Histiocytic and dendritic cell neoplasms of the mediastinum	
Langerhans cell lesions Thymic Langerhans cell histiocytosis Langerhans cell sarcoma Histiocytic sarcoma	Follicular dendritic cell sarcoma Interdigitating dendritic cell sarcoma Fibroblastic reticular cell tumor Indeterminate dendritic cell tumor

(continued)

Table 6.12 (continued)

Myeloid sarcoma and extramedullary acute myeloid leukemia	
Soft tissue tumors of the mediastinum	

Thymolipoma
Lipoma
Liposarcoma
  Well-differentiated
  Dedifferentiated
  Myxoid
  Pleomorphic
Solitary fibrous tumor
  Malignant
Synovial sarcoma
  Synovial sarcoma, NOS
  Synovial sarcoma, spindle cell
  Synovial sarcoma, epithelioid cell
  Synovial sarcoma, biphasic
	Vascular neoplasms
	  Lymphangioma
	  Hemangioma
	  Epithelioid hemangioendothelioma
	  Angiosarcoma
	Neurogenic tumors
	  Tumors of peripheral nerves
	  Ganglioneuroma
	  Ganglioneuroblastoma
	  Neuroblastoma

Ectopic tumors of the thymus	
Ectopic thyroid tumors Ectopic parathyroid tumors Other rare ectopic tumors	

Used with permission from Travis WD, Brambilla E, Burke AP, Marx A, Nicholson A. WHO classification of tumors of the lung, pleura, thymus, and heart. Lyon, France: IARC; 2015

Differential Diagnosis

- Thymic carcinoma
- Thymic hyperplasia
- T-cell lymphoblastic lymphoma
- Neuroendocrine neoplasm

Histology

- Type A thymoma:
  1. Complete or incomplete fibrous capsule may display coarse lobulation with thick fibrous bands.
  2. Microcystic pattern is most common, more prominent in subcapsular areas.
  3. Other patterns: rosettes (with or without a central lumen), glandular or glomeruloid structures, Masson's hemangioma-like papillary projections in cystic spaces, meningioma-like whorls, fascicular growth, and storiform growth.
  4. Hassall corpuscles are absent.
  5. The tumor cells are spindled and/or oval-shaped with bland nuclei, finely dispersed powdery chromatin, and inconspicuous nucleoli.
  6. Low mitotic activity, usually <4 mitoses/per 2 mm^2.
  7. No or very few immature lymphocytes.
  8. When hypercellularity, increased mitotic counts, and focal necrosis are present, designate as atypical type A thymoma variant.
  9. Representative images are shown in Fig. 6.34a, b.
- Type AB thymoma:
  1. Well-demarcated and encapsulated tumor showing a lobulated growth pattern.
  2. Highly variable mixture of a lymphocyte-poor type A component and a more lymphocyte-rich type B-like component including a prominent infiltrate (often in dense clusters) of immature, TdT+ T cells. Infiltrate of TdT+ lymphocytes in >10% of the tumor area is a feature used to distinguish from type A thymoma.
  3. The tumor cells are small, oval to plump, spindled, or polygonal shaped, containing round to oval pale-staining nuclei showing dispersed chromatin and inconspicuous nucleoli.
  4. Medullary islands are very rare; Hassall corpuscles are absent.
  5. Summary of three distinctive features of type AB thymoma: (a) an admixed spindle cell-predominant, lymphocyte-poor component and lymphocyte-rich component; (b) bland, spindly, oval, and focally polygonal thymic epithelial cells; and (c) a focal or diffuse abundance of immature T cells.
- Type B1 thymoma:
  1. Thymus-like architecture with predominance of cortical areas.
  2. Either absence of lobulation or lobulated with larger lobules traversed by hypocellular, collagenous septa.
  3. The neoplastic epithelial cells are individually embedded in densely packed nonneoplastic immature lymphocytes; the epithelial cells have poorly defined, pale

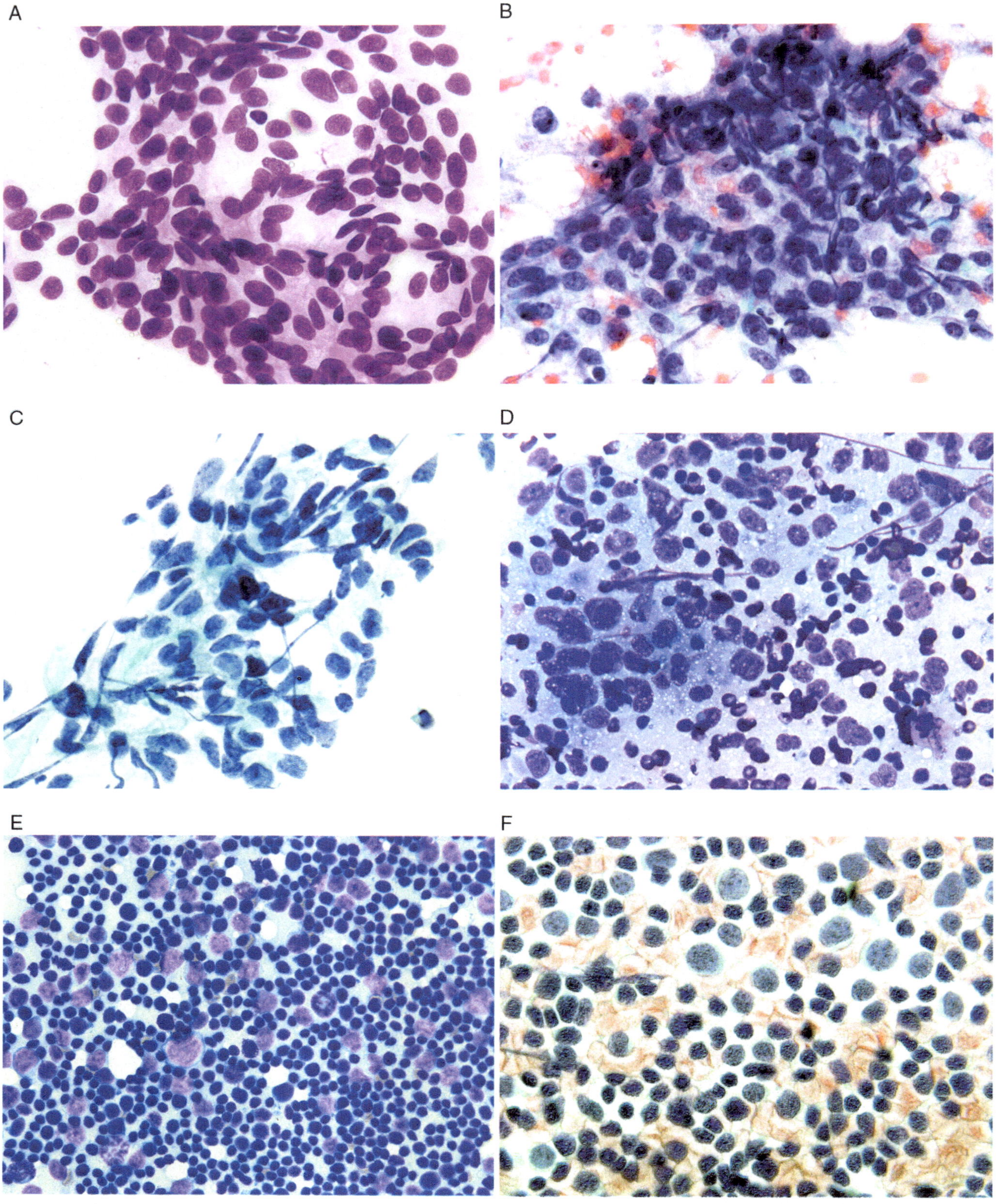

Fig. 6.33 Thymoma, cytology. (**a**, **b**) Epithelial prominence, showing round to slightly oval nuclei with vesicular chromatin and small but prominent nucleoli, Diff-Quik (**a**) and Pap (**b**) stains; (**c**) spindle cell predominant, bland-appearing, Pap stains; (**d**) mixed epithelial and lymphocytes, Diff-Quik; (**e**, **f**) lymphocyte predominant, Diff-Quick (E) and Pap (F) stains

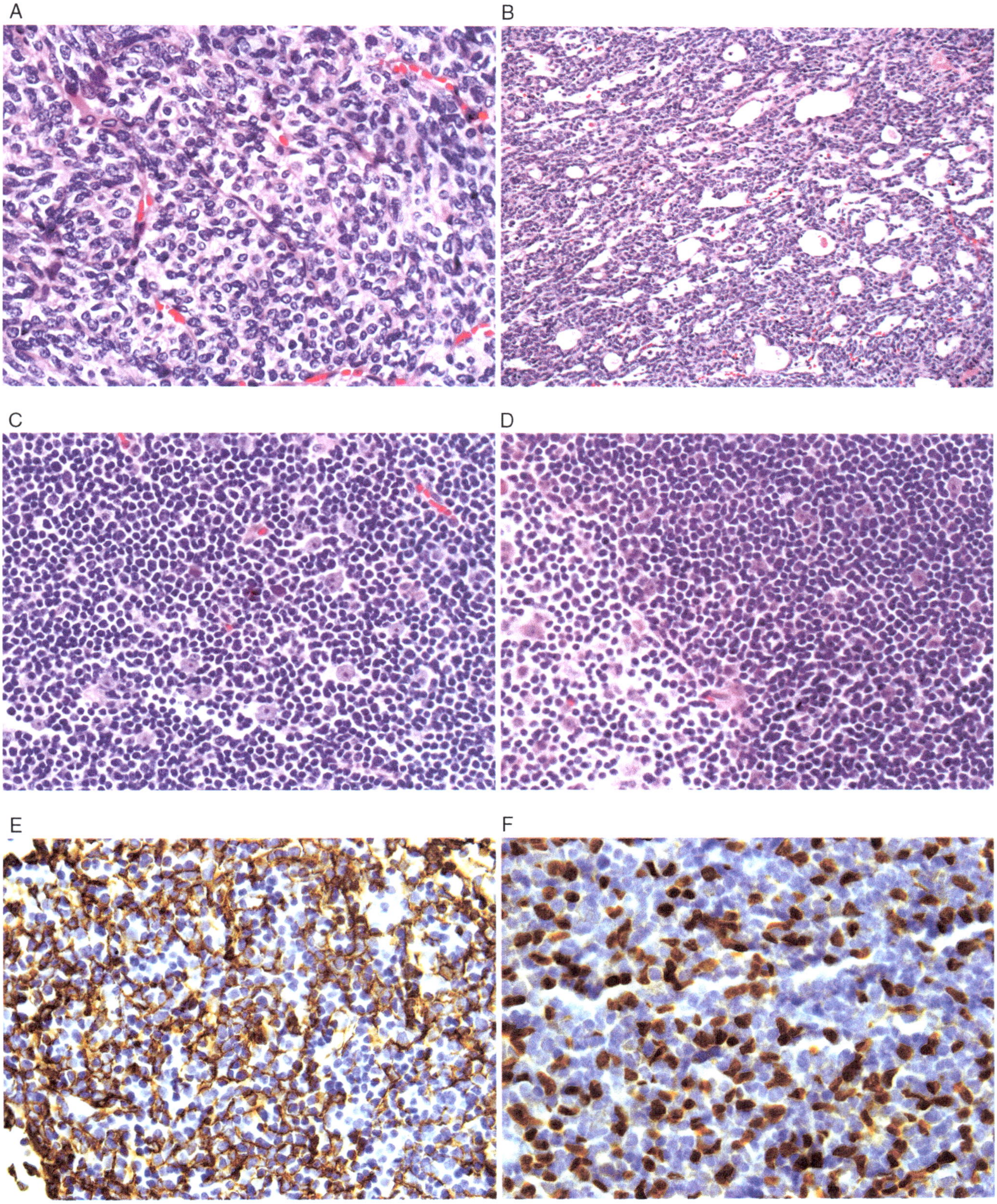

Fig. 6.34 Thymoma, histopathology. (**a**) Spindle cell predominant, type A, H&E; (**b**) type A, microcystic growth pattern, H&E; (**c**) lymphocyte-predominant, individual embedded epithelial tumor cells, type B1, H&E; (**d**) type B1, pale-stained medullary island left lower corner), H&E; (**e**) cytokeratin AE1/3 decorates tumor epithelial cells, IHC; (**f**) p63 positive in epithelial tumor cells, IHC; (**g**) TdT-positive mature T lymphocytes, IHC; (**h**) positive for CD5, mature T lymphocytes, IHC

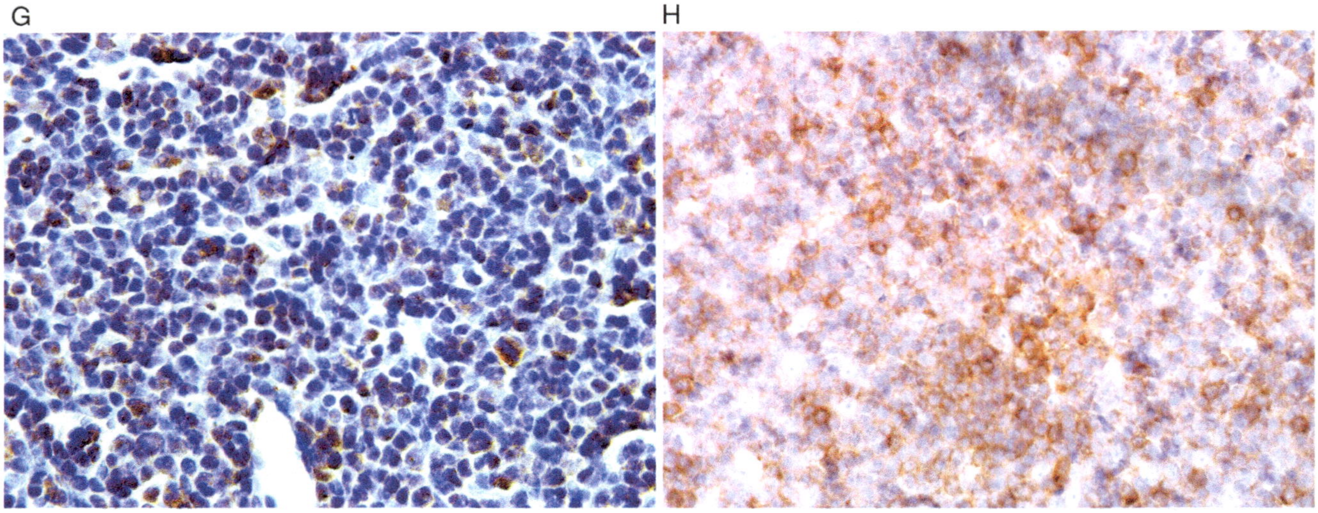

Fig. 6.34 (continued)

eosinophilic cytoplasm, and relatively uniform, oval to slightly irregular round nuclei, showing pale chromatin, distinct nuclear membranes, and small central nucleoli.

4. Medullary islands are always present and may contain Hassall corpuscles and myoid cells; perivascular spaces are often seen.
5. Summary of two distinctive features of type B1 thymoma: (a) close resemblance to the normal, non-involuted thymic cortex; (b) the consistent presence of medullary islands.
6. Representative images are shown in Fig. 6.34c, d.

- Type B2 thymoma:
  1. Encapsulated tumor, composed of lymphocyte- predominant, irregular size and shape tumor lobules surrounded by delicate fibrous septa, giving a lobular architecture and blue appearance on hematoxylin and eosin (H&E) stain.
  2. Interspersed among the lymphoid cells are single or poorly defined clusters of epithelial cells (≥ 3 cells).
  3. The epithelial cells have round or slightly oval nuclei with vesicular chromatin and small but prominent nucleoli; rare focal anaplasia may be seen.
  4. Perivascular spaces composed of a central venule surrounded by a clear space containing proteinaceous fluid or lymphocytes.
  5. Hassall corpuscles are rare; medullary islands are uncommon.
  6. Summary of distinctive features of type B2 thymoma: (a) polygonal (non-spindle shaped) neoplastic thymic epithelial cells in clusters; (b) high content of intermingled immature T cells.
- Type B3 thymoma:
  1. Tumor lobules separated by fibrous septa, pushing borders at the invasion front, prominent perivascular spaces with epithelial palisading, rare Hassall corpuscles.
  2. Tumor cells are polygonal with eosinophilic or clear cytoplasm and slightly/moderately atypical, round to elongated, grooved, or raisinoid nuclei.
  3. Summary of distinctive features of type B3 thymoma: (a) predominance of polygonal epithelial cells forming solid sheets, resulting in a pink appearance on H&E; (b) paucity of admixed nonneoplastic immature T cells.

Immunohistochemistry

- Epithelial cells: usually positive for AE1/3, CK7, CK19, p63, PAX8, forkhead box N1 (FOXN1), CD57, and CD205; negative for EMA, CD117, and CD5.
- Small lymphocytes (thymocytes) are mature T-cells, but positive for CD3, CD5, TdT, CD99, with a high MIB1 (Ki-67) proliferative index.
- Representative images are shown in Fig. 6.34e–h.

Thymic Carcinomas

Thymic carcinomas include of a variety of histological types of tumors, accounting for approximately 22% of all thymic epithelial neoplasms. The squamous cell carcinomas are the most common type, accounting for approximately 70% of all thymic carcinoma cases. Lymphoepithelioma-like carcinomas are rare, accounting for 6–32% of all thymic carcinomas; sarcomatoid carcinomas account for 5–10%; and basaloid carcinomas account for <5%. Other types, such as mucoepidermoid carcinomas, clear cell carcinomas, ADCs,

Table 6.13 Features of thymic carcinomas of the most common types

	Squamous cell carcinoma	Lymphoepithelioma-like carcinoma	Sarcomatoid carcinoma
Clinical features	1. 70% of all cases 2. Most common in sixth decade 3. Men slightly more than women 4. <5% associated with myasthenia gravis	1. 6–32% of all cases 2. Median age: 41; bimodal peaks at 14 and 48 years 3. Male/female: 2:1 4. Association with EBV in ~50% of cases, especially in children and young adults	1. 5–10% of all cases 2. In late adulthood, fourth–eighth decades, mean 47 years 3. Unknown etiology
Radiographic features	Usually an anterior mediastinal mass, often with poorly defined, irregular lobular margins, or with necrotic/cystic changes, which on CT appear as low-attenuation regions, on MRI with greater tumor heterogeneity	1. a large mass in the anterior mediastinum with necrosis (low-attenuation on CT) 2. Often invading surrounding tissues: pleura, lung, diaphragm, and pericardium	1. Usually a large, lobulated mass in the anterior mediastinum with necrosis (low-attenuation on CT) 2. Often invading surrounding tissues: pleura, lung, diaphragm, and pericardium; with encroachment on the major vessels
Cytologic features	Single or clusters of large atypical cells with enlarged nuclei showing coarse chromatin and macronucleoli and a moderate amount of cytoplasm (Fig. 6.35)	1. Malignant epithelial cells: clusters of large, relatively uniform cells with vesicular nuclei, one or more distinct nucleoli, indistinct cell borders; polygonal squamoid cells in some 2. Many lymphocytes and plasma cells	1. Type A thymoma component: spindled epithelial cells with bland nuclei, powdery chromatin, and inconspicuous nucleoli 2. Malignant spindle cells: coarse chromatin, prominent nucleoli, and frequent mitoses; may show heterologous sarcomatous fragments
Histology	1. Infiltrative, usually smooth contoured sheets, islands, and cords of large polygonal cells accompanied by broad zones of desmoplastic to sclerohyaline stroma 2. Polygonal tumor cells: large vesicular or hyperchromatic nuclei, distinct nucleoli, eosinophilic cytoplasm, and vague to obvious intercellular bridges; may be keratinized with keratin whorls mimic Hassall corpuscles 3. Foci of coagulative necrosis are common	1. Anastomosing sheets, nests, and cords of CA cells accompanied by dense lymphocytes and plasma cells 2. CA cells: large vesicular nuclei, one or more distinct nucleoli, and indistinct cell borders; the nuclei are relatively uniform, crowded, overlapping 3. Focal squamous differentiation 4. Coagulative necrosis 5. Many lymphocytes and plasma cells; may see germinal center, eosinophils, and granulomas	1. Usually a mixture of conventional type A thymoma and areas of malignant spindle cells 2. Gradual or abrupt transition between the two 3. Malignant cells: coarse chromatin. Prominent nucleoli, frequent mitoses 4. May see small areas of lymphoepithelioma-like CA or prominent squamous differentiation 5. May have heterologous mesenchymal elements
IHC	1. Positive for CKs, p63 (83%), PAX8 (~75%); CD5, CD117, GLUT1, and MUC1 (~80%); FOXN1 (68–76%), CD205 (10–59%) 2. Focal expression of NE markers: 64% cases 3. Lack TdT+ lymphocytes	1. for panCKs, p63, CD117, and CD5 (variable) 2. Negative for CK7 and CK20 3. Admixed CD3+/TdT- T cells and B cells; the plasma cells are polytypic for Ig.	1. Type A thymoma component: same as conventional 2. Malignant spindle cells: positive for CK, EMA; may or may not be CD5-positive 3. The heterologous sarcomatous elements express markers for their differentiation
Molecular Genetics	1. Chromosomes loss (16q, 6, 3p, and 17p); gain (1q, 17q, and 18) 2. Mutations of *KIT* (11%), *TP53* (~20%) 4. Copy number gain of *Bcl2*, loss of *p16 (CDKN2A)* 5. Missense mutation of *GTF2I* gene: <10%	1. EBV is almost always positive in children and young adults, uncommon positive in adults >30 years 2. The most reliable test: in situ hybridization for EBV-encoded small RNA	Information limited

EBV Epstein-Barr virus, *CT* computed tomography, *MRI* magnetic resonance imaging, *CA* carcinoma, *IHC* immunohistochemistry, *CK(s)* cytokeratin(s), *CD* cluster of differentiation, *GLUT1* glucose transporter 1, *MUC1* mucin 1, *FOXN1* forkhead box N1, *NE* neuroendocrine, *TdT* terminal deoxynucleotidyl transferase, *Ig* immunoglobulin, *EMA* epithelial membrane antigen, *KIT* a type III transmembrane receptor tyrosine kinase, *TP53* tumor protein 53, *Bcl2* B-cell CLL/lymphoma 2, *CDKN2A* cyclin-dependent kinase inhibitor 2A, *GTF2I* general transcription factor IIi, *RNA* ribonucleic acid

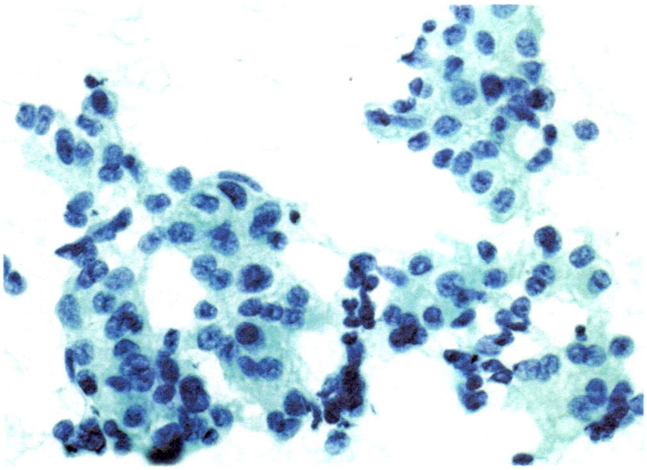

Fig. 6.35 Thymic carcinoma, showing single and clusters of large atypical cells with enlarged nuclei, coarse chromatin, macronucleoli, and moderate amount of cytoplasm, Pap stain

NUT carcinomas, and undifferentiated carcinomas, are very few. The characteristic features of the three most common types are summarized in Table 6.13.

Thymic Neuroendocrine Tumors

Thymic neuroendocrine tumors are categorized into two major groups: (1) low-grade typical carcinoids and intermediate-grade atypical carcinoids, which always show characteristic morphological and immunohistochemical neuroendocrine features, and (2) high-grade LCNECs and small cell carcinomas, which may lack some neuroendocrine features.

Key Clinical Features

- No established association with smoking.
- More aggressive clinical course: propensity for recurrence, lymph node or distant metastases, and tumor-associated death.
- Atypical carcinoids account for the majority of the tumors.
- Only carcinoids reported in setting of multiple endocrine neoplasia type 1 (MEN1).
- Average age at presentation: 49 years.
- Carcinoids show a strong male predominance.

Key Radiological Features

- Typically a lobulated, heterogeneous mass in the anterior mediastinum

Cytological Features

- Same as pulmonary neuroendocrine tumors; please refer that section in this chapter.
- Representative images are shown in Fig. 6.36a–i.

Differential Diagnosis

- Pulmonary neuroendocrine tumors: careful clinical and radiological correlation is the primary way to distinguish pulmonary from thymic neuroendocrine tumors.
- Thymoma, especially type A, to distinguish from carcinoids.
- Thymic carcinoma usually shows focal and/or weak expression of neuroendocrine markers.

Histology

The same as pulmonary neuroendocrine tumors, respectively.

Immunohistochemistry

Same as the pulmonary neuroendocrine tumors, respectively.

Germ Cell Tumors of the Mediastinum

Key Clinical Features

- Accounts for 3–4% of all germ cell tumors; up to 16% of all mediastinal tumors
- In prepubertal patients (mean <8 years): teratomas (58%), yolk sac tumors +/− teratoma (42%)
- In postpubertal female patients: teratoma (93%), seminoma (dysgerminoma) (4%), embryonal carcinoma (2%), and others (<1%)
- In postpubertal male patients (mean 25–29 years): teratoma (35%), seminoma (32%), mixed (16%), yolk sac tumor (10%), embryonal carcinoma (4%), and choriocarcinoma (3%)
- In patients with Klinefelter syndrome: mediastinal non-seminomatous germ cell tumors particularly common but not seminomas or testicular germ cell tumors
- Depending on tumor type, may have increased serum levels of the β-subunit of human chorionic gonadotropin (βhCG), α-fetoprotein (AFP), and lactate dehydrogenase

Key Radiological Features

- Anterior mediastinal mass: uncalcified and homogeneous for seminomas, heterogeneous with central attenuation, and a frond-like periphery for non-seminomatous germ cell tumors.
- Multilocular cystic lesions can accompany any type of mediastinal germ cell tumor (particularly seminomas), also others, such as thymomas, thymic carcinomas, Hodgkin or non-Hodgkin lymphomas, and metastases.

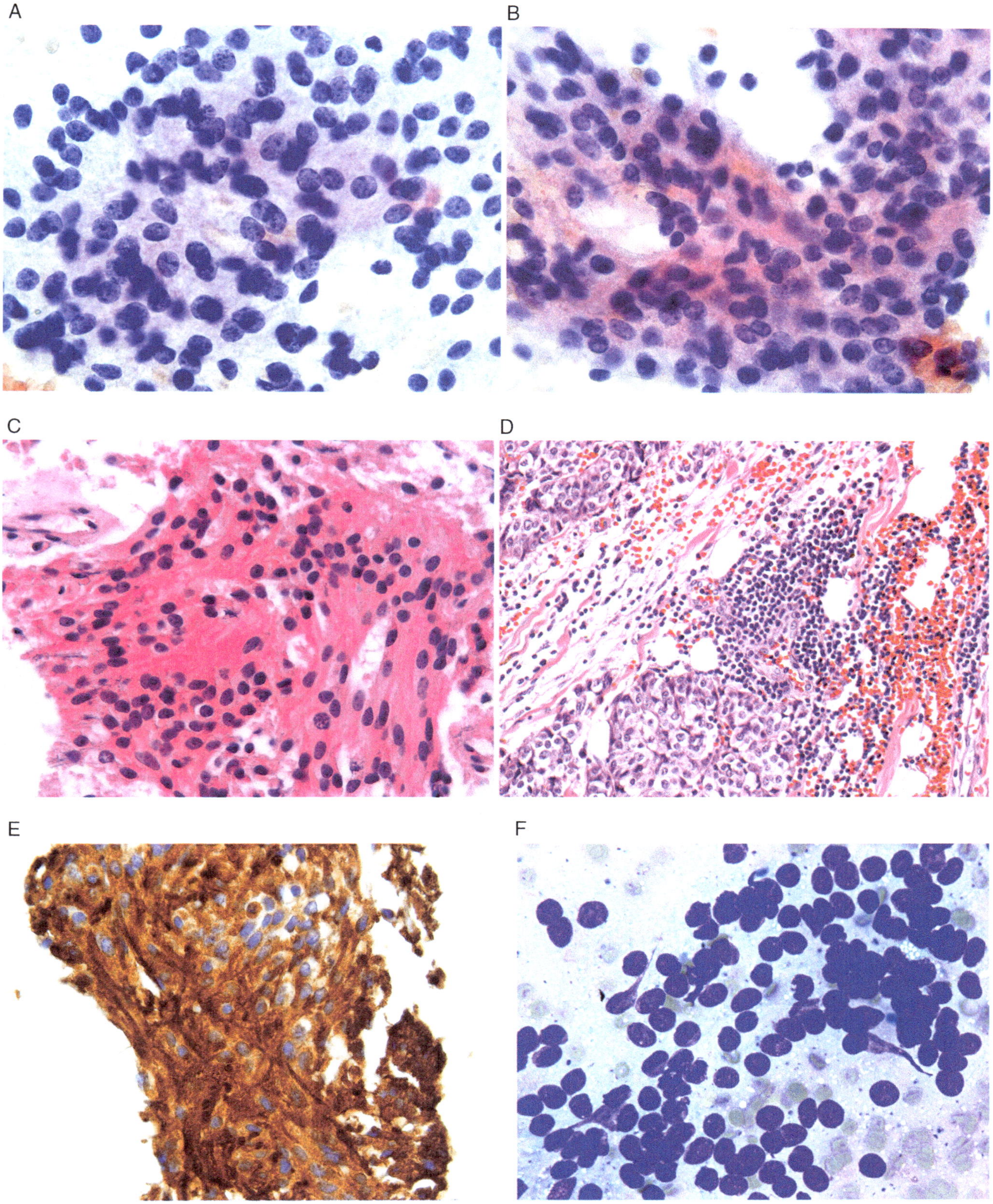

Fig. 6.36 Thymic neuroendocrine tumors. (**a**, **b**) Typical carcinoid, showing loosely cohesive and single of uniform cells with powdery chromatin pattern and discernible nucleoli, Pap stain; (**c**) atypical carcinoid, cellblock material, showing tumor cells forming rosette-like structure, H&E; (**d**) atypical carcinoid, tissue section showing nests of tumor cells, H&E; (**e**) atypical carcinoid, diffuse staining for chromogranin, IHC; (**f**, **g**) high-grade neuroendocrine carcinoma showing discohesive cells with moderate nuclear pleomorphism, prominent nucleoli and frequent mitoses, most compatible with large cell type, Diff-Quik (**f**) and Pap (**g**) stains; (**h**, **i**) high-grade neuroendocrine carcinoma showing discohesive small cells with nuclear molding, inconspicuous nucleoli and frequent mitoses, most compatible with small cell type, Diff-Quik (**h**) and Pap (**i**) stains

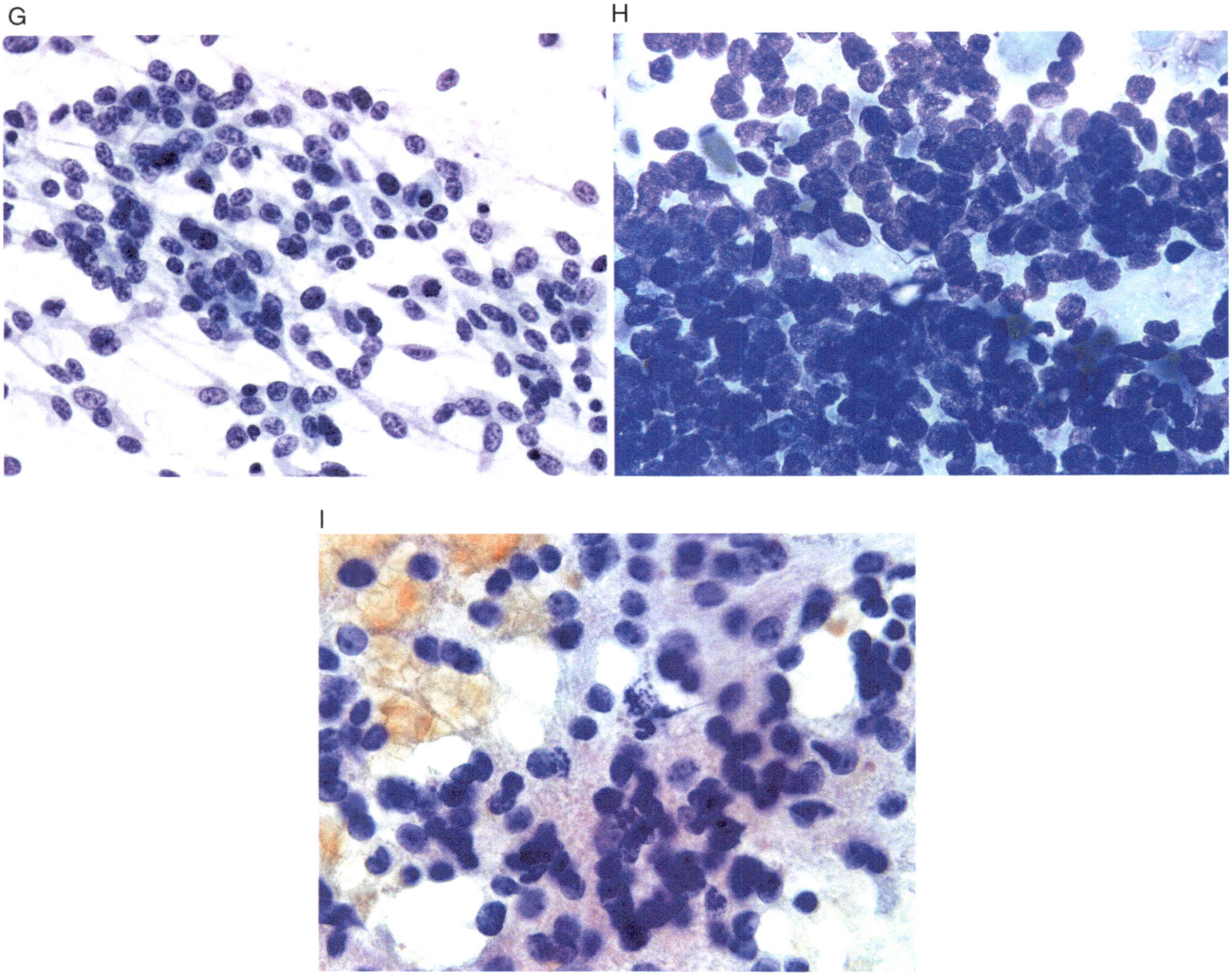

Fig. 6.36 (continued)

Cytological Features

- Seminomas:
  1. Highly cellular smears composed of small loose syncytium-like clusters or isolated large tumor cells with centrally located round nuclei containing one or more prominent, irregular nucleoli, and clear to granular cytoplasm.
  2. Mitoses present.
  3. Admixed with polymorphous lymphocytes, occasional epithelioid histiocytes.
  4. A characteristic tigroid background.
  5. Representative images are shown in Fig. 6.37a–h.
- Embryonal carcinomas:
  1. Highly cellular smears
  2. Three-dimensional clusters or sheets of large, pleomorphic tumor cells with high nuclear-to-cytoplasmic ratio, irregular nuclear contours, coarse chromatin, and several nucleoli
  3. Indistinct pale cytoplasm
  4. Bizarre-shaped cells, mitoses, and necrosis frequent
- Yolk sac tumors:
  1. Clusters of medium to large pleomorphic tumor cells with irregular nuclear contours, vesicular nuclei, prominent nucleoli, and eosinophilic or vacuolated cytoplasm.
  2. Some tumor cells contain intracytoplasmic dense hyaline globules.
  3. Granular debris and mucoid or metachromatic material in background.
  4. No lymphocytes or epithelioid histiocytes.
- Choriocarcinomas:
  1. Cellular smears
  2. Malignant cytotrophoblasts: mononucleated, medium-size cells with vacuolated, basophilic cytoplasm, and eccentric nuclei
  3. Malignant syncytiotrophoblasts: very large tumor cells with one or several nuclei, distinct nucleoli, and eosinophilic cytoplasm

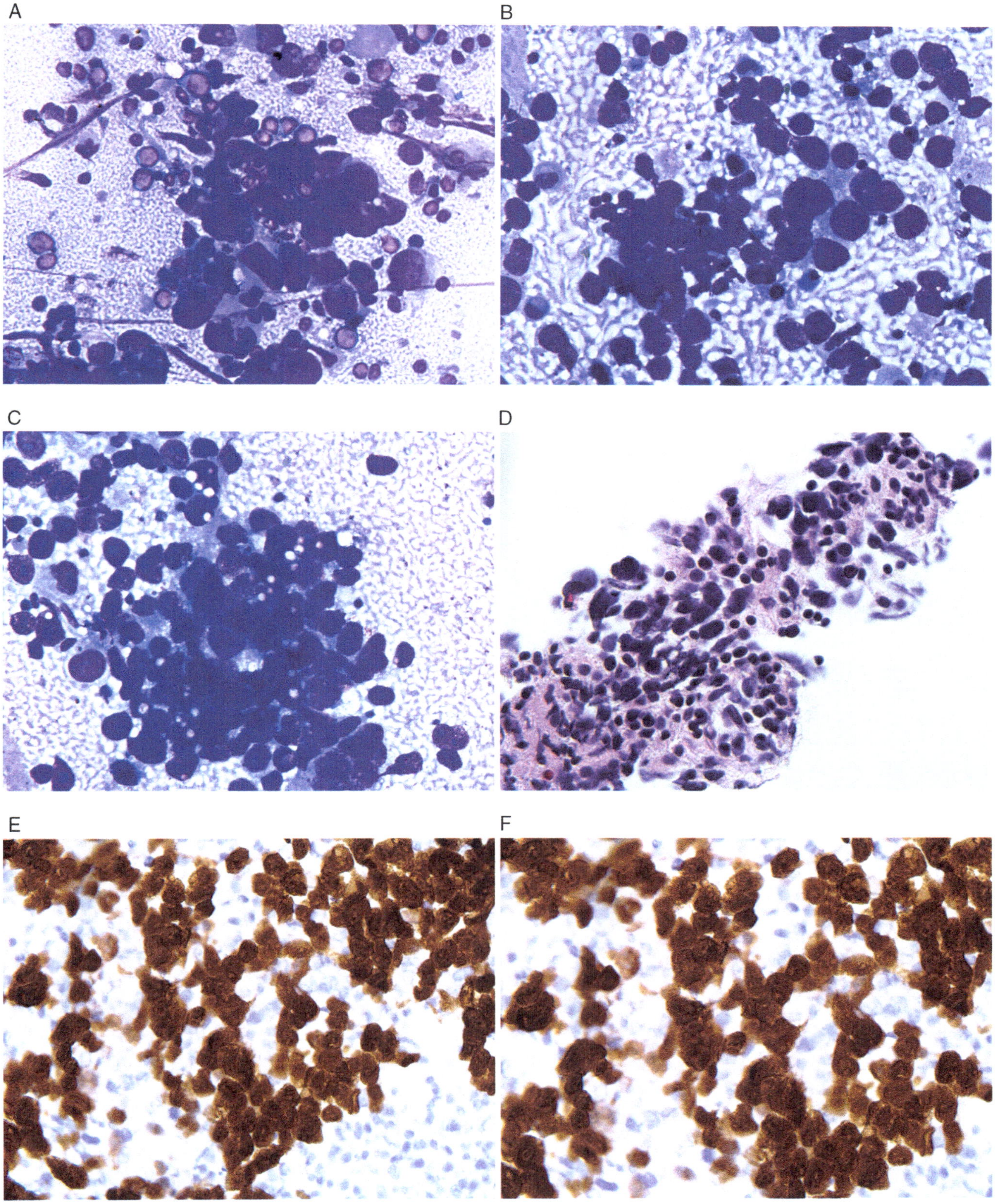

Fig. 6.37 Seminoma, mediastinum. (**a–c**) The smears reveal small loose syncytium-like clusters and isolated large tumor cells with centrally located round nuclei containing one or more prominent, irregular nucleoli, and clear to granular cytoplasm, with admixed polymorphous lymphocytes, in a characteristic tigroid background, Diff-Quik; (**d**) cell block preparation reveals thin core of tumor tissue showing small clusters of atypical cells with prominent nucleoli admixed with lymphocytes, H&E; (**e**) positive for SALL4, IHC; (**f**) positive for OCT4, IHC; (**g**) positive for CD117, IHC; (**h**) negative for CD30, IHC

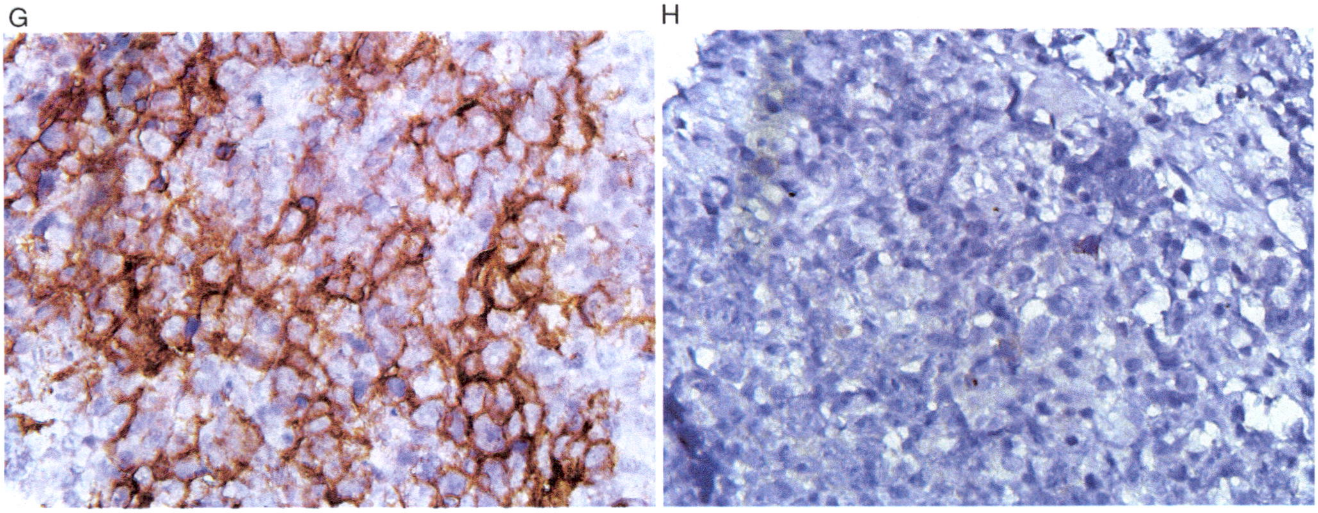

Fig. 6.37 (continued)

4. Atypical mitoses
5. Significant hemorrhage and necrosis in the background

- Teratoma:
  1. Mature teratoma: cytology diagnosis is difficult; may be paucicellular with few anucleated squamous cells and macrophages in a proteinaceous background; ciliated bronchial cells, smooth muscle, and cartilage are present; a mucoid background with bland-looking signet ring cell-like mucus cells may be seen.
  2. Immature teratoma: may be cellular, composed of aggregates or individual small, round, hyperchromatic cells with high nuclear-to-cytoplasmic ratio, and inconspicuous nucleoli; rare rosettes with neuropils, rhabdomyoblasts, immature cartilage, and blastema-like stromal cells may be identified.

Differential Diagnosis

- Metastatic gonadal germ cell tumors
- Metastatic carcinomas
- Small round blue cell tumors
- Sarcomas

Histology

- Seminoma:

1. Sheets, cords, or irregular lobules of monotonous, round to polygonal tumor cells with central nuclei, macronucleoli, and abundant clear to lightly eosinophilic cytoplasm.
2. Delicate fibrous septa, with infiltrates of lymphocytes, may form germinal centers.
3. Granulomatous reaction and fibrosis.
4. Syncytiotrophoblastic cells may be scattered throughout.

- Embryonal carcinoma:

1. Sheets, tubules, and papillary structures of large polygonal or columnar cells with round to oval, vesicular, hyperchromatic nuclei containing one or multiple nucleoli and a moderate amount of cytoplasm.
2. Numerous mitoses, apoptotic bodies, and coagulated necrosis are common.
3. Scattered single or small clusters of syncytiotrophoblasts in one third of cases.

- Yolk sac tumor:

1. Various patterns: reticular-microcystic, spindle cell, solid, macrocystic, papillary, forming Schiller-Duval bodies, polyvesicular vitelline, glandular-alveolar, and hepatoid patterns.
2. The tumor cells may be flat or columnar, with intracellular and extracellular hyaline globules, as well as basement membrane-like material deposition between the cells.

- Choriocarcinoma:

1. Two cell components, syncytiotrophoblasts and cytotrophoblasts, arranged in solid nests or sheets, occasionally in a villus-like arrangement.
2. The syncytiotrophoblasts are large, vacuolated, multinucleated giant cells with dark eosinophilic cytoplasm.
3. The cytotrophoblasts are uniform, medium-size, polygonal cells with abundant clear cytoplasm and distinct cytoplasmic borders.
4. Hemorrhage and necrosis are frequently observed.

- Teratoma:

1. Mature teratoma: solid or multicystic; cysts may be filled with clear, keratinous, gelatinous, or mucinous material; cartilage, spicules of bone, patches of pigmented tissue, or brain tissue may be discernible; an admixture of ectoderm, endoderm, and mesoderm is seen, assembled in either a disorganized or organized pattern.

Table 6.14 Immunophenotypic features of mediastinal germ cell tumors

Tumors/Antibody	CK	OCT3/4	SALL4	CD117	CD30	AFP	βhCG	Gly-3
Seminoma	−/+	+	+	+	−	−	−[e]	−
Embryonal CA	+	+	+	−/+	+	−/+	−[e]	−/+
Yolk Sac Tumor	+	−	+	+/−	−	+	−	+
Choriocarcinoma	+	−	+[b]	−	−	−	+	+/−[f]
Teratoma	+[a]	−	−/+[c]	−/+	−	−/+[d]	−	+/−

CK cytokeratin, *OCT3/4* octamer-binding transcription factor 3/4, *SALL4* Sal-like protein 4, *CD* cluster of differentiation, *AFP* α-fetoprotein, *βhCG* B subunit of human chorionic gonadotropin, *Gly-3* glypican 3, *CA* carcinoma
[a]Epithelial component
[b]Mononuclear trophoblast
[c]Focal staining in enteric glands, primitive neuroepithelium, and blastema-like stroma of immature teratoma
[d]AFP can be positive in fetal gut, liver, or neuroepithelium in immature teratoma
[e]Positive in scattered syncytiotrophoblasts
[f]Positive in syncytiotrophoblasts

2. Immature teratoma: the immature teratomatous elements are mostly cellular spindle mesenchymal components, but immature neural and epithelial elements can be seen; frequent mitoses; embryonic rhabdomyoblastic tissue, blastomatous tissue resembling embryonic kidney or lung, primitive neuroectodermal tumor (PNET), and other epithelial or mesenchymal malignant transformations can be seen.

Immunohistochemistry

The immunophenotypes of mediastinal germ cell tumors are summarized in Table 6.14.

Lymphomas of the Mediastinum

Primary Mediastinal Large B-Cell Lymphoma

Key Clinical Features

- An aggressive large B-cell lymphoma, of putative thymic B-cell origin
- Accounting for 2–3% of all non-Hodgkin lymphomas
- Predominantly in young adults, third to fourth decades
- Female predominance
- No known risk factors

Key Radiographic Features

- Anterior-superior mediastinal mass, often bulky, invading adjacent structures
- The mass typically shows a regular contour.

Cytological Features

- Atypical medial to large-size, monomorphic lymphoid cells with irregular, round to oval nuclei, small nucleoli and clear to eosinophilic cytoplasm
- Background of lymphoglandular bodies and abundant necrosis

Differential Diagnosis

- Diffuse large B-cell lymphoma
- Hodgkin lymphoma

Histology

- Diffuse, sheets, or clusters of medium to large, monomorphic tumor cells with irregular, round to oval nuclei, small nucleoli, and clear or eosinophilic cytoplasm; some cases show cells with pleomorphic nuclei and abundant amphophilic cytoplasm resembling Hodgkin lymphoma or nonlymphoid tumors.
- Admixed, especially at the periphery, are reactive lymphocytes, macrophages, and granulocytes.
- Distinct fibrosis to form irregular collagen bands dividing tumor into variable size compartments.

Immunohistochemistry

- Express CD19, CD20, CD22, and CD79a.
- Express PAX5, B-cell Oct-binding protein 1 (BOB1), OCT2, and PU.1.
- Lack expression of immunoglobulin; CD10 is often negative.
- CD30 expression in >80% of cases, but usually weak and heterogeneous.
- Positive for interferon regulatory factor 4/multiple myeloma oncogene 1 (IRF4/MUM1) (75%), CD23 (70%), and variable to Bcl2 and Bcl6.
- Positive for myelin and lymphocyte (MAL) antigen, CD54, CD95, tumor necrosis factor receptor 1 (TRAF1), p63, and nuclear REL.

Other Types of Lymphomas

Refer to Chap. 4 on lymph nodes.

Case Presentations

Case Scenario 1: Reactive Metaplastic Changes in Viral Infection

Learning Objectives

1. To describe the cytological features of this entity
2. To become aware of its cytologic atypia, a potential mimic of malignancy
3. To become familiar with the utility of lab tests in the diagnosis of this entity

Case

A 14-year-old female with a medical history of Rett syndrome presented with respiratory illness, fatigue, and pneumonia for 2–3 months. Respiratory secretion for culture and RT-PCR and bronchial washing for cytology and differential cell count were received.

The bronchial washing specimen revealed scattered atypical squamoid cells with large nuclei, high nuclear-to-cytoplasmic ratio, and hyperchromatic, smudged chromatin with a suggestion of nuclear inclusions in background of intense acute inflammation, reactive respiratory epithelial cells, and pulmonary macrophages. The cellblock material showed similar findings. Immunohistochemically, the scattered atypical cells were decorated by CK7, but nonreactive to p40; the profile suggested that those cells are pneumocytes. Representative images are shown in Fig. 6.38a–d.

SARS, a new human emergent infectious disease mainly involving the lower respiratory tract, became a worldwide outbreak in 2003, affecting more than 8000 patients, with a fatality rate of 9.2%. A novel coronavirus (SARS-CoV), a member of a family of large, positive, single-stranded RNA viruses, was identified as the etiological agent for this disease. The key pulmonary pathology is that of DAD, featured by pronounced pulmonary edema and hyaline membrane formation. There are interstitial thickening, fibrosis, and intra-alveolar exudates with granulation tissue formation, as well as sparsely inflammatory cell infiltrates, including macrophages (often multinucleated forms) and lymphocytes. Depending on different phases in the disease progression, the degree of fibrosis and the composition of inflammatory cells may vary. Other pathologic findings, such as prominent vascular injury, hemophagocytosis, squamous metaplasia, apoptosis, and atypical pneumocytes, including multinucleated giant pneumocytes with irregularly distributed nuclei or pneumocytes with large atypical nuclei, prominent eosinophilic nucleoli, and granular amphophilic cytoplasm, were reported. However, distinct viral inclusions were not apparent. Ancillary tests, such as in situ hybridization, immunohistochemistry, viral isolation, or RT-PCR are necessary to confirm the viral infection.

For the index case, serology testing and culture of the respiratory secretion were positive for coronavirus OC43. Electron microscopy (EM) revealed viral-like particles in pneumocytes, but not in macrophages or other cell types of lung. The findings confirmed the viral infection.

The atypical pneumocytes, metaplastic squamous cells, and apoptosis may mimic malignancy. Caution should be exercised in the interpretation of specimens from patients with a history of SARS and coronavirus infection. The awareness of clinical history and the limited amount of atypical cells should alert the pathologists to avoid overdiagnosis in this clinical setting.

Case Scenario 2: Metastatic Melanoma

Learning Objectives

1. To describe the cytological features of this entity
2. To become aware of the common differential diagnoses of this tumor
3. To become familiar with the potential utility of the immunohistochemical markers in the diagnosis of this tumor

Case

An 81-year-old gentleman with no documented past history of malignancy presented with dizziness and difficulty of breathing. CT imaging of the chest revealed multiple lung nodules and lymphadenopathy. In addition, a possible brain lesion was noted on imaging. An ultrasound-guided FNA of the hilar lymph node was performed. The smears were highly cellular, composed of clusters, aggregated cell groups, and abundant single spindled to plump cells with hyperchromatic nuclei without prominent nucleoli. Some rosette-like structures were seen, as well as scattered pigment-laden macrophages. The pigments were dusky and brown granules on Pap stain and blue-black on Diff-Quik stain. Abundant necrosis was noted. Representative images of the FNA smears and cell-block material were shown in Fig. 6.39a–d.

The cytological features raise a differential diagnosis that includes neuroendocrine tumor, spindle cell tumors, including sarcomatoid carcinoma and metastatic melanoma of the spindle cell type. A limited panel of immunoassays was performed, revealing tumor cells with strong and diffuse nuclear staining for

(continued)

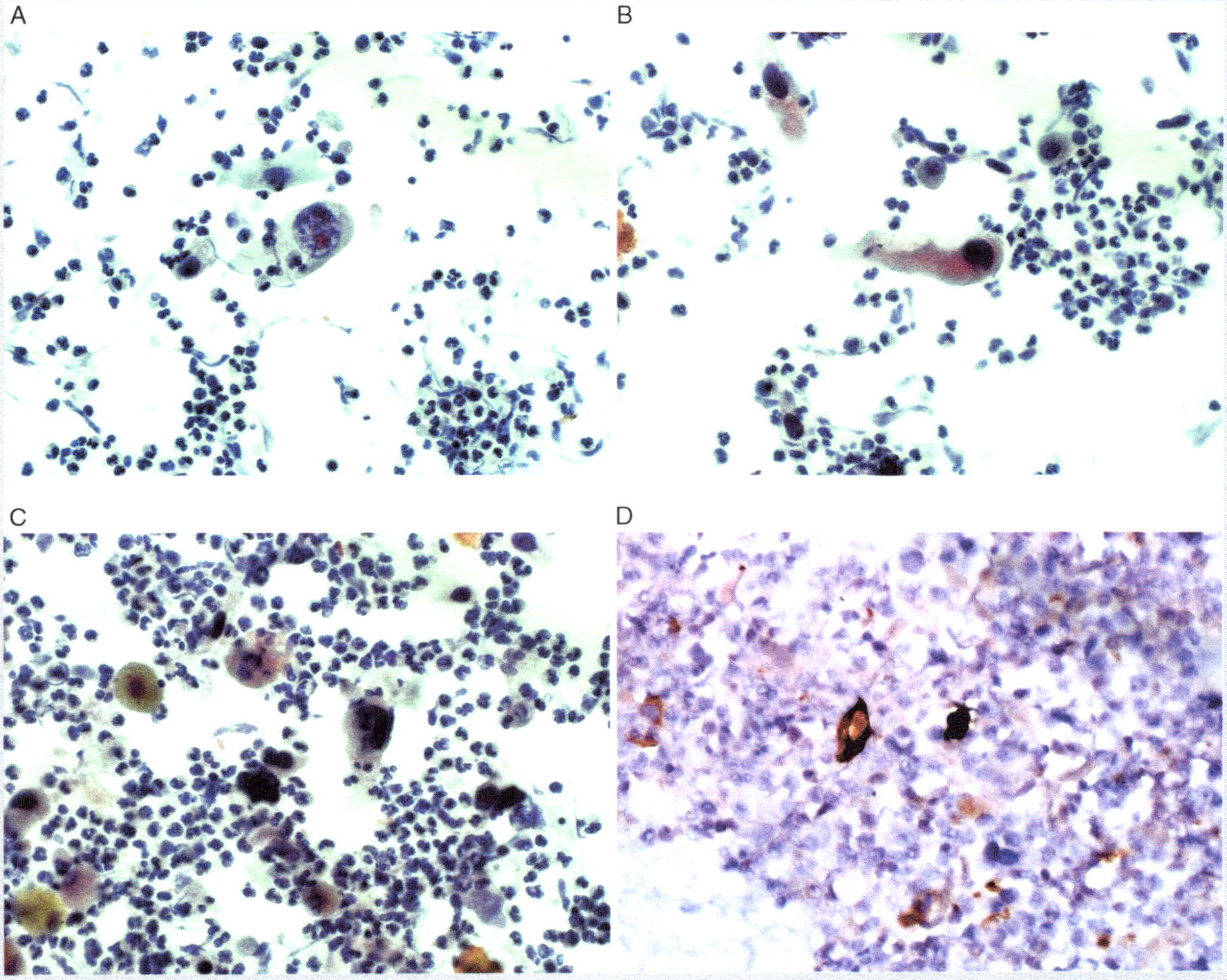

Fig. 6.38 Bronchial washing, in patient with coronavirus infection. (**a**) Atypical pneumocytes with large atypical nuclei, prominent eosinophilic nucleoli, and granular amphophilic cytoplasm, Pap stain; (**b**, **c**) scattered atypical metaplastic squamous cells with smudged chromatin, Pap stain; (**d**) CK7 highlights the atypical pneumocytes, IHC

sex determining region Y box 10 (SOX10) and cytoplasmic staining for vimentin and human melanoma black 45 (HMB45), focally for melanoma antigen recognized by T cells (MART1) and S100 (both nuclear and cytoplasmic), while CK AE1/3 and neuroendocrine markers (synaptophysin, chromogranin and CD56) were nonreactive. Representative images are illustrated in Fig. 6.39e–h. The overall findings are those of a metastatic spindle cell melanoma.

The diagnosis of metastatic spindle cell melanoma can be challenging on FNA specimens. The spindled tumor cells can display a wide range of morphologies, from deceptively bland-appearing reactive fibroblast-like cells to highly pleomorphic, high-grade sarcomatous spindle cells. The diagnostic cytological features of conventional melanoma, such as a dispersed single cell pattern, eccentric nuclei, cytoplasmic melanin pigments, intranuclear pseudoinclusions, prominent macronucleoli, and bi- or multinucleations, are often subtle or even lacking. For the index case, the presence of melanin pigments is a valuable clue to raise the suspicion for melanoma which, in conjunction with the immunophenotype, justified the diagnosis of spindle cell melanoma. The presence of cytoplasmic melanin

(continued)

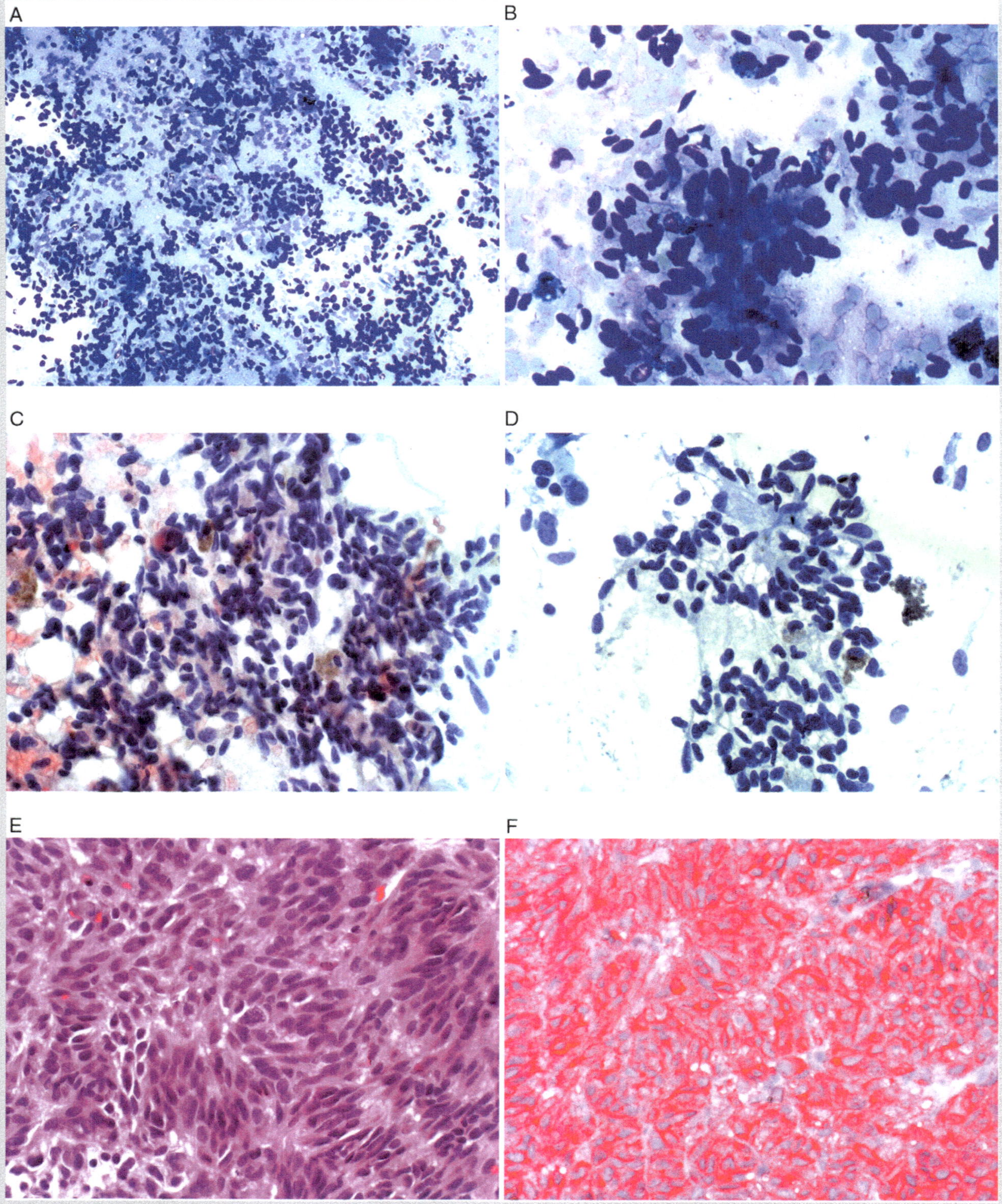

Fig. 6.39 Metastatic spindle cell melanoma. (**a**) Highly cellular smears, comprised of clusters and abundant singly spindle to plump cells with hyperchromatic nuclei without discernible nucleoli, Diff-Quik; (**b**) some rosette-like structures are seen, as well as scattered pigment laden macrophages; the pigments are dusky, blue-black, Diff-Quik; (**c**, **d**) same as **b**, the pigments are brown, granular, Pap stain; (**e**) cellblock preparation reveals spindled cells with perivascular palisading; scattered pigment-laden macrophages are seen, but not shown, H&E; (**f**) diffuse positive for HMB-45, IHC; (**g**) strong, diffuse SOX10 nuclear staining, IHC; (**h**) no CK AE1/3 expression, IHC

(continued)

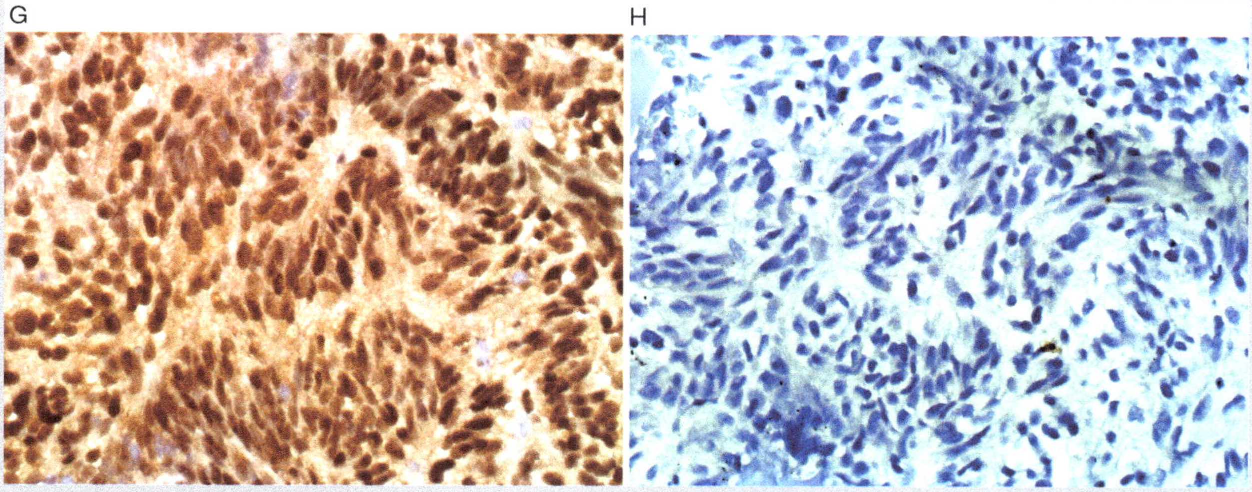

Fig. 6.39 (continued)

pigments in FNA samples varies, reported in the range of 30–80%. However, these pigments can occasionally be identified in melanotic schwannomas and melanotic malignant peripheral nerve sheath tumors (MPNSTs).

Immunohistochemistry plays a critical role in the diagnosis of spindle cell melanoma, especially in the clinical scenario of metastasis. Metastatic spindle cell melanomas tend to lose expression of some melanoma markers. Piao and colleagues reported that spindle cell melanomas express S100, HMB45, and MART1 in 67%, 50%, and 18% of cases, respectively. Although the sensitivity of S100 for melanoma in general is very high (~93–100%), its specificity is low. The expression of S100 can be seen in a variety of tumors. HMB45 is expressed in melanocytic tumors, also in clear cell sarcomas, perivascular epithelial cell tumors (PEComas), melanocytic schwannomas, meningeal melanocytomas, some ovarian steroid tumors, and renal cell carcinomas with the t(6;11)(p29;q12) translocation. The sensitivity of HMB45 for melanoma in general is in the range of 70–90%, but only 0–30% for desmoplastic melanomas. MART1 has a sensitivity of ~85–97% for primary and ~57–92% for metastatic melanomas, but only 0–33% for desmoplastic melanomas; its specificity for melanoma is 95–100%. MART1 expression is also seen in PEComas and clear cell sarcomas.

SOX10 is a transcription factor that is essential for the survival of neural crest-derived cells and for the maintenance of the multipotency of neural crest cells. The cells derived from neural crest multipotential cells include neurons and glial cells in the peripheral nervous system, melanocytes of the skin, C cells of the thyroid, catecholaminergic cells of the adrenal gland, and cartilage and bone of the face. Studies have shown that, among tumors, SOX10 is commonly expressed in melanomas, including desmoplastic melanomas, tumors with Schwann cell differentiation, myoepithelial cell tumors of the soft tissue and some salivary gland neoplasms, particularly those with myoepithelial differentiation, and acinic cell carcinomas. When compared with other melanocytic-associated markers, SOX10 is highly sensitive and specific and can assist in the differential diagnosis of melanomas. Even in desmoplastic melanomas, SOX10 expression was reported in 100% of cases. Studies of SOX10 expression in tumors of the nervous system reported that SOX10 is commonly expressed in schwannomas (100%), neurofibromas (98–100%), and, less frequently, MPNSTs (~50–55%).

The differential diagnosis of this case is summarized in Table 6.15.

Table 6.15 Immnohistochemical differential diagnosis of spindle cell melanoma

	MSM	NET	SC	MPNST
SOX10	+	−	−	−/+
S100	+	−	−	−/+
CK AE1/3	−	+	+	−
SYN	−	+	−	−
CHR	−	+	−	−
HMB45	−/+	−	−	−
MART1	−/+	−	−	−

MSM malignant spindle cell melanoma, *NET* neuroendocrine tumor, *SC* sarcomatoid carcinoma, *MPNST* malignant peripheral nerve sheath tumor, *SOX10* sex determining region Y box 10, *CK* cytokeratin, *SYN* synaptophysin, *CHR* chromogranin, *HMB45* human melanoma black 45, *MART1* melanoma antigen recognized by T cells

(continued)

Case Scenario 3: Metastatic Carcinoma

Learning Objectives

1. To describe the cytological features of this entity
2. To become aware of the subtle differences in cytology and to raise the question of a metastasis
3. To become familiar with the potential utility of immunohistochemical markers in the diagnosis of this tumor

Case

A 72-year-old female with a past medical history of noninvasive low-grade papillary urothelial carcinoma a year ago presented with coughing and chest pain for month. CT imaging of the chest revealed multiple lung nodules and lymphadenopathy. An ultrasound-guided FNA and biopsy of the hilar lymph node were performed. The smears were highly cellular, composed of loosely cohesive clusters and single spindle to plump cells with hyperchromatic nuclei, coarse chromatin, occasional discernible to prominent nucleoli, and abundant delicate cytoplasm without defined borders. Some of the cells appeared spindled, columnar or racket-shaped, with eccentrically located nuclei and cytoplasmic tails, also called cercariform cells. Abundant necrosis was noted in the background. Representative images of the FNA smears and biopsy are shown in Fig. 6.40a–f.

The cytological features raise a differential diagnosis that includes a non-small cell carcinoma of lung, especially squamous cell carcinoma, a sarcomatoid carcinoma, and metastatic carcinoma, especially metastatic urothelial carcinoma. A panel of immunoassays was performed, revealing that the tumor cells were positive for CK7, CK20 (focal), CK5/6, uroplakin II, p40, and placental S100 (S100P) while negative for TTF1, napsin A, synaptophysin, and chromogranin. Representative images are illustrated in Fig. 6.40g–j. The final diagnosis is metastatic carcinoma with urothelial differentiation

There are limited reports in literature regarding the cytology of metastatic urothelial carcinomas. The following features were reported: (1) loosely cohesive cells occurring singly and in syncytial clusters; (2) large hyperchromatic nuclei with irregularly distributed granular chromatin and abundant granular or fibrillar cytoplasm; (3) distinct cell borders; (4) multilayered papillary fragments; (5) cells with eccentric nuclei, multiple nucleoli, and intracytoplasmic vacuoles; and (6) cercariform cells, "bipolar" cells, and spindled-shaped cells. Among those, multilayered papillary fragments and cercariform cells are the most helpful features in the distinction of urothelial carcinoma from others. The cercariform cells, first described in 1993 by Johnson and Kini and further defined in 1995 by Powers and Elbadawi, are fusiform, pyramidal, or racket-like cells with eccentric nuclei that form non-tapering, flattened, bulbous, or fishtail-like cytoplasmic extensions in varying lengths. The presence of a small vacuole in the bulbous tail was also a helpful criterion. These cells, which are encountered in 57–100% of metastatic urothelial carcinomas, are interpreted in favor of urothelial carcinoma, particularly when they are observed in large numbers. However, they are not specific and must be considered alongside other clinical and morphological characteristics and immunohistochemical phenotypes. The cytological features of metastatic urothelial carcinomas are very difficult to differentiate from mesenchymal tumors and squamous cell carcinomas. Immunohistochemical analyses play a crucial role.

Urothelial cell carcinomas express both CK7 and CK20. In addition, they express HMWCKs (CK5/6, CK903), p63, GATA binding protein 3 (GATA3), uroplakin II, and S100P. GATA3 is a zinc finger transcription factor with a diverse range of biologic roles. GATA3 is a newer generation of urothelial specific marker. GATA3 expression was reported in approximately 80% of urothelial carcinomas, over 90% of breast carcinomas, 100% of parathyroid gland tissue or tumors, salivary gland tumors, especially the salivary ductal carcinomas (~90%), and transitional proliferations of the gynecological tract. In addition, 0–12% of pulmonary squamous cell carcinomas and approximately 10% of pancreatic carcinomas were also reported to be positive for GATA3, although weakly and focally in the majority of positive cases.

The immunohistochemical differential diagnosis of metastatic urothelial carcinomas is summarized in Table 6.16.

(continued)

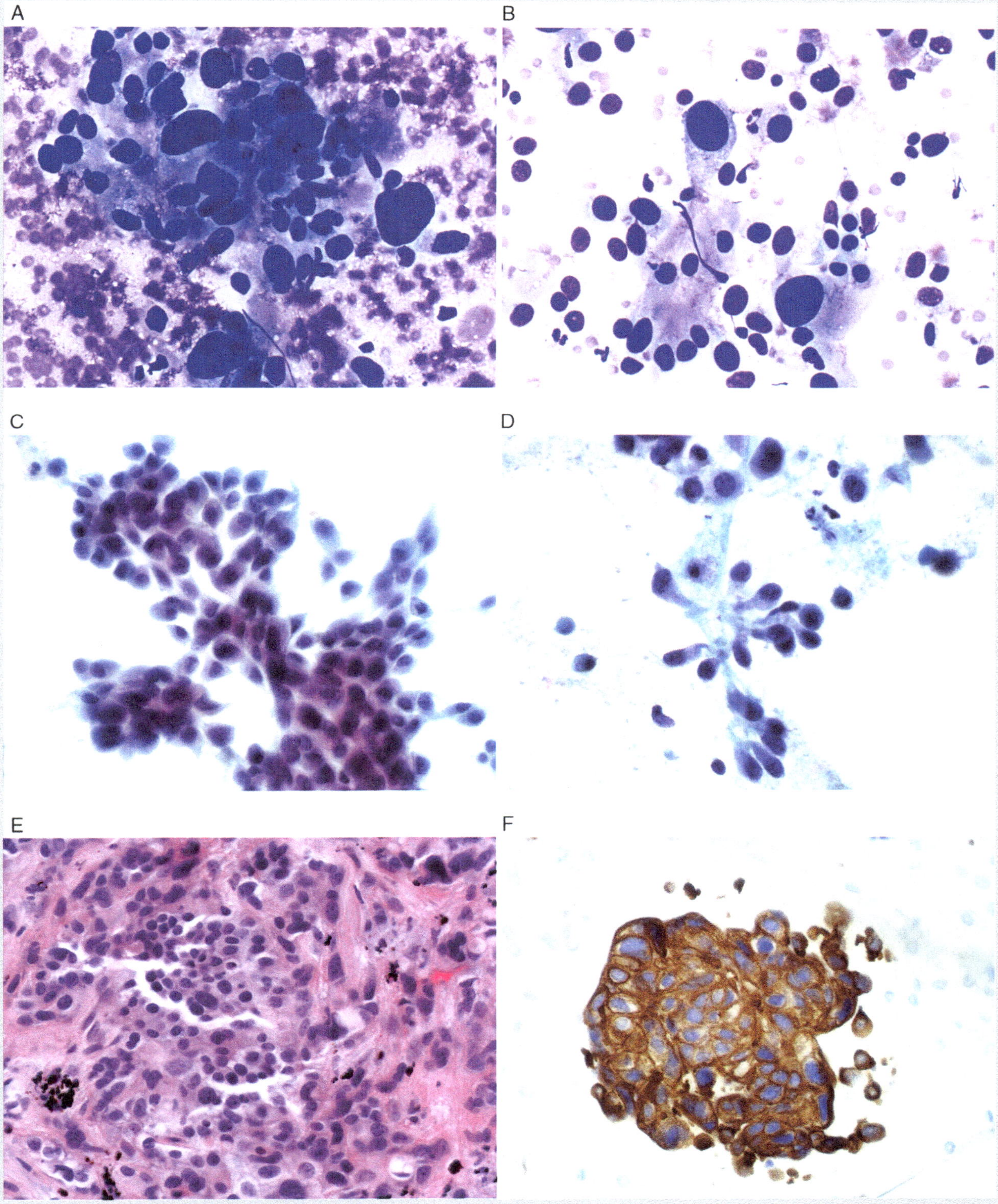

Fig. 6.40 Metastatic urothelial carcinoma, hilar lymph node, fine needle aspiration with biopsy. (**a**) Loosely cohesive atypical cells with pleomorphic and hyperchromatic nuclei, Diff-Quik; (**b**) the tumor cells show eccentrically placed, oval-shaped nuclei, and abundant cytoplasm, Diff-Quik; (**c**) multilayered papillary fragments, Pap stain; (**d**) many racket-shaped cells, also called cercariform cells showing eccentrically located nuclei with cytoplasmic tails, Pap stain; (**e**) biopsy, H&E; (**f**) positive for CK7, IHC; (**g**) positive for CK20, IHC; (**h**) positive for GATA3, IHC; (**i**) positive for uroplakin II, IHC; (**j**) positive for S100P, IHC

(continued)

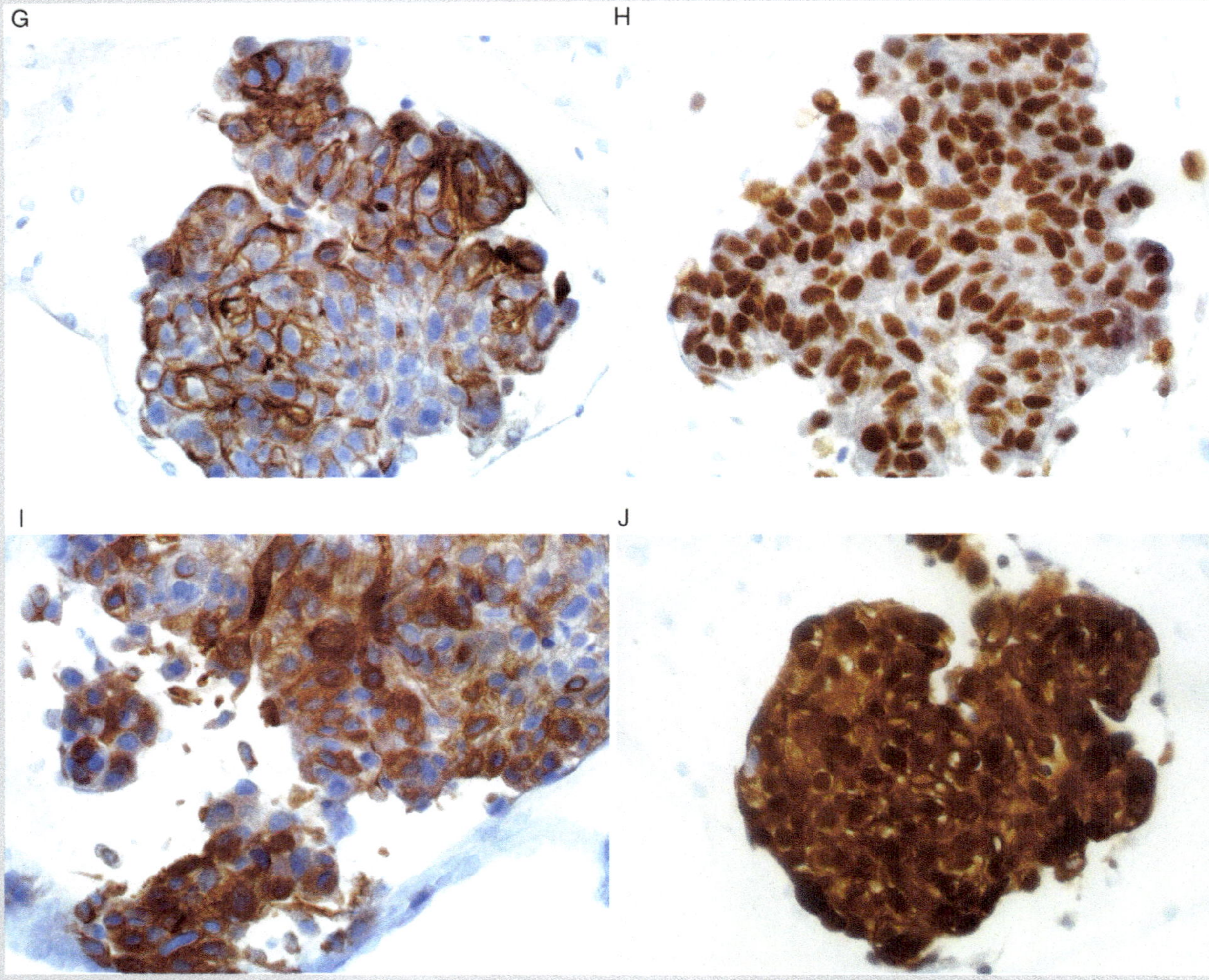

Fig. 6.40 (continued)

Table 6.16 Immunohistochemical differential diagnosis of metastatic urothelial carcinoma

	Met UCA	SqCC	Sarcomatoid CA
CK7	+	–	–/+
CK20	+/–	–	–
CK5/6	+	+	+/–
TTF1	–	–	–/+
GATA3	+	–/+[a]	–
Uroplakin II	+	–	–
p63	+/–	+	–/+
S100P	+	–	–

Met UCA metastatic urothelial carcinoma, *SqCC* squamous cell carcinoma, *CA* carcinoma, *CK* cytokeratin, *TTF1* thyroid transcription factor 1, *GATA3* GATA binding protein 3, *S100P* placental S100

[a]GATA3 expression in squamous cell carcinoma of lung was reported in 0–12% of cases; when positive, it is usually weak and focal.

Abbreviations List

Abbreviation	Full Text
ADC	Adenocarcinoma
AFP	Alpha-fetoprotein (α-fetoprotein)
AIDS	Acquired immunodeficiency syndrome
AIS	Adenocarcinoma in situ
AKT	Protein kinase B
ALCL	Anaplastic large cell lymphoma
ALK	Anaplastic lymphoma kinase
ATS	American Thoracic Society
B72.3	Tumor-associated glycoprotein (TAG)72
BAC	Bronchioloalveolar carcinoma
BAP1	BRCA1 associated protein 1
Bcl (Bcl2, Bcl6)	B-cell CLL/lymphoma 2, 6
BerEP4	Epithelial cell adhesion molecule
BOB1	B-cell Oct-binding protein 1
BRD	Bromodomain containing (BRD3, BRD4)
CA	Carcinoma
CCNE1	Cyclin E1
CD	Cluster of differentiation
CDKN2	Cyclin-dependent kinase inhibitor 2 (CDKN2A, CDKN2B)
CEA	Carcinoembryonic antigen
CHR	Chromogranin (table only)
CK	Cytokeratin
CREB1	CAMP responsive element binding protein
CT	Computed tomography
CTNNB1	Catenin beta 1
CUL3	Cullen 3
DAD	Diffuse alveolar damage
EBV	Epstein-Barr virus
EGFR	Epithelial growth factor receptor
EM	Electron microscopy
EMA	Epithelial membrane antigen
EML4	Echinoderm microtubule-associated protein-like 4
ERS	European Respiratory Society
EWSR1	Ewing sarcoma break point region 1
F	Focal (table)
FDG	fluorodeoxyglucose
FGFR1	Fibroblast growth factor receptor 1
FNA	Fine needle aspiration
FOXN1	Forkhead box N1
GATA3	GATA binding protein 3
GI	Gastrointestinal

Abbreviation	Full Text
GLUT1	Glucose transporter 1
Gly3	Glypican 3
GMS	Grocott's methenamine silver
GTF2I	General transcription factor IIi
GYN	Gynecologic
H&E	Hematoxylin and eosin
HMB45	Human melanoma black 45
HMGA2	High-mobility group AT-hook 2
HMWCK	High molecular weight cytokeratin
IASCL	International Association for the Study of Lung Cancer
Ig	Immunoglobulin
IHC	Immunohistochemistry (only in table)
IMP3	Insulin-like growth factor II messenger RNA protein
IRF4	Interferon regulatory factor 4
KEAP1	Kelch-like ECH-associated protein 1
KIT	
KRAS	Kirsten rat sarcoma viral oncogene
LCNEC	Large cell neuroendocrine carcinoma
LCNEM	Large cell carcinoma with neuroendocrine morphology (in table only)
LeuM1	Cluster of differentiation (CD)15
LG	Low grade (table only)
LMWCK	Low molecular weight cytokeratin
LPP	Lipoma preferred partner
MAL	Myelin and lymphocyte
MALT	Mucosa-associated lymphoid tissue
MART1	Melanoma antigen recognized by T cells
MDM2	Mouse double minute 2 homolog
Med	Median (table)
MEN1	Multiple endocrine neoplasia type 1
Met UCA	Metastatic urothelial carcinoma
MIA	Minimally invasive adenocarcinoma
MIB1	Mindbomb E3 ubiquitin protein ligase 1
MPNST	Malignant peripheral nerve sheath tumor
MRI	Magnetic resonance imaging
MSA	Muscle-specific actin
MSM	Malignant spindle cell melanoma
MUC	Mucin (e.g., MUC1)
MUM1	Multiple myeloma oncogene 1
N/C	Nuclear-to-cytoplasmic ratio
NATB2	NGFI-A binding protein 2
NE	Neuroendocrine
NET	Neuroendocrine tumor
NF2	Neurofibromin 2
NFE2L2	Nuclear factor, erythroid 2 like 2
NK	Natural killer

Abbreviation	Full Text
NKX3.1	NK3 homeobox 1
NOS	Not otherwise specified
NOTCH1	Notch (Drosophila) homolog 1
NSCC	Non-small cell carcinoma (in tables only)
NSCLC	Non-small cell lung carcinoma
NUT	Nuclear protein in testis
OCT3/4	Octamer-binding transcription factor 3/4
OT2	
Pap	Papanicolaou
PAS	Periodic acid-Schiff
PAX	Paired box gene (PAX5, PAX8)
PEComa	Perivascular epithelioid cell tumor
PEComatous	Perivascular epithelioid cell (PEC) omatous tumors
PET	Positron emission tomography
PNET	Primitive neuroectodermal tumor
PU.1	
RB1	Retinoblastoma 1
REL	
RNA	Ribonucleic acid
RT-PCR	Reverse transcription polymerase chain reaction
S100P	Placental S100
SALL4	Sal-like protein 4
SARS	Severe acute respiratory syndrome
SARS-CoV	Severe acute respiratory syndrome caused by coronavirus (SARS coronavirus)
SATB2	Special AT-rich sequence-binding protein 2
SC	Sarcomatoid
SCNC	Small cell neuroendocrine carcinoma
SMA	Smooth muscle actin
SOX	Sex-determining region Y box (SOX1, SOX10, etc.)
spp.	Species (many)
SqCC	Squamous cell carcinoma (in tables only)
STAT6	Signal transducer and activator of transcription 6
SYN	Synaptophysin
TdT	Terminal deoxynucleotidyl transferase
TP	Tumor protein (TP53, TP63)
TRAF	Tumor necrosis factor receptor
TTF1	Thyroid transcription factor 1
WHO	World Health Organization
WT1	Wilms tumor 1
βhCG	Β subunit of human chorionic gonadotropin

Suggested Reading

Cytology/Fine Needle Aspiration

Bibbo M, Wilbur DC. Comprehensive cytopathology. 4th ed. Philadelphia: Elsevier, Saunders; 2015.

Cibas ES, Ducatman BS. Cytology: diagnostic principles and clinical correlates. 2nd ed. Philadelphia: Saunders; 2003.

DeMay RM. The art & science of cytopathology. 2nd ed. Chicago: American Society for Clinical Pathology (ASCP) Press; 2012.

Kaur G, Verma K. Fine needle aspiration cytology of metastatic urothelial carcinoma: study of seven cases with review of literature. J Cytol. 2012;29(2):116–20.

Vural C, Yildiz K, Çabuk D, Akgül A. Transthoracic fine-needle aspiration cytology of non-invasive, low-grade urothelial carcinoma with lung metastasis: a case report with review of the literature. J Cytol. 2015;32(2):132–5.

Histology

Cancer Genome Atlas Research Network. Comprehensive genomic characterization of squamous cell lung cancers. Nature. 2012;489(7417):519–25.

Franks TJ, Chong PY, Chui P, Galvin JR, Lourens RM, Reid AH, et al. Lung pathology of severe acute respiratory syndrome (SARS): a study of 8 autopsy cases from Singapore. Hum Pathol. 2003;34(8):743–8.

Gokmen-Polar Y, Cano OD, Kesler KA, Loehrer PJ, Badve, S. NUT midline carcinomas in the thymic region. Mod Pathol. 2014;27(12):1649–56.

Gu J, Korteweg C. Pathology and pathogenesis of severe acute respiratory syndrome. Am J Pathol. 2007;170(4):1136–47.

Nicholls JM, Poon LL, Lee KC, Ng WF, Lai ST, Leung CY, et al. Lung pathology of fatal severe acute respiratory syndrome. Lancet. 2003;361(9371):1773–8.

Suster S, Moran CA. Tumors of the lung and pleura. In: Fletcher CDM, editor. Diagnostic histopathology of tumors. 4th ed. Philadelphia: Saunders; 2013. p. 207–45.

Travis WD, Brambilla E, Burke AP, Marx A, Nicholson A. WHO classification of tumours of the lung, pleura, thymus and heart. Lyon: IARC; 2015a.

Travis WD, Brambilla E, Nicholson AG, Yatabe Y, Austin JH, Beasley MB, et al. WHO panel. The 2015 World Health Organization classification of lung tumors: impact of genetic, clinical and radiologic advances since the 2004 classification. J Thorac Oncol. 2015b;10(9):1243–60.

Travis WD, Brambilla E, Noguchi M, Nicholson AG, Geisinger K, Yatabe Y, et al. Diagnosis of lung cancer in small biopsies and cytology: implications of the 2011 International Association for the Study of Lung Cancer/American Thoracic Society/European Respiratory Society classification. Arch Pathol Lab Med. 2013a;137(5):668–84.

Travis WD, Brambilla E, Noguchi M, Nicholson AG, Geisinger K, Yatabe Y, et al. Diagnosis of lung adenocarcinoma in resected specimens: implications of the 2011 International Association for the Study of Lung Cancer/American Thoracic Society/European Respiratory Society classification. Arch Pathol Lab Med. 2013b;137(5):685–705.

Tse GM, To KF, Chan PK, Lo AW, Ng KC, Wu A, et al. Pulmonary pathological features in coronavirus associated severe acute respiratory syndrome (SARS). J Clin Pathol. 2004;57(3):260–5.

Ancillary Tests

Chang A, Amin A, Gabrielson E, Illei P, Roden RB, Sharma R, et al. Utility of GATA3 immunohistochemistry in differentiating urothelial carcinoma from prostate adenocarcinoma and squamous cell carcinomas of the uterine cervix, anus, and lung. Am J Surg Pathol. 2012;36(10):1472–6.

Dupin E, Calloni G, Real C, Gonçalves-Trentin A, Le Douarin NM. Neural crest progenitors and stem cells. C R Biol. 2007;330(6–7):521–9.

Esheba GE, Longacre TA, Atkins KA, Higgins JP. Expression of the urothelial differentiation markers GATA3 and placental S100 (S100P) in female genital tract transitional cell proliferations. Am J Surg Pathol. 2009;33(3):347–53.

Gershon TR, Oppenheimer O, Chin SS, Gerald WL. Temporally regulated neural crest transcription factors distinguish neuroectodermal tumors of varying malignancy and differentiation. Neoplasia. 2005;7(6):575–84.

Gruver AM, Amin MB, Luthringer DJ, Westfall D, Arora K, Farver CF, et al. Selective immunohistochemical markers to distinguish between metastatic high-grade urothelial carcinoma and primary poorly differentiated invasive squamous cell carcinoma of the lung. Arch Pathol Lab Med. 2012;136(11):1339–46.

Higgins JP, Kaygusuz G, Wang L, Montgomery K, Mason V, Zhu SX, et al. Placental S100 (S100P) and GATA3: markers for transitional epithelium and urothelial carcinoma discovered by complementary DNA microarray. Am J Surg Pathol. 2007;31(5):673–80.

Huang X, Saint-Jeannet JP. Induction of the neural crest and the opportunities of life on the edge. Dev Biol. 2004;275(1):1–11.

Kang Y, Pekmezci M, Folpe AL, Ersen A, Horvai AE. Diagnostic utility of SOX10 to distinguish malignant peripheral nerve sheath tumor from synovial sarcoma, including intraneural synovial sarcoma. Mod Pathol. 2014;27(1):55–61.

Kelsh RN. Sorting out Sox10 functions in neural crest development. BioEssays. 2006;28:788–98.

Lin F, Liu H. Unknown primary/undifferentiated neoplasm. In: Lin F, Prichard JW, Liu H, Wilkerson M, Chen ZE, editors. Handbook of practical immunohistochemistry: frequently asked questions. 2nd ed. New York: Springer Science+Business Media; 2015. p. 119–63.

Liu H, Shi J, Prichard J, Gung Y, Lin F. Immunohistochemical evaluation of GATA-3 expression in ER-negative breast carcinomas. Am J Clin Pathol. 2014;141(5):648–55.

Liu H, Shi J, Wilkerson ML, Lin F. Immunohistochemical evaluation of GATA3 expression in tumors and normal tissues: a useful immunomarker for breast and urothelial carcinomas. Am J Clin Pathol. 2012;138(1):57–64.

Miettinen M, PA MC, Sarlomo-Rikala M, Biernat W, Czapiewski P, Kopczynski J, et al. Sox10-a marker for not only schwannian and melanocytic neoplasms but also myoepithelial cell tumors of soft tissue: a systematic analysis of 5134 tumors. Am J Surg Pathol. 2015;39(6):826–35.

Nonaka D, Chiriboga L, Rubin BP. Sox10: a pan-schwannian and melanocytic marker. Am J Surg Pathol. 2008;32(9):1291–8.

Ordóñez NG. Value of GATA3 immunostaining in tumor diagnosis: a review. Adv Anat Pathol. 2013a;20(5):352–60.

Ordóñez NG. Value of melanocytic-associated immunohistochemical markers in the diagnosis of malignant melanoma: a review and update. Hum Pathol. 2014;45(2):191–205.

Ordóñez NG. Value of SOX10 immunostaining in tumor diagnosis. Adv Anat Pathol. 2013b;20(4):275–83.

Paratore C, Goerich DE, Suter U, Wegner M, Sommer L. Survival and glial fate acquisition of neural crest cells are regulated by an interplay between the transcription factor Sox10 and extrinsic combinatorial signaling. Development. 2001;128:3949–61.

Wilkerson ML, Cheng L. Urinary bladder and urachus. In: Lin F, Prichard JW, Liu H, Wilkerson M, Chen ZE, editors. Handbook of practical immunohistochemistry: frequently asked questions. 2nd ed. New York: Springer Science+Business Media; 2015. p. 421–37.

Wilkerson ML, Lin F, Liu H, Cheng L. The application of immunohistochemical biomarkers in urologic surgical pathology. Arch Pathol Lab Med. 2014;138(12):1643–65.

Yang GG, Minasyan A, Gordon J, Lacey M, Lundquist K. Rabbit polyclonal anti-SOX10 is a reliable IHC marker for melanoma and its mimics [abstract]. Mod Pathol. 2013;26(S2):124A–5A.

Zhang K, Deng H, Cagle PT. Pleuropulmonary and mediastinal neoplasms. In: Lin F, Prichard JW, Liu H, Wilkerson M, Chen ZE, editors. Handbook of practical immunohistochemistry: frequently asked questions. 2nd ed. New York: Springer Science+Business Media; 2015. p. 313–41.

7 Liver

Fan Lin, Haiyan Liu, and Jun Zhang

Summary of Pearls and Pitfalls

- Fine needle aspiration (FNA) and small needle core biopsies of the liver under a guidance of computed tomography (CT) or ultrasound (US) are popular procedures to obtain a diagnosis from a mass lesion. It is a very useful approach in the diagnosis of malignant liver neoplasms, with sensitivity ranging from 75% to 94% and specificity ranging from 87% to 100%.
- Approximately 95% of malignant liver tumors are metastasis, and the majority of other malignant tumors are hepatocellular carcinoma (HCC).
- In order to obtain a definitive diagnosis, a cellblock preparation or thin needle core biopsy in conjunction with immunohistochemical (IHC) stains is strongly encouraged for every FNA of the liver.
- FNA of the liver cannot differentiate among the benign lesions of hepatocellular adenoma (HCA), focal nodular hyperplasia, and regenerative nodule in cirrhosis.
- Two important diagnostic issues are frequently encountered in the FNA of the liver. One is to differentiate well-differentiated HCC from benign/reactive hepatic lesion, and the other is to distinguish poorly differentiated HCC from cholangiocarcinoma or metastatic carcinomas or even sarcomas.
- Glypican-3, heat-shock protein 70 (HSP70), glutamine synthetase (GS), and clusterin are useful markers in diagnosing a well-differentiated HCC.
- Alpha-fetoprotein (AFP) is a specific, after exclusion of germ cell tumors and other tumors, but insensitive marker (about 25%) in the detection of HCC on tissue section.
- Arginase-1 is a more specific marker than hepatocyte paraffin-1 (HepPar-1) in confirming a hepatocellular origin when working on a tumor of unknown origin.
- Approximately 70% of intrahepatic cholangiocarcinomas (IHCCs) are positive for von Hippel-Lindau tumor suppressor gene protein (pVHL); in contrast, metastatic adenocarcinomas, including those from the pancreas and extrahepatic biliary tract, are negative for pVHL.
- Albumin by ribonucleic acid (RNA) in situ hybridization has been reported to be detectable in nearly 100% of HCCs and IHCCs and the majority of hepatoid carcinomas.
- Vascular tumors of the liver tend to have a bloody and hypocellular smear; therefore, avoid calling a smear non-diagnostic before excluding a vascular tumor. Bland spindled endothelial cells may be mistaken for other mesenchymal lesions.
- When working on a spindle cell lesion, even if no lipomatous component is seen, an angiomyolipoma should be included in the differential diagnoses. The epithelioid variant of angiomyolipoma can mimic other tumors, such as HCC, clear cell renal cell carcinoma (RCC), adrenocortical carcinoma, and melanoma.

Liver Lesions, Neoplasms, and Tumors in the 2010 World Health Organization (WHO) Classification, Modified[1]

Normal/reactive liver
Infection
  Hepatic abscess
  Granulomatous inflammation
  Echinococcal (hydatid) cyst

[1]Modified with permission from Bosman et al. (2010).

© Springer International Publishing AG 2018
F. Lin et al., *Handbook of Practical Fine Needle Aspiration and Small Tissue Biopsies*, DOI 10.1007/978-3-319-57386-1_7

Benign neoplasms/lesions
- HCA
- Focal nodular hyperplasia
- Cirrhosis
- Regenerative nodules
- Bile duct adenoma and hamartoma
- Cavernous hemangioma
- Angiomyolipoma (perivascular epithelioid cell tumor [PEComa])
- Lymphangioma
- Lymphangiomatosis
- Infantile hemangioma
- Mesenchymal hamartoma
- Solitary fibrous tumor

Premalignant lesions
- Intraductal papillary neoplasm with low-, intermediate-, or high-grade dysplasia
- Mucinous cystic neoplasm with low-, intermediate-, or high-grade dysplasia

Malignant neoplasms
- Hepatocellular carcinoma (HCC)
- HCC, fibrolamellar variant
- Hepatoblastoma
- Intrahepatic cholangiocarcinoma (IHCC)
- Combined hepatocellular-cholangiocarcinoma
- Intraductal papillary neoplasm with an associated invasive carcinoma
- Mucinous cystic neoplasm with an associated invasive carcinoma
- Angiosarcoma
- Epithelioid hemangioendothelioma
- Other sarcomas
- Germ cell tumors
- Lymphomas

Rare primary lesions/tumors

Secondary tumors

Normal Cytology of the Liver

Hepatocytes (Figs. 7.1, 7.2, 7.3, 7.4, 7.5, 7.6, 7.7, and 7.8)

- Large polygonal cells singly, in ribbons, or in large tissue fragments.
- Round and centrally located nuclei with prominent nucleoli.
- Binucleation and intranuclear inclusion are common.
- Low nuclear-to-cytoplasmic ratio with abundant granular cytoplasm.
- Pigments can be lipofuscin (Fig. 7.4), bile (Figs. 7.5 and 7.6), or hemosiderin (Fig. 7.7).

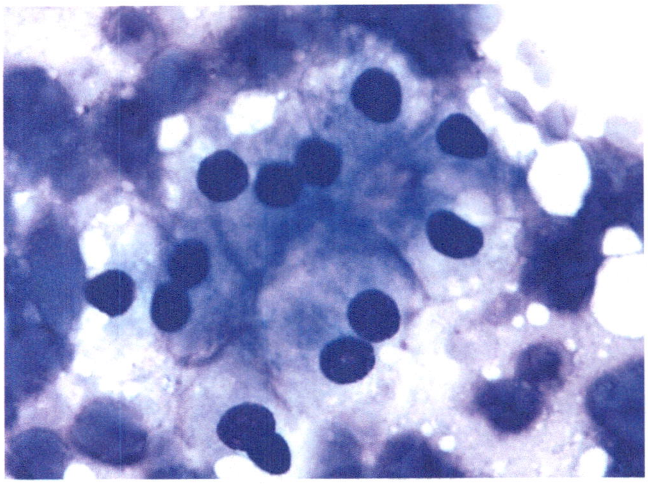

Fig. 7.1 Normal hepatocytes with round and centrally located nuclei with prominent nucleoli (Diff-Quik)

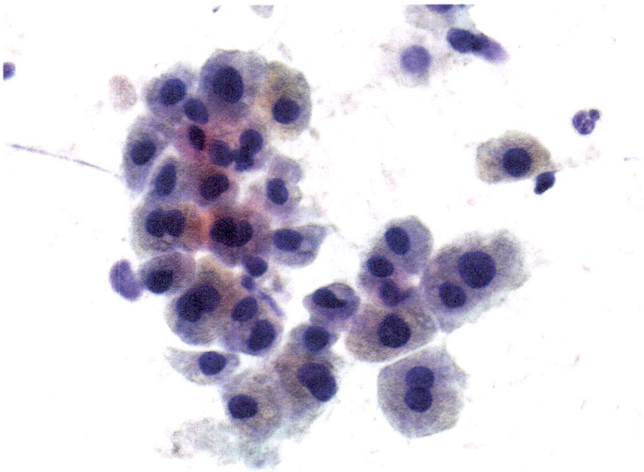

Fig. 7.2 Normal hepatocytes (Papanicolaou [Pap] stain)

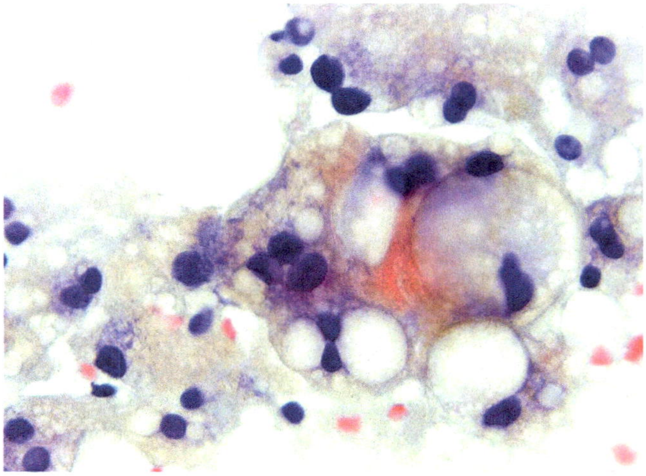

Fig. 7.3 Hepatocytes with steatosis

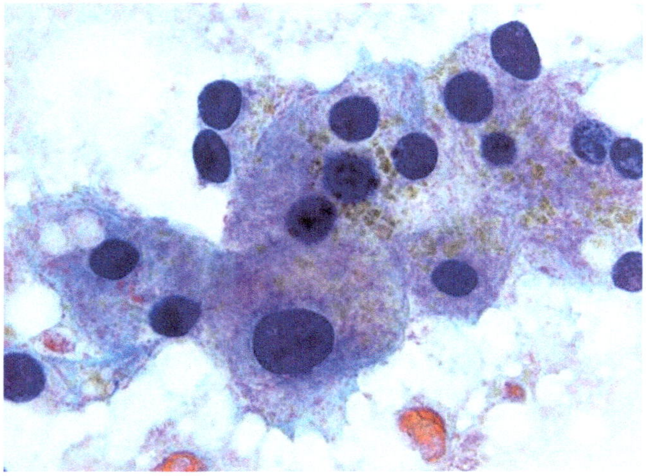

Fig. 7.4 Hepatocytes with lipofuscin

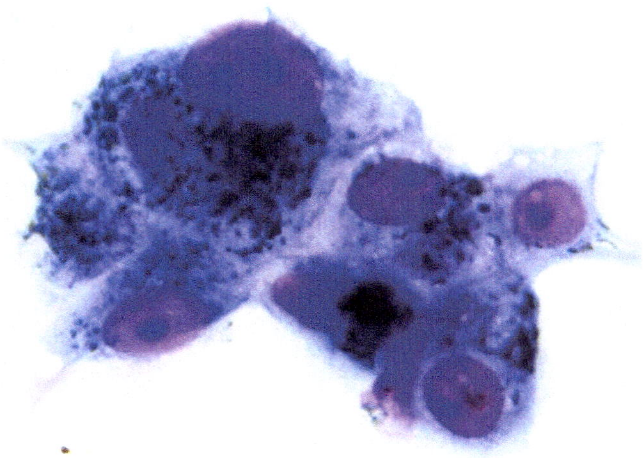

Fig. 7.5 Hepatocytes with bile (Diff-Quik)

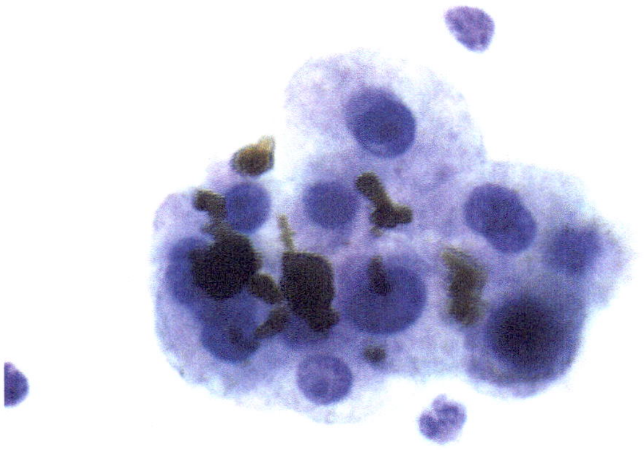

Fig. 7.6 Hepatocytes with bile (Pap stain)

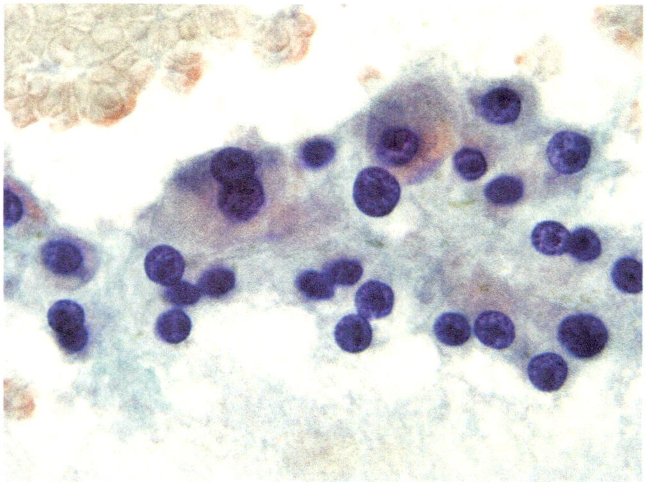

Fig. 7.7 Reactive hepatocytes with prominent nucleoli

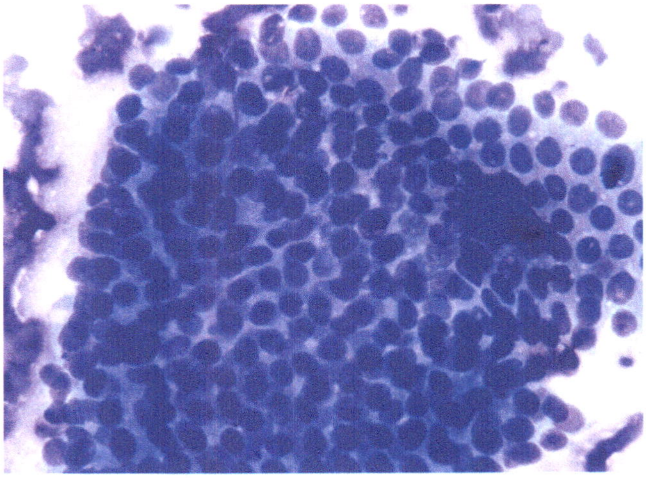

Fig. 7.8 Two-dimensional sheets of benign duct epithelium cells. The nuclei are round to ovoid, same size or slightly larger than one red blood cell, evenly distributed nuclear chromatin, smooth nuclear membranes, and indistinct nucleoli (Diff-Quik)

Bile Duct Epithelial Cells

- Two-dimensional sheets of variable sizes, with a scant amount of cytoplasm and poorly defined cytoplasmic borders.
- The cell borders may be prominent, forming an orderly honeycomb appearance.
- The nuclei are round to ovoid, the same size or slightly larger than one red blood cell, evenly distributed nuclear chromatin, smooth nuclear membranes, and indistinct nucleoli (Fig. 7.9a, b).

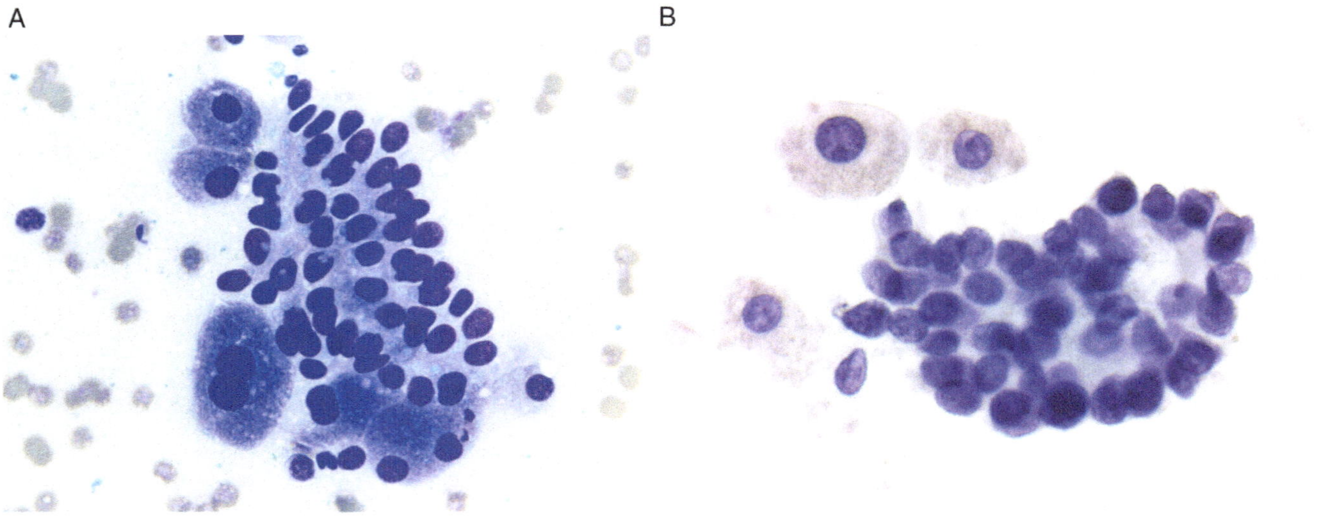

Fig. 7.9 (**a**, **b**) Benign duct cells and hepatocytes on Diff-Quik (**a**) and Pap stain (**b**)

Hepatic Abscess

Cytological Features

- Numerous acute inflammatory cells and necrotic debris as shown in Fig. 7.10.
- Culture is needed.
- Cellblock preparation for special stains.

Differential Diagnosis

- Bacteria, amoeba, fungus, or neoplasms

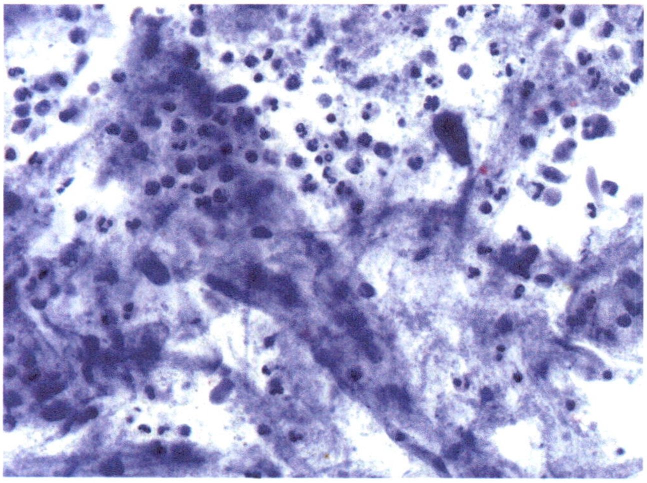

Fig. 7.10 Hepatic abscess with acute inflammatory cells and necrotic debris

Granulomatous Inflammation

Cytological Features

- Aggregates of epithelioid histiocytes, multinucleated giant cells, and chronic inflammatory cells with or without necrosis, as shown in Fig. 7.11

Histology

- Aggregates of epithelioid histiocytes, multinucleated giant cells, and chronic inflammatory cells with or without necrosis

Differential Diagnosis

- Infection, such as tuberculosis, fungus, parasites
- Sarcoidosis
- Reaction to foreign materials
- Neoplasms, Hodgkin's lymphoma, T-cell lymphoma, and seminoma

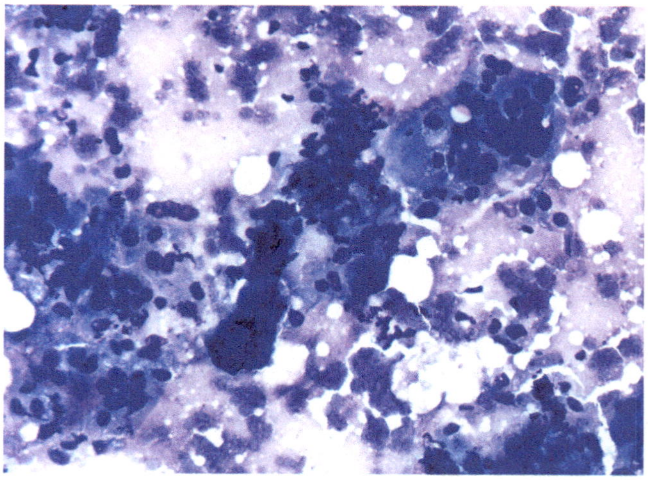

Fig. 7.11 Granulomatous inflammation

Echinococcal (Hydatid) Cyst

Clinical Features

- Anaphylactic shock has been reported as an occasional complication of the FNA.

Cytological Features (Fig. 7.12)

- Fragments of the laminated membrane
- Scolices
- Hooklets

Hepatocellular Adenoma

Clinical Features

- Young female, usually under age 30.
- Long-term use of oral contraceptives or androgenic steroids.
- Other nonhormonal risk factors such as glycogenosis type 1 and 3, galactosemia, familial polyposis coli, obesity, etc.
- Sizes are variable from microscopic focus to 20 cm.

Cytological Features

- Normal-appearing or mildly atypical hepatocytes, singly or in groups or sheets (Fig. 7.13a–c)
- Normal nuclear-to-cytoplasmic ratio with abundant granular cytoplasm
- Decreased numbers or lack of bile duct epithelial cells

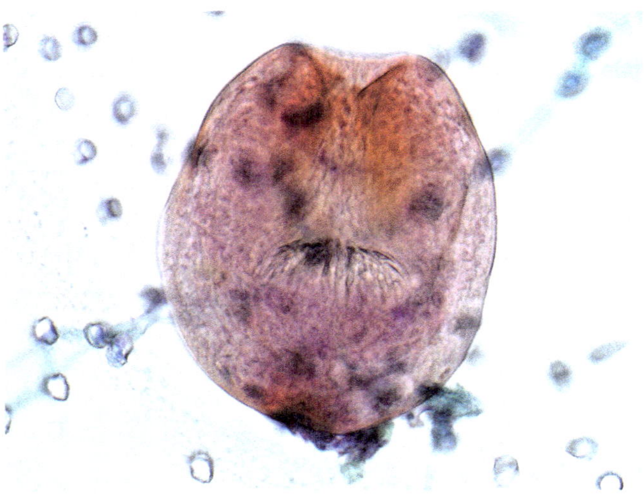

Fig. 7.12 Hydatid cyst showing hooks

Histology

- Benign hepatocytes arranged in plates, one or two cells thick (Fig. 7.14a–d).
- Absence of portal tracts with presence of isolated arteries.
- Tumoral hepatocytes may show steatotic, clear, or pigmented cytoplasm.
- Focal pseudoglandular formation can be seen.
- Minimal nuclear atypia and no mitosis.
- Biopsy of adjacent nontumoral liver to determine the presence of absence of cirrhosis is important.
- HCA has been recently subclassified into several groups: hepatocyte nuclear factor 1-alpha (HNF-1a)-inactivated HCA (35–40%), beta-catenin-activated HCA (10–15%), inflammatory HCA (>50%), and unclassified HCA (<10%).
- Beta-catenin-activated HCA has an increased risk of malignant transformation.

Immunohistochemistry

- A panel of IHC markers including liver fatty acid-binding protein (L-FABP), HNF-1a, serum amyloid A (SSA)/C-reactive protein (CRP), beta-catenin, and GS has been reported to be useful in this subclassification. The immunoreactivity to each IHC marker for each subtype of HCA is summarized in Table 7.1.

Differential Diagnosis

- Normal liver
- Focal nodular hyperplasia
- Regenerative nodules
- Cirrhosis

Focal Nodular Hyperplasia

Clinical Features

- Nodule usually contains a central scar.

Cytological Features

- Normal-appearing or mildly atypical hepatocytes in singly or in groups or sheets
- Normal nuclear-to-cytoplasmic ratio with abundant granular cytoplasm
- Increased numbers of bile duct epithelial cells

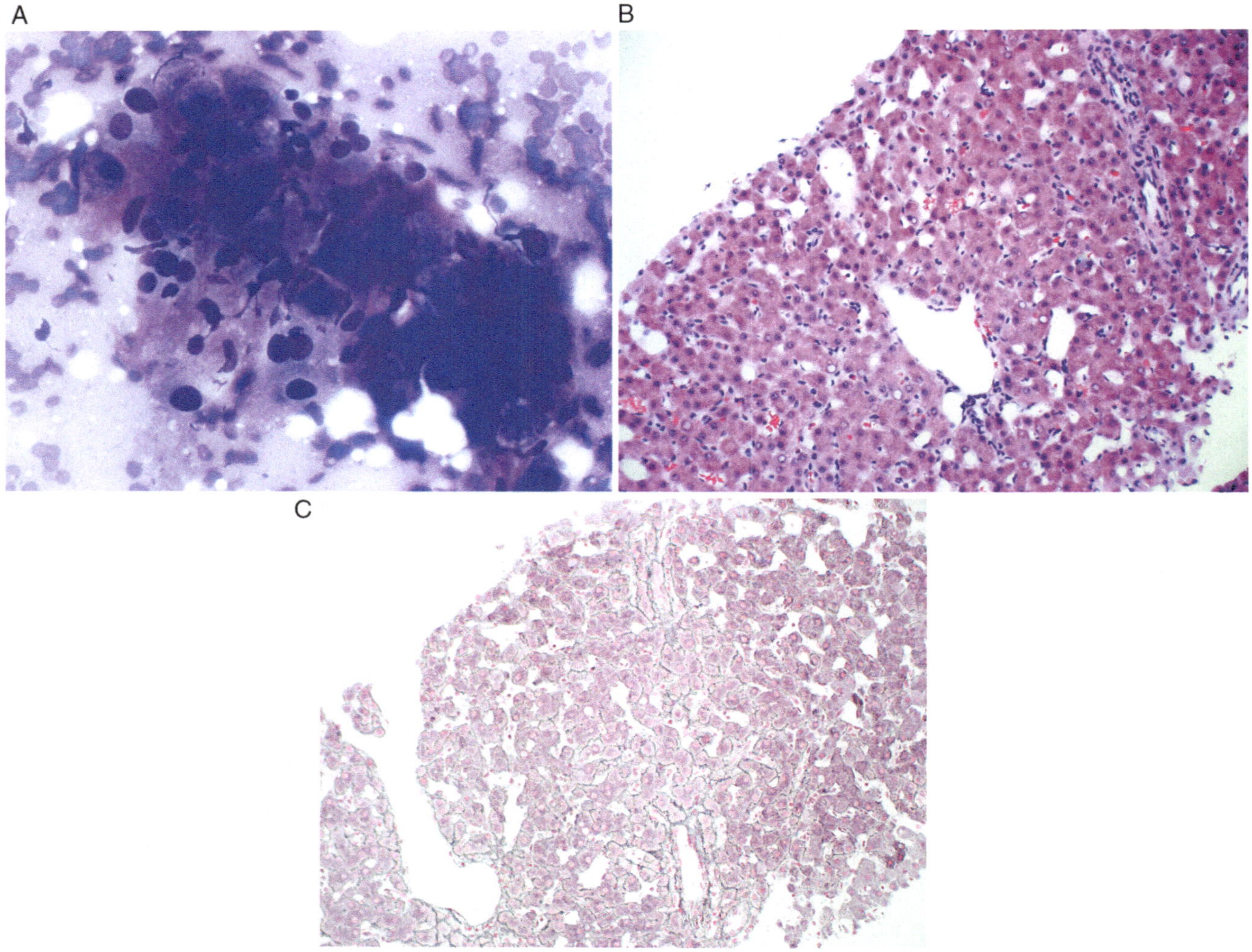

Fig. 7.13 (**a**–**c**) HCA with benign hepatocytes and no ductal cells on an FNA smear (**a**), on cellblock (**b**), and reticulin showing hepatocytes of 1–2 cells in thickness (**c**)

Histology

- Benign hepatocellular nodules arranged in plates no more than two cells thick (Figs. 7.15a–d and 7.16a–d).
- Central scar containing one or more large dystrophic vessels and many small arterioles.
- Portal-like structures with arteries only, absence of veins or bile ducts.
- Stromal inflammatory infiltration, cholate stasis, and ductular reaction at the parenchymal-stromal interface.
- Cytokeratin (CK)7 highlights the prominent ductular reaction.
- Sinusoids adjacent to arteries are lined by cluster of differentiation (CD)34-positive endothelium.

Differential Diagnosis

- Normal liver
- HCA
- Regenerative nodules
- Cirrhosis

Bile Duct Adenoma/Hamartoma

Clinical Features

- Usually multiple small nodules

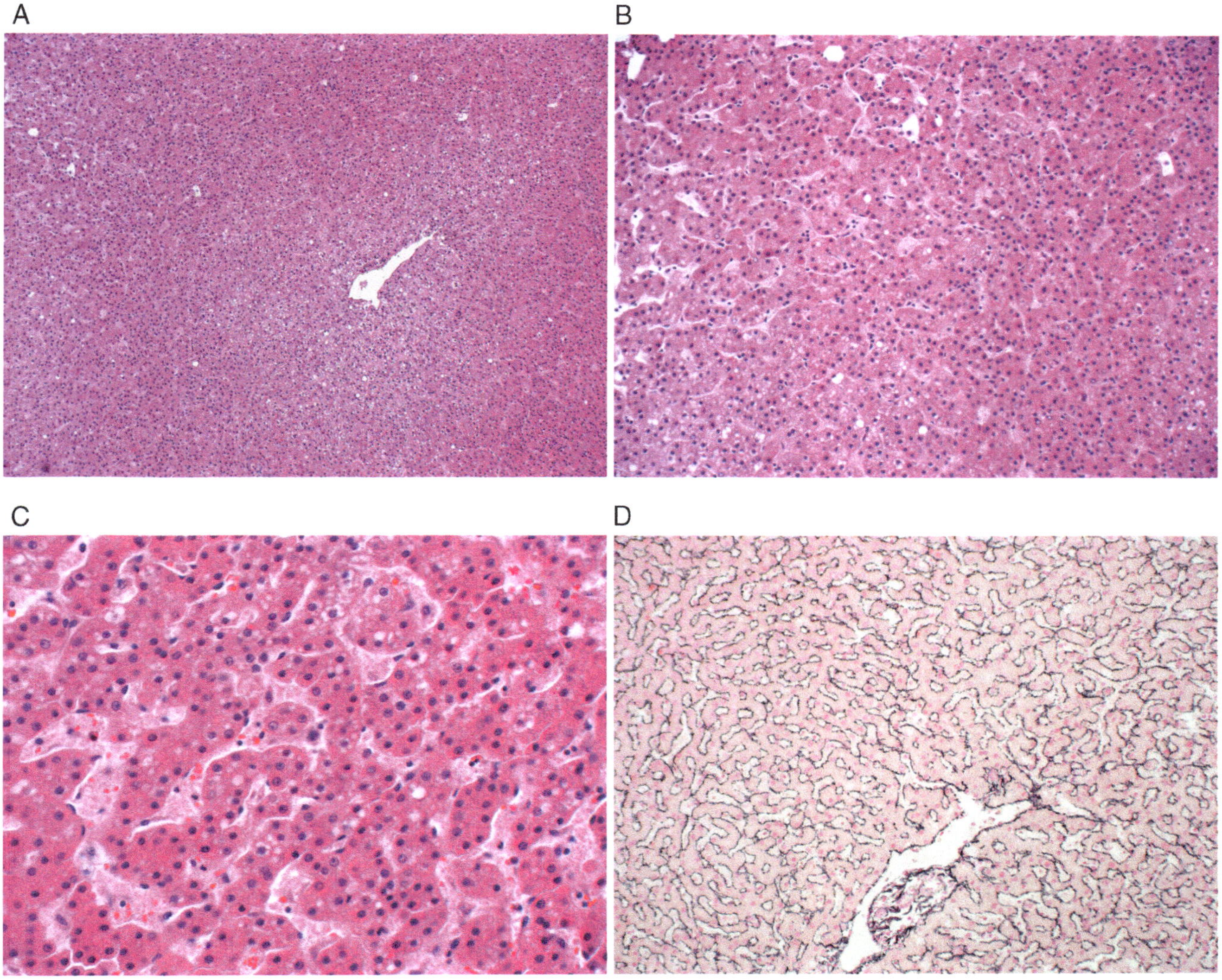

Fig. 7.14 (**a–d**) HCA showing hepatocytes arranged in layers of one to two cells in thickness and absence of portal tracts (**a–c**) and reticulin highlighting hepatocytes of 1–2 cells in thickness (**d**)

Table 7.1. Summary of useful IHC markers in subclassification of HCA

Markers/diagnosis	HNF-1a-inactivated HCA	Beta-catenin-activated HCA	Inflam-matory HCA	Unclassified HCA
L-FABP	–	+	+	+
GS	–	+	–	–
Beta-catenin (N+)	–	+	–	–
SAA/CRP	–	–	+	–

Note: *N* nuclear

Cytological Features

- Hypocellular specimen with increased numbers of benign to mildly atypical bile duct epithelial cells
- Normal hepatocytes

Histology (Fig. 7.17a, b)

- Bile duct adenoma is characterized by a proliferation of normal-appearing small bile ducts surrounded by connective tissue with entrapped portal tract forming a nodule or multiple nodules, usually in a subcapsular location. Nuclear atypia, mitosis, and intraluminal bile are usually absent.
- Hamartoma is formed by a proliferation of bile ducts in anastomotic channels containing bile in a fibrotic stroma.

Differential Diagnosis

- Cirrhosis
- Focal nodular hyperplasia
- Cholangiocarcinoma
- Metastatic well-differentiated adenocarcinoma

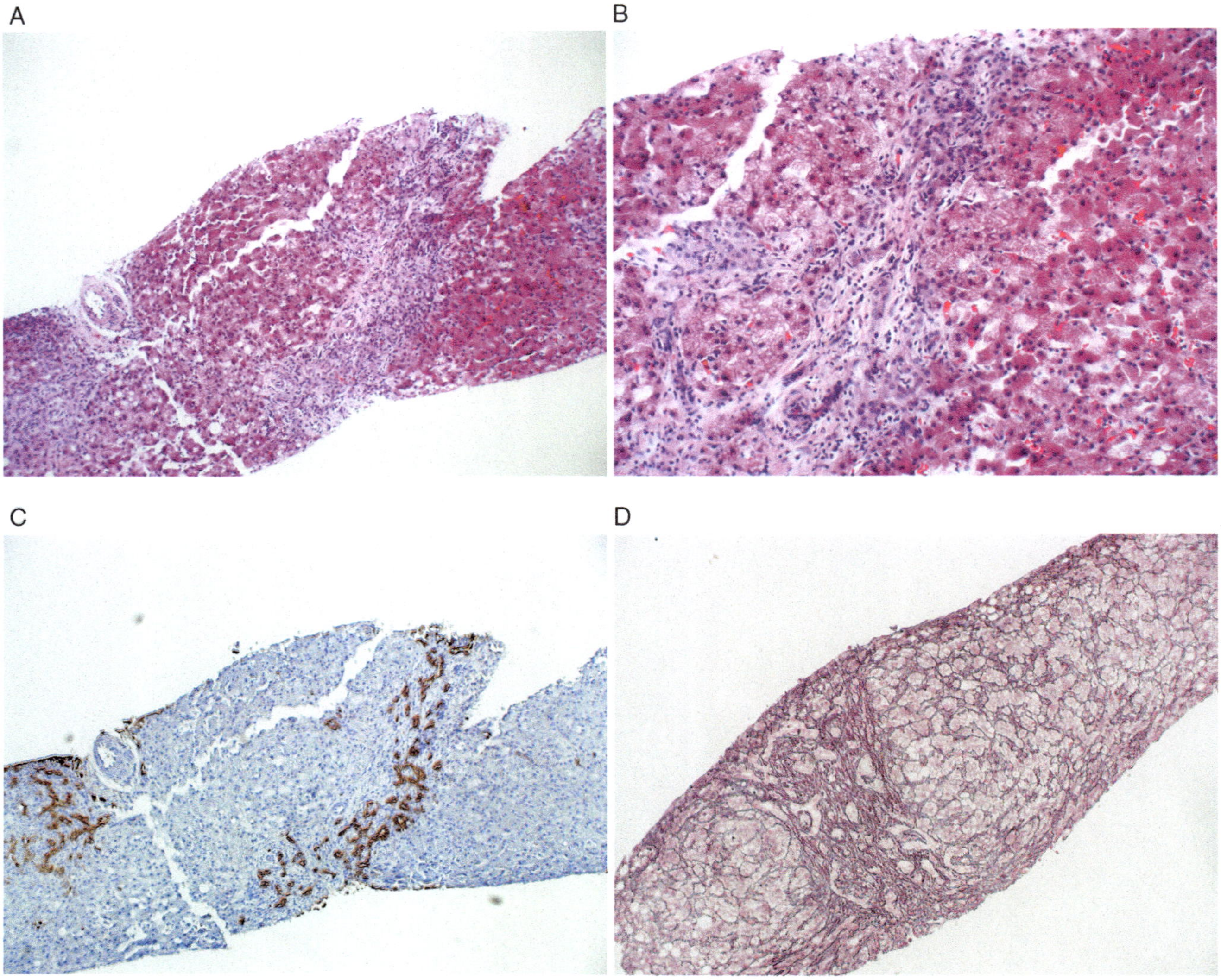

Fig. 7.15 (a–d) Focal nodular hyperplasia with benign hepatocytes arranged in layers of less than two cells in thickness, lack of portal tract, stromal inflammatory infiltrate, and ductular reaction on a core biopsy

Angiomyolipoma (PEComa)

Clinical Features

- Most common benign tumor of the kidney

Cytological Features (Figs. 7.18 and 7.19)

- Cluster of spindle cells or epithelioid smooth muscle cells.
- Adipocytes.
- Thickened wall blood vessels.
- The ratio of the above three components is variable from one case to another.
- Extramedullary hematopoiesis.

Histology

- Smooth muscle proliferation admixed with various proportions of adipose tissue and thick-walled hyalinized blood vessels.
- Smooth muscle cells can be spindled or epithelioid. The epithelioid cells can have clear or oncocytic cytoplasm.

Immunohistochemistry

- Positive for smooth muscle actin (SMA), human melanoma black 45 (HMB45), and melanoma antigen recognized by T cells-1 (Mart-1)
- Can be positive for CD117 and desmin
- Usually negative for S100

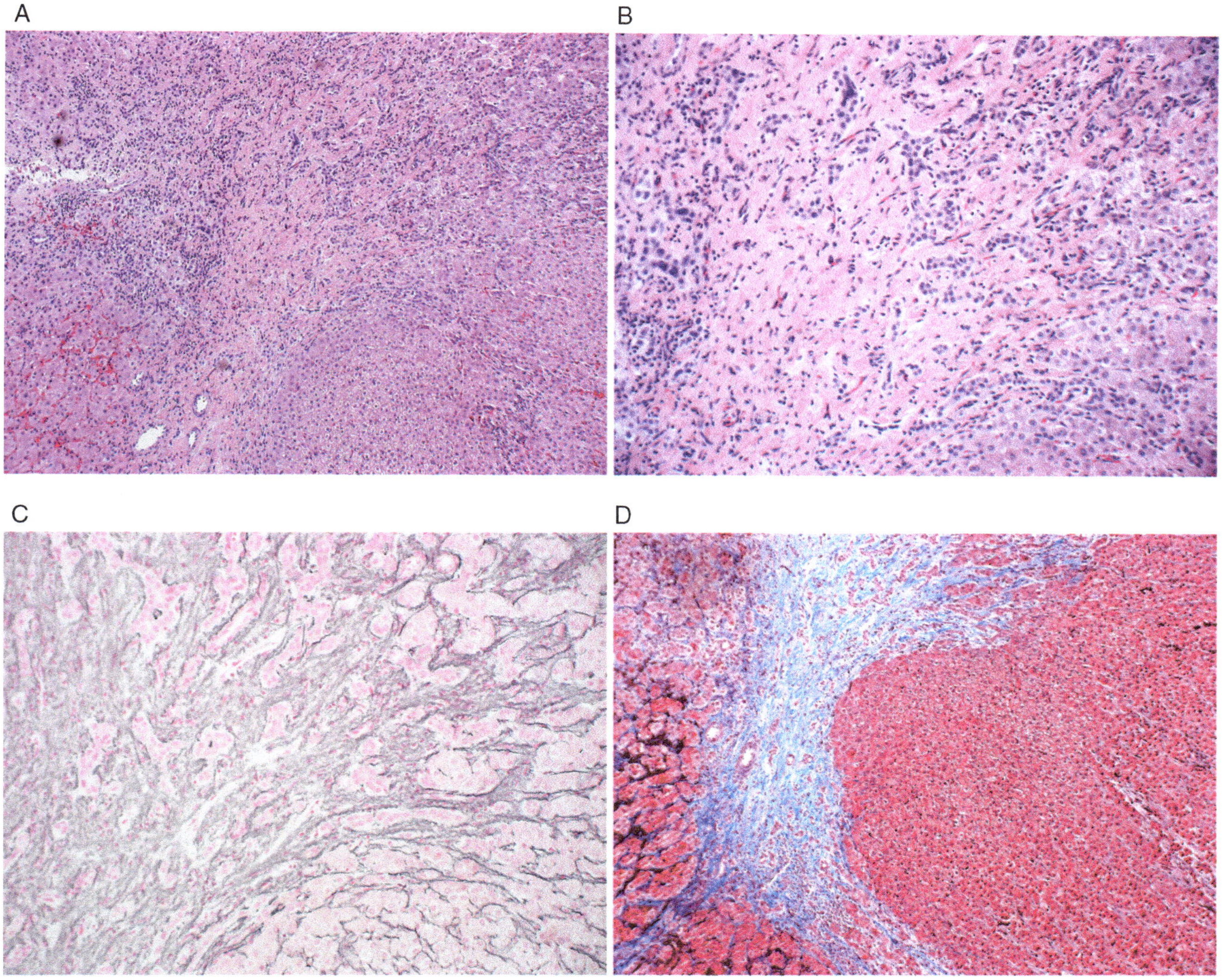

Fig. 7.16 (**a–d**) Focal nodular hyperplasia with benign hepatocytes arranged in layers of less than two cells in thickness, lack of portal tract, stromal inflammatory infiltrate, and ductular reaction on a resection specimen. Note the reticulin stain (**c**) and trichrome stain (**d**)

Differential Diagnosis

- HCC
- RCC
- Adrenocortical carcinoma
- Sarcoma
- Carcinoma
- Granulomatous inflammation

Hemangioma

Clinical Features

- The most common benign neoplasm of the liver
- Reported in up to 20% of autopsy studies
- More common in young adult females
- May increase in size or even rupture during pregnancy

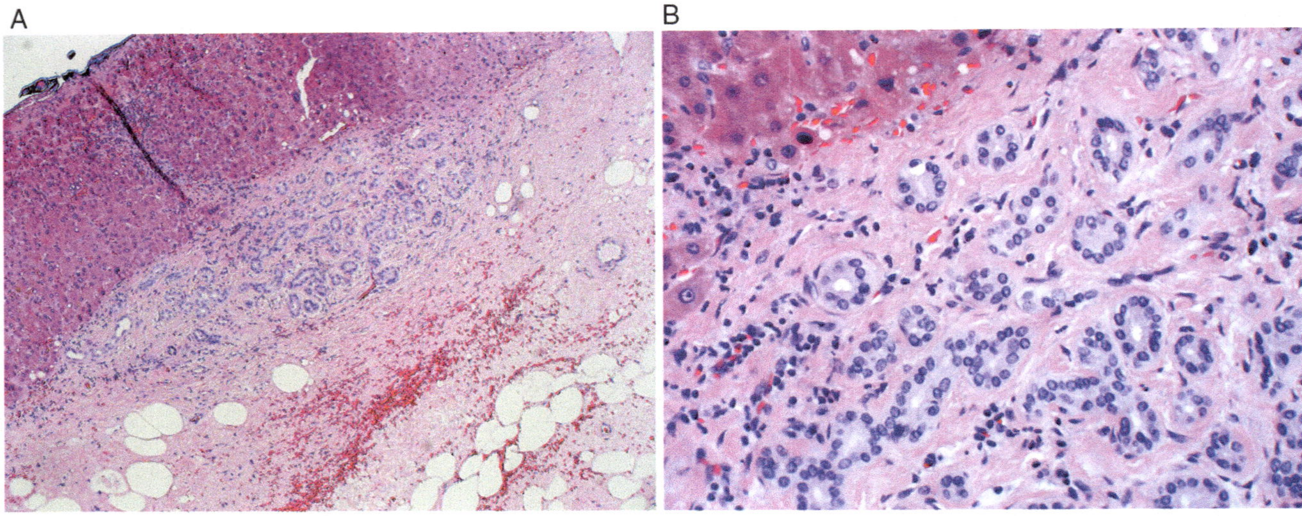

Fig. 7.17 (**a**, **b**) Bile duct adenoma

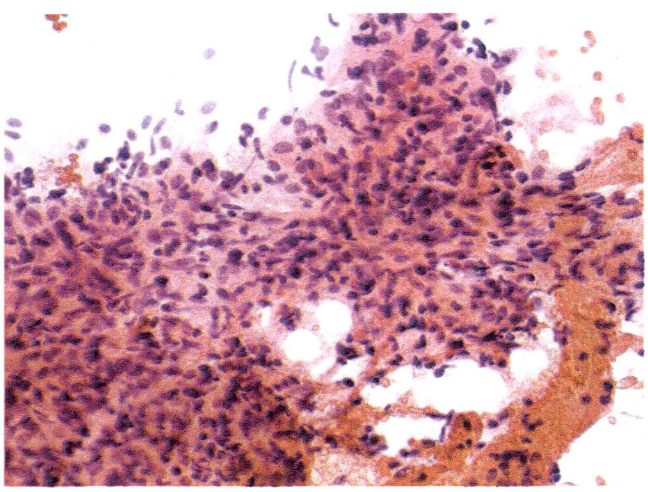

Fig. 7.18 Angiomyolipoma with spindle cells and fat cells

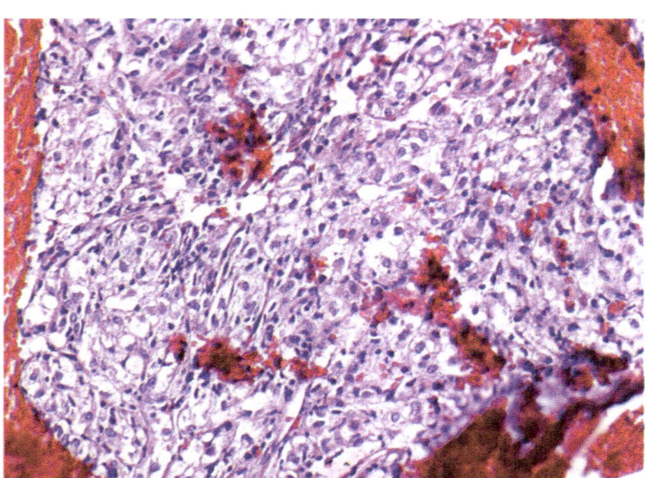

Fig. 7.19 Angiomyolipoma on cellblock section

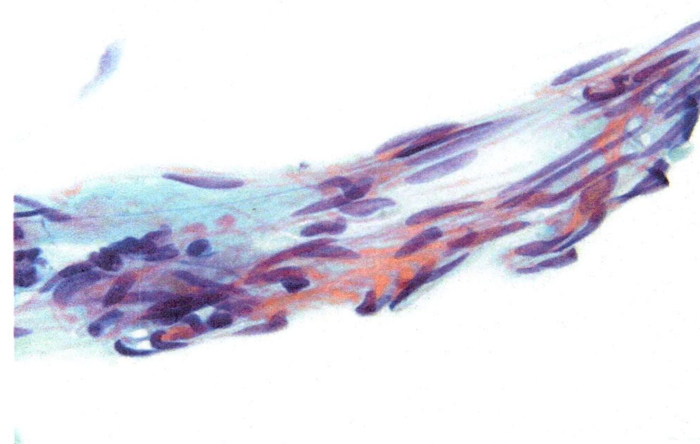

Fig. 7.20 Hemangioma with few benign elongated spindle cells

Cytological Features (Figs. 7.20, 7.21, and 7.22)

- Bloody sample with low cellularity and normal hepatocytes in the background
- Scattered, isolated cytologically bland spindle cells
- Small clusters of three-dimensional coiled elongated spindle cells

Histology

- Most benign vascular tumors are cavernous hemangiomas.
- Various-sized blood-filled vascular channels lined by a single layer of flat endothelial cells separated by fibrous septa of various thicknesses.

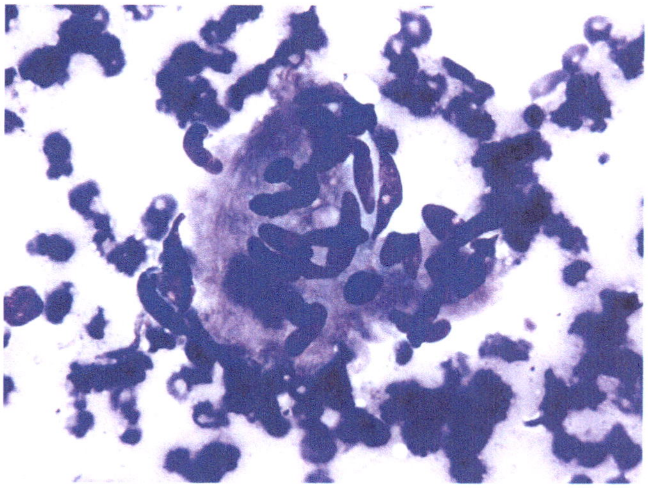

Fig. 7.21 Hemangioma with small cluster of three-dimensional coiled elongated spindle cells

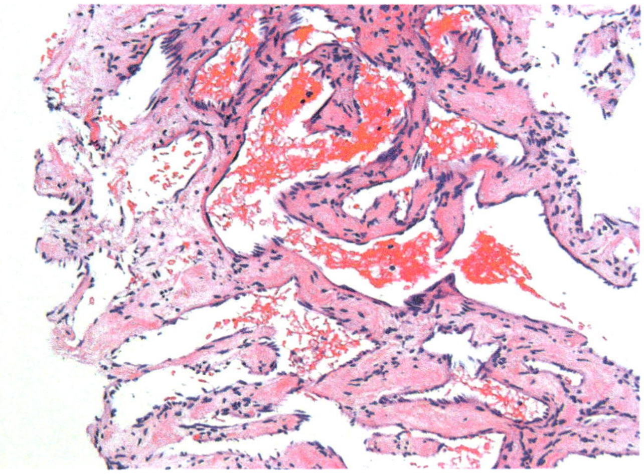

Fig. 7.22 Tissue section of hemangioma

Differential Diagnosis

- Spindle cell tumor if a highly cellular sample is obtained
- Granulomatous inflammation
- Lymphangioma and lymphangiomatosis

Hepatocellular Carcinoma (HCC)

Clinical Features

- Over 90% of primary malignant tumors of the liver are HCCs.
- Can be solitary or multiple nodules or even a diffuse infiltrate.
- Serum AFP is not a very sensitive or specific marker.
- Frequently associated with cirrhosis.
- Fibrolamellar-type HCC is not associated with cirrhosis; mean age of patients is 23; normal serum AFP.

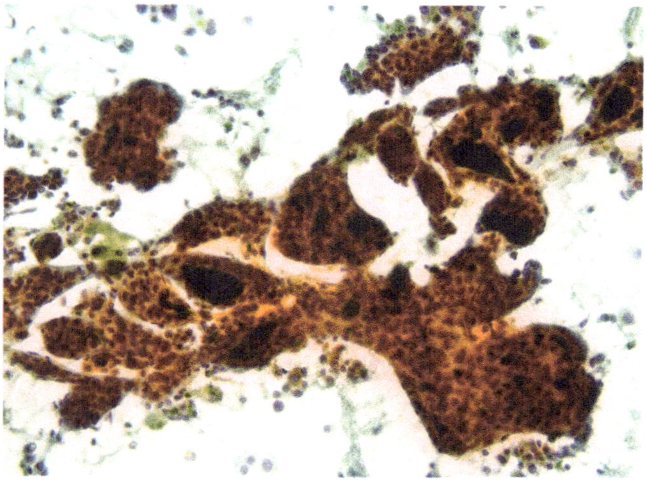

Fig. 7.23 Hypercellular smears of HCC, low power; hypercellular samples with many single cells, thick cores, nets, and sheets

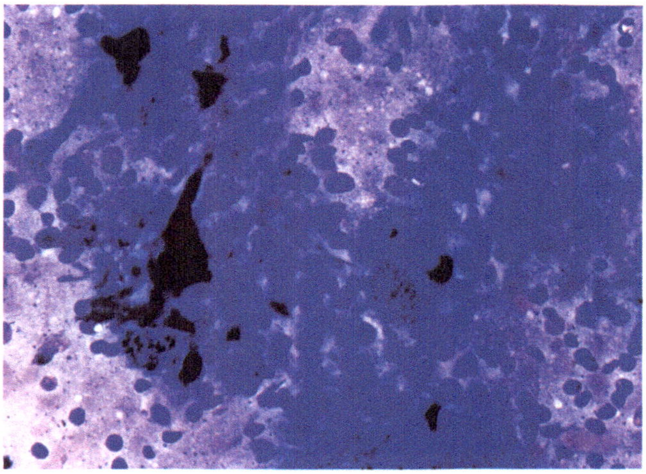

Fig. 7.24 Well-differentiated HCC with trabeculae (Diff-Quik)

Cytological Features for Well-Differentiated HCC (Figs. 7.23, 7.24, 7.25, 7.26, 7.27, 7.28, 7.29, 7.30, 7.31, 7.32, 7.33, 7.34, 7.35, 7.36, 7.37, 7.38, 7.39, 7.40, and 7.41a–d)

- Hypercellular samples with many single cells, thick cores, nets, and sheets.
- Hepatocytes more than three cell layers thick wrapped by spindle-shaped endothelial cells are the key to a final diagnosis.
- Pseudoglandular formation with bile is another diagnostic feature.
- Many naked, large/pleomorphic nuclei.
- Hepatocytes with high nuclear-to-cytoplasmic ratio, large nuclei, prominent nuclei, and intranuclear inclusions.
- Clear cell changes.
- Steatosis.
- Fibrolamellar HCC.

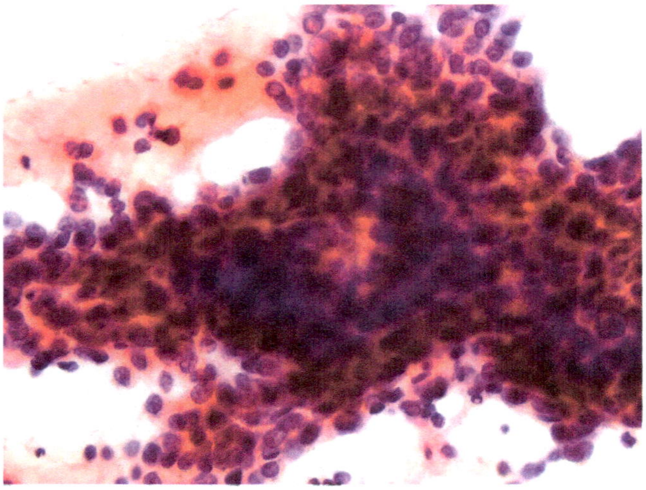

Fig. 7.25 Well-differentiated HCC with trabeculae (Pap stain)

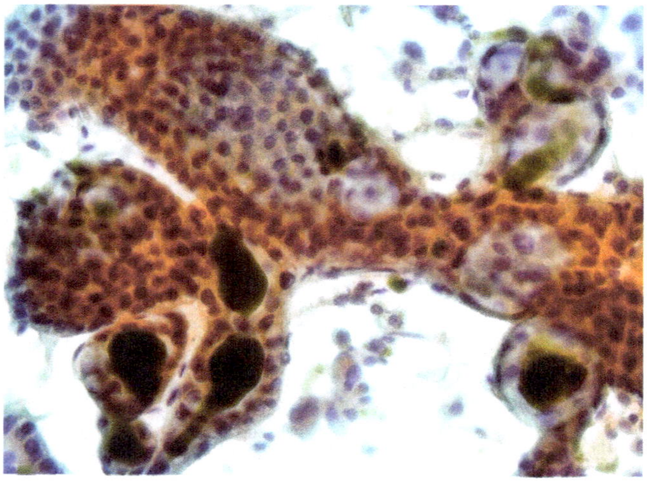

Fig. 7.26 Well-differentiated HCC with bile

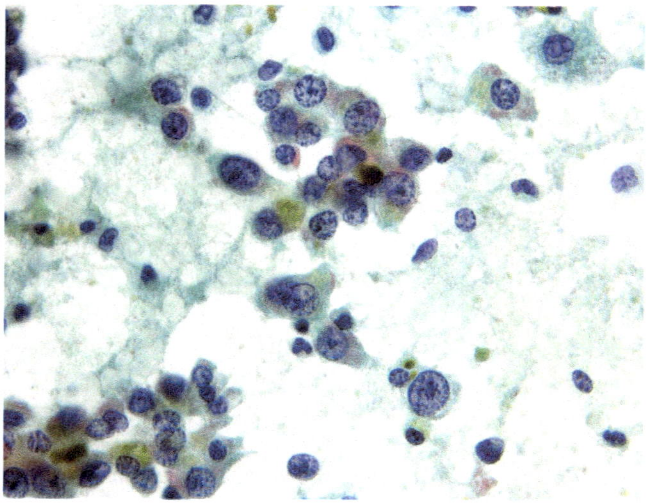

Fig. 7.27 Well-differentiated with high nuclear-to-cytoplasmic ratio (Pap stain)

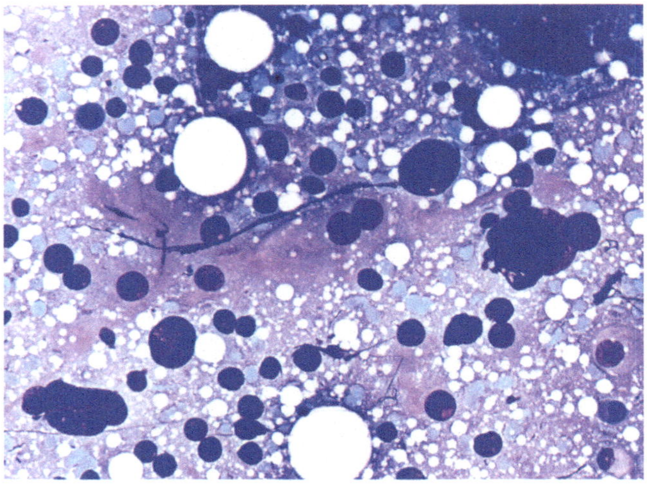

Fig. 7.28 Numerous naked nuclei

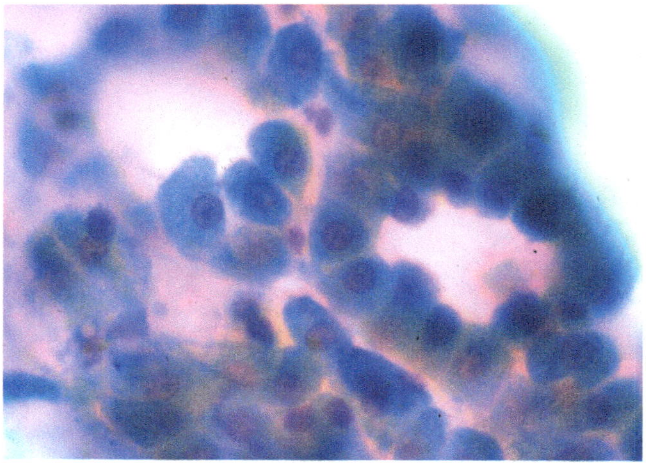

Fig. 7.29 Well-differentiated with pseudoglandular formation (Pap stain)

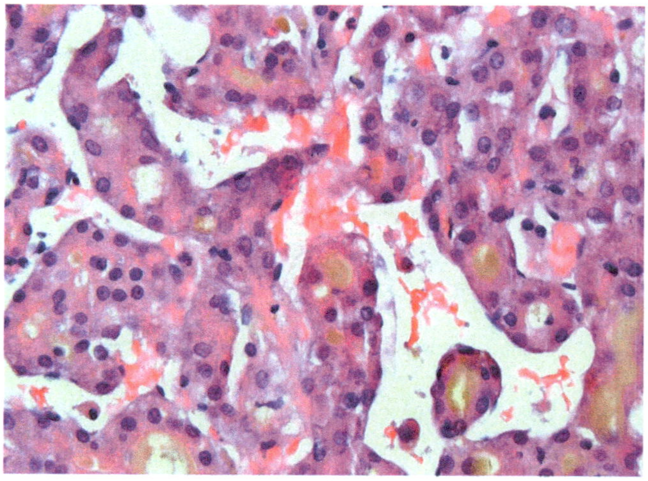

Fig. 7.30 Tissue with pseudoglands

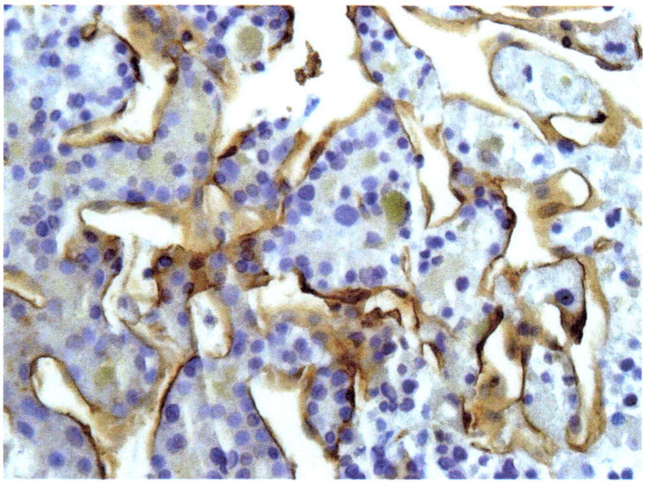

Fig. 7.31 Well-differentiated HCC; CD34 highlighting the trabecular growth pattern

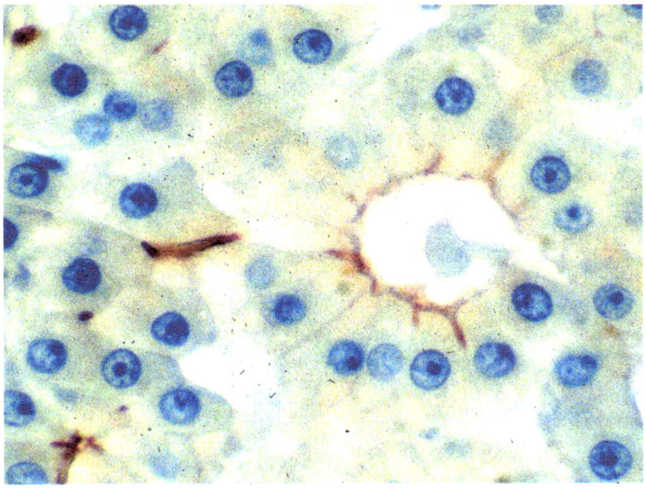

Fig. 7.32 Well-differentiated HCC; polyclonal CEA showing canalicular staining pattern

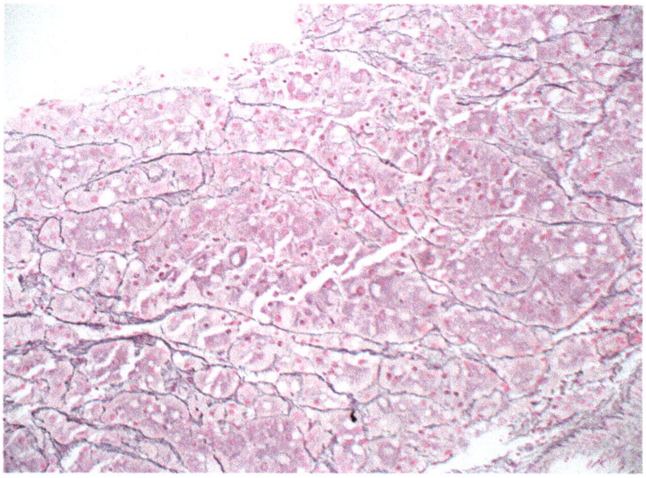

Fig. 7.34 Well-differentiated HCC; lack of reticulin stain

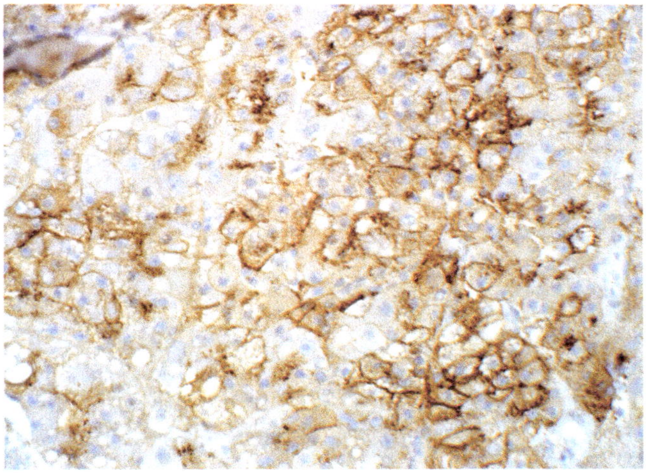

Fig. 7.35 Well-differentiated HCC; positive for glypican-3

A B

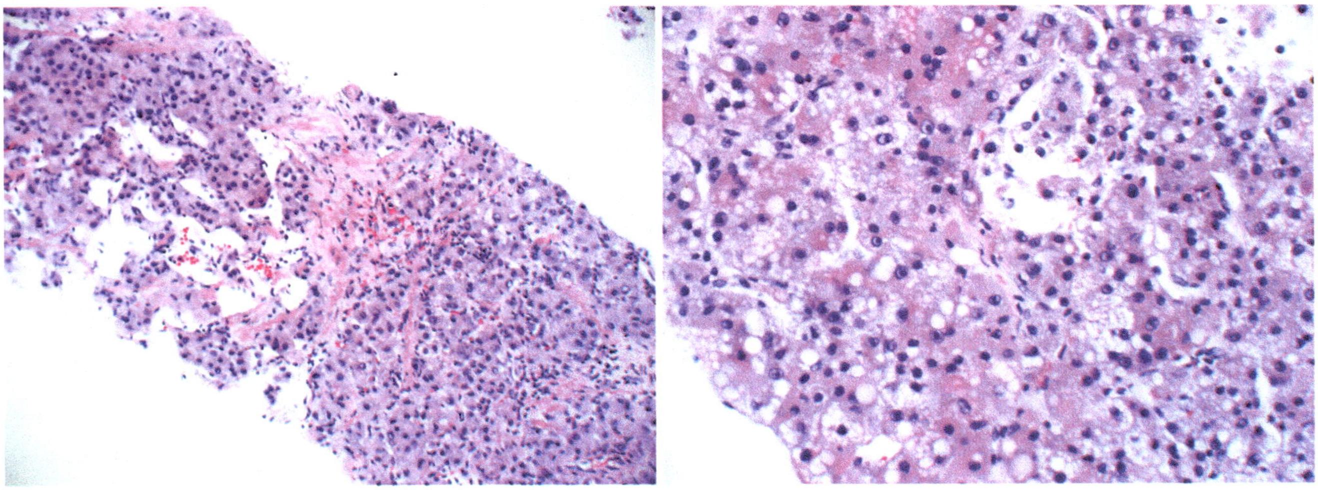

Fig. 7.33 (**a**, **b**) Well-differentiated HCC on tissue sections

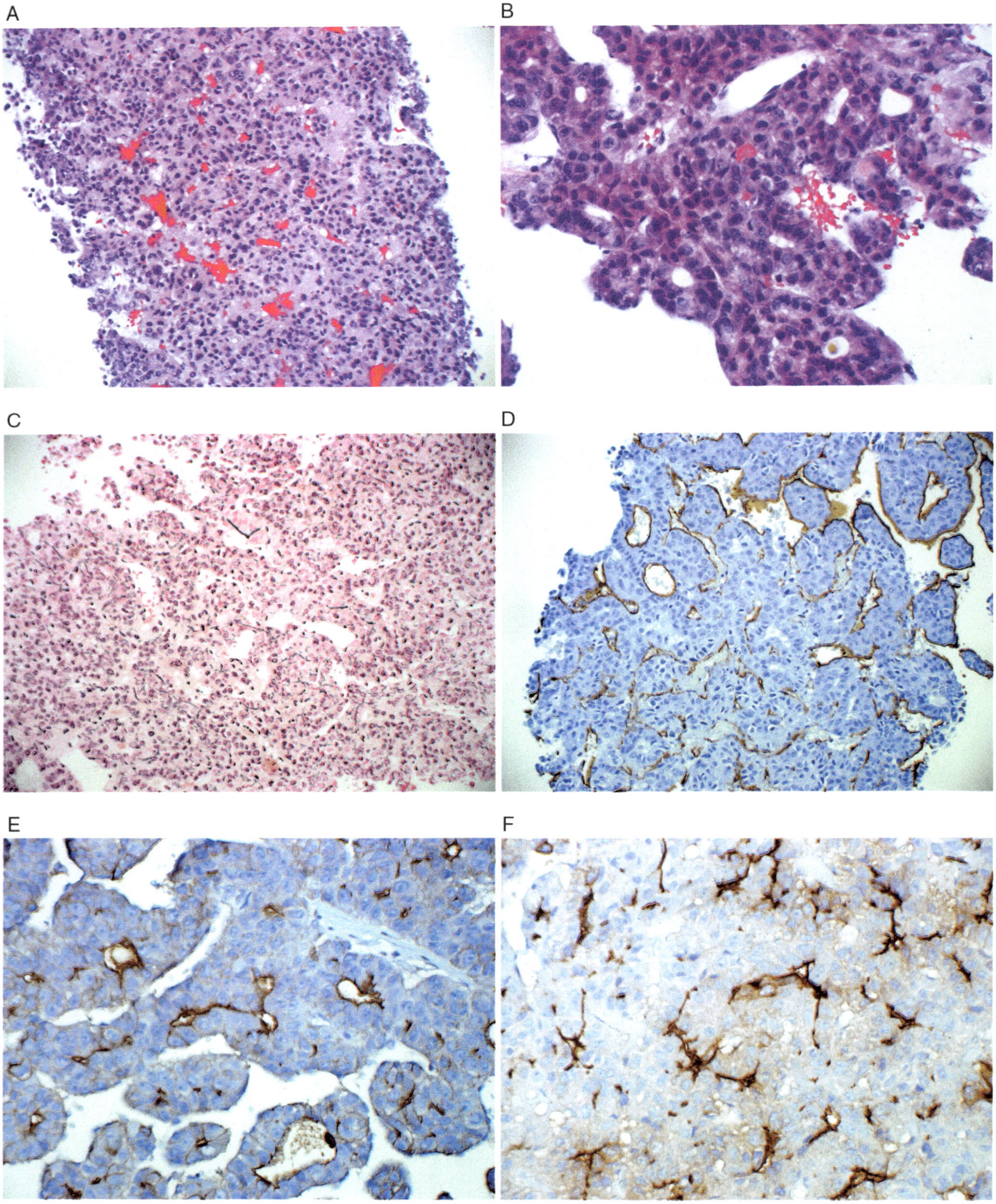

Fig. 7.36 (**a**–**f**) Moderately differentiated HCC with pseudoglandular formation on (**a**) and (**b**). Note the loss of reticulin in the tumor cells (**c**), CD34 (**d**), CD10 (**e**), and polyclonal CEA (**f**)

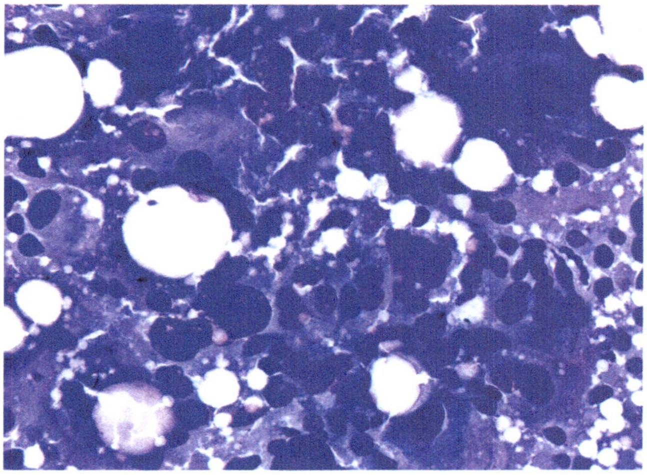

Fig. 7.37 Poorly differentiated HCC showing marked nuclear atypia with giant cells, spindle cells, and atypical mitoses and many pleomorphic naked nuclei

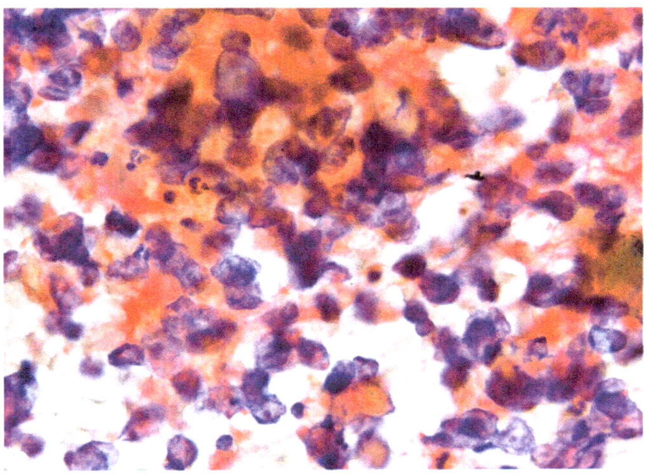

Fig. 7.38 Poorly differentiated HCC (Pap stain)

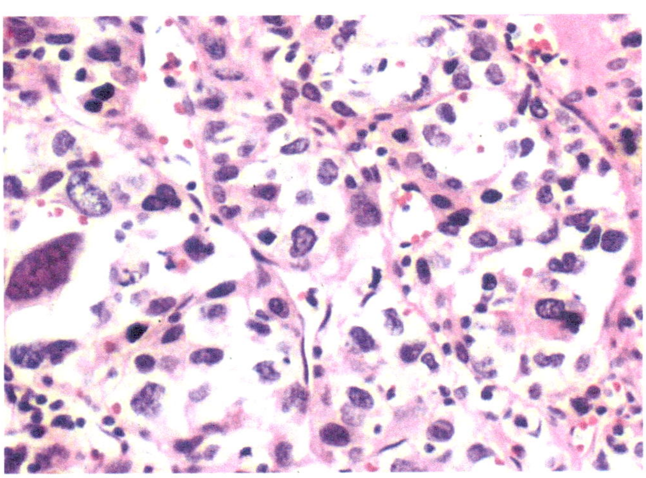

Fig. 7.39 Poorly differentiated HCC on cellblock

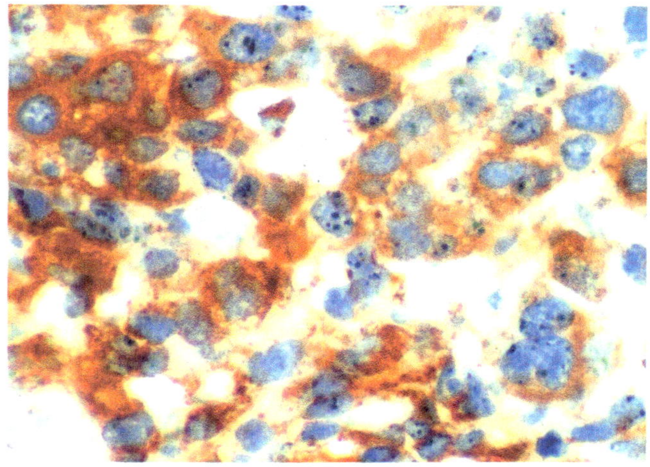

Fig. 7.40 AFP positivity on cellblock

Histology

- Architectural patterns: Trabecular pattern, pseudoglandular or acinar pattern, and compact/solid pattern
- Cytological variants: Pleomorphic cells, clear cells, fatty changes, spindle cells

Immunohistochemistry and Special Stains

- Arginase-1 is positive in both benign and neoplastic liver tissues. It is the most sensitive and specific marker available to identify hepatocellular origin when working on tumor of unknown primary.
- HepPar1 is similar to arginase-1 with a lower specificity. It can be positive in other carcinomas.
- Glypican-3 is expressed in fetal liver, reactivated in about 80% of HCCs, including a small HCC and poorly differentiated HCC, and usually negative in normal liver, cirrhosis, benign hepatic lesions, and dysplastic nodules.
- GS is frequently positive in HCC (defined as positive in >10% of tumor cells).
- HSP70 is upregulated in HCCs, including early HCC (defined as positive in at least 10% of tumor cells), but usually negative in normal hepatocytes and expressed in bile ducts (as an internal positive control).
- Glypican-3, GS, and HSP70 can serve as a diagnostic panel in the workup of a difficult case.
- Clusterin has been reported to be overexpressed in HCC.
- AFP is positive in only about 25% of HCC cases.
- CD34 highlights neovascular spaces/sinusoidal capillarization; usually no immunoreactivity seen in normal liver and benign hepatic lesions; some immunoreactivity can be seen in the peripheral portion of a cirrhotic nodule.

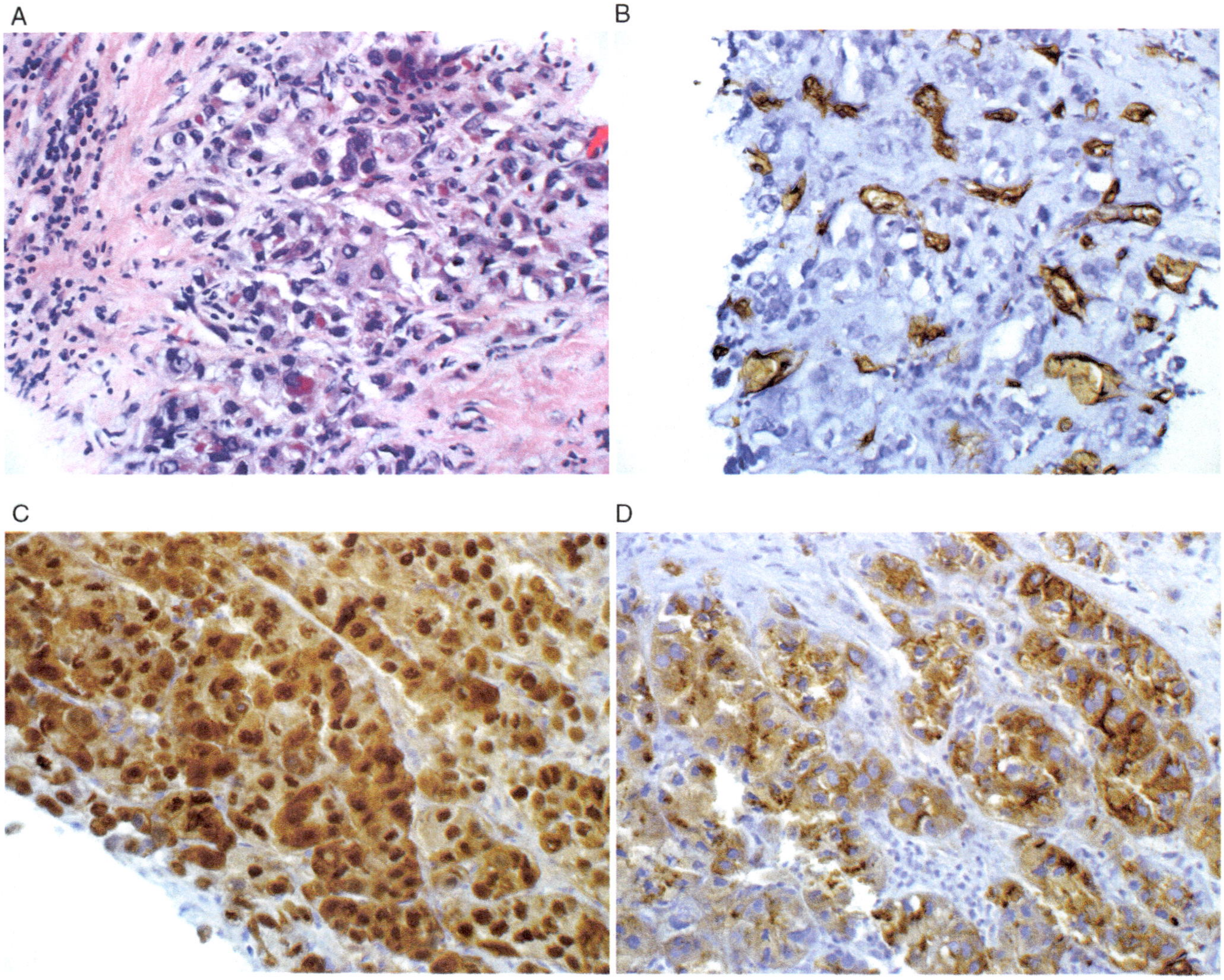

Fig. 7.41 (**a**–**d**) Poorly differentiated HCC on core biopsy specimen (**a**), CD34 (**b**), arginase-1 (**c**), and glypican-3 (**d**)

- CD10 and polyclonal carcinoembryonic antigen (CEA) show a canalicular staining pattern.
- Albumin by RNA in situ hybridization.

Differential Diagnosis for Well-Differentiated HCC

- Regenerative nodules in cirrhosis
- Focal nodular hyperplasia
- HCA

Cytological Features for Moderate and Poorly Differentiated HCC

- Hypercellular samples with many singles, thick cores, nets, and sheets
- Marked nuclear atypia with giant cells, spindle cells, and atypical mitoses
- Many pleomorphic naked nuclei

Table 7.2. Useful markers in the distinction between HCC and IHCC

Marker	HCC	IHCC
CK7	Negative or focally +	+
Arginase-1	+ (90%)	–
MOC31	–	+
pVHL	–	+ (70%)

Note: MOC31 – EpCAM/epithelial specific antigen

Differential Diagnosis for Moderately and Poorly Differentiated HCC

- Cholangiocarcinoma
- Metastatic carcinoma
- Table 7.2 summarizes some useful markers in the distinction between HCC and IHCC.

Variants of HCC

Fibrolamellar Variant (Figs. 7.42, 7.43, 7.44, and 7.45)

- Accounts for 0.5–9.0% of HCCs in various studies.
- More common in North America and European countries.
- Most frequently occurs in patients aged 35 years or younger with a peak at age 25.
- Non-cirrhotic background.
- Central scar in radiologic finding and gross examination.
- Nests and bands of large polygonal tumor cells with abundant, granular oncocytic cytoplasm, large vesicular nuclei, and prominent nucleoli, in a distinctive lamellar fibrotic background.
- Pseudoglandular formation and cytoplasmic "pale bodies" or "hyaline bodies" can be seen.
- CK7 is frequently positive.
- Better prognosis than typical HCC.

Scirrhous HCC

- Accounts for 5% of HCCs.
- Marked fibrotic background, sinusoid-like blood space, and atrophic tumor trabeculae.
- Better prognosis than typical HCCs has been reported.

Clear Cell HCC and Sarcomatoid HCC

- Clear cell HCC (Figs. 7.46a, b, 7.47, and 7.48)

Lymphoepithelioma-Like Carcinoma

- A very rare type of HCC
- Epstein-Barr virus (EBV)-positive

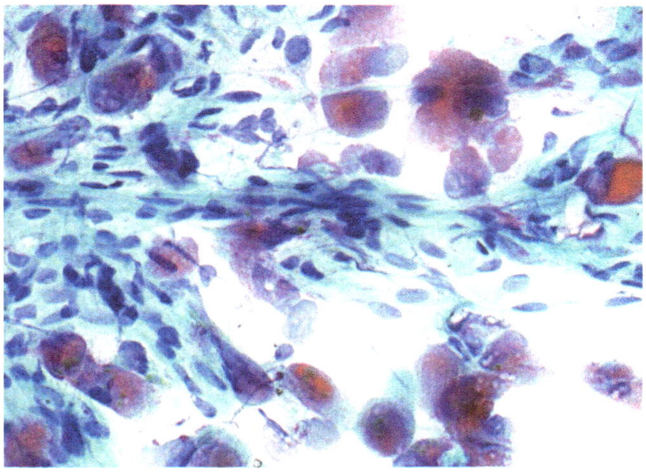

Fig. 7.42 Fibrolamellar HCC

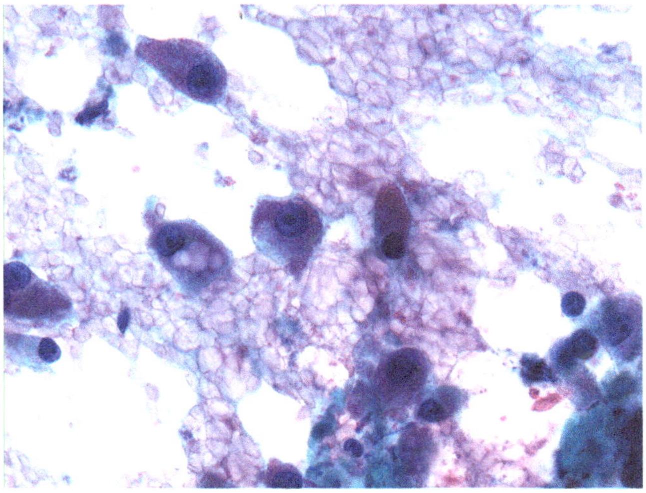

Fig. 7.43 Fibrolamellar HCC – intracytoplasmic pale body

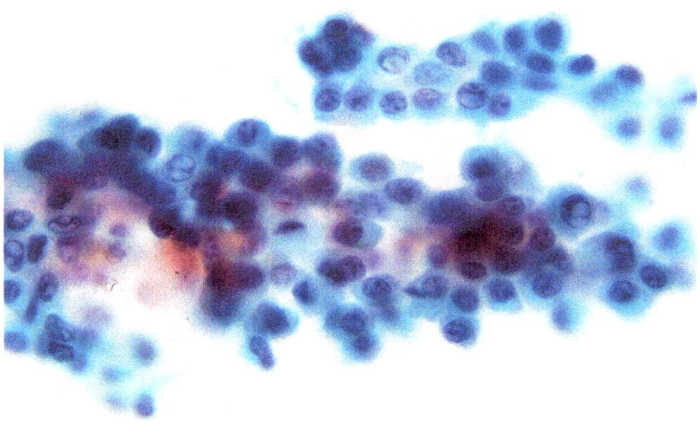

Fig. 7.44 Fibrolamellar HCC – intranuclear inclusion

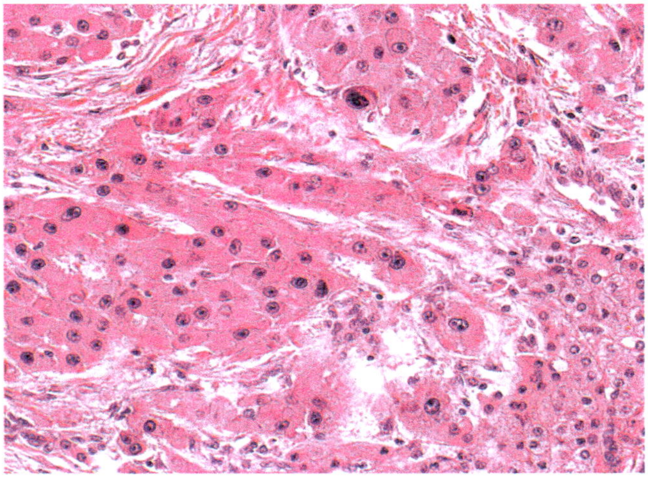

Fig. 7.45 Fibrolamellar HCC tissue section

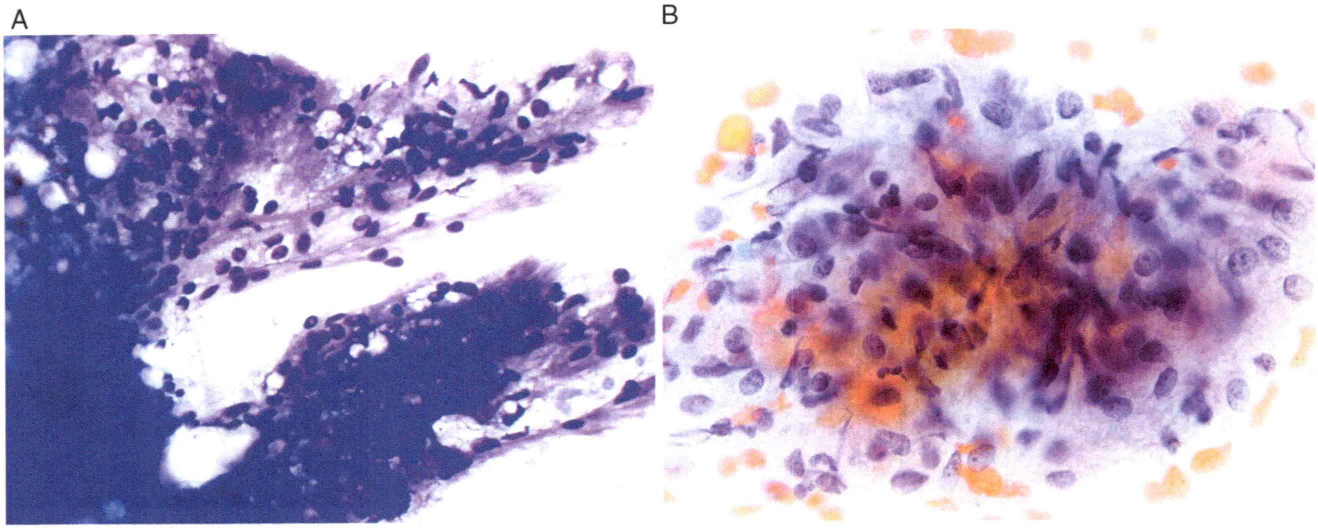

Fig. 7.46 (**a**, **b**) Clear cell HCC on the smear (**a**, DQ; and **b**, Pap stain)

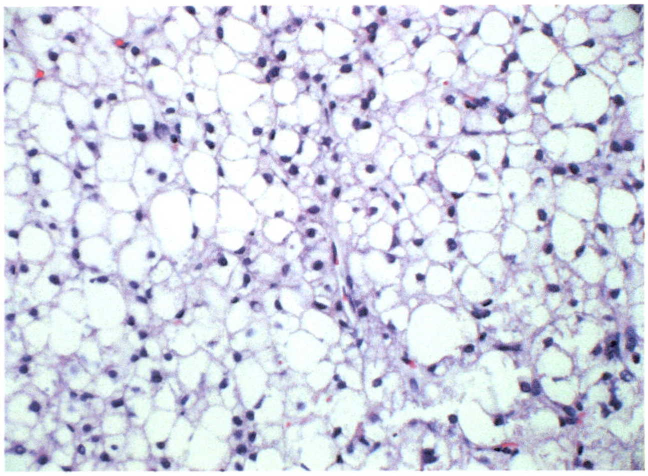

Fig. 7.47 Clear cell HCC on small core biopsy

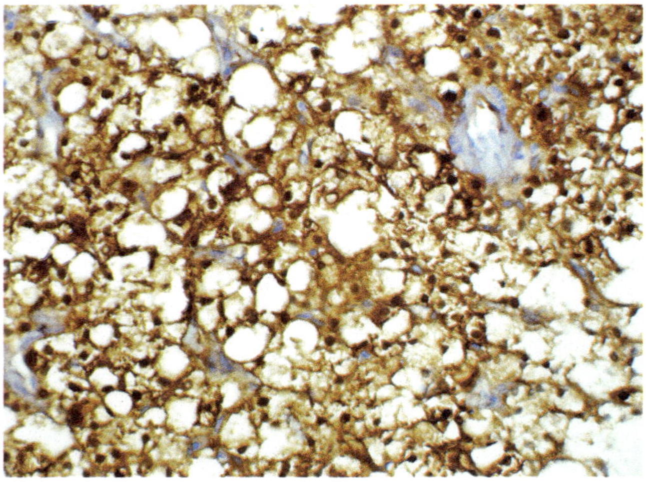

Fig. 7.48 Clear cell HCC positive for arginase-1

Intrahepatic Cholangiocarcinoma (IHCC)

Clinical Features

- Second most common primary malignant tumor of the liver
- Accounting for 5–15% in various study series
- Arising from any portion of intrahepatic biliary tree except the right and left hepatic ducts (usually referred to as hilar cholangiocarcinoma or "Klatskin tumor")
- May be associated with sclerosing cholangitis, inflammatory bowel disease, Caroli disease, parasitic infection, hepatolithiasis, non-biliary cirrhosis including hepatitis C, alcoholic liver disease, human immunodeficiency virus (HIV), and diabetic mellitus
- Radiologic findings similar to HCC

Cytological Features (Fig. 7.49a, b)

- Single and crowded groups of atypical epithelial cells
- Nuclear enlargement, loss of nuclear polarity, and variation in nuclear sizes
- Nuclear contour irregularities, high nuclear-to-cytoplasmic ratio, and mitoses

Gross and Histology (Figs. 7.50a, b and 7.51a, b)

- In non-cirrhotic liver.
- Three types by gross examination, mass-forming type, periductal-infiltrating type, and intraductal growth type, or mixture of these three types.
- Resembling adenocarcinoma of the pancreas and other biliary tract tumors.
- Tubular, papillary, acinar, and cord-like growth pattern.

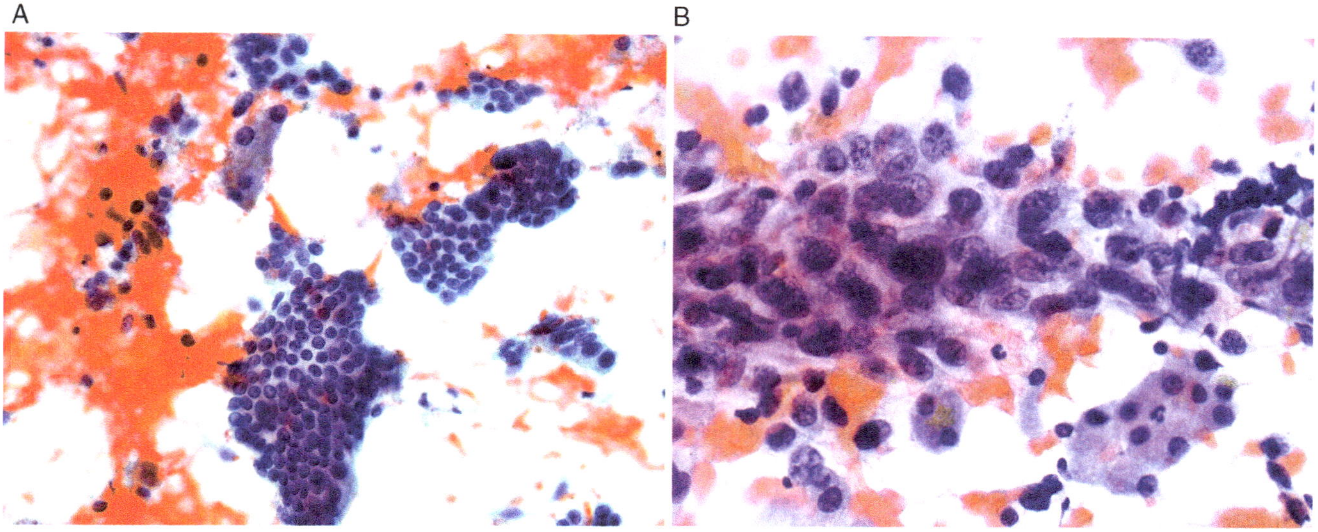

Fig. 7.49 (**a**, **b**) Cholangiocarcinoma – single and crowded groups of atypical epithelial cell nuclear enlargement, loss of nuclear polarity, and variation in nuclear sizes

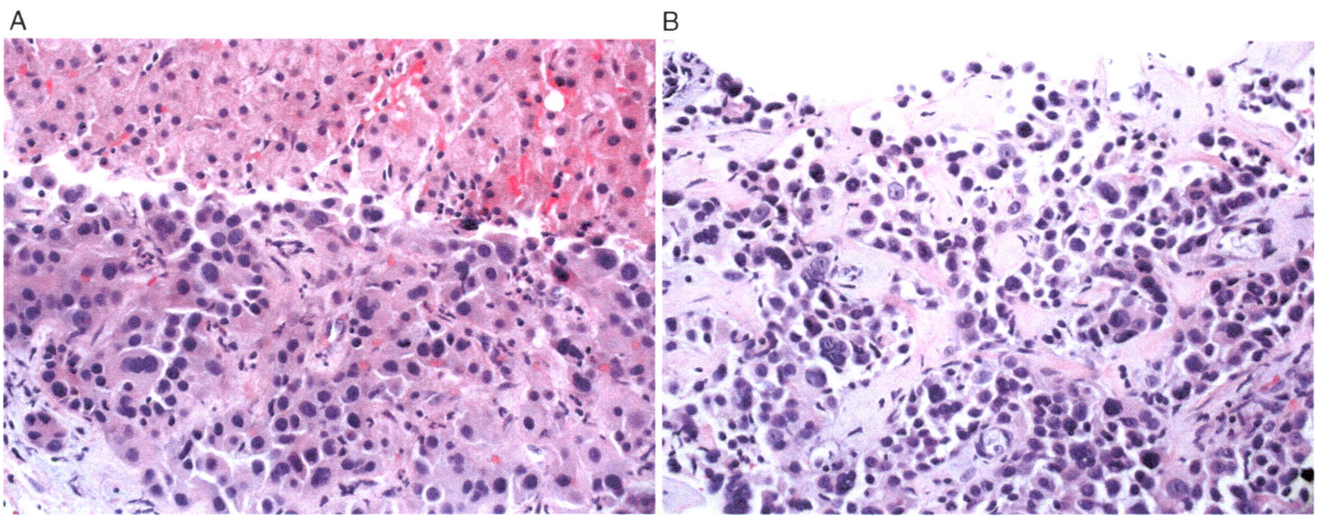

Fig. 7.50 (**a**, **b**) Cholangiocarcinoma – well differentiated

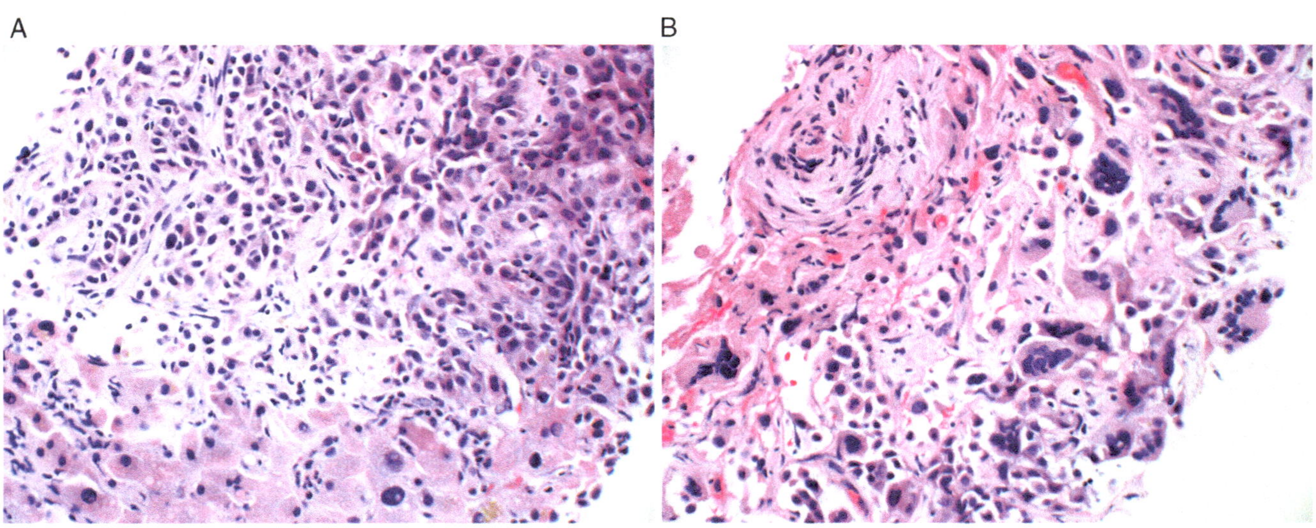

Fig. 7.51 (**a**, **b**) Cholangiocarcinoma – poorly differentiated

- Most of tumor cells with eosinophilic to pale cytoplasm, but can be clear or abundant cytoplasm.
- May have abundant fibrous stroma.
- Many histologic variants have been reported, such as adenosquamous, mucinous, signet cell, clear cell, mucoepidermoid, lymphoepithelioma-like, and sarcomatoid IHCC.

Immunohistochemistry

- Positive for MOC31, CEA, CK7, CK19, epithelial membrane antigen (EMA), and mucin (MUC)1.
- Negative for CD10, arginase-1, and AFP.
- Small percentages are positive for CK20 and caudal type homeobox 2 (CDX2).
- 70% of IHCCs are positive for pVHL; in contrast, other pancreatobiliary tract adenocarcinomas are usually negative for pVHL. Additionally, S100P is expressed in only 20% of IHCCs and over 90% of other pancreatobiliary adenocarcinomas. MUC5AC and CK17 are reported in 60% of adenocarcinomas of the pancreas and are usually negative in IHCCs.
- Albumin RNA in situ hybridization has been shown to be positive in 100% of IHCCs.

Differential Diagnosis

- Metastatic carcinomas
- HCC

Combined Hepatocellular-Cholangiocarcinoma

- Defined by WHO as a tumor containing unequivocal, intimately mixed HCC and cholangiocarcinoma.
- HCC and cholangiocarcinoma in the same liver are defined as a collision tumor.
- Accounts for less than 1% of all liver tumors.
- Morphologic and immunophenotypic features of typical HCC and typical cholangiocarcinoma in the same tumor.
- The transitional zone between the two components often demonstrates mixed features with intermediate morphology and immunophenotype.
- Subtypes of combined hepatocellular-cholangiocarcinoma with stem cell features may be positive for CK19, CD56, c-Kit (CD117), and epithelial cell adhesion molecule (EpCAM).
- An example is shown in Fig. 7.52a–d.

Intraductal Papillary Neoplasm with an Associated Invasive Carcinoma

- See Chap. 8, Pancreas and Biliary Tract.

Mucinous Cystic Neoplasm with an Associated Invasive Carcinoma

- See Chap. 8, Pancreas and Biliary Tract.

Hepatoblastoma

Clinical Features

- 90% under the age of 5, 68% under the age of 2, and 4% at birth.
- May be associated with congenital anomalies.
- Marked elevation of AFP is seen in 90% of cases.
- Low or normal serum AFP is associated with an aggressive course.
- Tumors with small-cell or rhabdoid features are associated with an aggressive clinical course as well.
- May be associated with familial adenomatous polyposis due to the germ line mutation of the adenomatous polyposis coli (APC) gene.

Cytological Features

- Cytomorphology is dependent on the histologic types.
- Mixed epithelial type, including fetal pattern, embryonal pattern and fetal pattern, macrotrabecular pattern, or small-cell undifferentiated pattern.
- Mixed epithelial and mesenchymal type.
- Figure 7.53a shows a small-cell pattern resembling other small blue cell tumors, and Figure 7.53b shows an embryonal pattern with prominent nucleoli.

Histology (Fig. 7.54a–c)

- Pure epithelial type, including fetal pattern, mixed embryonal pattern and fetal pattern, macrotrabecular pattern, or small-cell undifferentiated pattern
- Mixed epithelial and mesenchymal type
- Mixed epithelial and mesenchymal type with teratoid features

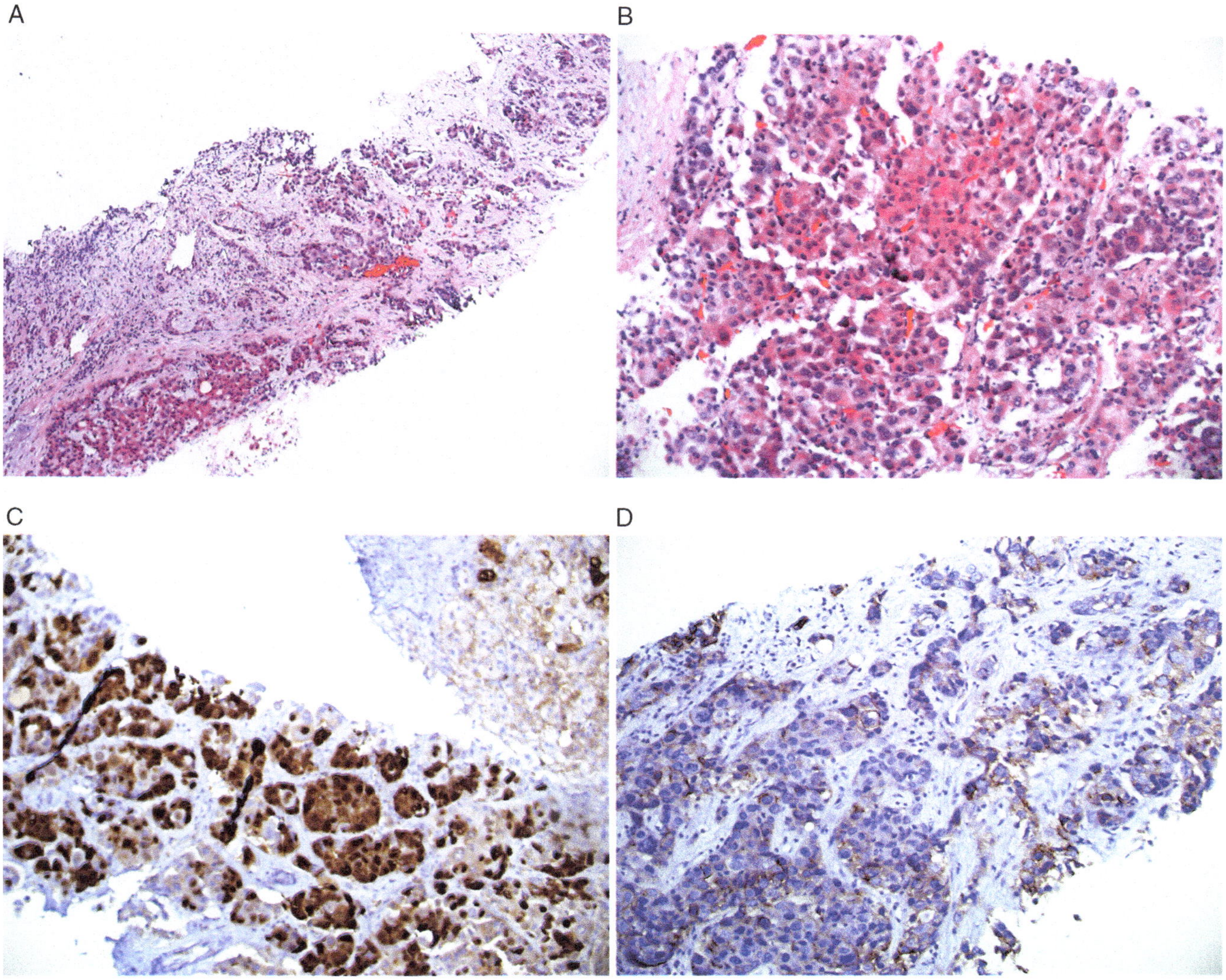

Fig. 7.52 (**a**–**d**) Combined HCC – cholangiocarcinoma positive for arginase-1 (**c**) and MOC-31 (d)

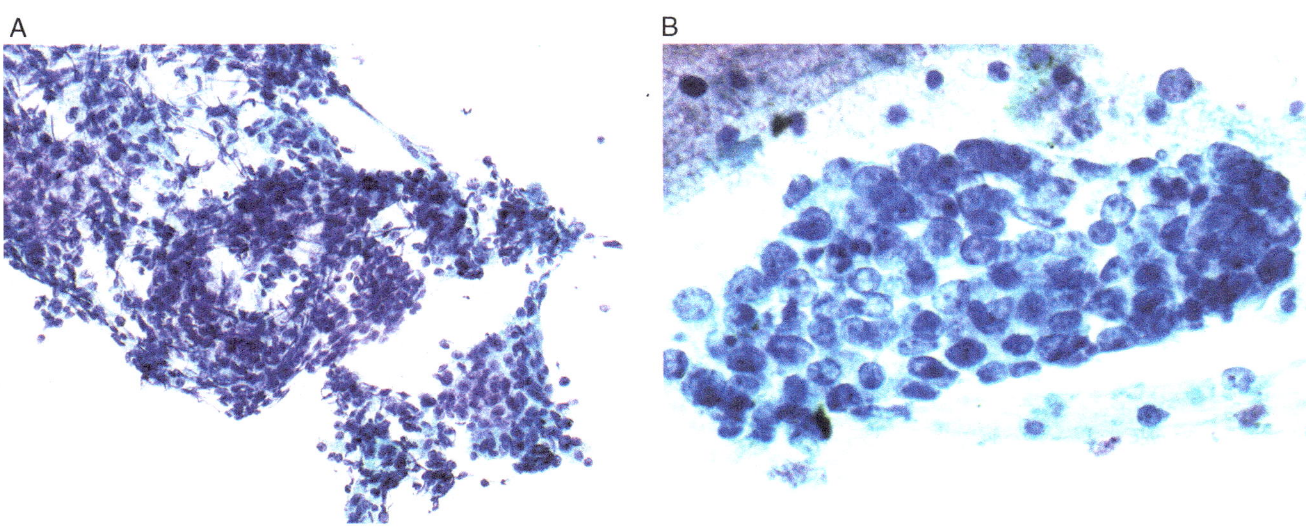

Fig. 7.53 (**a**, **b**) Hepatoblastoma on the smear

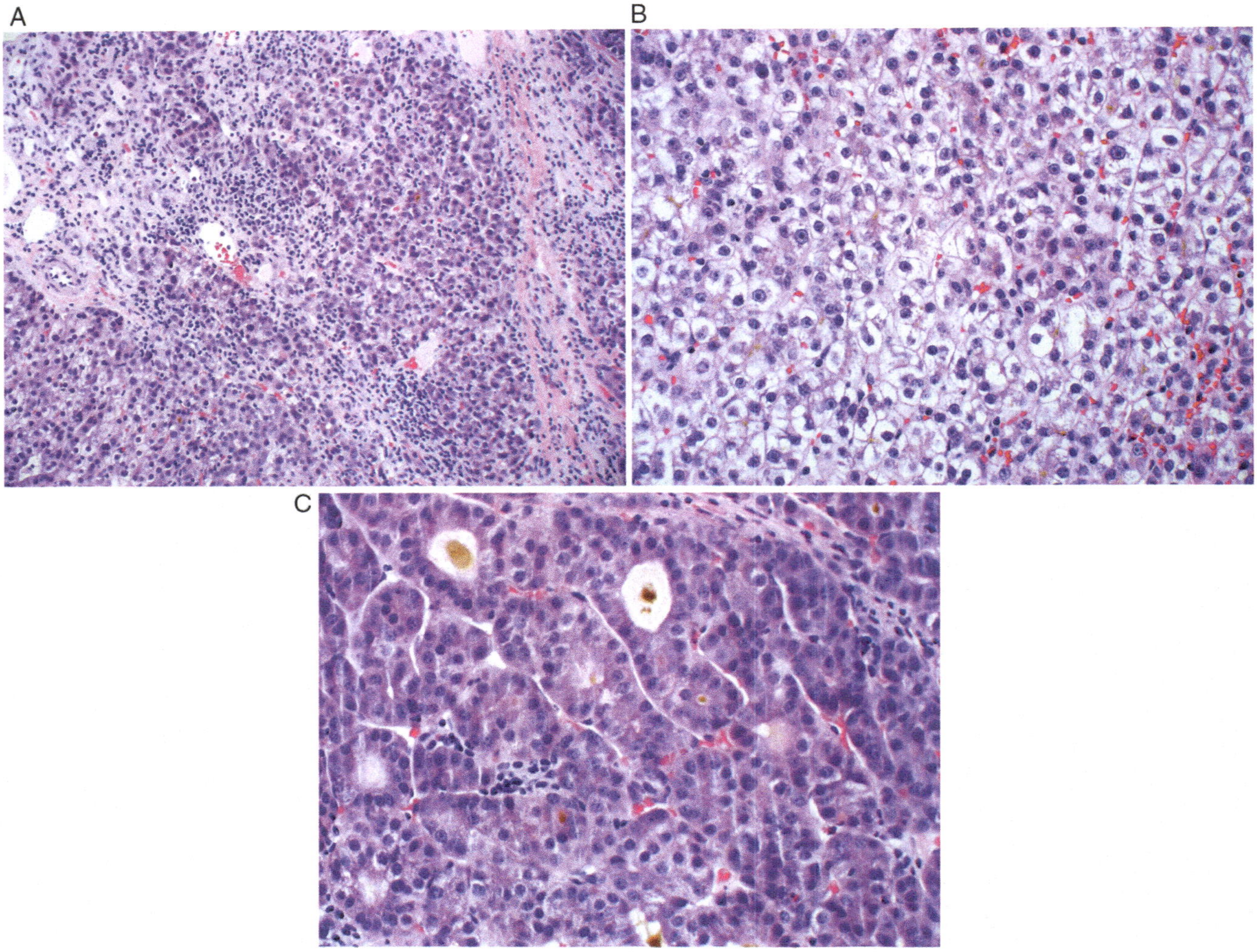

Fig. 7.54 (a–c) Hepatoblastoma on tissue sections

Immunohistochemistry

- AFP-positive in 90% of cases
- Beta-catenin nuclear positivity in 70% of cases

Differential Diagnosis

- Other small blue cell tumors

Angiosarcoma

Clinical Features

- Associated with exposure to polyvinyl chloride, iatrogenic thorium dioxide (Thorotrast), radium, androgenic-anabolic steroids, and arsenic compounds
- Usually multiple nodules
- Normal serum AFP
- Frequently seen in males older than 60

Cytological Features (Figs. 7.55, 7.56, and 7.57)

- Elongated spindle cells and epithelioid cells with pleomorphic nuclei
- Small clusters of cohesive atypical cells
- Vacuolated and granular cytoplasm
- Abnormal mitoses in high-grade angiosarcoma

Histology (Figs. 7.58 and 7.59a, b)

- Irregular vascular spaces lined by highly atypical endothelial cells
- Mitosis and tumor necrosis
- Solid and pseudopapillary growth patterns

Immunohistochemistry

- Immunostains for ETS-related gene (ERG), CD31, and CD34 performed on cellblock or thin core biopsy are useful.
- Focal cytokeratin positivity can be seen.

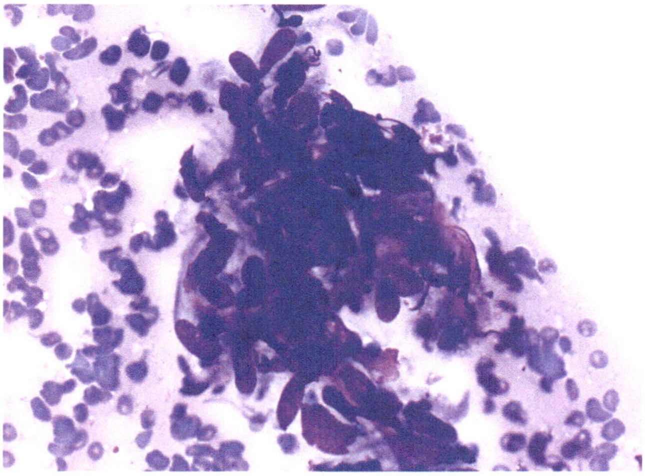

Fig. 7.55 Angiosarcoma showing elongated spindle cells, epithelioid cells with pleomorphic nuclei, and small clusters of cohesive atypical cells

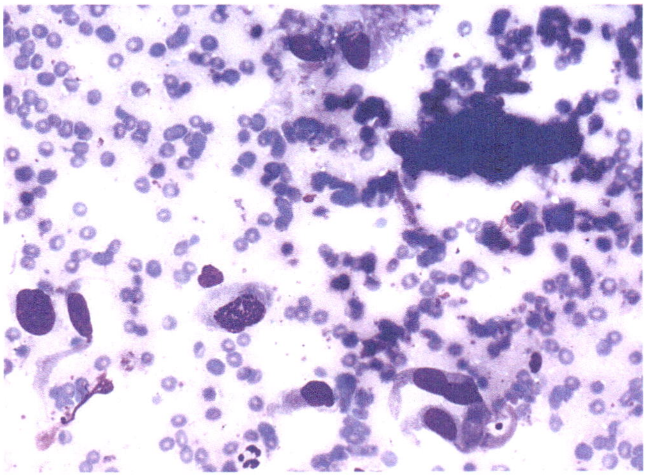

Fig. 7.56 Angiosarcoma with abnormal mitoses

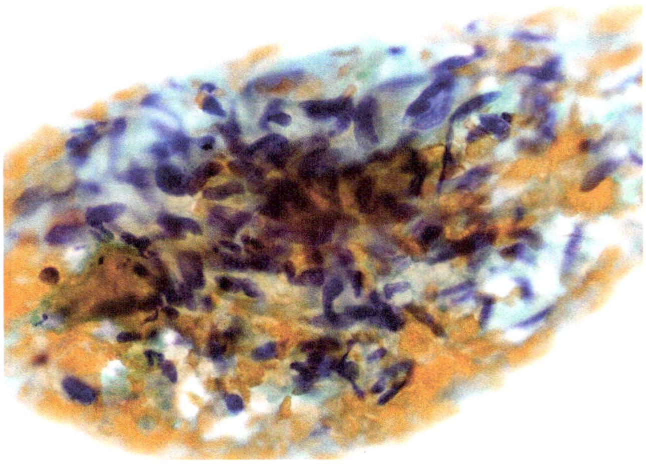

Fig. 7.57 Angiosarcoma – Pap stain

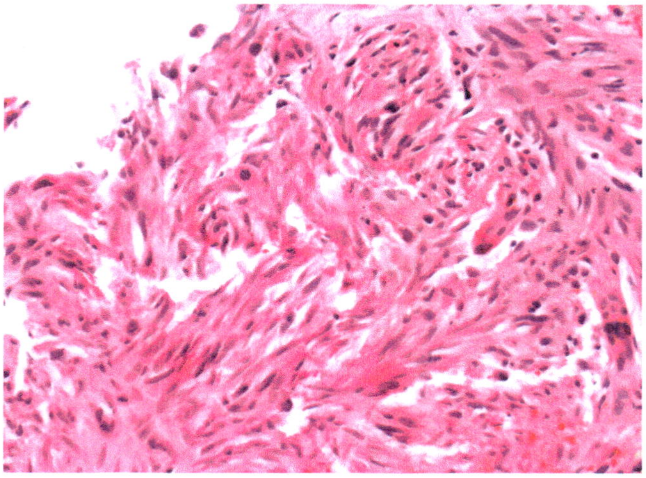

Fig. 7.58 Angiosarcoma – cellblock

Differential Diagnosis

- Other malignant carcinomas or sarcomas
- Epithelioid hemangioendothelioma

Epithelioid Hemangioendothelioma

Clinical Features

- A tumor of varying malignant potential with spindle and epithelioid vascular cell proliferation
- More common in females than males and frequently seen in young adults but reported in ages ranging from 12 to 86
- Can be solitary or multiple lesions

Cytological Features (Fig. 7.60a, b)

- Single or small groups of loosely cohesive, large, atypical cells with irregular nuclear contour
- Binucleation and multinucleation
- Prominent nucleoli and intracytoplasmic inclusion
- Abundant lacy cytoplasm

Histology (Fig. 7.61a, b)

- A mixture of epithelioid cells, dendritic/spindle cells, and intermediate cells in a fibrotic stroma or myxoid stroma.
- Epithelioid cells show vacuolated cytoplasm with signet ring cell features.
- Some cytoplasmic vacuoles may contain red blood cells.
- Mitotic rate is variable; no mitosis found in 58% of tumors.

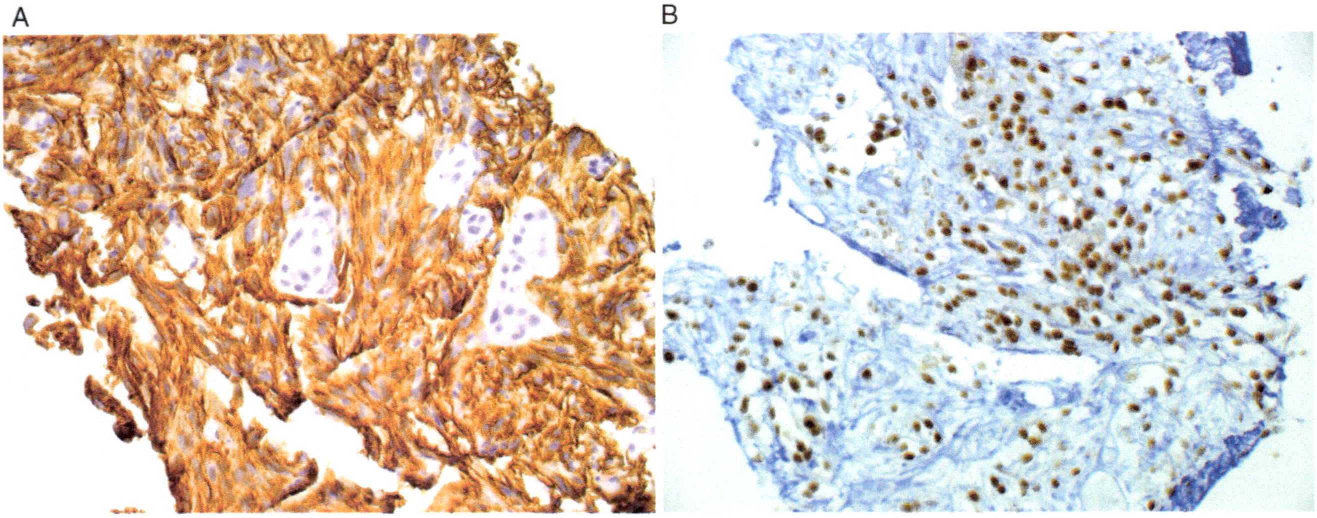

Fig. 7.59 (**a**, **b**) Angiosarcoma with CD34 (**a**) and ERG positivity (**b**)

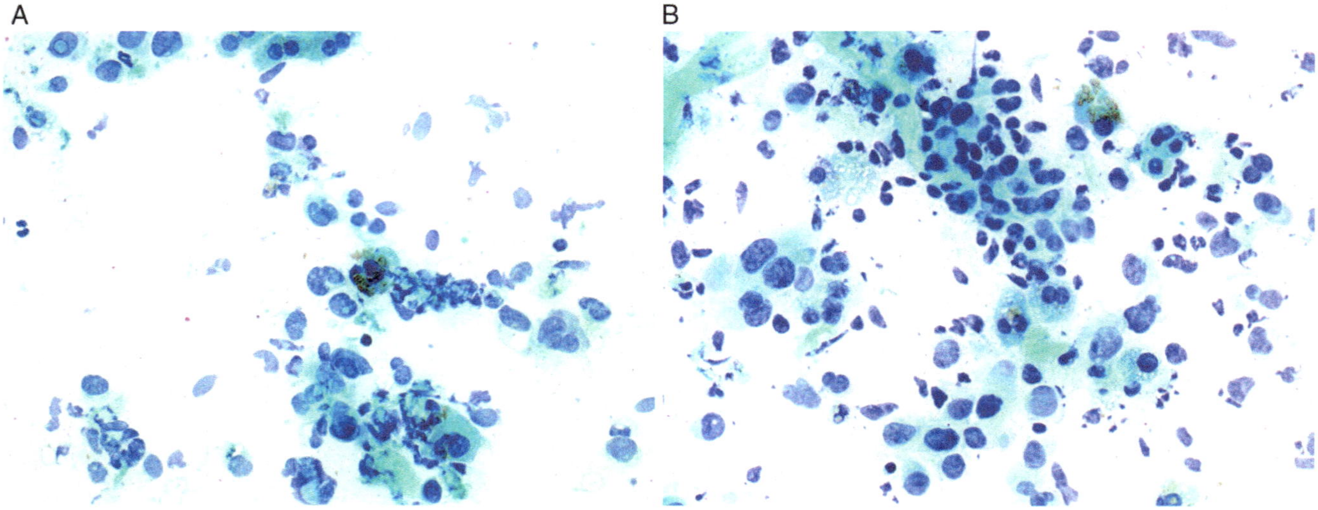

Fig. 7.60 (**a**, **b**) Epithelioid hemangioendothelioma with single or small groups of loosely cohesive large atypical cells with irregular nuclear contour, prominent nucleoli and intracytoplasmic inclusion, and abundant lacy cytoplasm

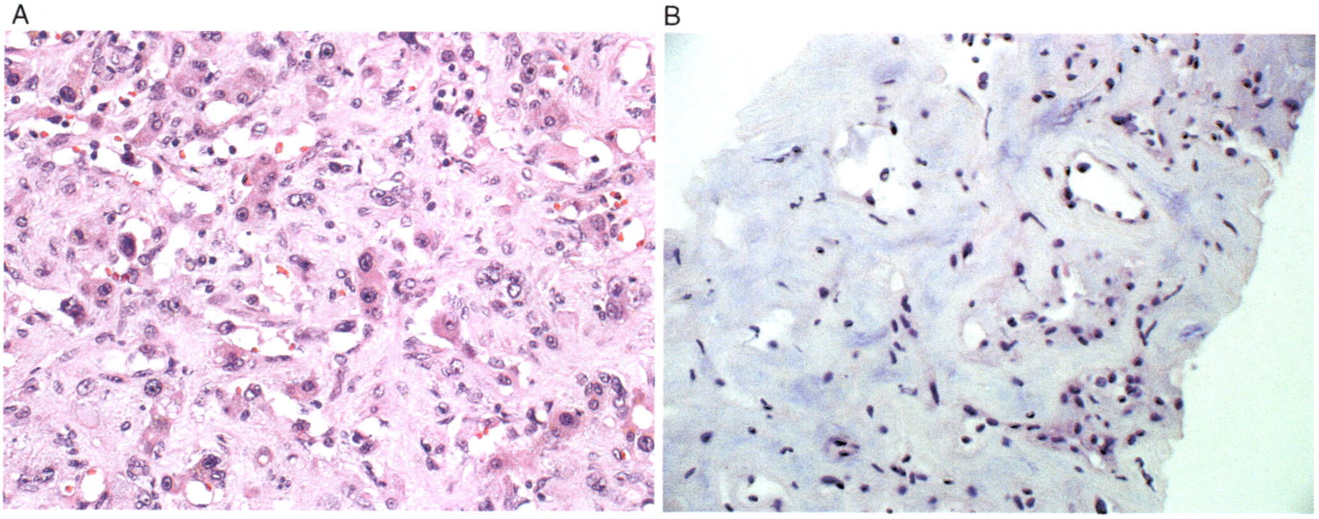

Fig. 7.61 (**a**, **b**) Epithelioid hemangioendothelioma tissue section

Immunohistochemistry

- ERG, CD31, CD34, and podoplanin (D2-40)
- Can be focally positive for cytokeratin, especially CK18

Differential Diagnosis

- Other carcinomas and sarcomas
- Angiosarcoma

Rare Primary Lesions/Tumors of the Liver

Some mesenchymal lesions/tumors and primary lymphomas of the liver are rarely encountered. The clinical, cytologic, and histologic features of these lesions/tumors and useful ancillary studies are summarized in Table 7.3.

Secondary Tumors

- Over 90% of malignant liver tumors are metastases.
- Most metastases are carcinomas, followed by melanomas.
- Most frequent tumors with a liver metastasis are testicular tumors, ocular melanomas, pancreatobiliary carcinomas, breast carcinomas, lung carcinomas, and colorectal carcinomas.
- Most common metastases by absolute numbers are breast, colorectal, and gastric carcinomas.
- Neuroendocrine tumors/carcinomas frequently metastasize to the liver.
- Lymphomas, myelomas, myeloid sarcomas, and sarcomas with liver involvement are uncommon.
- A summary of useful IHC for the differential diagnosis of HCC, IHCC, and mimics is listed in Table 7.4.

Table 7.3. Summary of rare primary lesions/tumors of the liver

Diagnosis	Clinical features	Cytological features	Histologic features	Ancillary studies
Mesenchymal hamartoma	A benign tumorlike condition, most frequently seen under age 2	Bland spindle cells and benign ductal epithelial cells	Loose connective tissue and epithelial bile duct or ductule-like in varying proportions	Some chromosomal aberrations have been reported, such as the breakpoint 19q13.4
Inflammatory pseudotumor	Benign, nonneoplastic condition, mean age 37, male-to-female ratio 3:1	Spindle cells, lymphocytes, plasma cells, histiocytes, eosinophils, and granulation	A mixture of myofibroblasts, fibroblasts, collagen bundles, and dense inflammatory cells, including plasma cells and eosinophils	Numerous IgG4-positive plasma cells in IgG4-related disease
Solitary fibrous tumor	Adult, female-to-male ratio, 2:1. May cause hypoglycemia	Spindle cells	Bland uniform fibroblast-like spindle cells in a collagenized stroma with mixed hypocellular and hypercellular areas	Positive for STAT6, CD34, Bcl2, and CD99
Embryonal (undifferentiated) sarcoma	Commonly seen in older children, 6–15 years. No evidence of specific differentiation	Pleomorphic spindle, stellate, and giant tumor cells	A loose myxoid tissue containing immature-looking tumor cells with spindle, stellate, giant, and pleomorphic appearance. Intracellular or extracellular hyaline globules	Consistently positive for vimentin and negative for AFP. Inconsistent results with other markers including keratin, SMA, alpha-antitrypsin, desmin, MyoD1, CD10, and CD68
Extrarenal malignant rhabdoid tumor	Highly aggressive tumor	Small round cell tumor features	Loosely cohesive tumor cells with high N/C ratio and rhabdoid features	Consistently positive for vimentin with a dot-like staining pattern; loss of INI-1
Follicular dendritic cell tumor	Aggressive EBV-associated tumor of the liver and spleen	Spindle cells, lymphocytes, and plasma cells; similar to inflammatory pseudotumor	Fascicles of spindle cells with bland vesicular nuclei and small nucleoli. Reed-Sternberg-like cells may be seen	Positive for CD21 and CD35. EBV-positive by in situ hybridization
Lymphomas	Rare. Most are diffuse large B-cell lymphoma, followed by MALT lymphomas, hepatosplenic T-cell lymphoma, and EBV-positive lymphoproliferative disease of childhood	Similar to the involvement of a secondary lymphoma	A monotonous population of large lymphoid cells or abnormal lymphoid cells infiltrating hepatic sinusoids	IHC, flow cytometry, and molecular tests as for other nodal lymphomas

Note: *Bcl2* B-cell CLL/lymphoma 2, *IgG4* immunoglobulin 4, *INI-1* integrase interactor-1, *MALT* mucosa-associated lymphoid tissue, *N/C* nuclear-to-cytoplasmic, *STAT6* signal transducer and activator of transcription 6

Table 7.4. Summary of useful IHC markers for the common metastases in the liver

Marker/diagnosis	HCC	IHCC	Breast	Colon	Pancreas	Upper GI	Lung	Mel	CRCC	Testis
*Albumin	+	+	−	−	−	−	−	−	−	−
Arg-1	+	−	−	−	−	−	−	−	−	−
pVHL	−	+	−	−	−	−	−	−	+	−
PAX8	−	−	−	−	−	−	−	−	+	−
GATA3	−	−	+	−	−	−	−	−	−	+/−
ER	−	−	+	−	−	−	−	−	−	−
MOC31	−	+	+	+	+	+	+	−	−	−/+
SOX10	−	−	−	−	−	−	−	+	−	−
HMB45	−	−	−	−	−	−	−	+	−	−
TTF1	−	−	−	−	−	−	+	−	−	−
CDX2	−	−/+	−	+	−	+/−	−	−	−	−
SALL4	−	−	−	−	−	−	−	−	−	+
CK7	−	+	+	−	+	+/−	+	−	−	−
CK20	−	−/+	−	+	−/+	−/+	−	−	−	−

Note: *Arg-1* arginase-1, *CRCC* clear cell renal cell carcinoma, *GATA3* GATA binding protein 3, *Mel* melanoma, *TTF1* thyroid transcription factor 1, *PAX8* paired box gene 8
* By RNA in situ hybridization

Table 7.5. Summary of useful markers for identifying the origin of neuroendocrine neoplasms

Marker/organ	Lung	Pancreas	Duodenum	Stomach	Ileum	Appendix	Rectum
CK7	+/−	+/−	+/−	+/−	−	−	−
CK20	−	−	−	−	+	+	+
CDX2	−	−	−	−	+	+	+
SATB2	−	−	−	−	−/+	−/+	+
TTF1	+/−	−	−	−	−	−	−
PR	−	+/−	−	−	−	−	−
PAX8	−	+/−	−	−	−	−	−
ATRX/DAXX	+	Loss in 50%	+	+	+	+	+

Note: *ATRX/DAXX* alpha-thalassemia/mental retardation syndrome/death domain-associated protein, *PR* progesterone receptor, *SATB2* special AT-rich sequence-binding protein 2

- A summary of useful IHC markers in identifying the origin of metastatic neuroendocrine neoplasms in the liver is listed in Table 7.5.

Key Cytologic and Histologic Features of Common Metastatic Tumors

Colorectal Adenocarcinoma

- Atypical glandular cells in the background of dirty necrosis (Fig. 7.62a, b)
- Positive for CK20, CDX2, and SATB2

Pancreas/Extrahepatic Biliary Tract

- Sheets of epithelial cells with various degrees of nuclear atypia (Fig. 7.63)
- Gastric-type mucinous differentiation frequently seen

Breast

- Neoplastic cells with plasmacytoid features or intracytoplasmic lumen/signet ring cells (Figs. 7.64, 7.65, 7.66, and 7.67a–c)
- Single or loosely cohesive tumor cells with variable nuclear atypia
- Positive for estrogen receptor (ER), GATA3, and gross cystic disease fluid protein 15 (GCDFP15) (40–50% cases)

Lung Adenocarcinoma

- A spectrum of histomorphology from well-formed glands in a well-differentiated adenocarcinoma to solid sheets of high-grade tumors in a poorly differentiated adenocarcinoma.
- Positive for TTF1 and napsin A.
- Mucinous type may be positive for CDX2 and CK20.

A B

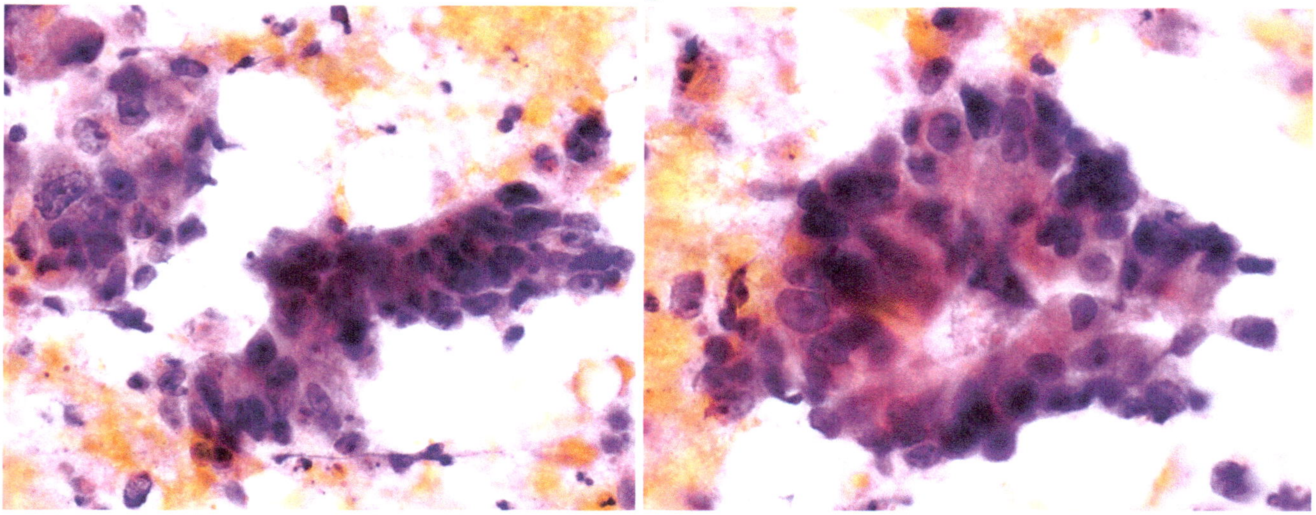

Fig. 7.62 (**a**, **b**) Colorectal adenocarcinoma, atypical glandular cells in the background of dirty necrosis – Pap stain

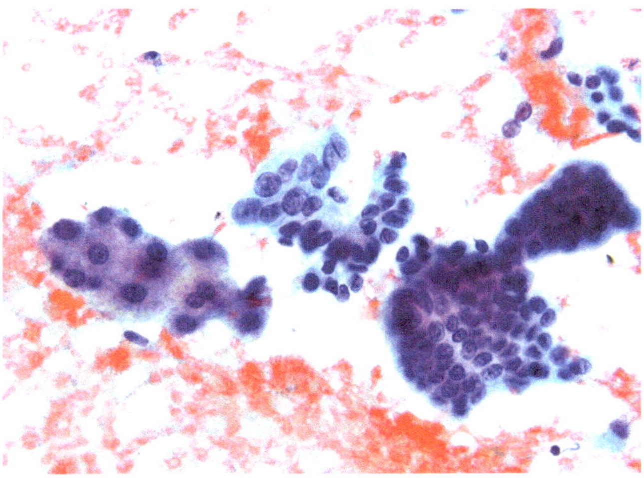

Fig. 7.63 Metastatic pancreatic cancer – Pap stain

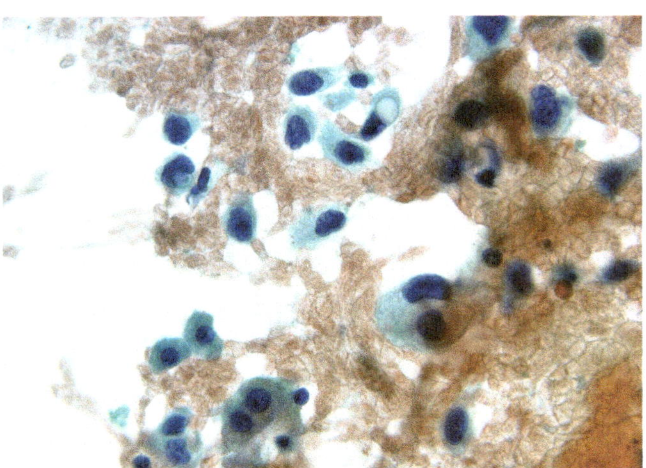

Fig. 7.64 Metastatic breast with intracytoplasmic lumen – Pap stain

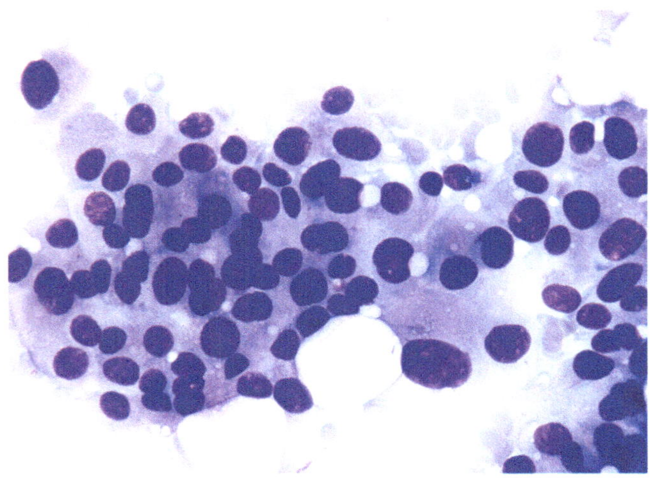

Fig. 7.65 Metastatic breast – similar to HCC (Diff-Quik)

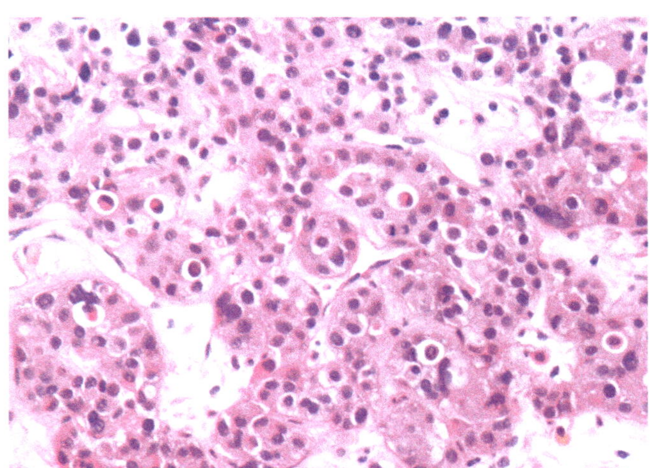

Fig. 7.66 Metastatic breast – cellblock

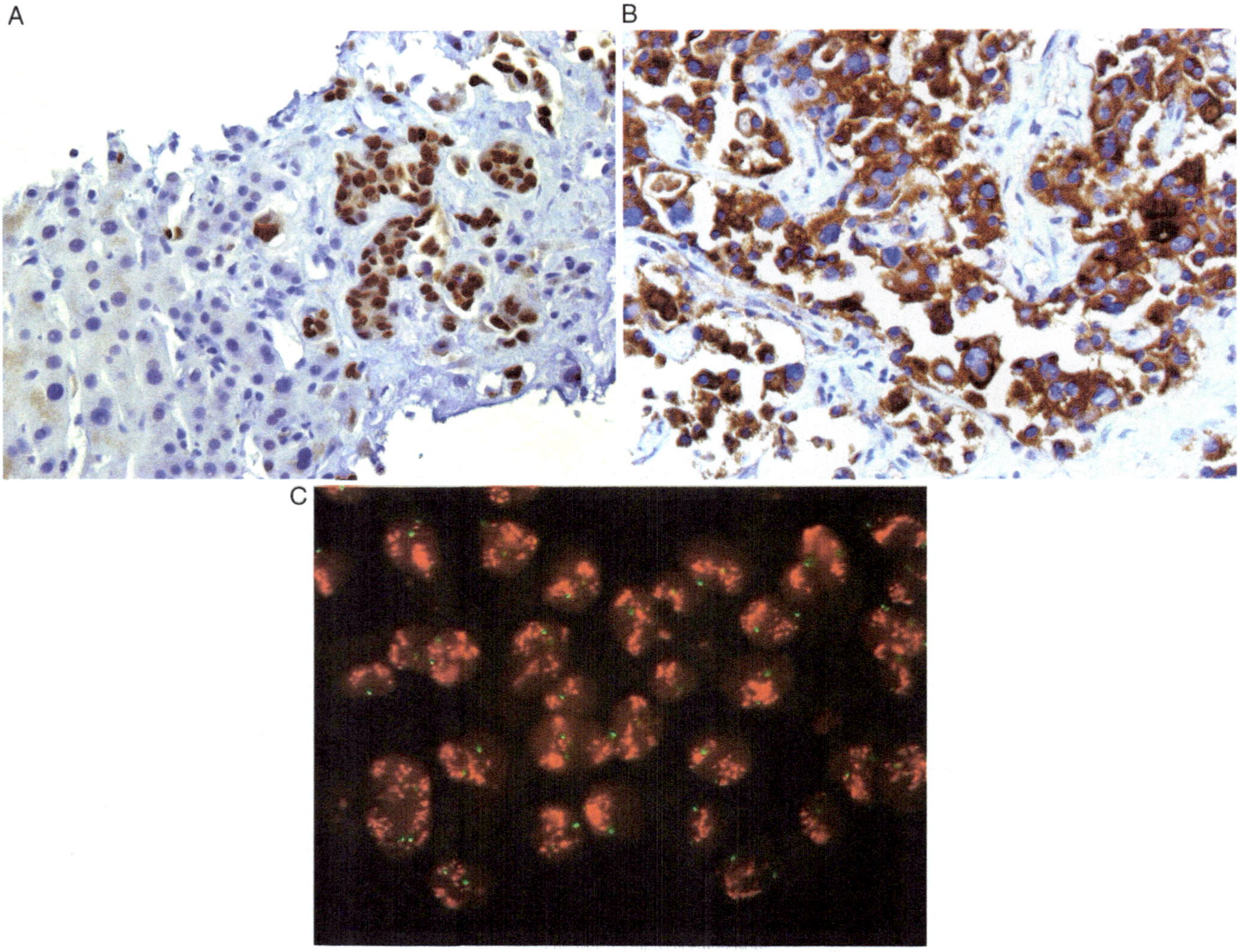

Fig. 7.67 (**a–c**) Metastatic breast carcinoma positive for ER (**a**) and GCDFP15 (**b**) and HER2 overexpression by FISH (**c**)

Stomach and Upper Gastrointestinal Tract

- Signet ring cells.
- CK7, CK20, and CDX2 can be useful.

Kidney

Cytological Features (Figs. 7.68, 7.69, 7.70, and 7.71a, b)

- Large neoplastic cells with large nuclei, prominent nucleoli, and clear to foamy cytoplasm.
- Low nuclear-to-cytoplasmic ratio.
- Binucleation and intranuclear pseudoinclusion.
- Thin vascular networks.
- Mixed inflammatory cells with neoplastic cells and vessels.
- PAX 8, PAX2, renal cell carcinoma marker (RCCma), CD10, vimentin, and EMA are useful markers in diagnosing clear cell RCC.

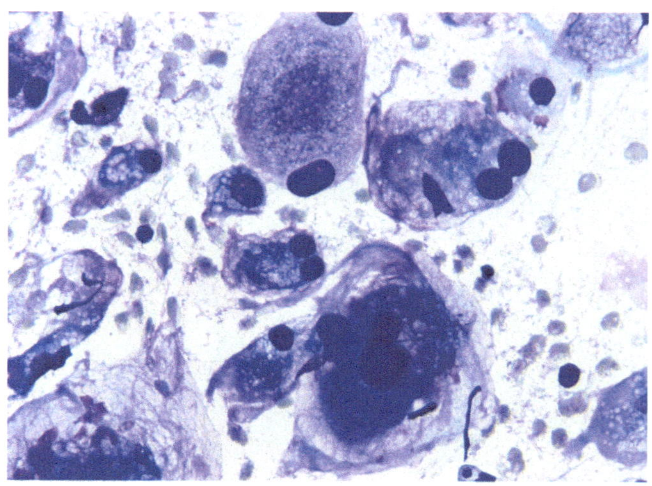

Fig. 7.68. Metastatic RCC with large neoplastic cells with large nuclei, prominent nucleoli, and clear to foamy cytoplasm, low nuclear-to-cytoplasmic ratio, binucleation and intranuclear pseudoinclusion, thin vascular networks, and mixed inflammatory cells with neoplastic cells and vessels – (Diff-Quik)

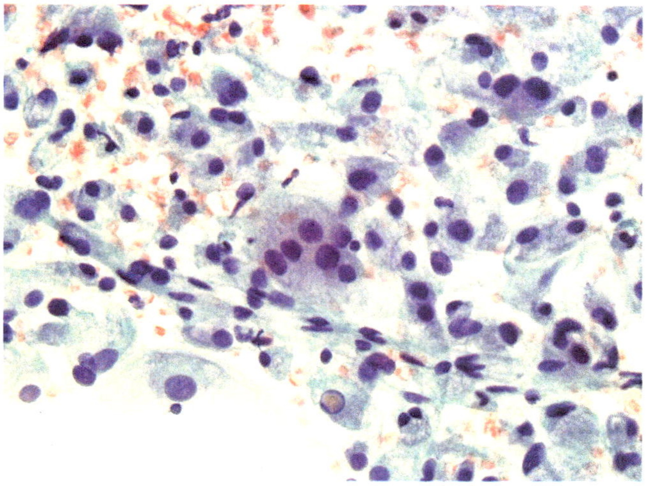

Fig. 7.69 Metastatic RCC – Pap stain

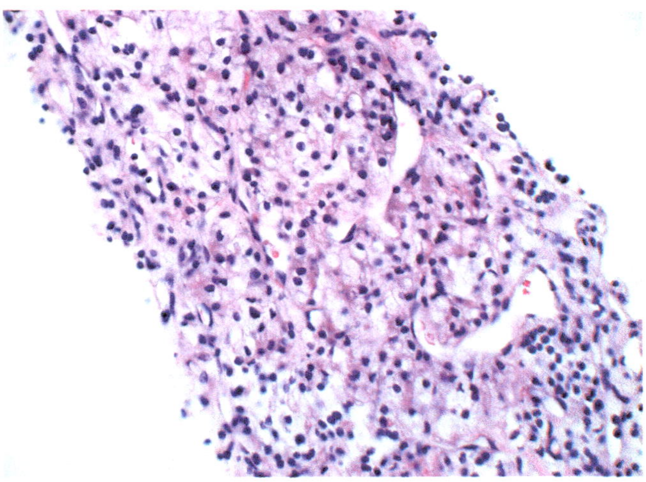

Fig. 7.70 Metastatic RCC – cellblock section

Small-Cell Carcinoma

- Neoplastic cells with high nuclear-to-cytoplasmic ratio, nuclear pleomorphism, neuroendocrine chromatin, tumor necrosis, and many mitoses (Figs. 7.72, 7.73, 7.74, and 7.75a, b)

Neuroendocrine Tumor, Grades I and II (Figs. 7.76a, b, 7.77, and 7.78a, b)

- Mixed population of single and cohesive epithelial cells.
- Plasmacytoid cells, binucleation, neuroendocrine chromatin, small nucleolus, intranuclear inclusion.
- A panel of useful IHC markers is summarized in Table 7.4.

Adenoid Cystic Carcinoma

- Small cohesive groups of epithelial cells with hyaline globules (Fig. 7.79).
- CD117, sex-determining region Y box 10 (SOX)10, S100, and p63 are useful markers.

Testicular Tumors

- Seminoma with relatively uniform large atypical cells with prominent nucleoli and small lymphoid cells in the background.
- Embryonal carcinoma with large pleomorphic cells and tumor necrosis.
- Yolk sac tumor with varying histomorphology.
- Spalt-like transcription factor 4 (SALL4), octamer-binding transcription factor 4 (OCT4), CD30, glypican-3, AFP, and CD117 are useful markers.

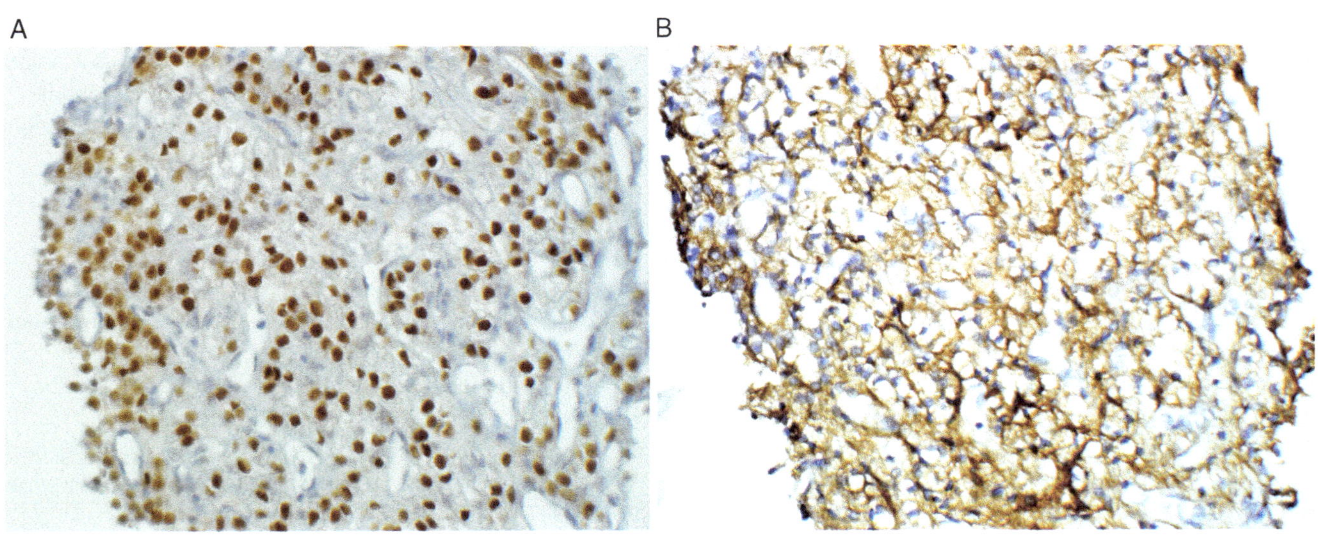

Fig. 7.71 (**a**, **b**) Metastatic RCC; PAX8 (**a**) and RCC-positive (**b**)

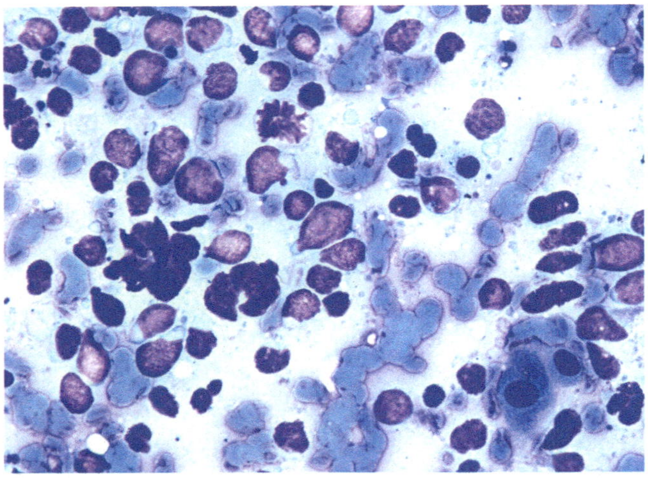

Fig. 7.72 Metastatic small-cell undifferentiated carcinoma, neoplastic cells with high nuclear-to-cytoplasmic ratio, nuclear pleomorphism, neuroendocrine chromatin, tumor necrosis, and many mitoses

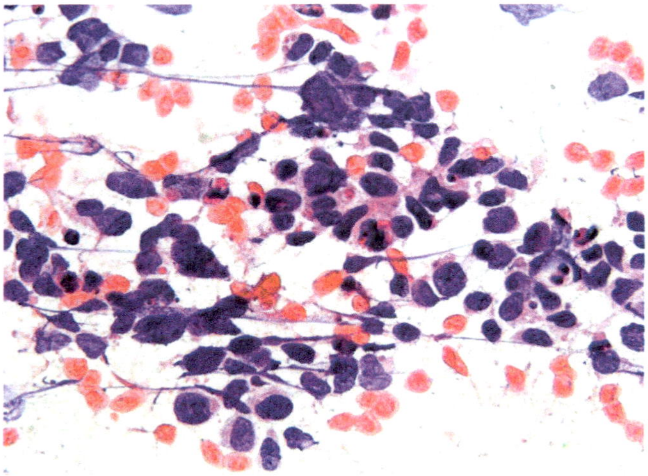

Fig. 7.73 Metastatic small-cell carcinoma – Pap stain

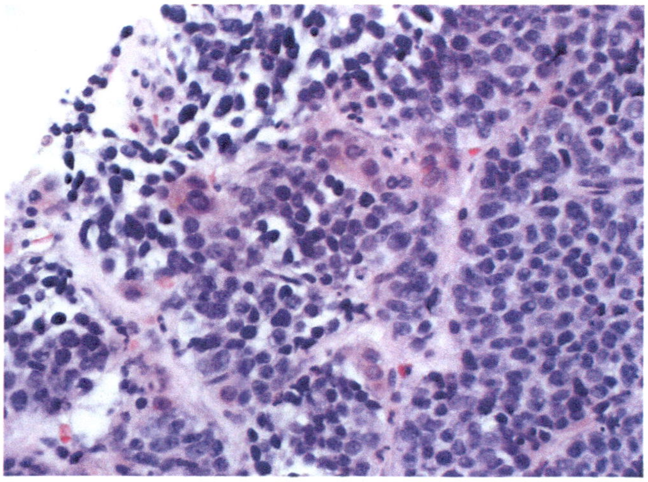

Fig. 7.74 Metastatic small-cell carcinoma – cellblock

Melanoma

Cytological Features (Fig. 7.80a, b)

- Epithelioid cells in loosely cohesive groups or single cells.
- Large nuclei, prominent nucleoli, and intranuclear inclusion.
- Abundant cytoplasm with low nuclear-to-cytoplasmic ratio.
- Marked nuclear pleomorphism and abnormal mitoses can be seen.
- May have a spindle cell population.
- Dusty pigments.
- Positive for S100, SOX10, HMB45, Mart-1, and microphthalmia transcription factor (MiTF).

Prostatic Adenocarcinoma (Figs. 7.81, 7.82, and 7.83a, b)

- Gleason pattern 3 carcinoma will show repeat acinar structures.
- Most metastases are Gleason pattern 4 or 5 with sheets of relatively uniform tumor cells with vaguely formed rosette-like structures, large nuclei and prominent nucleoli, and pale, vacuolated, or even clear cytoplasm.
- Positive for prostate-specific antigen (PSA), NK3 homeobox 1 (NKX3.1), alpha methylacyl-CoA racemase (AMACR, P504S), and prostatic acid phosphatase (PAP).

Bladder/Urothelial Carcinoma (Figs. 7.84, 7.85, and 7.86a, b)

- Typically showing a mixed epithelioid tumor cells with squamous changes and spindled tumor cells on an FNA sample
- Sheets of epithelial tumor cells with squamous features and various nuclear pleomorphisms on tissue sections
- Positive for CK7, CK20 (50%), high molecular weight CK, uroplakin II, p63, and S100P

Gynecologic Carcinomas (Figs. 7.87 and 7.88a–c)

- Can be a metastasis from the endocervix, endometrium, or ovary.
- Glandular, tubular, or papillary structures.
- Clear cell changes or squamous differentiation.
- Estrogen receptor (ER), PAX8, Wilms tumor gene-1 (WT-1), p53, p16, vimentin, and human papilloma virus (HPV) in situ hybridization can be useful.

A B

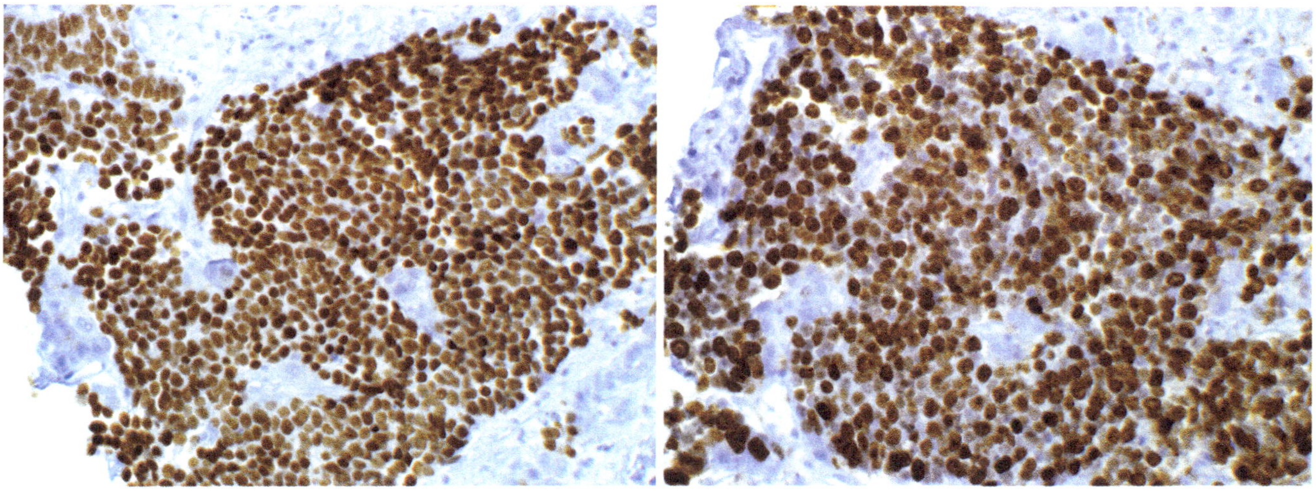

Fig. 7.75 (**a**, **b**) Metastatic small-cell carcinoma, TTF1 (**a**), and over 90% MIB-1 proliferative index (**b**)

A B

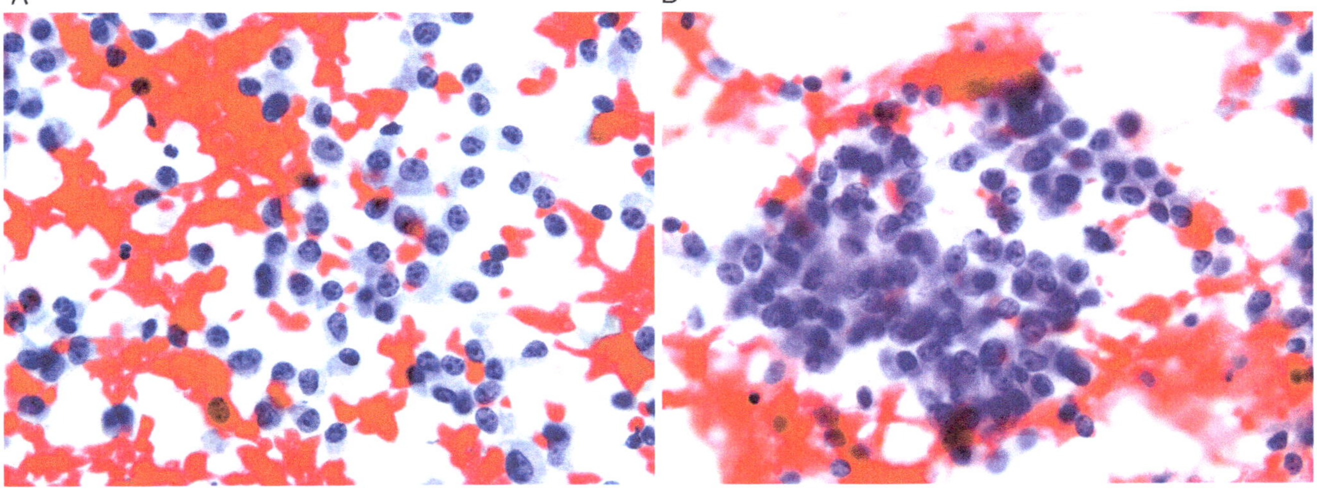

Fig. 7.76 (**a**, **b**) Neuroendocrine tumor grade II, mixed population of single and cohesive epithelial cells, plasmacytoid cells, binucleation, neuroendocrine chromatin, and small nucleolus

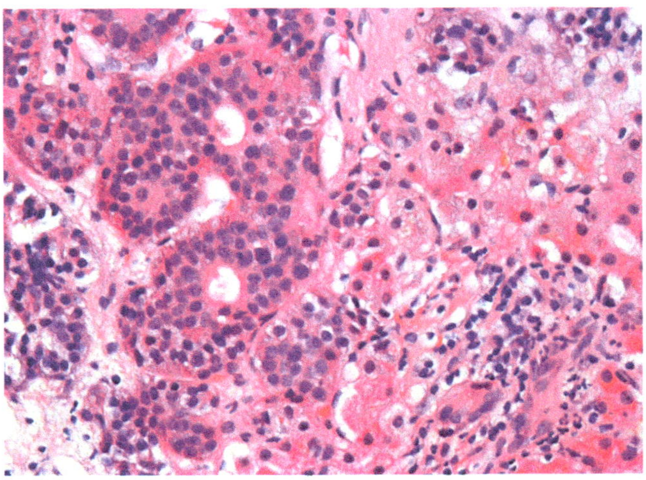

Fig. 7.77 Tissue core showing neuroendocrine tumor

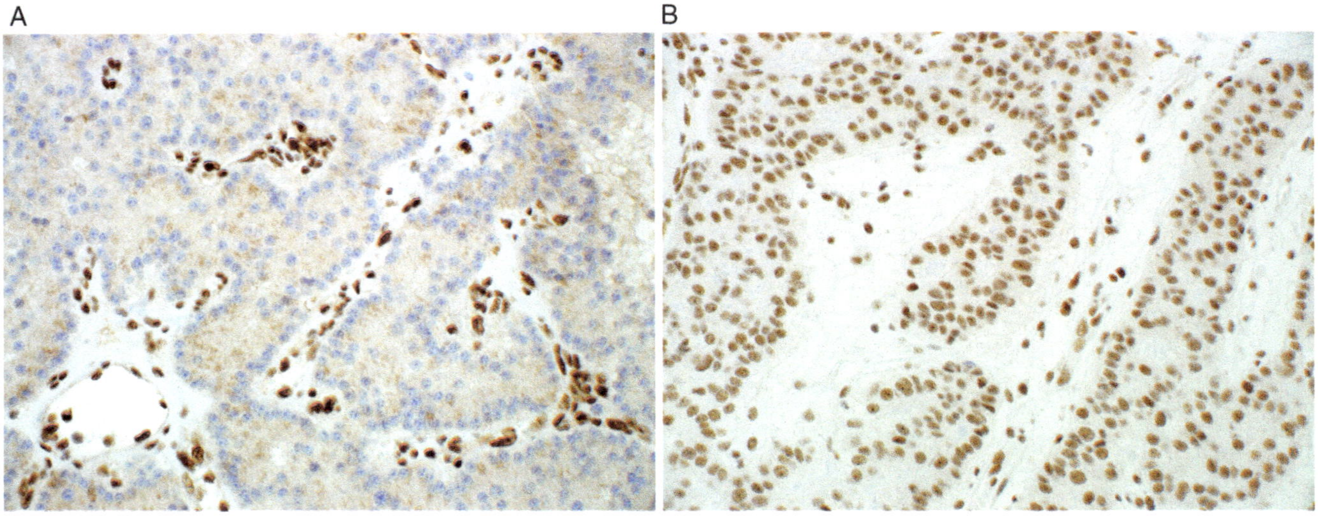

Fig. 7.78 (**a**, **b**) Loss expression of ATRX (**a**) and/or DAXX (**b**), suggestive of pancreatic primary

Fig. 7.79 Metastatic adenoid cystic carcinoma, small cohesive groups of epithelial cells with hyaline globules

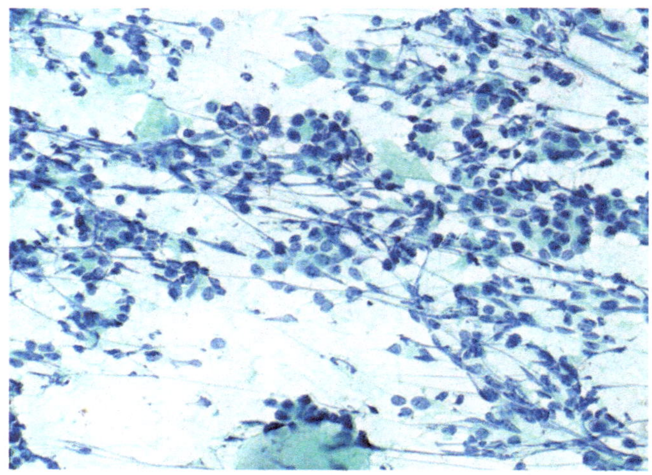

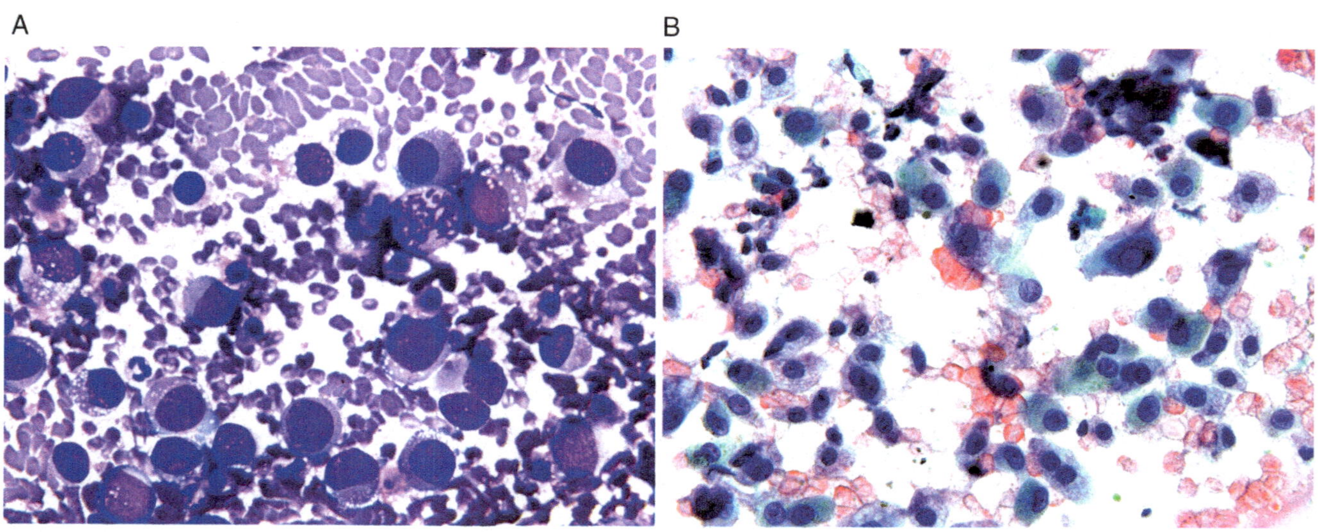

Fig. 7.80 (**a**, **b**) Metastatic melanoma with epithelioid cells in loosely cohesive groups or single cells

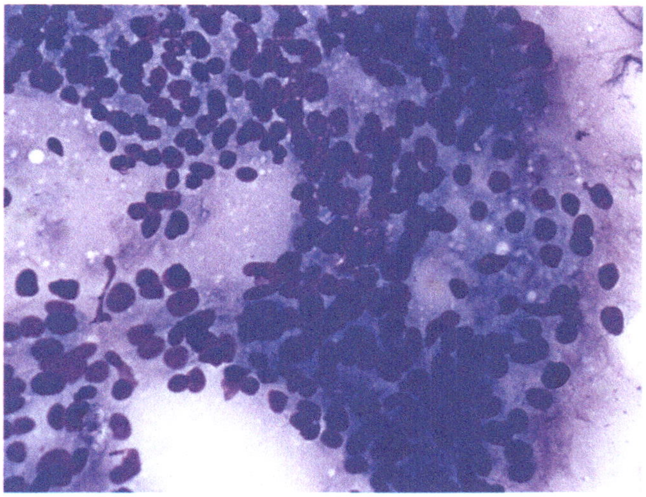

Fig. 7.81 Metastatic prostatic acinar adenocarcinoma on FNA smear

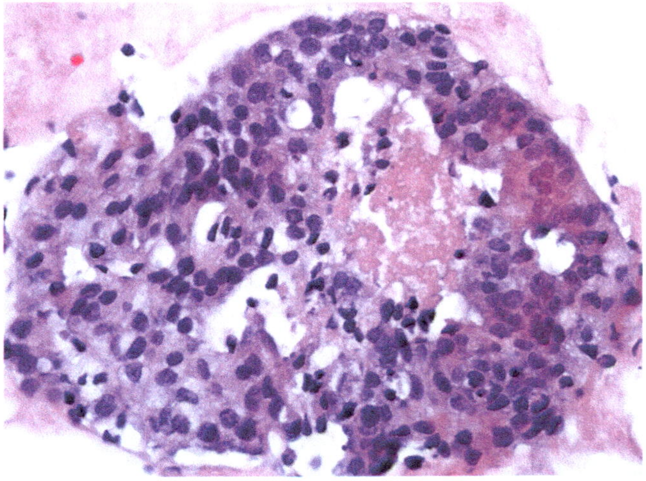

Fig. 7.82 Metastatic prostatic acinar adenocarcinoma – cellblock

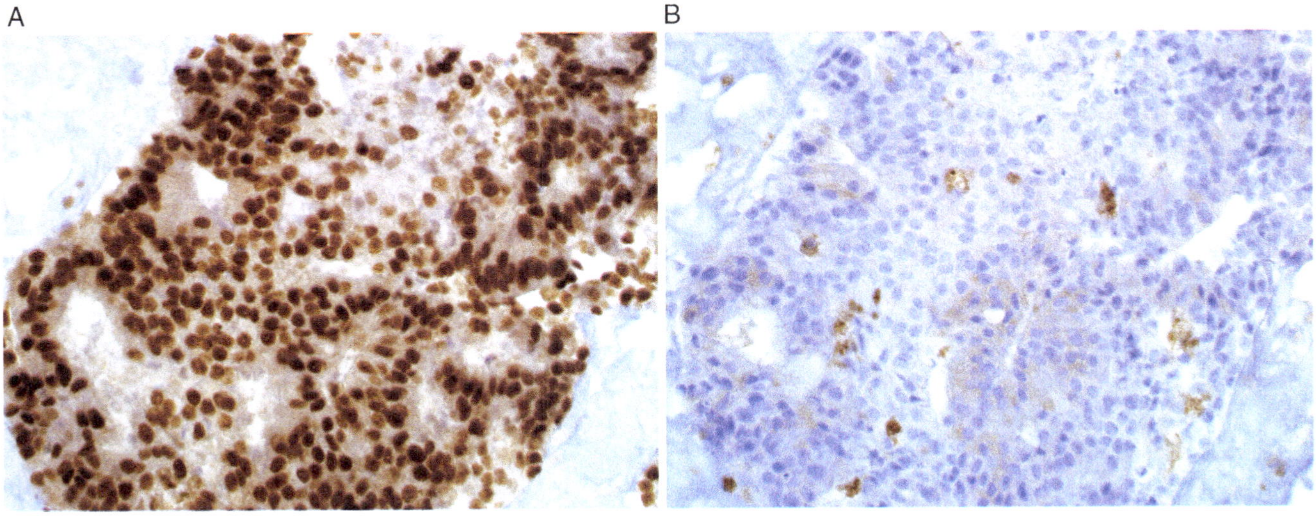

Fig. 7.83 (**a**, **b**) Metastatic prostatic acinar adenocarcinoma positive for NKX3.1 (**a**) and PSA (**b**)

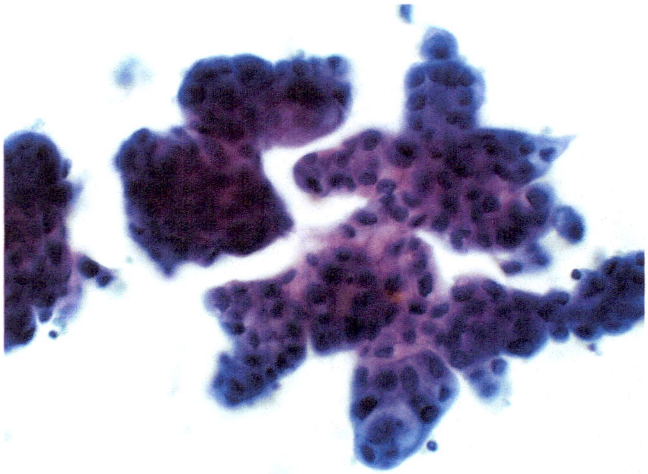

Fig. 7.84 Metastatic urothelial carcinoma on FNA smear

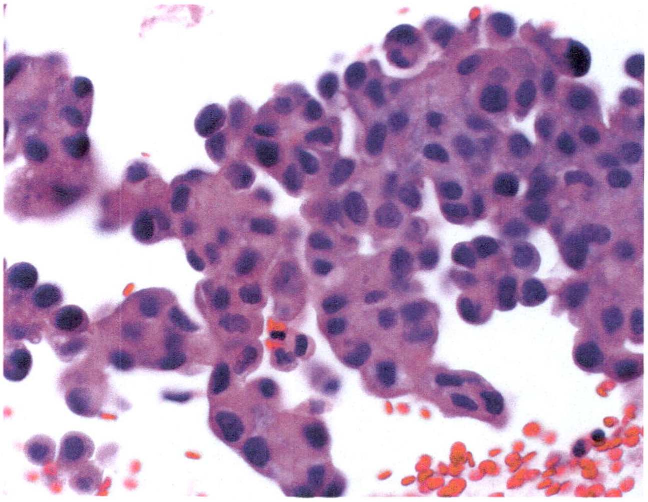

Fig. 7.85 Metastatic urothelial carcinoma – cellblock

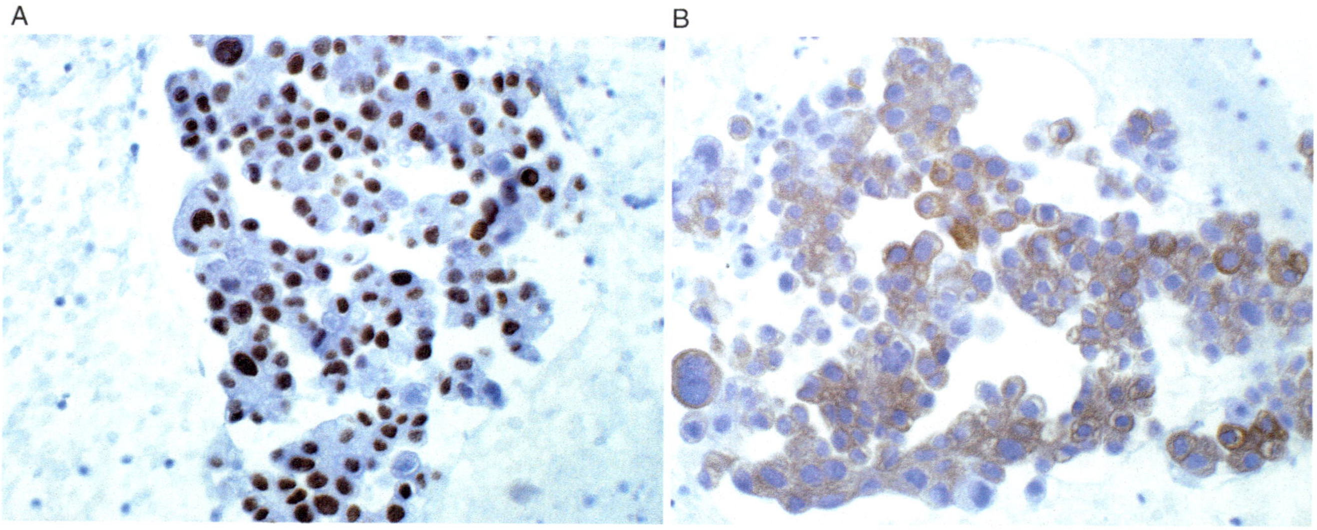

Fig. 7.86 (**a**, **b**) Metastatic urothelial carcinoma positive for GATA3 (**a**) and uroplakin II (**b**)

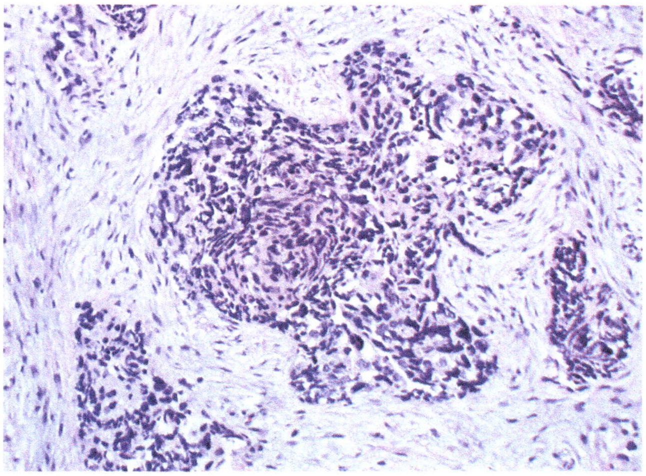

Fig. 7.87 Metastatic ovarian serous carcinoma on tissue section

Sarcoma (Gastrointestinal Stromal Tumor [GIST]) (Figs. 7.89, 7.90, and 7.91)

- Spindle neoplastic cells, or mixed with epithelioid cells
- Positive for CD117 (c-kit), discovered on GIST1 (DOG1), and CD34 (50%)

Multiple Myeloma, Lymphoma, or Myeloid Sarcoma (Figs. 7.92, 7.93, and 7.94a, b)

- Many single cells with plasmacytoid features, binucleation, may have intranuclear or intracytoplasmic inclusions.
- Perinuclear clearing is a key to identify the origin of plasma cells, which is not usually seen in other neoplasms with plasmacytoid features, such as melanoma and neuroendocrine tumor.
- Immunostains for CD38 and CD138 and in situ hybridization for kappa and lambda light chains are useful.

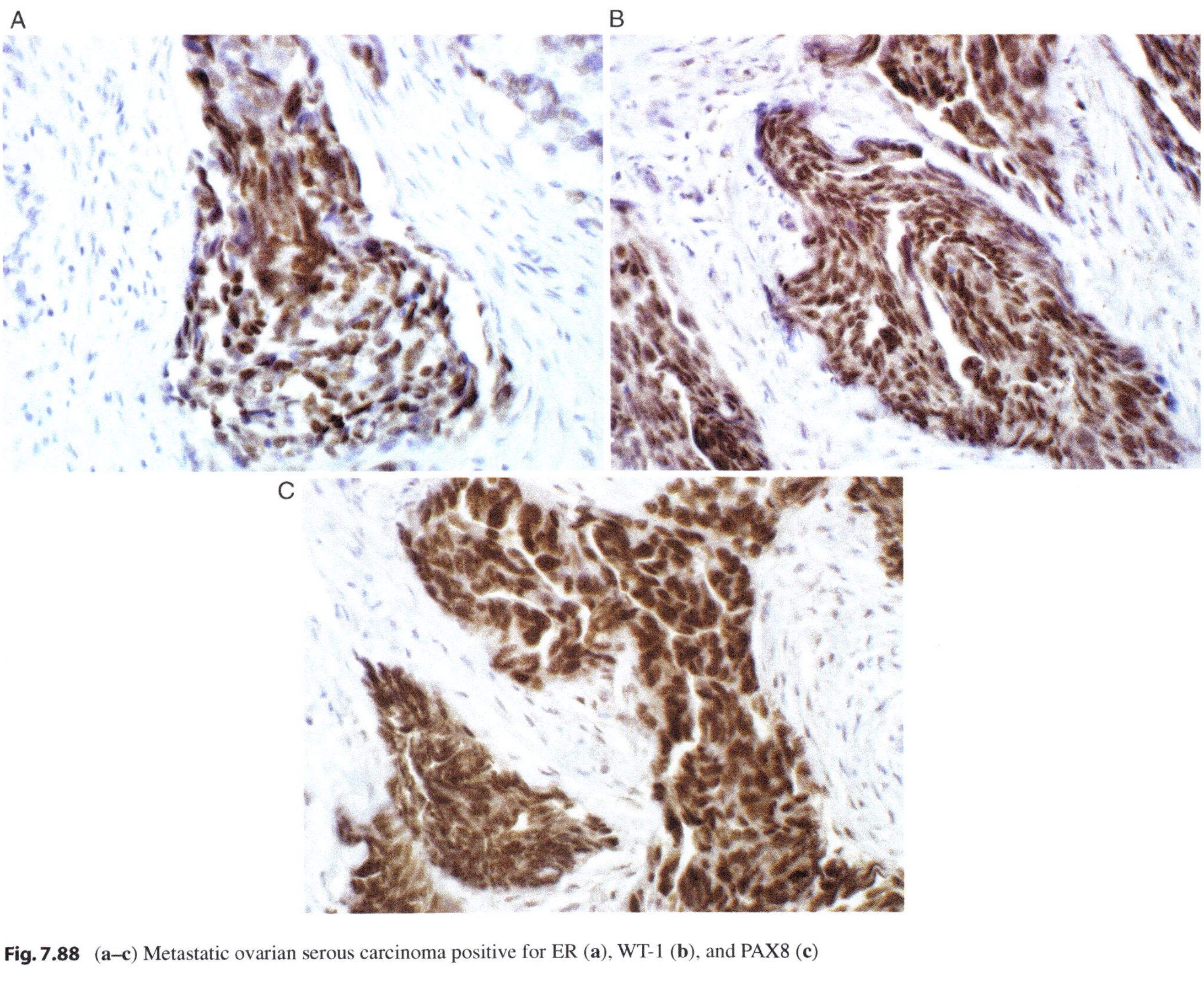

Fig. 7.88 (**a–c**) Metastatic ovarian serous carcinoma positive for ER (**a**), WT-1 (**b**), and PAX8 (**c**)

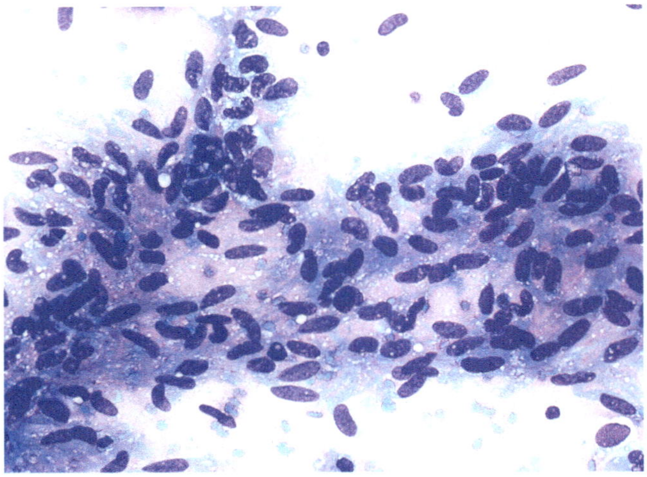

Fig. 7.89 Metastatic GIST – spindle neoplastic cells

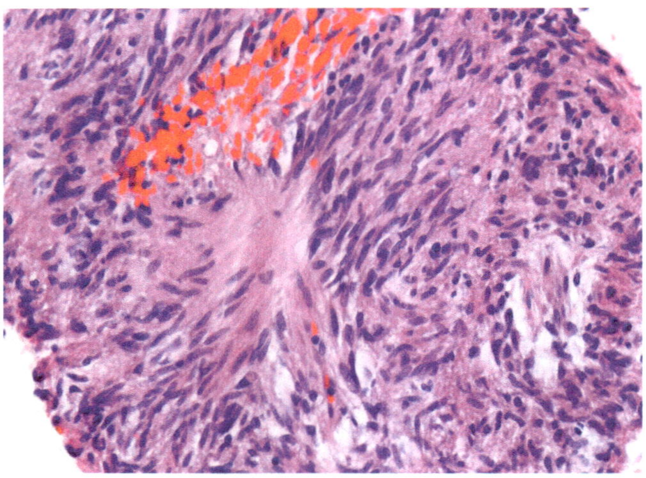

Fig. 7.90 Cellblock section of GIST

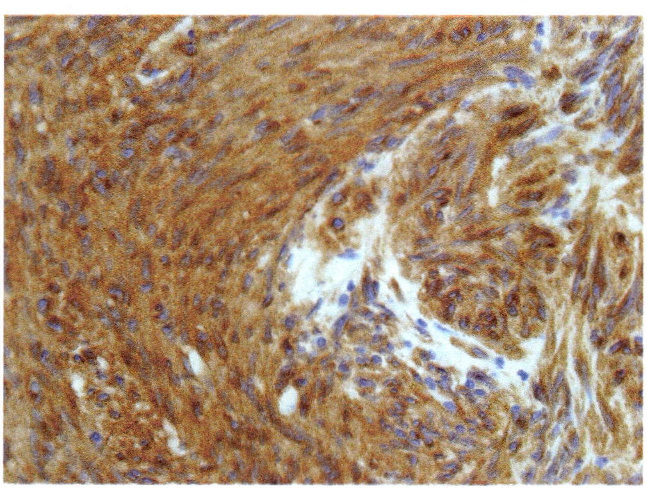

Fig. 7.91 Metastatic GIST – immunostain for CD117 (c-kit)

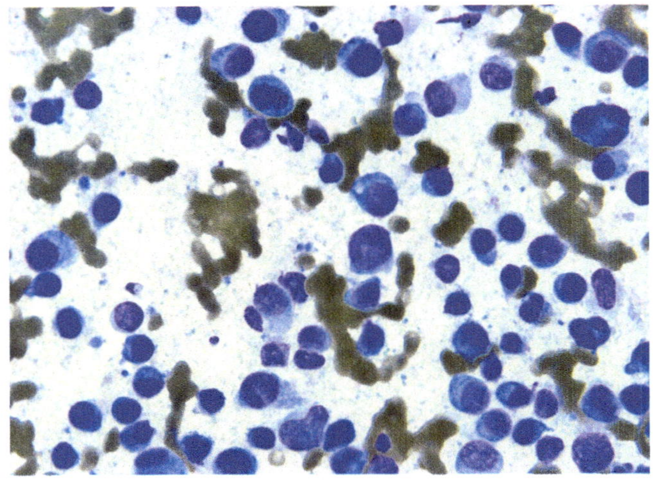

Fig. 7.92 Multiple myeloma – Diff-Quik

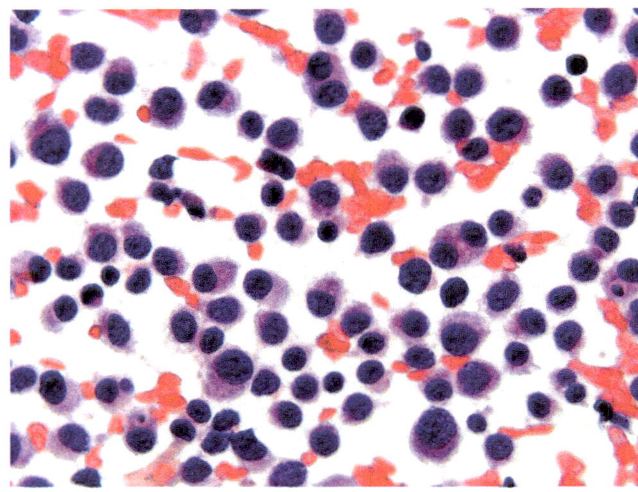

Fig. 7.93 Multiple myeloma – Pap stain

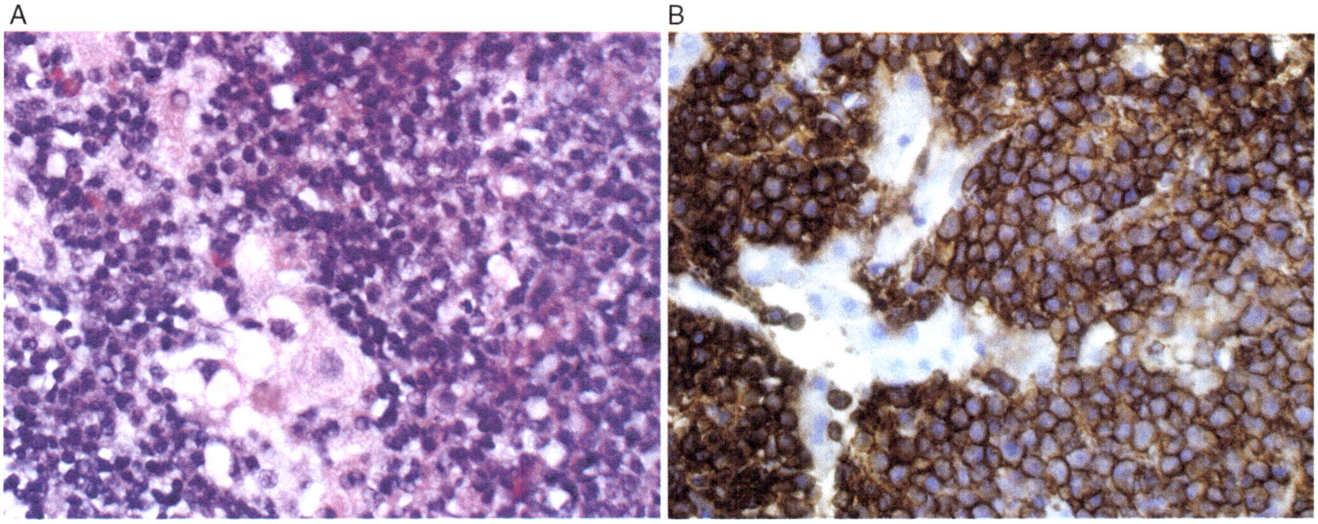

Fig. 7.94 (**a**, **b**) Diffuse large B-cell lymphoma (**a**) and positive for CD20 (**b**)

Case Presentations

There are three scenarios commonly encountered in daily practice when evaluating an FNA biopsy of a liver mass/focal lesion with or without a cellblock and/or thin tissue core biopsy. Case Scenario 1 is how to make a diagnosis of well-differentiated HCC from other hepatocellular lesions and metastatic carcinomas in a limited specimen; Case Scenario 2 is how to deal with an overt malignancy or neoplastic process in which cholangiocarcinoma, HCC, and a secondary tumor are included in the diagnostic consideration; and Case Scenario 3 is how to work on a small round cell tumor.

Case Scenario 1

Learning Objectives

1. Reiterate the diagnostic criteria for well-differentiated HCC on both FNA and small tissue biopsy specimens.
2. Review the most effective panel of immunomarkers for the diagnosis of HCC and its mimics.

Case

A 74-year-old man with no known history of malignancy presented with a 4.0 cm mass of the liver. A US-guided FNA and biopsy were performed. The FNA smear was hypocellular, with a few groups of mildly atypical epithelial cells with clear cytoplasm associated with fibrosis as shown in Fig. 7.95a. A cellblock preparation was also obtained, which contained thin tissue cores with a proliferation of epithelial cells with marked clear cell/steatotic changes as shown in Fig. 7.95b, c. There was surrounding fibrosis and a lymphoplasmacytic inflammatory infiltrate. Background cirrhosis was suspected.

At this point, the question is: Is this material sufficient to render a definitive diagnosis of malignancy such as HCC or a metastasis? If the answer is no, then why not? Can any special stain or IHC panel be helpful in this scenario?

Based on the cytomorphology and histology shown above, a definitive diagnosis cannot be rendered without additional special stains and immunohistochemical stains. A well-differentiated HCC with clear cell changes is the top diagnostic consideration. However, a few other entities should be included: 1) a benign hepatic lesion with steatotic changes/clear cell changes, such as an HCA; 2) a metastatic carcinoma with clear cell changes, including clear cell RCC; 3) a metastatic neuroendocrine tumor with clear cell changes; and 4) less likely, a metastatic melanoma with clear cell changes.

Focusing on the differential diagnosis mentioned above, a reticulin stain and a small panel of immunostains including CD34, arginase-1, CK7, MOC31, and PAX8 were performed. The results demonstrated a clear loss of reticulin network throughout the area of clear cell/steatotic hepatocytes, and CD34 highlighted a diffuse network of endothelialized sinusoidal spaces (Fig. 7.95d, e). There were frequent cell plates greater than three layers in thickness decorated by both reticulin and CD34 stains. The epithelial cells were positive

(continued)

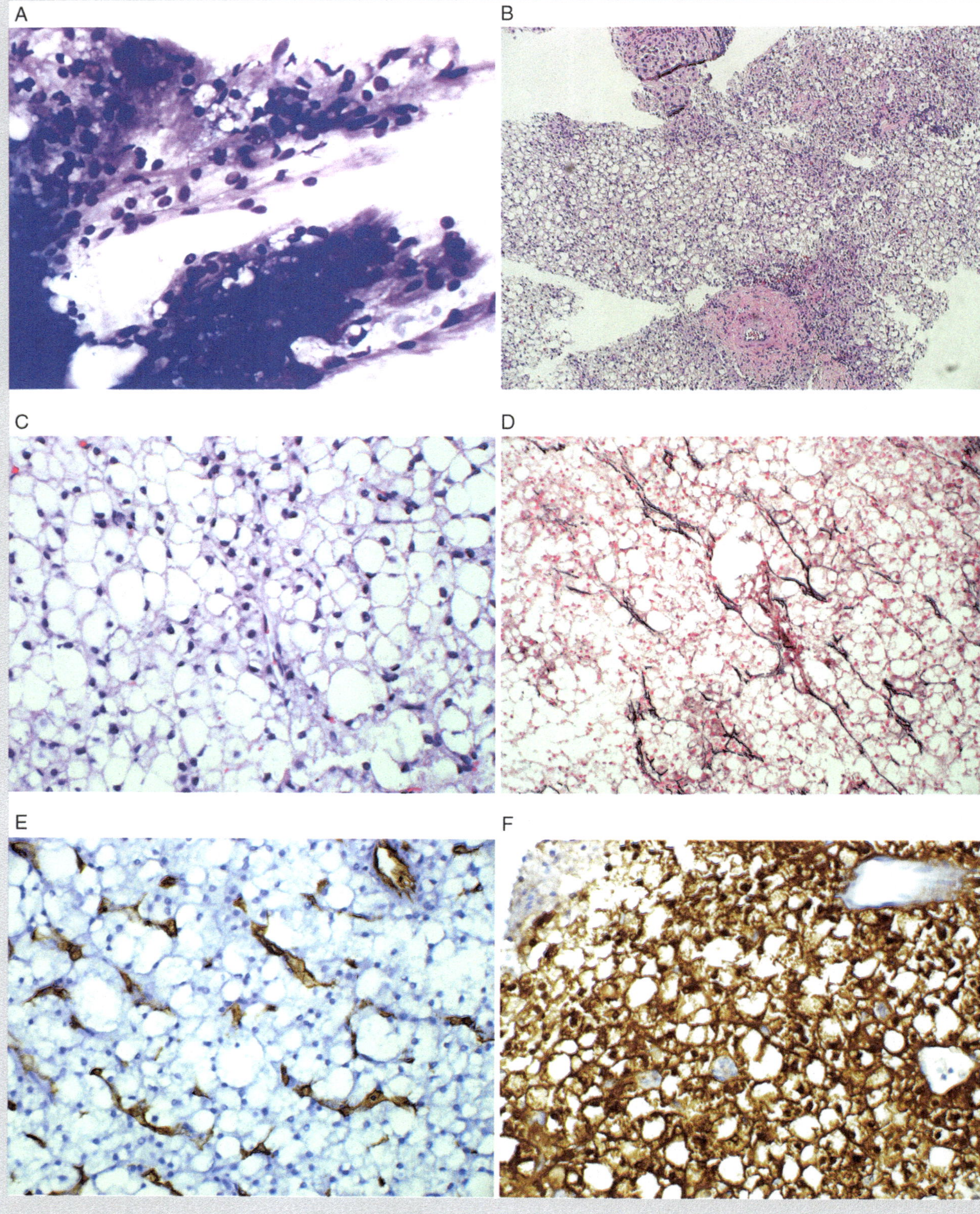

Fig. 7.95 (**a**–**f**) An example of HCC with clear cell changes. Note that mildly atypical epithelial cells have clear cytoplasm (**a**), thin tissue cores (**b**,**c**), clear loss of reticulin network (**d**), endothelialized sinusoidal spaces highlighted by CD34 (**e**), and positive immunostaining for arginase-1 (**f**)

(continued)

for arginase-1 immunostain (Fig. 7.95f) and negative for CK7, MOC31, and PAX8, confirming the hepatic origin. The negative staining for CK7, MOC31, and PAX8 largely excluded the possibility of a cholangiocarcinoma, a metastatic adenocarcinoma, and a clear cell RCC.

Final Diagnosis

HCC with clear cell changes.

Learning Points

The learning points from this staining panel included:

1. Reticulin and CD34 to differentiate well-differentiated HCC from benign hepatic lesion such as HCA
2. CK7, MOC31, and arginase-1 to distinguish HCC from cholangiocarcinoma
3. PAX8 to separate clear cell variant of HCC from clear cell RCC

Case Scenario 2

Learning Objectives

1. Review the most effective panel of immunomarkers for diagnosis of IHCC from other metastatic adenocarcinomas.
2. Review the differential diagnosis of a poorly differentiated neoplasm.

Case 1

A 68-year-old man with a history of alcoholic cirrhosis and known history of HCC treated with embolization presented with a mass of the liver. CT scans showed interval growth in a lesion which was previously believed to be a hemangioma but recently displayed an atypical appearance. A CT-guided fine needle aspiration and small tissue core biopsies were performed. The FNA smear revealed malignant epithelial cells in large groups and small clusters and scattered large atypical cells as shown in Fig. 7.96a, b. The core biopsy specimens showed benign liver tissue with infiltrating tumor in nesting and trabecular growth patterns. Some poorly formed glandular structures were suggested. The tumor cells showed large nuclei with conspicuous to prominent nucleoli and a moderate amount of eosinophilic cytoplasm as shown in Fig. 7.96c, d.

Based on the morphologic features above, a diagnosis of carcinoma can be established. The differential diagnosis may include HCC, IHCC, or metastatic carcinoma. A small panel of IHC markers including CK7, MOC31, and arginase-1 was performed; the results showed that the tumor cells were positive for CK7 and MOC31 and negative for arginase-1, which confirmed the diagnosis of moderately to poorly differentiated adenocarcinoma.

The question is: Is this a primary cholangiocarcinoma or a metastatic adenocarcinoma?

A few additional markers including pVHL, carbonic anhydrase 9 (CA9), TTF1, CDX2, and CK20 were performed; the result showed the tumor cells were diffusely positive for pVHL and CA9 (Fig. 7.96e, f) and negative for TTF1, CDX2, and CK20. These results supported the diagnosis of an IHCC.

Our previous studies demonstrated that the vast majority of adenocarcinomas of the pancreas, common bile duct, and gallbladder were negative for pVHL and overexpressed maspin, S100P, and insulin-like growth factor 2 mRNA-binding protein 3 (IMP3). Interestingly, Wang and colleagues reported that 71% of IHCCs were diffusely positive for pVHL. The expression of maspin and S100P was observed in 73% and 27%, respectively. Additionally, approximately 60% of adenocarcinomas of the pancreas were positive for MUC5AC and CK17, whereas only 12% and 12% of IHCCs were positive for MUC5AC and CK17, respectively. Our study also demonstrated that CA9 was a very sensitive marker for IHCC with a sensitivity of over 90%; however, it was not a very specific marker since other adenocarcinomas, including gynecologic, pancreatic, and those from the GI tracts, as well as clear cell RCCs, can be positive. The negative staining for CA9 made the diagnosis of IHCC unlikely.

Another example of IHCC was from a 69-year-old man who presented with a 5.0 cm liver mass. In this case, the tumor was composed of many multinucleated giant tumor cells as shown in Fig. 7.97a, b, which was morphologically challenging to render a diagnosis of IHCC. However, the small panel of IHC markers including CK7, MOC31, pVHL, and arginase-1 confirmed the diagnosis. The tumor cells, including multinucleated giant tumor cells, were diffusely positive for pVHL as shown in Fig. 7.97c.

Recently, some limited studies have shown that RNA in situ hybridization for albumin was highly sensitive and specific to confirm the diagnosis of HCC and IHCC. Some preliminary studies also suggested that over 80% of hepatoid carcinomas also express albumin by RNA in situ hybridization.

(continued)

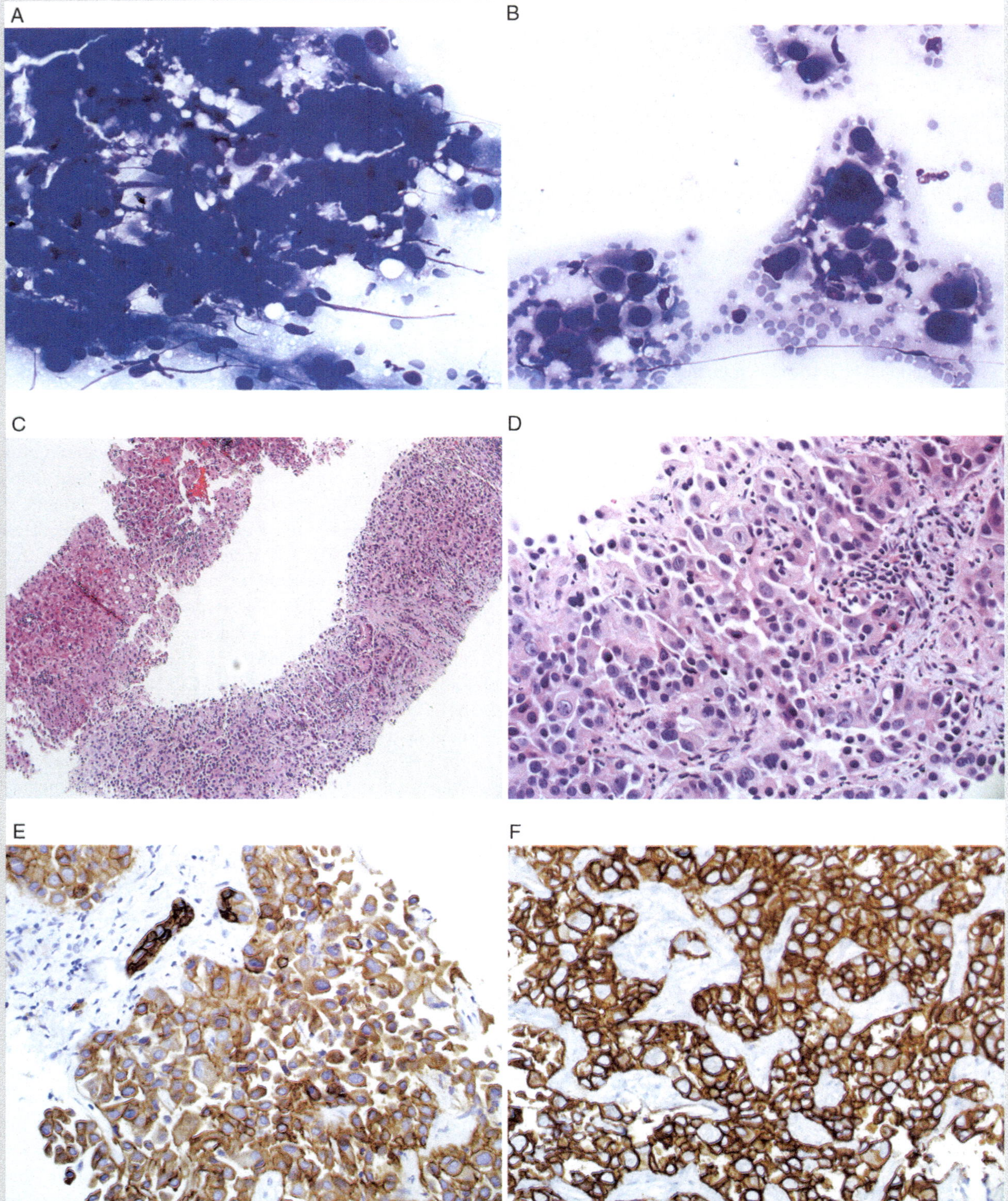

Fig. 7.96 (**a**–**f**) An example of intrahepatic cholangiocarcinoma Note the malignant epithelial cells in large groups and small clusters (**a**, **b**), benign liver tissue with infiltrating tumor (**c**, **d**), and tumor positive for pVHL and CA9 (**e**, **f**)

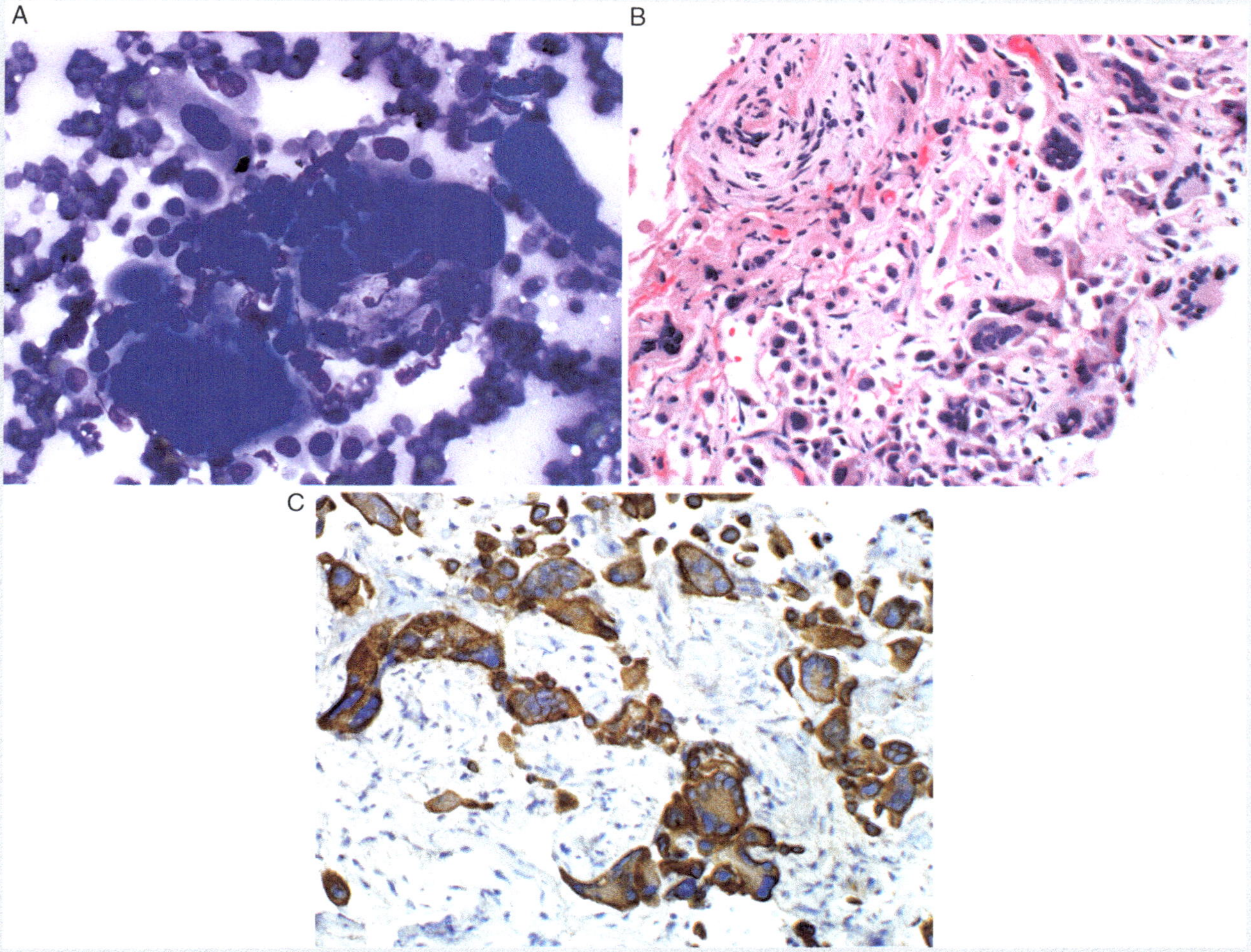

Fig. 7.97 (**a–c**) Another example of intrahepatic cholangiocarcinoma with predominately multinucleated giant tumor cells (**a**, **b**) and diffusely and strongly positive for pVHL (**c**)

Final Diagnosis

Intrahepatic cholangiocarcinoma.

Learning Points

The learning points from these two cases include:

1. pVHL and CA9 are useful markers to differentiate an IHCC from other metastatic adenocarcinomas, including metastatic adenocarcinomas from other pancreatobiliary tract adenocarcinomas.
2. Albumin RNA in situ hybridization has been reported as a highly sensitive and specific marker to distinguish an IHCC from other metastatic adenocarcinomas and HCCs.

Case 2

A 44-year-old man initially presented with right-sided flank pain. The subsequent workup revealed a 6.1x4.4x5.4 cm hepatic mass in the right lobe of the liver. He had no known history of malignancy. He underwent a CT-guided FNA and core biopsies. The FNA smear preparation demonstrated predominately isolated tumor cells with large pleomorphic nuclei, irregular nuclear contour, and high nuclear-to-cytoplasmic ratio as shown in Fig. 7.98a, b. The thin needle core biopsy samples showed nests and trabeculae of the atypical cells in the rich vascular networks. The stroma showed some myxoid changes with residual benign bile ducts and scattered benign hepatocytes.

(continued)

Focal tumor necrosis, hemorrhage, and rare mitosis were noted. Some of the vascular spaces appeared to be lined by atypical endothelial cells. Representative microscopic photos are shown in Fig. 7.98c, d.

Based on the morphologic features, a high-grade malignant tumor can be easily established. The differential diagnosis may include poorly differentiated carcinoma, HCC, melanoma, and high-grade sarcoma such as angiosarcoma. A panel of immunostains including low molecular weight cytokeratin (CAM5.2), CK7, MOC31, ERG, and CD31 was performed. The results demonstrated that the tumor cells were strongly positive for ERG and CD31 as shown in Fig. 7.98e, f and negative for CK and MOC31, which confirmed the diagnosis of angiosarcoma.

Final Diagnosis
Angiosarcoma.

Learning Points
A few learning points from this case include:

1. When working on a high-grade neoplasm from the liver, especially in the presence of rich vascular networks or vascular spaces and areas of hemorrhage, an angiosarcoma should be suspected.
2. Angiosarcoma, especially epithelioid angiosarcoma, is frequently positive for cytokeratin, and in some instances the positivity can be diffuse, which may potentially be misdiagnosed as a carcinoma.
3. ERG has proven to be the best vascular marker when compared to CD31, CD34, and others.

Case 3
A 68-year-old woman with remote history of melanoma of the face presented with periportal adenopathy and a liver lesion. A CT-guided core biopsy was performed. The core needle biopsy specimen contained fragments of liver tissue infiltrated by small- to medium-sized tumor cells with a very high nuclear-to-cytoplasmic ratio, irregular nuclei, vesicular chromatin, occasional intranuclear inclusions, eosinophilic cytoplasm, and focal spindle cell appearance. Representative microscopic photos are shown in Fig. 7.99a–c.

Based on the morphology and patient's history, neuroendocrine tumor, metastatic carcinoma, cholangiocarcinoma, and metastatic melanoma were considered. A screening panel of immunostains including pancytokeratin, S100, and synaptophysin was performed. The results showed that the tumor cells were negative for all three markers (negative for S100 shown in Fig. 7.99d). What was the differential diagnosis? The negative staining for pancytokeratin and synaptophysin made a diagnosis of carcinoma and neuroendocrine tumor very unlikely, especially with this epithelioid morphology. With the known history of melanoma, additional melanoma markers including SOX10 and HMB45 were performed; the results showed both markers were positive as shown in Fig. 7.99e, f, which confirmed the diagnosis of metastatic melanoma.

Final Diagnosis
Metastatic melanoma.

Learning Points
The important learning point from this case is that a very small percentage of melanomas, even with epithelioid morphology, can be negative for S100. S100 negativity does not entirely exclude the possibility of melanoma. With a known history, morphologic suspicion, or a biopsy sample fixed in alcohol solution, additional melanoma markers, including SOX10, HMB45, and Mart-1, should be performed.

Case Scenario 3

Learning Objectives
1. Review the differential diagnosis of malignant small round cell tumors in the liver.
2. Review the most effective panel of immunomarkers for diagnosis of malignant round cell tumors.

Case
A 75-year-old man with a known history of non-Hodgkin's lymphoma presented with multiple masses in the liver. A CT-guided FNA was performed. The FNA smear preparation showed sheets of single or loosely cohesive tumor cells with a markedly increased nuclear-to-cytoplasmic ratio, fine nuclear chromatin, small nucleoli, and many mitoses, as shown in Fig. 7.100a, b. Background lymphoglandular bodies were not presented. Plasmacytoid cells, binucleations, salt-and-pepper chromatin, and prominent nucleoli were not seen. At this point, lymphoma, myeloid sarcoma, and high-grade neuroendocrine carcinoma were considered. A panel of immunostains including CK,

(continued)

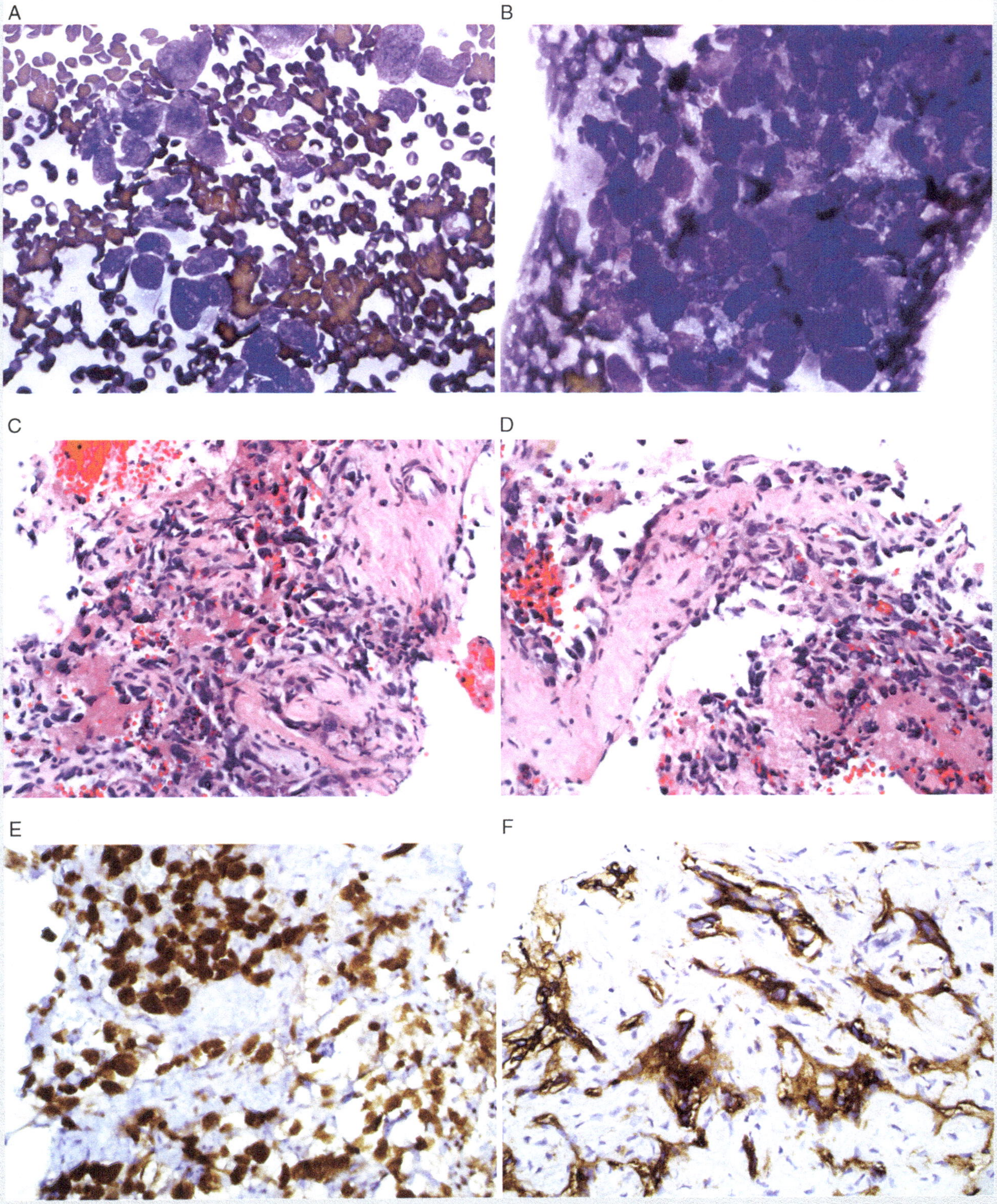

Fig. 7.98 (**a–f**) An example of angiosarcoma from a 44-year-old man Note the large pleomorphic tumor cells on the smear (**a**, **b**), infiltrating tumor cells in the vascular networks (**c**, **d**), and positive for ERG and CD31 (**e**, **f**)

(continued)

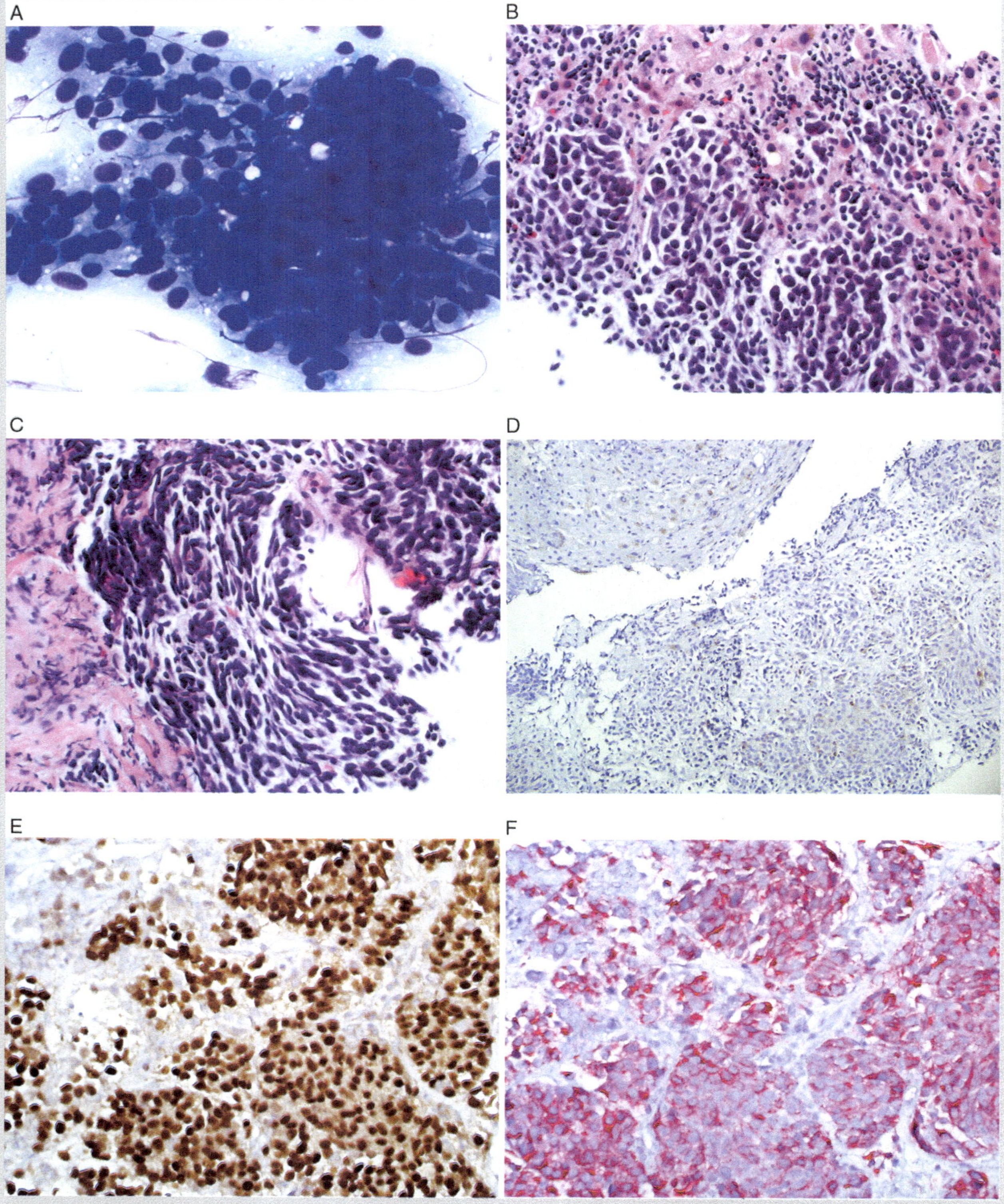

Fig. 7.99 (**a**–**f**) An example of metastatic melanoma with S100 negativity Note the infiltrating tumor with epithelioid on FNA smear (**a**), histology (**b**, **c**), negative for S100 (**d**) and positive for SOX10 (**e**) and HMB45 (**f**)

(continued)

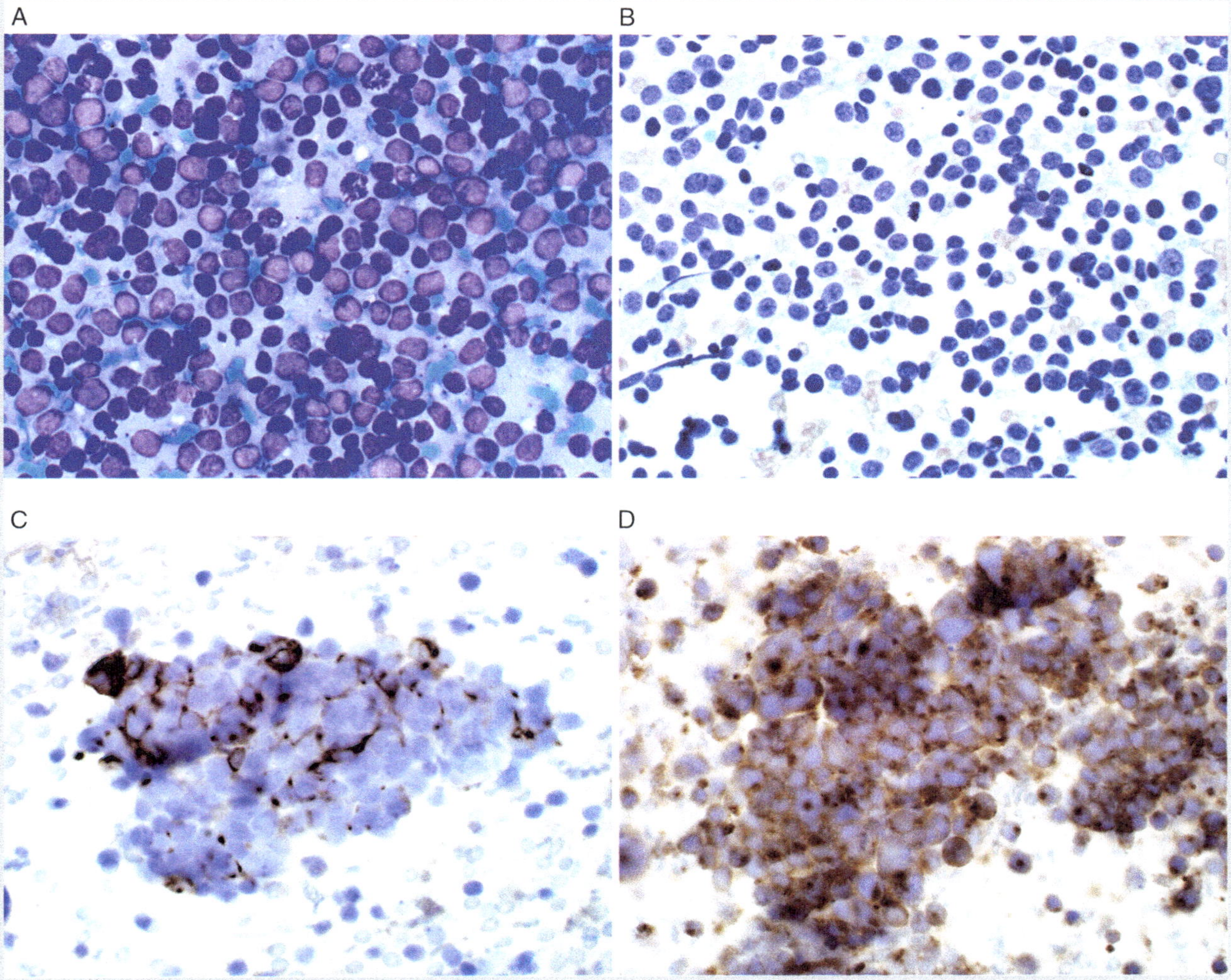

Fig. 7.100 (**a–d**) An example of metastatic Merkel cell carcinoma Note the small round cell tumor with fine nuclear chromatin and small nucleoli (**a**, **b**), perinuclear dot-like staining for CK20 (**c**) and synaptophysin (**d**), and negative for TTF1 and lymphoid markers (not shown)

CK7, CK20, MIB-1 (Ki-67), TTF1, synaptophysin, CD3, and CD20 was performed. The results demonstrated the tumor cells to be positive for CK20 and synaptophysin with perinuclear dot-like staining patterns as shown in Fig. 7.100c, d and negative for all other markers. The MIB-1 proliferative index was approximately 50%. The overall features were diagnostic for metastatic Merkel cell carcinoma.

Final Diagnosis

Metastatic Merkel cell carcinoma.

Learning Points

What are the learning points from this case?

1. Merkel cell carcinoma frequently shows fine nuclear chromatin instead of the salt-and-pepper chromatin seen in a small-cell carcinoma.
2. Most large cell lymphomas show background lymphoglandular bodies and tumor cells with prominent nucleoli.
3. Lack of plasmacytoid features and binucleation or multinucleation make a diagnosis of plasma cell tumor less likely.
4. Approximately 75% of Merkel cell carcinomas are positive for Merkel cell polyomavirus (negative in this case).
5. Small-cell carcinoma usually shows a much higher MIB-1 proliferative index (greater than 90%).

Abbreviation List

Abbreviation	Full text
AFP	Alpha-fetoprotein
APC	Adenomatous polyposis coli
Arg-1	Arginase-1
ATRX/DAXX	Alpha-thalassemia/mental retardation syndrome/death domain-associated protein
CA9	Carbonic anhydrase 9
CAM5.2	Low molecular weight cytokeratin
CD	Cluster of differentiation
CDX2	Caudal type homeobox 2
CEA	Carcinoembryonic antigen
CK	Cytokeratin
CRCC	Clear cell renal cell carcinoma
CRP	C-reactive protein
CT	Computed tomography
D2-40	Podoplanin
DOG1	Discovered on GIST1
EBV	Epstein-Barr virus
EMA	Epithelial membrane antigen
EpCAM	Epithelial cell adhesion molecule
ER	Estrogen receptor
ERG	ETS-related gene
FNA	Fine needle aspiration
GATA3	GATA binding protein 3
GCDFP15	Gross cystic disease fluid protein 15
GIST	Gastrointestinal stromal tumor
GS	Glutamine synthetase
HCA	Hepatocellular adenoma
HCC	Hepatocellular carcinoma
HepPar-1	Hepatocyte paraffin-1
HMB45	Human melanoma black 45
HNF-1a	Hepatocyte nuclear factor-1a
HPV	Human papilloma virus
HSP70	Heat-shock protein 70
IgG4	Immunoglobulin G4
IHC	Immunohistochemical, immunohistochemistry
IHCC	Intrahepatic cholangiocarcinoma
IMP3	Insulin-like growth factor 2 mRNA-binding protein
INI-1	Integrase interactor-1
L-FABP	Liver fatty acid-binding protein
MALT	Mucosa-associated lymphoid tissue
Mart-1	Melanoma antigen recognized by T cells-1
Mel	Melanoma
MIB-1	Mindbomb E3 ubiquitin protein ligase 1
MiTF	Microphthalmia transcription factor
MOC31	EpCAM/epithelial membrane antigen
MUC (MUC5AC, etc.)	Mucin
N/C	Nuclear-to-cytoplasmic
NKX3.1	NK3 homeobox 1
OCT4	Octamer-binding transcription factor 4
P504S (AMACR)	Alpha methylacyl-CoA racemase
PAP	Prostatic acid phosphatase
Pap	Papanicolaou
PAX (e.g., PAX8)	Paired box gene
PEComa	Perivascular epithelioid cell tumor
PR	Progesterone receptor
PSA	Prostate-specific antigen
pVHL	von Hippel-Lindau tumor suppressor gene protein
RCCMa	Renal cell carcinoma marker
RNA	Ribonucleic acid
SALL4	Spalt-like transcription factor 4
SATB2	Special AT-rich sequence-binding protein 2
SMA	Smooth muscle actin
SOX10	Sex-determining region Y box 10
SSA	Serum amyloid A
STAT6	Signal transducer and activator of transcription 6
TTF1	Thyroid transcription factor 1
US	Ultrasound
WHO	World Health Organization
WT-1	Wilms tumor gene-1

Suggested Reading

Cytology/Fine Needle Aspiration

Bottles K, Cohen MB, Holly EA, Chiu SH, Abele JS, Cello JP, et al. A step-wise logistic regression analysis of hepatocellular carcinoma. An aspiration biopsy study. Cancer. 1988;62(3):558–63.

Cohen MB, Haber MM, Holly EA, Ahn DK, Bottles K, Stoloff AC. Cytologic criteria to distinguish hepatocellular carcinoma from nonneoplastic liver. Am J Clin Pathol. 1991;95(2):125–30.

Das DK. Cytodiagnosis of hepatocellular carcinoma in fine-needle aspirates of the liver: its differentiation from reactive hepatocytes and metastatic adenocarcinoma. Diagn Cytopathol. 1999;21(6):370–7.

Davenport RD. Cytologic diagnosis of fibrolamellar carcinoma of the liver by fine-needle aspiration. Diagn Cytopathol. 1990;6(4):275–9.

DeMay RM. Liver. In: The Art and Science of Cytopathology, vol. 3. 2nd ed. Chicago: ASCP Press; 2010. p. 1249–1296,chapter 18.

Donat EE, Anderson V, Tao LC. Cytodiagnosis of clear cell hepatocellular carcinoma. A case report. Acta Cytol. 1991;35(6):671–5.

Greene CA, Suen KC. Some cytologic features of hepatocellular carcinoma as seen in fine needle aspirates. Acta Cytol. 1984;28(6):713–8.

Gupta RK, AlAnsari AG, Fauck R. Aspiration cytodiagnosis of clear cell hepatocellular carcinoma in an elderly woman. A case report. Acta Cytol. 1994;38(3):467–9.

Kondo F, Wada K, Kondo Y. Morphometric analysis of hepatocellular carcinoma. Virchows Arch A Pathol Anat Histopathol. 1988;413(5):425–30.

Mansouri D, Van Nhieu JT, Couanet D, Terrier-Lacombe MJ, Brugières L, Cherqui D, et al. Fibrolamellar hepatocellular carcinoma: a case report with cytological features in a sixteen-year-old girl. Diagn Cytopathol. 2006;34(8):568–71.

Pérez-Guillermo M, Masgrau NA, García-Solano J, Sola-Pérez J. De Agustín y de Agustín P. Cytologic aspect of fibrolamellar hepatocellular carcinoma in fine-needle aspirates. Diagn Cytopathol. 1999;21(3):180–7.

Pitman MB. Fine needle aspiration biopsy of the liver. Principal diagnostic challenges. Clin Lab Med. 1998;18(3):483–506. vi

Renshaw AA, Haja J, Wilbur DC, Miller TR; Cytology Committee, College of American Pathologists. Fine-needle aspirates of adenocarcinoma/metastatic carcinoma that resemble hepatocellular carcinoma: correlating cytologic features and performance in the College of American Pathologists Nongynecologic Cytology Program. Arch Pathol Lab Med 2005;129(10):1217–21.

Suen KC, Magee JF, Halparin LS, Chan NH, Greene CA. Fine needle aspiration cytology of fibrolamellar hepatocellular carcinoma. Acta Cytol. 1985;29(5):867–72.

Tao LC, Ho CS, McLoughlin MJ, Evans WK, Donat EE. Cytologic diagnosis of hepatocellular carcinoma by fine-needle aspiration biopsy. Cancer. 1984;53(3):547–52.

Vecchio FM, Fabiano A, Ghirlanda G, Manna R, Massi G. Fibrolamellar carcinoma of the liver: the malignant counterpart of focal nodular hyperplasia with oncocytic change. Am J Clin Pathol. 1984;81(4):521–6.

Wee A. Fine needle aspiration biopsy of hepatocellular carcinoma and hepatocellular nodular lesions: role, controversies and approach to diagnosis. Cytopathology. 2011;22(5):287–305.

Wee A, Nilsson B, Chan-Wilde C, Yap I. Fine needle aspiration biopsy of hepatocellular carcinoma. Some unusual features. Acta Cytol. 1991;35(6):661–70.

Yang GC, Yang GY, Tao LC. Cytologic features and histologic correlations of microacinar and microtrabecular types of well-differentiated hepatocellular carcinoma in fine-needle aspiration biopsy. Cancer. 2004;102(1):27–33.

Histology

Bosman FT, Carneiro F, Hruban RH, Theise ND, editors. WHO Classification of Tumours of the Digestive System. 4th ed. Lyon: IARC Press; 2010. p. 195–254.

Ferrell L. Liver pathology: cirrhosis, hepatitis, and primary liver tumors. Update and diagnostic problems. Mod Pathol. 2000;13(6):679–704.

Rowland JM. Hepatoblastoma: assessment of criteria for histologic classification. Med Pediatr Oncol. 2002;39(5):478–83.

Ancillary Tests

Abenoza P, Manivel JC, Wick MR, Hagen K, Dehner LP. Hepatoblastoma: an immunohistochemical and ultrastructural study. Hum Pathol. 1987;18(10):1025–35.

Bioulac-Sage P, Rebouissou S, Thomas C, Blanc JF, Saric J, Sa Cunha A, et al. Hepatocellular adenoma subtype classification using molecular markers and immunohistochemistry. Hepatology. 2007;46(3):740–8.

Capurro M, Wanless IR, Sherman M, Deboer G, Shi W, Miyoshi E, et al. Glypican-3: a novel serum and histochemical marker for hepatocellular carcinoma. Gastroenterology. 2003;125(1):89–97.

Chen ZE, Lin F. Application of immunohistochemistry in gastrointestinal and liver neoplasms: new markers and evolving practice. Arch Pathol Lab Med. 2015;139(1):14–23.

Chu PG, Ishizawa S, Wu E, Weiss LM. Hepatocyte antigen as a marker of hepatocellular carcinoma: an immunohistochemical comparison to carcinoembryonic antigen, CD10, and alpha-fetoprotein. Am J Surg Pathol. 2002;26(8):978–88.

Chuma M, Sakamoto M, Yamazaki K, Ohta T, Ohki M, Asaka M, et al. Expression profiling in multistage hepatocarcinogenesis: identification of HSP70 as a molecular marker of early hepatocellular carcinoma. Hepatology. 2003;37(1):198–207.

Di Tommaso L, Destro A, Seok JY, Balladore E, Terracciano L, Sangiovanni A, et al. The application of markers (HSP70 GPC3 and GS) in liver biopsies is useful for detection of hepatocellular carcinoma. J Hepatol. 2009;50(4):746–54.

Di Tommaso L, Franchi G, Park YN, Fiamengo B, Destro A, Morenghi E, et al. Diagnostic value of HSP70, glypican 3, and glutamine synthetase in hepatocellular nodules in cirrhosis. Hepatology. 2007;45(3):725–34.

Ferrone CR, Ting DT, Shahid M, et al. The ability to diagnose intrahepatic cholangiocarcinoma definitively using novel branched DNA-enhanced albumin RNA in situ hybridization technology. Ann Surg Oncol. 2016;23(1):290–6.

Gonzalez-Crussi F. Undifferentiated small cell ("anaplastic") hepatoblastoma. Pediatr Pathol. 1991;11(1):155–61.

Gray SG, Hartmann W, Eriksson T, Ekstrom C, Holm S, Kytola S, et al. Expression of genes involved with cell cycle control, cell growth and chromatin modification are altered in hepatoblastomas. Int J Mol Med. 2000;6(2):161–9.

Jeannot E, Poussin K, Chiche L, Bacq Y, Sturm N, Scoazec JY, et al. Association of CYP1B1 germ line mutations with hepatocyte nuclear factor 1alpha-mutated hepatocellular adenoma. Cancer Res. 2007;67(6):2611–6.

Lai JP, Chen ZM, Lok T, Chan OT, Himmelfarb E, Zhai Q, et al. Immunohistochemical stains of proliferating cell nuclear antigen, insulin-like growth factor 2 and clusterin help distinguish malignant from benign liver nodular lesions. J Clin Pathol. 2014;67(6):464–9.

Laumonier H, Bioulac-Sage P, Laurent C, Zucman-Rossi J, Balabaud C, Trillaud H. Hepatocellular adenomas: magnetic resonance imaging features as a function of molecular pathological classification. Hepatology. 2008 Sep;48(3):808–18.

Lin F, Abdallah H, Meschter S. Diagnostic utility of CD10 in differentiating hepatocellular carcinoma from metastatic carcinoma in fine-needle aspiration biopsy (FNAB) of the liver. Diagn Cytopathol. 2004;30(2):92–7.

Lin F, Chen ZE, Wang HL. Utility of immunohistochemistry in the pancreatobiliary tract. Arch Pathol Lab Med. 2015;139(1):24–38.

Lin F, Liu H. Immunohistochemistry in undifferentiated neoplasm/tumor of uncertain origin. Arch Pathol Lab Med. 2014;138(12):1583–610.

Liu H, Shi J, Anandan V, Wang HL, Diehl D, Blansfield J, et al. Reevaluation and identification of the best immunohistochemical panel (pVHL, Maspin, S100P, IMP-3) for ductal adenocarcinoma of the pancreas. Arch Pathol Lab Med. 2012;136(6):601–9.

Lin F, Shi J, Liu H, Hull ME, Dupree W, Prichard JW, et al. Diagnostic utility of S100P and von Hippel-Lindau gene product (pVHL) in pancreatic adenocarcinoma-with implication of their roles in early tumorigenesis. Am J Surg Pathol. 2008a;32(1):78–91.

Lin F, Shi J, Liu H, Zhang J, Zhang PL, Wang HL, et al. Immunohistochemical detection of the von Hippel-Lindau gene product (pVHL) in human tissues and tumors: a useful marker for metastatic renal cell carcinoma and clear cell carcinoma of the ovary and uterus. Am J Clin Pathol. 2008b;129(4):592–605.

Lin F, Wang HL. Liver, bile ducts and gallbladder. In: Lin F, Prichard JW, Liu H, Wilkerson M, Chen ZM, editors. Handbook of practical immunohistochemistry – frequently asked questions. 2nd ed. New York: Springer Science+Business Media; 2015a. p. 503–23.

Lin F, Wang HL. Pancreas and ampulla. In: Lin F, Prichard JW, Liu H, Wilkerson M, Chen ZM, editors. Handbook of practical immunohistochemistry – frequently asked questions. 2nd ed. New York: Springer Science+Business Media; 2015b. p. 481–502.

Lok T, Chen L, Lin F, Wang HL. Immunohistochemical distinction between intrahepatic cholangiocarcinoma and pancreatic ductal adenocarcinoma. Hum Pathol. 2014;45(2):394–400.

Nguyen TB, Roncalli M, Di Tommaso L, Kakar S. Combined use of heat-shock protein 70 and glutamine synthetase is useful in the distinction of typical hepatocellular adenoma from atypical hepatocellular neoplasms and well-differentiated hepatocellular carcinoma. Mod Pathol. 2016;29(3):283–92.

Osada T, Sakamoto M, Nagawa H, Yamamoto J, Matsuno Y, Iwamatsu A, et al. Acquisition of glutamine synthetase expression in human hepatocarcinogenesis: relation to disease recurrence and possible regulation by ubiquitin-dependent proteolysis. Cancer. 1999;85(4):819–31.

Shahid M, Mubeen A, Tse J, Kakar S, Bateman AC, Borger D, et al. Branched chain in situ hybridization for albumin as a marker of hepatocellular differentiation: evaluation of manual and automated in situ hybridization platforms. Am J Surg Pathol. 2015;39(1):25–34.

Timek DT, Shi J, Liu H, Lin F. Arginase-1, HepPar-1, and Glypican-3 are the most effective panel of markers in distinguishing hepatocellular carcinoma from metastatic tumor on fine-needle aspiration specimens. Am J Clin Pathol. 2012;138(2):203–10.

Wachter DL, Schlabrakowski A, Hoegel J, Kristiansen G, Hartmann A, Riener MO. Diagnostic value of immunohistochemical IMP3 expression in core needle biopsies of pancreatic ductal adenocarcinoma. Am J Surg Pathol. 2011;35(6):873–7.

Wee A. Diagnostic utility of immunohistochemistry in hepatocellular carcinoma, its variants and their mimics. Appl Immunohistochem Mol Morphol. 2006;14(3):266–72.

Yan BC, Gong C, Song J, Krausz T, Tretiakova M, Hyjek E, et al. Arginase-1: a new immunohistochemical marker of hepatocytes and hepatocellular neoplasms. Am J Surg Pathol. 2010;34(8):1147–54.

Zucman-Rossi J, Jeannot E, Nhieu JT, Scoazec JY, Guettier C, Rebouissou S, et al. Genotype-phenotype correlation in hepatocellular adenoma: new classification and relationship with HCC. Hepatology. 2006;43(3):515–24.

Pancreas and Biliary Tract

8

Fan Lin, Haiyan Liu, and Jun Zhang

Summary of Pearls and Pitfalls

- Clinical information such as age, sex, location of a lesion, solid versus cystic, and serum tumor markers, should be taken into consideration.
- Well-differentiated adenocarcinoma of the pancreas may only show subtle cytological atypia; therefore, variation of nuclear sizes (4:1 ratio), loss of nuclear polarity, and nuclear membrane irregularities are the key criteria to make a diagnosis.
- Gastrointestinal or mesothelial cell contamination should be excluded before a diagnosis of mucin-producing tumor or well-differentiated adenocarcinoma is rendered.
- Some pancreatic neuroendocrine neoplasms may show prominent nucleoli and focal significant nuclear atypia, which may mislead one to call it adenocarcinoma or even poorly differentiated carcinoma.
- Aspirate from an intraductal papillary mucinous neoplasm (IPMN) or mucinous cystic neoplasm (MCN) may contain mainly thick mucinous material and few benign-appearing columnar epithelial cells.
- Serous cystadenoma may contain only a few groups of benign-appearing epithelial cells in a clear, watery background or bloody background with hemosiderin-laden macrophages; correlation with a radiological finding is important.
- In addition to pancreatitis, acute inflammatory cells are frequently seen in IPMN, MCN, and high-grade ductal adenocarcinoma.
- When a markedly cellular specimen with a spectrum from bland to high-grade nuclear atypia is present, a mucin-producing cystic neoplasm, especially an IPMN, should be considered.
- When a markedly cellular specimen with frankly malignant cells and many single malignant cells and no mucin in the background is present, a metastasis such as a lung or breast primary should be excluded.
- Cellblock preparation in conjunction with appropriate immunostains is useful in assisting diagnosis of a difficult case.
- von Hippel gene product (pVHL), S100P, and maspin are a panel of useful immunomarkers to confirm a diagnosis of well-differentiated adenocarcinoma in cellblock and small tissue core biopsy specimens, but caution should be taken since a mucin-containing cystic neoplasm will demonstrate a similar staining profile. Additionally, gastric contamination will also show positivity for S100P and maspin, and duodenal mucosa will show weakly positive for maspin.
- Carcinoembryonic antigen (CEA), mucin (MUC)5 AC, p53, DPC4/SMAD4, and insulin-like growth factor 2 mRNA-binding protein 3 (IMP3)(K homology domain containing protein overexpressed in cancer [KOC]) are also helpful immunomarkers in confirming the diagnosis of adenocarcinoma. Strong immunoreactivity for three of these markers (p53, CEA, IMP3) is usually not observed in gastric and duodenal contaminants.
- Cytokeratin (CK)7 is usually strongly positive in an MCN/IPMN of the pancreas; in contrast, gastric and duodenal mucosal contamination tends to be negative or only very focally positive for CK7.
- IPMNs and MCNs are indistinguishable on fine needle aspiration (FNA) samples. This is because the subepithelial ovarian stroma of an MCN is unlikely to be sampled or recognizable on smears or cellblocks.

© Springer International Publishing AG 2018
F. Lin et al., *Handbook of Practical Fine Needle Aspiration and Small Tissue Biopsies*, DOI 10.1007/978-3-319-57386-1_8

Common Pancreatic Lesions in the 2010 World Health Organization (WHO) Classification, Modified[1]

I. Epithelial neoplasms
   A. Exocrine neoplasms
      1. Acinar cell cystadenoma
      2. Microcystic serous cystadenoma
      3. MCNs, with low-, intermediate-, or high-grade dysplasia
      4. IPMNs with low-, intermediate, or high-grade dysplasia
      5. Intraductal tubulopapillary neoplasm
      6. Pancreatic intraepithelial neoplasia, grade 3 (PanIN-3)
      7. Invasive ductal adenocarcinoma
         (a) Tubular adenocarcinoma
         (b) Adenosquamous carcinoma
         (c) Colloid carcinoma (CC, mucinous noncystic carcinoma)
         (d) Hepatoid carcinoma
         (e) Medullary carcinoma
         (f) Signet ring cell carcinoma
         (g) Undifferentiated carcinoma
         (h) Undifferentiated carcinoma with osteoclast-like giant cells
      8. Acinar cell carcinoma
      9. Mixed carcinoma with two or three components (acinar, neuroendocrine, and ductal)
      10. Pancreatoblastoma
      11. Solid-pseudopapillary neoplasm
      12. Serous cystadenocarcinoma
   B. Neuroendocrine neoplasms
      Neuroendocrine microadenoma (<0.5 cm)
      Neuroendocrine tumor (NET)
         Nonfunctional NET, grade I and grade II
         Functional NET
      Neuroendocrine carcinoma (NEC)
         Large cell NEC
         Small cell NEC
II. Nonneoplastic lesions
   A. Chronic pancreatitis
   B. Pseudocyst
   C. Autoimmune pancreatitis (lymphoplasmacytic sclerosing pancreatitis)
   D. Lymphoepithelial cyst
III. Metastasis and Rare Lesions

[1]Modified with permission from Bosman FT, Carneiro F, Hruban RH, and Theise ND, editors. WHO Classification of Tumours of the Digestive System. 4th ed. Lyon, France: IARC Press; 2010.

Normal Cytology of the Pancreas

- Normal pancreas consists of a dominant exocrine component and small endocrine component. The exocrine component is composed of approximately 80% acini and a minor component of ductal cells as shown in Fig. 8.1.
- Acinar cells are present in small, cohesive groups, or singly, and commonly with naked nuclei in the background. The nuclei are eccentrically located, round to ovoid, about the size of a red blood cell, with evenly distributed nuclear chromatin, smooth nuclear contours, and distinct nucleoli. Prominent nucleoli may be present in some acinar cells. The acinar cells usually have well-defined cell borders and moderate to abundant granular cytoplasm. Clear or vacuolated cytoplasm secondary to degeneration may be seen. Normal acinar cells are illustrated in Fig. 8.2.
- The ductal cells tend to form two-dimensional sheet of variable sizes, with a scant amount of cytoplasm and

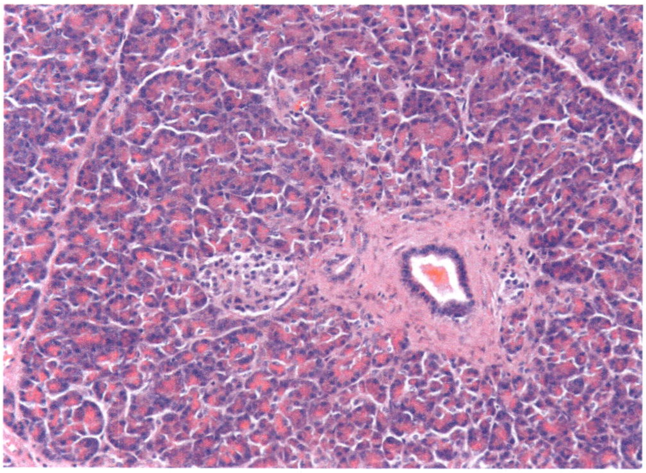

Fig. 8.1 Histological section of normal pancreatic tissue. H&E stain

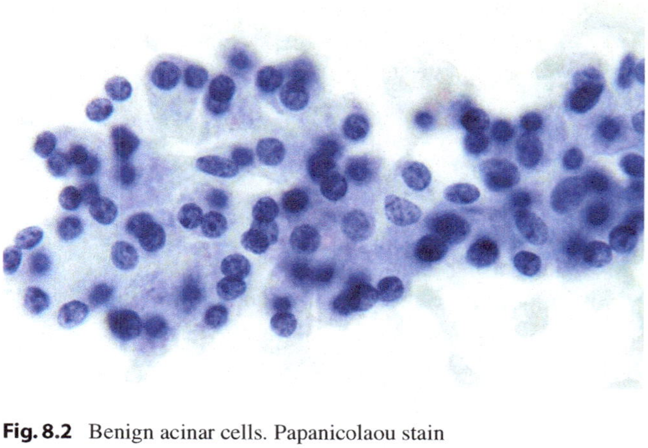

Fig. 8.2 Benign acinar cells. Papanicolaou stain

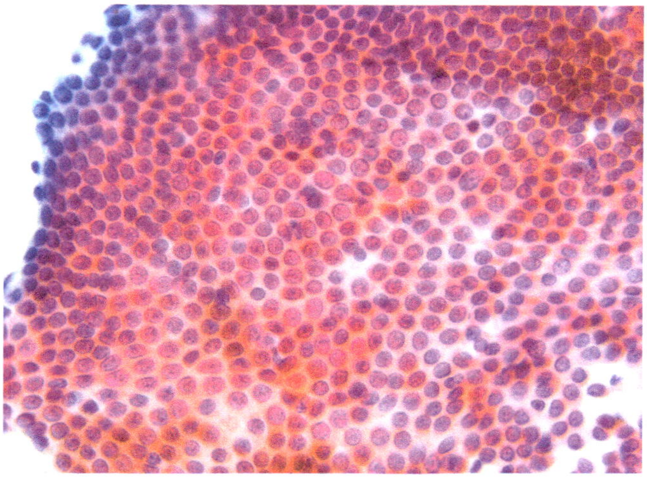

Fig. 8.3 Benign ductal cells. Cohesive, flat sheet of benign ductal cells with small, uniform nuclei and smooth nuclear membranes. Note that folding of the ductal epithelium is present. Papanicolaou stain

poorly defined cytoplasmic borders. The cell borders may be prominent, forming an orderly honeycomb appearance. The nuclei are round to ovoid, the same size or slightly large than one red blood cell, with evenly distributed nuclear chromatin, smooth nuclear membranes, and indistinct nucleoli. Figure 8.3 illustrates normal ductal cells.

- Islet cells are usually not present or not easily recognizable in fine needle aspiration biopsy (FNAB) smears. They form small, loosely cohesive clusters or may be present singly. The nuclei are small, round, with fine, granular chromatin and small to indistinct nucleoli.
- Mesothelial cells, endothelial cells, hepatocytes, and small intestinal and gastric glandular cells may be seen in FNAB smears. Benign glandular epithelium with goblet cells and gastric glandular epithelial cells usually seen in an endoscopic ultrasound-guided (EUS)-FNA sample is shown in Fig. 8.4a–h.

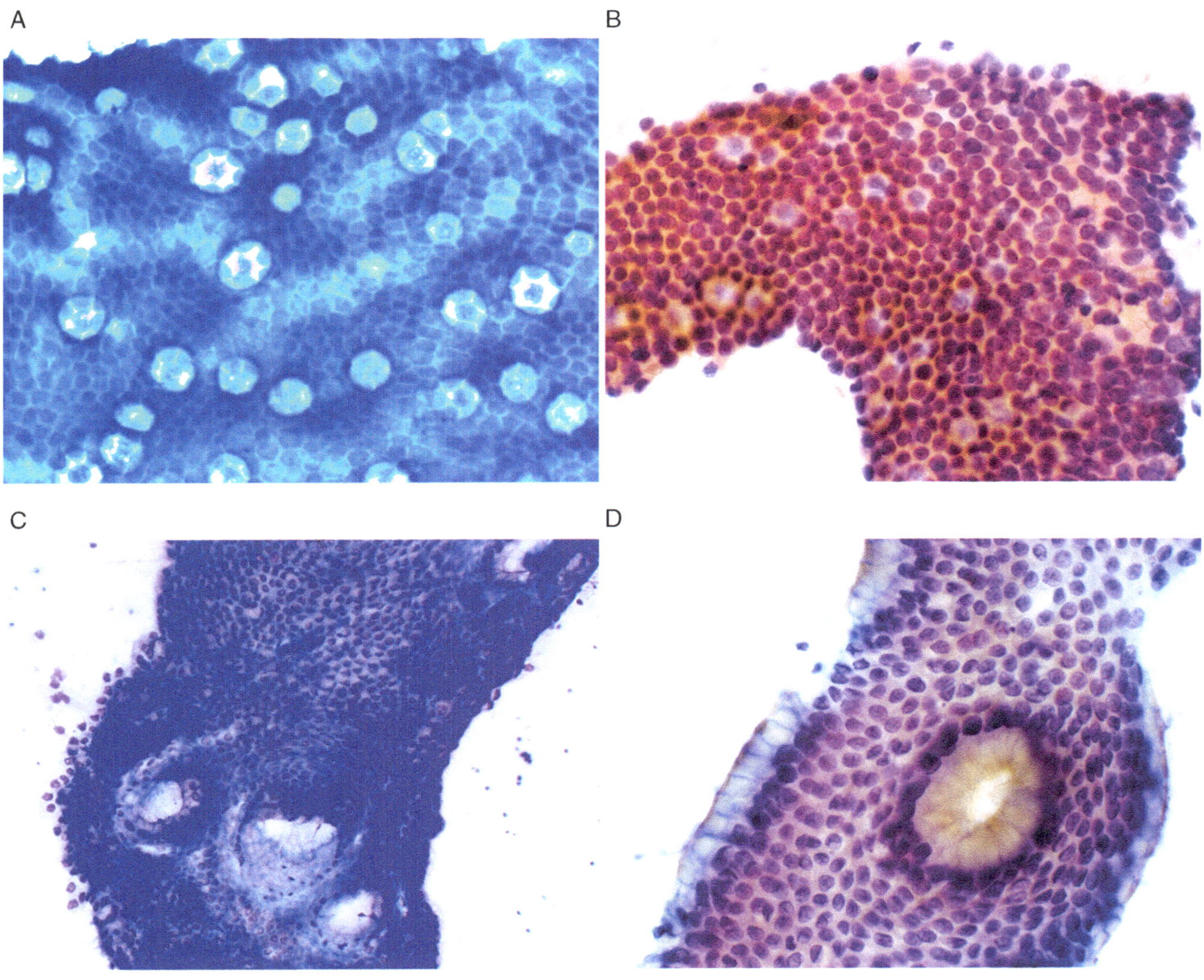

Fig. 8.4 Benign glandular epithelium with many mucin-containing goblet cells (**a**, **b**), gastric foveolar epithelium (**c–e**), gastric body mucosa (**f**), and gastric mucosa on cellblock sections (**g**, **h**) are frequently present in an EUS-guided FNAB specimen

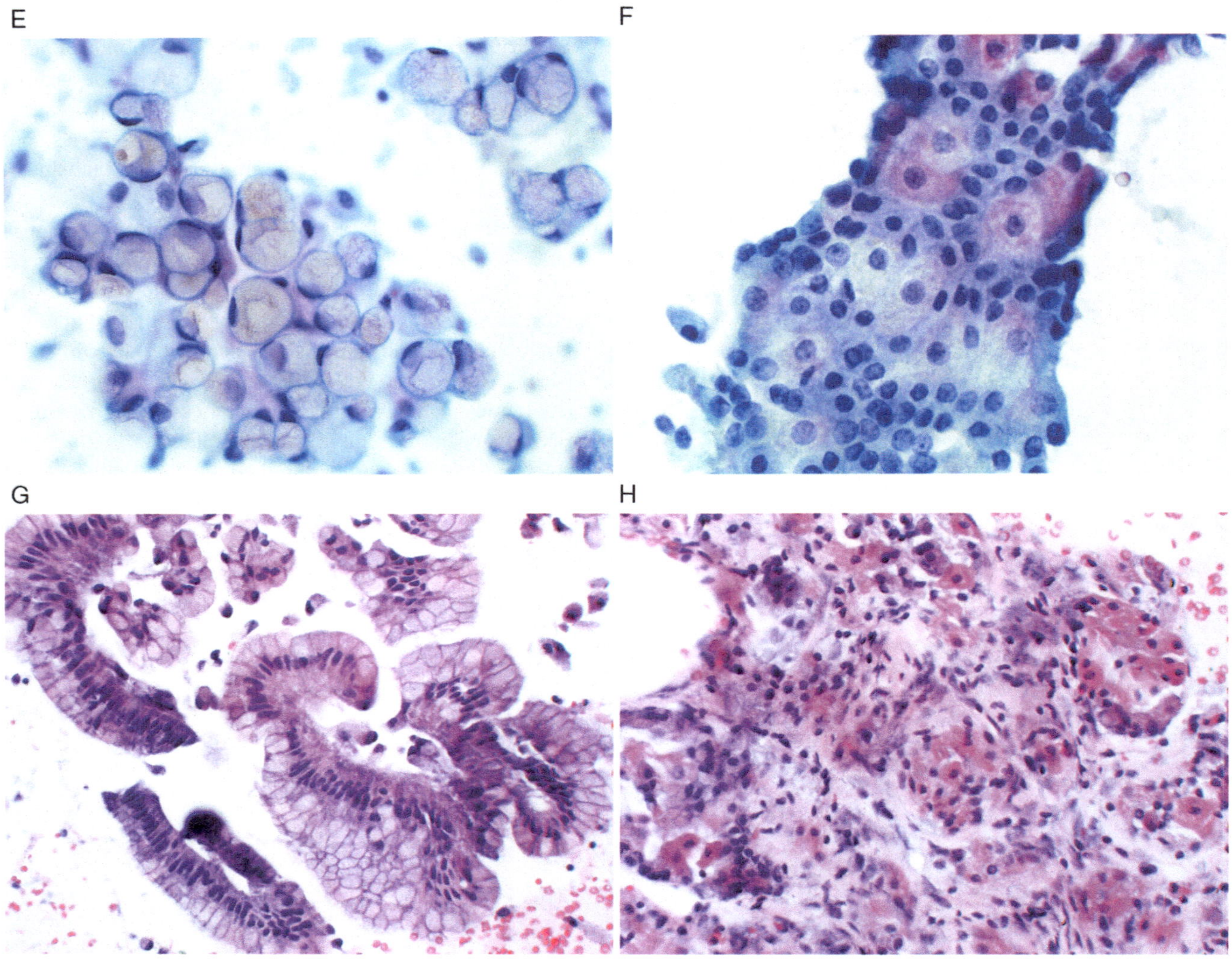

Fig. 8.4 (continued)

Chronic Pancreatitis

Key Clinical Features

- Obstructive jaundice, pain, and weight loss may be present.

Key Radiological Findings

- A mass lesion or diffuse involvement of the pancreas may be seen radiographically.

Major Cytologic Features

- Chronic inflammation, acinar atrophy, fibrosis, calcifications, ductal hyperplasia, and relatively increased numbers of islet cells.
- In the early stage, evidence of acute and chronic inflammation, fat necrosis, and granulation tissue may be the dominant features as shown in Fig. 8.5.
- In the late stage, due to an extensive acinar atrophy, the smear may be composed predominately of ductal epithelial cells, fibrosis, chronic inflammatory cells, and islet cells.
- If the inflammatory component is rich in lymphocytes, plasma cells, and eosinophils, lymphoplasmacytic sclerosing pancreatitis should be suspected.
- Squamous metaplasia has been described. Ductal epithelial cells associated with significant cytologic atypia may be present.
- Figure 8.6 shows a sheet of ductal cells with mild-moderate nuclear atypia. The nuclear atypia more frequently shows a combination of nuclear enlargement and prominent nucleoli. In contrast, marked anisonucleosis and/or nuclear membrane irregularity are rare findings.

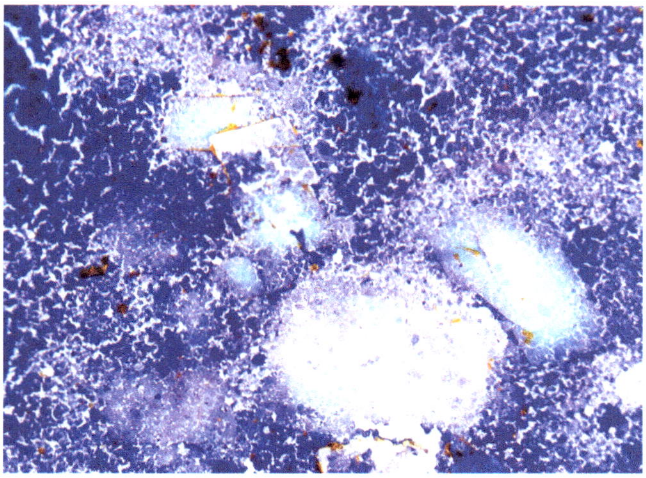

Fig. 8.5 Chronic pancreatitis

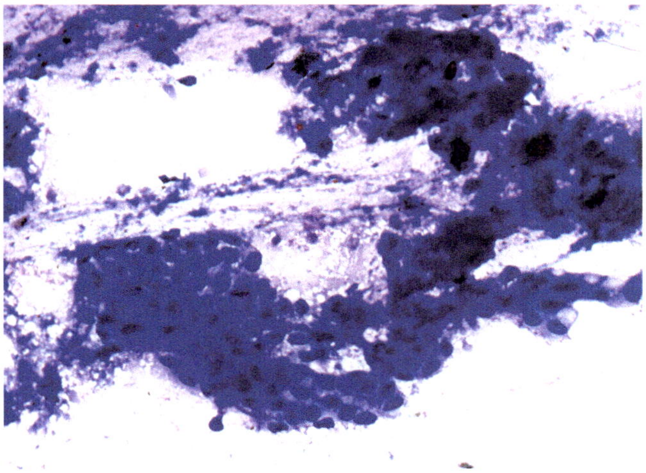

Fig. 8.6 Chronic pancreatitis with mild to moderate nuclear atypia. Diff-Quik stain

Differential Diagnosis

- Well-differentiated adenocarcinoma

Histology

- Depending on the stage of chronic pancreatitis, histology may show various degrees of perilobular and intralobular fibrosis, sclerosis, acinar atrophy, ductal proliferation, dilatation, squamous metaplasia, and chronic inflammation to include eosinophils and plasma cells. Langerhans' islets may show atrophy and distortion; conversely, it may show a marked proliferation of islet cells growing in small cords, clusters, and lobules. Perineurial extension of the proliferative islet cells can be seen, which may simulate a malignant process. An example of a marked proliferation of islet cells in a chronic pancreatitis adjacent to a ductal adenocarcinoma is shown in Fig. 8.7a, b. Immunohistochemical (IHC) stains have demonstrated the presence of all major types of islet cells in a case like this.
- In an autoimmune pancreatitis, the infiltrating plasma cells are predominately immunoglobulin G4 (IgG4)-positive plasma cells. An immunostain for IgG4 may be helpful in diagnosing a difficult case. It should be cautioned, however, that the presence of abundant IgG4-positive plasma cells does not preclude the diagnosis of pancreatic adenocarcinoma because in a small subset of pancreatic adenocarcinoma cases the cancer-adjacent tissue may show features of autoimmune pancreatitis. Examples of autoimmune pancreatitis with many IgG4-positive plasma cells are shown in Fig. 8.8a–c.

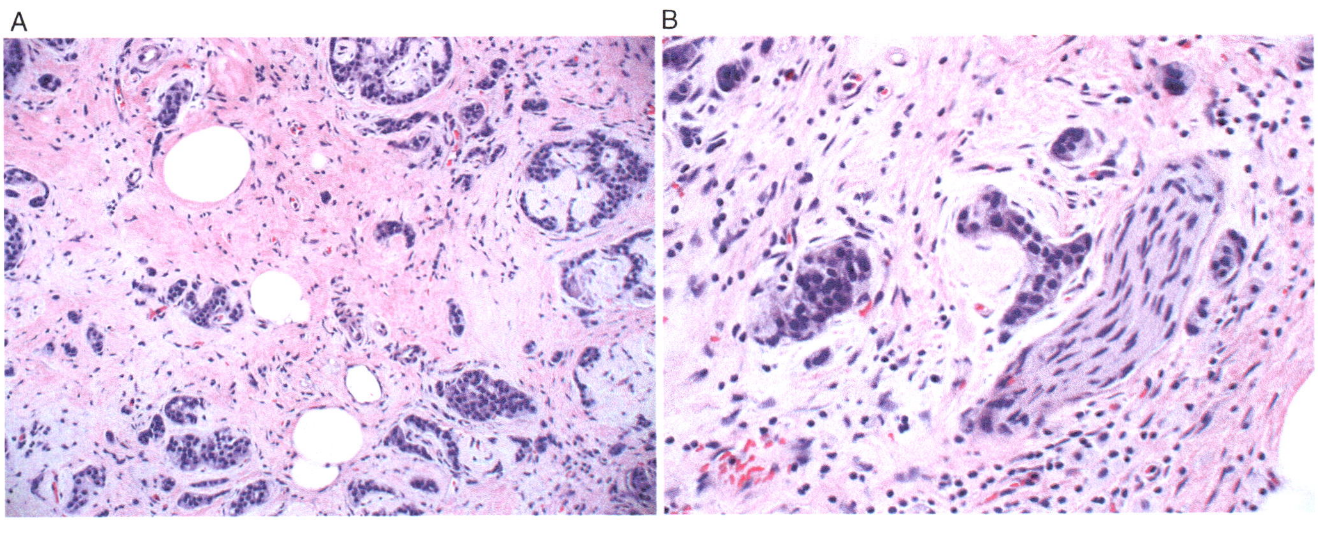

Fig. 8.7 Marked proliferation of islet cells in a case of chronic pancreatitis which may mimic a malignant process or a pancreatic neuroendocrine tumor

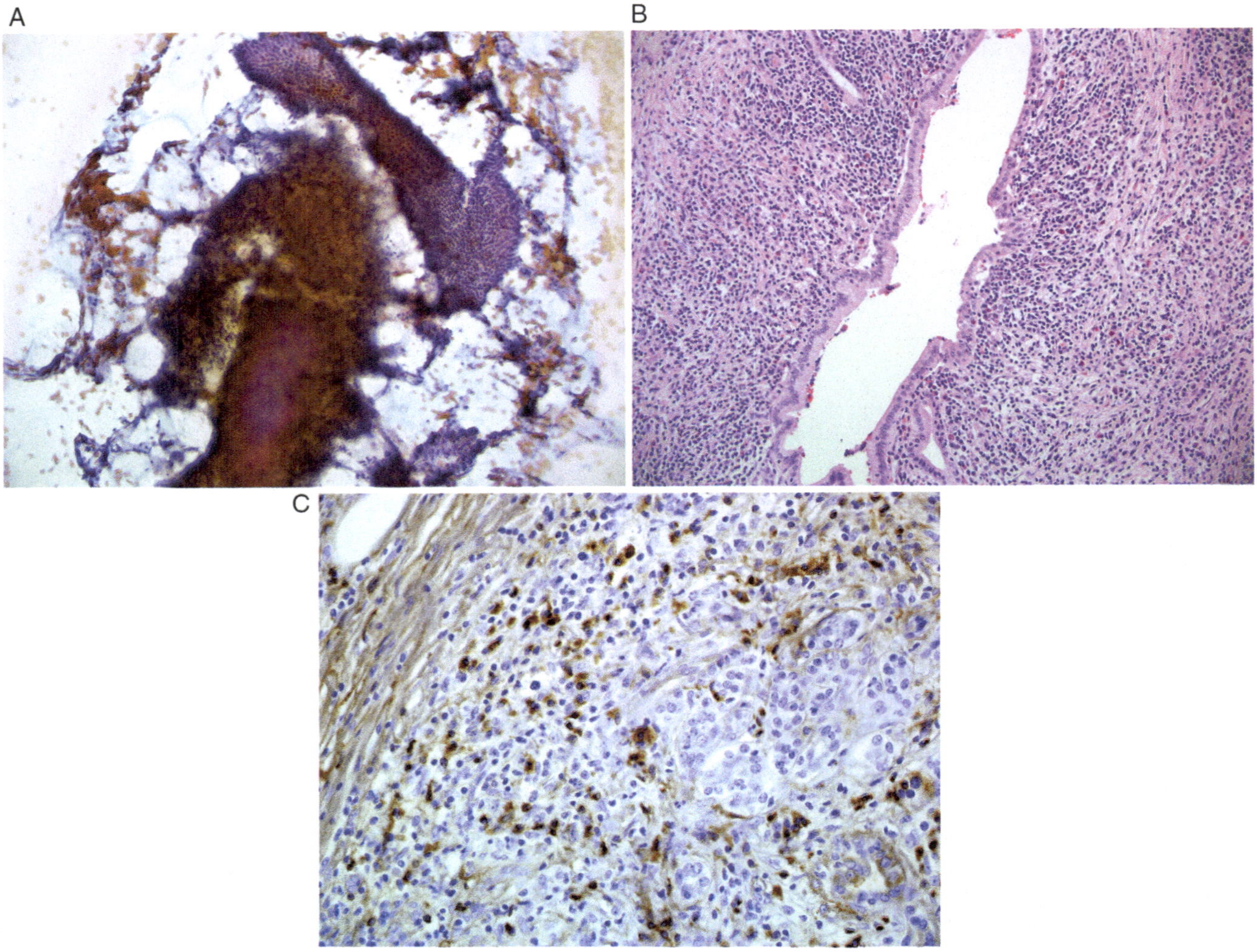

Fig. 8.8 Autoimmune pancreatitis on smear with groups of mildly atypical ductal cells, fibrous tissue, and inflammatory cells (**a**), histologic section (**b**) and many IgG4-positive plasma cells (**c**)

Immunohistochemistry

- Maspin and S100P have been shown to be positive in over 90% of ductal adenocarcinomas of the pancreas (with nuclear or both nuclear and cytoplasmic staining) and negative in normal ducts and reactive ducts (lack of nuclear staining).
- Immunostain for pVHL is positive in benign and reactive pancreatic ducts and negative in nearly 100% of ductal adenocarcinomas.
- CEA, CK17, and MUC5AC are usually negative in normal and reactive ducts, and the expression of these three markers in ductal adenocarcinomas was reported as approximately 80%, 60%, and 60%, respectively.
- Strong and diffuse p53 positivity was reported in approximately 50% of ductal carcinomas and usually negative or only weakly positive in benign/reactive ducts.
- Clusterin, mesothelin, and prostate stem cell antigen (PSCA) may provide some valuable information. All three markers are much more frequently positive in adenocarcinomas than in reactive ducts.

Well-Differentiated Ductal Adenocarcinoma

Key Clinical Features

- Epigastric pain radiating to the back, painless jaundice, weight loss, and other general symptoms
- The average sensitivity of computed tomography (CT)-guided FNAB and EUS-guided FNAB of the pancreas is about 80–90%, and specificity approaches 100%.
- The main advantages of EUS-guided over CT-guided FNAB are the ability to detect smaller lesions, to identify

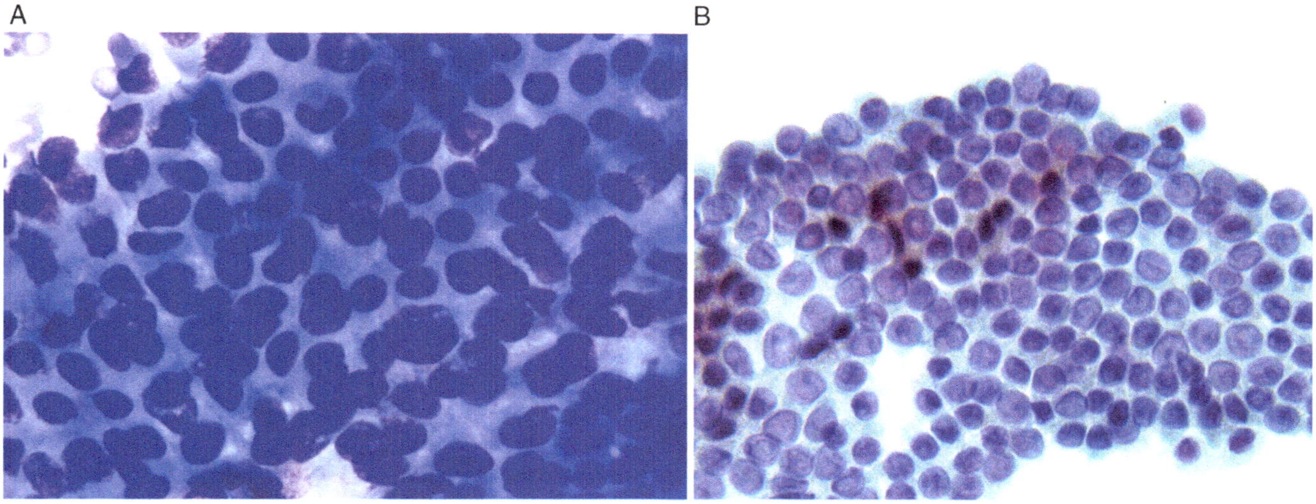

Fig. 8.9 Well-differentiated adenocarcinoma. Nuclear enlargement, nuclear crowding/loss polarity, anisonucleosis, and nuclear membrane irregularities. Papanicolaou stain, ×600

a possible local invasion of the tumor, and to simultaneously sample the adjacent lymph node for cancer staging.

Key Radiological Findings

- Hypointense masses on magnetic resonance imaging (MRI) and hypodense masses on CT scans

Major Cytologic Features (Fig. 8.9a, b)

- Anisonucleosis (variation in nuclear size of greater than a 4:1 ration within an epithelial group)
- Nuclear membrane irregularity
- Nuclear crowding/overlapping/three-dimensionality
- Nuclear enlargement (if more than two red blood cells)

Minor Cytologic Features

- Gap versus confluent cell spacing
- Hyperchromasia
- Macronucleoli
- Mitosis
- Chromatin clearing
- Necrosis
- Single malignant cells

Differential Diagnosis

- Chronic pancreatitis/autoimmune pancreatitis
- Acinar cell carcinoma
- Pancreatic neuroendocrine neoplasm
- Solid-pseudopapillary neoplasm of the pancreas
- Metastasis

Histology

- Haphazardly arranged infiltrating duct-like structures; small, medium-sized, or large duct variant
- Duct-like structures with angular or irregular contours
- Desmoplastic stroma with mucin production
- Perineural and vascular invasion
- Cytologic bland duct-like structures adjacent to muscular vessels
- Ruptured and incomplete ducts
- Single atypical cells

Figure 8.10a–e shows ductal adenocarcinoma with intensive desmoplastic stromal reaction (a), large duct type (b), perineural invasion (c), atypical glands adjacent to muscular vessels (d), and single malignant cells (e).

Immunohistochemistry

- Upregulation of maspin and S100P and downregulation of pVHL have been shown to be the highly sensitive and specific markers for diagnosis of adenocarcinoma of the pancreas. Examples are shown in Fig. 8.11 (double immunostaining of S100P and pVHL) and Fig. 8.12 (double immunostaining of maspin and pVHL).
- Expression IMP3 (KOC) has been demonstrated in over 90% of ductal adenocarcinomas; it is negative/very weakly positive in normal ductal epithelium and chronic pancreatitis.
- SMAD4/DPC4 is negative in 55% of adenocarcinomas.
- Kirsten rat sarcoma viral oncogene homolog (K-ras) gene mutation was detected in 43–77% of ductal adenocarcinomas of the pancreas in FNAB specimens but was rarely positive in benign conditions.

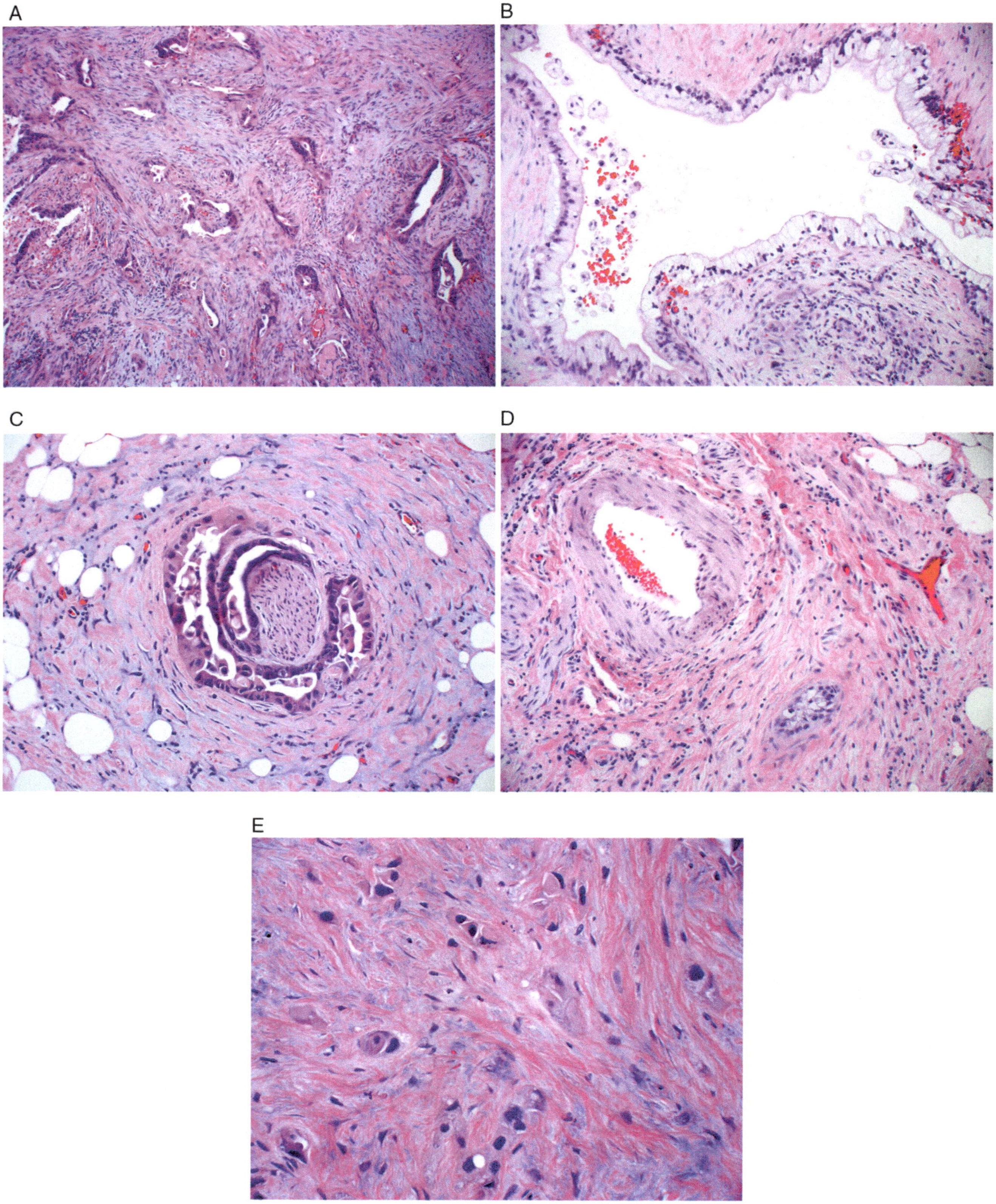

Fig. 8.10 Ductal adenocarcinoma with intensive desmoplastic stromal reaction (**a**), large-duct type (**b**), perineural invasion (**c**), atypical glands adjacent to muscular vessels (**d**), and single malignant cells (**e**)

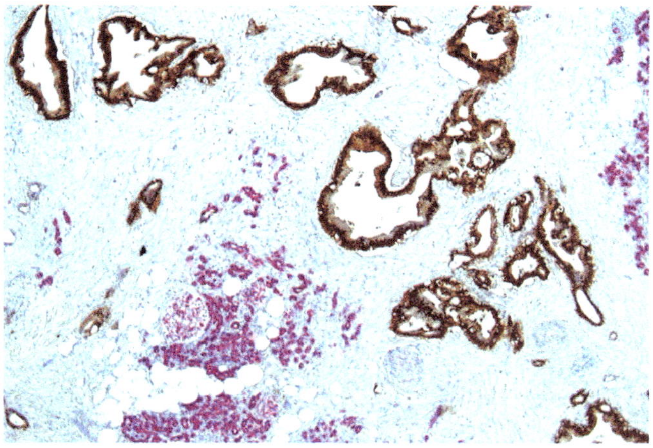

Fig. 8.11 Double immunostaining of pVHL and S100P in a case of adenocarcinoma. Carcinoma is positive for S100P (*brown*) and normal duct and acinar cells are positive for pVHL (*red*)

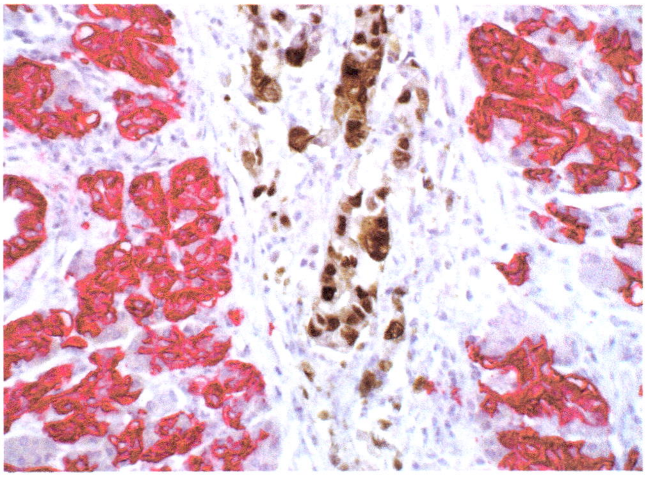

Fig. 8.12 Double immunostaining of pVHL and maspin in a case of adenocarcinoma. Carcinoma is positive for maspin (*brown*) and normal duct and acinar cells are positive for pVHL (*red*)

- MUC1 has been shown to be positive in the majority of ductal adenocarcinomas and rarely positive in chronic pancreatitis and benign conditions in FNAB specimens.
- A strong and diffuse expression of claudin 4 protein predominately in a membranous distribution in over 90% of ductal adenocarcinomas of the pancreas, metastatic pancreatic adenocarcinomas, and PanINs. In contrast, most benign ductal epithelium showed focal and weak immunoreactivity.
- Table 8.1 summarizes the useful IHC markers for the differential diagnosis between pancreatic ductal adenocarcinoma and chronic pancreatitis. Examples of staining for other IHC markers are shown in Fig. 8.13a–d: a (IMP3), b (DPC4/SMAD4), c (p53), and d (MUC5AC).

Table 8.1 Useful immunomarkers for differential diagnosis between pancreatic ductal adenocarcinoma and chronic pancreatitis

Markers	Adenocarcinoma	Chronic pancreatitis
pVHL	Negative	Positive
Maspin	>90% positive	Negative
S100P	>90% positive	Negative or cytoplasmic staining
IMP3	>80% positive	Negative
MUC5AC	60% positive	Negative
P53	50% diffusely and strongly positive	Weak or negative
DPC4/SMAD4	50% loss	Positive

Treatment and Prognosis

- 5-year survival rate is less than 5%. Most patients die within 1 year following the diagnosis.

Moderately and Poorly Differentiated Adenocarcinoma

- In general, a diagnosis of moderately and poorly differentiated adenocarcinoma tends to be straightforward on both FNA and tissue biopsy specimens.
- Abnormal cytologic features are more pronounced than in well-differentiated adenocarcinoma.
- In addition to marked nuclear pleomorphism and nuclear membrane irregularities, single malignant cells, tumor necrosis, mitoses, and prominent nucleoli are frequently present. Figure 8.14a, b show examples of moderately and poorly differentiated adenocarcinoma, respectively.

Adenosquamous Carcinoma

- Adenosquamous carcinoma accounts for approximately 1–4% of all exocrine malignant tumors of the pancreas.
- Pure squamous cell carcinoma of the pancreas is very rare. A metastasis such as from the lung should be excluded first.
- An FNAB smear generally shows moderate to high cellularity with a dual population of malignant squamous and glandular epithelial cells.
- Tumor necrosis frequently presents. Rare cytoplasmic vacuoles may be the only evidence of glandular differentiation. Keratin pearls may be present. Keratinization may be absent; instead, the tumor cells display dense cytoplasm. Sometimes malignant squamous cells become a predominant cell population.

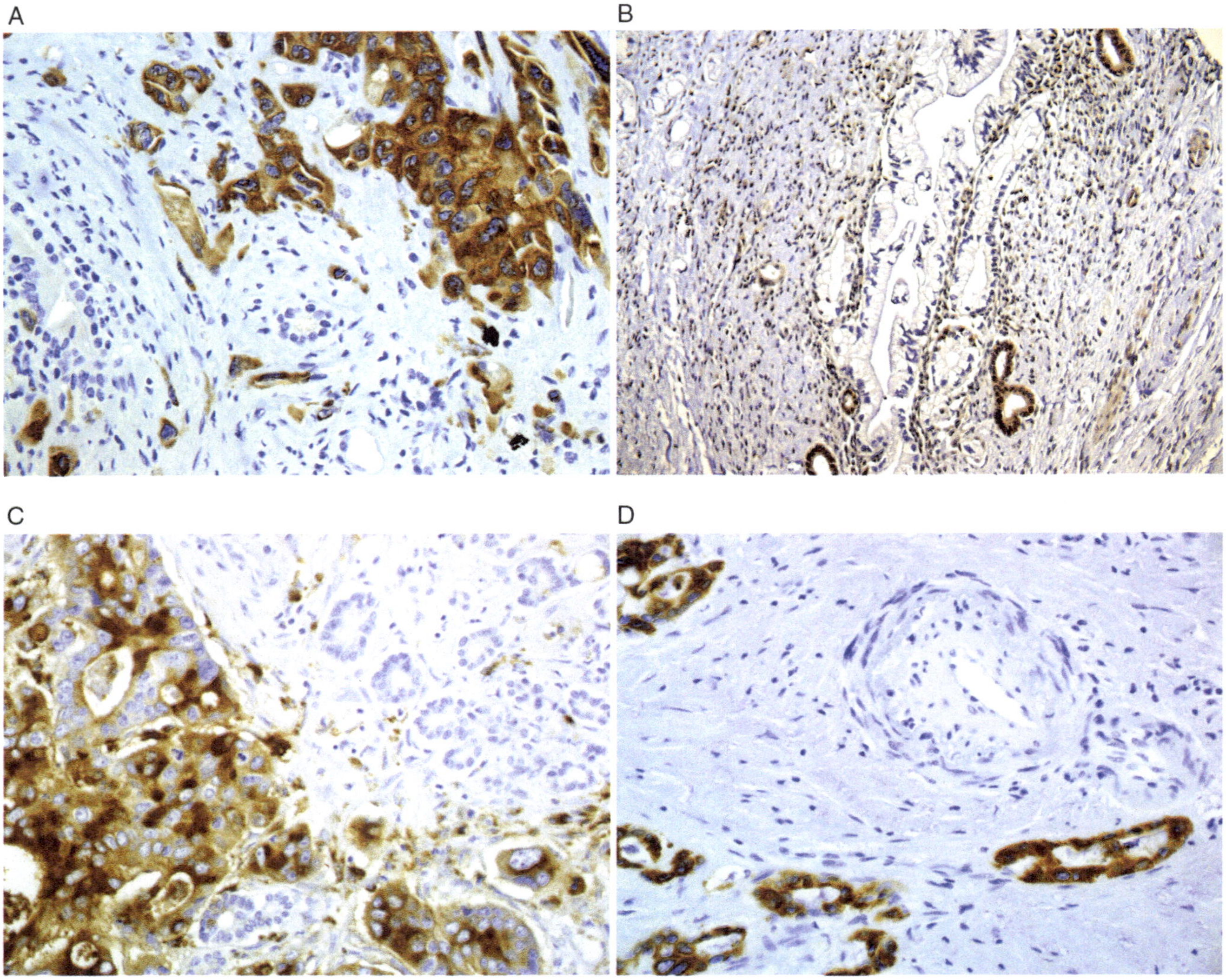

Fig. 8.13 Other useful immunohistochemical markers in ductal adenocarcinoma such as IMP3 (**a**), loss of DPC4/SMAD4 (**b**), monoclonalCEA (**c**), and MUC5AC (**d**)

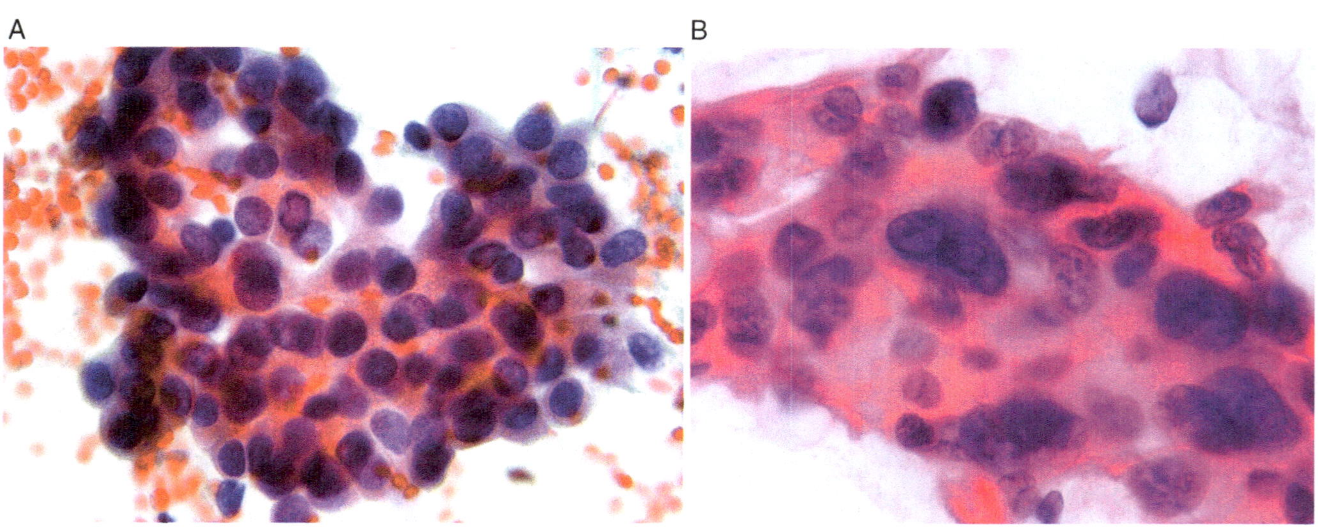

Fig. 8.14 Moderately differentiated adenocarcinoma (**a**) and poorly differentiated adenocarcinoma (**b**). Papanicolaou stain

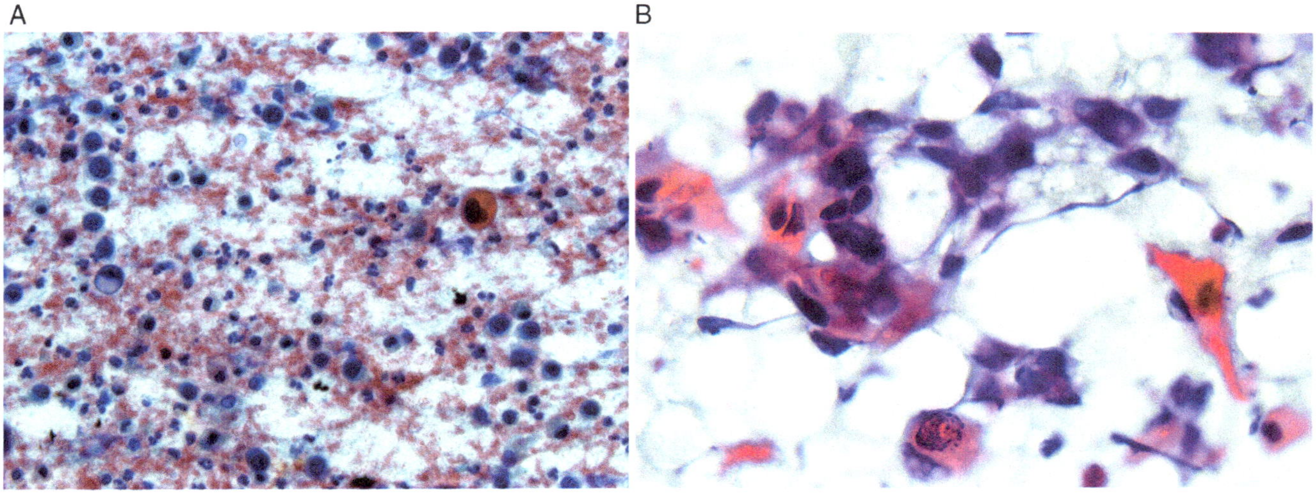

Fig. 8.15 Adenosquamous carcinoma. Intracytoplasmic mucin vacuoles in (**a**) and malignant keratinizing squamous cells in (**b**). Papanicolaou stain, ×600

- However, careful search may find signet ringlike glandular cells. Figure 8.15a, b reveal some characteristic cytologic features of adenosquamous carcinoma.

Histology

- Histologically, it shows both gland-forming adenocarcinoma with intracellular/extracellular mucin and squamous differentiation of prominent intercellular junctions and varying degrees of keratinization.
- Immunohistochemically, a tumor is frequently negative for p16 and SMAD4/DPC4 with strong p53 expression.
- Most cases show K-ras mutation at codon 12.

Colloid Carcinoma (CC)

- CC, mucinous noncystic carcinoma, characterized by stromal mucinous nodules containing scant malignant epithelial cells that is morphologically similar to CC of the breast and skin, had been previously regarded as a histologic variant of ductal adenocarcinoma as shown in Fig. 8.16a, b.
- Mean age of CC is 61 without gender predominance.
- The average size of the tumor at the time of diagnosis is 6.0 cm.
- Approximately half of the cases are associated with an IPMN, intestinal type.
- Studies of molecular phenotypes of CC show expression of MUC2 and lack of mutation of K-ras gene. In contrast, ductal adenocarcinoma of the pancreas is usually positive for MUC1 and associated with k-ras gene mutation in codon 12. See Fig. 8.17a, b.
- More recently, Caudal type homeobox 2 (CDX2) is much more frequently positive in CC than in ductal adenocarcinoma. Conversely, galactin 3 displayed a strong positivity in the majority of ductal adenocarcinoma but only positive in 15–20% of CC.
- Most importantly, the clinical course of CC appears to be significantly better than that of conventional ductal adenocarcinoma of the pancreas, with a 5-year survival rate of 55% in CC vs. 5% in ductal adenocarcinoma of the pancreas.

Other Variants of Ductal Carcinoma

- These include medullary carcinoma, hepatoid carcinoma, undifferentiated (anaplastic) carcinoma, signet ring cell carcinoma, and mixed ductal-endocrine carcinoma.
- An example of medullary carcinoma of the pancreas is shown in Figs. 8.18a, b and 8.19a, b. Medullary carcinoma of the pancreas has a similar morphology to medullary carcinoma of the colon and other organs characterized by poor differentiation with limited gland formation, syncytial growth pattern, and pushing growth border with lymphoid infiltration. Most medullary carcinomas are microsatellite unstable (MSI +) and wild type for K-ras gene. Immunostains demonstrate loss of one or two of the mismatch repair (MMR) proteins (MutL homolog 1 [MLH1], postmeiotic segregation increased 2 [PMS2], MutS protein homolog 2 [MSH2], and MutS protein homolog 6 [MSH6]). Despite poor differentiation, the prognosis for patients with a medullary carcinoma is better than ductal adenocarcinoma.

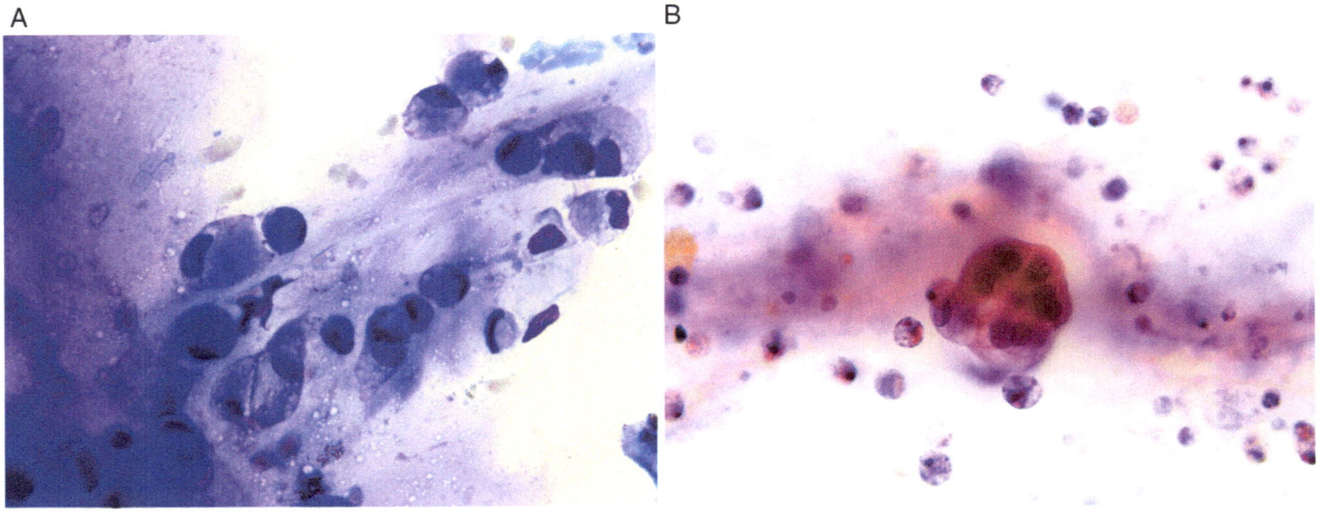

Fig. 8.16 (**a**, **b**) Colloid carcinoma with groups of atypical epithelial cells in the background of thick mucin

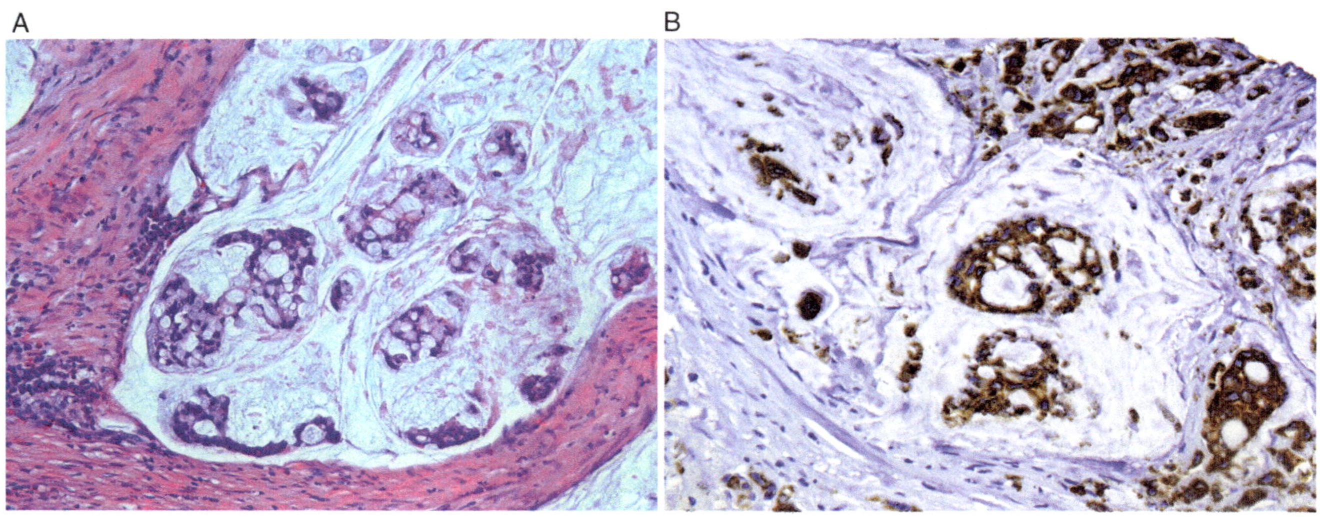

Fig. 8.17 (**a**, **b**) Histological section of colloid carcinoma (**a**) and tumor cells are positive for MUC2 (B) which is usually negative in ductal/tubular adenocarcinoma

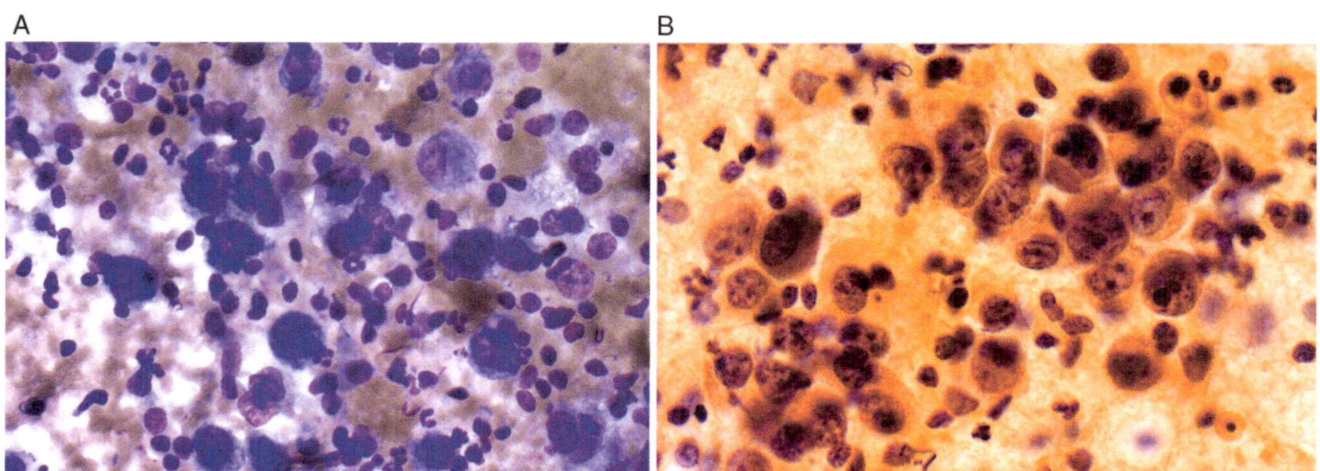

Fig. 8.18 (**a**, **b**) Medullary carcinoma with large tumor cells singly or in small clusters in the background of numerous lymphoid cells

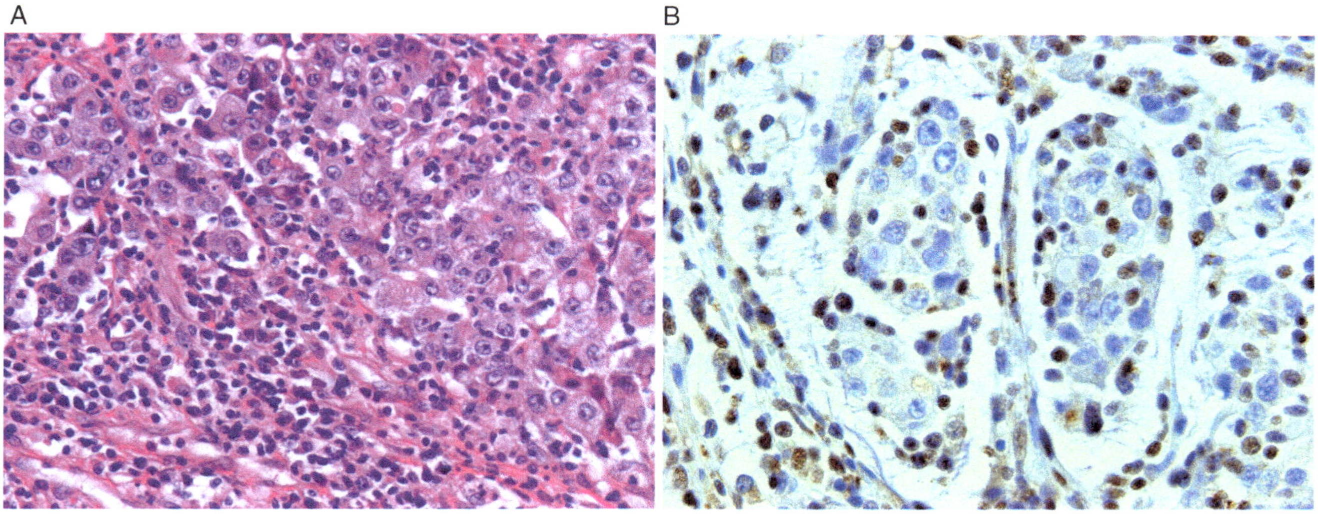

Fig. 8.19 Histological section of medullary carcinoma (**a**) and immunostain showing loss of MSH2 expression on tumor cells with positive internal control (**b**)

Pancreatic Neuroendocrine Neoplasms

Key Clinical Features

- Pancreatic neuroendocrine neoplasms are relatively rare tumors, accounting for less than 5% of all pancreatic neoplasms.
- The neoplasms frequently occur in adults and rarely in children.
- The majority of pancreatic neuroendocrine neoplasms are functional. Nonfunctional tumors account for 15–30% of reported cases.
- In the new WHO classification (2010), pancreatic neuroendocrine neoplasms encompass a spectrum of lesions, including microadenoma (<0.5 cm); NET, grade I, and grade II; and NEC, large cell NEC and small cell NEC. The proposed grading is based on counting mitoses or Ki-67 index as summarized in Table 8.2. The grading system requires mitotic count in at least 50 high-power fields (HPFs) and Ki67 index using the MIB antibody as a percentage of 500–2000 tumor cells counted in the areas of strongest nuclear labelling. If a grade differs for mitotic count compared with Ki67 index, it is suggested the higher grade be assumed.

Table 8.2 Pancreatic neuroendocrine neoplasms classified based on mitotic rates and Ki67 proliferative index

Grade	Mitotic count	Ki67 index
NET, grade 1	< 2/per 10 HPF	≤ 2% Ki67 index
NET, grade 2	2–20/per 10 HPF	3–20% Ki67 index
NEC, grade 3	>20/per 10 HPF	>20% Ki67 index

- Caution should be taken in grading a NET on a cellblock preparation or a small tissue biopsy specimen. An accurate grading can be even more challenging in the presence of a large amount of lymphoid cells/inflammatory cells.
- Our experience shows that most NECs, especially small cell carcinomas, have a greater than 50% Ki67 index. Caution should be taken when dealing with a small cell carcinoma/high-grade NEC with a Ki67 index marginally over 20% on cytologic specimens.

Key Radiological Findings

- CT scans reveal solid, circumscribed, enhanced masses. Cystic change and calcification may occur.

Major Cytologic Findings

- Hypercellular smears with a mixture of loosely cohesive clusters and single cells as shown in Figs. 8.20a, b and 8.21a–c. Acinar-like formation, perivascular tumor growth, or trabecular pattern can be seen.
- The neoplastic cells are typically monotonous, with focal nuclear pleomorphism. Individual cells with well-defined cytoplasm or even plasmacytoid appearance are common findings.
- The nuclei tend to be round to ovoid with smooth nuclear membrane and salt-and-pepper nuclear chromatin pattern. Binucleated and multinucleated neoplastic cells are usually seen.

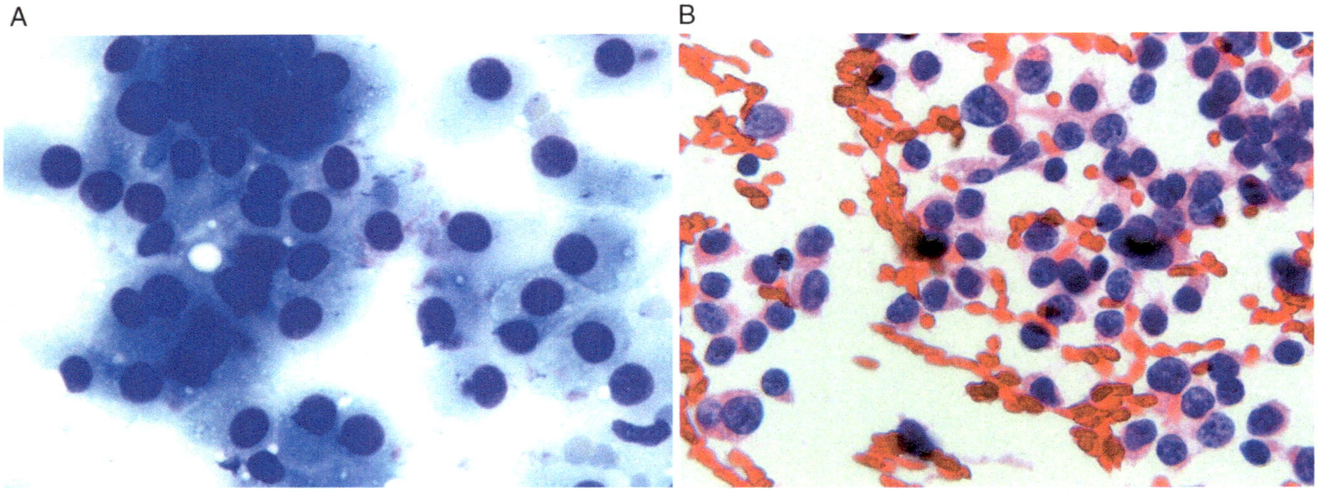

Fig. 8.20 (**a**, **b**) Pancreatic endocrine neoplasm. Loosely cohesive clusters and single cells with salt-pepper nuclear chromatin pattern, abundant cytoplasm, and plasmacytoid appearance. Papanicolaou stain

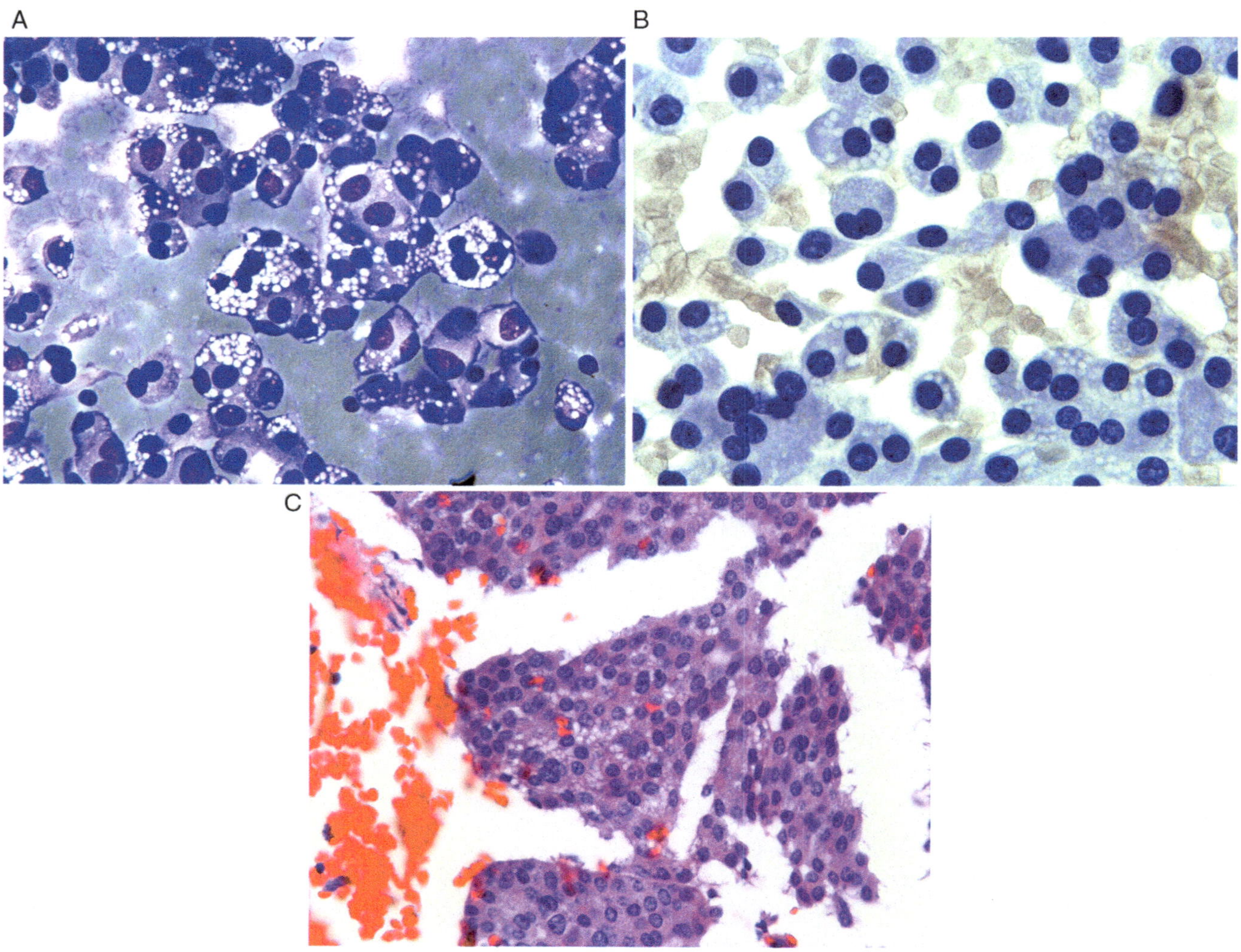

Fig. 8.21 Pancreatic neuroendocrine tumor with prominent cytoplasmic vacuoles and prominent nucleoli in some tumor cells (**a**, **b**) and on cell-block section (**c**)

- In less differentiated tumors, predominant single cells with high nuclear-to-cytoplasmic ratio, prominent nucleoli, and mitoses are characteristic features.
- Pancreatic NEC is relatively rare and shows cytologic features similar to high-grade NECs in other organs.

Differential Diagnosis

- Acinar cell carcinoma
- Ductal adenocarcinoma
- Solid-pseudopapillary tumor (SPT)
- Islet cell hyperplasia

Histology

- Various histologic patterns such as nesting, trabecular, glandular, gyriform, tubuloacinar, and pseudorosette arrangements.
- Granular amphophilic to eosinophilic granular cytoplasm, but can be clear, lipid-rich, oncocytic, or have "rhabdoid" features.
- Salt-and-pepper nuclear chromatin frequently with distinct or even prominent nucleolus.
- Foci of nuclear pleomorphism can be seen.
- Tumor necrosis is infrequent and often limited.
- Amyloid deposition and calcification can be present.
- In NEC, prominent nuclear atypia, necrosis, a high Ki67 index (>20%), and >20/10 HPFs mitotic rates. Primary small cell carcinoma of the pancreas can be positive for thyroid transcription factor 1 (TTF1).
- Figure 8.22a, b highlights a lipid-rich variant.

Immunohistochemistry

- Positive for chromogranin (over 90%) and synaptophysin (100%).
- Cluster of differentiation (CD)56 is the most sensitive neuroendocrine marker for lung small cell carcinoma, which is only positive in approximately 60% of pancreatic NETs.
- CK7 and CK20 are frequently negative.
- Positive for progesterone receptors (PR, 60%), paired box gene (PAX)8 (60%, polyclonal antibody), islet-1(82%), and pancreas/duodenum homeobox-1 (PDX-1, 72%). None of these markers is entirely specific for a pancreatic NET.
- An example of pancreatic NET positive for PR, PAX8, and islet-1 is shown in Fig. 8.23a–d.

Indication of Malignancy

- Reliable histological criteria, as well as cytologic criteria, to predict the malignant potential are not available.
- Tumor necrosis is a good indicator for malignancy. The unequivocal indicators for malignancy are metastasis and invasion of adjacent organs.
- Quantitative fluorescence in situ hybridization (FISH) technique indicates that telomere shortening is a feature of malignant tumor.
- The term neuroendocrine carcinoma is reserved for small cell carcinoma or large NEC only.

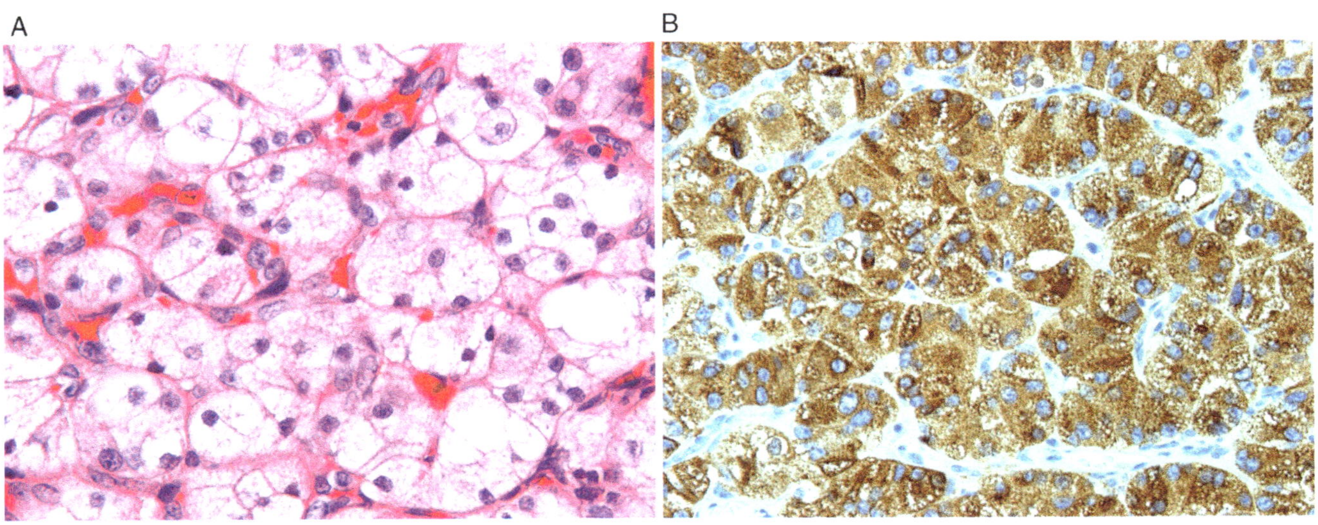

Fig. 8.22 Lipid-rich variant of neuroendocrine tumor (**a**) and positive for chromogranin (**b**)

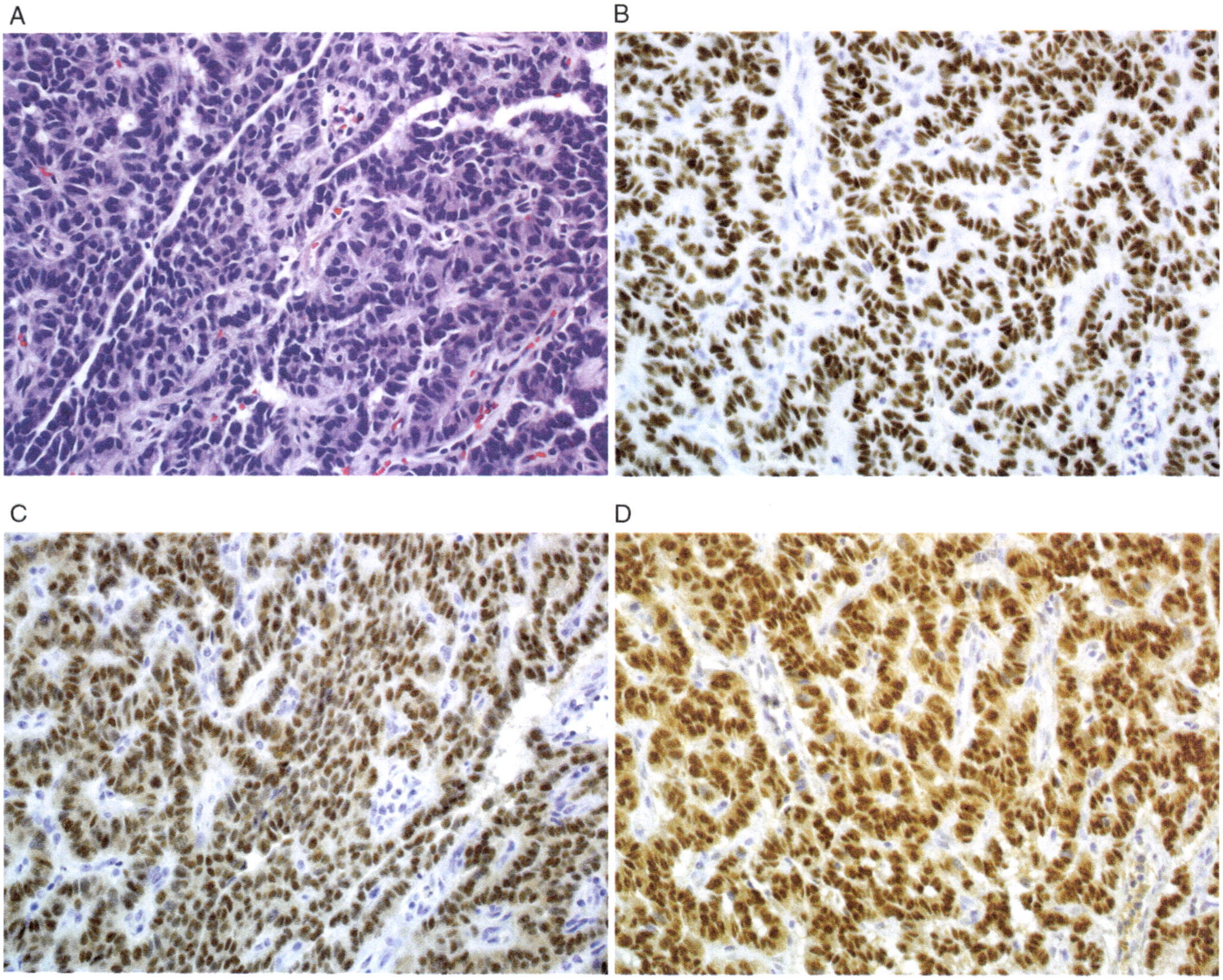

Fig. 8.23 An example of pancreatic neuroendocrine tumor on H&E section (**a**), positive for PR (**b**), PAX8 (**c**), and islet-1 (**d**)

Treatment and Prognosis

- Depends on the clinical behavior of the tumor

Acinar Cell Carcinoma

Key Clinical Features

- A rare tumor, accounting for less than 1% of all pancreatic malignancies.
- The tumor has been reported in a wide age distribution, from 3 to 90 years, more frequently in males.
- Approximately 15% of patients may have an associated clinical syndrome characterized by extrapancreatic fat necrosis, polyarthralgia, and eosinophilia.

Key Radiological Features

- CT and MRI reveal a well-marginated, large, round to oval mass.

Major Cytologic Features

- Typically highly cellular with a mixture of cohesive groups and single acinar cells as shown in Fig. 8.24a, b.
- The neoplastic cells tend to have high nuclear-to-cytoplasmic ratio, irregular nuclear contour, and prominent nuclei.
- Many naked nuclei may be present in the background.
- Well-differentiated tumor may resemble benign acinar tissue. Ductal epithelial cells are usually absent.
- Mitotic figures are variable.
- Significant nuclear pleomorphism will be exceptional.

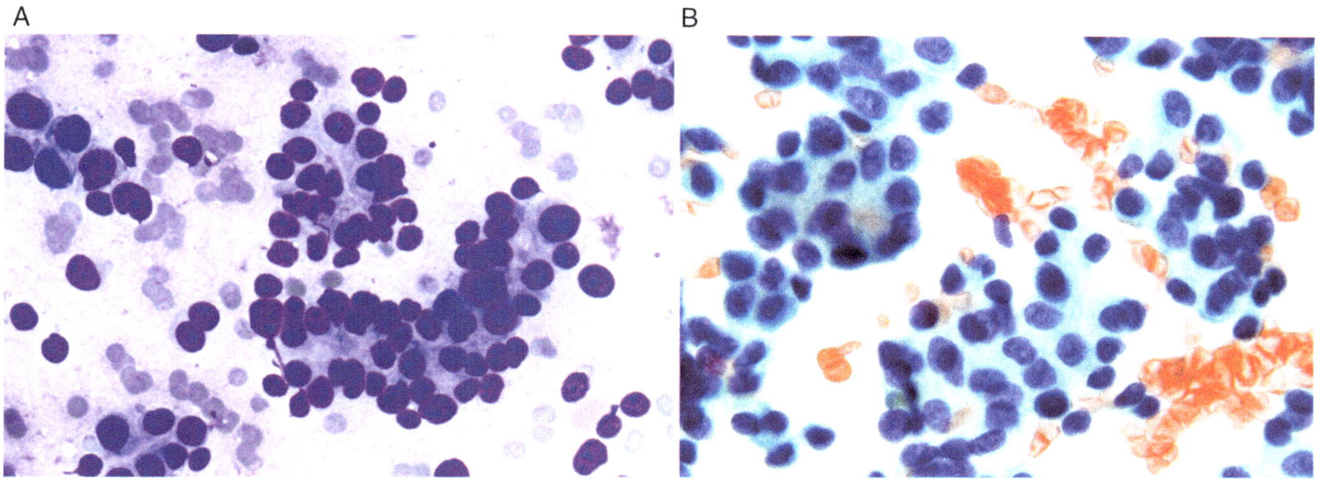

Fig. 8.24 (**a**, **b**) Acinar cell carcinoma. Loosely cohesive groups with high nuclear-to-cytoplasmic ratio and prominent nucleoli. Diff-Quik and Papanicolaou stain

Differential Diagnosis

- Neuroendocrine neoplasm
- Ductal adenocarcinoma
- SPT of pancreas
- Benign acinar tissue

Histology

- Highly cellular tumor with little stroma. Desmoplastic stroma frequently seen in ductal adenocarcinoma is often absent.
- Several histologic patterns with acinar and solid patterns are most commonly seen. Other growth patterns include trabecular arrangement, gyriform appearance, and intraductal and papillary variant. Figure 8.25a–f demonstrates a few growth patterns.
- Round to oval nuclei, minimal to moderate amount fine granular cytoplasm, and single, prominent nucleolus.
- Mitotic rate is variable from 0 to greater than 50/10 HPFs with a mean of 14/HPF.
- Tumor necrosis can be seen.
- Mixed acinar-ductal carcinoma or mixed acinar-NEC when greater than 25% of second component is present.
- It is called acinar cell cystadenocarcinoma when many cystic spaces are formed.

Immunohistochemistry

- Usually positive for cytokeratins 8 and 18 (AE1/3 and CAM5.2) and negative for CK7 and CK20.
- Chromogranin tends to label scattered individual tumor cells, and synaptophysin can be focally positive.
- Most cases are positive for trypsin and chymotrypsin.
- B-cell lymphoma/leukemia 10 (BCL10), glypican-3, and carboxyl ester lipase (CEL) have been reported in 85%, 59%, and 91% of acinar cell carcinomas, respectively.
- β-catenin nuclear staining has been reported.
- Rarely, expression of alpha-fetoprotein (AFP) has been reported especially in younger patients.
- pVHL, S100P, and maspin are usually negative.

Treatment and Prognosis

- The prognosis of acinar cell carcinoma is somewhat less poor than stage-matched invasive ductal adenocarcinoma. The most important prognostic factor is stage. Patients with no nodal or distant metastases survive longer.

Solid-Pseudopapillary Tumor (SPT) of the Pancreas

Key Clinical Features

- WHO defines this as a low-grade malignant neoplasm composed of poorly cohesive monomorphic epithelial cells forming solid and pseudopapillary structures.
- Rare cases with high-grade malignant transformation and metastasis have been reported.
- Predominately occurs in adolescent girls and young women.

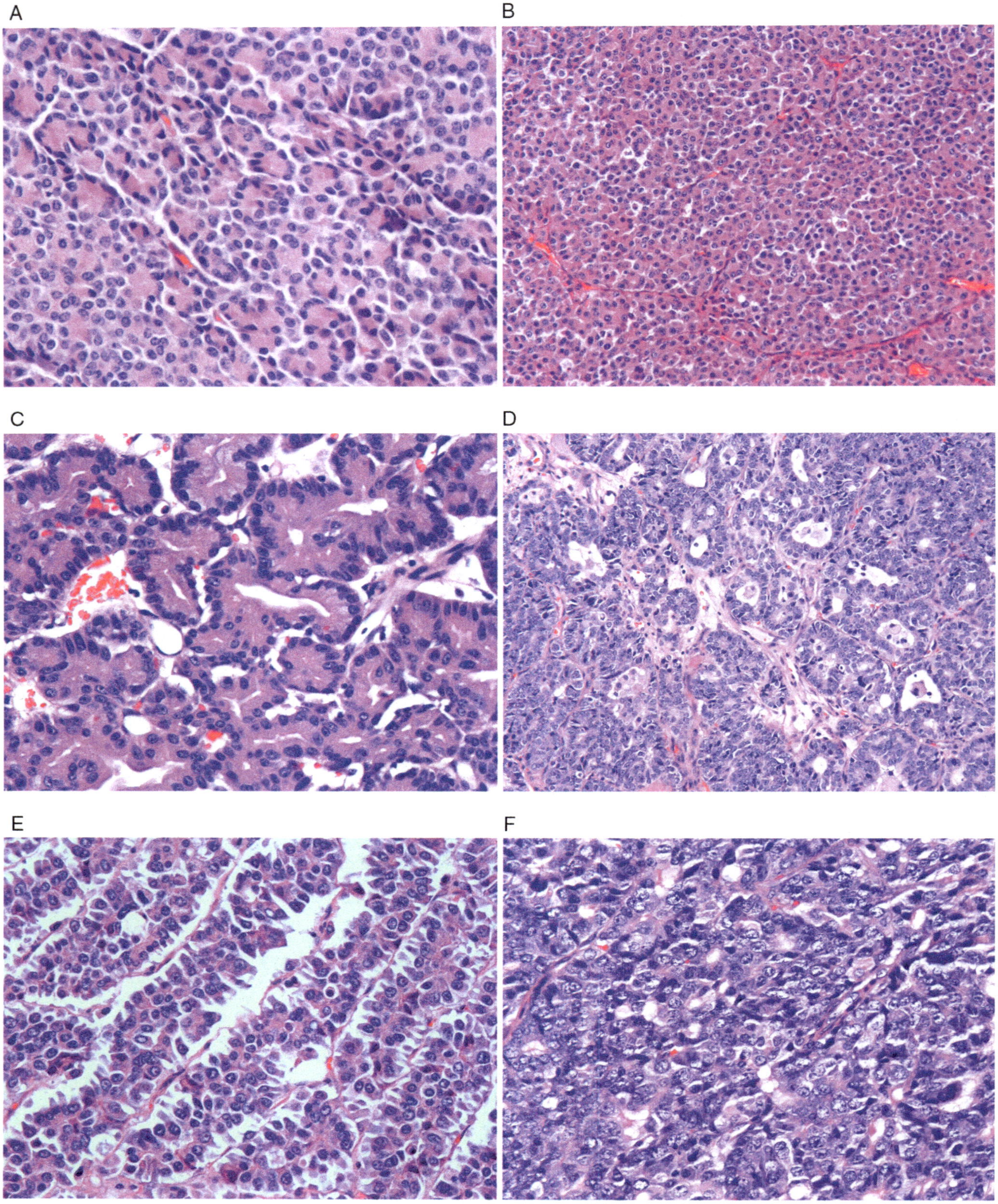

Fig. 8.25 (a–f) Histological section of acinar cell carcinoma with histologic variants

- The cell origin of these neoplasms is uncertain; however, the neoplasm has been shown to express epithelial, mesenchymal, and neuroendocrine markers.
- No evidence of overexpression of p53 and absence of k-ras mutation in SPT has been reported.
- β-catenin gene mutation was identified in SPT, leading to accumulation of cytoplasmic and nuclear β-catenin. The finding raises the possibility of its being associated with familial adenomatous polyposis.

Key Radiological Features

- CT and ultrasonography usually reveal a well-circumscribed, mixed solid and cystic mass with or without internal septa as shown in Fig. 8.26.

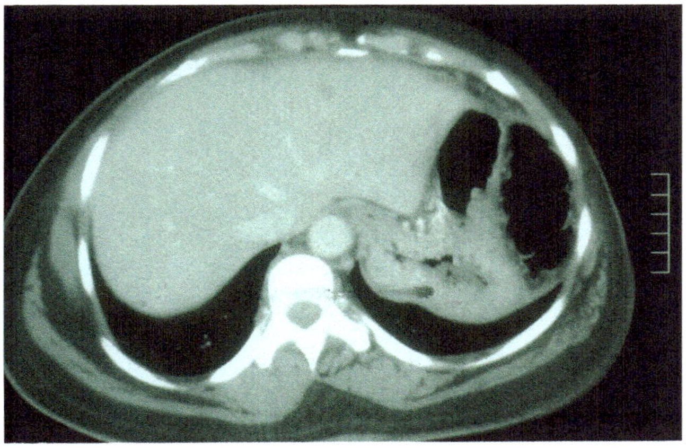

Fig. 8.26 Solid-pseudopapillary tumor of the pancreas. CT scan showing a large solid and cystic mass

Major and Minor Cytologic Features

- A highly cellular smear with clusters of papillary fronds and dissociated single cells as shown in Fig. 8.27a, b.
- The papillary fronds are composed of a delicate fibrovascular core covered by one to two layers of bland neoplastic cells.
- The tumor cells are monomorphic, with bland nuclei, evenly distributed nuclear chromatin, and frequent nuclear grooves.
- Nuclear pleomorphism, mitosis, and prominent nucleoli are consistently absent.
- Cytoplasmic processes and hyaline globules may be present.
- Foamy histiocytes, multinucleated giant cells, and cystic background are the common features.

Differential Diagnosis

- MCN
- IPMN
- Pseudocyst
- Cystic NET of the pancreas
- Cystic acinar cell carcinoma

Histology

- A mixture of solid, pseudopapillary, hemorrhagic-necrotic, and cystic components in variable proportions.
- Poorly cohesive monomorphic tumor cells admixed with hyalinized to myxoid stroma containing thin-walled blood vessels.

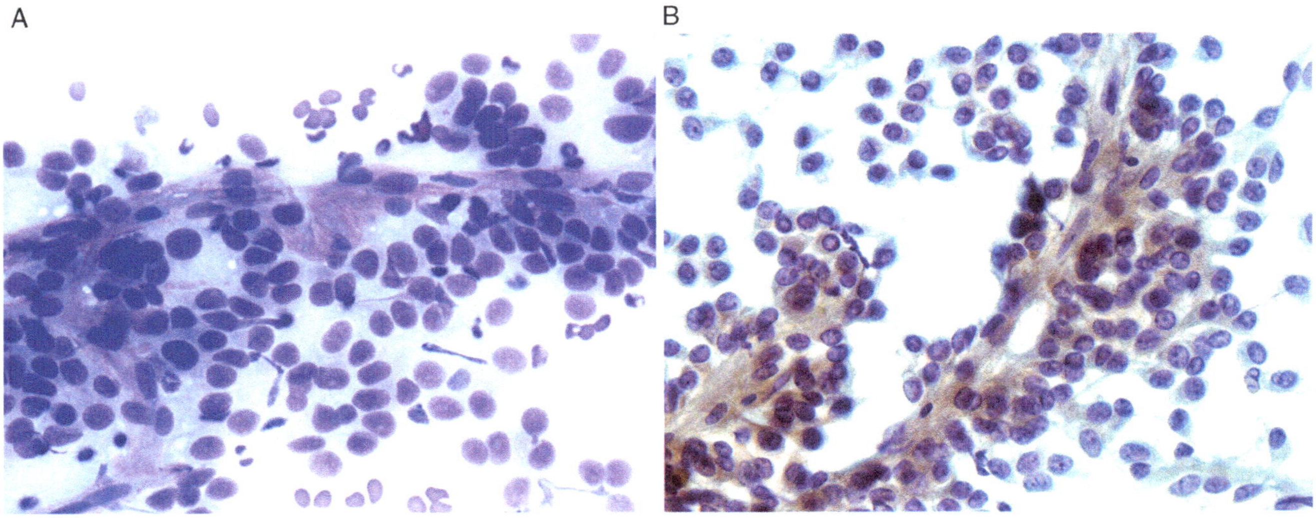

Fig. 8.27 (**a**, **b**) SPT. Papillary fronds lined by one to multiple layers of monomorphic, bland nuclei with evenly distributed nuclear chromatin and nuclear grooves. Singly, bland, uniform neoplastic cells, some with elongated cytoplasmic process are shown in (**b**)

- Foci of calcification and ossification can be seen.
- Neoplastic cells with eosinophilic to clear vacuolated cytoplasm, some containing periodic acid-Schiff (PAS)-positive cytoplasmic globules in variable sizes.
- Foreign body giant cells containing cholesterol crystals are frequently seen.
- Mucin, mitosis, and significant nuclear pleomorphism are not seen.
- Examples are shown in Fig. 8.28a–e.

Immunohistochemistry

- Vimentin and alpha-1 antitrypsin are positive in all of the reported cases.
- PR is positive in some cases.
- Focal pancytokeratin positivity.
- Strong immunohistochemical positivity for neuron-specific enolase (NSE), CD56, and CD10 and focal reactivity for synaptophysin in some cases have been documented, suggesting a neuroendocrine differentiation. Tumor is usually negative for chromogranin.
- Nuclear β-catenin positivity was reported in >90% of cases.
- CD99 shows a cytoplasmic dot-like stain.
- E-cadherin is negative.
- A small panel of IHC markers composed of β-catenin, vimentin, chromogranin, and CD10, and E-cadherin is recommended. An example is shown in Fig. 8.29a–d.

Treatment and Prognosis

- The long-term prognosis following an adequate local surgery is generally excellent, although local recurrence or even metastasis has been reported. An accurate preoperative diagnosis in FNAB specimen is crucial because it should lead to a more conservative surgery.

Serous Cystadenoma

Major Clinical Features

- An uncommon benign cystic tumor with a striking predilection for elderly women.
- A rare case of serous cystadenocarcinoma of the pancreas has been reported. A combined serous cystadenoma and pancreatic neuroendocrine neoplasm may occur.
- Frequently occur in the head of the pancreas, with an average size of 10 cm.

Key Radiological Features

- Sharply demarcated, multilocular cyst; may have a central stellate scar and a sunburst-type calcification on a CT scan

A

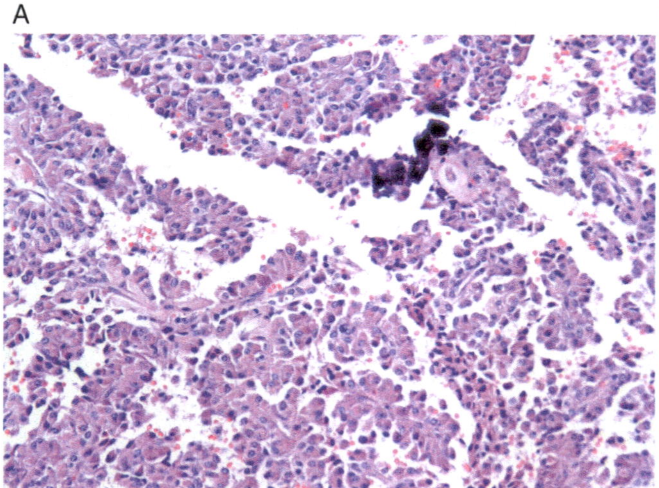

B

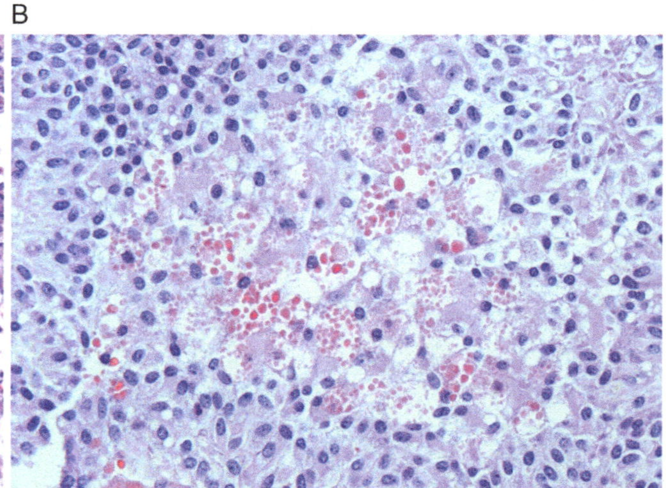

Fig. 8.28 SPT. Histologic section of the same case showing both solid and papillary growth patterns with bland neoplastic cells. Note that eosinophilic, hyaline, intracellular, and extracellular globules (**b**), multinucleated giant cell reaction (**c**), nuclear grooving (**d**), and intracytoplasmic vacuoles (**e**) are present. H&E stain

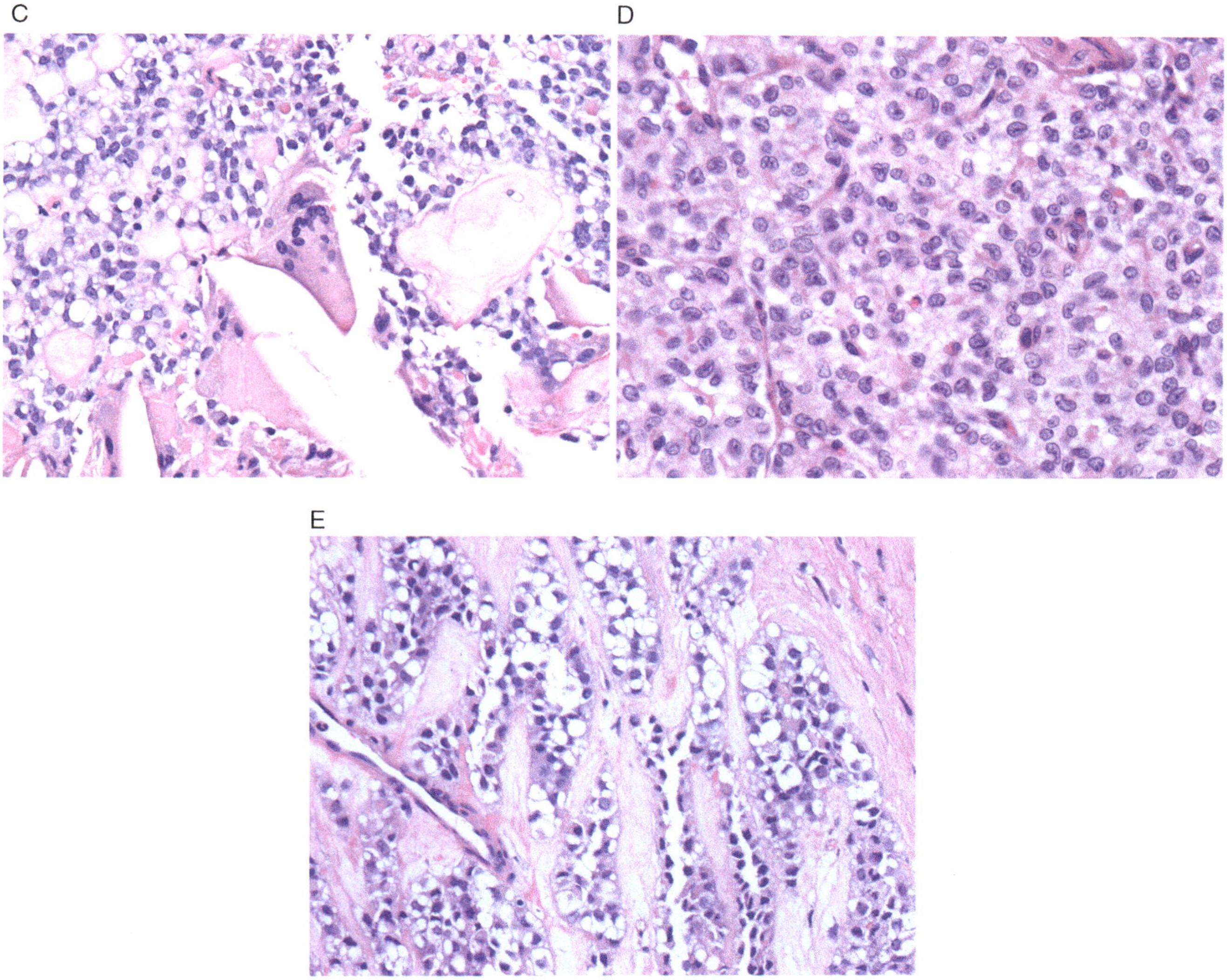

Fig. 8.28 (continued)

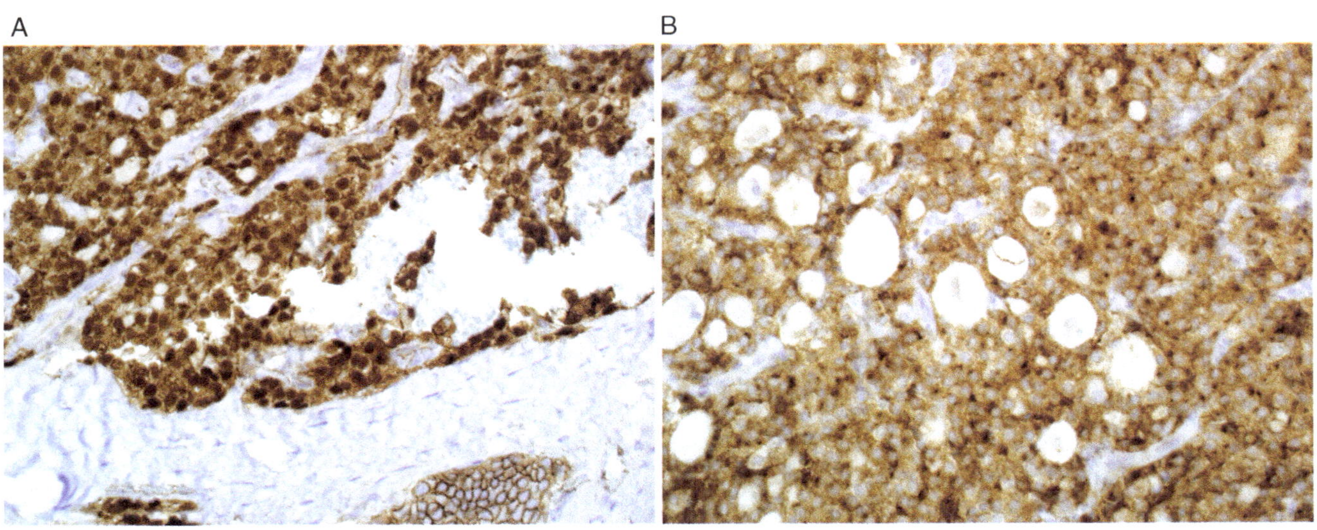

Fig. 8.29 Solid-pseudopapillary tumor positive for β-catenin (**a**), CD10 (**b**), vimentin (**c**), and PR (**d**)

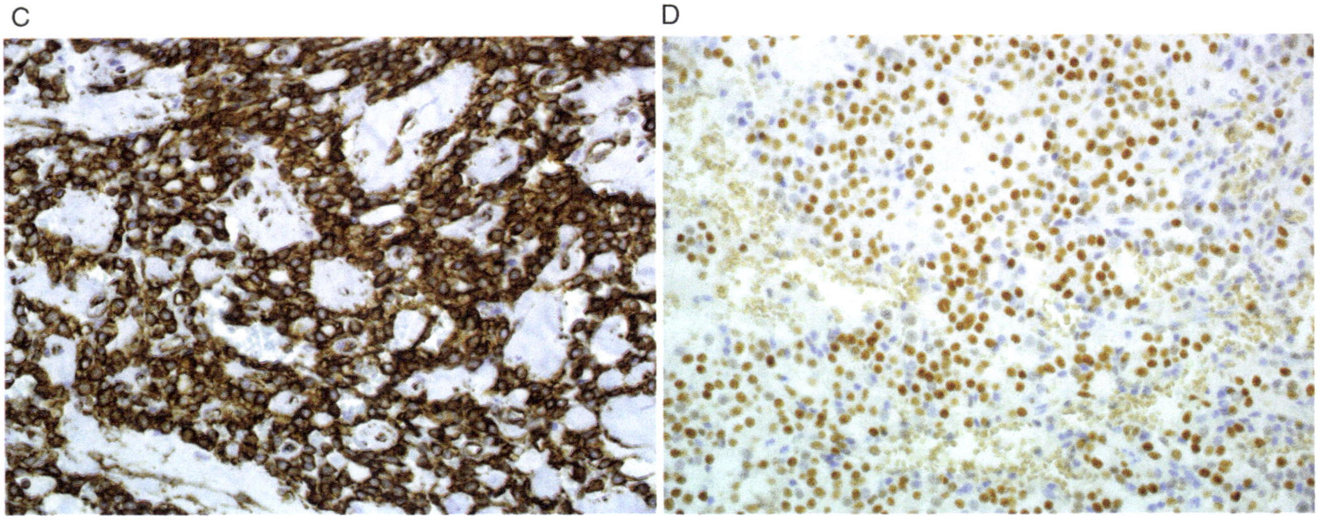

Fig. 8.29 (continued)

Major Cytologic Features

- Hypocellular smear with the presence of few groups of ductal-like cells in a background of clear, watery fluid as shown in Fig. 8.30.
- Hemosiderin-laden histiocytes are frequently seen.
- The epithelial cell groups are usually tightly cohesive, with mild nuclear pleomorphism. Occasional well-defined papillary fronds with bland epithelial cells may be present.
- Single atypical cells, marked nuclear pleomorphism, prominent nucleoli, and mitoses are not the characteristic cytologic features.
- PAS stain demonstrates positive reactivity for cytoplasmic glycogen. Mucicarmine stain for intracytoplasmic mucin is uniformly negative.

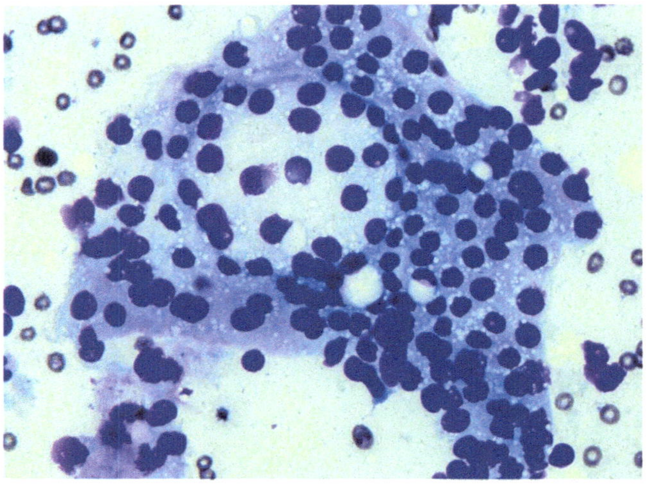

Fig. 8.30 Serous cystadenoma. Cohesive group of ductal-like cells with some atypical cytologic features, mimicking a well-differentiated adenocarcinoma. Papanicolaou stain

Differential Diagnosis

- Pseudocyst
- Acinar cell cystadenoma
- MCN
- IPMN
- Cystic NET

Histology

- Cysts in various sizes lined by a single layer of cuboidal or flattened epithelial cells with clear cytoplasm as shown in Fig. 8.31a.
- Oval to round nuclei with inconspicuous nucleolus.
- Nuclear atypia and mitosis are absent.
- Intracystic papillary projections can be seen.
- In a solid variant, similar cells are arranged in small acini with no central lumina as shown in Fig. 8.31b.

Immunohistochemistry

- Positive for CK7 and frequently positive for pVHL (Fig. 8.31c), MUC6, inhibin-α, and NSE

Treatment and Prognosis

- Surgical resection with an excellent prognosis

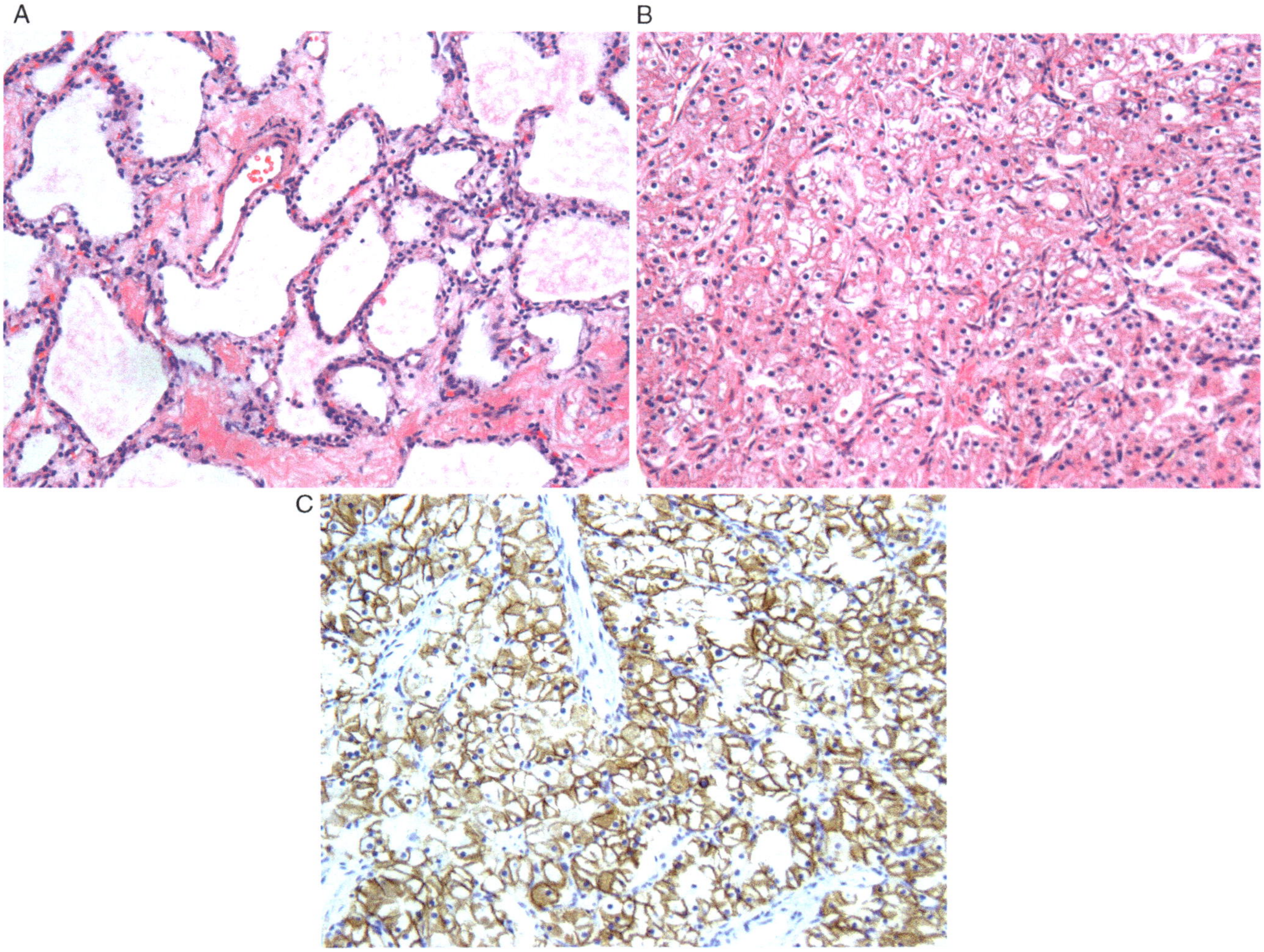

Fig. 8.31 Histological section of serous cystadenoma. Microcystic spaces lined by a single layer of low cuboidal, benign-appearing cells (**a**). The lining cells are positive for PAS and negative for mucin. (**a**) solid variant is shown in (**b**) and positive for pVHL immunostain (**c**)

Mucinous Cystic Neoplasms (MCNs)

Key Clinical Features

- Uncommon tumors of the pancreas, accounting for approximately 2–2.5% of total pancreatic tumors.
- Usually occur in middle-age patients, almost exclusively in female.
- The average size of tumors is 10 cm (ranging from 2 to 20 cm); frequently located in the body or tail of the pancreas. It usually does not communicate with the pancreatic ductal system.
- Mucinous cystic tumors of the pancreas can be classified into MCN with low-grade dysplasia, MCN with moderate dysplasia, MCN with severe dysplasia, and mucinous cystadenocarcinoma.

Key Radiological Features

- CT scans usually demonstrate a well-demarcated, thick-walled, multilocular cystic mass, sometimes with peripheral calcification.
- Mural nodules and papillary excrescences into the cysts are more common in MCNs with an associated invasive carcinoma.
- Larger pancreatic ducts do not communicate with the cysts.

Major Cytologic Features

- Grossly, specimens contain watery or viscid mucoid material. Mucoid material tends to be metachromatic on Diff-Quik stain, but it may not be very apparent on the Papanicolaou stain.

- The cellularity of an FNAB specimen is variable depending on the amount of mucin obtained or if the solid area is aspirated. The finding of columnar, mucin-containing cells is the key diagnostic feature, as illustrated in Fig. 8.32a, b.
- Groups of ductal cells with cytologic atypia may be present.
- The degree of architectural and nuclear atypia may be variable depending on the nature of the lesion. Papillary clusters may be present.
- Unequivocal cytologic features of malignancy are diagnostic for mucinous cystadenocarcinoma. However, mucinous cystadenocarcinoma may be noninvasive or invasive. Unfortunately, no reliable cytologic criteria are available to differentiate invasive vs. noninvasive mucinous cystadenocarcinoma.

Differential Diagnosis

- IPMN
- Serous cystadenoma
- Pseudocyst
- Gastrointestinal contamination

Histology

- Columnar mucin-producing epithelium associated with ovarian-type subepithelial stroma as shown in Fig. 8.33.
- The lining columnar cells can be pseudopyloric, gastric foveolar, and intestinal type, rarely with squamous differentiation.
- Low-grade dysplasia, minimal to mild architectural and cytologic atypia with no papillary projection or mitosis.
- Intermediate-grade dysplasia, moderate cytologic atypia and papillary projection; mitosis can be seen.
- High-grade dysplasia, severe cytologic atypia, nuclear stratification, papillae, and mitosis.
- Up to one-third of MCNs may be associated with an invasive component, which is usually infiltrating ductal carcinoma, but can be other variants of ductal carcinoma.

Immunohistochemistry

- DPC-4/SMAD4 protein is usually positive in noninvasive MCNs but negative in invasive mucinous carcinomas. In contrast, MUC1 is usually expressed in invasive ductal carcinoma and negative in MCN.
- The lining epithelium, even in low-grade dysplasia, is usually negative for pVHL and positive for S100P and maspin.
- The subepithelial ovarian-like stroma is positive for PR (60–90%) and estrogen receptor (ER, 30%).

Treatment and Prognosis

- Complete resection with an excellent prognosis if no invasive carcinoma is identified

Intraductal Papillary Mucinous Neoplasms (IPMNS) and Intraductal Tubulopapillary Neoplasms (ITPNS)

Key Clinical Features

- In the WHO 2010 classification, intraductal neoplasms of the pancreas include IPMNs and intraductal tubulo-

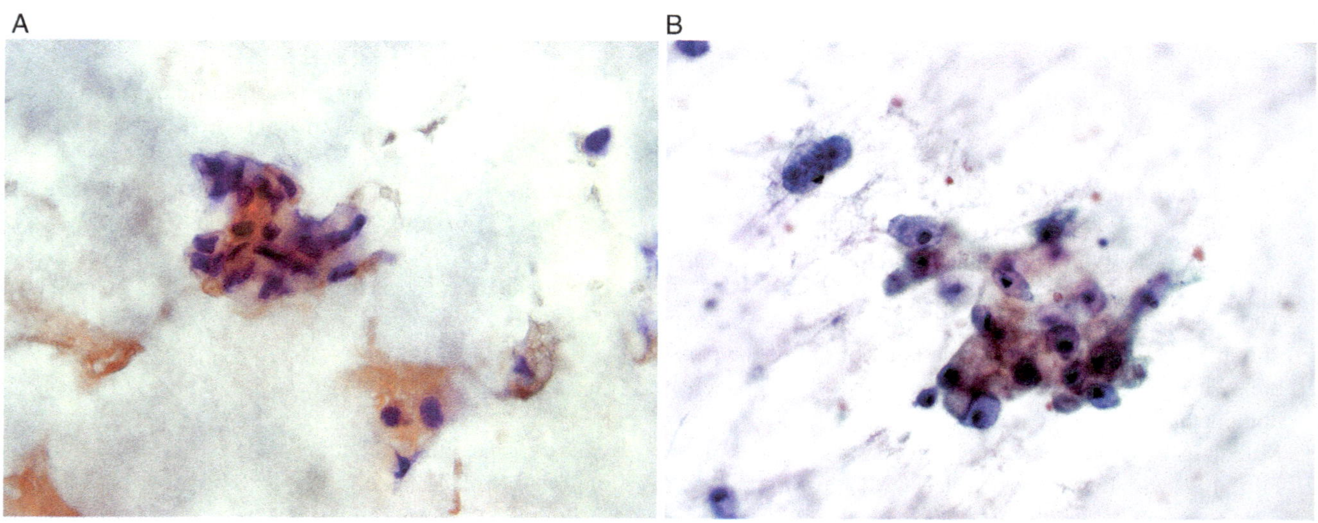

Fig. 8.32 Mucinous cystic neoplasm. Columnar, mucin containing epithelial groups in a background of mucinous macrophages and mucoid material (**a**). Flat sheet of epithelial cells with cytologic atypia (**b**). Papanicolaou stain, ×600

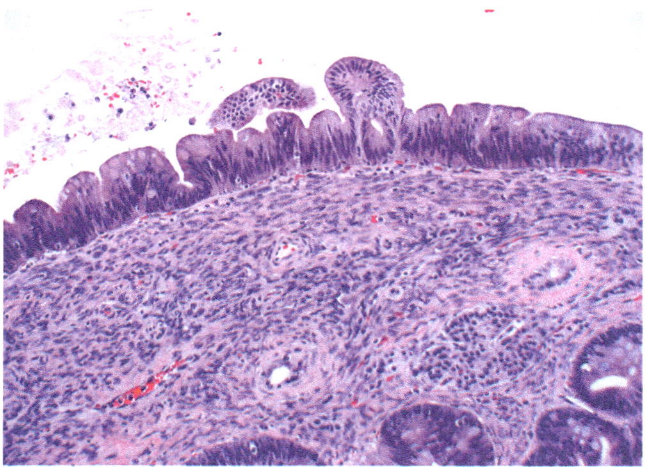

Fig. 8.33 Histological section of MCN. H&E, ×200

papillary neoplasms (ITPNs). Tumor is usually larger than 1.0 cm.

- In IPMN, the tumor is characterized as having tall, columnar, mucin-producing epithelium with or without papillary projections, according to the WHO criteria.
- The main differences between IPMN and ITPN are: IPMN is associated with a significant amount of intracellular mucin, with a predominately papillary growth pattern, and positive for MUC5AC immunostain; in contrast, ITPN lacks intracellular mucin, has a predominately tubular growth pattern, with evidence of necrosis, and is negative for MUC5AC immunostain.
- It has been proposed that IPMN can be classified into IPMN with low-grade dysplasia, IPMN with intermediate-grade dysplasia, and IPMN with high-grade dysplasia. About 30% of IPMNs are associated with invasive carcinoma, and half of them are CCs.
- Morphologically, IPMN can be further classified into three subtypes based on the ductal location of the tumor involvement: main pancreatic duct involvement, side branches of the main pancreatic duct, and a combination of the two. IPMNs arising from the main pancreatic duct or a combination of main duct and side branches are usually located in the head of the pancreas, whereas side branch disease most commonly occurs in the uncinate process, followed by the tail of the pancreas.
- IPMN of the pancreas accounts for approximately 10–24% of pancreatic cysts and 1% of all exocrine tumors of the pancreas.
- IPMN more frequently affects men, with a mean age of 65.
- Symptoms may include abdominal pain, back pain, obstructive jaundice, and diabetes mellitus.
- Acute pancreatitis is most frequently associated with the main duct type of IPMN. Chronic pancreatitis with diabetes and steatorrhea is a common clinical presentation.

Key Radiological Findings

- Endosonographically, IPMN typically appears as small, thin-walled cysts without septations, which actually represent dilated side branches. This appearance has been described as "clusters of grapes."
- EUS imaging may also show a dilated main pancreatic duct associated with intraductal mucin, mural nodules, or a mass lesion. The finding of mural nodules or a mass lesion correlates with an increased likelihood of malignancies.

Major Cytologic Features

- Typically low cellularity with an abundant amount of very viscid mucus. The thick mucus may be difficult to express from the needle, making it hard to make thin smears. This is quite different from the thin, watery, dirty-appearing or bile-stained normal upper gastrointestinal (GI) luminal mucus.
- A few glandular epithelial cells either singly or in small clusters, foamy histiocytes, neutrophils, and lymphocytes. Papillary groups may be present but infrequently. Goblet cells and bland columnar epithelial cells with abundant cytoplasmic mucin may be present in some cases. Cytologic features are illustrated in Fig. 8.34a–c. Various degrees of dysplasia on both smear and cellblock preparations are shown in Fig. 8.35a–f.
- IPMNs and MCNs are indistinguishable on FNA samples. This is because the subepithelial ovarian stroma of MCN is unlikely to be sampled or recognizable on smears or cellblock.
- Table 8.3 summarizes the main differential diagnoses of the pancreatic cystic lesions.

Differential Diagnosis

- MCN
- Serous cystadenoma
- Pseudocyst
- PanIN

Histology

- IPMN is characterized by intraductal proliferation of columnar mucin-producing cells with various degrees of nuclear and architectural dysplasia.

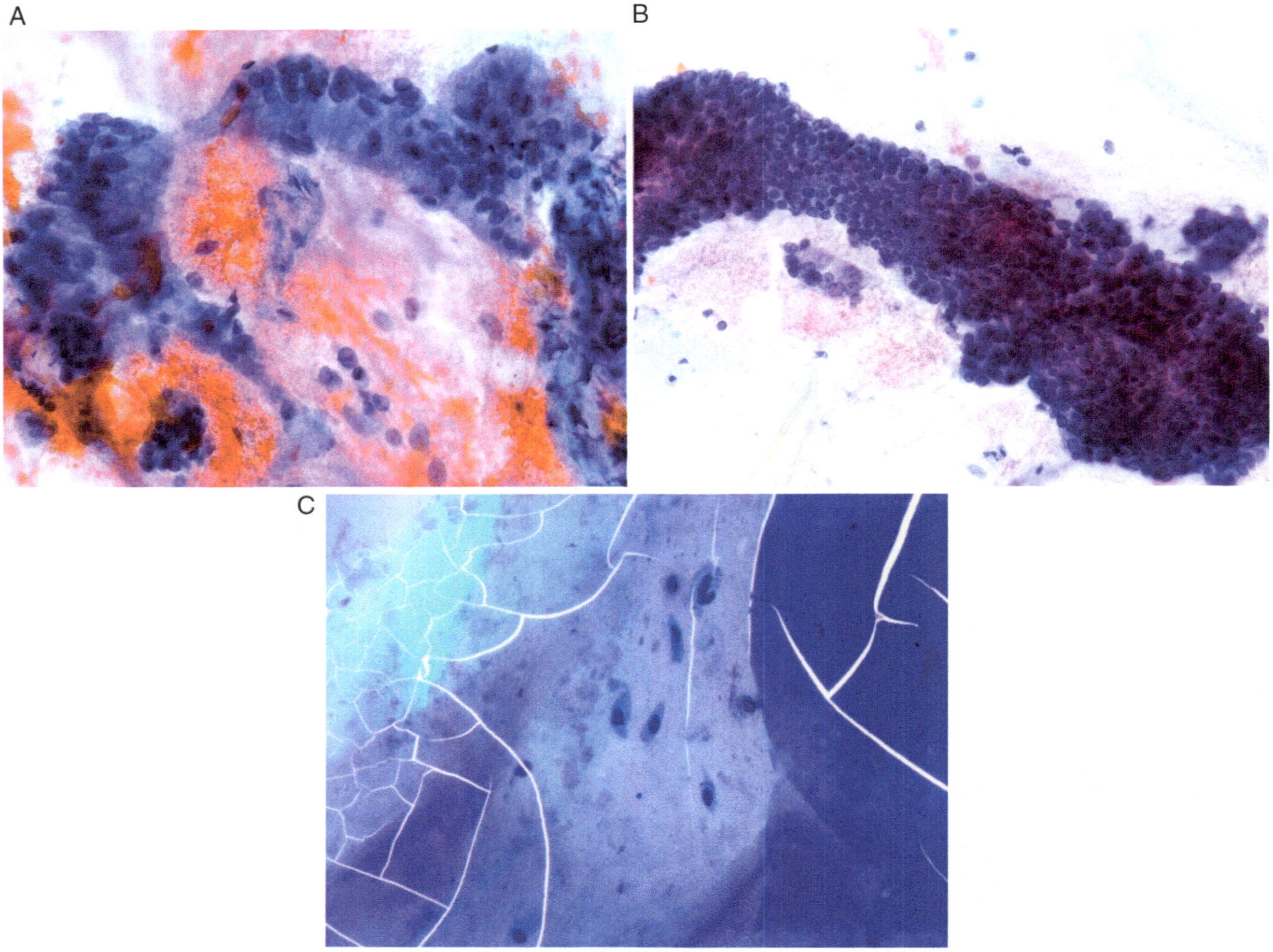

Fig. 8.34 IPMN. Mucin-containing glandular cells and mucinous macrophages in a background of thick mucin (**a**); papillary structure and columnar cells (**b**); thick mucin with limited cells (**c**)

- Can be subclassified into four types: gastric type, intestinal type, pancreatobiliary type, and oncocytic type.
- Gastric-type IPMN tends to show low- or intermediate-grade dysplasia; intestinal type tends to show intermediate- to high-grade dysplasia; pancreatobiliary type and oncocytic type tend to show high-grade dysplasia. Representative examples of histologic variants of IPMN are shown in Fig. 8.36a–e.
- ITPN is characterized by back-to-back tubular glands resulting in large cribriform structures, with an occasional papillary growth pattern and lack of intracellular mucin. ITPN tends to show high-grade dysplasia with complex architecture, nuclear atypia, mitosis, and tumor necrosis. An invasive component is found in 40% of cases.

Immunohistochemistry

- IPMN – intestinal type: positive for CDX2, MUC2, and MUC5AC.
- IPMN – gastric type: positive for MUC5AC.
- IPMN – pancreatobiliary type: positive for MUC1 and MUC5AC.
- IPMN – oncocytic type: MUC6, MUC1, and MUC5AC.
- ITPN – positive for MUC6 and MUC1.
- SMAD4/DPC4 is positive in most IPMNs and ITPNs.
- pVHL has been shown to be negative in all types of IPMNs, including the ones with low-grade epithelial dysplasia.

Treatment and Prognosis

- Good prognosis if no invasive carcinoma is identified and clear surgical margin.
- For IPMNs, about 30% of cases may show invasive carcinoma; half are CC, which carries a 50–60% 5-year survival rate.
- For ITPNs, invasive carcinoma is found in 40% of cases.

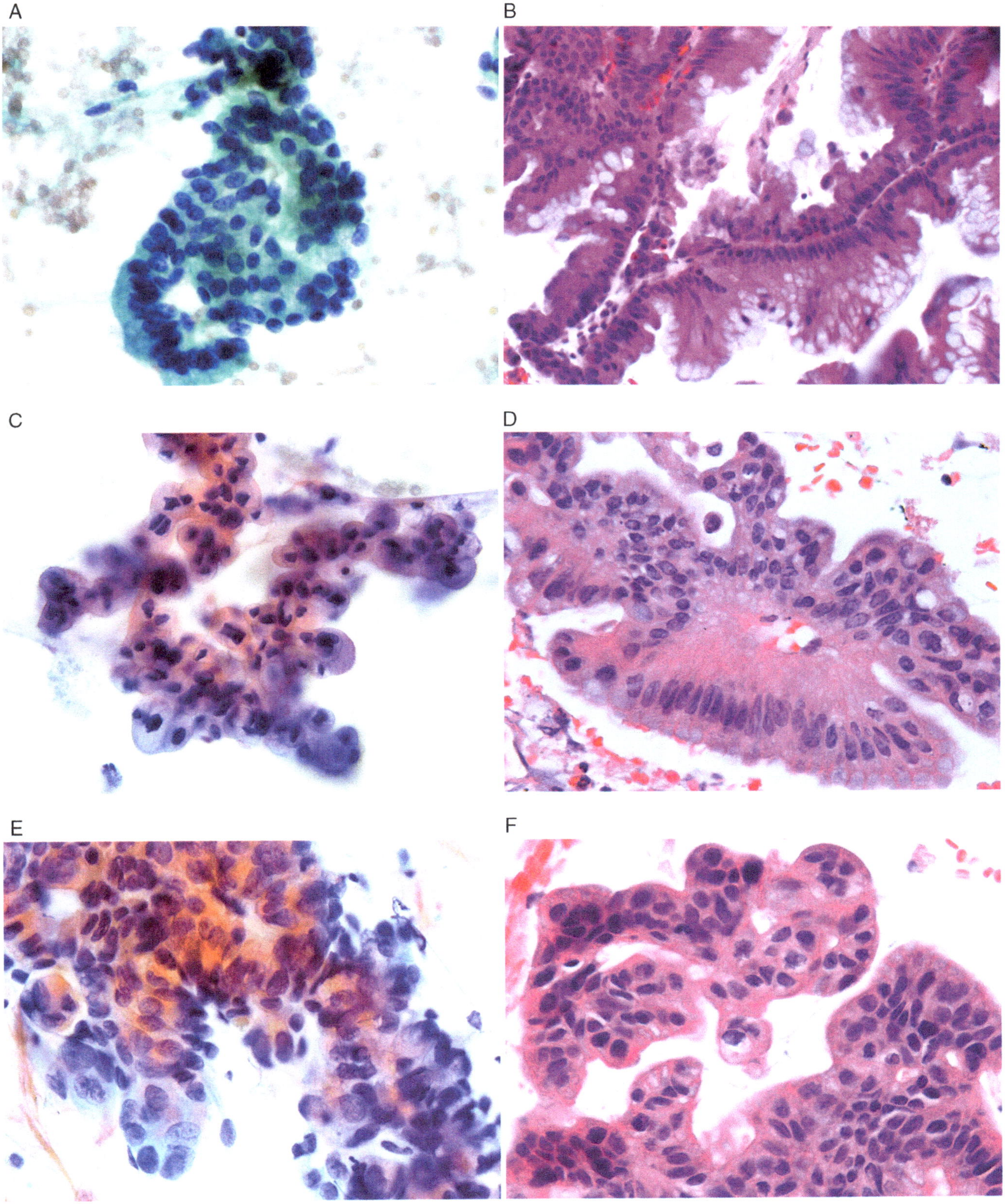

Fig. 8.35 IPMN with low-grade dysplasia on smear (**a**) and cellblock (**b**), intermediate grade dysplasia on smear (**c**) and cellblock (**d**), and high-grade atypia/dysplasia on smear (**e**) and cellblock (**f**)

Table 8.3 Differential diagnosis of cystic lesions of the pancreas

Diagnosis	Clinical features	Radiologic features	Cytologic findings	Special stains and cyst fluid findings
Pseudocyst	Body and tail. Acute and chronic pancreatitis, trauma	Solitary or multilocular cyst, thick wall	Fluid and debris, histiocytes, bile pigments, inflammatory cells, rare or no epithelial cells and mesenchymal cells	High amylase; low CEA, viscosity, CA 72-4, and CA 125. PAS (−), Mucin (−)
SCA	Elderly, F>>M Head > tail, body	Complex multicystic lesion, with a mean diameter of 10 cm; 30% with central calcification, some with central stellate scar	Hypocellular smears with few groups of epithelial cells, clear background, minimal nuclear pleomorphism, occasional papillary groups	Low CEA, viscosity, and CA 72-4; variable CA 125. PAS (+), Mucin (−) IHC: CK7, pVHL, MUC6, Inhibin-α-positive
SPT	F>>M, Adolescent girls, young women. Tail, body > head	Multicystic, well-demarcated mass with solid areas, necrosis and calcifications	Hypercellular smear with groups of papillary fronds and single monomorphic cells in a cystic background	Mucin (−), PAS (±); IHC: Beta-catenin nuclear and cytoplasmic positive in >90%, E-cadherin (-), CD10 (+), vimentin (+), chromogranin (-)
IPMN	M:F, about same, mean age 65. Main duct type – head and uncinate process. Side branch type – body, tail	Single or multiple small, thin-walled cysts without septations, referred to as "clusters of grapes." Finding of mural nodule or mass lesion correlating with an increased chance of malignancy	Low cellularity, very thick mucin; a few single or small clusters of columnar epithelial cells; histiocytes and neutrophils. Papillary clusters may be present. Variable nuclear atypia	High CEA; very high viscosity; variable CA 72-4, CA 19-9, CA 15-3. Mucin (+), PAS (−). IHC: MUC2 and MUC5AC positive in 80% of cases, DPC4/SMAD4 (+)
MCN	F>>M, middle age. Body, tail	Multilocular cyst with mean diameter of 7 cm; each cyst >2.0 cm in diameter; smooth external border; calcifications in 19% of cases	Watery or viscid mucoid material, metachromatic on Diff-Quik stain; columnar mucin-containing epithelial cells; papillary groups may be present; variable nuclear atypia	High CEA and viscosity; low CA 15-3, CA 72-4; variable CA 125 and CA 19-9. Mucin (+), PAS (−)
MCA	F>M Body, tail	Multiple cysts with solid areas, local invasion or hepatic metastasis may be seen	High cellularity. Atypical glandular epithelial cells in a background of mucin and necrosis. Single pleomorphic tumor cells or signet ring cells	High CEA, viscosity, CA 15-3, CA 72-4, and variable CA 19-9, CA 125. Mucin (+), PAS (−). IHC: MUC1 positive, 95%
CPNET	Adults, rare in children. Body, tail.	Well-defined, very vascular, calcification and cystic changes. Only 30–40% seen on CT scan with contrast	Small, uniform, single cells and loosely cohesive groups, plasmacytoid appearance; binucleation; salt-and-pepper chromatin; small nucleoli; no reliable cytologic criteria to predict the malignant potential	IHC: CK (+), chromogranin (+), synaptophysin (+), Ki-67 variable

CPNET Cystic pancreatic neuroendocrine tumor

Metastases and Uncommon Lesions

- Metastasis accounts for 4–5% of all malignancies of the pancreas found at autopsies.
- The most common metastases are renal cell carcinomas, melanomas, colorectal carcinomas, breast carcinomas, lung adenocarcinomas, and sarcomas.
- Distinction of primary ductal adenocarcinoma of the pancreas from metastatic carcinoma may be impossible, especially on FNA samples or small core biopsy specimens.
- The most common sources of metastatic malignant tumors of the pancreas are the lung, kidney, breast, liver, gastrointestinal tract, sarcoma, and melanoma. Some tumors may present as an initial presentation.
- Eleven cases of metastatic malignant tumors were identified in our study, including renal (four cases), stomach (three cases), prostate (one case), squamous cell carcinoma (one case), liver (one case), and sarcoma (one case).
- Most metastatic carcinomas demonstrate extremely high cellularity, many single malignant cells, and significant nuclear pleomorphysim. In our experience, when a diagnosis of pancreatic malignancy is getting "too easy," a metastasis should be entertained.
- If a cellblock is available, a panel of IHC markers may provide some useful information. The IHC staining profiles for the common pancreatic metastases are summarized in the Table 8.4.

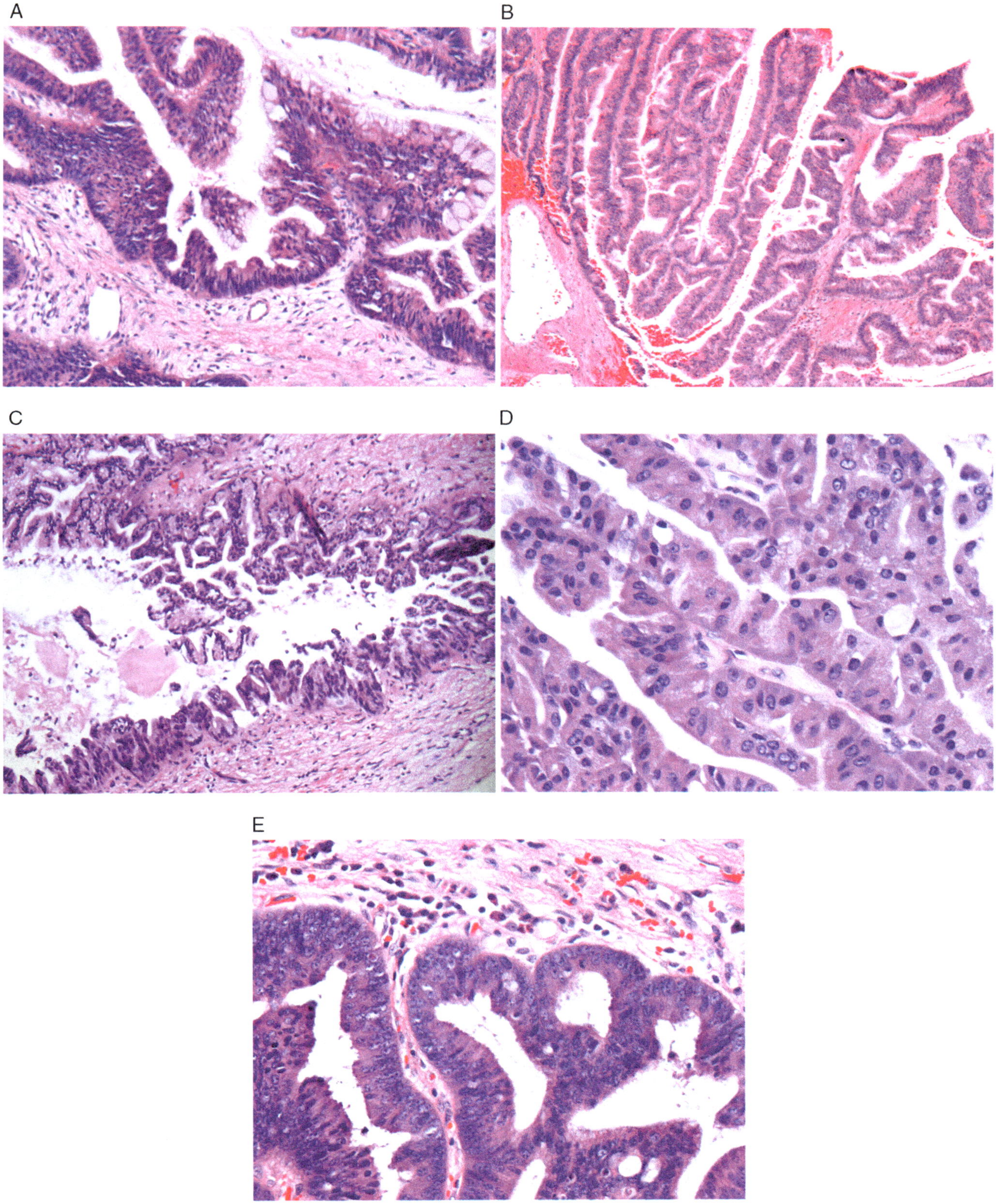

Fig. 8.36 Histological variants of IPMN with gastric type (**a**), intestinal type (**b**), pancreatobiliary type (**c**), oncocytic type (**d**), and with high-grade dysplasia (**e**). H&E stain

Table 8.4 Summary of IHC markers for workup of common pancreatic metastases

Marker/diagnosis	Pancreas	Kidney	Breast	Colon	Lung	Melanoma
CK7	+	–	+	–	+	–
CK20	–/+	–	–	+	–	–
CDX2	–/+	–	–	+	–	–
ER	–	–	+	–	–	–
GATA3	–/+	–	+	–	–	–
TTF1	–	–	–	–	+	–
PAX8	–	+	–	–	–	–
SOX10	–	–	–	–	–	+
SMAD4	–/+	+	+	+	+	+

Note: *GATA3* GATA binding protein 3, *SOX 10* sex-determining region Y box 10

Case Presentations

There are three scenarios commonly encountered in a daily practice when evaluating an FNAB of the pancreas with or without a cellblock and/or thin tissue core biopsy. Case scenario 1 is how to make a diagnosis of well-differentiated adenocarcinoma in a limited specimen; Case scenario 2 is how to deal with an overt malignancy or neoplastic process in which a secondary malignancy or non-ductal neoplasm is included in the diagnostic consideration; and Case scenario 3 is how to effectively work on a cystic lesion of the pancreas.

Case Scenario 1

Learning Objectives

1. Reiterate the diagnostic criteria for well-differentiated adenocarcinoma of the pancreas on both FNA and small tissue core biopsy specimens;
2. Review the most effective panel of immunomarkers for diagnosis of ductal adenocarcinoma of the pancreas;
3. Emphasize how to correctly interpret the immunostaining results to avoid diagnostic pitfalls.

Case

A 60-year-old woman presented with jaundice, abdominal pain, and a 3.0 cm mass at the head of the pancreas. An EUS-FNA was performed. The FNA smear was hypocellular with a few groups of moderately atypical epithelial cells associated with air-dried artifacts as shown in Fig. 8.37a. A cellblock preparation was also obtained, which contained a small thin tissue core with a few atypical glands and scattered single cells embedded in a desmoplastic stroma as shown in Fig. 8.37b.

At this point, the question is: Is this material sufficient to render a definitive diagnosis of adenocarcinoma? If the answer is no, then why not? Can any IHC panel be helpful at this scenario?

Based on our experience, we preferred to designate this as suspicious for adenocarcinoma because of the moderate degree of nuclear atypia and the limited sample. In general, when dealing with an FNA of the pancreas from a younger patient, one should be more conservative and tend to raise the threshold for making a definitive diagnosis. The question that should be kept in mind is: Is it prudent to call this cancer? For a well-differentiated pancreatic adenocarcinoma, the key criteria to confirm a malignant diagnosis include (1) variations in nuclear sizes of greater than a 4:1 ratio in the same group of atypical epithelial cells, (2) nuclear contour irregularities, and (3) loss of nuclear polarities. When observing this atypical group closely, it was felt insufficient to make a definite call based on the above criteria. Significant nuclear pleomorphism, perineural invasion, and large muscular vessels adjacent to the atypical glands were not seen on the thin tissue core, which made it challenging to render a malignant diagnosis as well.

In this scenario, a panel of IHC markers including pVHL, maspin, S100P, and IMP3 can be helpful. As reported previously, the vast majority of adenocarcinoma cases are positive for maspin, S100P, and IMP3 and negative for pVHL. As shown in Fig. 8.37c below, a double staining for pVHL/maspin showed that the atypical glands were strongly positive for maspin (both nuclear and cytoplasmic) and negative for pVHL. Also, the atypical glands were strongly positive for S100P (Fig. 8.37d, both nuclear and cytoplasmic) and cytoplasmic IMP3 (Fig. 8.37e). At this point, we felt comfortable calling this case adenocarcinoma. A few caveats should be emphasized here to better utilize this diagnostic IHC panel and avoid potential pitfalls:

1. When pVHL is positive, it shows a diffuse and strong membranous staining pattern. Weak and focal membranous staining or only cytoplasmic staining should be regarded as negative. Adenocarcinoma of the pancreas diffusely and strongly positive for pVHL has not been seen in our practice. Approximately 5% of pancreatic ductal adenocarcinomas, 10% of gallbladder

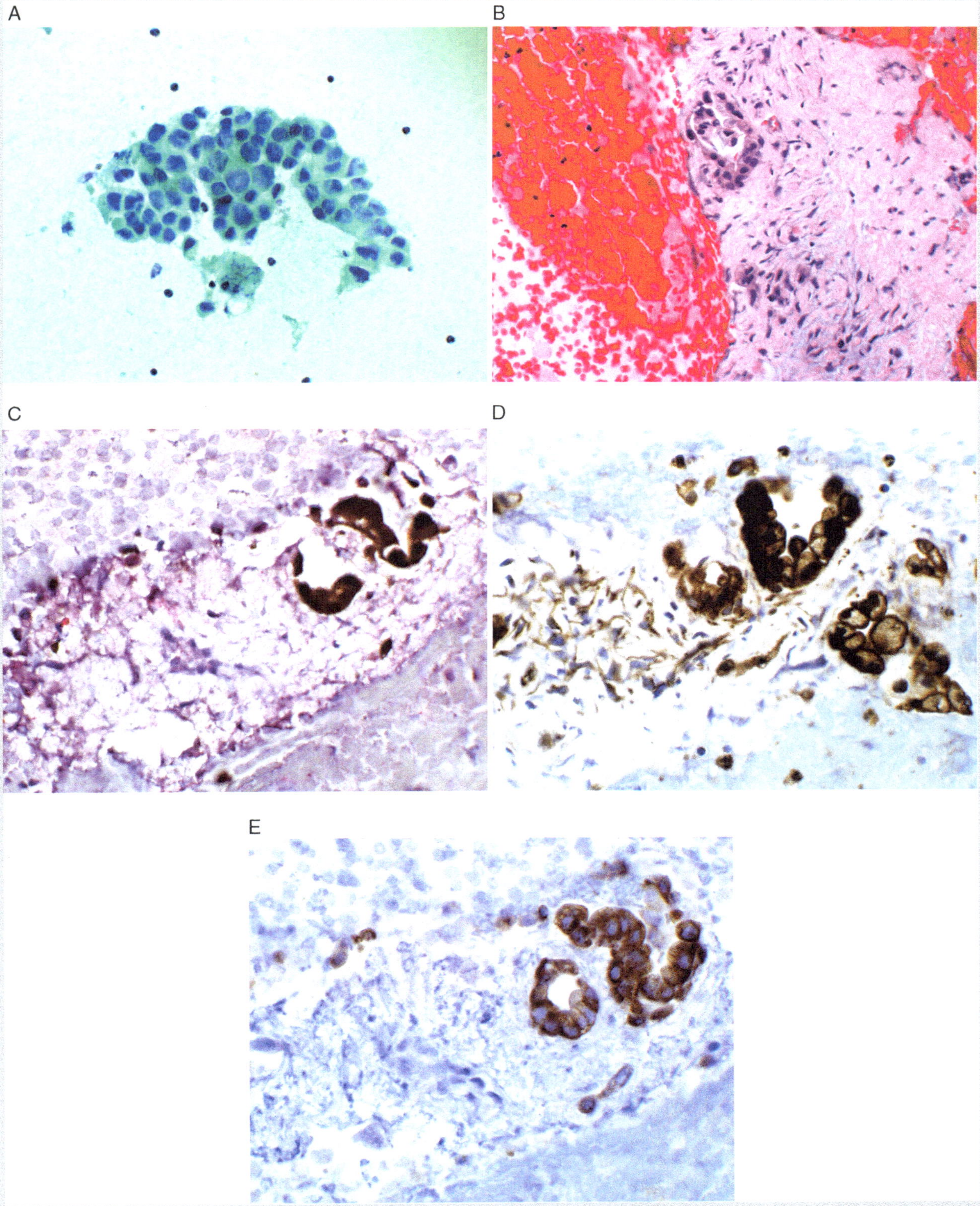

Fig. 8.37 FNA smear and thin tissue core biopsy from a 60-year-old woman with a 3.0 cm mass at the head of the pancreas. Atypical ductal cells and glands are shown in (**a**, **b**), respectively, which are suspicious but not diagnostic for a malignancy. Positive immunostaining for maspin/pVHL (**c**), S100P (**d**), and IMP3 (**e**) confirms the malignant diagnosis

(continued)

adenocarcinomas, and 10% of common bile duct adenocarcinomas can be focally positive for pVHL. Interestingly, approximately 70% of intrahepatic cholangiocarcinomas are diffusely and strongly positive for pVHL, which is potentially useful when the diagnostic consideration has included an intrahepatic cholangiocarcinoma vs. other pancreatobiliary tract carcinomas.

2. Both maspin and S100P are positive in over 90% of pancreatic ductal adenocarcinomas, but staining should be considered positive only when diffusely and strongly positive in both the nuclear and cytoplasmic compartments of the atypical cells/glands. Weak staining, especially cytoplasmic staining, can be seen in a reactive condition. More importantly, gastric and duodenal mucosa are positive for maspin and can be strongly positive. Gastric mucosa is also positive for S100P. This usually is not a problem when dealing with a small tissue biopsy or a needle core biopsy specimen because the benign gastric or duodenal mucosa is easily recognizable.

   However, when working on a cellblock specimen containing an EUS-FNA sample, one needs to be aware of this potential pitfall since gastric or duodenal mucosal contamination is frequently present in an EUS-FNA sample of the pancreas. One way to avoid this pitfall is to match the atypical groups on the hematoxylin and eosin (H&E)-stained slide to the maspin-positive groups on the IHC-stained slide if possible. Both maspin and S100P are also expressed in both IPMN and MCN, regardless of the degree of epithelial dysplasia; however, a high-grade dysplasia tends to demonstrate strong and diffuse positivity. Additionally, PanIN is also positive for maspin and S100P. If an EUS-FNA sample was obtained from a cystic or solid and cystic mass, atypical epithelial groups with maspin or S100P positivity may only represent the dysplastic epithelia from the PanIN. In other words, maspin and S100P are not useful when the diagnostic consideration is between invasive adenocarcinoma and epithelial dysplasia.
3. IMP3 is a highly specific diagnostic marker for some adenocarcinomas, including pancreatobiliary tract adenocarcinomas. Benign, reactive, and gastric and duodenal contamination are generally negative for IMP3. The sensitivity was reported in some literature to be over 90%; however, in our experience, the sensitivity is relatively low, in the range of 70%.
4. A few more immunomarkers may be helpful, including p53, MUC5AC, and DPC4/SMAD4. Diffuse and strong p53 and MUC5AC positivity was seen in 50% and 60% of pancreatic ductal adenocarcinomas, respectively. Lack of expression of DPC4/SMAD4 was observed in approximately 50% of pancreatic ductal adenocarcinomas.
5. Significant ductal cell atypia can be seen in chronic pancreatitis, especially in an autoimmune pancreatitis. In a case of autoimmune pancreatitis, extensive fibrosis, many inflammatory cells, including plasma cells and eosinophils, can be seen. Serum IgG4 may be elevated as well. If a cellblock or thin tissue core is available, this small panel of immunomarkers can be useful as well.

Case Scenario 2

Learning Objectives

1. Recognize the cytologic features that raise concerns for a secondary tumor;
2. Recognize an unusual variant of pancreatic ductal adenocarcinoma;
3. Review the diagnostic criteria and features for non-ductal pancreatic neoplasms.

Case

A 53-year-old man presented with a 3.5 cm mass in the tail of the pancreas, abdominal discomfort, and weight loss. He had no known history of prior cancer. An EUS-FNA biopsy of the pancreatic mass was performed, and both smear and cellblock preparations were obtained. The FNA smears revealed a markedly cellular specimen with numerous groups and sheets of pleomorphic epithelial cells and many single atypical cells as shown in Fig. 8.38a–c. Some atypical cells contained large cytoplasmic vacuoles, and some contained intracytoplasmic lumina with a targetoid mucin. Many mitoses and some tumor necrosis were noted in the background. Mucinous material was not seen. The cellblock preparation is shown in Fig. 8.38d. Based on these cytologic features, a diagnosis of adenocarcinoma can be easily established. But the question that one should raise is: Is this a primary ductal adenocarcinoma of the pancreas? Or is this a variant of ductal adenocarcinoma of the pancreas? Or is this a metastatic carcinoma?

Some useful cytologic features which may suggest a secondary malignancy, variant of ductal carcinoma, or non-ductal neoplasm rather than a typical ductal adenocarcinoma of the pancreas are summarized in Table 8.5.

(continued)

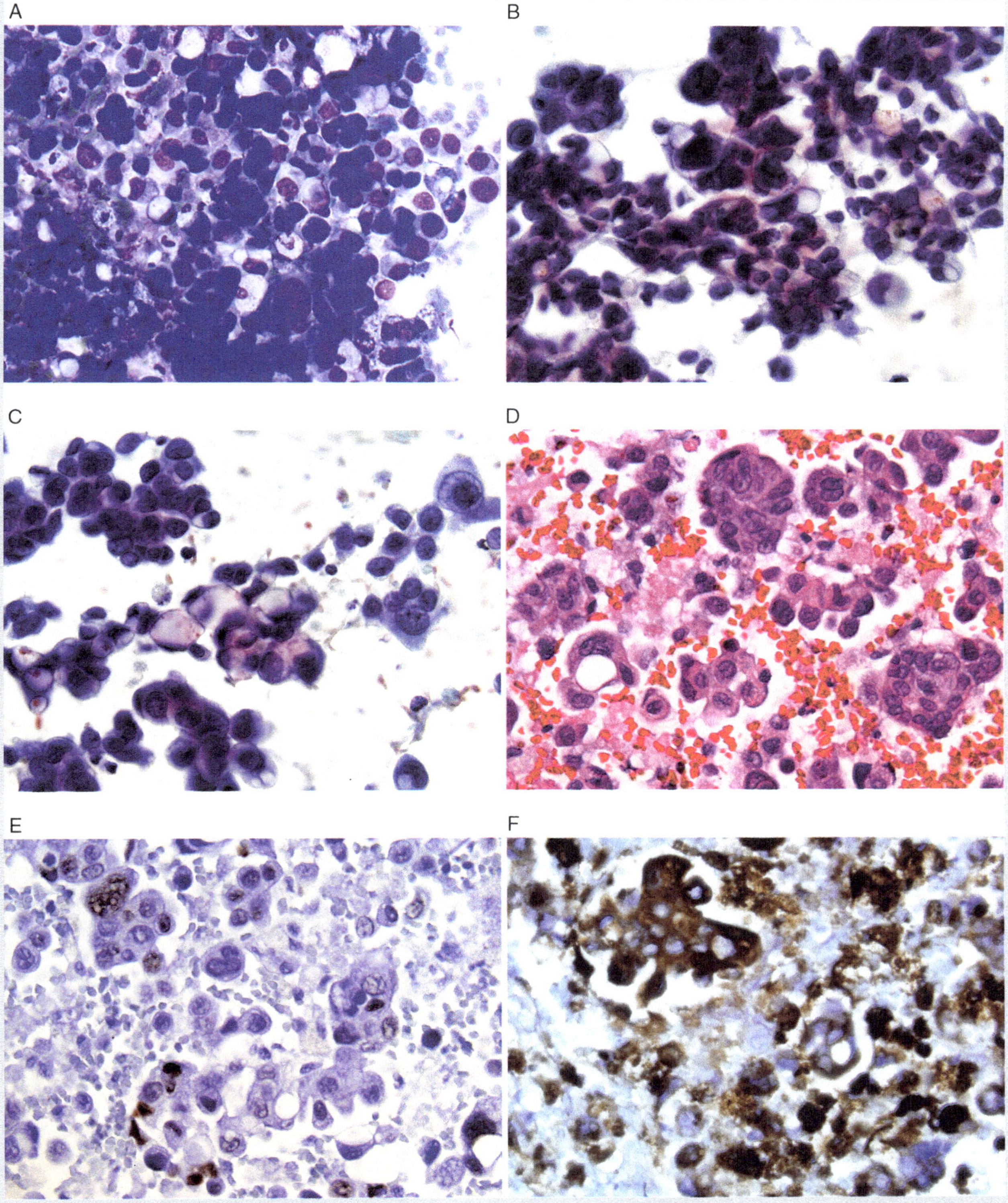

Fig. 8.38 Metastatic lung adenocarcinoma in the tail of the pancreas from a 53-year-old man. Hypercellular FNA smears with pleomorphic malignant cells with cytoplasmic vacuoles and many single tumor cells are shown in (**a–c**). Immunostains performed on the cellblock (**d**) show that the tumor cells are positive for TTF1 (**e**) and napsin A (**f**)

(continued)

Table 8.5 Useful clinical and cytologic features in the distinction of primary ductal adenocarcinoma from secondary tumors, variants of ductal carcinomas, and non-ductal neoplasms

Clinical and cytologic features	Primary ductal ADC	Secondary tumors/variants of ductal carcinomas/ non-ductal neoplasms
Age of patient	Usually over age 60	Can be any ages with the highest incidence in the sixth and seventh decades for a metastasis
Cellularity	Intermediate to low	Usually very cellular
Background mucin	More frequently seen	Less commonly seen
Glands with tall columnar cells	Unusual; unless in the background of intestinal IPMN	Colorectal or GI primary
Acinar structures	Unusual	Concern for acinar cell carcinoma or a metastasis such as prostatic adenocarcinoma
Nuclear pleomorphism	Moderate	Marked atypia
Chromatin and nuclear membrane	Fine or open chromatin with membranous irregularities	Hyperchromasia
Brisk mitoses	Less frequent	Frequent
Cellular cohesion	More cohesive groups	Loosely cohesive
Single tumor cells	Few single tumor cells; unless a poorly differentiated one	Can be many single cells especially a metastasis from the breast or lung; or a melanoma, sarcoma or lymphoid/hematopoietic tumors
Binucleated tumor cells	Infrequently seen	Melanoma, NET
Plasmacytoid cells	Infrequently seen	Melanoma, NET, plasmacytomas
Tumor necrosis and hemorrhage	Less frequent	More common
Large cytoplasmic vacuoles	Infrequently seen	Lung, GI
Signet ring tumor cells	Infrequently seen	Lung, GI, or breast primary
Clear cells	Clear cells changes in the background of mucin	Clear cells with rich vascular networks such as metastatic renal cell carcinoma
Spindle tumor cells	Uncommonly seen	GIST, sarcoma or sarcomatoid carcinoma

Note: *GIST* gastrointestinal stromal tumor

From Fig. 8.38a, b, the cytologic features described above, and a review of Table 8.5, a metastasis was suspected. Therefore, a panel of immunomarkers including CK7, CK20, TTF1, napsin A, S100P, and CDX2 was performed on the cellblock sections. The results demonstrated that the tumor cells were positive for CK7, napsin A, and TTF1 as shown below in Fig. 8.38e, f, and negative for CK20, S100P and CDX2, which suggested a lung primary. Subsequent CT scans revealed a lung mass. In short, this patient presented with a metastatic lung adenocarcinoma in the pancreas as the initial presentation.

Another example of a 51-year-old woman with metastatic ductal carcinoma of the breast in the head of the pancreas is shown in Fig. 8.39a–f. As shown in these figures, it was a highly cellular FNA specimen with loosely cohesive groups of tumor cells and many single tumor cells in the background. Tumor cells were very hyperchromatic with high nuclear-to-cytoplasmic ratios, and no mucin was observed in the background. Immunostains performed on the cellblock sections showed the tumor cells to be positive for ERs and GATA3, which confirmed the diagnosis of metastatic breast carcinoma.

Secondary malignancies of the pancreas account for less than 5% of malignant tumors of the pancreas. The most common metastases include renal cell carcinoma; melanoma; lung adenocarcinomas, breast carcinomas, and colon carcinomas. Any of these tumors can potentially present with a pancreatic mass as the initial presentation and mimic a primary ductal adenocarcinoma.

Additionally, non-epithelial neoplasms, such as melanoma, plasmacytoma/multiple myeloma, lymphoma, and myeloid sarcoma, can involve the pancreas as a primary or secondary presentation. Examples of melanoma and plasmacytoma are shown in Figs. 8.40a, b and 8.41a, b, respectively. Caution should be taken as many plasmacytomas, especially poorly differentiated ones, are diffusely positive for

(continued)

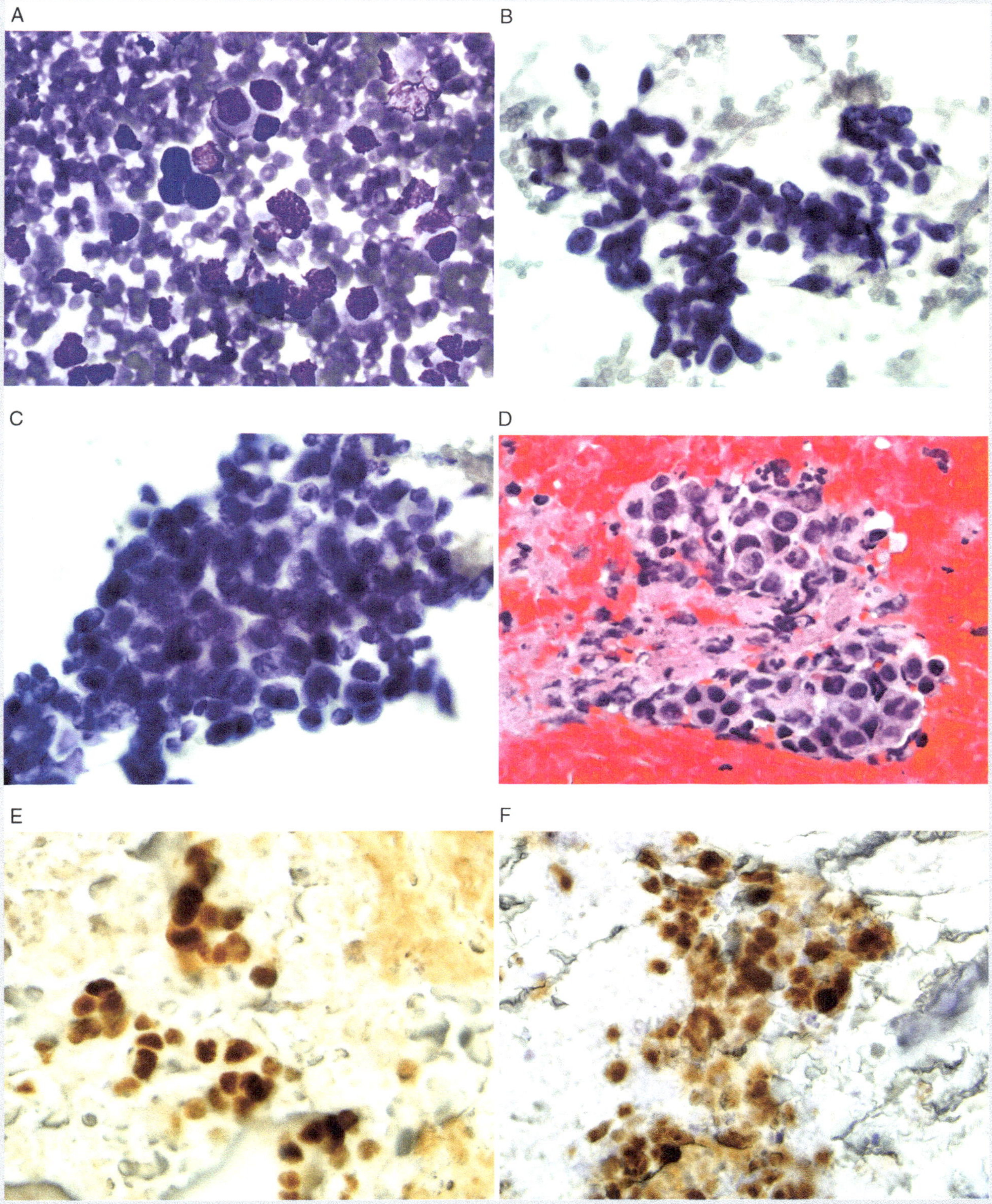

Fig. 8.39 Metastatic breast ductal carcinoma in the head of the pancreas from a 51-year-old woman. Hypercellular FNA smears with loosely cohesive groups of tumor cells and many single tumor cells are shown in (**a–c**). Immunostains performed on the cellblock (**d**) show that the tumor cells are positive for ER (**e**) and GATA3 (**f**)

(continued)

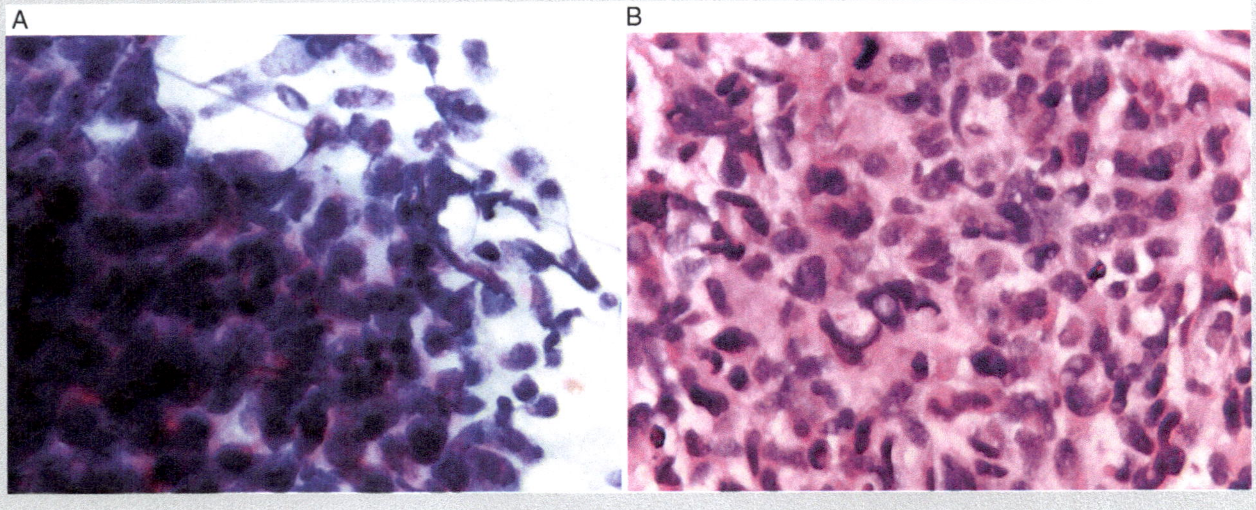

Fig. 8.40 Metastatic melanoma in the pancreas

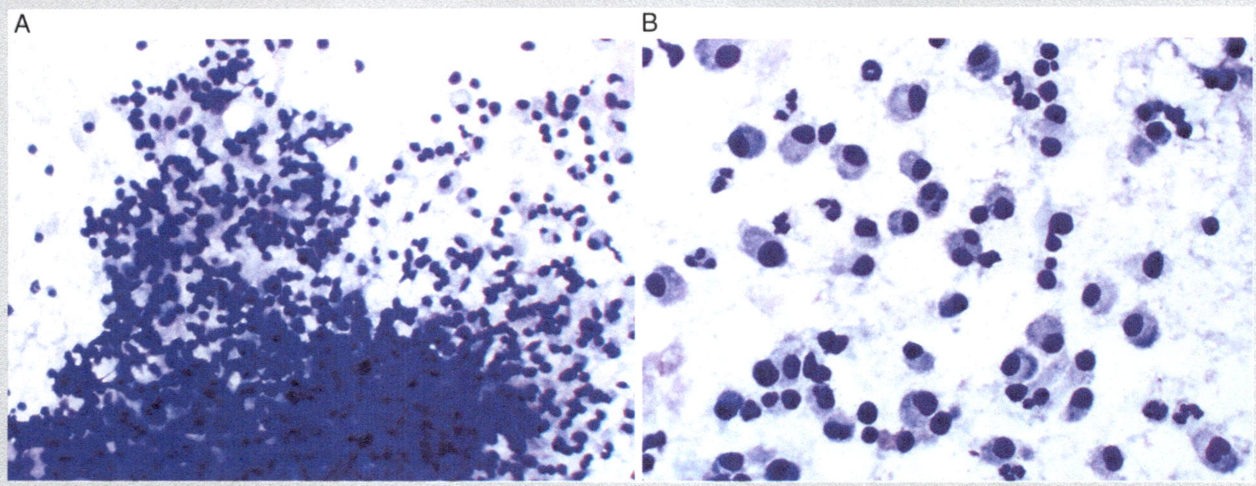

Fig. 8.41 Plasmacytoma involving the head of the pancreas

epithelial membrane antigen (EMA), but usually negative for CK7. Some melanoma cases, especially when an FNA sample is fixed in alcohol (which will dissolve S100 protein), or spindle cell melanoma, or ocular melanoma, can be negative for S100. In this case, SOX10 would be a better screening immunomarker.

Conversely, some variants of pancreatic ductal adenocarcinomas, such as medullary carcinoma, adenosquamous cell carcinoma, hepatoid carcinoma, giant cell carcinoma, sarcomatoid carcinoma, and signet ring cell carcinoma, may be mistakenly considered as a secondary tumor. An example of medullary carcinoma of the pancreas from a 63-year-old man (Figs. 8.18a, b and 8.19a, b), which revealed a very cellular specimen with large, loosely cohesive groups and single tumor cells intermixed with small lymphoid cells. The cellblock preparation and resected tumor sections showed a sheet of large tumor cells with a moderate amount of cytoplasm, large nuclei with open/vesicular nuclear chromatin, and prominent nucleoli. Many intra-tumorous lymphoid cells were noted. Hepatoid carcinoma of the pancreas is extremely rare and demonstrates essentially the same cytologic, histologic, and immunophenotypic features of a hepatocellular carcinoma as illustrated in Fig. 8.42a–g, which show a hepatoid carcinoma of the pancreas from a

(continued)

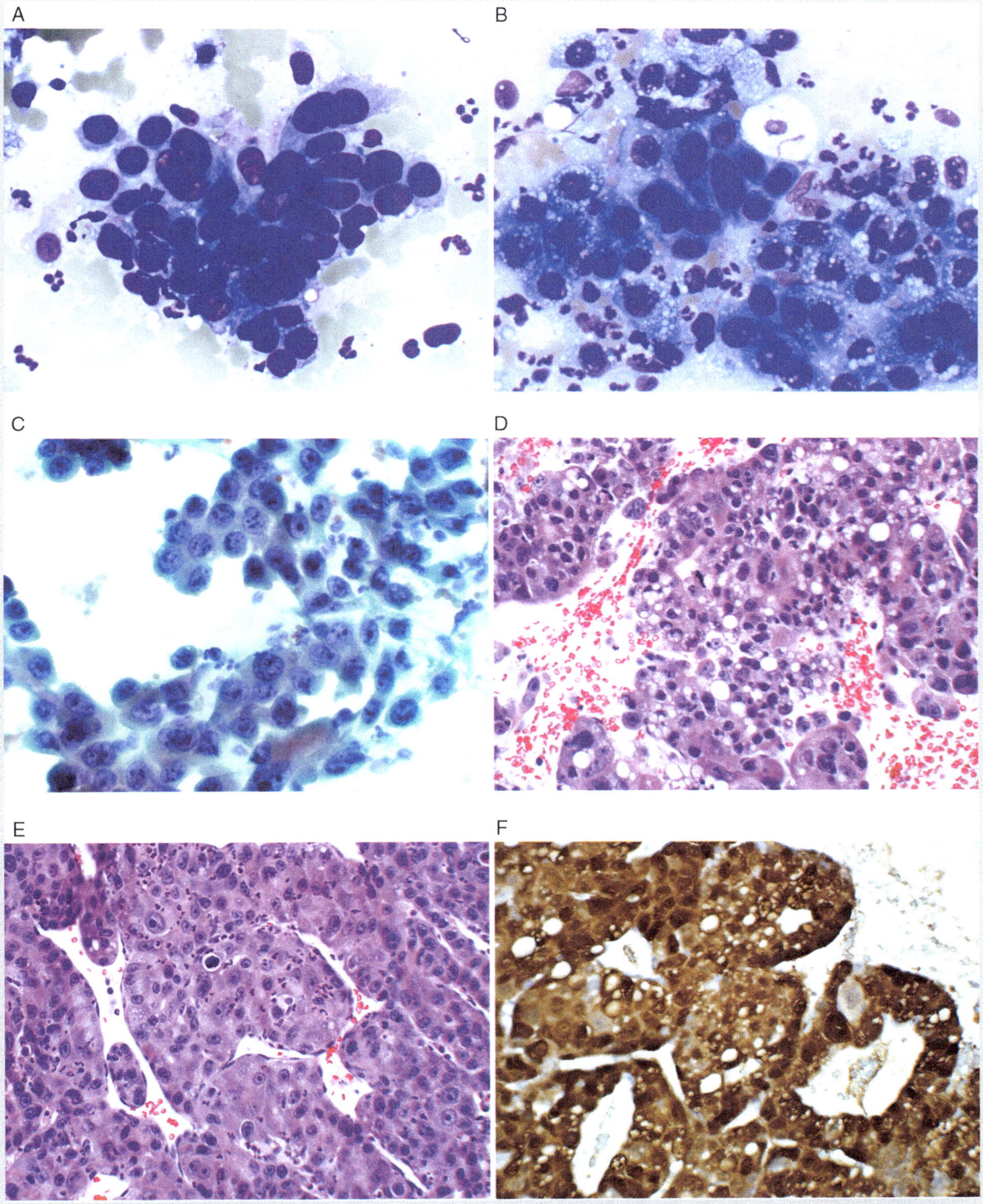

Fig. 8.42 Hepatoid carcinoma of the pancreas. Note that large neoplastic cells with granular and vacuolated cytoplasm on FNA smear (**a–c**), cellblock containing core biopsy specimen (**d**, **e**), and positive for arginase-1 (**f**), and focally positive for glypican-3 (**g**)

(continued)

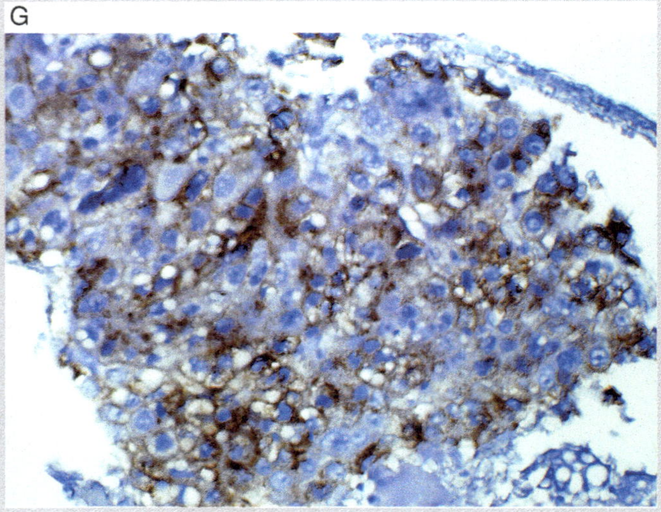

Fig. 8.42 (continued)

71-year-old man with a 7.6 × 3.8 cm pancreatic mass, elevated CA19-9 (1122), and no evidence of mass in other organs, including the liver.

Finally, some non-ductal neoplasms, including neuroendocrine neoplasm, acinar cell carcinoma, and SPT of the pancreas, may be diagnosed as a ductal carcinoma. Many neuroendocrine neoplasms of the pancreas demonstrate conspicuous or prominent nucleoli, which is not a typical finding in neuroendocrine neoplasms from other organs such as the lung and GI tract. In addition, some may also show focal significant nuclear pleomorphism. The combination of nuclear pleomorphism and prominent nucleoli may potentially mislead one to render a diagnosis of poorly differentiated carcinoma. Careful evaluation of other features, including mitoses, necrosis, and neuroendocrine nuclear chromatin, binucleations, and plasmacytoid tumor cells, will prevent one from making this mistake. If a cellblock or thin tissue core is available, immunostains for chromogranin and synaptophysin will resolve this problem. CD56 is not the best neuroendocrine marker for pancreatic neuroendocrine neoplasms since approximately 50% can be negative for CD56. Another potential pitfall is calling an acinar cell carcinoma a ductal carcinoma or a neuroendocrine neoplasm. Acinar cell carcinoma is rare and accounts for less than 1% of pancreatic malignancies. There is a wide spectrum of cytomorphology associated with acinar cell carcinoma, from well-differentiated resembling normal acini to poorly differentiated losing typical morphologic features. An example of acinar cell carcinoma is shown in Fig. 8.43a, b. An immunohistochemical stain for CK7 tends to show very focal positivity as shown in Fig. 8.43c or negativity; in contrast, the vast majority of ductal adenocarcinomas of the pancreas are diffusely positive for CK7. Other immunomarkers, including BCL10, antitrypsin, glypican-3, and lipase, have been reported to be useful.

Case Scenario 3

Learning Objectives

1. Evaluate a cystic lesion of the pancreas;
2. Determine the most effective IHC panel for a serous cystadenoma;
3. Determine the best way to approach a mucin-producing cystic neoplasm:
   A. Three diagnostic categories: definitive diagnosis, descriptive terms, and inconclusive ones;
   B. What needs to be mentioned in a final report?
   C. How to differentiate mucinous cyst lining epithelia from GI contaminants;
   D. Are there good criteria to separate an IPMN from an MCN on EUS-FNA samples?

Case

When evaluating a cystic lesion of the pancreas, a few relevant questions should be asked. Is this a mucin-producing cystic neoplasm? If the answer is yes, what

(continued)

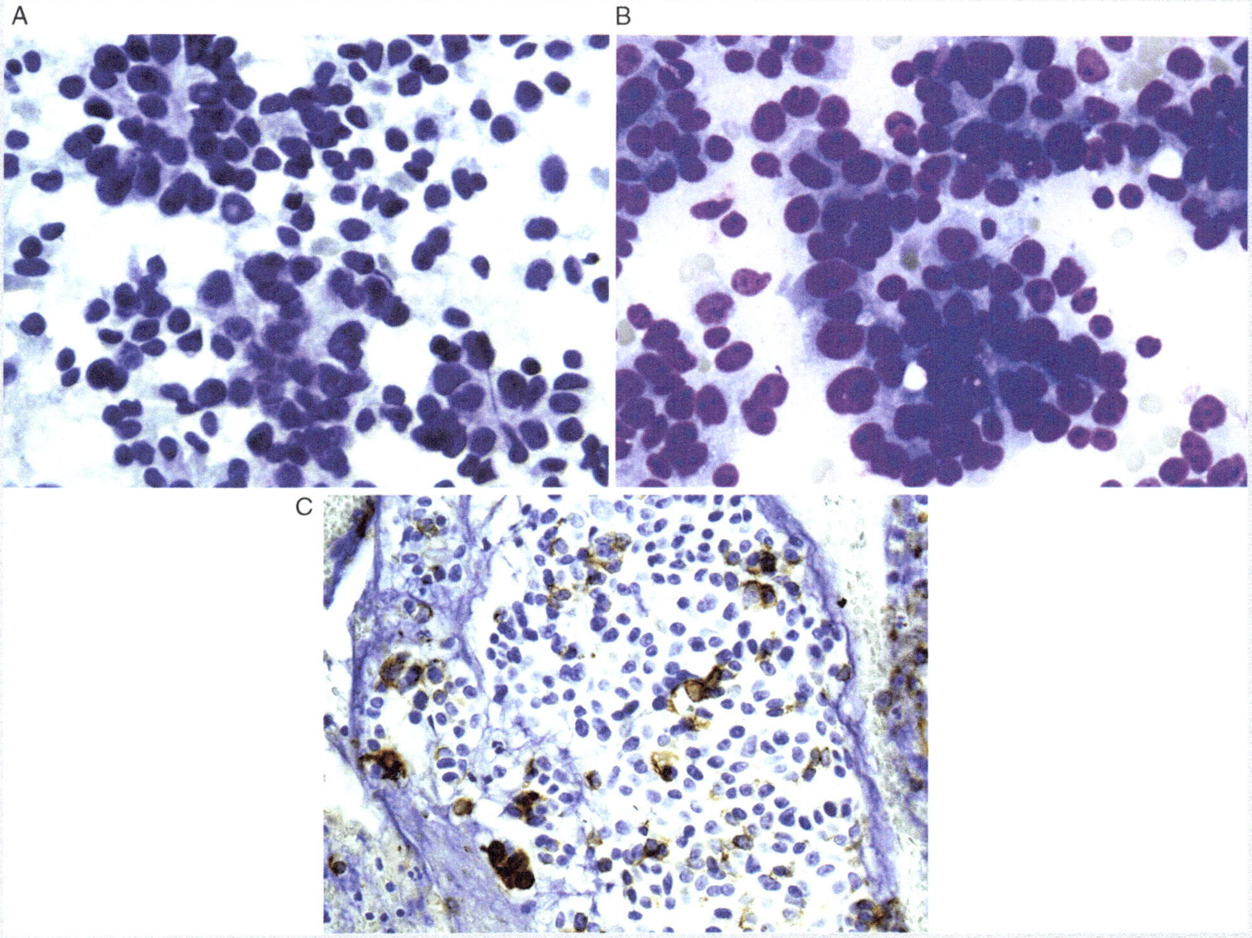

Fig. 8.43 (**a**, **b**) Show an acinar cell carcinoma, and (**c**) is very focally positive for CK7 on the cellblock

is the degree of epithelial atypia/dysplasia? If it is not a mucinous lesion, is this a pseudocyst? Or is this a serous cystadenoma? Or is this a rare cystic lesion such as lymphoepithelial cyst or other squamous epithelial cell lining cysts? Or is this a non-MCN, such as a cystic neuroendocrine neoplasm or an SPT? In the standardized terminology and nomenclature for pancreatobiliary cytology proposed by the Papanicolaou Society of Cytopathology, in addition to the traditional five diagnostic categories for cytologic specimens (nondiagnostic, benign, atypical, suspicious, and malignant), a new category called "neoplastic" or "category IV" was added to this scheme. This new category was further separated into "benign/category A" for serous cystadenoma and "other/category B" for premalignant mucinous cysts, NETs, and SPTs.

A 68-year-old woman presented with a 2.5 cm cystic lesion of the body of the pancreas. An EUS-FNA was performed, and both smear and cellblock preparations were obtained. The FNA smears were nearly acellular and had no mucinous material in the background. The cellblock section revealed a thin tissue core with non-neoplastic pancreatic lobules with small clefts, suggestive of cystic spaces. Some of the spaces appeared to be lined by a single layer of epithelial cells with clear cytoplasm. Significant nuclear atypia, goblet cells, or tall columnar mucinous cells were not seen. Based on the findings shown in Fig. 8.44a, b, a serous cystadenoma was suspected. For the confirmation of this diagnosis, a panel of IHC markers was performed, which showed that the lining cells were positive for CK7, pVHL, and MUC6 as shown in Fig. 8.44c–e.

(continued)

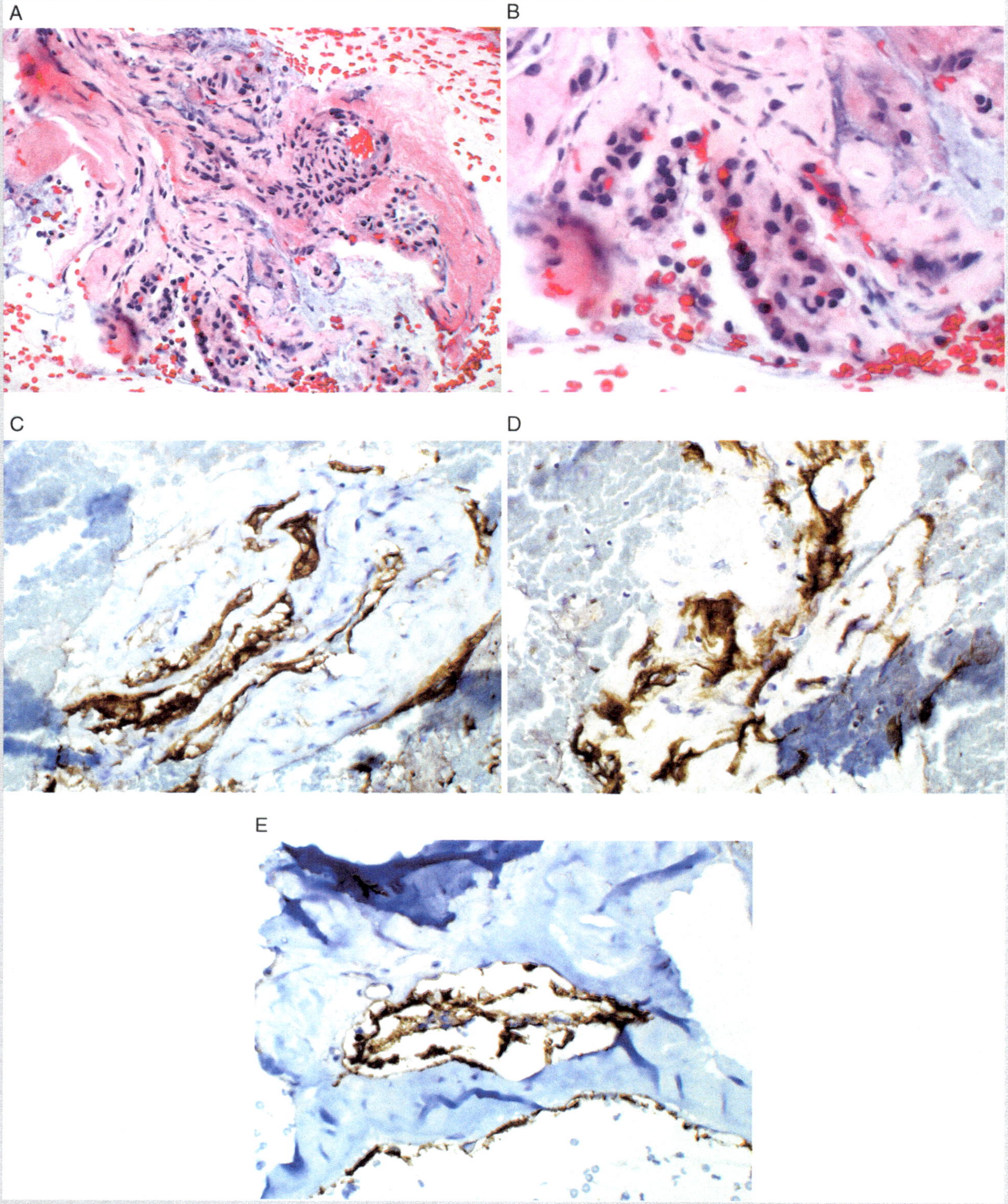

Fig. 8.44 Serous cystadenoma on thin tissue core biopsy (**a, b**) and positive immunostains for CK7 (**c**), pVHL (**d**), and MUC6 (**e**)

(continued)

We have found, and others have agreed, that making a diagnosis of serous cystadenoma of the pancreas on an FNA sample is problematic because of the inadequate cellularity of most specimens. Most of the smears were acellular or contained only rare groups of epithelial cells with bland cytology in a watery background. Many of these samples were regarded as nondiagnostic. In many instances, especially when the cystic lesions had been repeatedly sampled, the FNA smears usually contained many hemosiderin-laden histiocytes and debris, with or without epithelial cells. In this scenario, a diagnostic consideration of a pseudocyst may be included as well. Hemosiderin-laden histiocytes are infrequently seen in an MCN. When GI contamination and thin mucin are present in the background of a serous cystadenoma, a mucin-producing neoplasm may also be suggested. A cellblock preparation or thin tissue core biopsy is highly recommended and will be very helpful in reaching a final diagnosis. If a cellblock or thin tissue core is available, a panel of IHC markers including CK7, pVHL, MUC6, and inhibin-α can be helpful, since the vast majority of serous cystadenomas are diffusely positive for these four markers.

Another example of benign cystic lesion is a squamous cell-lined cyst such as lymphoepithelial cyst, dermoid cyst, and epidermoid cyst. A sample obtained from this type of cyst is frequently considered a nondiagnostic specimen or even a mucin-producing cyst due to the presence of only a few benign squamous cells/squames, debris, or GI contamination and thin mucin. Figure 8.45a, b shows a case of lymphoepithelial cyst

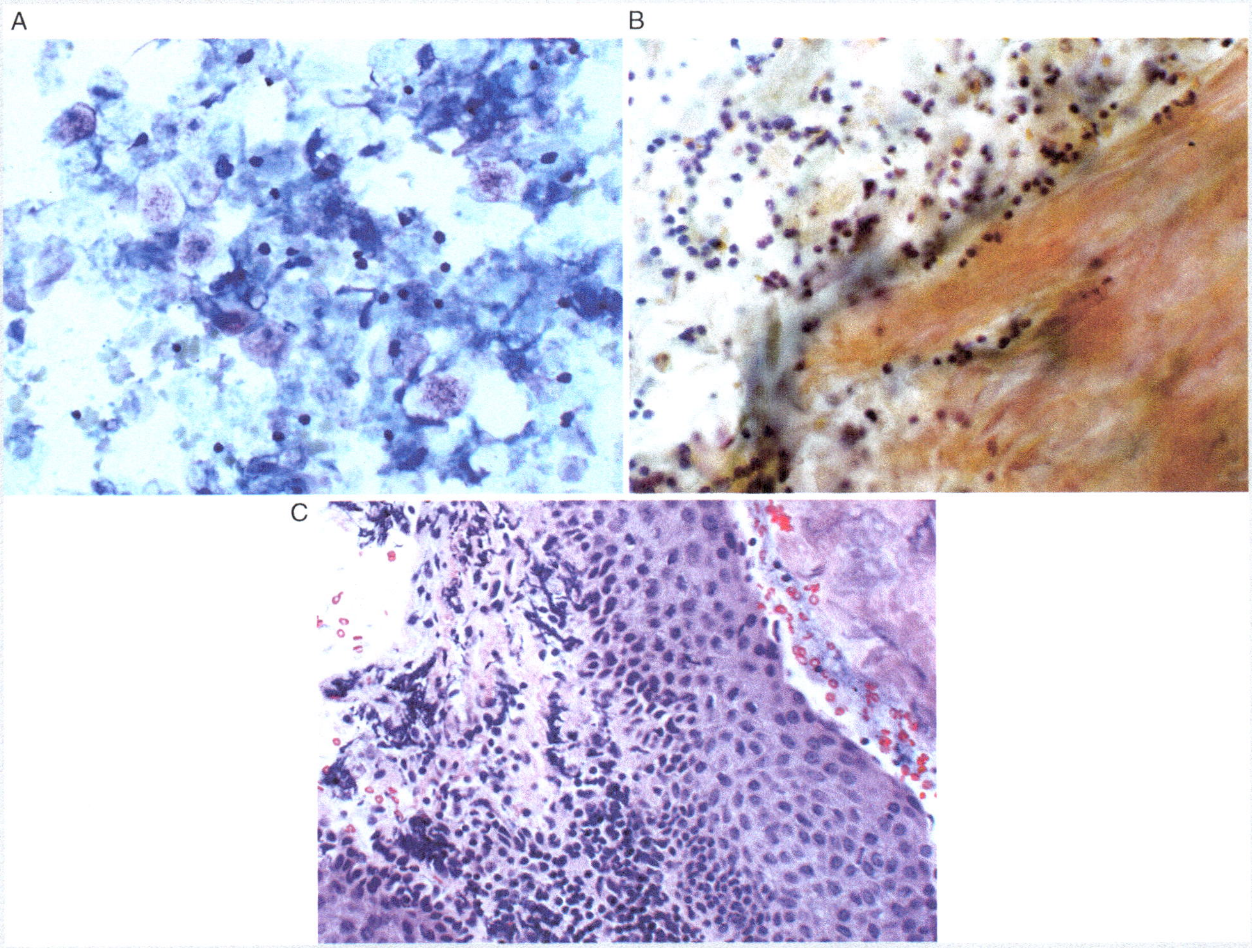

Fig. 8.45 Lymphoepithelial cyst on FNA smear (**a**, **b**) and cellblock (**c**)

(continued)

from a 55-year-old man presenting with a 3.0 cm mass at the tail of the pancreas. The cellblock preparation demonstrated a fragment of cystic wall which was composed of benign squamous epithelium and the underlining lymphoid tissue and keratin debris as shown in Fig. 8.45c.

Perhaps the most challenging task is to determine whether or not the cystic lesion is a mucin-producing cystic neoplasm and the degree of epithelial atypia/dysplasia. A 38-year-old woman presented with a 5.8 cm cystic lesion at the body of the pancreas. An EUS-FNA was performed. The FNA smears were very hypercellular, with numerous papillary groups and sheets of epithelial cells, with a spectrum of nuclear atypia, and mild to high-grade dysplasia in the background of mucin as shown in Fig. 8.46a–d. The cellblock section demonstrated findings similar to those shown in Fig. 8.46e, f. Based on these cytologic features, the diagnosis was "mucin-producing cystic neoplasm with high-grade dysplasia; invasion cannot be excluded." The subsequent resection of the tail of the pancreas was done, and representative areas of the histology of the tumor are illustrated in Fig. 8.46g, h. Invasive adenocarcinoma was not identified after thoroughly examining the entire cystic tumor. The final histologic diagnosis was "MCN with high-grade dysplasia. No invasive carcinoma identified."

So, what did we learn from this example? We tend to group a mucin-producing cystic neoplasm into three diagnostic categories: (a) definitive diagnosis, (b) descriptive diagnosis, and (c) nondiagnostic. For the definitive diagnosis category, one expects to see (1) a highly cellular specimen with papillary groups of various degrees of epithelial atypia/dysplasia, in the background of thick colloid-like mucus as shown in the above example; (2) low cellularity with small clusters or papillary groups of epithelial cells with various degrees of epithelial atypia/dysplasia and background mucin; and (3) a very hypocellular specimen with thick/colloid-like, gelatinous mucus and tall mucinous columnar cells in singles or small groups and histiocytes/muciphages. For a descriptive diagnosis case, one expects to see a mixture of small epithelial groups with degenerative changes/cellular debris and significant GI contaminants in the background of thin mucin. For the nondiagnostic category, one expects to see predominately GI contamination or a nearly acellular specimen without thick background mucus.

Are there good criteria to separate an IPMN from an MCN on an EUS-FNA sample? The answer is no. IPMN was defined as a mucinous cystic tumor involving main and/or side branch pancreatic ducts; an MCN generally does not involve the pancreatic duct system. Identification of ovarian-like stroma on the cystic wall is the hallmark of an MCN. In addition, an MCN nearly always occurs in a woman, usually in middle-age, and in the body or tail of the pancreas. In general, an FNA sample obtained from an IPMN tends to be more cellular and more frequently contains papillary clusters than an MCN specimen. In fact, it is more common to

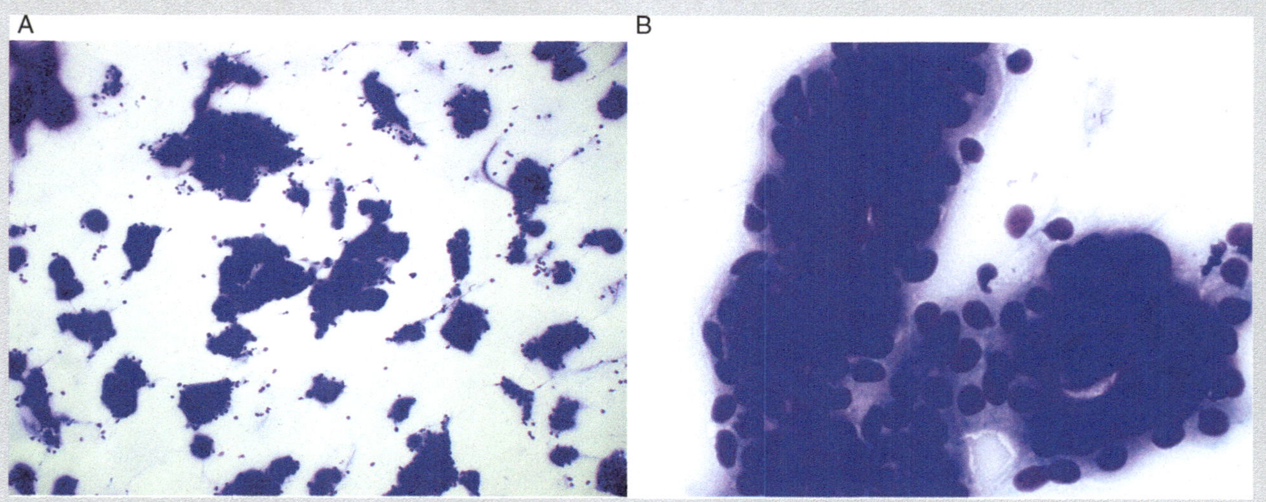

Fig. 8.46 Mucinous cystic neoplasm with high-grade atypia/dysplasia on FNA smears (**a–d**) and histologic sections (**e–h**)

(continued)

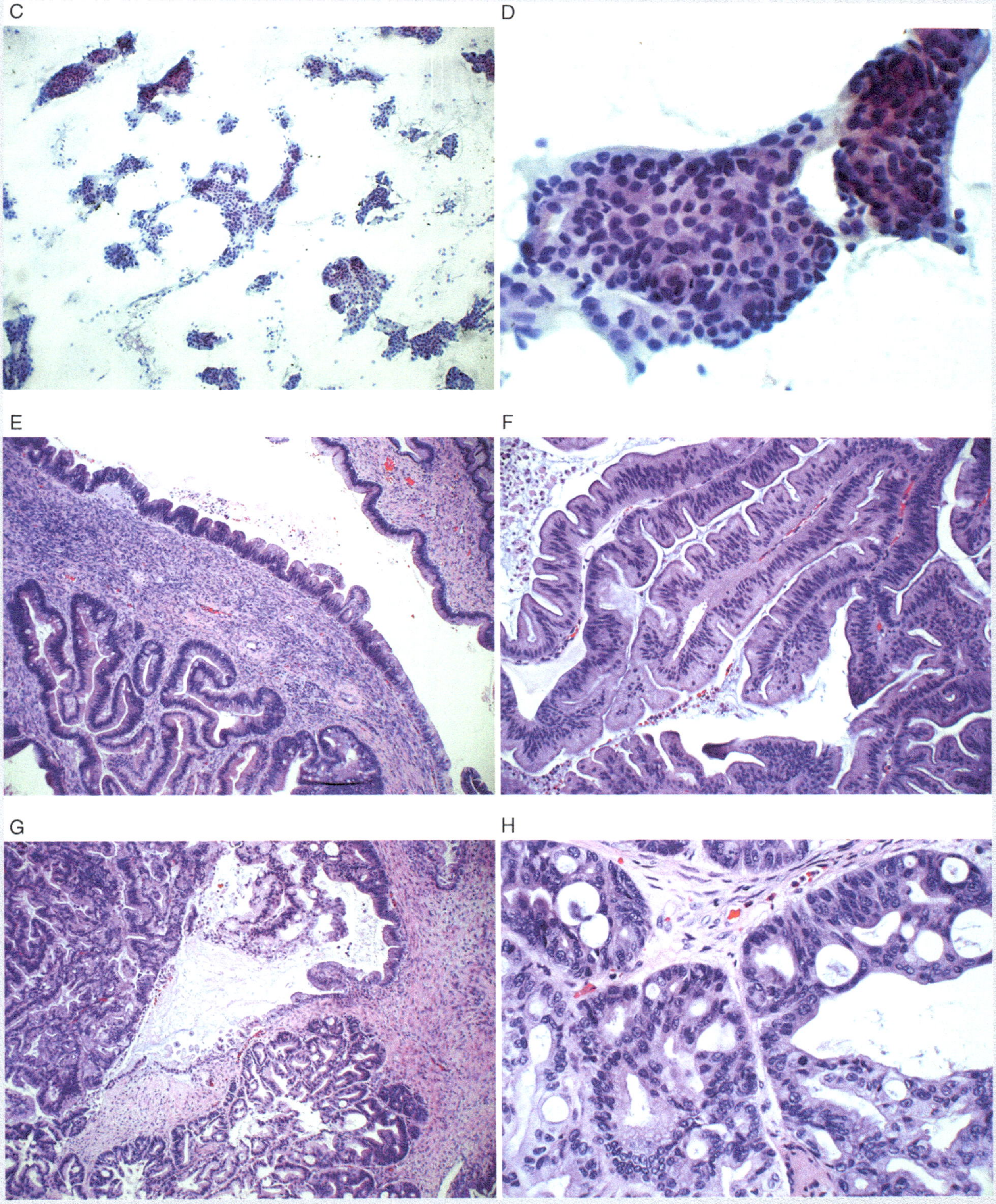

Fig. 8.46 (continued)

(continued)

render a definitive diagnosis from an IPMN sample than from an MCN specimen because there is a higher percentage of acellular or paucicellular specimens obtained from MCN cases. Another important observation from this case is that one should have a high threshold for diagnosing a pancreatic cancer when an FNA sample is very hypercellular with a spectrum of epithelial dysplasia. Extremely high cellularity suggests an intraductal or an intracystic growth of the lesion and lack of desmoplastic stroma. As well known, most invasive pancreatic ductal adenocarcinomas demonstrate invasive malignant glands in the desmoplastic stroma. As a result, an FNA sample from a ductal adenocarcinoma of the pancreas tends to show moderate to low cellularity. In a final cytology report, the degree of epithelial dysplasia must be included. For a cystic lesion with descriptive diagnosis, the presence or absence of epithelial cells, thick mucus, and epithelial dysplasia should be stated in the final report. Since about 25% of mucinous tumors of the pancreas may demonstrate invasive tubular/ductal carcinoma on the resected specimens, an extensive sampling (if not complete) of the cystic mass is strongly recommended.

Another important consideration is how to differentiate mucinous cyst lining epithelia from GI contaminants. The recognition of duodenal epithelial contaminant is less problematic since the duodenal mucosa presents with two-dimensional, honeycomb sheets with no nuclear atypia, scattered clear-appearing goblet cells, and intraepithelial lymphoid cells. The challenge is to differentiate gastric epithelial contaminant from gastric-type IPMN or MCN with only low-grade epithelial atypia. Unfortunately, there are no reliable cytologic criteria for making this distinction. In general, gastric contamination shows large sheets of epithelial cells in the background of thin mucin; in contrast, a low-grade gastric type IPMN or MCN tends to show small groups of epithelial cells with some degenerative changes or some cellular debris in a mucinous background. If parietal cells are present, then gastric contamination is favored. Our recent study demonstrated that CK7 was diffusely positive in gastric-type IPMN or MCN but tended to be negative or only focally positive in gastric epithelial contaminant. Analysis of the cystic fluid from these types of pancreatic cysts can be useful. CEA levels of 200 ng/mL or above are strongly supportive of a neoplastic mucinous cyst. However, a low CEA level does not exclude a mucinous cyst. In addition, molecular analysis of K-ras, loss of heterozygosity (LOH), DNA contents, and GNAS may provide additional value in diagnosing an MCN of the pancreas, especially the ones with very hypocellular specimens and lack of significant epithelial atypia/dysplasia.

Abbreviations List

Abbreviation	Full text
CC	Colloid carcinoma
CD	Cluster of differentiation
CDX2	Caudal type homeobox 2
CEA	Carcinoembryonic antigen
CK	Cytokeratin
Computed tomography	CT
CPNET	Cystic pancreatic neuroendocrine tumor
ER	Estrogen receptor
EUS	Endoscopic ultrasound-guided
EUS-FNA	Endoscopic ultrasound-guided fine needle aspiration
FISH	Fluorescence in situ hybridization
FNA	Fine needle aspiration
FNAB	Fine needle aspiration biopsy
GI	Gastrointestinal
GIST	Gastrointestinal stromal tumor
H&E	Hematoxylin and eosin
HPF	High-power field

Abbreviation	Full text
IgG4	Immunoglobulin G4
IHC	Immunohistochemical
IMP3	Insulin-like growth factor 2 mRNA-binding protein 3
IPMN	Intraductal papillary mucinous neoplasm
ITPN	Intraductal tubulopapillary neoplasm
KOC	K homology domain containing protein overexpressed in cancer
K-ras	Kirsten rat sarcoma viral oncogene homolog
LOH	Loss of heterozygosity
MCN	Mucinous cystic neoplasm
MLH1	MutL homolog 1
MMR	Mismatch repair
MRI	Magnetic resonance imaging
MSH2	MutS protein homolog 2
MSH6	MutS protein homolog 6
MSI	Microsatellite instability
MUC	Mucin (MIC1, MUC2, MUC4, MUC5AC, and MUC6)
NEC	Neuroendocrine carcinoma
NET	Neuroendocrine tumor

Abbreviation	Full text
PanIN	Pancreatic intraepithelial neoplasia
PAS	Periodic acid-Schiff
PAX8	Paired box gene 8
PDX-1	Pancrease/duodenum homeobox-1
PMS2	Postmeiotic segregation increased 2
PR	Progesterone receptor
pVHL	von Hippel-Lindau gene product
SPT	Solid-pseudopapillary tumor
TTF1	Thyroid transcription factor 1
WHO	World Health Organization

Suggested Reading

Abraham SC, Klimstra DS, Wilentz RE, Yeo CJ, Conlon K, Brennan M, et al. Solid-pseudopapillary tumors of the pancreas are genetically distinct from pancreatic ductal adenocarcinomas and almost always harbor beta-catenin mutations. Am J Pathol. 2002;160(4):1361–9.

Adsay NV, Pierson C, Sarkar F, Abrams J, Weaver D, Conlon KC, et al. Colloid (mucinous noncystic) carcinoma of the pancreas. Am J Surg Pathol. 2001;25(1):26–42.

Adsay NV. Cystic neoplasia of the pancreas: pathology and biology. J Gastrointest Surg. 2008;12(3):401–4.

Bellizzi AM, Stelow EB. Pancreatic cytopathology: a practical approach and review. Arch Pathol Lab Med. 2009;133(3):388–404.

Bosman FT, Carneiro F, Hruban RH, Theise ND. WHO classification of tumours of the digestive system. 4th ed. Lyon: IARC Press; 2010. p. 279–334.

Brugge WR, Lewandrowski K, Lee-Lewandrowski E, Centeno BA, Szydlo T, Regan S, et al. Diagnosis of pancreatic cystic neoplasms: a report of the cooperative pancreatic cyst study. Gastroenterology. 2004;126(5):1330–6.

Cao D, Zhang Q, Wu LS, Salaria SN, Winter JW, Hruban RH, et al. Prognostic significance of maspin in pancreatic ductal adenocarcinoma: tissue microarray analysis of 223 surgically resected cases. Mod Pathol. 2007;20(5):570–8.

Cizginer S, Turner BG, Bilge AR, Karaca C, Pitman MB, Brugge WR. Cyst fluid carcinoembryonic antigen is an accurate diagnostic marker of pancreatic mucinous cysts. Pancreas. 2011;40(7):1024–8.

Crippa S, Salvia R, Warshaw AL, Domínguez I, Bassi C, Falconi M, et al. Mucinous cystic neoplasm of the pancreas is not an aggressive entity: lessons from 163 resected patients. Ann Surg. 2008;247(7):571–9.

DeMay RM. Chapter 19. Pancreas. In:The art and science of cytopathology, vol. 3. 2nd ed. Chicago: ASCP Press; 2010. p. 1298–327.

Deng H, Shi J, Wilkerson M, Meschter S, Dupree W, Lin F. Usefulness of S100P in diagnosis of adenocarcinoma of pancreas on fine-needle aspiration biopsy specimens. Am J Clin Pathol. 2008;129(1):81–8.

Findeis-Hosey JJ, Xu H. The use of insulin like-growth factor II messenger RNA binding protein-3 in diagnostic pathology. Hum Pathol. 2011;42(3):303–14.

Hruban RH, Pitman MB, Klimstra DS. Tumors of the pancreas. In:AFIP atlas of tumor pathology. 4th series, fascicle 6, 6th ed. Washington, DC: American Registry of Pathology; 2007. p. 103–64.

Hruban RH, Takaori K, Klimstra DS, Adsay NV, Albores-Saavedra J, Biankin AV, et al. An illustrated consensus on the classification of pancreatic intraepithelial neoplasia and intraductal papillary mucinous neoplasms. Am J Surg Pathol. 2004;28(8):977–87.

Khalid A, Zahid M, Finkelstein SD, LeBlanc JK, Kaushik N, Ahmad N, et al. Pancreatic cyst fluid DNA analysis in evaluating pancreatic cysts: a report of the PANDA study. Gastrointest Endosc. 2009;69(6):1095–102.

Klimstra DS. Pathology reporting of neuroendocrine tumors: essential elements for accurate diagnosis, classification, and staging. Semin Oncol. 2013;40(1):23–36.

Levy M, Lin F, Xu H, Dhall D, Spaulding BO, Wang HL. S100P, von Hippel-Lindau gene product, and IMP3 serve as a useful immunohistochemical panel in the diagnosis of adenocarcinoma on endoscopic bile duct biopsy. Hum Pathol. 2010;41(9):1210–9.

Lin F, Chen ZE, Wang HL. Utility of immunohistochemistry in the pancreatobiliary tract. Arch Pathol Lab Med. 2015;139(1):24–38.

Lin F, Liu H. Immunohistochemistry in undifferentiated neoplasm/tumor of uncertain origin. Arch Pathol Lab Med. 2014;138(12):1583–610.

Liu H, Shi J, Anandan V, Wang HL, Diehl D, Blansfield J, et al. Reevaluation and identification of the best immunohistochemical panel (pVHL, Maspin, S100P, IMP-3) for ductal adenocarcinoma of the pancreas. Arch Pathol Lab Med. 2012a;136(6):601–9.

Lin F, Shi J, Liu H, Hull ME, Dupree W, Prichard JW, et al. Diagnostic utility of S100P and von Hippel-Lindau gene product (pVHL) in pancreatic adenocarcinoma-with implication of their roles in early tumorigenesis. Am J Surg Pathol. 2008a;32(1):78–91.

Lin F, Shi J, Liu H, Zhang J, Zhang PL, Wang HL, et al. Immunohistochemical detection of the von Hippel-Lindau gene product (pVHL) in human tissues and tumors: a useful marker for metastatic renal cell carcinoma and clear cell carcinoma of the ovary and uterus. Am J Clin Pathol. 2008b;129(4):592–605.

Liu H, Shi J, Wang HL, Zhang J, Brown RE, Wilkerson M, et al. Expression of von Hippel-Lindau gene product (pVHL) and S100P in cystic neoplasms of the pancreas – with an implication for their roles in tumorigenesis. Ann Clin Lab Sci. 2012b;42(2):109–17.

Lin F, Staerkel G. Cytologic criteria for well differentiated adenocarcinoma of pancreas in fine-needle aspiration specimens. Cancer Cytopathol. 2003;99(1):44–50.

Lin F, Wang HL. Pancreas and ampulla. In: Lin F, Prichard JW, Liu H, Wilkerson M, Chen E, editors. Handbook of practical immunohistochemistry – frequently asked questions. 2nd ed. New York: Springer Science + Business Media; 2015. p. 481–502.

Lok T, Chen L, Lin F, Wang HL. Immunohistochemical distinction between intrahepatic cholangiocarcinoma and pancreatic ductal adenocarcinoma. Hum Pathol. 2014;45(2):394–400.

Lüttges J, Galehdari H, Bröcker V, Schwarte-Waldhoff I, Henne-Bruns D, Klöppel G, et al. Allelic loss is often the first hit in the biallelic inactivation of the p53 and DPC4 genes during pancreatic carcinogenesis. Am J Pathol. 2001;158(5):1677–83.

Pitman MB, Centeno BA, Ali SZ, Genevay M, Stelow E, Mino-Kenudson M, et al. Standardized terminology and nomenclature for pancreatobiliary cytology: the Papanicolaou Society of Cytopathology Guidelines. Cytoournal. 2014a;11(Suppl 1):3.

Pitman MB, Centeno BA, Daglilar ES, Brugge WR, Mino-Kenudson M. Cytological criteria of high-grade epithelial atypia in the cyst fluid of pancreatic intraductal papillary mucinous neoplasms. Cancer Cytopathol. 2014b;122(1):40–7.

Pitman MB, Genevay M, Yaeger K, Chebib I, Turner BG, Mino-Kenudson M, et al. High-grade atypical epithelial cells in pancreatic mucinous cysts are a more accurate predictor of malignancy than "positive" cytology. Cancer Cytopathol. 2010;118(6):434–40.

Sato N, Fukushima N, Matsubayashi H, Goggins M. Identification of maspin and S100P as novel hypomethylation targets in pancreatic cancer using global gene expression profiling. Oncogene. 2004;23(8):1531–8.

Schmidt MT, Himmelfarb EA, Shafi H, Lin F, Xu H, Wang HL. Use of IMP3, S100P, and pVHL immunopanel to aid in the interpretation of bile duct biopsies with atypical histology or suspicious for malignancy. Appl Immunohistochem Mol Morphol. 2012;20(5):478–87.

Shen J, Brugge WR, Dimaio CJ, Pitman MB. Molecular analysis of pancreatic cyst fluid: a comparative analysis with current practice of diagnosis. Cancer. 2009;117(3):217–27.

Shi J, Liu H, Wang HL, Prichard JW, Lin F. Diagnostic utility of von Hippel-Lindau gene product, maspin, IMP3, and S100P in adenocarcinoma of the gallbladder. Hum Pathol. 2013;44(4):503–11.

Tanaka Y, Kato K, Notohara K, Hojo H, Ijiri R, Miyake T, et al. Frequent beta-catenin mutation and cytoplasmic/nuclear accumulation in pancreatic solid-pseudopapillary neoplasm. Cancer Res. 2001;61(23):8401–4.

Wachter DL, Schlabrakowski A, Hoegel J, Kristiansen G, Hartmann A, Riener MO. Diagnostic value of immunohistochemical IMP3 expression in core needle biopsies of pancreatic ductal adenocarcinoma. Am J Surg Pathol. 2011;35(6):873–7.

Wilentz RE, Goggins M, Redston M, Marcus VA, Adsay NV, Sohn TA, et al. Genetic, immunohistochemical, and clinical features of medullary carcinoma of the pancreas: a newly described and characterized entity. Am J Pathol. 2000;156(5):1641–51.

Winner M, Sethi A, Poneros JM, Stavropoulos SN, Francisco P, Lightdale CJ, et al. The role of molecular analysis in the diagnosis and surveillance of pancreatic cystic neoplasms. JOP. 2015;16(2):143–9.

Yantiss RK, Woda BA, Fanger GR, Kalos M, Whalen GF, Tada H, et al. KOC (K homology domain containing protein overexpressed in cancer): a novel molecular marker that distinguishes between benign and malignant lesions of the pancreas. Am J Surg Pathol. 2005;29(2):188–95.

9 Kidney and Adrenal Glands

Jun Zhang, Fan Lin, and Haiyan Liu

Summary of Pearls and Pitfalls

- Up to 30% of aspirates are nondiagnostic; a scant specimen containing only small number of atypical cells is not reliable for a positive diagnosis; even if it is called suspicious, it is likely the kidney will be resected.
- The diagnosis of a cystic renal cell carcinoma (RCC) has very low sensitivity on FNA.
- RCCs can be subclassified by FNA.
- It may be difficult to distinguish oncocytoma from chromophobe RCC, especially for the hybrid oncocytic chromophobe tumor.
- When evaluating an FNA from a radiographically visible mass, renal adenoma is not a diagnostic consideration.
- It is difficult to make a diagnosis of an angiomyolipoma on FNA in practice because only the radiographically the low fat masses are selected for FNA.
- Metanephric adenomas are benign and negative for EMA and may be difficult to distinguish from a Wilms tumor (nephroblastoma) but mostly in children under 6 years old.
- Urothelial carcinoma (UC) cells often have hyperchromatic angulated nuclei and squamoid cytoplasm, such as cercariform cells, and are frequently immunoreactive for CEA, GATA3, and CK20.
- Metastatic tumor cells usually have different cytomorphologic features and usually have known primary elsewhere, except collecting duct RCC, which can mimic metastatic tumors.
- Hepatocytes can be accidently sampled, usually have abundant granular cytoplasm with patterns in groups and singly placed cells, may have bile, or show nuclear and cellular size variation.
- Adrenal cortical lesions are immunoreactive for inhibin, calretinin, and melan A.
- Fine-needle aspiration (FNA) of the kidney is a useful technique for the diagnosis of selected renal lesions. Most renal lesions are not candidates for FNA.
  - Resected with a presumptive diagnosis based on imaging studies, without a preoperative FNA.
  - In adults, the great majority of renal lesions are either radiologically benign cysts requiring no treatment or radiologically suspicious masses requiring a resection regardless of the result of an FNA.
  - Only a small percentage of adult renal lesions, perhaps less than 10%, are candidates for FNA, but in these cases, an FNA can be very helpful.
- Recently a more conservative treatment of a small renal mass (less than 7.0 cm) has been introduced:
  - Cryotherapy
  - Radiofrequency
  - Ethanol injections
- As the result, a preoperative diagnosis is often required. So FNA or thin-needle core biopsy may gradually gain its popularity.

FNA Indications

When radical nephrectomy is contraindicated:

- Unresectable renal cell carcinoma.
- Possible metastasis to the kidney (e.g., history or suspicion of cancer elsewhere).
- Patient has coincident medical problems and cannot tolerate the operation.

© Springer International Publishing AG 2018
F. Lin et al., *Handbook of Practical Fine Needle Aspiration and Small Tissue Biopsies*, DOI 10.1007/978-3-319-57386-1_9

- Patient desires an investigational treatment (lesion ablation in vivo); an FNA is obtained for tissue diagnosis before the ablation procedure.

When radiologic findings are equivocal:

- Atypical cysts; FNA is used to triage patients for either surgery or clinical observation. Advances in radiographic assessment of cystic renal lesions have made FNA less useful in this setting.
- Fat-free angiomyolipomas.

When a partial nephrectomy is considered:

- Some papillary RCC and chromophobe RCC with a good prognosis.
- Smaller lesions and lesions in younger patients as the incidence increases.
- Patients with the von Hippel-Lindau syndrome at risk for bilateral tumors.
- Patients with decreased renal function are candidates for nephron-sparing surgery.
- Although the ultimate decision to treat by partial nephrectomy depends on the size and location of the lesion as well as other clinical factors, FNA is valuable because it discloses whether or not the tumor is one of the "good prognosis" neoplasms amenable to conservative treatment.

When an abscess is suspected:

- Patient with a renal abscess, needle placement permits both diagnosis and therapeutic drainage.

An equivocal case is best diagnosed as "oncocytic neoplasm: oncocytoma, chromophobe RCC, and clear cell RCC with eosinophilic granular cytoplasm." With a note, if clinically indicated, a partial nephrectomy should be considered. Finally one must consider inadvertent sampling of the liver.

Specimen Collection and Preparation

- All aspirations are virtually carried out by radiologists: They rarely are performed intraoperatively by surgeons.
- Complications are uncommon and include bleeding, hematuria, pneumothorax, infection, arteriovenous fistula, and urinoma.
- Needle-tract seeding is extremely rare with the use of small (less than 18-gauge) needles.
- Slides may be air-dried and stained with a Romanowsky stain and/or alcohol fixed and stained with the Papanicolaou or hematoxylin and eosin stains.
- Cell blocks are particularly helpful for identifying architectural features such as papillae and provide an ideal platform for immunohistochemical studies (e.g., HMB-45 to confirm the diagnosis of an angiomyolipoma).

Accuracy and Adequacy

The true accuracy of renal FNA in routine practice is uncertain. Investigators with experience find:

- Renal FNA accurately distinguishes benign from malignant lesions in 73–94% of cases.
- Correct subclassification of RCC is achieved in 74% of cases.
- In the 1998 College of American Pathologists Non-Gynecologic Cytology Program, renal FNA had the highest false-positive rate (30.4%) of any FNA specimen and the second highest false-negative rate (13.9%).

False-positive results occur with FNA:

- Xanthogranulomatous pyelonephritis
- Angiomyolipoma
- Benign hepatocytes
- Benign tubular cells
- Benign adrenal cortical cells

This disappointing accuracy is likely a reflection of the difficulty in obtaining experience in general practice, however, which better reflects the spectrum of routine practice, because so few kidney lesions are aspirated.

There is no consensus on adequacy:

- Up to 30% of renal aspirates are nondiagnostic (inadequate).
- A repeat aspiration is unhelpful in over 40% of cases.

It is reasonable to consider a specimen adequate if a specific (benign or malignant) diagnosis can be made or if there is sufficient cellularity to suggest a limited differential diagnosis. A specimen composed exclusively of macrophages is best reported as "nondiagnostic" rather than negative, because a cystic RCC cannot be excluded.

Table 9.1 lists the new version of the classification of renal neoplasia. This chapter will mainly focus on the common renal and adrenal tumors which often can be diagnosed on FNA specimens.

The Kidney

Normal cytology of the kidney:

- Glomeruli
- Proximal tubular cells
- Distal tubular cells

Table 9.1 ISUP Vancouver modification of WHO (2004) histologic classification of kidney tumors

Renal cell tumors
Papillary adenoma
Oncocytoma
Clear cell renal cell carcinoma
Multilocular cystic clear cell renal cell neoplasm of low malignant potential[a]
Papillary renal cell carcinoma[b]
Chromophobe renal cell carcinoma
Hybrid oncocytic chromophobe tumor[a]
Carcinoma of the collecting ducts of Bellini
Renal medullary carcinoma
MiT family translocation renal cell carcinoma[a]
Xp11 translocation renal cell carcinoma
t(6;11) renal cell carcinoma[a]
Carcinoma associated with neuroblastoma
Mucinous tubular and spindle cell carcinoma
Tubulocystic renal cell carcinoma[a]
Acquired cystic disease associated renal cell carcinoma[a]
Clear cell (tubulo) papillary renal cell carcinoma[a]
Hereditary leiomyomatosis renal cell carcinoma syndrome-associated
renal cell carcinoma[a]
Renal cell carcinoma, unclassified
Metanephric tumors
Metanephric adenoma
Metanephric adenofibroma
Metanephric stromal tumor
Nephroblastic tumors
Nephrogenic rests
Nephroblastoma
Cystic partially differentiated nephroblastoma
Mesenchymal tumors
Occurring mainly in children
Clear cell sarcoma
Rhabdoid tumor
Congenital mesoblastic nephroma
Ossifying renal tumor of infants
Occurring mainly in adults
Leiomyosarcoma (including renal vein)
Angiosarcoma
Rhabdomyosarcoma
Malignant fibrous histiocytoma
Hemangiopericytoma
Osteosarcoma
Synovial sarcoma[a]
Angiomyolipoma
Epithelioid angiomyolipoma[a]
Leiomyoma
Hemangioma
Lymphangioma
Juxtaglomerular cell tumor
Renomedullary interstitial cell tumor
Schwannoma
Solitary fibrous tumor
Mixed mesenchymal and epithelial tumors
Cystic nephroma/mixed epithelial stromal tumor
Neuroendocrine tumors
Carcinoid (low-grade neuroendocrine tumor)
Neuroendocrine carcinoma (high-grade neuroendocrine tumor)
Primitive neuroectodermal tumor
Neuroblastoma
Pheochromocytoma
Hematopoietic and lymphoid tumors
Lymphoma
Leukemia
Plasmacytoma
Germ cell tumors
Teratoma
Choriocarcinoma
Metastatic tumors
Other tumors

Used with permission from Srigley JR, Delahunt B, Eble JN, et al. The International Society of Urological Pathology (ISUP) Vancouver Classification of Renal Neoplasia. Am J Surg Pathol. 2013;37:1469–1489

[a]Additions and changes in terminology or position in classification

[b]The majority of consensus attendees subtype papillary carcinoma (type 1, type 2, or not otherwise specified)

Benign lesions:

- Oncocytoma
- Renal cortical adenoma
- Angiomyolipoma
- Metanephric adenoma
- Cystic nephroma/mixed epithelial and stromal tumor
- Xanthogranulomatous pyelonephritis
- Renal abscess
- Renal infarct
- Renal cysts

Renal cell carcinoma:

- Clear/conventional renal cell carcinoma
- Papillary renal cell carcinoma
- Chromophobe renal cell carcinoma
- Sarcomatoid renal cell carcinoma
- Mucinous tubular and spindle cell carcinoma
- Xp11.2 translocation-associated renal cell carcinoma
- Collecting duct carcinoma (Bellini tumor)

Urothelial carcinoma

Metastatic tumors

Normal Elements

Glomeruli

Cytological Features

- Large papillary structures
- Capillary loops (Fig. 9.1)

Differential Diagnosis

- Papillary RCC
- Clear cell RCC

Proximal Tubular Cells

Cytological Features

- Rare cells with abundant granular cytoplasm (Figs 9.1 and 9.2)

Differential Diagnosis

- Oncocytoma
- Chromophobe RCC

Distal Tubular Cells

Cytological Features

- Rare cells with scant cytoplasm and minimal atypia (Fig. 9.1)

Differential Diagnosis

- Low-grade clear cell or papillary RCC

Normal elements are occasionally encountered and may be misinterpreted as tumor cells. The cells in a glomerulus are not evenly distributed, but rather are much more dense in the center than at the periphery. Most importantly, endothelial cells lining capillary loops are seen at the edges. In RCCs, the nucleus is atypical, not as flat as that of an endothelial cell, and has size variations. See Fig. 9.1.

Proximal tubular cells have abundant granular cytoplasm and poorly demarcated cell membranes, and the granules often appear to be spilling out of the cells. They are similar to the cells of an oncocytoma and chromophobe RCC. Usually the cell borders of tumor cells are well defined, while those of proximal tubular cells are torn and irregular. See Figs. 9.1 and 9.2.

Distal tubular cells are smaller cells with less clear to granular cytoplasm and small round nuclei without nucleoli. The cell borders are well defined, and the cytoplasm is not vacuolated. These cells are very similar to those of a low-grade clear cell or papillary RCC. However, the tumor cells of low-grade papillary RCC form papillae and spherules. See Fig. 9.1.

Benign Lesions

Oncocytoma

Key Clinical Findings

- Benign and comprise 3–5% of all renal tumors
- Usually adults
- Predominantly male
- May be bilateral or multicentric

Key Radiologic Findings

Imaging findings substantially overlap those of common subtypes of clear cell and non-clear cell renal cell carcinomas.

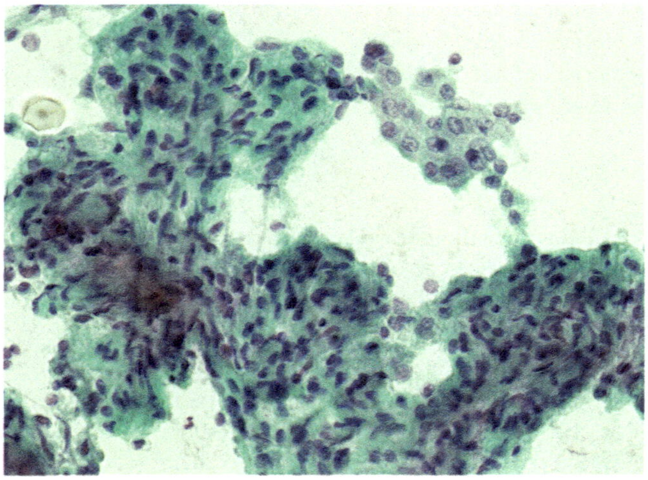

Fig. 9.1 Normal glomerulus. Dense cohesive spherical structures with small nuclei and scalloped borders, the capillary loops with spindle endothelial cells. Proximal tubular cells with abundant granular cytoplasm and ill-defined cell borders. Rare smaller distal tubular cells with scant cytoplasm (Papanicolaou stain)

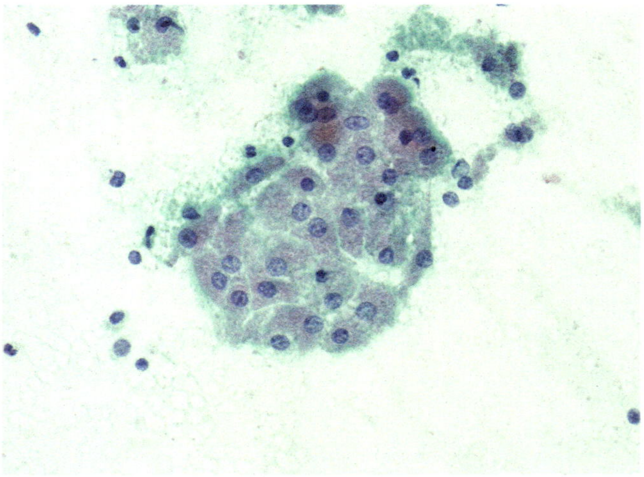

Fig. 9.2 Proximal tubular cells with abundant granular cytoplasm and ill-defined cell borders and smaller distal tubular cells with scant cytoplasm (Papanicolaou stain)

Multifocal renal oncocytomas are not rare, and making the diagnosis of oncocytoma with concomitant renal cell carcinoma is difficult. In addition, renal oncocytomas that demonstrate interval growth or develop in the setting of end-stage renal disease may be mistaken for malignancy.

Cytological Features

- Hypercellular with mainly isolated uniform cells and cohesive nests
- Abundant eosinophilic and granular cytoplasm
- Well-demarcated cell borders
- Frequent binucleation, round nuclei with prominent nucleoli
- Figure 9.3a, b

Differential Diagnosis

- Chromophobe RCC
- Clear cell RCC with granular cytoplasm
- Hepatocytes

Renal (Cortical) Adenoma

Except for their size, renal cortical adenomas are histologically, immunohistochemically, and cytogenetically indistinguishable from low-grade papillary RCCs. Renal adenomas account for 20% of adult kidneys and are by definition very small lesions, always in the cortex and less than 0.5 cm and usually less than 0.2 cm. They are too small to be aspirated, and therefore, the diagnosis "renal cell adenoma" is inappropriate for an FNA specimen.

Angiomyolipoma

Key Clinical Findings

- Accounts for 0.07–2% of renal tumors.
- Average is 40 years (30 years in tuberous sclerosis patients). Range is 12–72 years.
- Predominantly female, up to 80% bilateral and multifocal in tuberous sclerosis (TS) patients. Usually unilateral and solitary in patients without TS.
- About half occur in young patients with TS. Most are benign, large lesions, can bleed, and are often resected to prevent this from occurring. A very small proportion of the epithelioid subtype does metastasize, but predicting malignant behavior is not possible by FNA. The tumor has three neoplastic components: blood vessels, mature fat, and an atypical smooth muscle cell that can be spindled or epithelioid.
- Asymptomatic lesions incidentally detected on CT scan or ultrasound. Symptomatic lesions greater than 4 cm have higher risk of spontaneous rupture and hemorrhage.
- Pleomorphism and mitoses not associated with more aggressive behavior.

Key Radiologic Findings

- The typical lesion with abundant adipose tissue is diagnosed confidently radiologically and as a result is rarely aspirated. Most FNAs are from radiologically atypical lesions, usually those with scant adipose tissue.

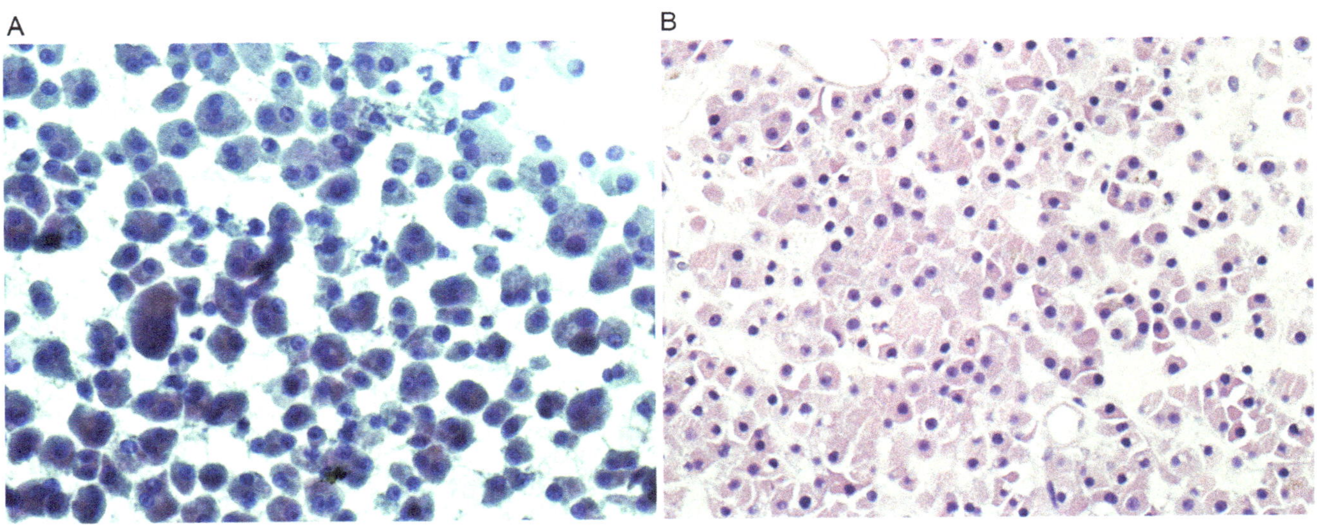

Fig. 9.3 (**a**) Single uniform cells with abundant granular cytoplasm and distinctive cell borders, binucleation, and small prominent nucleoli (Papanicolaou stain). (**b**) Single uniform cells and small round nests with edematous stroma (cell block H&E)

Cytomorphology

- Fragments of spindle cells with vacuolated cytoplasm
- Mature fat cells
- Eccentrically thick-walled blood vessels
- Often nuclear atypia
- Most cases immunoreactive for HMB-45
- Figure 9.4a-d

Differential Diagnosis

- Clear cell RCC when epithelioid cells predominate
- Sarcomatoid RCC or sarcoma when spindle cells predominate

Metanephric Adenoma

Key Clinical Findings

- A benign lesion most commonly occurs as an incidental finding predominantly in women with a mean age of 41 years.
- 10% of patients with polycythemia.
- May have abdominal or flank pain, hematuria, fever, and hypertension.

Key Radiologic Findings

- CT shows moderate enhancement of a mass with mean tumor size of 5.5 cm. Cystic areas along with hemorrhage and necrosis are common.

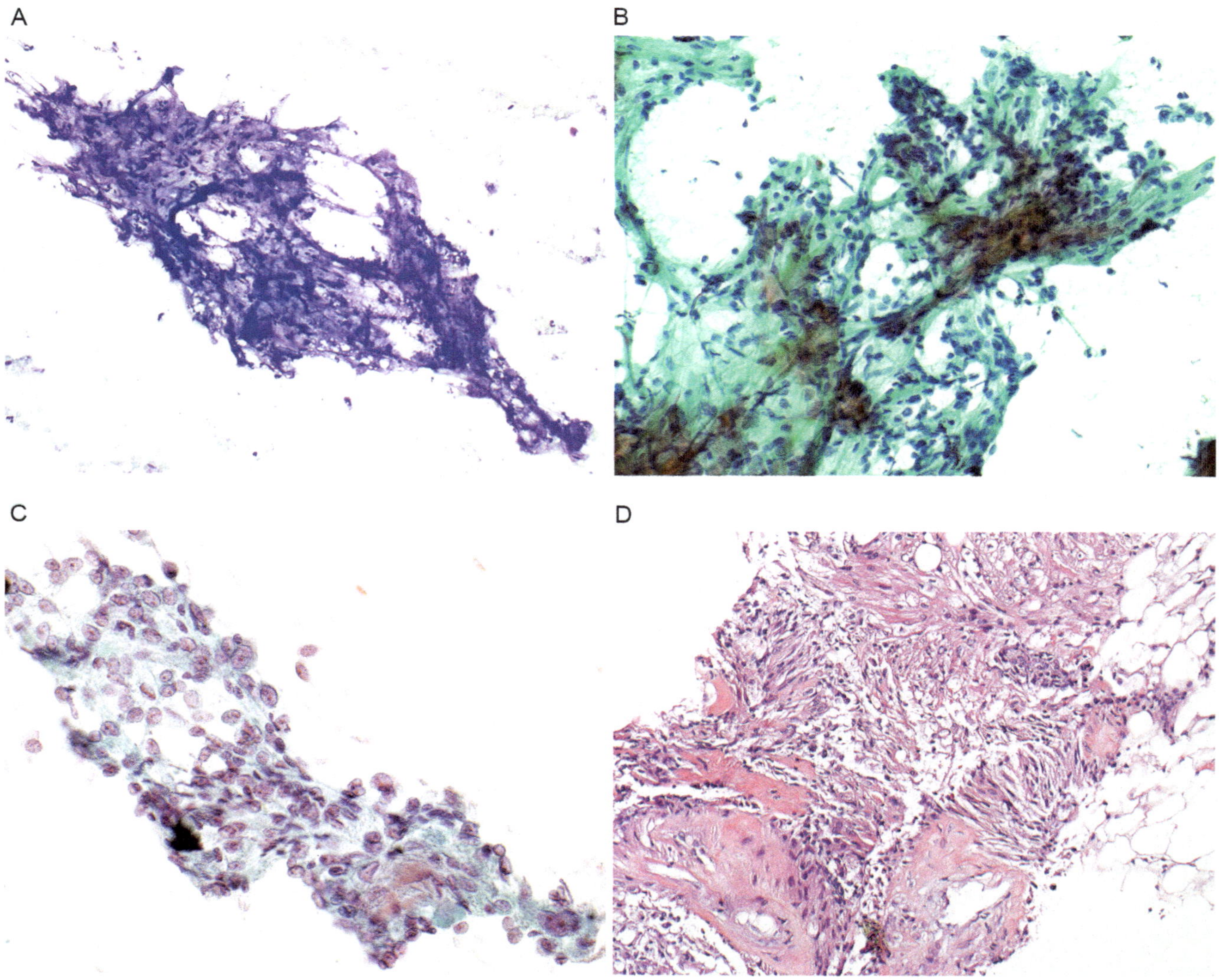

Fig. 9.4 (**a**) Cohesive tissue fragments comprised of vacuolated spindle cells and mature adipocytes (Romanowsky stain). (**b**) More spindle-shaped, smooth muscle cells and interspersed mature adipocytes (Papanicolaou stain). (**c**) Epithelioid AML with atypical nuclei and small prominent nucleoli mimics clear cell RCC (Papanicolaou stain). (**d**) Classic AML with vacuolated spindle cells, eccentrically thickened vessel wall, and scant mature adipose tissue (H&E)

Cytomorphology

- Cellular smear with tight, short papillae and loose sheets
- Round monotonous nuclei, fine chromatin, rare small nucleoli, and scant cytoplasm
- Occasional psammoma bodies
- Negative for EMA and CK7 and positive for WT-1, CD56, and CD57
- BRAF V600E mutations found in ~90% of tumor
- Figure 9.5a–c

Differential Diagnosis

- Wilms tumor (epithelial predominant type)
- Papillary RCC (low grade)
- Metastasis or small cell carcinoma

Renal Abscess

Radiologically renal abscess may appear as a mass. Aspirates contain necrotic material and numerous neutrophils with rare atypical epithelial cells, which may be confused with those of a clear cell RCC. The atypical cells are few in number, however, and such aspirates should be diagnosed as suspicious rather than positive.

Xanthogranulomatous Pyelonephritis

Key Clinical Findings

- 8% of kidneys removed for inflammation
- Usually adults, predominantly female
- UTI symptoms, almost always associated with urinary outflow obstruction

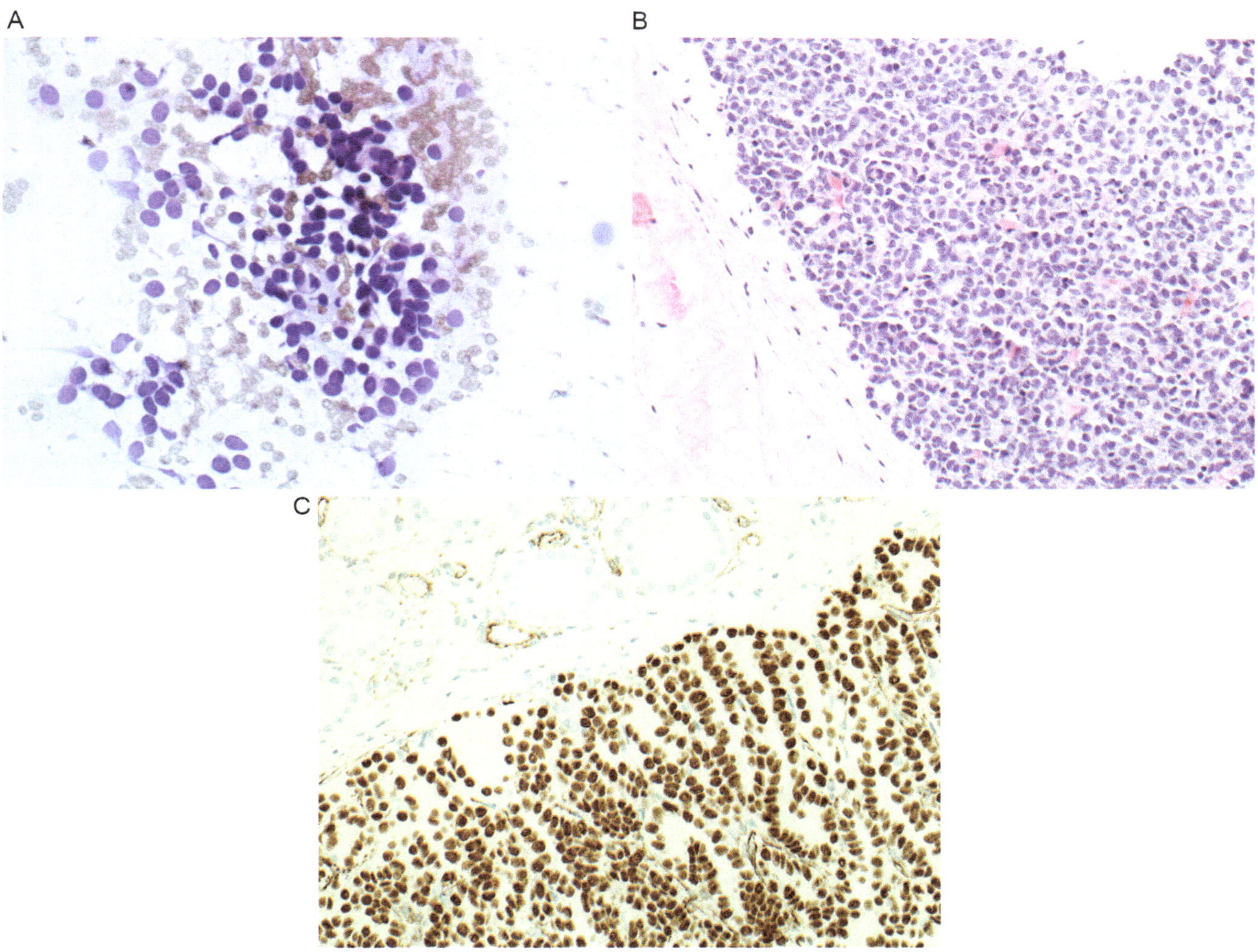

Fig. 9.5 (**a**) Loose sheets or small clusters of round cells with monotonous nuclei, fine chromatin, rare small nucleoli, and scant cytoplasm (Romanowsky stain). (**b**) Well-circumscribed tumor with crowded small acini of primitive blue cells in paucicellular intervening stroma. (**c**) Diffuse nuclear stain for WT-1

Key Radiologic Findings

- Solid nodules centered upon pyramids

Cytomorphology

- Single and clusters of histiocytes
- No nuclear atypia
- Multinucleated giant cells
- CD68 positivity and negative for cytokeratin and EMA
- Figure 9.6

Differential Diagnosis

- Clear cell RCC

Renal Infarct

Rarely, renal infarcts present as a mass suspicious for malignancy. Specimens are sparsely cellular and composed of necrotic material, which can contain rare atypical cells resembling those of clear cell RCC. A diagnosis of malignancy should be avoided when the atypical cells are few in numbers, which is usually the case with renal infarcts.

Renal Cysts

- Cysts are common and most are benign.
- Renal cell carcinomas can be cystic.
- Adequate sampling difficult.
- Some benign cysts are difficult to distinguish from RCC, such as cysts due to renal failure, adult polycystic kidney disease, and cystic nephroma.
- The value of a negative diagnosis is limited.
- If an FNA is performed and even a few atypical cells are seen, a "suspicious" diagnosis is appropriate.
- If the result is nondiagnostic (macrophages only), an explanatory note can be helpful, such as "the findings are consistent with a cystic renal lesion. Because parenchymal elements have not been sampled, the possibility of a neoplasm cannot be excluded."

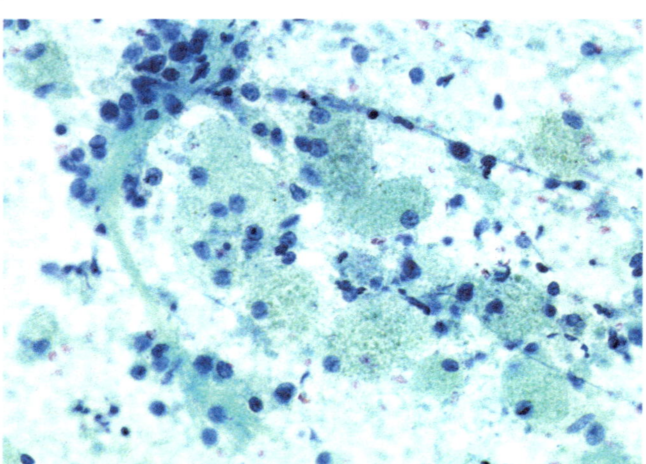

Fig. 9.6 Single or clusters of histiocytes with uniform small nuclei and abundant foamy granular cytoplasm (Papanicolaou stain)

Benign Entities that Sometimes Have Atypical Cells

- Proximal tubular cells
- Renal abscess
- Xanthogranulomatous nephritis
- Renal infarct
- Atypical cysts
- Angiomyolipoma

Best Diagnostic Clue

- Hypocellular

Best Diagnostic Terminology

- Suspicious rather than positive

Renal Cell Carcinoma

RCC is the most common tumor of the kidney. Patients may present with hematuria, flank pain, or a palpable mass, but the tumor is often discovered incidentally. RCCs are graded using the Fuhrman system; because it is based on nuclear features, it is easily applied to cytologic preparations, with good cytological-histologic correlation. With heterogeneous RCCs, the highest grade is assigned. The most recent histologic classification system, strongly influenced by cytogenetic data on the various subtypes, is shown in Table 9.2. Many immunohistochemical markers are proven to be useful in distinction among the subtypes of renal cell neoplasms. Table 9.3 summarizes the frequently used markers.

Cytologists should be familiar with these subtypes, which differ in their morphological features and prognosis. When performed on a portion of the cytologic specimen, cytogenetic analysis, whether fluorescence in situ hybridization or karyotyping, is helpful as an adjunct in subclassifying renal neoplasms.

Table 9.2 Cytogenetic data on subtypes of renal neoplasms

Type of RCC	% of all RCCs	Cytogenetics	Other
Clear cell/ conventional	75	del 3p	–
Papillary	15	Trisomies 7, 16, 17	Good prognosis, multifocal
Chromophobe	3–5	Markedly hypodiploid, multiple chromosomes lost	Good prognosis
Collecting duct	<1	Not well characterized	–
Sarcomatoid	3	Complex karyotypes	Poor prognosis

Table 9.3 Summary of useful immunohistochemical markers in renal epithelial neoplasms

Markers	CRCC	PRCC	ChRCC	Onco	CDC	MTSCC	UC
CK7	–	+	+	–	+	+	+
CK20	–	–	–	–	–	–	+ or –
CK903	–	–	–	–	+	–	+
p63	–	–	–	–	–	–	+
CD10	+	+	– or +	– or +	–	–	–
KIM-1	+	+	–	–	–	N/A	–
PAX8	+	+	+ or –	+	+	–	–
RCCMa	+	+	– or +	–	–	–	–
CD117	–	–	+	+	+or –	–	–
S100A1	+	+ or –	–	+	–	–	–
S100P	–	–	–	–	–	–	+
UP II	–	–	–	–	–	–	+ or –
GATA3	–	–	–	–	–	–	+
CD15	–	–	–	+ or –	–	–	+ or –
Vimentin	+	+ or –	–	–	+	–	–
Ksp-cadherin	– or +	–	+	+	–	–	–
AMACR (P504S)	– or +	+	–	–	–	+ or –	–
CA IX	+	+	–	–	– or +	N/A	+
UEA1	–	–	–	–	+	–	+

Note: "+" usually greater than 70% of cases are positive, "–" less than 5% of cases are positive, "+ or –" usually more than 50% of cases are positive "– or +" less than 50% of cases are positive. N/A data not available

CRCC clear cell renal cell carcinoma, *PRCC* papillary renal cell carcinoma, *ChRCC chromophobe renal cell carcinoma*, *Onco* oncocytoma, *CDC* collecting duct carcinoma, *MTSCC* mucinous tubule and spindle cell carcinoma, *UC* urothelial carcinoma, *KIM-1* Kidney injury molecule-1, *UP II* uroplakin II

Clear Cell/Conventional RCC

Key Clinical Findings

- Clear cell RCC comprises 75–80% of all RCCs and is strongly associated with a deletion of chromosome 3p, the site of the von Hippel-Lindau gene.

Cytomorphology

- Hypercellular with large cohesive sheets and isolated cells
- Abundant clear, vacuolated, or granular cytoplasm
- Large, round eccentrically placed nucleus/extruded nucleus
- Pink, strand-like fibrillary material/basement membrane material (DQ)
- Mixed inflammatory cells in the background
- Figure 9.7a–g

Differential Diagnosis

- Distal tubular cells
- Macrophages
- Adrenal cortical cells
- Hepatocytes
- Other types of RCC

Papillary RCC

Key Clinical Findings

- Account for 7% and 15% of all RCCs.
- It is associated with trisomies of chromosomes 7, 16, and 17.
- It may be associated with renal cortical adenomas and multifocality.
- Large tumors can be cystic and necrotic.
- Patients with type 1 (low grade/low stage) papillary RCC have an excellent prognosis, whereas those with type 2 (high grade/high stage) papillary RCC have a poor prognosis.

Key Radiologic Findings

- Although it is rarely performed nowadays, angiography classically shows an avascular or hypovascular lesion.

Cytomorphology

- True papillae, spherules, and tubules
- Foamy macrophages (smears or cell block)
- Uniform cells with prominent nucleoli (type 1)
- Large cells with large nuclei and grade prominent nucleoli (type 2)
- Some intracytoplasmic hemosiderin
- Positive for CK7, P504S, CD10, and vimentin
- Figure 9.8a–c

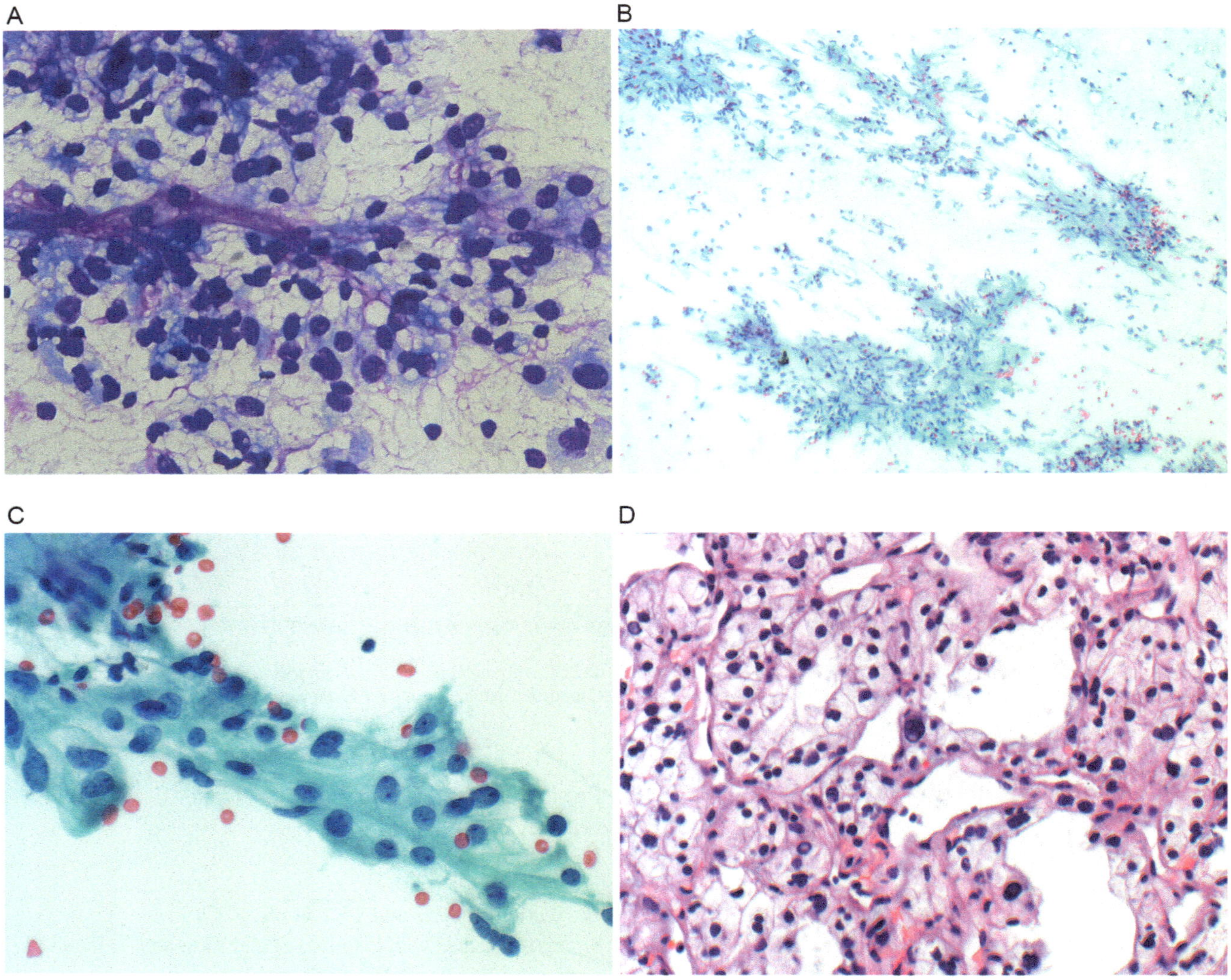

Fig. 9.7 (**a**) Clear cell RCC. Large cohesive sheets cells with clear cytoplasm (Romanowsky stain). (**b**) Clear cell RCC. Hypercellular with large loosely cohesive clusters (tissue fragments) and isolated cells (Papanicolaou stain). (**c**) Clear cell RCC. Large cohesive sheet of cells with vacuolated cytoplasm (Papanicolaou stain). (**d**) Clear cell RCC. Typical alveolar arrangement and nests of clear cells with thin-walled blood vessels (H&E). (**e**) Clear cell RCC. Cohesive clusters with abundant granular eosinophilic cytoplasm (Papanicolaou stain). (**f**) Clear cell RCC with eosinophilic features and lymphoid infiltrate (H&E). (**g**) Clear cell RCC. Strong and diffuse positive membrane and cytoplasmic staining for KIM-1

Differential Diagnosis

- Distal tubular cells
- Clear cell/conventional RCC

Chromophobe RCC

Key Clinical Findings

- It comprises 3–5% of all RCCs and is associated with characteristic chromosomal deletions.
- Patients have an excellent prognosis, unless their tumor is large or multifocal.
- In the appropriate clinical setting, a partial nephrectomy is the preferred treatment for both lesions.

Cytomorphology

- Discohesive cells with trabecular arrangement
- Koilocytoid cells with abundant clear to eosinophilic cytoplasm, distinct accentuated cell borders
- Frequent binucleation/dark chromatin
- Irregular nuclear outlines/nuclear grooves
- Positive for cytokeratin 7 and negative for KIM-1
- Figure 9.9a–c

Differential Diagnosis

- Clear/conventional RCC
- Oncocytoma

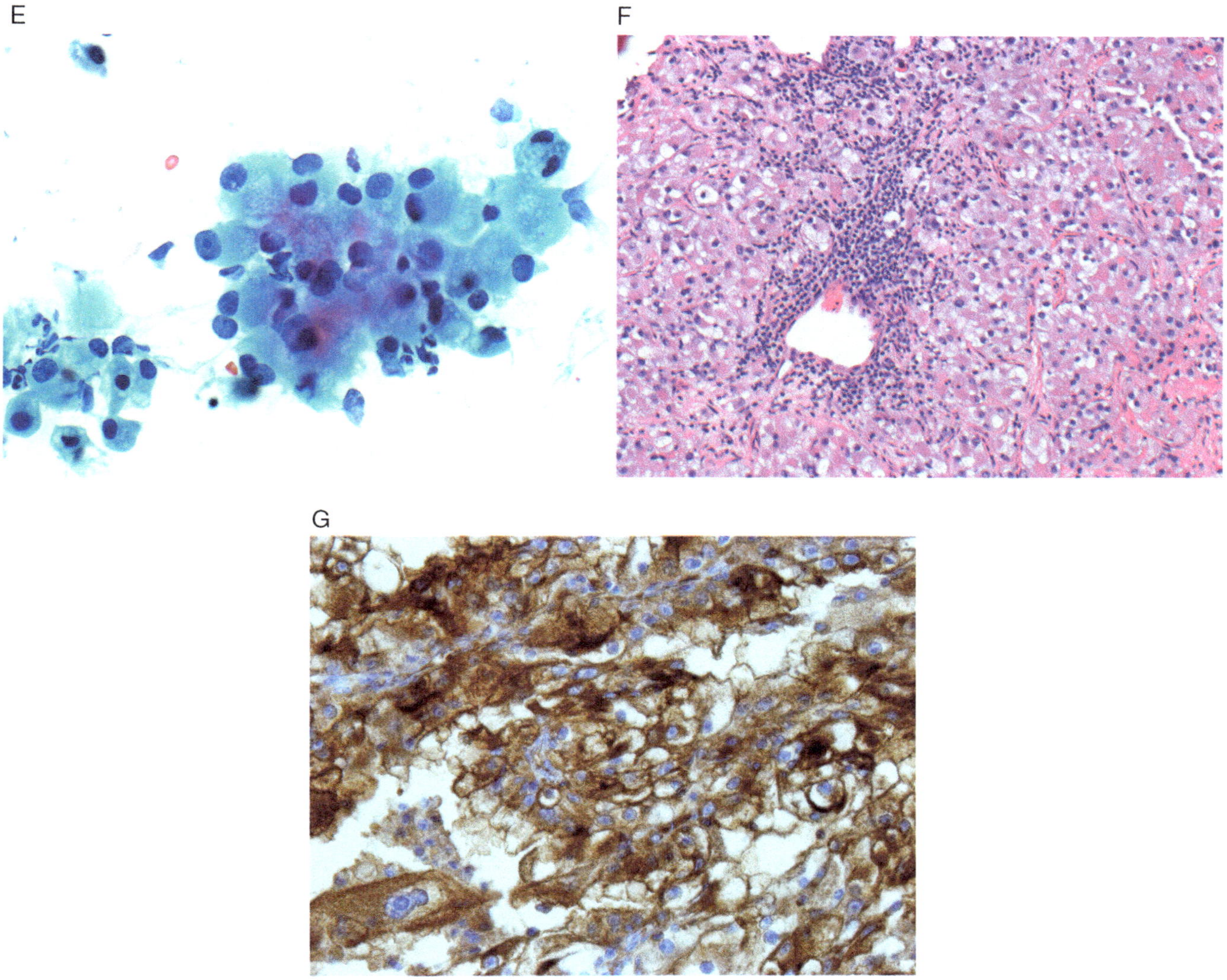

Fig. 9.7 (continued)

In some cases, the distinction between oncocytoma and chromophobe RCC is impossible by cytologic stains alone; a reasonable approach is to defer the distinction to extensive histologic sampling of the resected tumor and interpret the FNA specimen as oncocytic neoplasm (oncocytoma vs. chromophobe RCC), with comment that a partial nephrectomy should be considered if clinically appropriate.

Special Stains and Immunohistochemistry

- Diffuse cytoplasmic stains of Hale's colloidal iron contrasting with focal cell membrane staining in some oncocytomas.
- Characteristic microvesicles are seen by electron microscopy.

Sarcomatoid RCC

Key Clinical Findings

Sarcomatoid RCC comprises 3% of all RCCs. It is a high-grade tumor with a poor prognosis: many are unresectable at presentation and therefore candidates for FNA, although more and more are being identified at a lower stage. They are probably a form of dedifferentiated carcinoma. Most are found in association with clear cell RCC, but sarcomatoid transformation of chromophobe, collecting duct, and papillary RCCs also occurs.

Cytomorphology

- Hypercellular smears with clusters and singly placed cells.
- Pleomorphic, malignant spindle, or epithelioid cells.

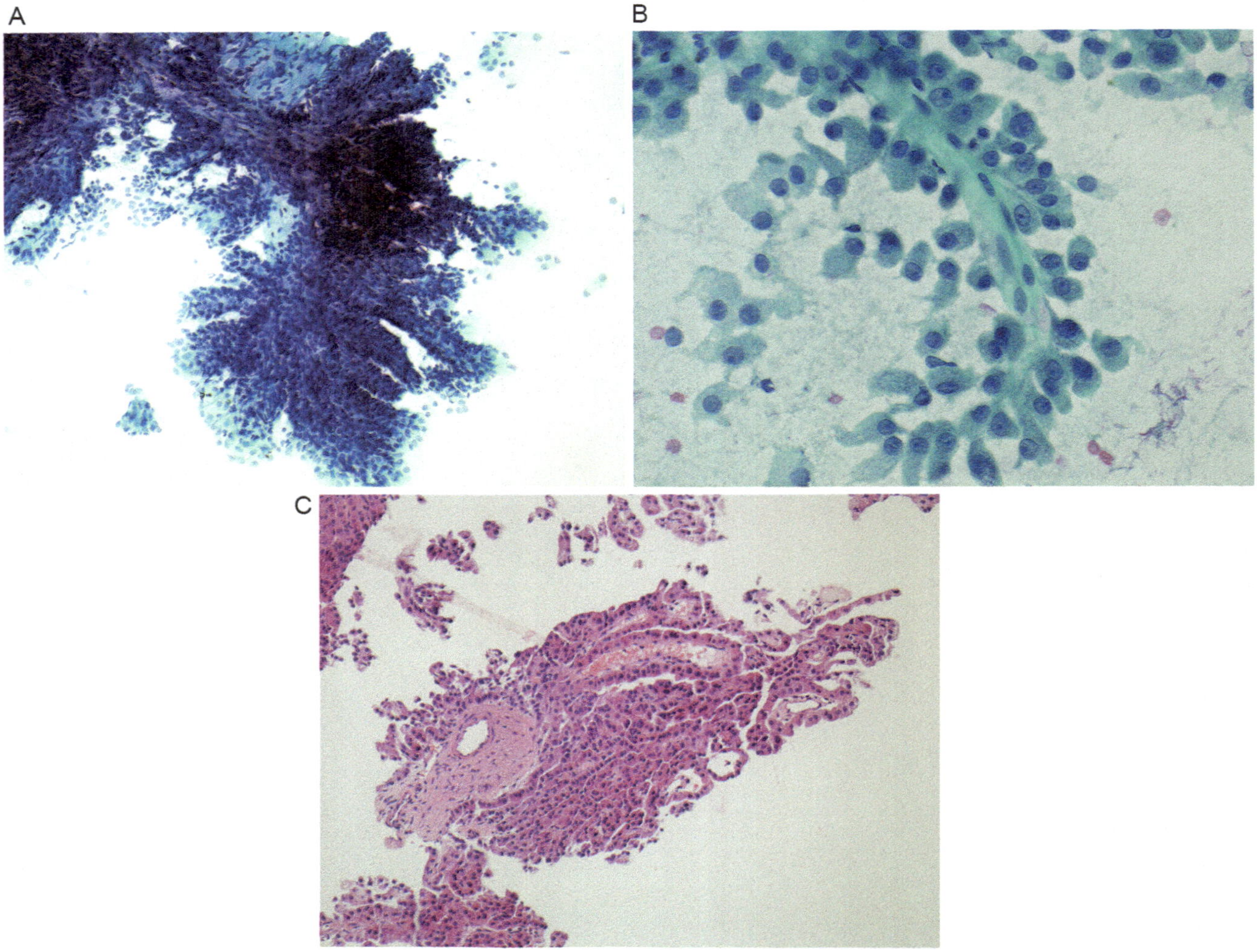

Fig. 9.8 (**a**) Papillary RCC. True papillae with uniform cells with conspicuous nucleoli (type1) (Papanicolaou stain). (**b**) Papillary RCC. True papillae with large cells, large nuclei, and prominent nucleoli (type2) (Papanicolaou stain). (**c**) Papillary RCC. True papillae and tubules with uniform cells with conspicuous nucleoli (H&E)

- Spindle cells must be immunoreactive to keratin or EMA.
- Figure 9.10a, b.

Differential Diagnosis

- Sarcoma or angiomyolipoma if spindle cells only

Mucinous Tubular and Spindle Cell Carcinoma

Key Clinical Findings

Mucinous tubular and spindle cell carcinoma is a rare and newly described type of renal cell carcinoma (RCC) with a relatively indolent behavior. Its morphological features as well as a strong preferential expression of proximal tubule markers suggest that this tumor is a type of RCC with proximal tubular differentiation, which appears closely related to or represents a morphological variant of papillary RCC. Loss of chromosomes has been reported.

Cytomorphology

- Relatively uniform, oval to spindle-shaped cells
- Abundant myxoid matrix

Differential Diagnosis

- Low-grade clear RCC
- Papillary RCC
- Some metastatic tumors

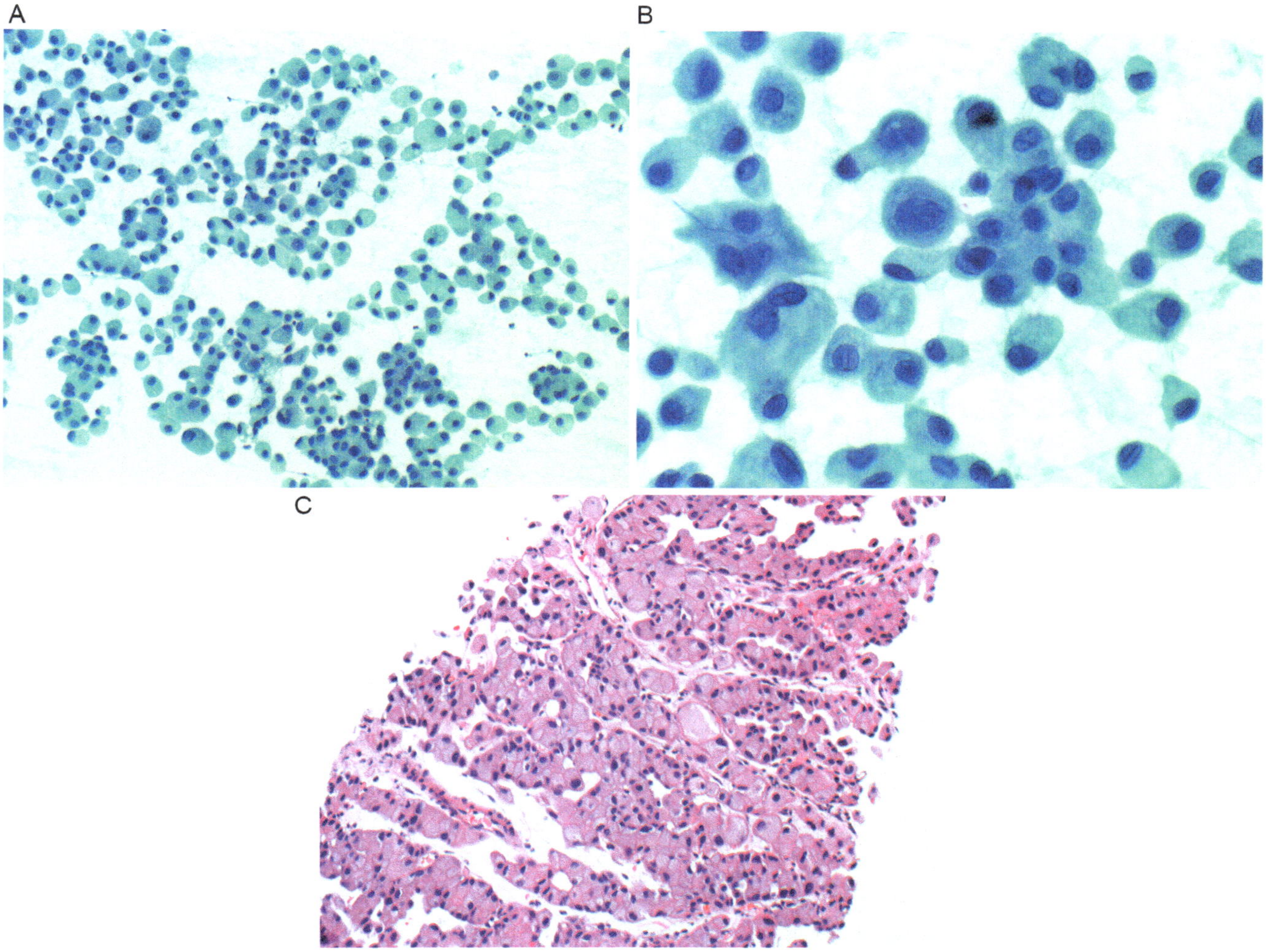

Fig. 9.9 (**a**) Chromophobe RCC. Discohesive cells with trabecular arrangement (Papanicolaou stain). (**b**) Chromophobe RCC. Koilocytoid cells with abundant clear to eosinophilic cytoplasm, distinct accentuated cell borders, frequent binucleation/dark chromatin, and irregular nuclear outlines/nuclear grooves (Papanicolaou stain). (**c**) Chromophobe RCC. Core biopsy with trabecular pattern, abundant clear to eosinophilic cytoplasm, distinct cell borders, frequent binucleation, and nuclear grooves (H&E)

Special Stains and Immunohistochemistry

- Tumor cells are immunoreactive for CK7, AMACR, and EMA
- Figure 9.11a–c

Xp11.2 Translocation-Associated RCC

Key Clinical Findings

Xp11.2 translocation renal cell carcinomas (RCCs), a recently recognized distinct subtype, are rare tumors predominantly reported in young patients. They comprise at least one-third of pediatric RCCs, and only few adult cases have been reported. They are characterized by various translocations involving chromosome Xp11.2, all resulting in gene fusions involving the transcription factor E3 (TFE3) gene. In recent years, at least six different Xp11.2 translocation RCCs have been identified and characterized at the molecular level. These include a distinctive RCC that bears a translocation with the identical chromosomal breakpoints (Xp11.2, 17q25) and identical resulting ASPL-TFE3 gene fusion as alveolar soft part sarcoma. Only limited data are available so far; they are believed to be rather indolent, but there have been increasing, recent reports of an aggressive clinical course in adult cases.

Cytomorphology

- Papillary or nested architecture
- Cells with voluminous, clear, or eosinophilic cytoplasm

Differential Diagnosis

- Clear cell RCC
- Papillary RCC

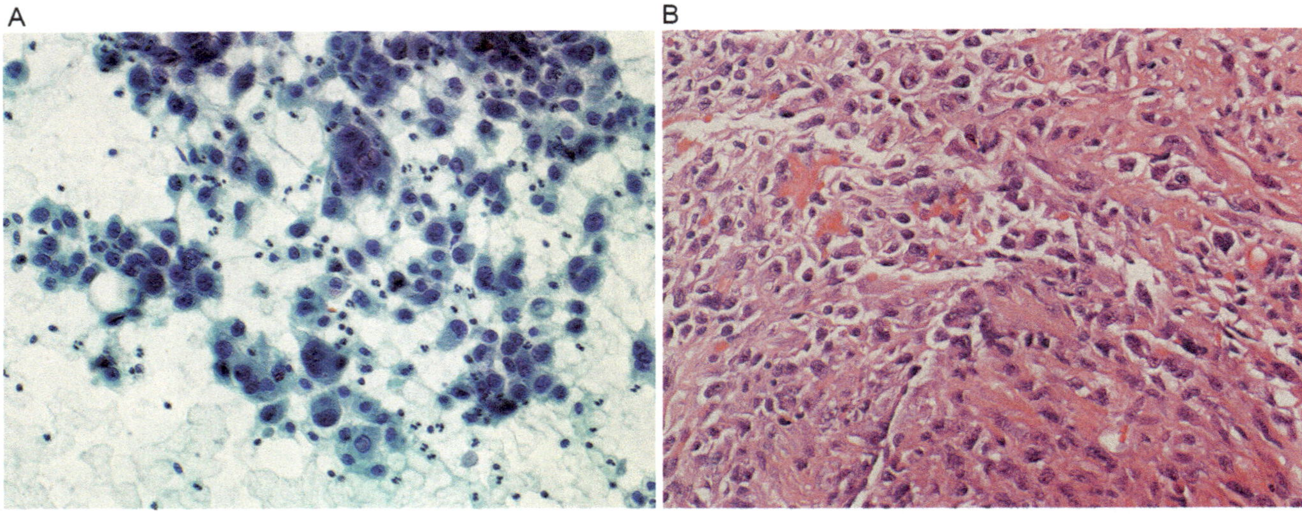

Fig. 9.10 (a) Sarcomatoid RCC. Hypercellular smears with clusters and singly placed pleomorphic spindle or epithelioid cells (Papanicolaou stain). (b) Sarcomatoid RCC. Pleomorphic spindle or epithelioid cells (H&E)

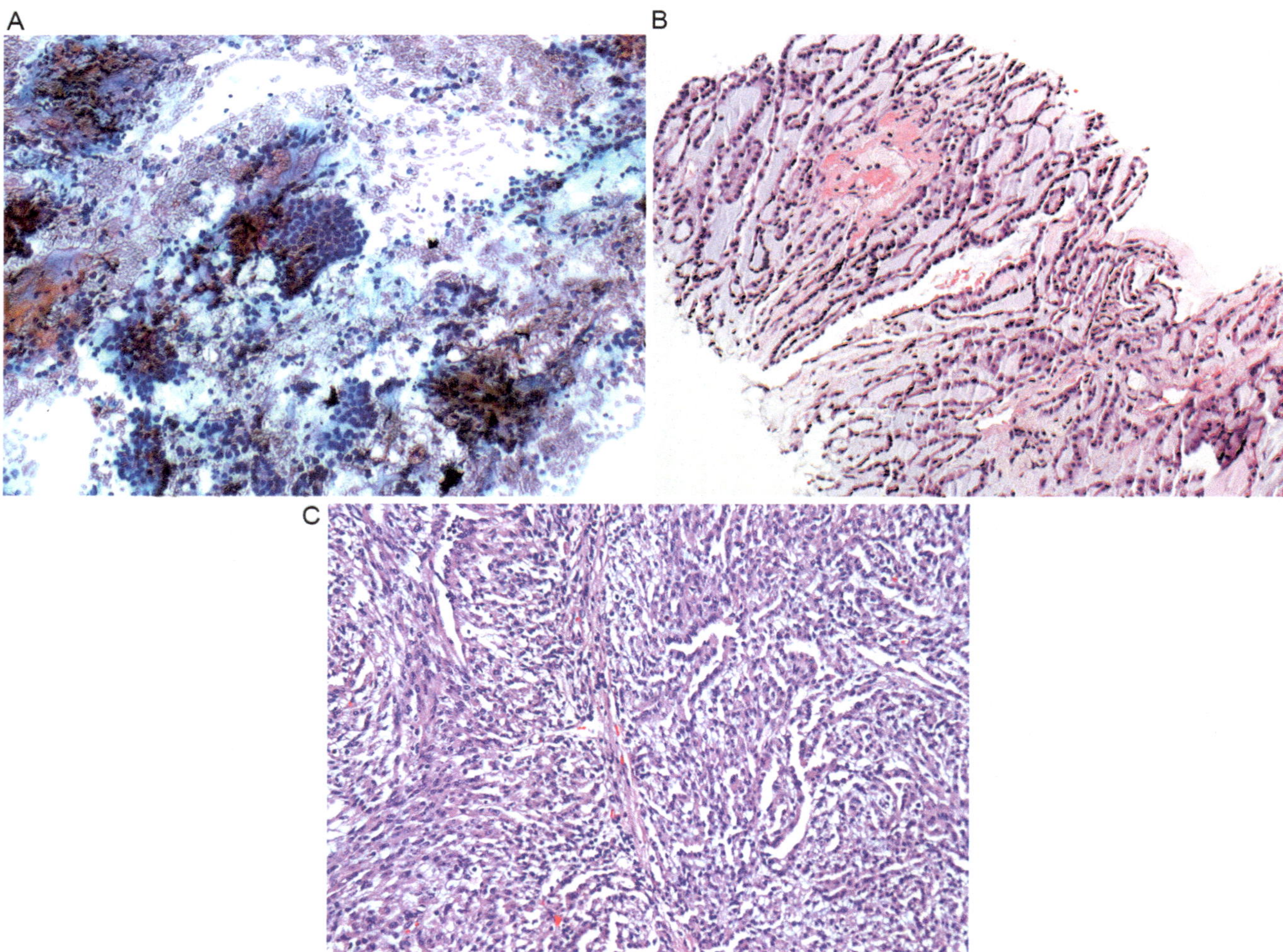

Fig. 9.11 (a) Mucinous tubular and spindle cell carcinoma (Papanicolaou stain). (b) Mucinous tubular and spindle cell carcinoma (H&E). (c) Mucinous tubular and spindle cell carcinoma (H&E)

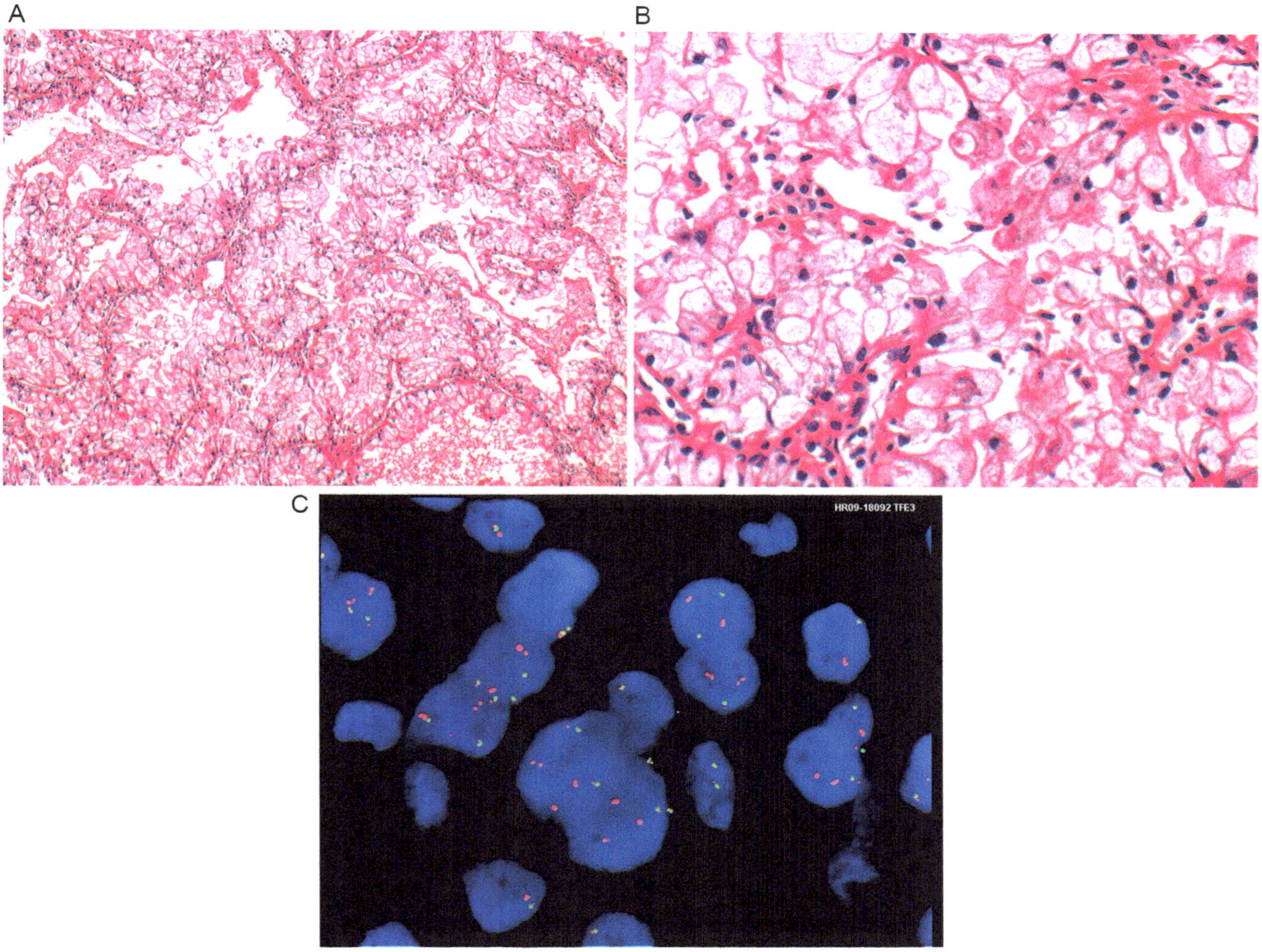

Fig. 9.12 (**a**) Xp11.2 translocation-associated RCC. Papillary architecture, alveolar pattern, and clear cells (H&E). (**b**) Xp11.2 translocation-associated RCC. Feature cells with granular and eosinophilic cytoplasm (H&E). (**c**) Xp11.2 translocation-associated RCC. Positive rearrangement of the TFE3 gene by using TFE3 break apart FISH probe which comes labeled in green and pink

Special Stains and Immunohistochemistry

- Their most distinctive immunohistochemical feature is nuclear labeling for TFE3 protein in all RCC with unusual histology.
- Figure 9.12a–c.

Collecting Duct Carcinoma (Bellini Tumor)

Key Clinical Findings

- A rare tumor, characterized by its medullary location
- Thought to arise from collecting ducts rather than proximal tubules
- Worse prognosis than ordinary renal cell carcinoma

Cytomorphology

- High-grade, large, malignant cells
- Hyperchromatic nuclei and scant cytoplasm
- Mimicking metastatic tumors

Special Stains and Immunohistochemistry

- Immunoreactive to CK903 (HMW keratin, 34BE12) and EMA
- Figure 9.13a–c

Differential Diagnosis

- Medullary carcinoma of the kidney

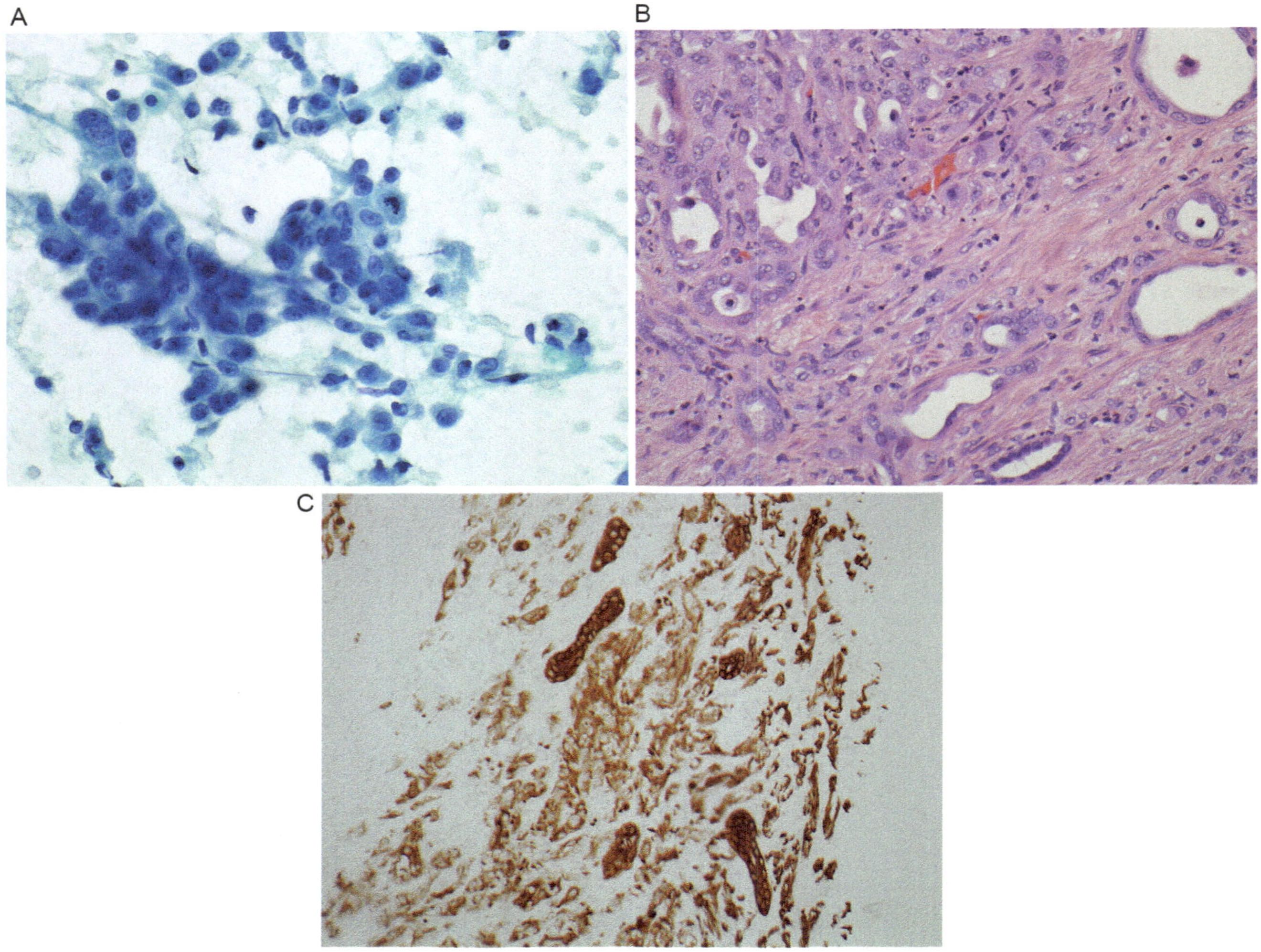

Fig. 9.13 (**a**) Collecting duct carcinoma. High-grade, large, malignant cells and cell clusters with hyperchromatic nuclei and scant cytoplasm mimicking metastatic tumors (Papanicolaou stain). (**b**) Collecting duct carcinoma. Invasive ducts with hobnail-like lining epithelial cell, desmoplasia, and neutrophils in the background. There are entrapped benign renal tubules between the malignant ducts (H&E). (**c**) Collecting duct carcinoma. Immunoreactive to CK903 (HMW keratin, 34BE12)

- Papillary RCC
- High-grade urothelial carcinoma

Urothelial Carcinoma

Key Clinical Findings

- It accounts for 5–10% of all renal tumors.
- The most common presentation is painless hematuria.
- Distinguishing UCs from RCCs is important because the urologist will resect the ureters with the kidney if the tumor is UC.

Cytomorphology

- Hypercellular smears with sheets, papillae, or large singly placed cells
- Scant squamoid/opaque cytoplasm without vacuolization
- Hyperchromatic irregular nuclei with granular chromatin
- Single cell with a long cytoplasmic tail

Special Stains and Immunohistochemistry

- Positive for CK903 (keratin 34BE12), CK7, CK20, CEA, and mucin
- Figure 9.14a–e

Differential Diagnosis

- High-grade RCC
- Metastatic tumors
- Collecting duct carcinoma

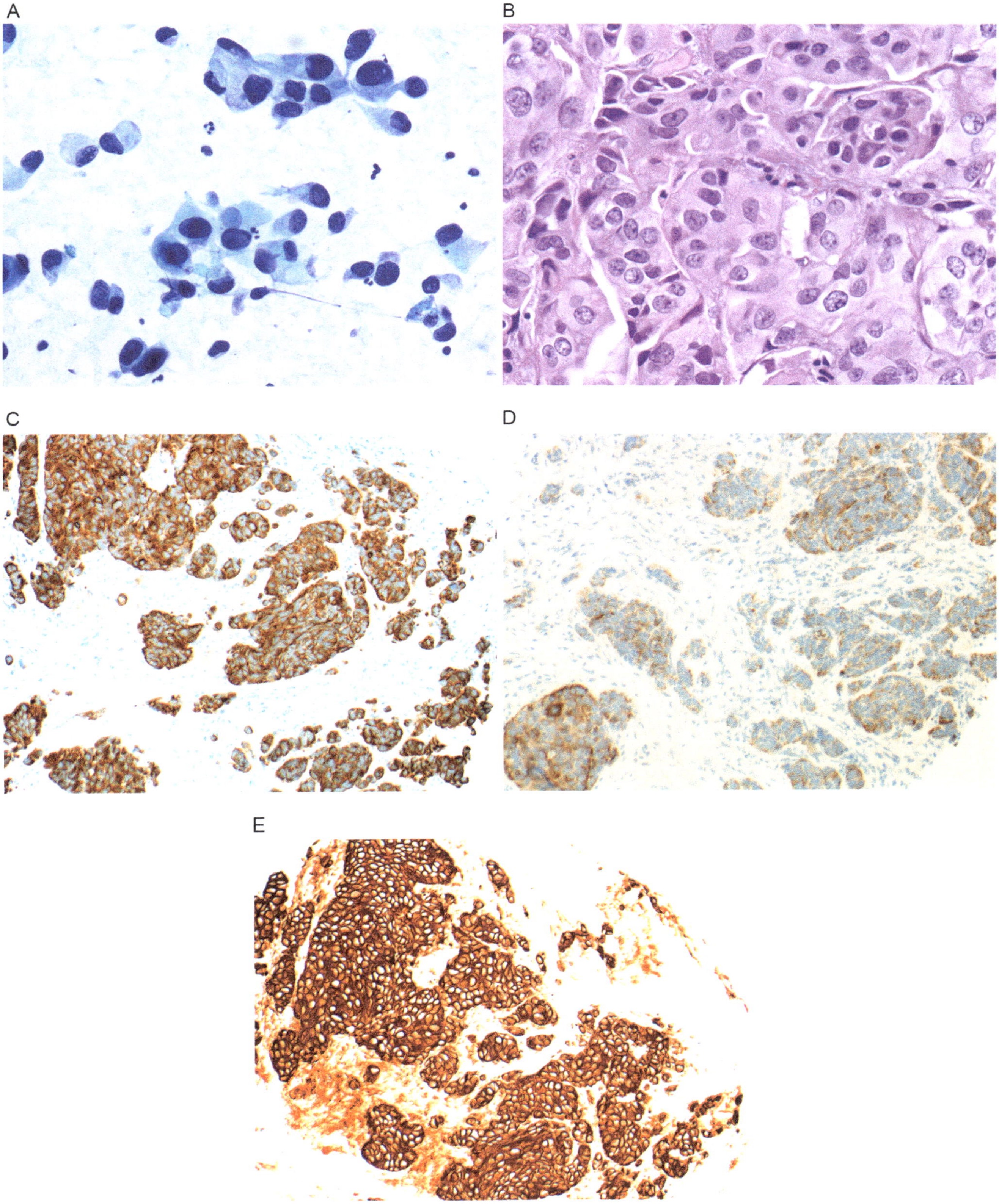

Fig. 9.14 (**a**) Urothelial carcinoma of the kidney. Large singly placed cells with hyperchromatic irregular nuclei, granular chromatin, and scant squamoid/opaque cytoplasm. Single cell with a long cytoplasmic tail (Papanicolaou stain). (**b**) Urothelial carcinoma of the kidney. Solid nest and sheets of cells with hyperchromatic irregular nuclei, granular chromatin, and squamoid/opaque cytoplasm (H&E). (**c**) Urothelial carcinoma of the kidney. Positive CK7 stain. (**d**) Urothelial carcinoma of the kidney. Positive CK20 stain. (**e**) Urothelial carcinoma of the kidney. Positive membrane staining for CK903

Metastatic Tumors

Key Clinical Findings

Metastases to the kidney are present in about 7% of all cancer patients at autopsy, but most are clinically silent. It is extremely rare for a metastasis to the kidney to be the initial manifestation of malignancy. Most metastases without a known primary probably represent unusual primary tumors. The lung is the most common primary site. See Fig. 9.15.

Differential Diagnosis of Lung Metastases

- Primary RCCs
- Collecting duct carcinoma
- Medullary carcinoma of the kidney
- Lymphoma of the kidney
- Urothelial carcinoma
- Figure 9.16a, b

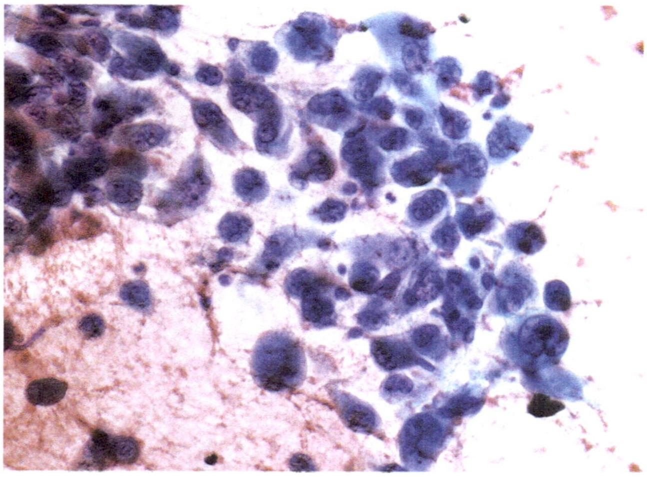

Fig. 9.15 Metastatic lung carcinoma to the kidney. These high-grade and poorly differentiated carcinoma cells are not typical RCC. A patient with a history of lung carcinoma, the findings are most consistent with a lung primary (Papanicolaou stain)

Fine-Needle Aspiration in Pediatric Patients

Wilms Tumor

Key Clinical Findings

Wilms tumor, also called Wilms' tumor or nephroblastoma, is the most common type of kidney cancer in children. It is named after Max Wilms, a German doctor who wrote one of the first medical articles about the disease in 1899. About 85–90% of Wilms tumor patients with favorable histology can be cured. Cure rates for patients with anaplastic histology, a more aggressive form of Wilms tumor, are lower. Beckwith-Wiedemann syndrome is associated with Wilms tumor.

Key Radiologic Findings

Imaging tests that create images of a child's kidneys can help determine whether your child has a kidney *tumor*. Imaging tests may include ultrasound, computerized tomography (CT), and magnetic resonance imaging (MRI). When Wilms tumor is suspected, a sonogram and CT scan are usually performed to examine a child's chest, abdomen, and pelvis for cancer staging.

Cytomorphology

- Three components more or less present
- Blastemal cells with small round cells
- Round/oval stripped nuclei
- Fine powdery chromatin, mitotic figures, and apoptosis
- Scant to no cytoplasm, rarely glomeruloid bodies
- Tubules
- Stroma

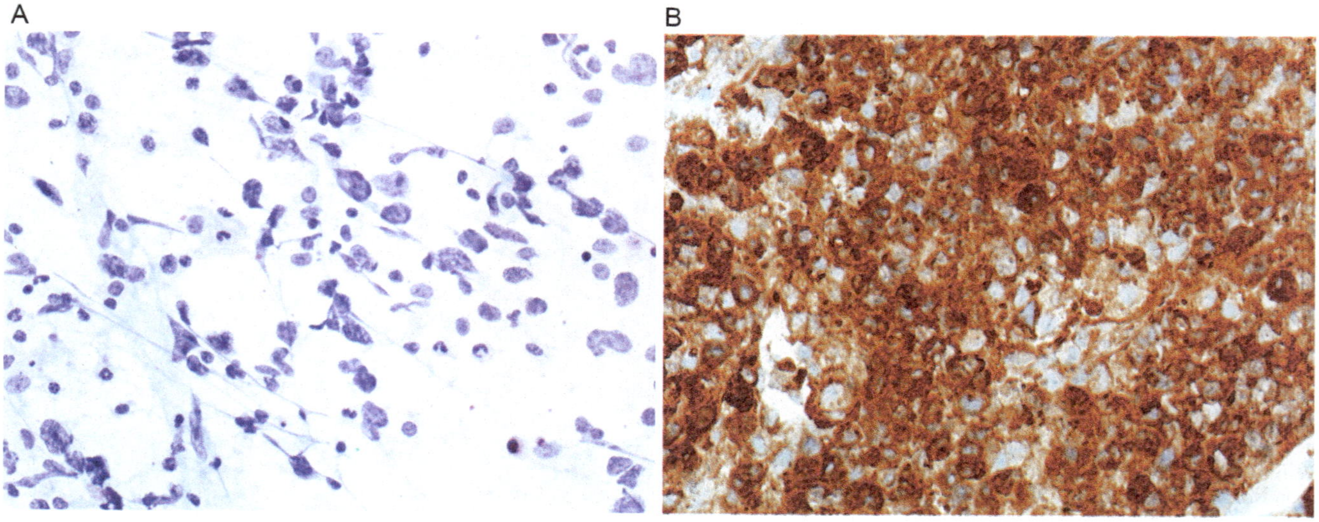

Fig. 9.16 (**a**) Diffuse large B cell lymphoma of the kidney. Singly placed larger naked nuclei with prominent nucleoli and smearing artifact (Papanicolaou stain). (**b**) Diffuse large B cell lymphoma of the kidney. Immunostain for CD20 shows diffuse strong membrane and cytoplasmic staining

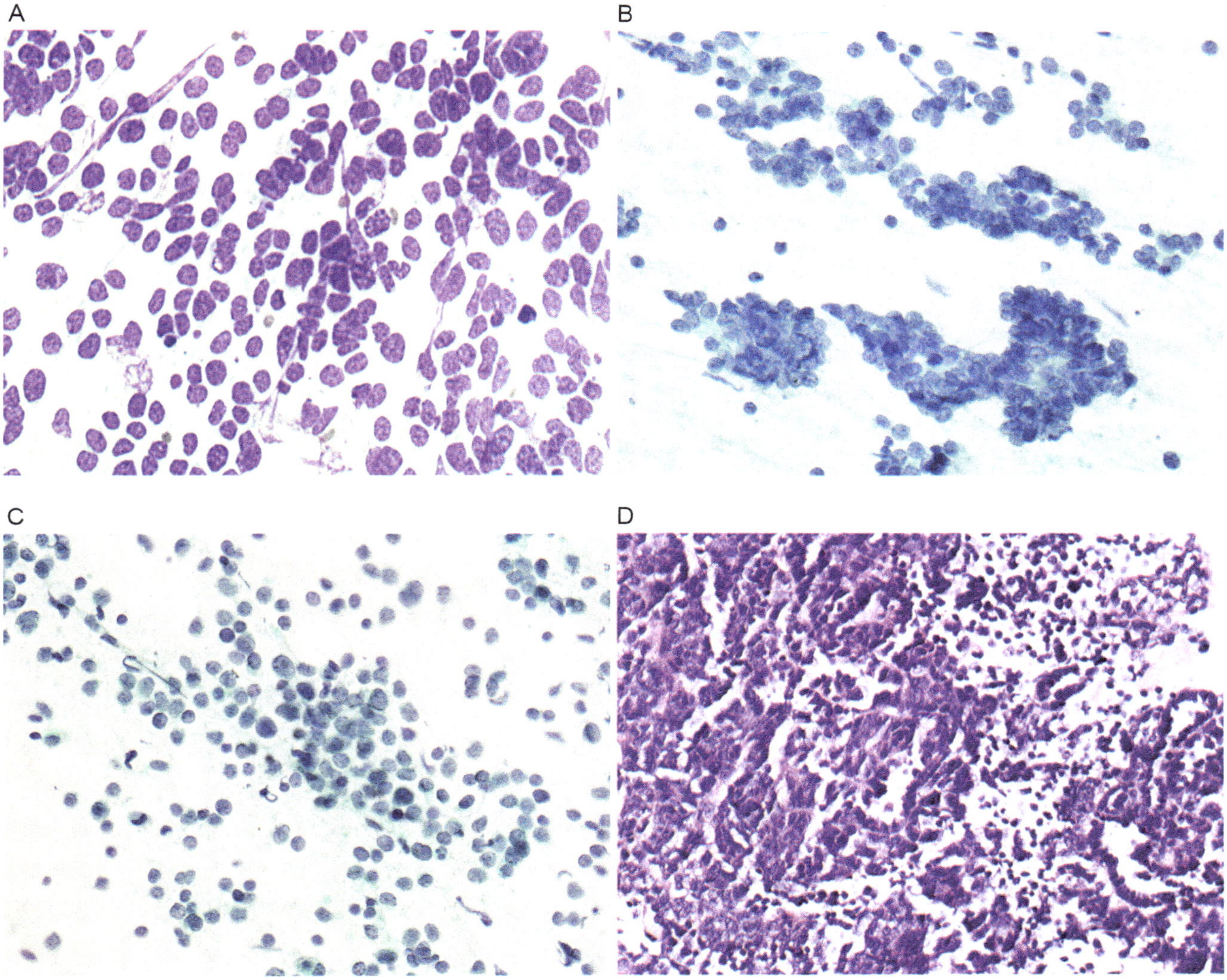

Fig. 9.17 (**a**) Wilms tumor. Blastemal cells with round/oval stripped nuclei and scant to no cytoplasm (Romanowsky stain). (**b**) Wilms tumor. Primitive epithelial cells with open nuclear chromatin, mitotic figures, and apoptosis (Papanicolaou stain). (**c**) Wilms tumor. Dispersed blastemal cells with round/oval stripped nuclei, fine powdery chromatin, and scant to no cytoplasm (Papanicolaou stain). (**d**) Wilms tumor. Classic three components: blastemal cells, primitive epithelial cells, and stroma (H&E)

Differential Diagnosis

- Malignant germ cell tumor
- Retiform Sertoli-Leydig cell tumor
- Figure 9.17a–d

Adrenal Gland

The adrenal gland:

- Malakoplakia
- Adrenal cortical neoplasms/hyperplastic nodules
- Pheochromocytoma
- Metastatic tumors

Malakoplakia

Key Clinical Findings

- Thought to be unusual with ineffective response to *E. coli* infection and form granulomatous inflammation
- May form a mass and organisms usually not identifiable

Cytomorphology

- Granulomatous inflammation
- Cellular smears with singly placed foamy macrophages and Michaelis-Gutmann bodies inside and outside
- Roughly nuclear size, basophilic, concentrically laminated round bodies
- Figure 9.18a, b

Special Stains and Immunohistochemistry

- Stains for PAS, iron, and Von Kossa's (calcium) are positive in Michaelis-Gutmann bodies; intracellular bacilli by immunohistochemistry electron microscopy.
- If no Michaelis-Gutmann bodies, call granuloma.

Differential Diagnosis

- Xanthogranuloma

Myelolipoma

Key Clinical Findings

- A rare benign tumor of the adrenal gland is composed of adipose tissue and benign hematopoietic elements. The tumor is usually an incidental finding, although it can grow to a sizable mass.

Cytomorphology

- Mature fat with normal marrow elements
  Nucleated RBC
  Megakaryocytes
  Granulocytes and their precursors
- Figure 9.19a, b

Differential Diagnosis

- Angiomyolipoma

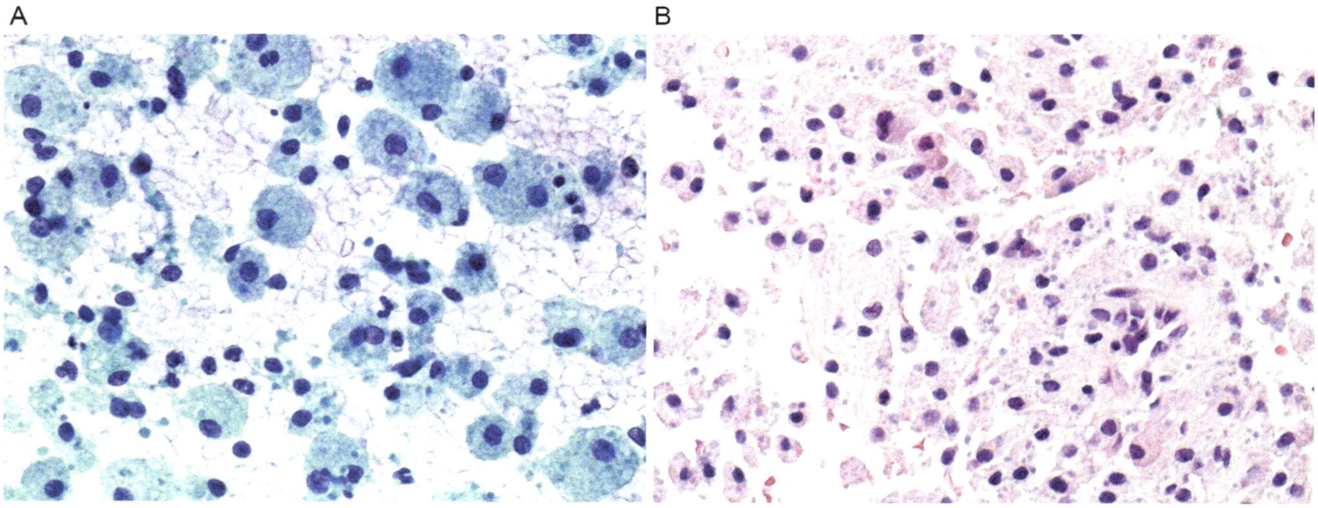

Fig. 9.18 (**a**) Malakoplakia. Cellular smears with singly placed foamy macrophages and Michaelis-Gutmann bodies inside and outside (Papanicolaou stain). (**b**) Malakoplakia. Fine-needle aspiration cell block H&E: roughly nuclear size, basophilic, concentrically laminated round bodies inside and outside foamy macrophages

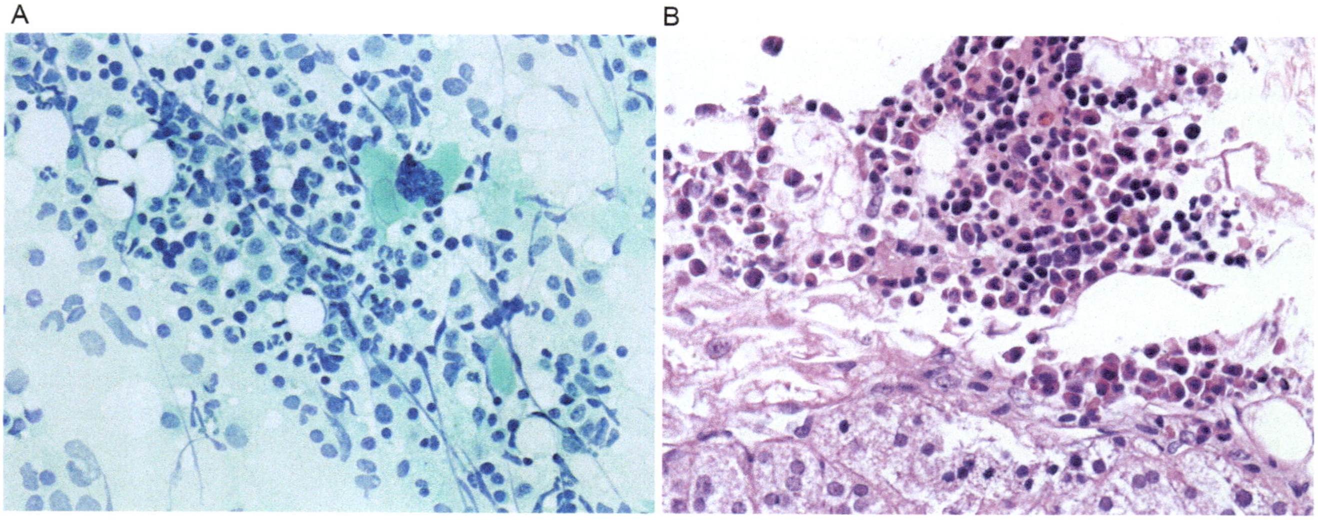

Fig. 9.19 (**a**) Myelolipoma. Mature fat with normal marrow elements: nucleated RBC, megakaryocytes, and granulocytes (Papanicolaou stain). (**b**) Myelolipoma. Normal adrenal cortical cells, adipose tissue, and benign hematopoietic elements (H&E)

Adrenal Cortical Neoplasms/Hyperplastic Nodules

Key Clinical Findings

- Occur in 5% of adults, and most are benign adenomas.
- It is not always possible to distinguish adrenal cortical adenoma from adrenal cortical carcinoma by FNA. Adrenal cortical adenomas tend to be smaller, but small carcinomas have been identified, particularly with the increased use of CT imaging.

Key Radiologic Findings

- Usually unilateral, solitary mass, in contrast to adrenal cortical hyperplasia, which is a bilateral, diffuse, or multinodular enlargement

Cytomorphology

- Cellular smears with numerous isolated stippled nuclei
- Frothy, granular background and no mitotic figures
- Occasional intact cells with bubbly cytoplasm
- Occasional cells with abundant intracellular lipofuscin pigment
- Figure 9.20a–d

A B C D

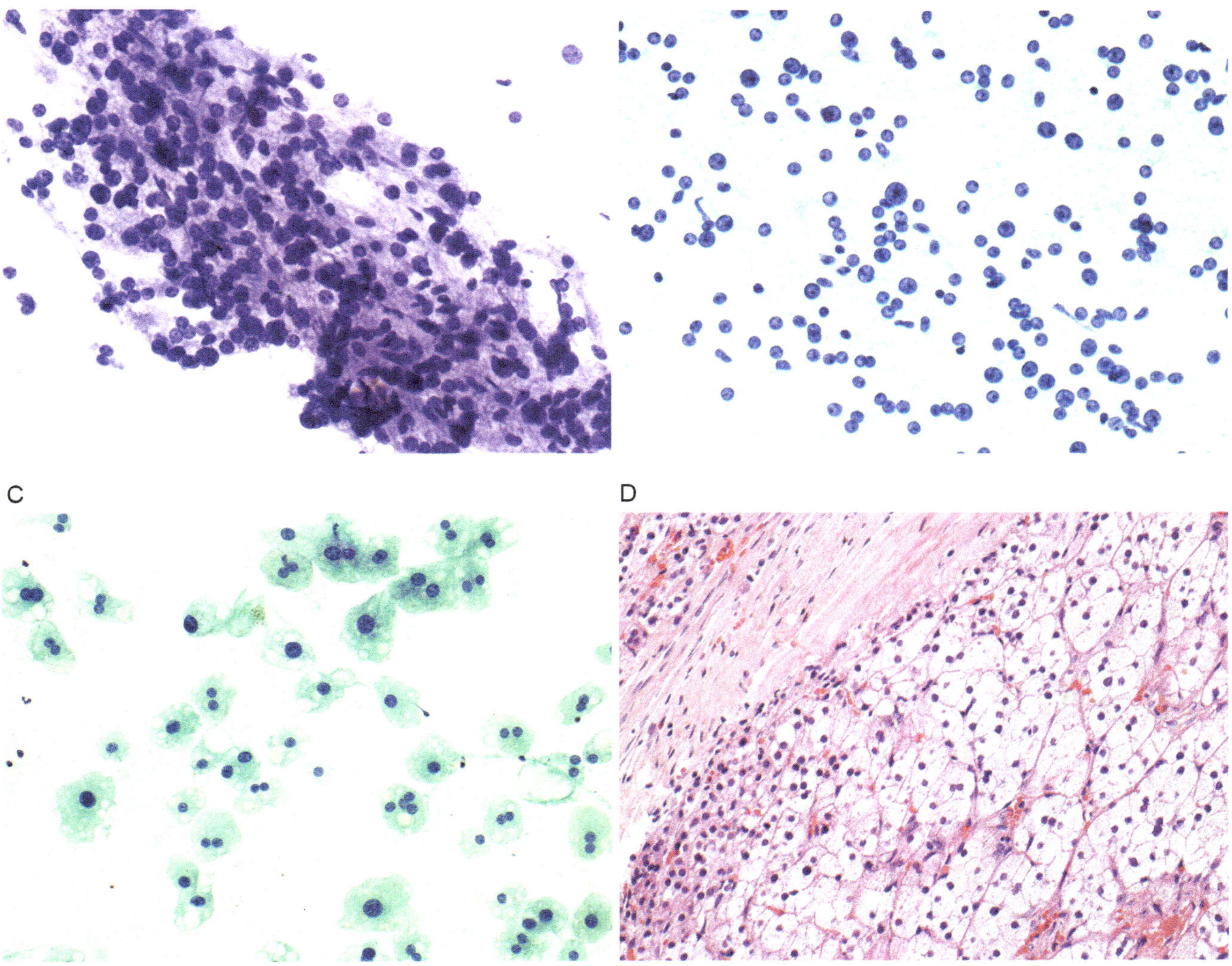

Fig. 9.20 (**a**) Adrenal cortical adenoma/hyperplastic nodule. Cellular smears with frothy, granular background and no mitotic figures (Romanowsky stain). (**b**) Adrenal cortical adenoma/hyperplastic nodule. Cellular smears with numerous isolated stippled nuclei (Papanicolaou stain). (**c, d**). Adrenal cortical adenoma/hyperplastic nodule. Occasional intact cells with bubbly cytoplasm and intracellular lipofuscin pigment (Papanicolaou stain)

Differential Diagnosis

- Cannot differentiate from normal adrenal cortical cells

Adrenal Cortical Carcinoma

Key Clinical Findings

- Range from well- to poorly differentiated tumors.
- Distinguishing between adrenal adenoma and carcinoma can be perplexing, however, in cases that show only mild or moderate nuclear atypia. When the findings are ambiguous, then surgical excision is advised.

Cytomorphology

- Numerous isolated cells with intact granular/vacuolated cytoplasm
- Enlarged, pleomorphic nuclei
- Mitotic figures and necrotic debris
- Figure 9.21a–e

Special Stains and Immunohistochemistry

- Positive for inhibin and melan A and negative for EMA and cytokeratin (including CK7 and CK20) (Table 9.4)
- Can be weakly positive for CAM 5.2

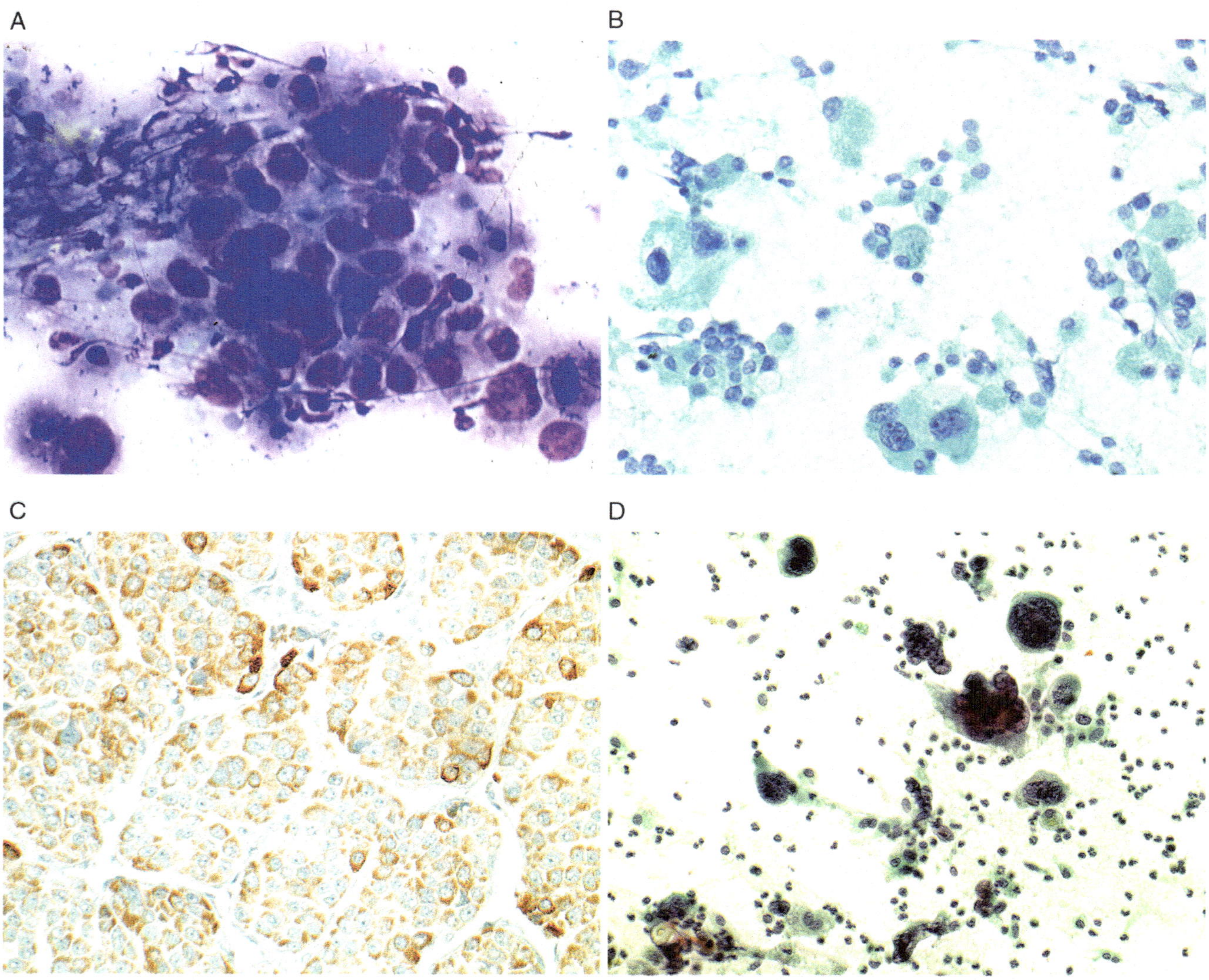

Fig. 9.21 (**a**). Adrenal cortical carcinoma. Large cells with enlarged, hyperchromatic nuclei and necrotic debris in the background (Romanowsky stain). (**b**) Adrenal cortical carcinoma. Numerous isolated cells with intact granular/vacuolated cytoplasm (Papanicolaou stain). (**c**) Adrenal cortical carcinoma. Positive immunostain for inhibin. (**d**) Adrenal cortical carcinoma. Large cells with enlarged, pleomorphic nuclei and necrotic debris in the background (Papanicolaou stain). (**e**) Adrenal cortical carcinoma. Large cells with enlarged, pleomorphic nuclei, macronucleoli, and necroinflammatory debris in the background (cell block H&E)

E

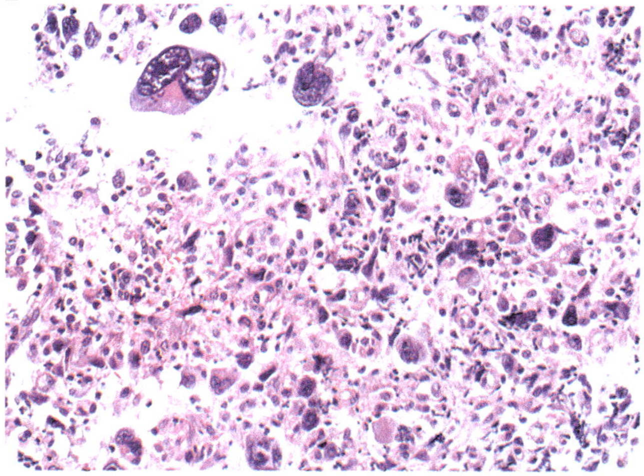

Fig. 9.21 (continued)

Table 9.4 Distinction of adrenal cortical carcinoma from clear cell renal cell carcinoma

Markers	Adrenal cortical carcinoma	Renal cell carcinoma
Cytokeratin 7	–	–
Cytokeratin 20	–	–
EMA	–	+
Vimentin	+	+
Inhibin-alpha	+	–
Melan A	+	–
KIM-1	–	+
pVHL	–	+

KIM-1 Kidney injury molecule-1, *pVHL* von Hippel-Lindau gene product

Differential Diagnosis

- Small cell carcinoma of the lung
- Adenocarcinoma of the lung
- Solitary metastatic RCC
- Melanoma
- Undifferentiated pleomorphic sarcoma

Pheochromocytoma

Key Clinical Findings

- Usually in adults and rare in childhood (more likely bilateral and multicentric).
- Familial tumors occur at younger ages.
- 10–20% of cases, they are associated with familial neoplastic syndromes such as the MEN syndrome 2a and 2b, neurofibromatosis, and the von Hippel-Lindau syndrome.
- 10–20% of tumors are bilateral, most often in familial cases.
- 10% extra-adrenal gland; a small percentage occurs in the urinary bladder.

Key Radiologic Findings

- Well-circumscribed mass, usually between 3 and 5 cm in size; hemorrhage and cyst formation are common.

Cytomorphology

- Cellular smears with loose clusters and isolated cells
- Small polygonal cells admixed with large spindle-shaped cells
- Pleomorphic and irregular nuclei with fine chromatin
- Intranuclear holes and prominent nucleoli
- Abundant fibrillary granular cytoplasm
- Positive for chromogranin, neurofilament protein, and S100
- Figure 9.22a–e

Differential Diagnosis

- Adrenal cortical neoplasms
- Metastasis

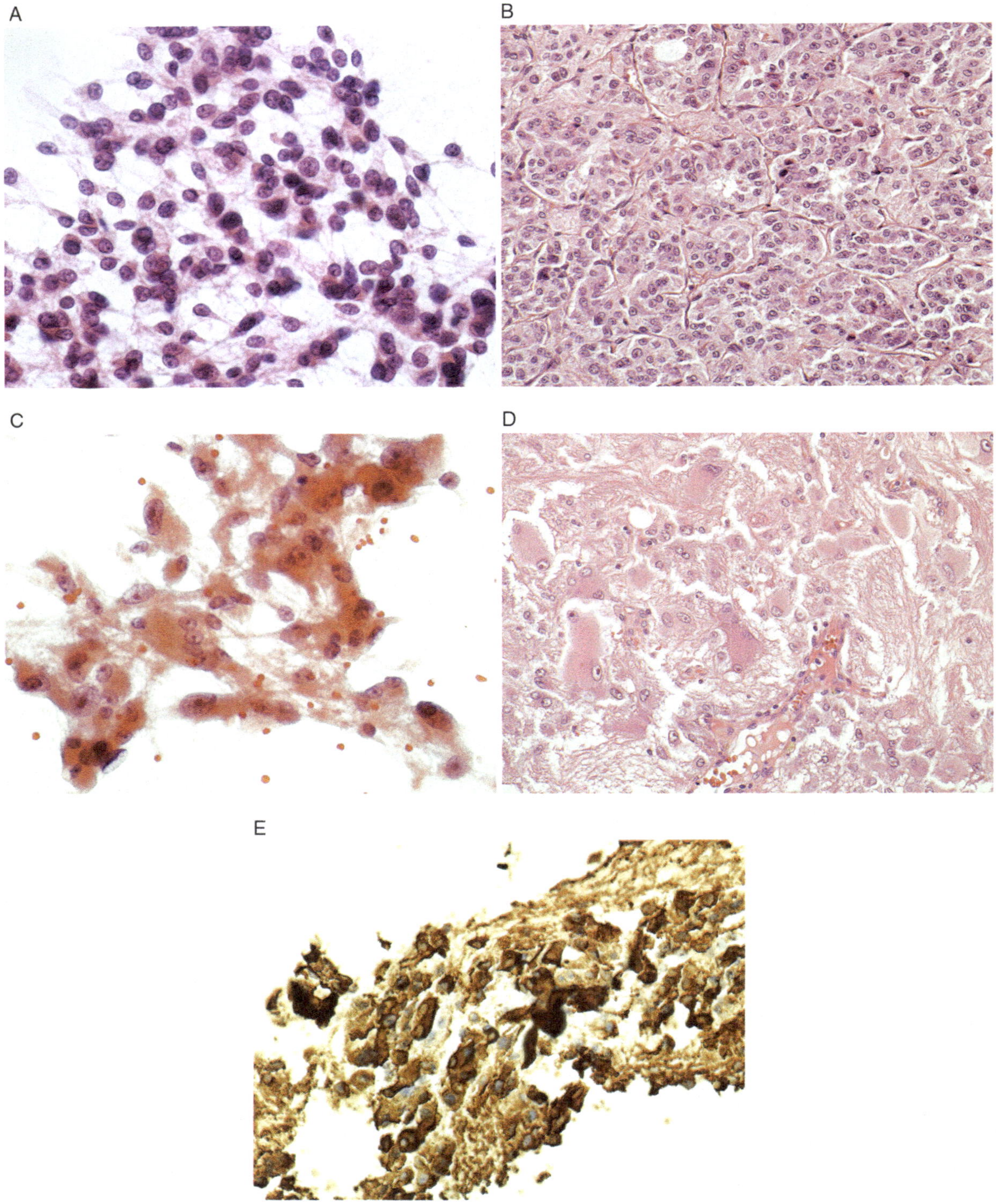

Fig. 9.22 (**a**) Pheochromocytoma. Cellular smears with loose clusters and isolated cells, small polygonal cells admixed with spindle-shaped cells (Papanicolaou stain). (**b**) Pheochromocytoma. Uniform cells arranged in nests and alveolar structures with round-ovoid and vesicular nuclei, single prominent nucleoli. Cytoplasm is faintly basophilic and granular (H&E). (**c**) Pheochromocytoma with ganglion differentiation. Loose clusters of ganglion-like cells (Papanicolaou stain). (**d**) Pheochromocytoma with ganglion differentiation. Ganglion-like cells (H&E). (**e**) Pheochromocytoma. Positive immunostain for chromogranin

Fig. 9.23 (continued) gland. Three dimensional pseudostratified columnar cells with hyperchromatic nuclei and necrosis (Papanicolaou stain). (**f**) Metastatic endometrial carcinoma to adrenal gland. Low cuboidal cells with vague acinar formation in a patient with history of endometrioid endometrial carcinoma (Papanicolaou stain). (**g**) Metastatic hepatocellular carcinoma to adrenal gland. Thick hepatocyte plate with lining endothelial cells wrapping around is diagnostic of hepatocellular carcinoma (Papanicolaou stain). (**h**) Metastatic hepatocellular carcinoma to adrenal gland. Hepatocellular carcinoma invading into adrenal gland (H&E)

Metastatic Tumors

Metastatic malignancies to the adrenal gland are diagnosed about four times more frequently than primary adrenal tumors. The most common primaries are lung and breast cancers, melanoma, and RCC. Certain tumors have tendency to produce a solitary nodule that mimics a primary adrenal lesion on imaging studies. Fine-needle aspiration with minimal invasiveness can help confirm or rule out an adrenal metastasis in a patient with history of cancer. See Fig. 9.23a–h.

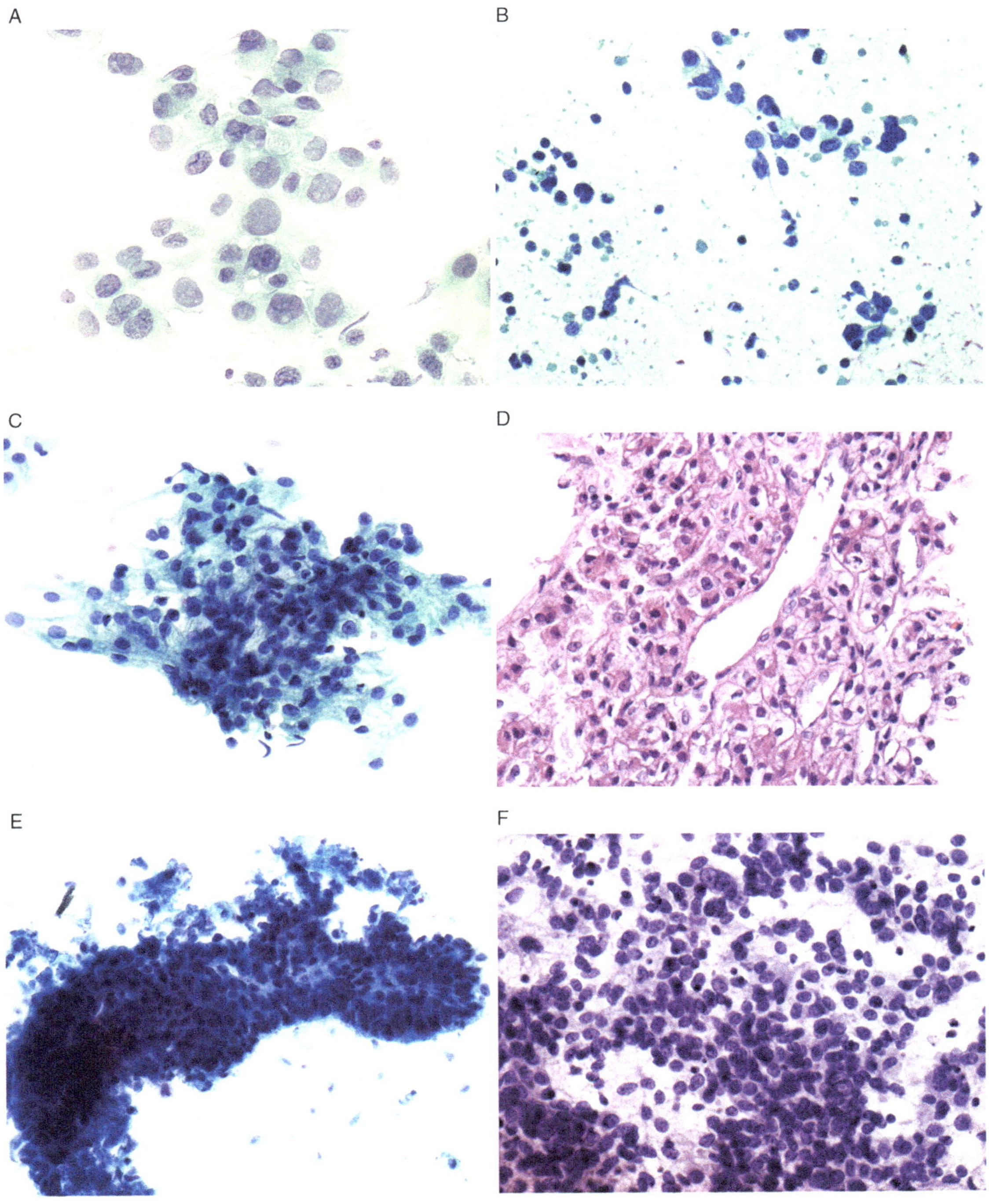

Fig. 9.23 (**a**) Metastatic lung adenocarcinoma to adrenal gland. Loose cohesive clusters of adenocarcinoma cells mimic adrenal cortical neoplasms or pheochromocytoma (Papanicolaou stain). (**b**) Metastatic lung small cell carcinoma to adrenal gland. Discohesive small cell carcinoma cells showing nuclear molding, smearing artifact, and apoptotic bodies (Papanicolaou stain). (**c**) Metastatic clear RCC to adrenal gland. Cohesive tissue cluster of cells with clear cells and small nucleoli (Papanicolaou stain). (**d**) Metastatic clear RCC to adrenal gland. Typical clear cell RCC with focal eosinophilic cytoplasm (H&E). (**e**) Metastatic colorectal adenocarcinoma to adrenal

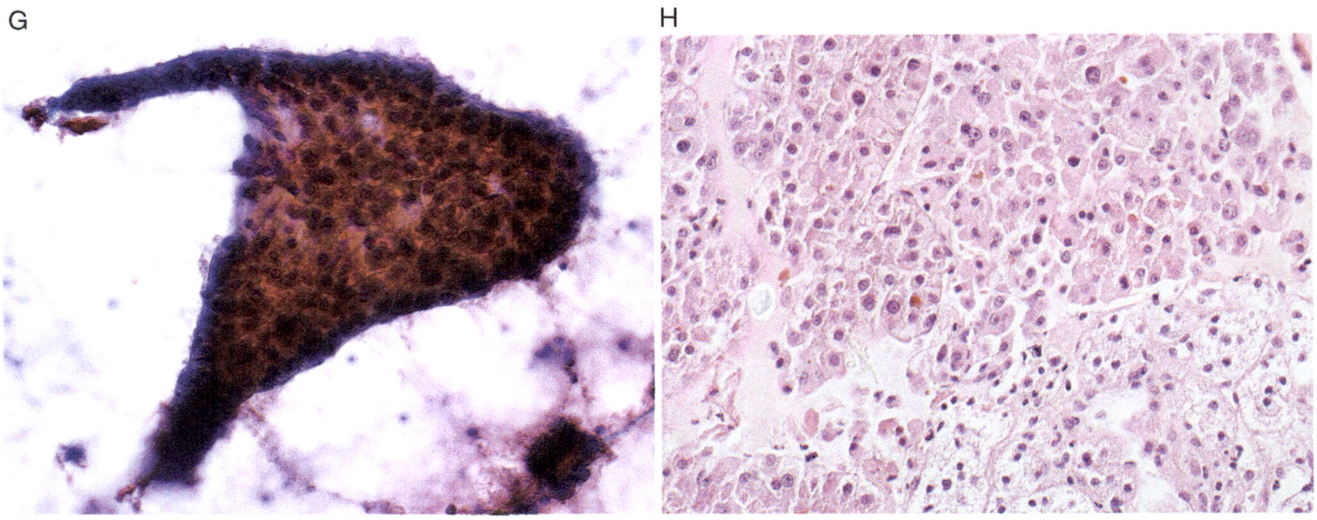

Fig. 9.23 (continued)

Case Presentation

Diagnosis of oncocytic epithelial neoplasms of the kidney, such as normal renal components (proximal renal tubular cells), renal oncocytoma, chromophobe RCC, papillary RCC, eosinophilic variant of clear cell RCC, or papillary urothelial carcinoma of the renal pelvis, has become a common practice of renal fine-needle aspiration biopsy. Sometime even in adequately sampled FNA specimens, the diagnosis can be very challenging, and very often, a cell block material or tissue core biopsy is needed to perform immunohistochemistry studies for further classifying the tumors. See Figs. 9.24a–g, 9.25, 9.26, 9.27, and 9.28a–e.

Case Scenario 1

Learning Objectives

1. Reiterate the diagnostic criteria for renal oncocytoma/oncocytic epithelial neoplasm, chromophobe RCC, papillary RCC, and papillary urothelial carcinoma of the renal pelvis.
2. Review the most effective panel of immunomarkers for diagnosis of renal oncocytoma/oncocytic epithelial neoplasm, chromophobe RCC, papillary RCC, and papillary urothelial carcinoma of the renal pelvis.

Case

A 52-year-old man presented with flank pain and found a 5-cm mass in the mid-pole of the kidney on CT scan. He has no known history of a prior malignancy and no significant family history for cancer.

A CT-guided FNA was performed. The FNA smear showed a cellular specimen with loose clusters and discohesive oncocytic epithelial cells in small groups. The cellular components showed small- to medium-size round nuclei with fine nuclear chromatin, small inconspicuous nucleoli, and abundant fine granular cytoplasm as shown in Fig. 9.24a–c. Occasional binucleation was noted. No nuclear grooves present. Based on the cytological features, the preliminary diagnosis was positive for neoplasm. Cytopathologic findings were consistent with oncocytic epithelial neoplasm. The diagnostic consideration included (1) renal oncocytoma, (2) chromophobe RCC, (3) clear cell RCC, (4) papillary RCC, and (5) papillary urothelial carcinoma of the renal pelvis.

If one strictly follows the diagnostic criteria of cytopathology on renal epithelial neoplasms, based on the pattern of recognition and the architectures of low magnification under the microscope, the renal oncocytoma and chromophobe RCC will have very similar patterns showing mainly single cells and dispersed small clusters (Figs. 9.3a, 9.9a, 9.24a, and 9.25a), rarely tissue fragments, or large sheets. On the other hand, the clear cell RCC and papillary RCC usually have cohesive clusters or tissue fragments with some degree of stromal tissue or fibrovascular cores (Figs. 9.7a, b, 9.8a, b, 9.27a, and 9.28a, b). The papillary urothelial carcinoma, however, can have both patterns under the low magnification (Figs. 9.14a and 9.26a).

(continued)

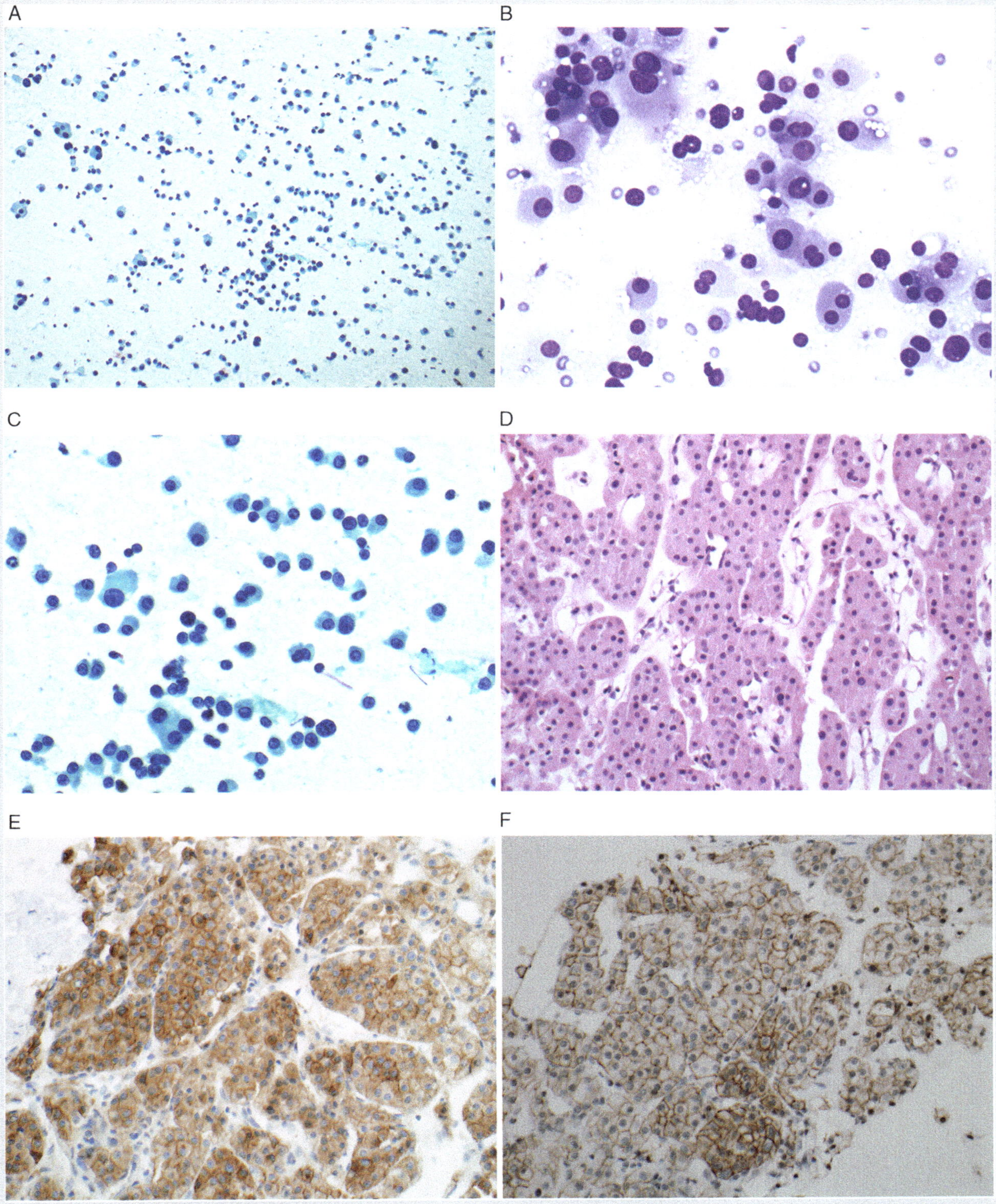

Fig. 9.24 (**a**) Renal oncocytoma (Papanicolaou stain). (**b**) Renal oncocytoma. (Romanowsky stain). (**c**) Renal oncocytoma (Papanicolaou stain). (**d**) Renal oncocytoma (H&E). (**e**) Renal oncocytoma. Positive membrane staining for C-KIT. (**f**) Renal oncocytoma. Positive membrane staining for E-cadherin. (**g**) Renal oncocytoma. Patchy positive membrane staining for CD15

(continued)

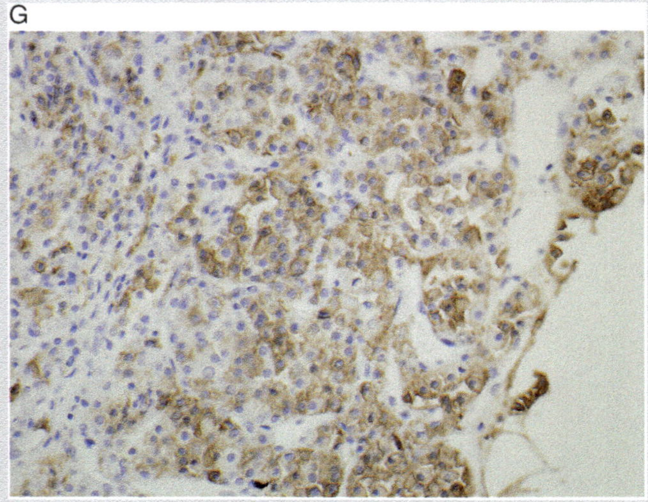

Fig. 9.24 (continued)

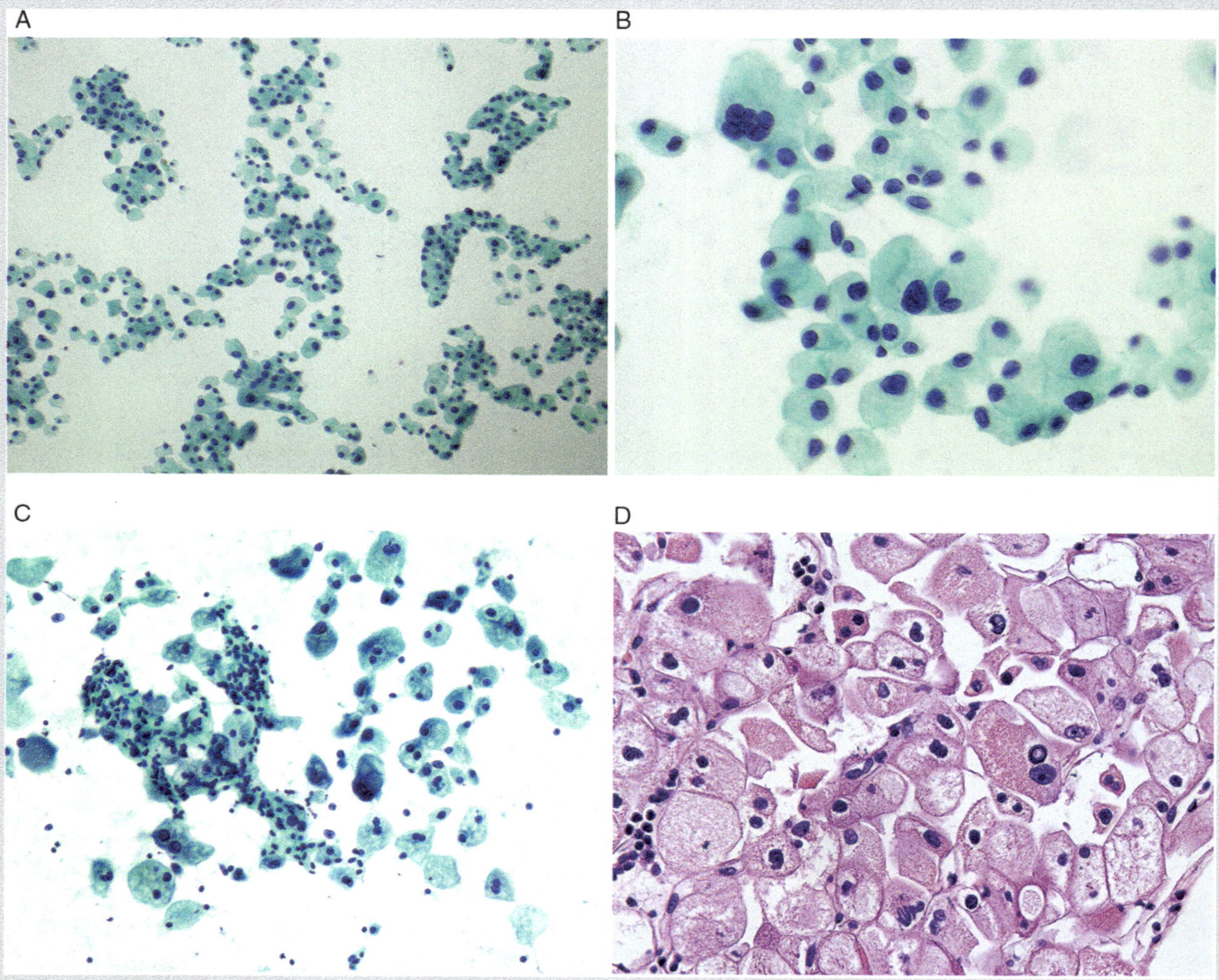

Fig. 9.25 (**a**) Chromophobe RCC (Papanicolaou stain). (**b**) Chromophobe RCC. (Papanicolaou stain). (**c**) Chromophobe RCC (Papanicolaou stain). (**d**) Chromophobe RCC (H&E). (**e**) Chromophobe RCC. Positive membrane staining for CK7. (**f**) Chromophobe RCC. Positive membrane staining for C-KIT. (**g**) Chromophobe RCC. Positive membrane staining for E-cadherin. (**h**) Chromophobe RCC (Papnicolaou stain)

(continued)

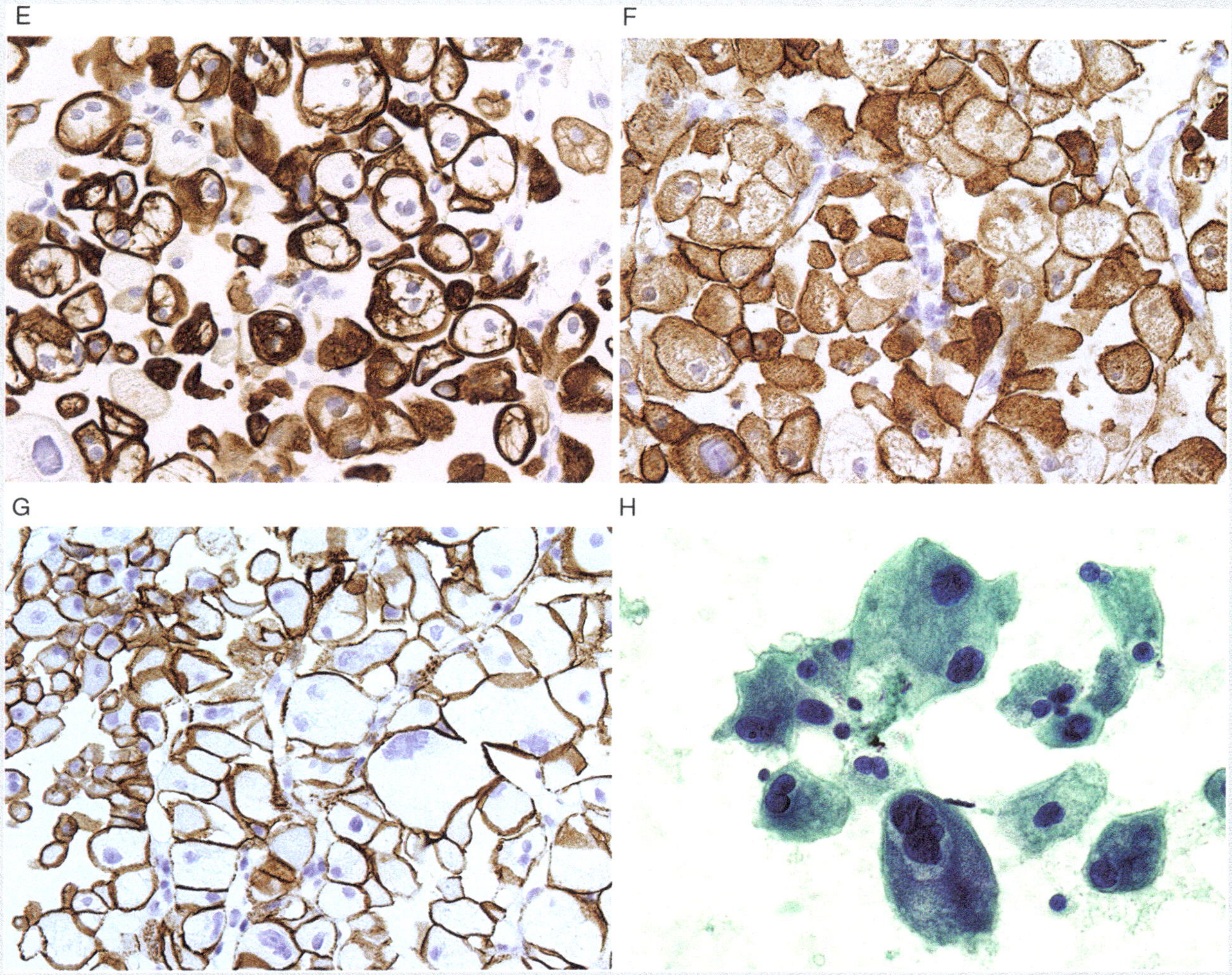

Fig. 9.25 (continued)

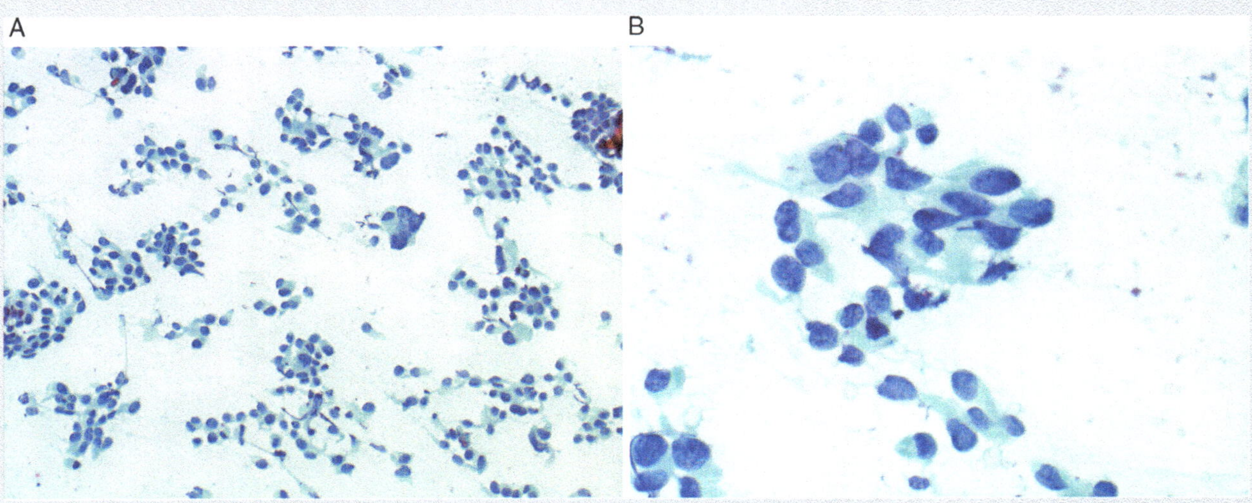

Fig. 9.26 (**a**) Urothelial carcinoma of the renal pelvis (Papanicolaou stain). (**b**) Urothelial carcinoma of the renal pelvis (Papanicolaou stain). (**c**) Urothelial carcinoma of the renal pelvis (H&E)

(continued)

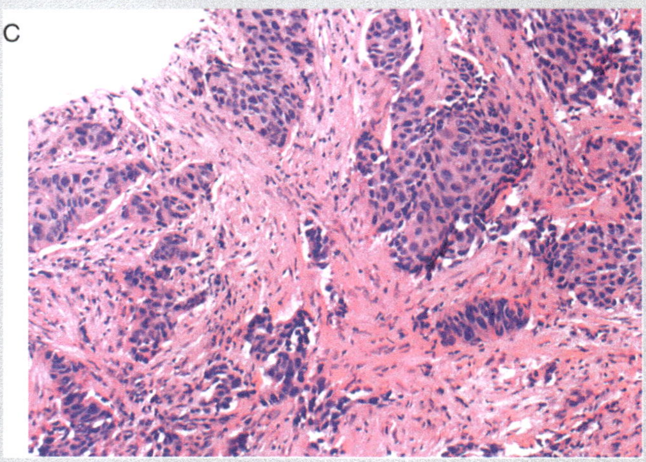

Fig. 9.26 (continued)

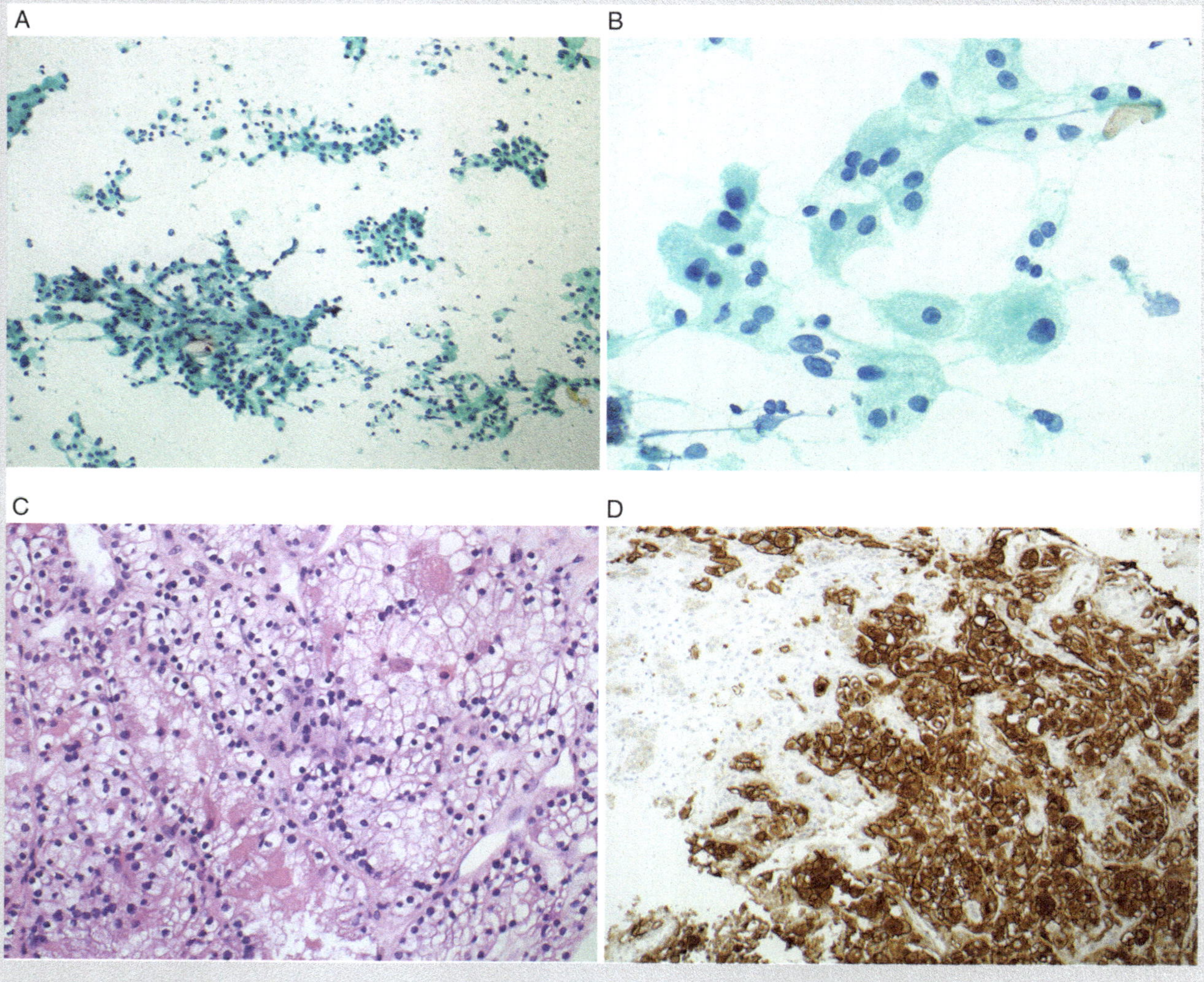

Fig. 9.27 (**a**) Clear cell RCC (Papanicolaou stain). (**b**) Clear cell RCC (Papanicolaou stain). (**c**) Clear cell RCC (H&E). (**d**) Clear cell RCC. Positive membrane staining for CD10

(continued)

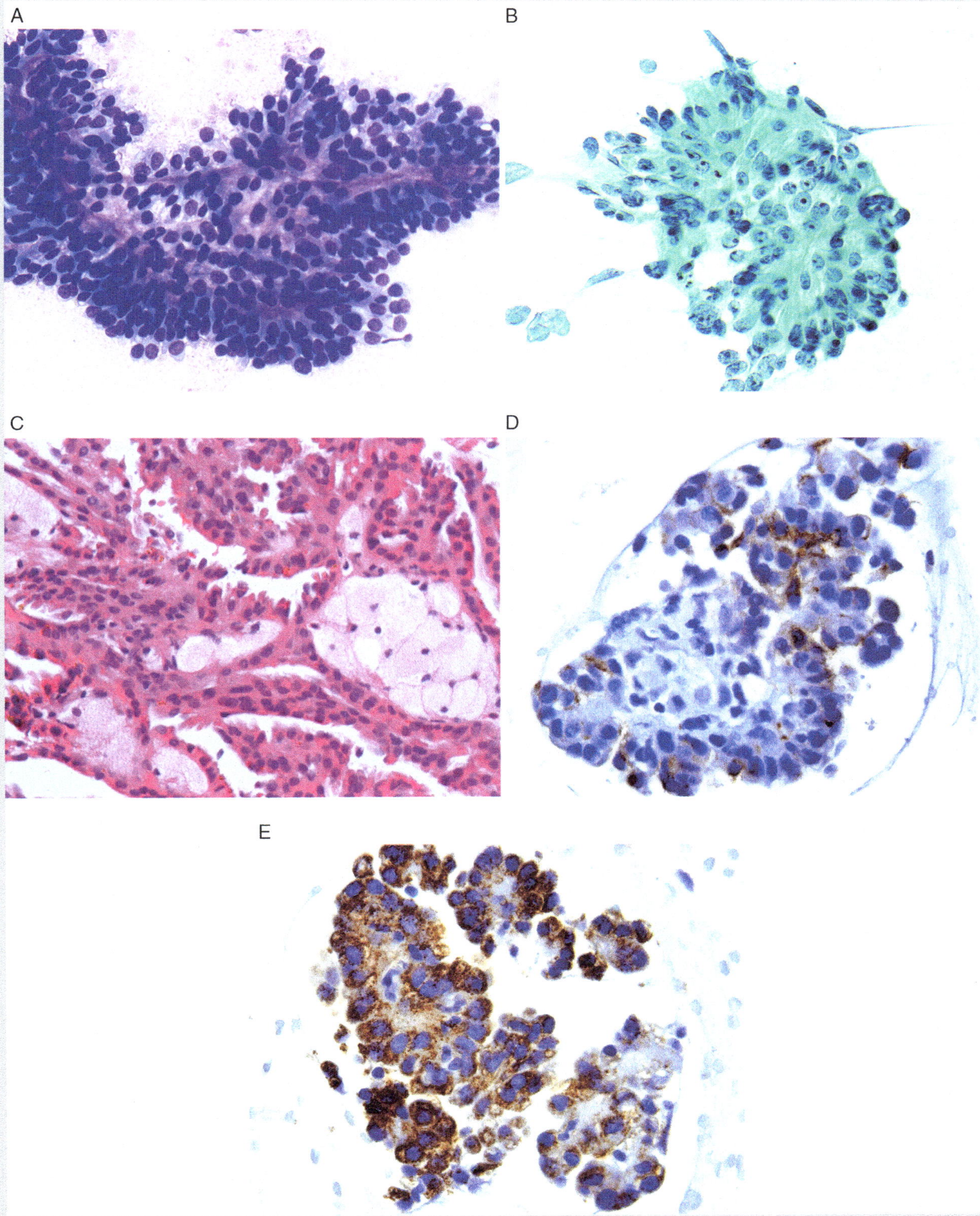

Fig. 9.28 (**a**) Papillary RCC (Romanowsky stain). (**b**) Papillary RCC (Papanicolaou stain). (**c**) Papillary RCC (H&E). (**d**) Papillary RCC. Focal membrane staining for KIM-1. (**e**) Papillary RCC. Strong cytoplasmic staining for p504S

(continued)

Then if one further combines the typical nuclear and cytoplasmic features of the high magnification under the microscopy, the definitive diagnosis can be made without

waiting for the tissue (cell block or tissue core biopsy) H&E slides: (1) Renal oncocytoma cells have round to oval nuclei, small prominent nucleoli, binucleation, abundant granular cytoplasm, and distinctive cell border (Figs. 9.3a and 9.24b, c). (2) Chromophobe RCC cells have classic raisinoid nuclei, binucleation, nuclear grooves, wrinkled nuclear contours, perinuclear haloes, and prominent cell membrane (Figs. 9.9b and 9.25e–g). (3) Clear cell: RCC cells usually have abundant clear, vacuolated, or granular cytoplasm and large, round eccentrically placed nucleus/extruded nucleus (Figs. 9.7c, e, and 9.27b). (4) Papillary: RCC cells have true papillae or spherules lined by uniform cells (type 1) or large cells with large nuclei, prominent nucleoli, and foamy macrophages in the background (Figs. 9.8b and 9.28a, b). (5) Papillary urothelial carcinoma of the renal pelvis can have single cell pattern or sheets or clusters of pleomorphic cells with hyperchromatic angulated nuclei, dark coarse chromatin, and cytoplasmic tails (Figs. 9.14a and 9.26b).

If the cytopathologic features are still insufficient for a definitive diagnosis, the H&E slides from cell block and tissue core (Figs. 9.3b, 9.7d, f, 9.8c, 9.14b, 9.24d, 9.25c, 9.26c, 9.27c, and 9.28c) can help make a final diagnosis.

Furthermore, immunohistochemistry studies can aid in classifying the diagnosis (Figs. 9.7g, 9.14d, e, 9.24g, 9.25e, 9.27d, and 9.28d, e).

Final Diagnosis on FNA Specimen

Positive for neoplasm. Renal oncocytic epithelial neoplasm consistent with renal oncocytoma.

Abbreviations List

Abbreviation	Full text
AMACR	α-Methylacyl CoA racemase(P504S)
CD	Cluster of differentiation (CD10, CD56, CD57, CD68, CD117)
CEA	Carcinoembryonic antigen
CK	Cytokeratin (CK7, CK20)
CT	Computed tomography
DQ	Diff-Quick (Romanowski)
EMA	Epithelial membrane antigen
FNA	Fine-needle aspiration
GATA3	GATA binding protein 3
GST-alpha	Glutathione S-transferase- alpha alpha
H&E	Hematoxylin and eosin
HMB45	Human melanoma black 45
HMWCK	High molecular weight cytokeratin
IHC	Immunohistochemistry
KIM-1	Kidney injury molecule-1
KIT	Tyrosine-protein kinase Kit
MIB1	Mindbomb E3 ubiquitin protein ligase 1
MPNST	Malignant peripheral nerve sheath tumor
MRI	Magnetic resonance imaging
N/C	Nuclear-to-cytoplasmic ratio
Pap	Papanicolaou
PAS	Periodic acid-Schiff
PAX	Paired box gene (PAX5, PAX8)
PET	Positron emission tomography
pVHL	von Hippel-Lindau tumor suppressor
RT-PCR	Reverse transcription polymerase chain reaction
TFE3	Transcription factor E3
STAT6	Signal transducer and activator of transcription 6
TTF1	Thyroid transcription factor 1
WHO	World Health Organization
WT1	Wilms tumor 1

Suggested Reading

Cibas E, Ducatman B. Kidney and adrenal. In:Text cytology diagnostic principles and clinical correlates. 4th ed. Philadelphia: Saunders Elsevier; 2014.

DeMay RM. Chapter 7. Introduction to FNA Biopsy. In:The art and science of cytopathology, vol. 2. 2nd ed. Chicago: ASCP Press; 2010. p. 536–61.

Gleeson FC, Kipp BR, Levy MJ, et al. Lung cancer adrenal gland metastasis: optimal fine-needle aspirate and touch preparation smear cellularity characteristics for successful theranostic next-generation sequencing. Cancer Cytopathol. 2014;122(11):822–32.

Neuzillet Y, Lechevallier E, Andre M, et al. Accuracy and clinical role of fine needle percutaneous biopsy with computerized tomography guidance of small (less than 4.0 cm) renal masses. J Urol. 2004;171(5):1802–5.

Perez-Ordonez B, Hamed G, Campbell S, et al. Renal oncocytoma: a clinicopathologic study of 70 cases. Am J Surg Pathol. 1997;21(8):871–83.

Saboorian MH, Katz RL, Charnsangavej C. Fine needle aspiration cytology of primary and metastatic lesions of the adrenal gland. A series of 188 biopsies with radiologic correlation. Acta Cytol. 1995;39(5):843–51.

Shen SS, Ro JY, Tamboli P, Truong LD, Zhai Q, Jung SJ, Tibbs RG, Ordonez NG, Ayala AG. Mucinous tubular and spindle cell carcinoma of kidney is probably a variant of papillary renal cell carcinoma with spindle cell features. Ann Diagn Pathol. 2007;11(1):13–21.

Wadih GE, Nance KV, Silverman JF. Fine-needle aspiration cytology of the adrenal gland, fifty biopsies in 48 patients. Arch Pathol Lab Med. 1992;116(8):841–6.

Soft Tissue

10

Jun Zhang, Haiyan Liu, and Fan Lin

Summary of Pearls and Pitfalls

- Benign STT outnumbers sarcomas by at least 100:1.
- Benign lesions are superficial and located in dermal or subcutaneous soft tissue.
- The most common benign tumor is lipoma, which often goes untreated.
- The desmoid-type fibromatosis or intramuscular hemangioma requires wide excision comparable to a sarcoma; otherwise local recurrence is very frequent.
- Excisional biopsy or shelling out of a sarcoma is inappropriate and often may cause difficulties in further patient management.
- Then it is generally advisable to obtain a diagnostic biopsy prior to definitive treatment for all soft tissue masses >5 cm.
- Unless a very obvious subcutaneous lipoma and for all subfascial or deep-seated masses, irrespective of size due to the high risk of being a sarcoma (about 10%).
- Such patients should ideally be referred to a specialized tumor center before surgery for optimal treatment.

Imaging of Soft Tissue Tumors

MRI is the modality of choice for detecting, characterizing, and staging STTs due to its ability to distinguish tumor tissue from adjacent muscle and fat, as well as to define relationships to key neurovascular bundles. It provides better tissue discrimination between normal and abnormal tissues than any other imaging modality. In addition, it aids in guiding biopsy, planning surgery, evaluating response to chemotherapy, restaging, and in the long-term follow-up for local recurrence. MRI accurately defines tumor size and provides information on hemorrhage, necrosis, edema, cystic and myxoid degeneration, and fibrosis. Soft tissue masses that do not demonstrate tumor-specific features on MRI should be considered indeterminate, and biopsy should always be obtained to exclude malignancy.

In *MRI-guided biopsy*, caution has to be excised in three respects for indeterminate STTs: selection of an appropriate pathway, coordination with the treating surgeon, and participation of a pathologist comfortable with interpreting percutaneous biopsies. The radiologist should undertake the biopsies only at the request of the treating surgeon and not necessarily at the request of the patient's initial physician. In collaboration with the treating surgeon, the needle tract (which needs to be excised with the tumor) can be established and the patient well served.

Spiral CT is preferable for examining sarcomas of the chest and abdomen, since air/tissue interface and motion artifacts often degrade MRI quality. A baseline chest CT scan at the time of the diagnosis for evidence of lung metastasis is important, particularly for sarcomas >5 cm, for accurate staging of patients.

Early studies suggest that *positron emission tomography (PET)* has clinical potential by determining biological activity of soft tissue masses. It can be used to distinguish benign tumors from high-grade sarcomas, pretreatment grading of sarcomas, and evaluation of local recurrence.

Biopsy

A biopsy is necessary and appropriate to establish malignancy, to assess histologic grade, and to determine the specific histological type of sarcoma given the prognostic and therapeutic importance of accurate diagnosis. A treatment plan, if it is possible, can be designed that is tailored to a lesion's predicted pattern of local growth, risk of metastasis, and likely sites of distant spread. A large enough sample from a viable area of sarcoma is usually required for definitive diagnosis and accurate grading. Most limb masses are generally best sampled

© Springer International Publishing AG 2018
F. Lin et al., *Handbook of Practical Fine Needle Aspiration and Small Tissue Biopsies*, DOI 10.1007/978-3-319-57386-1_10

Table 10.1 Accuracy of soft tissue tumor FNA

Sensitivity rates	Up to 95%
Specificity for sarcoma	54–98%
Positive predictive values	91–99%
False-positive rate	0–5%
False-negative rate	2–15%

through a longitudinally oriented incision, so that the entire biopsy tract can be completely excised at the time of definitive resection. An incisional biopsy with minimal extension into adjacent tissue planes is the ideal approach for most extremity masses. Excisional biopsy should be avoided, particularly for lesions greater than 2 cm in size, since such an approach will make definitive reexcision more extensive due to the contamination of surrounding tissue planes. For deep-seated lesions, a core biopsy approach may be used to establish a diagnosis; however, the limited tissue obtained with this technique may make definitive grading and prognostication difficult. FNA cytology of STTs might be desirable to large specialty centers with a well-integrated multidisciplinary team, since careful clinicoradiologic correlation and considerable experience are required in order to make accurate diagnoses, but most patients are first seen in smaller community practices. A systematic approach to differential diagnosis, specimen triage, recommendations, and referrals can enhance the efforts of the cytopathologist, regardless of level of experience.

Sampling error is a problem which FNA shares with core and even incisional biopsies. Rapid evaluation and triage for ancillary studies such as immunohistochemistry (IHC), flow cytometry, cytogenetics, and electron microscopy (EM) are often indispensable for definitive classification and can decrease the inadequate rate. Criteria for specimen adequacy can reduce the rate of false-negative cases, but any clinically suspicious lesion should be further evaluated by biopsy. The three main reasons for a false diagnosis are sampling error, technically inferior material, and misinterpretation. Concern over needle tract seeding, stemming from the era of larger needles, however, is unfounded. See Table 10.1.

FNA of STTs is cost-effective and the least invasive method of sampling a heterogeneous lesion and does not compromise tissue planes for a subsequent excision. The indications of FNA include (1) screening, (2) primary diagnosis (although not widely accepted by most soft tissue pathologists for primary classification of sarcomas), and (3) detection of recurrence.

Specimen Collection and Preparation

- 22- to 23-gauge needles
- Dedicated passes for ancillary studies
- Alcohol-fixed, Papanicolaou-stained smears for nuclear detail
- Air-dried, Romanowsky-type-stained smears for cytoplasmic and matrix details
- Limited use for thin-layer preparations

Ideally, one makes a separate pass for each desired ancillary study. Papanicolaou-stained slides highlight nuclear details, while Romanowsky-type stains highlight cytoplasmic details and matrix material. Thin-layer preparations offer good nuclear detail, optimize results from aspirates carried out without the benefit of rapid evaluation, and can be used for adjunct studies. However, cells appear smaller, rounder, and falsely epithelioid, and useful background information (e.g., vascular patterns) is sometimes lost.

Reporting Terminology

As with other cytologic specimens, there should be a general category: malignant, suspicious, atypical, benign, and nondiagnostic. Because most STTs are treated by wide surgical excision, lack of a specific histologic subtype may not affect management. When a histologic subtype is not possible, a descriptive diagnosis should be used.

The most important prognostic consideration is the histologic grade, and most neoplasms are amenable to grading. A two-tiered grading system of low versus high is probably sufficient in the majority of cases.

Low-grade lesions have mild nuclear atypia, minimal or absent necrosis, low cellularity with minimal nuclear overlap, and rare or absent mitoses (<3/10HPF). High- grade lesions have moderate to severe nuclear atypia, intermediate to high cellularity with conspicuous to prominent nuclear overlap, definite necrosis, and frequent mitoses.

The presence or absence of mitoses and necrosis is an objective finding worthy of separate mention in the report. When only smears are available, a statement such as "mitoses are absent" or "mitoses are numerous" suffices to avoid falsely high or low counts.

Finally, most cytology reports should include a comment to address the differential diagnosis, suggest ancillary studies in equivocal cases, or advise on appropriate subsequent management.

Ancillary Studies

Ancillary studies include electron microscopy (EM), immunohistochemistry (IHC) (Table 10.2), flow cytometry, and cytogenetics.

EM is especially helpful in classifying poorly differentiated high-grade lesions and small round blue cell tumors.

Table 10.2 Common soft tissue tumor immunomarker positive rate (%)

VIM	DES	MSA	SMA	CALD	S100	CD57	CD34	CD31	CD99	HMB-45	MI
95	95	96	25	Rare	Rare	17	–	–	20%	–	–
100	–	–	Rare	–	Rare	–	–	–	0	–	–
91	75	90	88	85	8	50	16	Rare	20	–	–
100	11	18	Rare	Rare	63	43	9	–	50	–	–
100	–	0	12	Rare	Rare	90	–	–	50	–	–
100	–	<10	Rare	Rare	Rare	–	80	80	–	–	–
100	–	–	12	0	30	Focal	–	–	Focal	–	–
100	10	39	33	25	Rare	–	52	–	N/A	–	–
100	–	30	–	–	90	17	4	–	N/A	85	70
50	20	<10	–	–	30	–	–	–	N/A	–	–
100	–	–	Rare	Rare	70	–	–	–	–	N/A	N/A
100	<10	17	18	Rare	Rare	–	–	–	–	N/A	N/A

KER AE1/3; *EMA* epithelial membrane antigen, *VIM* vimentin, *DES* desmin, *MSA* muscle-specific actin, *SMA* smooth muscle actin, *CALD* h-caldesmon, *HMB-45* melanomas marker, *M1* Malan-A, *RMS* rhabdomyosarcoma, *FS* fibrosarcoma, *LMS* leiomyosarcoma, *MPNST* malignant peripheral nerve sheath tumor, *SS* synovial sarcoma, *AS* angiosarcoma, *MFH* malignant fibrous histiocytoma, *EPS* epithelioid sarcoma, *CCS* clear cell sarcoma, *ASPS* alveolar soft part sarcoma, *PLPS/DLPS* pleomorphic and dedifferentiated liposarcoma, *DCHOR* dedifferentiated chordoma

Cell block sections are preferred for IHC stains, but air-dried or thin-layer preparations may also be used. Flow cytometry is useful when lymphoma is suspected on rapid on-site evaluation.

An increasing number of reproducible, relatively specific cytogenetic abnormalities are identified with routine chromosomal analysis, fluorescence in-situ hybridization (FISH), and reverse transcriptase-polymerase chain reaction (RT-PCR) techniques.

Conventional chromosomal analysis offers the advantages of a full karyotype counterbalanced by low sensitivity and long turnaround time.

FISH accurately labels targeted chromosomal regions. Cytologic specimens provide ideal substrates with intact cells and nuclei free of sectioning artifact and truncation. A moderately cellular, evenly spread preparation, such as cytocentrifuge or thin-layer preparations, is key. As only a specified chromosomal abnormality is targeted, a negative result provides little information.

Classification of Soft Tissue Tumors

In 2013, with the new genetic data, the World Health Organization (WHO) published an updated, more reproducible classification of tumors of the soft tissue. Based on the methods that the experts use and focus on visual pattern recognition to formulate a diagnosis by using concise text and an algorithmic method to make arriving at a diagnosis efficient, we put the common STTs into the following major practical categories for cytopathology of FNA specimens Table 10.3.

Table 10.3 Practical categories of STTs for cytopathology of FNA specimens based on 2013 World Health Organization (WHO) classification of tumors of the soft tissue

Epithelioid tumors
Clear cell sarcoma (malignant melanoma of soft parts)
Epithelioid sarcoma
Epithelioid angiosarcoma
Epithelioid hemangioendothelioma
Alveolar soft part sarcoma
Granular cell tumor
Spindle cell tumors
Inflammatory myofibroblastic tumor
Schwannoma
Malignant peripheral nerve sheath tumor
Synovial sarcoma
Leiomyosarcoma
Extrapleural solitary fibrous tumor
Fibromatoses
Dermatofibrosarcoma protuberans
Fibrosarcoma
Nodular fasciitis
Round cell tumors
Neuroblastoma
Extraosseous Ewing's sarcoma/primitive neuroectodermal tumor
Desmoplastic small round cell tumor
Alveolar and embryonal rhabdomyosarcoma
Extraskeletal mesenchymal chondrosarcoma
Adipocytic tumors
Hibernoma
Lipoma
Spindle cell/pleomorphic lipoma

(continued)

Table 10.3 (continued)

Atypical lipomatous tumors/well-differentiated liposarcoma
Pleomorphic liposarcoma
Myxoid tumors
Intramuscular myxoma
Lipoblastoma
Chordoma
Extraskeletal myxoid chondrosarcoma
Myxoid liposarcoma
Myxofibrosarcoma (low- and high-grade)
Myxofibrosarcoma-like dedifferentiated liposarcoma
Myxoinflammatory fibroblastic sarcoma/atypical myxoinflammatory fibroblastic tumor
Low-grade fibromyxoid sarcoma (Evans tumor)
Fibrohistiocytic tumors
Angiomatoid fibrous histiocytoma
Tenosynovial giant cell tumor
Pleomorphic tumors
Pleomorphic rhabdomyosarcoma (PRMS)
Undifferentiated pleomorphic sarcoma (UPS)
Dedifferentiated sarcomas (DDS)
Fibroblastic/myofibroblastic lesions
Elastofibroma
Idiopathic retroperitoneal fibrosis
Sarcomatoid carcinoma and melanoma involving soft tissue mimicking sarcomas
Sarcomatoid carcinomas – sarcomatoid renal cell carcinoma
Melanomas

Modified with permission from Fletcher et al. (Fletcher et al., 2013)

Epithelioid Tumors

- Epithelioid soft tissue tumors are composed of epithelioid cells with abundant cytoplasm.
- Metastatic carcinoma and melanoma are always in the differential diagnosis.
- Generally neoplasms in this category yield hypercellular aspirates composed of both cohesive aggregates and numerous singly placed cells.

Clear Cell Sarcoma (Melanoma of Soft Parts)

Key Clinical Findings

- Neural crest origin with melanocytic differentiation
- <1% of all soft tissue neoplasms
- Young adults, 20–40 years old
- Deep tissue of distal extremities, particularly foot and ankle
- Slowly growing, often painful mass associated with fascia and tendons
- Most lesions are less than 5 cm.
- Highly malignant, metastases and local recurrences common
- Spread to the lung, lymph nodes, and bone
- Prognosis mainly based on tumor size and necrosis

Key Radiologic Findings

- Present as soft tissue mass on CT scans and MRI
- Occasionally associated with calcification

Cytopathology

- Hypercellular smears
- Uniform single cells and small clusters
- Cells from round to polygonal to spindle
- Binucleated/multinucleated giant cells
- Intranuclear inclusions, prominent nucleoli
- Clear to pale staining cytoplasm
- Figure 10.1a, b

Histopathology

- Nests of rounded cells or fascicles of elongated cells, separated by delicate fibrovascular septa
- Cells usually have clear cytoplasm; some may be eosinophilic and granular.
- Nuclei usually vesicular, oval, and with prominent nucleoli
- Giant cells with a peripheral ring of nuclei are common.
- Overlying skin typically lacks melanocytic lesion.
- Figure 10.1c

Immunohistochemistry

- Most cases strongly positive for S100, HMB45, and melan-A
- Figure 10.1d–f

Cytogenetic Study

- >75% of the clear cell sarcomas revealed unique translocation t (12;22)(q13;q12) and carrying EWSR1-ATF1 and EWSR1-CREB1 fusion transcripts.
- Increased copies of chromosomes 7 and 8 have been reported.
- In contrast, the gene for cutaneous melanoma has been localized to 1p.
- Figure 10.1g.

Epithelioid Sarcoma (ES)

Key Clinical Findings

- Rare, usually adolescent to young adult.
- Predominantly male.
- Usually distal extremities, especially finger, hand, wrist, and forearm.

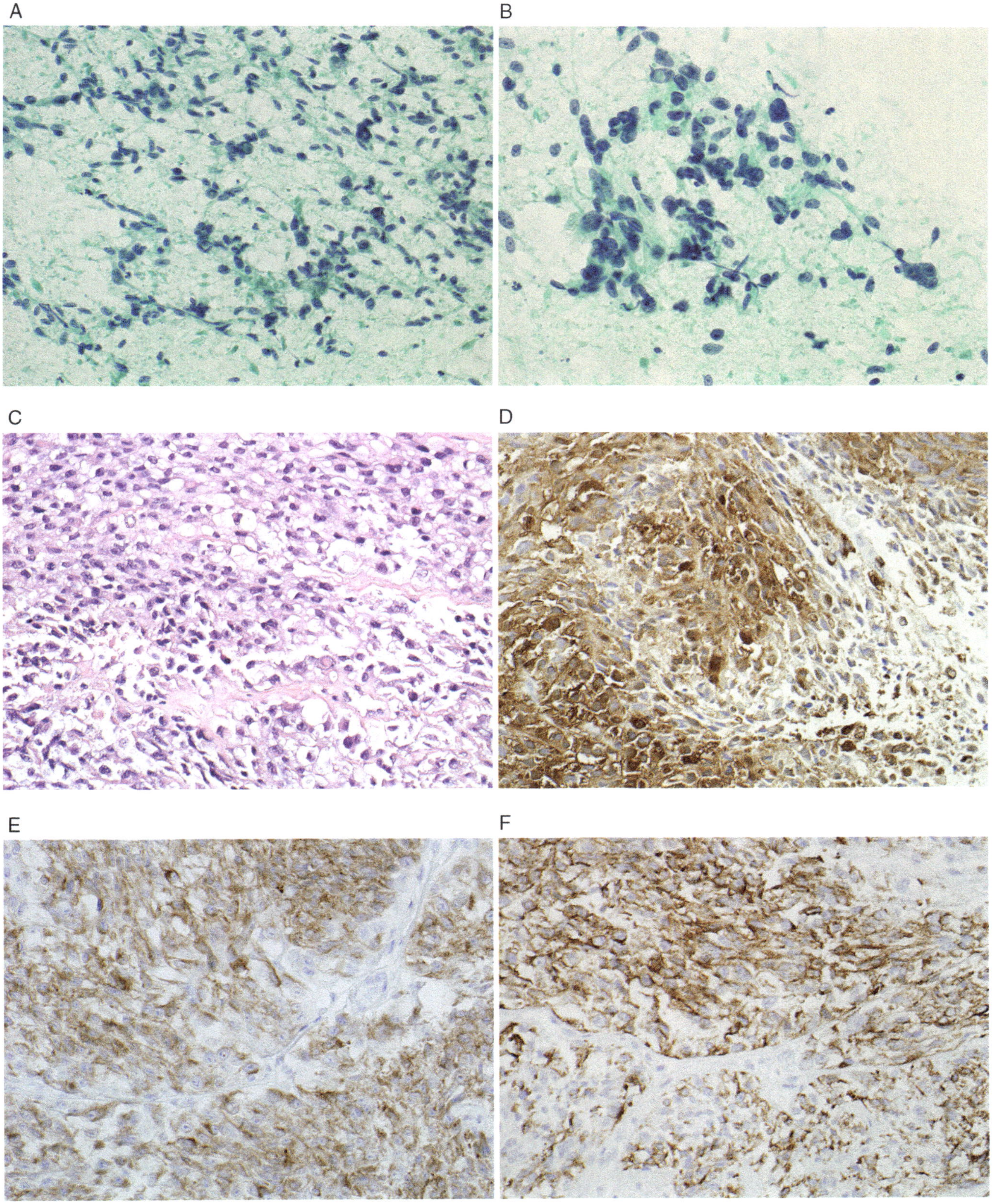

Fig. 10.1 (**a**–**g**) (**a**) Clear cell sarcoma. Cellular smears with uniform spindle cells and small clusters in a background of granular material. Occasional intranuclear inclusions (Papanicolaou stain). (**b**) Clear cell sarcoma. Clusters of spindle to polygonal cells, binucleated cells with prominent nucleoli (Papanicolaou stain). (**c**) Clear cell sarcoma. Nests of rounded or elongated cells with clear cytoplasm, some may be eosinophilic and granular, oval and vesicular, and prominent nucleoli. Occasional intranuclear inclusions separated by delicate fibrovascular septa (H&E). (**d**) Clear cell sarcoma. Strong and diffuse staining for S100. (**e**) Clear cell sarcoma. Strong and diffuse staining for melan-A. (**f**) Clear cell sarcoma. Strong and diffuse staining for HMB45. (**g**) Clear cell sarcoma. FISH performed on paraffin-embedded tissues revealed rearrangement of the EWS locus at 22q12 (Image demonstrated separation of EWSR1)

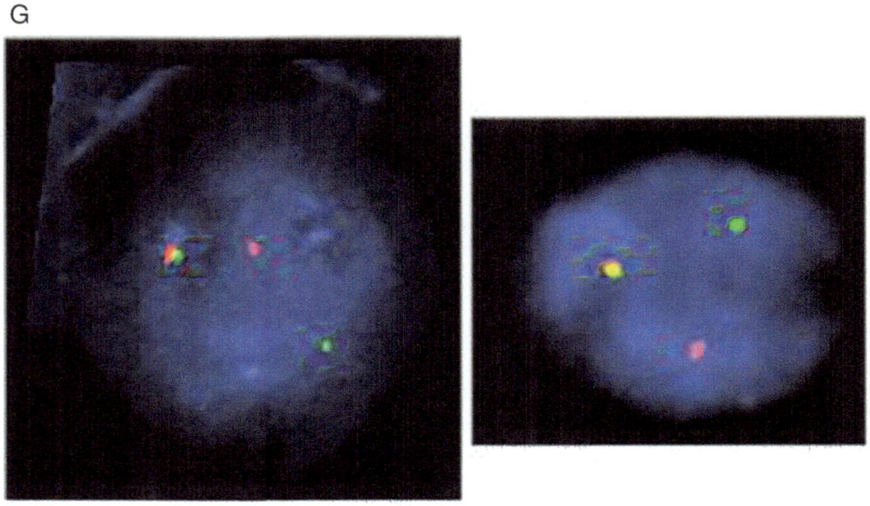

Fig. 10.1 (continued)

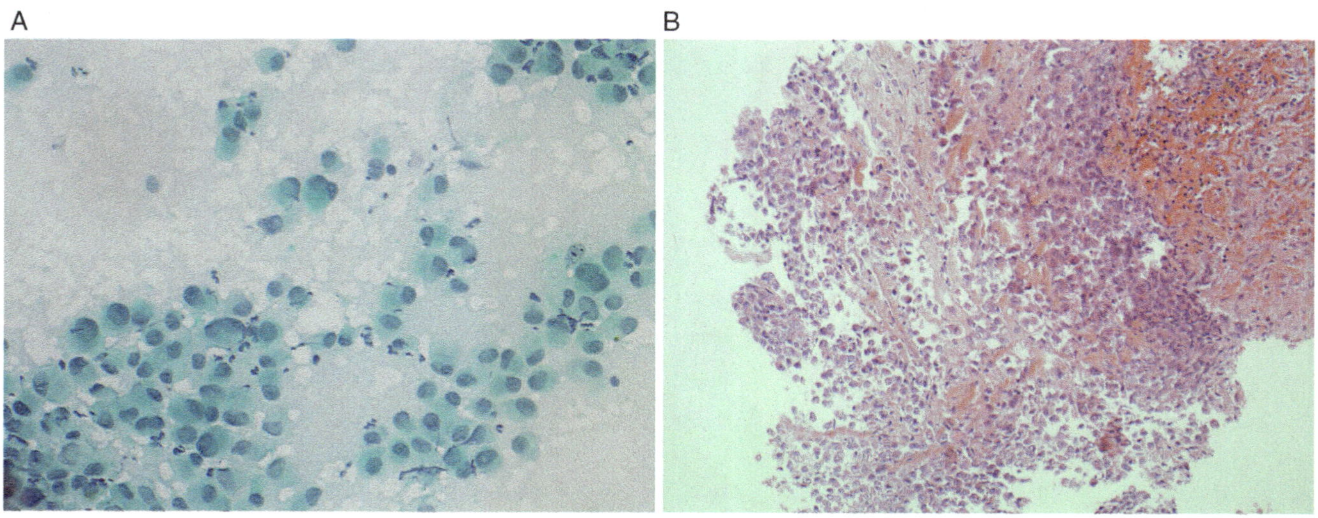

Fig. 10.2 (**a**, **b**) (**a**) Epithelioid sarcoma. Numerous singly placed round to polygonal cells with eccentric nuclei, dense cytoplasm (Papanicolaou stain). (**b**) Epithelioid Sarcoma. Nodular growth pattern with central necrosis, uniform plasmacytoid cells with eosinophilic cytoplasm embedded in visible collagen (H&E)

- Involving dermis and subcutis or attached to tendon or fascia.
- Slowly growing mass/pain and ulceration.
- Repeated local recurrences are common.
- Lymph node metastases are not uncommon.

Key Radiologic Findings

- Typically a soft tissue mass with occasional speckled pattern of calcification.
- Cortical thinning and erosion of underlying bone may be present, but invasion or destruction of adjacent bone is rare.
- MRI is useful for revealing the anatomic extent of the tumor.

Cytopathology

- Numerous dispersed round to polygonal cells
- Eccentrically placed nuclei
- Dense cytoplasm
- Granuloma-like structures
- Necro-inflammatory debris
- Figure 10.2a

Histopathology

- Nodular growth pattern with central necrosis.
- Cell types from rounded to spindled (but not biphasic, as in synovial sarcoma).

- Deeply eosinophilic cytoplasm, little to no pleomorphism, few to no giant cells.
- Visible collagen deposited between tumor cells.
- Calcification and ossification can occur.
- Central necrosis of nodules in skin may simulate a palisading granulomatous lesion.
- Figure 10.2b.

Immunohistochemistry

- Positive for cytokeratins and EMA
- Negative for S100 and HMB45
- Positive for CD34
- Negative for CD31 and factor VIII
- Loss of INI1 expression, characteristic of conventional and proximal-type ES, being detected in >90% of cases
- Immunostaining for INI1 can be used to confirm the diagnosis of ES in the appropriate context.

Epithelioid Angiosarcoma

Key Clinical Findings

- Usually adults, predominantly male.
- Lymphangiosarcoma predominantly female.
- Bone, breast, heart (most common sarcoma in heart), liver, orbit, pharynx, oral cavity, nose, and skin though mostly head and neck (scalp); rarely reported in soft tissue, spleen, and other organs.
- Clinical risk factors include vinyl chloride, arsenic, thorotrast, radiation, and chronic lymphedema.
- Breast angiosarcomas may be very well differentiated but almost always cause a mass lesion or symptoms (versus hemangioma).
- Lymphangiosarcoma typically arises 10 years after radical mastectomy for breast carcinoma. Possibly related to chronic lymphatic obstruction.
- Grossly ill-defined hemorrhagic areas; poor prognosis as cutaneous tumors frequently spread to lymph nodes.

Key Radiologic Findings

- CT showed a homogenous high-density mass with possible calcified foci.
- Intratumoral hemorrhage with juxtaposed hematoma and aggressive invasion to the surrounding tissue suggest angiosarcoma.
- MRI demonstrated a large heterogeneous mass on both T1-weighted images (T1WI) and T2-weighted images (T2WI).

Cytopathology

- Cellular sample with dyshesive large epithelioid cells
- Moderate to marked nuclear pleomorphism and prominent nucleoli
- Occasional intracytoplasmic vacuoles and hemosiderin pigments
- Mitotic figures common and bloody background
- Figure 10.3a–c

Histopathology

- Well differentiated, may resemble hemangioma.
- Moderately differentiated; anastomosing staghorn vascular channels lined by cytologically malignant, epithelioid endothelial cells.
- Cells have dusky pink cytoplasm and possibly hyaline cytoplasmic globules. Portion of cell with nucleus bulges into lumen (hobnail pattern).
- Nuclei large, hyperchromatic, mitotically active. Red cell extravasation. Little inflammation.
- Poorly differentiated. Similar cytology as in moderately differentiated, but blood vessels less well formed or unrecognizable. Architecture ranges from fascicles of spindle cells to sheets of more epithelioid cells.
- Figure 10.3d.

Special Stains/Studies

- Positive for factor 8, ulex, CD31, CD34, and other vascular markers, except in some poorly differentiated tumors.
- Especially epithelioid variants may express keratin.
- CD31 more sensitive than factor 8.
- Figure 10.3e, f.

Cytogenetic and Molecular Genetic Aberrations

- KDR mutation in mammary angiosarcoma
- MYC amplification and FLT4 co-amplification (25%) in secondary angiosarcoma

Epithelioid Hemangioendothelioma

Key Clinical Findings

- All ages, young adults in bone.
- Either sex, though with women usually occurs in the liver and lung.
- Soft tissue, bone, liver, and lung.

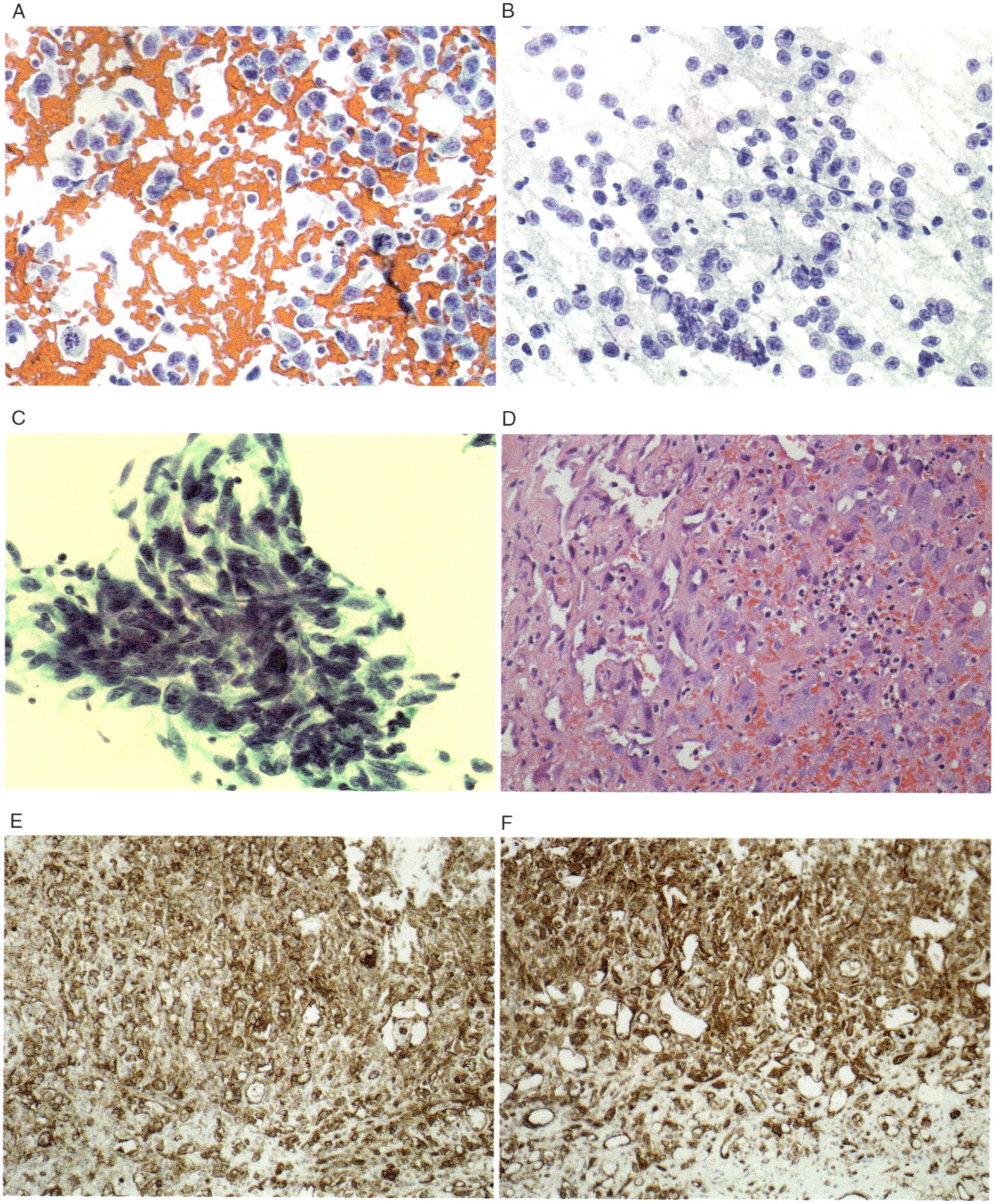

Fig. 10.3 (a–f) (**a**) Epithelioid angiosarcoma. Cellular sample with dyshesive large epithelioid cells, marked nuclear atypia, and a mitotic figure (Papanicolaou stain). (**b**) Epithelioid angiosarcoma. Dyshesive naked nuclei with moderate atypia, prominent nucleoli, scattered intracytoplasmic vacuoles (Papanicolaou stain). (**c**) Epithelioid angiosarcoma. Clusters of epithelioid and spindle cells with marked nuclear atypia and prominent nucleoli (Papanicolaou stain). (**d**) Epithelioid angiosarcoma. Poorly differentiated angiosarcoma showing blood vessels less well formed or unrecognizable. Architecture ranges from fascicles of spindle cells to sheets of more epithelioid cells. (H&E). (**e**, **f**) Strong CD31 and CD34 stain

- Clinically often associated with a blood vessel.
- Grossly may resemble organizing thrombus or appear nondescript white gray. In soft tissue, usually solitary. In the bone, liver, and lung, often multifocal.
- Potentially malignant. Lung tumor is usually fatal, while liver and soft tissue tumors are usually not.
- Commonly spreads to lymph nodes. Protracted but progressive course.

Key Radiologic Findings

- Present as a soft tissue mass with associated calcification; the adjacent bone may show erosion.

Cytopathology

- Moderate cellularity and bloody background
- Discohesive round to polygonal cells with abundant cytoplasm
- Slight nuclear pleomorphism
- Occasional intracytoplasmic vacuoles and few mitoses
- Figure 10.4a

Histopathology

- Arising from a vessel, tumor cells infiltrate outward from the endothelium to the surrounding tissue, while partially preserving the organization of the vessel.
- Neoplastic endothelial cells grow in cords and small nests within a myxoid, chondromyxoid, hyalinized, calcified, or sclerotic stroma.
- Areas of high and low cellularity are formed.
- The endothelial cells are small, round to slightly spindled, plump, eosinophilic, often vacuolated.
- Frank blood vessel structures are almost never formed, but many of the cells form single cell lumens that make them resemble signet cells.
- Nuclei are round, vesicular, and may be indented.
- About 1/4 of tumors have areas suggestive of malignant transformation: nuclear atypia, increased mitotic rate (greater than 1/10 HPF), spindle cells, or necrosis.
- Figure 10.4b.

Special Stains/Studies

- Endothelial cells are positive for vascular markers (factor 8, ulex, CD31).
- May also express keratin

Cytogenetic and Molecular Genetic Aberrations

- t(1;3)(p36.3;q25) and WWTR1-CAMTA1

Alveolar Soft Part Sarcoma

Key Clinical Findings

- Rare, <1% of all sarcomas.
- Adolescents and young adults.
- Predominantly female.

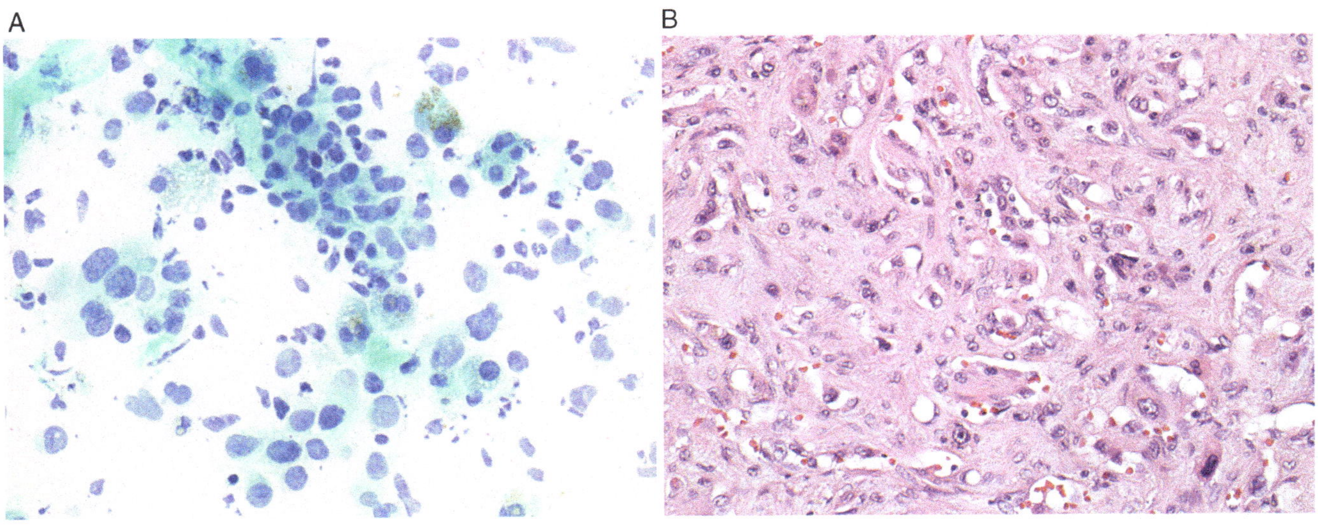

Fig. 10.4 (a, b) (a) Epithelioid hemangioendothelioma. Liver FNA showing cellular sample with discohesive round to polygonal cells, abundant cytoplasm, light nuclear pleomorphism in a background of benign hepatocytes with bile pigments (Papanicolaou stain). (b) Epithelioid hemangioendothelioma. Liver core biopsy showing neoplastic endothelial cells grow in cords and small nests within a myxoid, chondromyxoid, hyalinized, or sclerotic stroma. The endothelial cells are small, round to slightly spindled, plump, eosinophilic, often vacuolated. Frank blood vessel structures are almost never formed, but many of the cells form single cell lumens that make them resemble signet cells (H&E)

- Adults, typically the thigh.
- Children, typically the head and neck, and especially the orbit and tongue.
- Poorly circumscribed with necrosis, hemorrhage, many dilated veins at periphery.
- Most patients die of disease.
- Children have somewhat better prognosis than adults.

Key Radiologic Findings

- Hypervascularity with prominent draining veins and prolonged capillary staining, are usually seen with angiography and CT scans.
- On MRI, the tumor typically demonstrates high signal intensity on both T2- and T1-weighted images.

Cytopathology

- Moderate cellularity with abundant naked nuclei
- Discohesive large, round to polygonal cells
- Pseudoacinar or pseudoalveolar arrangements
- Round to oval nuclei with prominent nucleoli
- Abundant granular cytoplasm
- Intracytoplasmic and extracellular crystals
- Figure 10.5a

Histopathology

- Nests of round cells divided by thin-walled vascular channels.
- Cells are large, partially discohesive (especially in nest centers), eosinophilic, granular, possibly vacuolated.
- Nuclei are vesicular with small nucleoli and few mitoses.
- An architecture of sheets rather than nests is more common in children and has a better prognosis.
- Figure 10.5b.

Special Stains/Studies

- PASD-positive intracytoplasmic elongated crystals are pathognomonic, recognizable in 80% of tumors.
- Many of the remainder have PASD-positive granules.
- Glycogen in cells is PAS positive, NSE and S100 negative.

Granular Cell Tumor

Key Clinical Findings

- Also called granular cell myoblastoma; rare in children and common in middle-aged adults, derived from Schwann cells.
- Often found in anterior/posterior chest and upper extremities, can be found in anus, bile duct, larynx, oral cavity, pituitary, stomach, and vulva.
- Clinically 10–15% multiple sites, usually small (<3 cm) and poorly circumscribed.
- Recurrences are rare and malignant varieties are very rare. Malignant granular cell tumors are suggested by >2 mitoses/10 HPF, > 5 cm, more cellular and often more elongated cells.

Key Radiologic Findings

- Solid infiltrating soft tissue mass, suspicious for malignancy

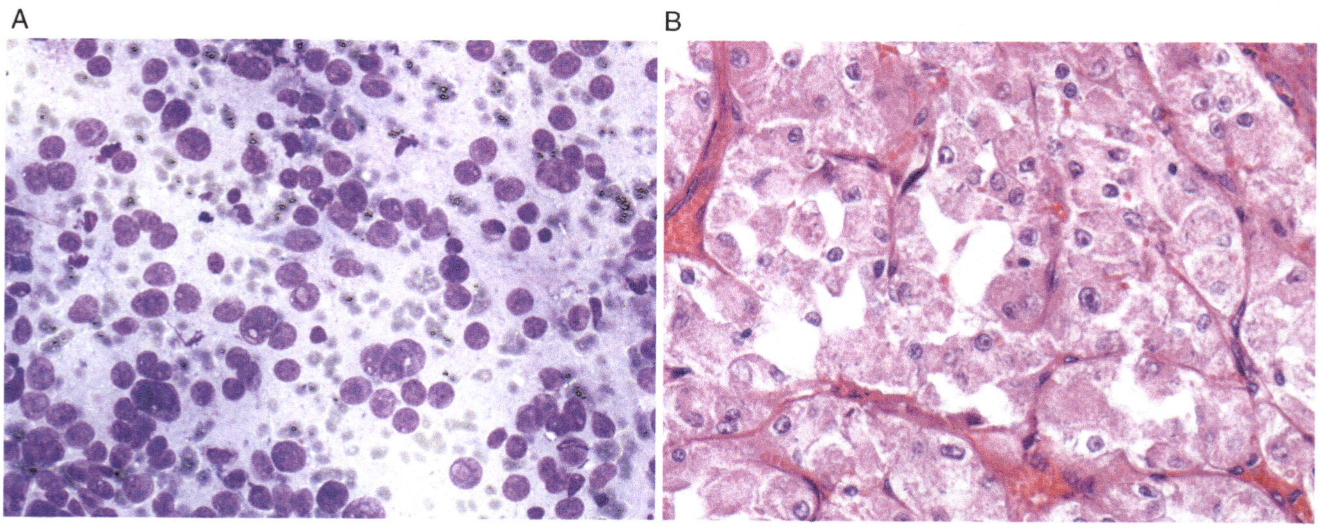

Fig. 10.5 (a, b) (a) Alveolar soft part sarcoma. Cellular smear with discohesive, large, naked round to oval nuclei, prominent nucleoli (Papanicolaou stain). (b) Alveolar soft part sarcoma. Nests of round cells divided by thin-walled vascular channels, vesicular nuclei and eosinophilic, granular, possibly vacuolated cytoplasm (H&E)

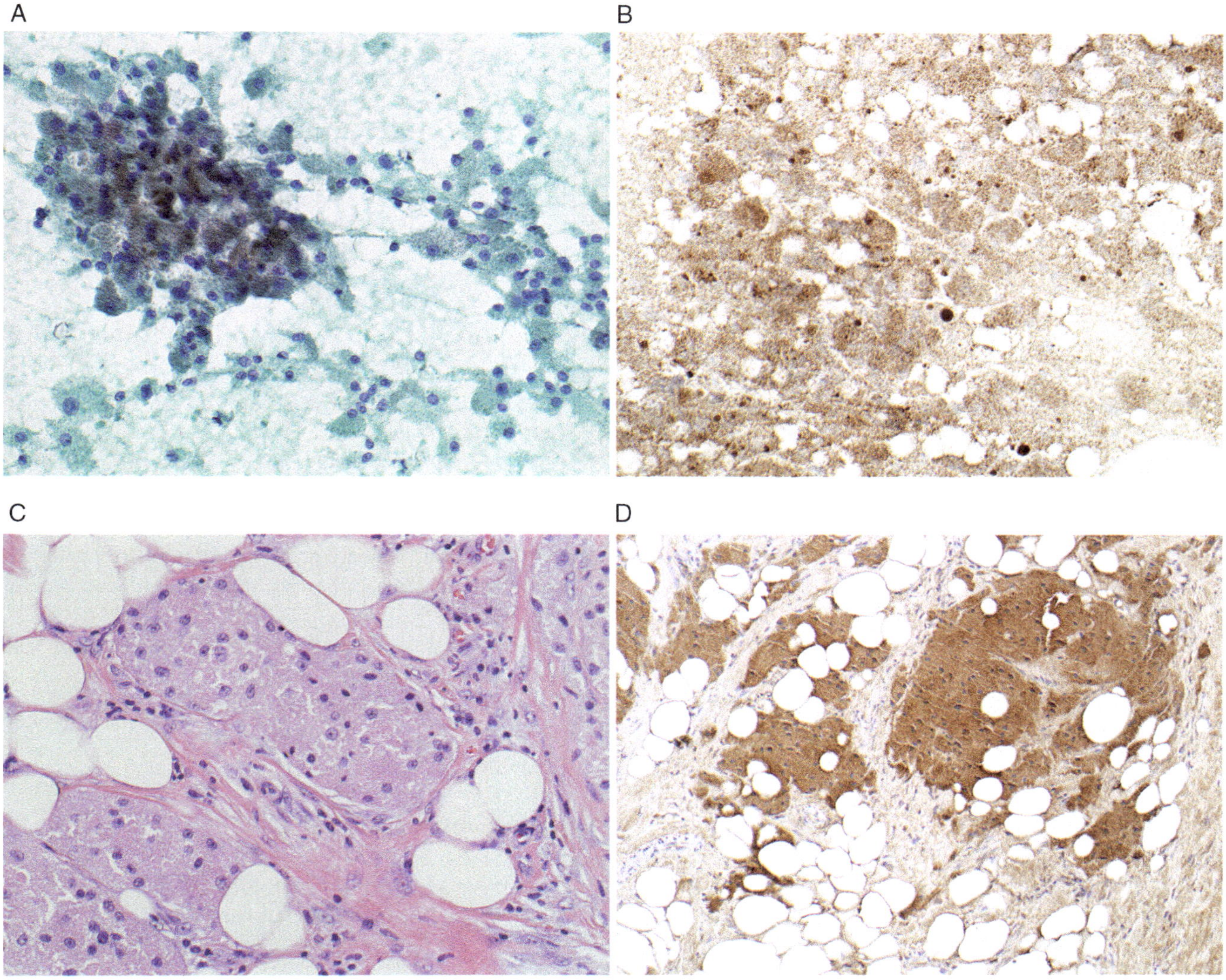

Fig. 10.6 (**a–d**) (**a**) Granular cell tumor. Abundant bare small nuclei with uniform cellular appearance in a granular background and abundant granular cytoplasm (Papanicolaou stain). (**b**) Granular cell tumor. Cytology prep showing strong and diffuse positive for S100. (**c**) Granular cell tumor. Nests or sheets of granular cells separated by collagen and fat. Cells with abundant granular eosinophilic cytoplasm, small central nuclei, and nucleoli (H&E). (**d**) Granular cell tumor. Strong and diffuse positive for S100

Cytopathology

- Cellular sample with abundant bare small nuclei
- Uniform cellular appearance
- Granular background and abundant granular cytoplasm
- Figure 10.6a

Histopathology

- Nests or sheets of cells separated by collagen
- Cells with abundant coarsely granular eosinophilic cytoplasm and small central nuclei. Nucleoli may be visible.
- Cases arising beneath squamous mucosa may be associated with marked pseudoepitheliomatous hyperplasia.
- Cells tend to surround nerves. Older lesions associated with more sclerosis.
- Figure 10.6b.

Special Stains/Studies

- Weak PAS-positive; S100 and NSE-positive
- Figure 10.6c, d

Spindle Cell Tumors

The benign lesions in this group produce cytologic specimens compromised of intact tissue fragments with few or no individual cells, while the malignant lesions features more discohesiveness, hypercellularity, necrosis, and mitotic activity. In addition to the distinction between benign and malignant, a frequent problem run into within this class is determining whether a lesion is of smooth muscle or nerve sheath origin. Sarcomatoid carcinoma and melanoma are always in the differential diagnosis.

Inflammatory Myofibroblastic Tumor (IMT)

Key Clinical Findings

- Wide age range for those lesions with no prior history of surgery. Somewhat older population for those with a history of surgery
- Occurs in the mesentery, bladder, central nervous system, cervix, eye (orbit), larynx, liver, lung (inflammatory pseudotumor of the lung), lymph node, oral cavity, prostate, salivary gland, spleen, uterus corpus, vagina, vulva
- Benign, but may recur

Key Radiologic Findings

- Ultrasound and CT scan mimicking infiltrating malignant mass

Cytopathology

- Hypercellular smears
- Clusters of plump, spindle fibroblastic, or myofibroblastic cells
- Large polygonal cells with variably atypical nuclei
- Prominent lymphocytes and plasma cells
- Fine cytoplasmic vacuoles and elongated cytoplasmic tails
- Figure 10.7a

Histopathology

- Intersecting fascicles of spindle cells with a delicate network of small blood vessels.
- Cells resemble reactive fibroblasts with uniformly elongated nuclei containing one or more distinct nucleoli. Mitotic figures may be numerous.
- Lesions contain scattered chronic inflammatory cells and prominent dilated capillaries similar to those seen in granulation tissue.
- Lesions lack significant nuclear pleomorphism and bizarre mitotic figures.
- Lesions tend to be small; however, they can infiltrate into muscle.
- Figure 10.7b

Special Stains/Studies

- Positive for vimentin, desmin, MSA
- Variable positive for cytokeratin and ALK1

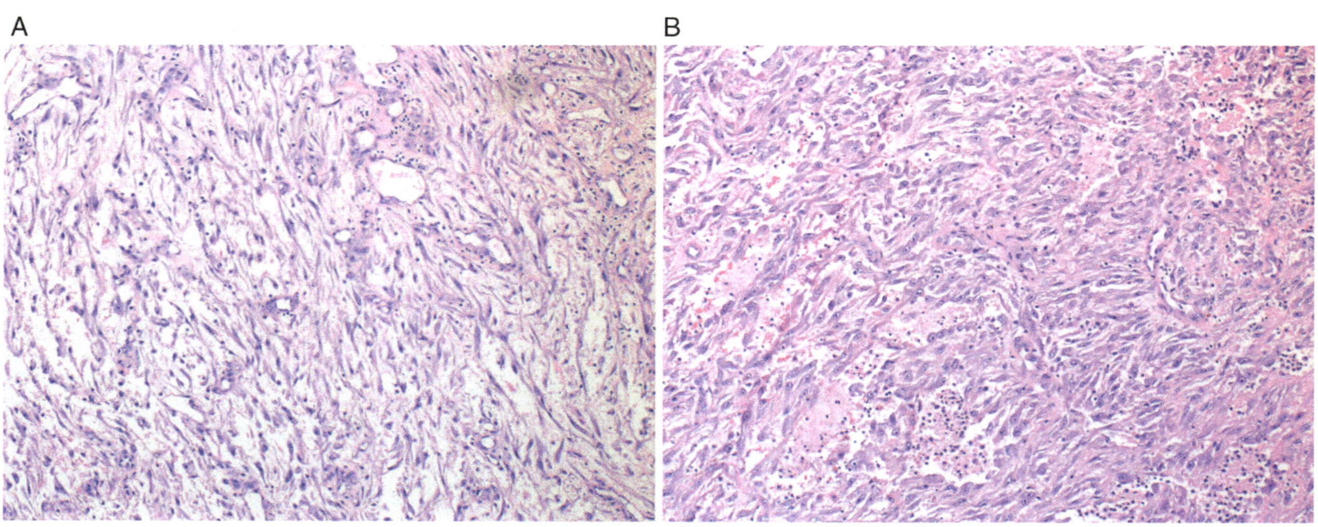

Fig. 10.7 (**a**, **b**) (**a**) Inflammatory myofibroblastic tumor (IMT). Well-circumscribed mass with intersecting fascicles of spindle fibroblastic cells and a delicate network of small blood vessels similar to those seen in granulation tissue (H&E). (**b**) Inflammatory myofibroblastic tumor (IMT). Spindle fibroblastic cells with prominent nucleoli and inflammatory cells in the background (H&E)

Schwannoma

Key Clinical Findings

- Common benign tumor of nerve sheath origin, usually adults.
- Soft tissue, extremities, neck, posterior mediastinum, retroperitoneum, posterior spinal roots, eighth cranial nerve, and other sites. Multiple organs are not commonly reported.
- Grossly attached to side of the nerve rather than infiltrating it like neurofibroma.
- Benign, cured by local excision.

Key Radiologic Findings

- Sonographically a well-circumscribed, hypoechoic, inhomogeneous solid mass.
- CT sharply demarcated, contrast-enhancing tumor.
- MR images; T1 signal from tumor was low, and T2 signal was high relative to white matter in all patients.

Cytopathology

- Clusters of cohesive spindle cells
- Oval to wavy nuclei, pointed nuclear ends
- Nuclear palisading, filamentous cytoplasm
- Myxoid background
- Figure 10.8a, b

Histopathology

- Showing both a cellular Antoni A area that palisades (Verocay bodies) and a loose myxoid paucicellular Antoni B area
- Old lesions showing cysts, hyalinized blood vessels, degenerative atypia
- Figure 10.8c

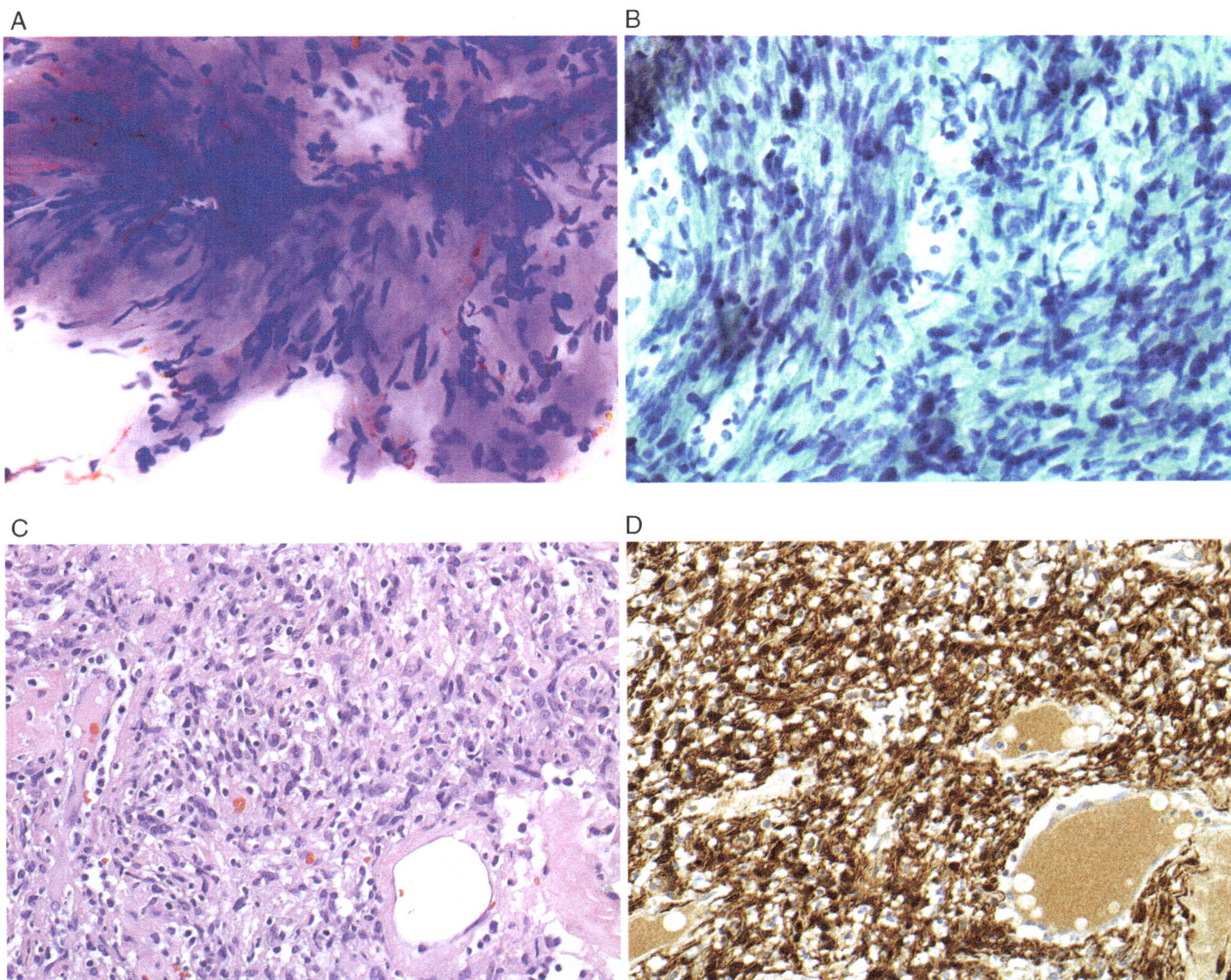

Fig. 10.8 (**a–d**) (**a**, **b**) Schwannoma. Clusters of cohesive spindle cells with oval to wavy nuclei, pointed nuclear ends (Romanowsky and Papanicolaou stain). (**c**) Schwannoma. hypercellular (Antoni A) spindle cells organized in fascicles with club-shaped nuclei, hyaline thick wall vessels and inflammatory cells in the background (H&E). (**d**) Schwannoma. Diffuse and strong S100 stain

Special Stains/Studies

- Can have melanin.
- Positive for S100; patchy GFAP positivity common.
- Silver stain shows no interspersed axons.
- Little stainable mucopolysaccharide.
- Cellular schwannomas show extensive S100 positivity in contrast to malignant peripheral nerve sheath tumors, in which staining is more focal.
- Figure 10.8d.

Malignant Peripheral Nerve Sheath Tumor

Key Clinical Findings

- Usually adults, rare in children.
- Soft tissue, neck, extremities, buttock, retroperitoneum, and posterior mediastinum. Almost all deep seated, rarely arising from superficial neurofibromas. Rarely reported in other organs.
- Clinically rapidly enlarging and painful.
- In about half the cases, the patient has neurofibromatosis 1 (Von Recklinghausen's disease).

Key Radiologic Findings

- CT scan obtained with oral and intravenous contrast material shows a large, heterogeneous, solid mass.

Cytopathology

- Cellular sample with single cells
- Fragments of variably sized fascicular tissue aggregates
- Naked nuclei with variable atypia
- Scant fibrillary cytoplasm and abundant mitotic figures
- Possible necrotic background
- Figure 10.9a, b

Histopathology

- Monomorphic spindle cells arranged in long fascicles or herringbone or whorled architecture.
- Nuclear features ranging from bland to anaplastic with mitoses, necrosis.
- May have features of schwannoma (palisading) or neurofibroma (serpentine cells).
- Blood vessels typically have large lumens. Ringed by several layers of larger, deeply staining cells.
- Connection with a nerve or nerve tumor (e.g., neurofibroma) helpful for diagnosis.
- Figure 10.9c.

Special Stains/Studies

- May have melanin.
- 50% S100 positive.
- Cytokeratin negative.
- 50% epithelioid MPNST and occasional myoepithelial carcinomas are negative for INI1.
- Loss of INI1 expression may also be helpful to distinguish epithelioid MPNST from metastatic melanoma in a subset of cases.
- Figure 10.9d.

Synovial Sarcoma

Key Clinical Findings

- Rare and affect young adults (10–34 years), up to 10% of all soft tissue sarcomas
- Near knee or ankle joint but can occur near other joints, retroperitoneum, and paravertebral with pharyngeal extension; associated with tendons and bursa
- Also occurs in the oral cavity, soft palate, and tongue, no particular relationship to synovia
- Prognosis better for heavily calcified lesions, younger patients (less than 15 years old), distal versus proximal extremity, smaller size (less than 5 cm)
- Conflicting studies as to whether monophasic type has worse prognosis
- Grossly varies from circumscribed to infiltrative
- Cystic formation also possible

Key Radiologic Findings

- On X-ray films as round or oval, lobulated mass of moderate density located in close proximity to a large joint.
- 15–20% of synovial sarcomas have multiple small, spotty radiopacities caused by focal calcification or bone formation.

Cytopathology

- Cellular sample with singly placed and clusters of cells
- Uniform oval to round, rare elongated nuclei
- Scant, delicate, and tapering cytoplasm
- Biphasic type
- Epithelioid cells mixed with spindled stroma
- Figure 10.10a–c

Special Stains/Studies

- Keratin and reticulin can help identify epithelial elements in biphasic type.

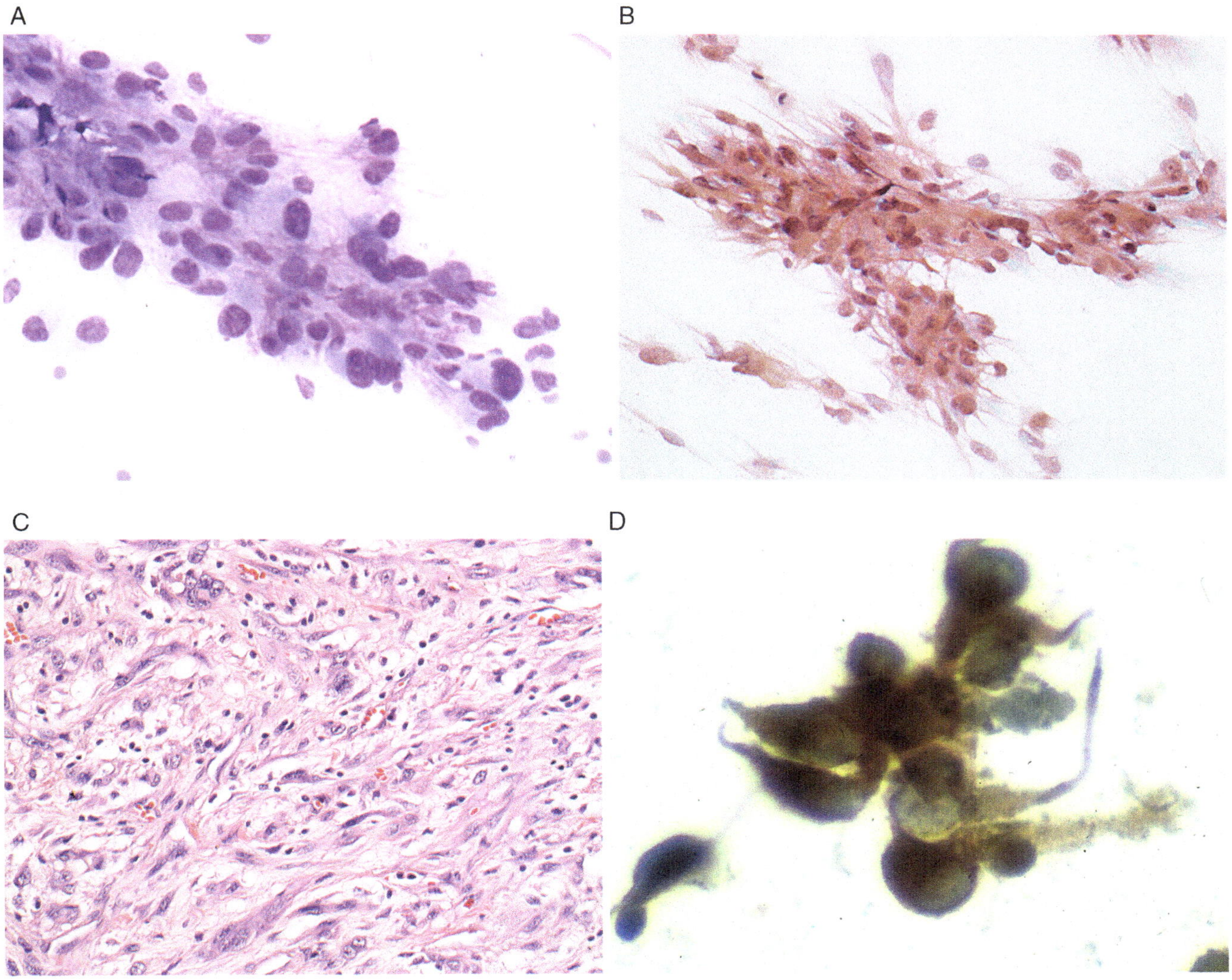

Fig. 10.9 (**a–d**) (**a**) Malignant peripheral nerve sheath tumor. Cellular sample with single cells, fascicular tissue aggregates, marked nuclear atypia in a background of scant fibrillary cytoplasm (Romanowsky stain). (**b**) Malignant peripheral nerve sheath tumor. Fragments of fascicular tissue aggregates with marked nuclear atypia in a background of scant fibrillary cytoplasm (Papanicolaou stain). (**c**) Malignant peripheral nerve sheath tumor. Monomorphic spindle cells arranged in long fascicles with bland to anaplastic nuclei, fibrillary cytoplasm, and scattered inflammatory cells in the background (H&E). (**d**) Malignant peripheral nerve sheath tumor. Strong S100 stain on smear slide

- Stromal cells can be weakly positive for keratin (although sometimes only in scattered cells) and possibly positive for EMA and CEA.
- Positive for TLE1, bcl-2, CD56, CD99.
- Almost all tumors have a characteristic chromosomal translocation (X:18).
- Figure 10.10d, e.

Leiomyosarcoma

Key Clinical Findings

- Any age, though typically elderly and either sex.
- Common in deep soft tissue, clinically superficial, and deep soft tissue lesions involve the extremities, particularly the thigh.
- Retroperitoneal lesions occur in older female.
- Vascular leiomyosarcomas occur particularly in the inferior vena cava or large veins of the lower limb in older adults. With lungs most are metastases.
- Grossly usually large and involves adjacent organs.

Key Radiologic Findings

- CT scans and angiography reveal hypovascular or moderately vascular soft tissue mass.
- Commonly involving other structures by direct extension.

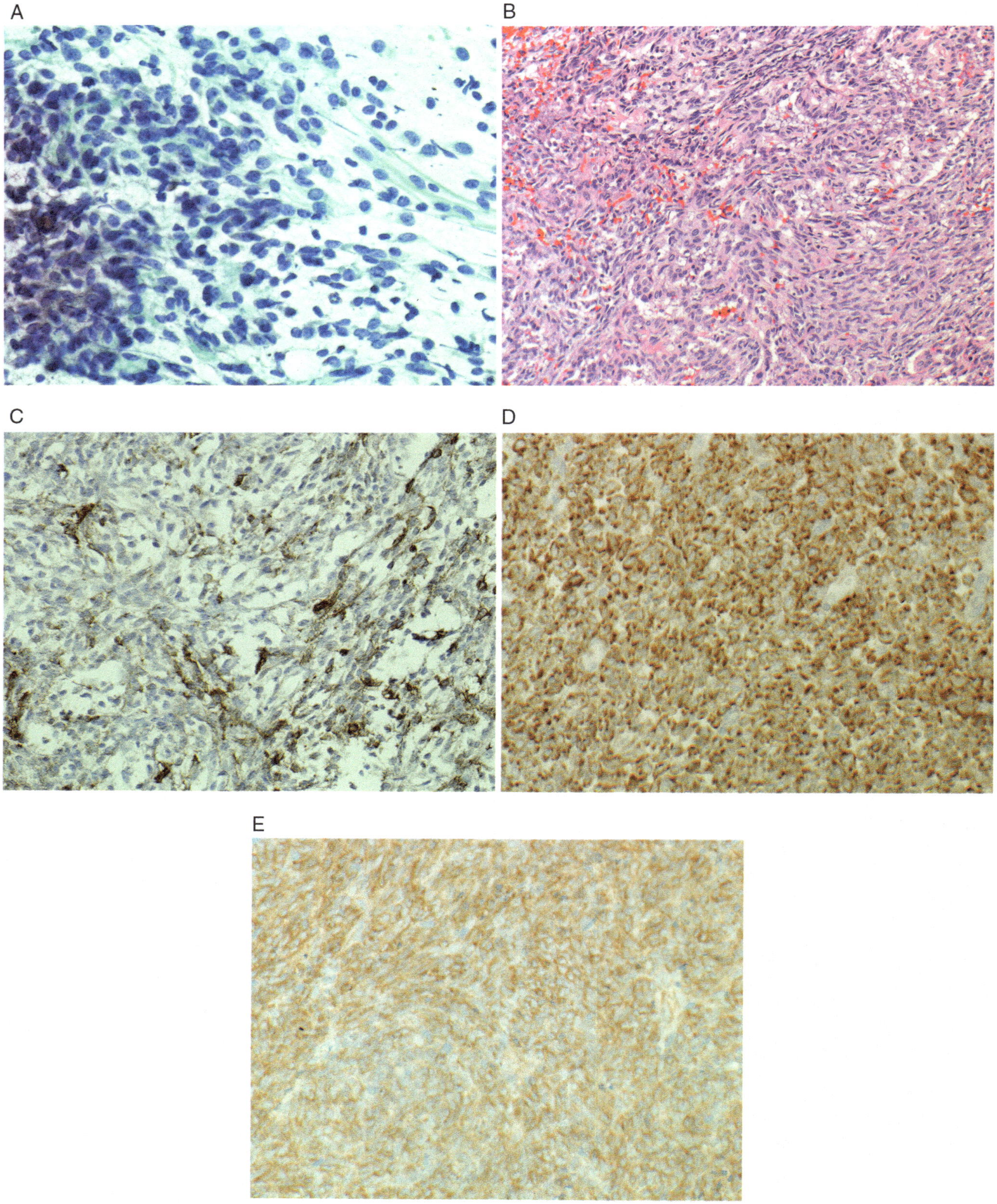

Fig. 10.10 (**a**–**e**) (**a**) Synovial sarcoma. Cellular sample with singly placed and clusters of cells, uniform round and elongated nuclei, scant, delicate, and tapering cytoplasm (Papanicolaou stain). (**b**) Synovial Sarcoma. Epithelioid cells mixed with spindled stroma in long eosinophilic fascicles (H&E). (**c**) Synovial sarcoma. The epithelioid cells are positive for EMA staining. (**d**, **e**) Synovial sarcoma. BCL2 and CD99 stains

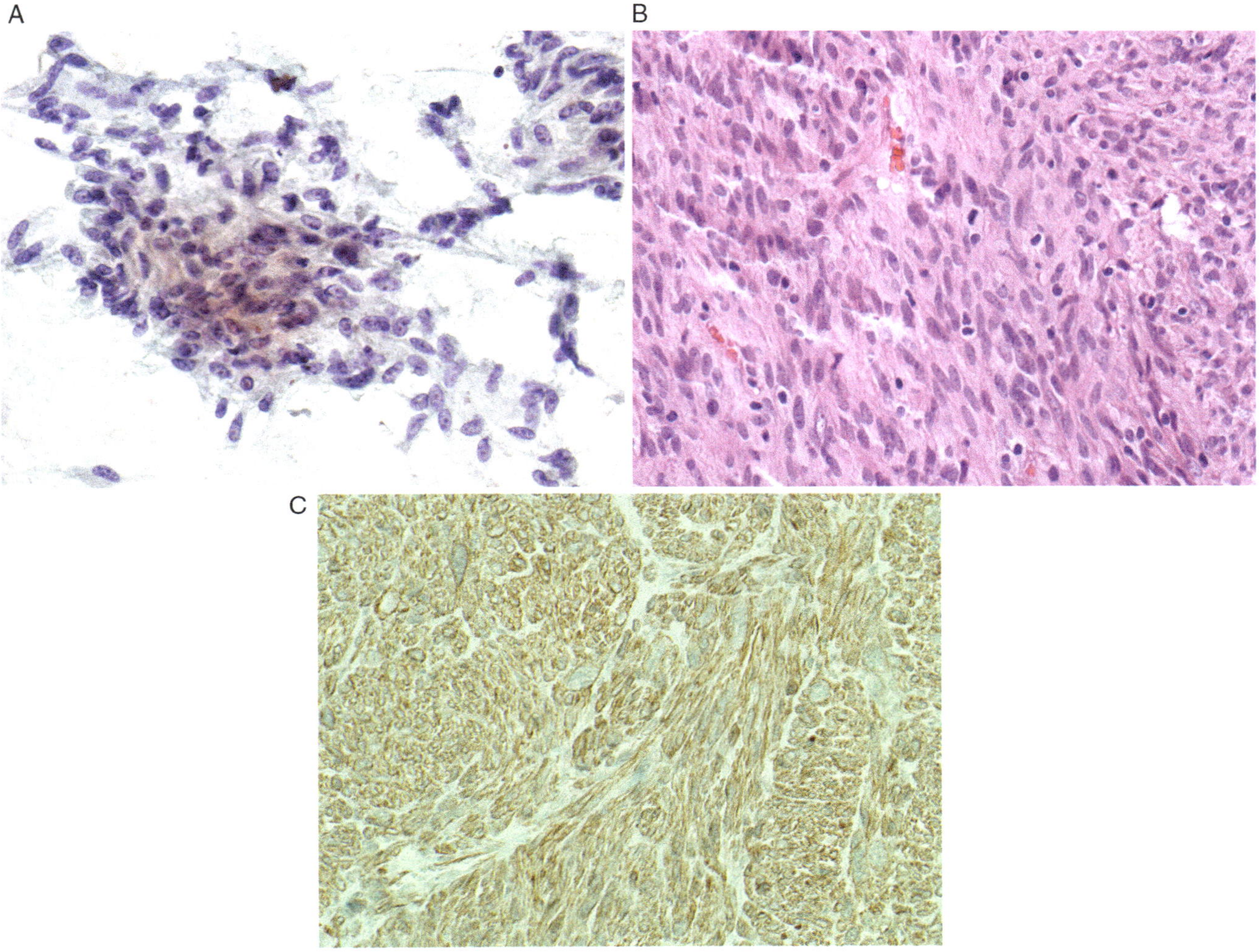

Fig. 10.11 (**a–c**) (**a**) Leiomyosarcoma. Loose clusters of spindle to cigar-shaped nuclei, rounded cells with abundant clear/amphophilic cytoplasm (Papanicolaou stain). (**b**) Leiomyosarcoma (high grade). Cellular spindle cell tumor with fascicles intersecting at wide angles. Cytoplasm deeply eosinophilic, nuclei vesicular, elongated, with blunt ends, may be indented by cytoplasmic vacuoles. Mitotic figures easily found (H&E). (**c**) Leiomyosarcoma. Strong and diffuse stain for SMA

Cytopathology

- Cellular sample with dyshesive naked nuclei
- Loose clusters of spindle to cigar-shaped nuclei
- Rounded cells with abundant clear/amphophilic cytoplasm
- Abundant cytoplasm and increased mitotic figures
- Figure 10.11a

Histopathology

- Cellular spindle cell tumor with fascicles intersecting at wide angles.
- Cytoplasm deeply eosinophilic, nuclei vesicular, elongated, with blunt ends, may be indented by cytoplasmic vacuoles.
- Vascularity may be prominent. Stroma may be myxoid.
- Grade 1 leiomyosarcoma hard to separate from leiomyoma. Malignant criteria (versus leiomyoma): greater than 5 mitoses/10HPF. Potentially malignant: 1–5 mitoses/10HPF especially if large (greater than 5 cm), necrotic, or cytologically atypical.
- Grade 2 leiomyosarcoma obviously malignant, yet not bizarre cytology.
- Grade 3 leiomyosarcoma has marked pleomorphism similar to that of malignant fibrous histiocytoma.
- Figure 10.11b, c.

Special Stains/Studies

- Positive for SMA, desmin, H-caldesmon, and calponin

Pleural and Extrapleural Solitary Fibrous Tumor (SFT)

Key Clinical Findings

- Mostly in pleural lesion, but increasingly recognized in other locations, subsumes most lesions that were previously termed hemangiopericytoma.
- Usually from middle age to elderly. Rare in infants and children (congenital/infantile hemangiopericytoma, now is categorized as part to the myofibroma spectrum).
- Common in the thigh, pelvic fossa, and retroperitoneum; deep seated
- Meningeal hemangiopericytoma (now regarded as SFT) occurs in adults and usually intracranial rather than intraspinal. Grossly lobulated, pink or gray, and fleshy. Vessels may be apparent on cut section. Clinically may be associated with hypoglycemia.
- Grossly well circumscribed, with wide size range. When found in infants, more superficial than adult SFT.
- Prognostically unfavorable: mitoses (greater than 4/10 HPF), necrosis, hemorrhage, and cellularity.
- In infants, mostly benign despite mitoses and necrosis.
- Meningeal SFT is aggressive with high rate of local recurrence and tendency to late distant metastases.
- Categorized as intermediate and rarely metastasizing.

Key Radiologic Findings

- Radiogically forming discrete mass
- No hyperostosis (as it is common with meningiomas)
- Non-calcification
- Highly vascular on angiographic study

Cytopathology

- Varying degrees of cellularity of spindle cells.
- Bloody background with small amounts of collagen.
- Nuclear pleomorphism, prominent nucleoli, and mitotic figures indicate aggressive behavior.
- Figure 10.12a, b.

Histopathology

- Spindle cells in hyper- and hypocellular zones, with variable architecture.
- Classic pattern is tissue culture – random orientation of fibroblasts.
- Focal area may resemble hemangiopericytoma or schwannoma or storiform or myxoid.
- Figure 10.12c–e.

Special Stains/Studies

- All cases stain positive for CD34, STAT6, variable for CD99 and bcl2, negative for keratins, S100, actin, and desmin
- Figure 10.12d, e

Molecular Studies

- Inv(12)(q13q13) and *NAB2-STAT6*

Fibromatoses

- A broad spectrum of lesions with an infiltrative growth pattern can recur but never metastasize.
- Two groups based on location:
  1. Superficial or fascial fibromatoses include the palmar, plantar, and penile variants.
  2. Deep or musculoaponeurotic fibromatoses include the extra-abdominal, abdominal, and intra-abdominal variants.

Fibromatoses, Superficial (Fascial) Types

Key Clinical Findings

- Palmar fibromatosis/Dupuytren's contracture is very common, occurring in 20% of elderly.
- Plantar and knuckle fibromatoses are less common and increase with age, but half of cases occur under age 30.
- Penile fibromatosis or Peyronie's disease is less common, does not occur in children, and increases with age though some patients have been under age 30.
- They occur predominantly in male.
- Clinically small and slow growing.
- Patients with one type of superficial fibromatosis are more likely to have another type.
- Associated with epileptic and diabetic patients, chronic alcoholics, and patients with increased serum lipids.
- Grossly small nodule or ill-defined thickening. Benign, though may recur.

Key Radiologic Findings

- Infiltrative growth mimicking a malignant lesion.
- These lesions reveal a low signal intensity on T1-weighted pulse sequences but may show low or high signal intensity on the T2-weighted sequences.
- Histologic correlation reveals that the lesion showing low signal intensity on T2-weighted sequences has a larger collagenous component and reduced cellularity compared with the lesion showing high signal intensity on T2-weighted sequences.

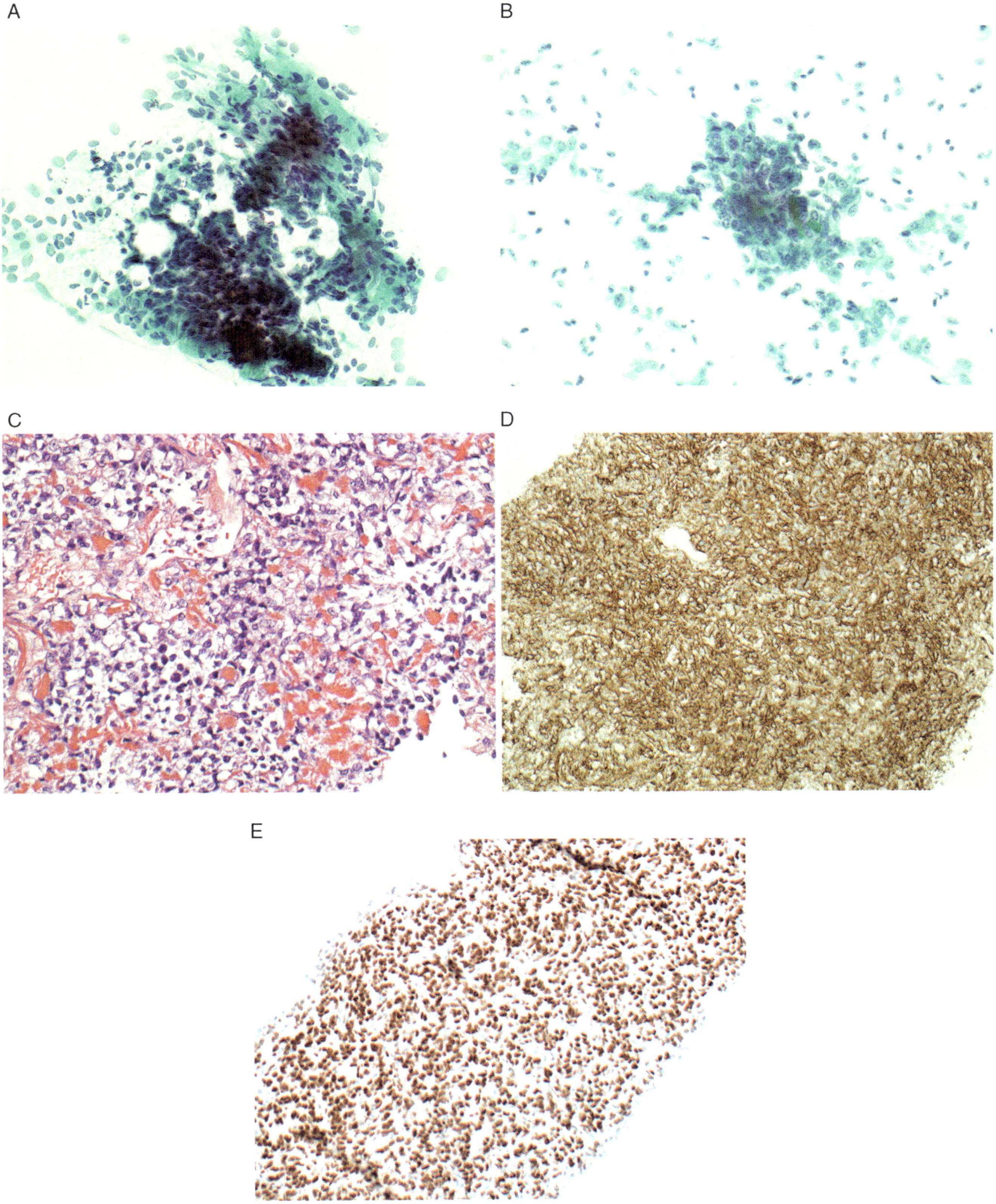

Fig. 10.12 (**a**–**e**) (**a**) SFT. Tissue clusters with bland spindle cells and ropy collagen (Papanicolaou stain). (**b**) SFT. Loose clusters and individual cells with nuclear pleomorphism, prominent nucleoli indicating aggressive biological behavior (Papanicolaou stain). (**c**) SFT. Cell block preparation with uniform bland spindle cells embedding in the ropy collagen (H&E). (**d**, **e**) SFT. CD34 and STAT6 strong and diffusely positive

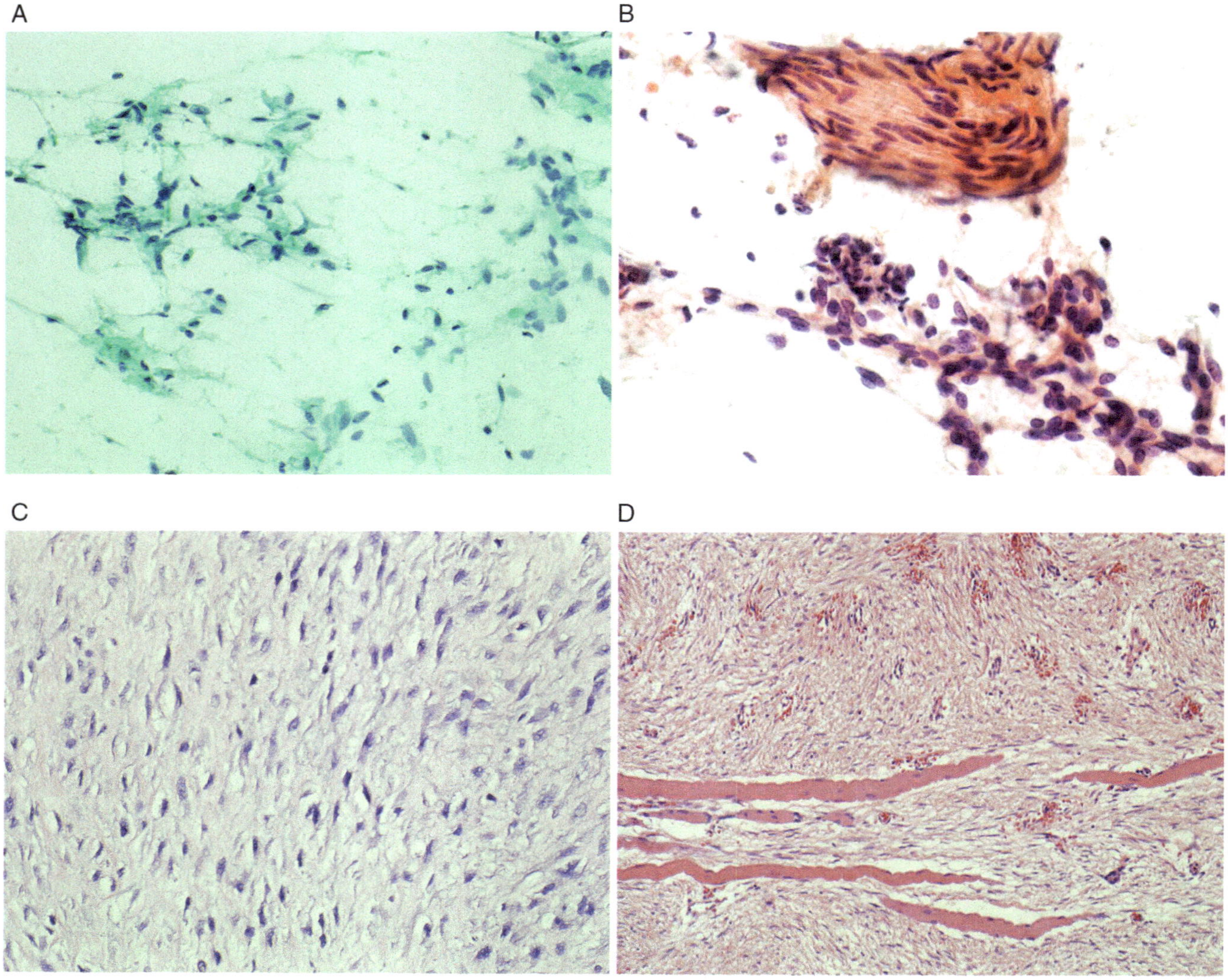

Fig. 10.13 (**a**–**d**) (**a**, **b**) Desmoid fibromatoses. Loose clusters and single uniform bland spindle or polygonal cells and rare dense collagenous stroma (Papanicolaou stain). (**c**, **d**) Desmoid fibromatoses. Uniform fibroblasts and dense collagen (H&E)

Cytopathology

- Hypercellularity
- Loose clusters and single uniform bland spindle or polygonal cells
- Oval to elongated nuclei
- No mitotic figures
- Figure 10.13a–d

Special Stains/Studies

- Positive for b-catenin
- Negative for SMA, CD34, and c-kit

Fibromatoses/Deep Fibromatosis (Musculoaponeurotic)

Key Clinical Findings

- Extra-abdominal, a few cases per million and occurs in adolescents and young adults of either sex.
- Extra-abdominal location, muscular aponeuroses of shoulder, pelvis, and thigh, clinically shows rapid growth.
- Abdominal, a few cases per 10,000 and common in reproductive age of women, typically during or just after pregnancy. Intra-abdominal, usually reproductive age in women though unrelated to pregnancy.
- Abdominal location, anterior wall muscles shows slow growth.

- Intra-abdominal locations, pelvic, mesenteric (latter may be associated with Gardner's syndrome and following surgery), and omentum.
- All sites may result in an area of previous trauma. Grossly extra-abdominal, typically 5–10 cm, abdominal, 3–10 cm and intra-abdominal, up to 15 cm.

Key Radiologic Findings

- Infiltrative growth mimicking a malignant lesion.
- These lesions reveal a low signal intensity on T1-weighted pulse sequences but may show low or high signal intensity on the T2-weighted sequences.

Cytopathology

- Variable cellularity
- Loose clusters and single uniform spindle and polygonal cells
- Oval to elongated nuclei
- No mitotic figures

Dermatofibrosarcoma Protuberans (DFSP)

Key Clinical Findings

- Young to middle-aged adults and rare in children, predominantly male.
- Occurs at any site, frequently in trunk and proximal extremities.
- Clinically presents as nodular, cutaneous mass with slow but persistent growth over a long period.
- Clinical and gross appearances determined by stage of disease.
- Clinically protuberant, gray-white mass involving subcutis and skin.
- Average size at surgery 5 cm.
- Locally aggressive with recurrence in up to half of patients.
- Risk of recurrence lower with wide local excision.
- Metastases are infrequent.

Cytopathology

- Moderately cellularity
- Clusters of dense uniform spindle cells
- Entrapped adipose tissue
- Variably sized oval nuclei with smooth and round membrane
- Occasional metachromatic fibrillary stroma

Special Stains/Studies

- CD34 positive

Molecular Studies

- DFSP and the related giant cells in children carrying characteristic COL1A1-PDGFB fusion gene

Fibrosarcoma

Key Clinical Findings

- Uncommon, adult – usually 30s–50s
- Adult – common in lower extremity, higher incidence years following radiation
- Infantile and congenital – usually first year of life, common in extremities
- Multiple organs, rarely reported
- Grossly >3 cm and deep-seated
- Adults – prognosis related to grade
- Infantile and congenital – more favorable with over 80% survival

Key Radiologic Findings

- Well circumscribed when it is small and infiltrative when it becomes a large one
- May encircle bone

Cytopathology

- Cytologically it lacks uniformly accepted diagnostic criteria.
- Given the vast clinical and pathologic heterogeneity, the term is regarded as a wastebasket diagnosis.
- Like adult fibrosarcoma, it is a diagnosis of exclusion and not reliably diagnosed by FNA.
- Figure 10.14a–c

Special Stains/Studies

- Negative for cytokeratin, EMA, and S100

Nodular Fasciitis

Key Clinical Findings

- Common for a soft tissue lesion, usually 20s–40s
- Occurs in arms or trunk in adults. Head and neck in children. Subcutaneous, intramuscular, fascial types.
- Clinically a new mass with very rapid growth (about 1 cm per week) but rarely larger than 3 cm.
- Lesions may persist for up to 1 year. Grossly round oval non-encapsulated mass.

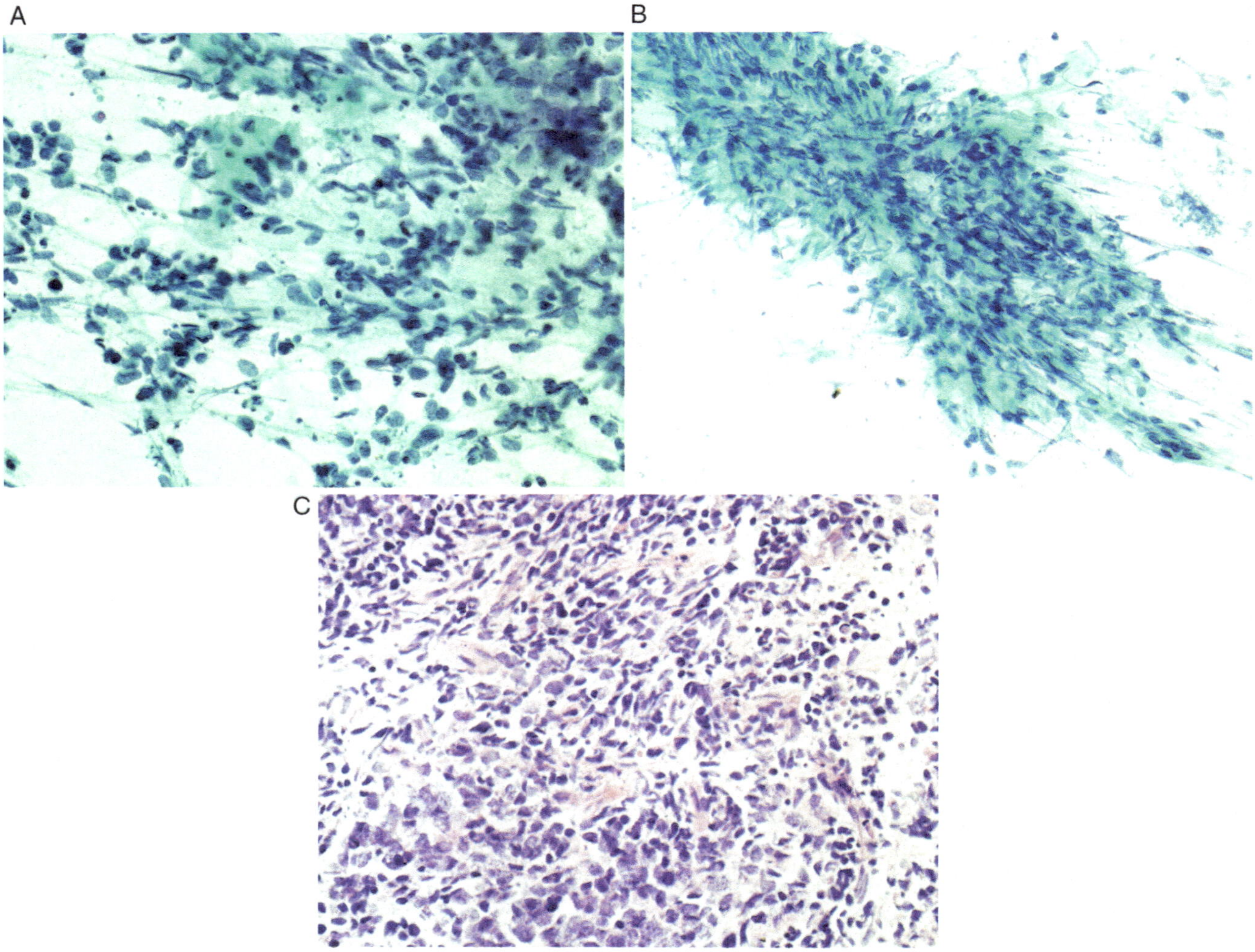

Fig. 10.14 (a–c) (a, b) Fibrosarcoma. Cellular sample with high-grade spindle cell malignancy (a diagnosis of exclusion) (Papanicolaou stain). (c) Fibrosarcoma. High-grade spindle cell malignant neoplasm (a diagnosis of exclusion) (H&E)

- It demonstrates the importance of careful correlation of clinical information with FNA aspiration findings.
- The diagnosis is often suggested just by the clinical presentation, and the FNA serves simply to confirm the clinical impression.
- Despite recent cytogenetic demonstration of clonality (*MYH9-USP6* gene fusion as a recurrent event in nodular fasciitis), nodular fasciitis is traditionally regarded as a reactive lesion. Benign, reactive rather than neoplastic.

Cytopathology

- Variable cellularity
- Loose clusters and discohesive spindle and stellate myofibroblasts
- Myxoid background and inflammatory cells
- Mitotic figures and no significant nuclear atypia
- Figure 10.15a, b

Molecular Studies

- t(17;22)(p13;q12.3) and carrying USP6-MYH9 fusion gene

Round Cell Tumors

Round cell tumor is a group of morphologically similar but high-grade malignant neoplasms with different origins, histogeneses, and biological behaviors and primarily tumors of young patients and accounts for the majority of pediatric solid malignancies. The sensitivity and specificity of FNA for round cell neoplasms exceed 90% and 93% with an adequate specimen; the accuracy is higher with the use of ancillary studies.

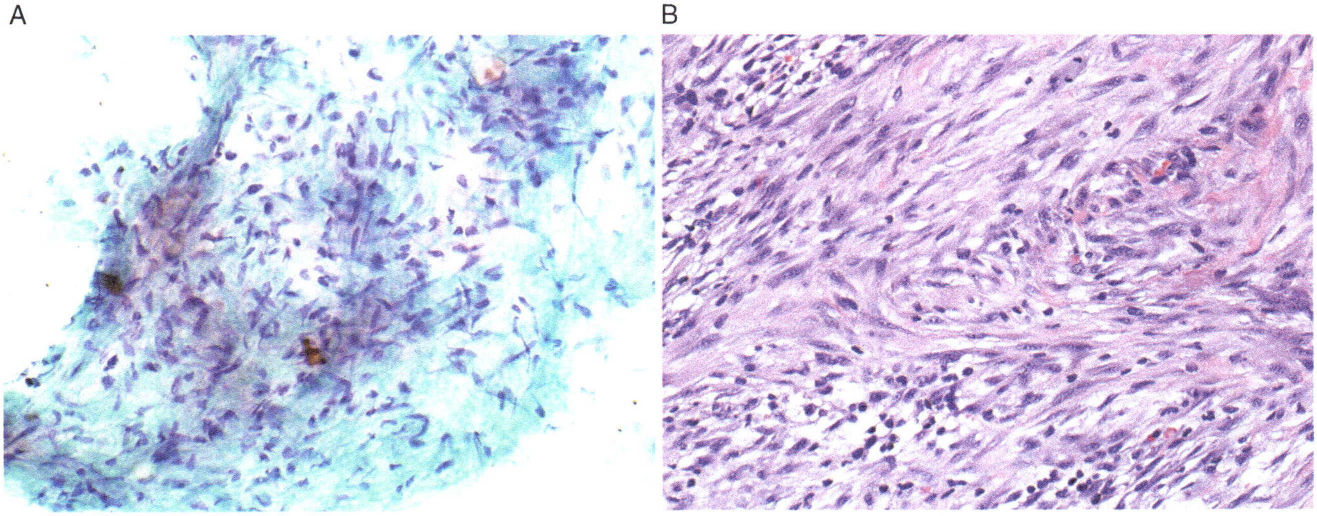

Fig. 10.15 (**a**, **b**) (**a**) Nodular fasciitis. Loose clusters and discohesive spindle and stellate myofibroblasts in a myxoid background and inflammatory cells (Papanicolaou stain). (**b**) Nodular fasciitis. Cells oriented in short fascicles and focal storiforming pattern with scattered lymphocytes and macrophages (H&E)

Ewing's Sarcoma/Primitive Neuroectodermal Tumor (ES/PNET)

Key Clinical Findings

- Malignant primitive neoplasm of neural crest origin.
- Occurs in children and young adults, 6% of sarcomas in children.
- Most common in soft tissue of the chest wall, lower extremities, and paravertebral region.
- All bones have been reported to be involved.
- Rapidly enlarging painful mass and rarely seen in blacks.

Key Radiologic Findings

- The imaging appearance of peripheral PNETs is nonspecific.
- These tumors should be considered in the differential diagnosis when one encounters a large retroperitoneal mass with aggressive feature.

Cytopathology

- Cellular smears with abundant single uniform cells.
- Nuclear molding and vacuolated cytoplasm.
- Arranged in variable numbers of pseudorosettes.
- Can have tigroid background on Romanowsky stain.
- Figure 10.16a.

Histopathology

- Undifferentiated small round cells lacking any specific differentiation.
- Abundant cytoplasmic glycogen can be demonstrated by PAS.
- Figure 10.16b.

Special Stains/Studies

- 50% contain pools of glycogen on PAS stain.
- Positive with MIC2 (CD99) antibody.
- Only rare neurosecretory granules and neurofilaments by electron microscopy.
- Figure 10.16c.

Molecular Studies

- 85% to 90% t(11.22) (24, q 12) translocation carrying *EWS-FLI-1* fusion gene.
- t(21.22) (q12q12) translocation involves the *ERG* gene, whereas t(7:22) t(q22:q12) involves the *ETV1* gene.

Neuroblastoma/Esthesioneuroblastoma (NB/ENB)

Key Clinical Findings

- The third most common malignancy of childhood and the most common malignancy of the neonate, 1 per 10,000 live births. Occurs under age 5.
- Olfactory neuroblastomas occur in a wide age range from childhood to elderly. The average age is middle aged adults, mainly male.
- Occurs in adrenal, brain, mediastinum, retroperitoneum, paraspinal.

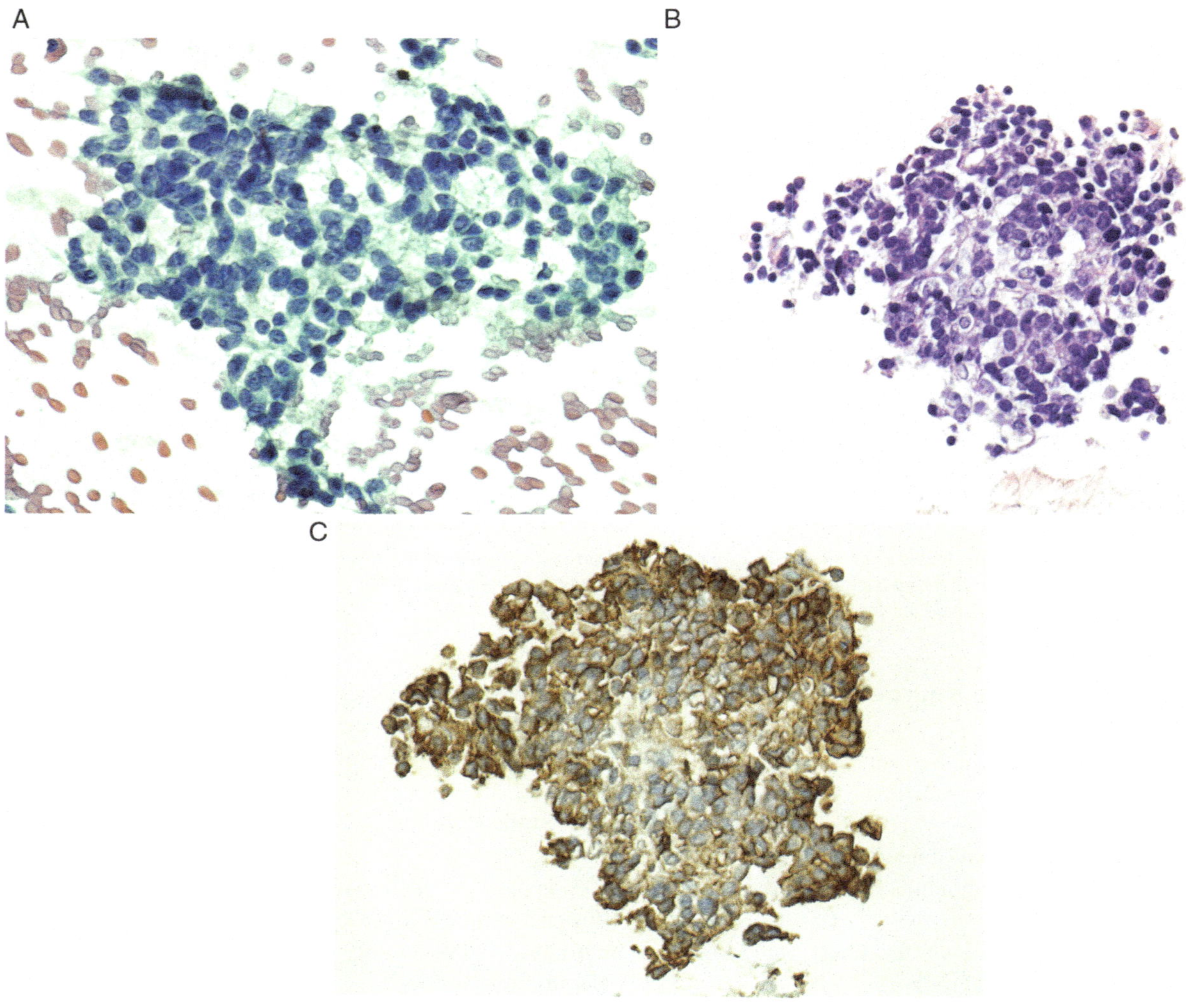

Fig. 10.16 (a–c) (a) Ewing's sarcoma (Papanicolaou stain). (b) Ewing's sarcoma (H&E). (c) Ewing's sarcoma. Positive CD99

- Lesions occurring in the roof of the nasal fossa are termed olfactory neuroblastoma (esthesioneuroblastoma).
- 90% of patients have increased catecholamines in urine.
- Malignant, survival rates based on a number of prognostic factors.
- Favorable factors include patient less than 2 years old, lack of N-myc amplification, low serum ferritin, hyperdiploidy, and high trk2 level (EGFR).

Key Radiologic Findings

- Half of the tumor has calcification; peripheral linear densities may be seen.
- Metastatic lesions commonly occur in the bone and result in osteolytic lesions that display a peculiar predilection for the skull, femur, and humerus; occasionally they are bilaterally symmetric in their distribution.
- Radiolabeled metaiodobenzylguanidine (MIBG) has been used to detect the bone and soft tissue involvement by neuroblastoma.

Cytopathology

- Cellular smear with discohesive small round blue cells
- Round to oval nuclei with fine nuclear chromatin
- Rare ganglion-like cells and neurogenic rosettes
- Figure 10.17a, b

Histopathology

- The cells are small and undifferentiated with a high nuclear cytoplasmic ratio.
- Small clusters of cells may be separated by pale blue to light purple fibrillar matrix.
- Structures corresponding to pseudorosettes are seen in histological sections.
- Figure 10.17c

Special Stains/Studies

- Positive for NSE, chromogranin, synaptophysin, and neurofilaments

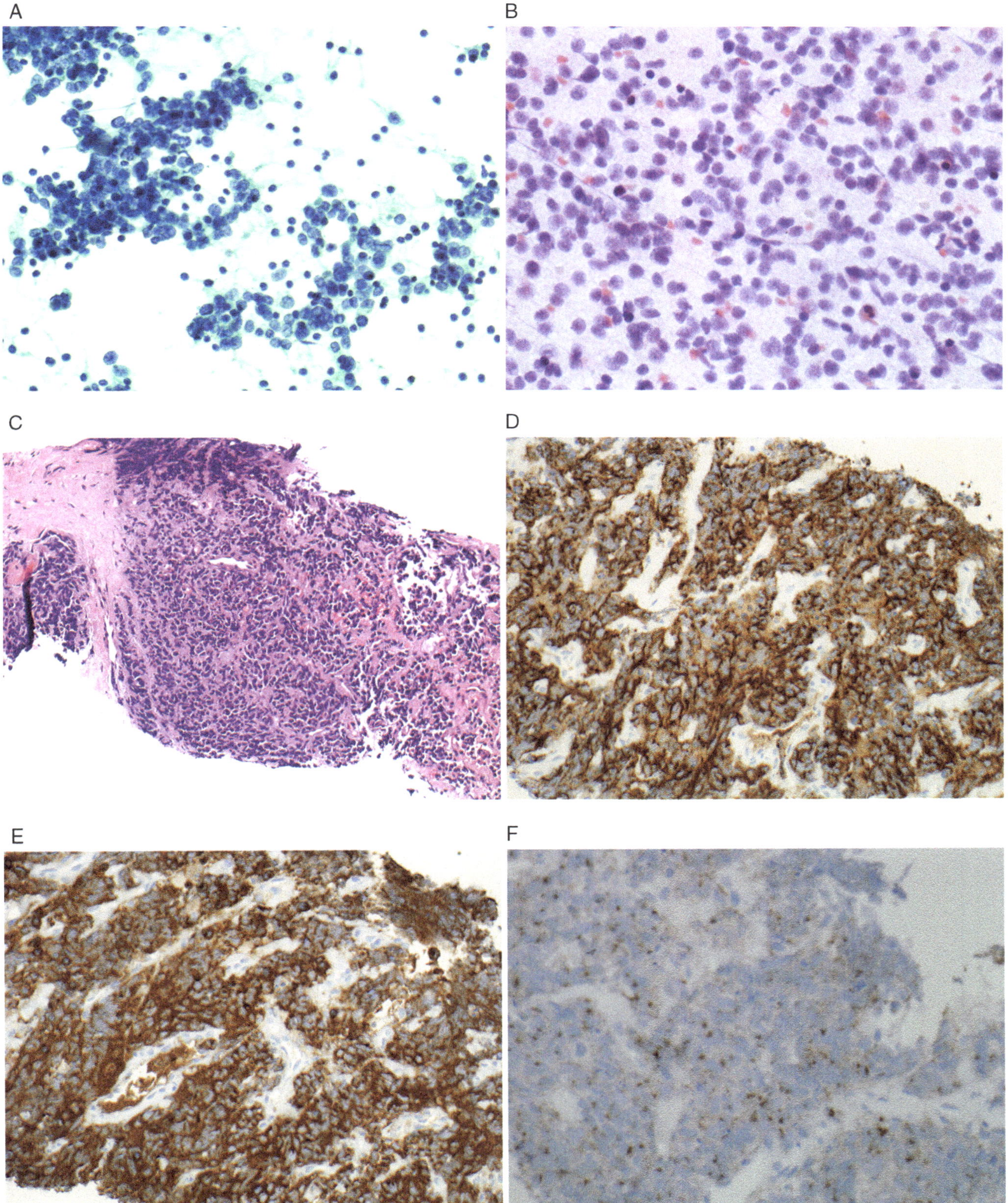

Fig. 10.17 (**a–g**) (**a**) Neuroblastoma/Esthesioneuroblastoma (Papanicolaou stain). (**b**) Neuroblastoma/Esthesioneuroblastoma (Papanicolaou stain). (**c**) Neuroblastoma/Esthesioneuroblastoma (H&E). (**d**) Neuroblastoma/Esthesioneuroblastoma. Positive stain for CD56. (**e**) Neuroblastoma/Esthesioneuroblastoma. Positive stain for synaptophysin. (**f**) Neuroblastoma/Esthesioneuroblastoma. Positive stain for chromogranin. (**g**) Extraskeletal mesenchymal chondrosarcoma. Hemangiopericytic vascular pattern is prominent (H&E)

G

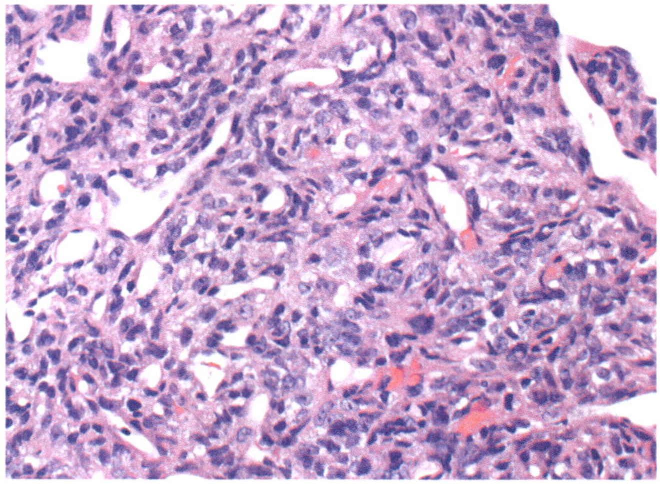

Fig. 10.17 (continued)

- S100 positive in ganglioneuromatous areas
- Numerous neurosecretory granules and processes evident on electron microscopy
- Figure 10.17d–f

Molecular Studies

- Deletion of the short arm of chromosome 1 (1p 36; 2–3) and amplification of the proto-oncogene N-myc abnormality of the chromosome number

Desmoplastic Small Round Cell Tumor/Intra-abdominal Desmoplastic Round Cell Tumor

Key Clinical Findings

- Rare malignant tumor of uncertain histogenesis.
- Mainly male adolescents.
- Often forming large tumor mass and smaller implants of the serosal surfaces
- Most cases intra-abdominal, such as peritoneum, omentum, pelvis, and ovary, also in scrotum and pleura.
- Poor prognosis with multiple peritoneal implants.
- Grossly large multilobulated mass.

Key Radiologic Findings

- CT: masses show variable enhancement due to vascularity and necrosis. Heterogeneity due to tumor hemorrhage may also be a feature of some lesions.
- MRI appearance of DSRCT is nonspecific. Relatively low signal intensity on T2-weighted imaging, due to the densely packed cellularity of small cell neoplasms in addition to a variable desmoplastic response within lesions, may suggest the diagnosis of a small cell histology based on imaging.
- Ultrasound: lesions are usually well-defined and hypo- or anechoic mimicking lymphoma, again as a result of the underlying small cell tumor histology.

Cytopathology

- Loose lusters and sheets of uniform cells
- Fragments of variably desmoplastic stroma
- Round to oval cells with nuclear molding

Histopathology

- Undifferentiated round cells arranged in sheets and sometimes surrounded by dense, collagenous stroma.
- When the desmoplastic stroma is not represented, a morphological diagnosis may be difficult.

Special Stains/Studies

- Positive for vimentin, keratin, and EMA
- Desmin positivity often paranuclear
- Variable positivity for NSE, S100, Leu 7, Leu-M1, and synaptophysin

Molecular Studies

- t(11:22) (p13q12) and carrying EWS-WT1 fusion gene

Extraskeletal Mesenchymal Chondrosarcoma/ Mesenchymal Chondrosarcoma

Key Clinical Findings

- Usually 20s–30s but teens through 50s possible. Either sex.
- Rare cartilaginous tumor accounting for 20–30% of chondrosarcomas.
- 50% occur in soft tissue of orbit, cranial, spinal meninges, and legs. Rest in medulla or cortex of diaphysis.
- Usually the jaw, pelvis, ribs, femur, spine.
- Usually fatal, but survival for many years before death is not uncommon.

Key Radiologic Findings

- A well-defined soft tissue mass with irregular radiopaque stipplings, arcs, flecks, or streaks as the result of focal calcification or bone formation in cartilaginous areas.
- CT scans, MRI, and angiography are helpful for outline the tumor prior to surgical therapy.

Cytopathology

- Clusters and uniform single small round cells
- Background cartilaginous matrix material
- Frequent mitoses

Histopathology

- Bimorphic malignant tumor composed of primitive small round cells and well-differentiated cartilage
- Figure 10.17g

Special Stains/Studies

- Undifferentiated stromal cells positive for leu7 but not S100

Alveolar and Embryonal Rhabdomyosarcoma (ARMS and ERMS)

Over one-half of pediatric soft tissue sarcomas are rhabdomyosarcomas: the head and neck (40% of cases), the male or female genitourinary tract (25% of cases), and the extremities (20% of cases). Four subtypes are recognized in current WHO classification:

1. Alveolar rhabdomyosarcoma (ARMS) in children
2. Embryonal rhabdomyosarcoma (ERMS) in children (60%)
3. Pleomorphic RMS exclusively in adults
4. Spindle cell/sclerosing RMS in children and adults

Key Radiologic Findings for ARMS and ERMS

- Ultrasound reveals a heterogeneous mass.
- CT and MRI scan reveal infiltrative and destructive manner, many invade bone.
- The enhancement pattern of CT is inhomogeneous with large low-attenuation areas suggesting necrosis.

Key Clinical Findings for ARMS

- ARMS occurs in the limbs and seen in the second and third decades of life. Clinically infiltrative and deep seated.
- ERMS occurs in the head, neck, and urogenital regions and common in the first decade of life. Those that arise in hollow viscera may be polypoid, whereas deep lesions are more infiltrative.
- Survival ranges from good to poor depending on stage and site, though ERMS has better prognosis than ARMS.
- ARMS and ERMS are fairly easy to distinguish based on histology results.
- Reliable distinction between ERMS and ARMS by cytology has been debated.
- Cytogenetic and molecular findings help the distinction.

Cytopathology for ARMS

- Small, single, uniformly round to polygonal cells
- Early undifferentiated rhabdomyoblasts
- Multinucleated giant tumor cells
- Figure 10.18a, b

Histopathology

- Nests of small round cells with scant cytoplasm separated by interwoven thick fibrous trabeculae to produce a pattern of reminiscent of lung alveoli

Special Stains/Studies for ARMS

- Positive for myoglobin, myogenin, desmin, MSA, and more specific marker MyoD1.
- Distinctive 2:13 chromosomal translocation.
- 90% shows t(2:13) q (35:Q14) and 10% shows variant t(1:13) (p36q14).
- Involving the *FKHR* gene on chr-13 and *Pax3/7* gene on chromosome 2 or 1.

Cytopathology for ERMS

- Cellularity with single cells and loose clusters
- Round to polygonal to spindle cells in myxoid stroma

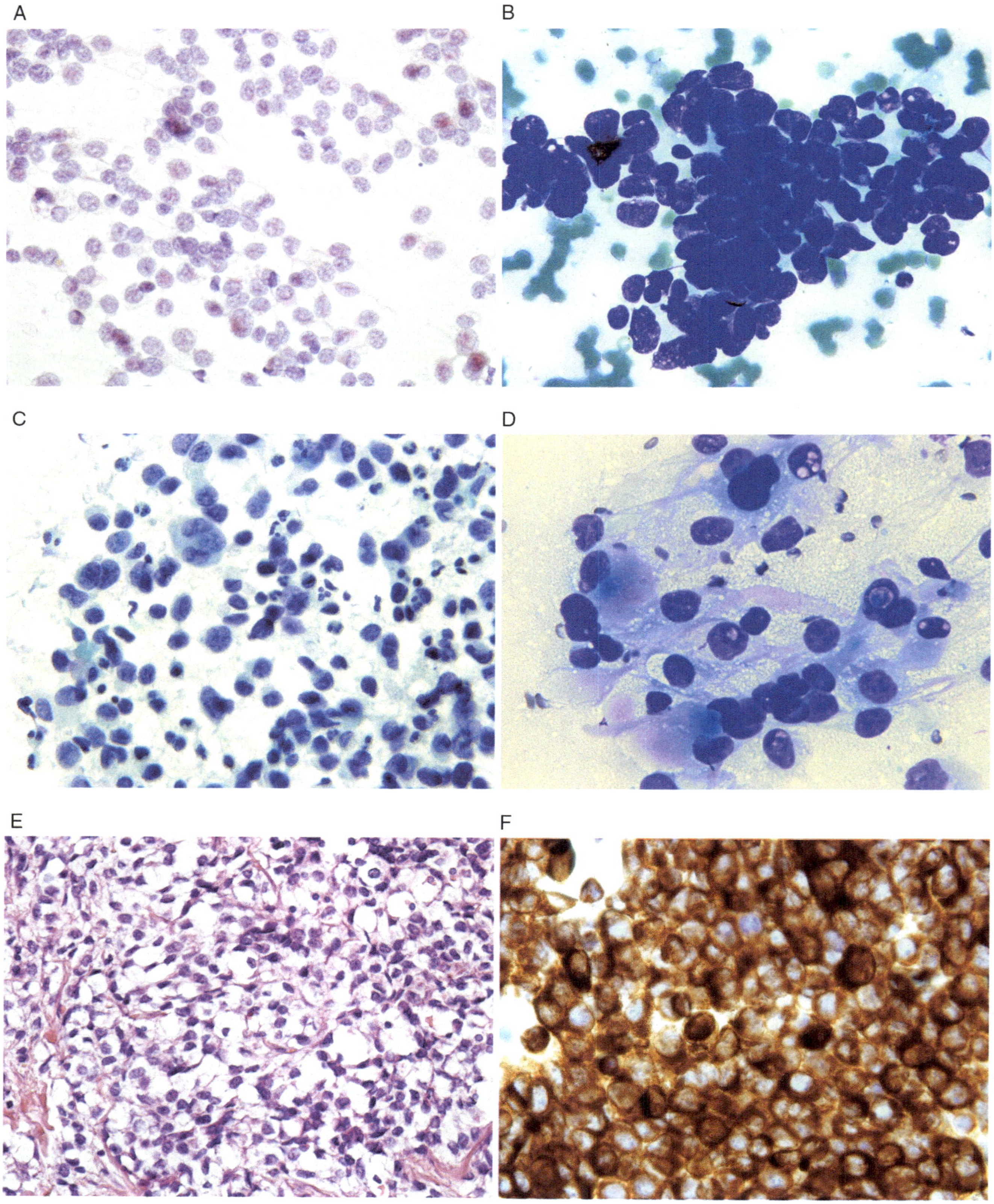

Fig. 10.18 (**a–g**) (**a**) ARMS. Uniform round to polygonal cells (Papanicolaou stain). (**b**) ARMS. Round to polygonal cells with scant cytoplasm and nuclear molding (Romanowsky stain). (**c**) ERMS. Round to polygonal cells, early undifferentiated rhabdomyoblasts, and rare multinucleated giant tumor cells (Papanicolaou stain). (**d**) ERMS. Rhabdomyoblasts with cytoplasmic inclusions (Romanowsky stain). (**e**) ERMS. Sheets of small round to spindled cells in myxoid stroma (H&E). (**f**) ERMS. Positive desmin stain. (**g**) ERMS. Positive myogenin stain

G

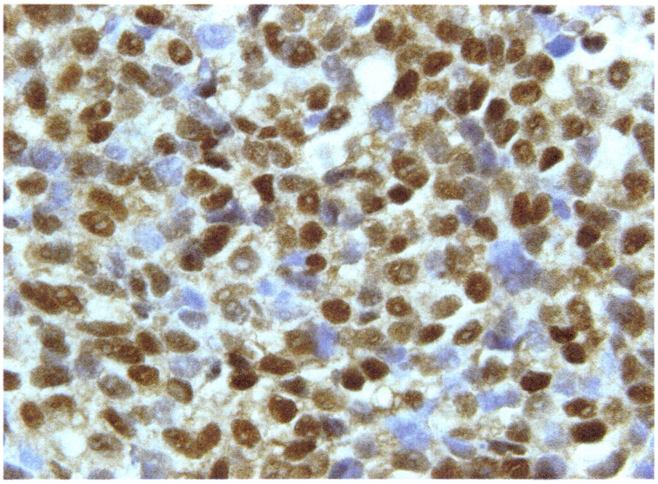

Fig. 10.18 (continued)

- Larger cell population with admixed pleomorphic rhabdomyoblasts
- Occasional deep eosinophilic cytoplasmic inclusions
- Figure 10.18c, d

Histopathology

- Sheets of small round to spindled cells in myxoid stroma
- Hypo- and hypercellular areas with varying numbers of admixed rhabdomyoblasts
- Figure 10.18e

Special Stains/Studies

- Positive for myoglobin, myogenin, desmin, MSA, and more specific marker MyoD1
- Figure 10.18f, g

Adipocytic Tumors

Adipocytic tumors represent the largest single group of mesenchymal tumors due to the high prevalence of lipomas and angiolipomas. Liposarcomas represent the single most common type of soft tissue sarcoma. Its principal histological subtypes (well differentiated, myxoid, and pleomorphic) are entirely separate diseases with different morphology, genetics, and natural history. Most types of adipocytic neoplasm have distinctive karyotypic aberrations which can be of considerable help in diagnosis. Principal changes and advances have been the recognition that atypical lipomatous tumor and well-differentiated liposarcomas (WDL) are essentially synonymous and that site-specific variations in behavior relate only to surgical resectability.

Lipogenic tumors occur over a wide age range, and malignant tumors occur exclusively in adults. Well-developed adipocytic lesion morphology is difficult to classify accurately. It is understandable some authorities discourage the use of FNA on deep-seated, large intramuscular, or retroperitoneal fatty lesions if the biopsy specimen is limited; the diagnosis of WDL can be missed. Therefore, a recommendation for lipogenic lesions needs to be excised and fully sampled for a definitive diagnosis. But this approach does not apply to pretreated lesions or for ancillary studies such as cytogenetics, which can aid in the diagnosis of most fatty lesions.

Hibernoma

Key Clinical Findings

- Rare benign tumor of brown fat
- Young adults, 20–50 years old, can be rarely seen in children
- Usually in interscapular region, upper thorax, mediastinum, retroperitoneum, thigh, or popliteal fossa

Key Radiologic Findings

- CT or MRI reveals a lipomatous tumor, often suggests liposarcoma.
- Well-defined, mobile mass in subcutis, with wide size range.

Cytopathology

- Moderately cellular aspirates
- Clusters and single uniform vacuolated mature adipocytes
- Small bland nuclei without atypia
- Figure 10.19a

Histopathology

- Organoid arrangement of large cells with central nuclei and small vacuolated cytoplasm containing neutral fat.
- Can be mixed with ordinary lipoma.
- Figure 10.19b.

Lipoma

Key Clinical Findings

- Benign tumor, 40–60 years of age. Rare in first two decades of life.
- Soft tissue – usually subcutaneous.
- Brain – midline or lateral with involvement of eighth cranial nerve. Midline often with structural abnormalities in adjacent tissue. Eighth nerve lipomas infiltrative.
- Spermatic cord – most are retraction of fat into hernia sac, not true neoplasms.

Key Radiologic Findings

- CT scans, like normal fat, have uniform density than liposarcomas.
- MRI (T1-weighted image): both benign and malignant lipomatous tumors exhibit a high signal density.
- MRI does not permit their distinction from old hematomas.
- Thinly encapsulated movable mass with wide size range.

Cytopathology

- Small clusters of uniform mature adipocytes
- Small, bland nuclei without atypia
- Figure 10.20a

Histopathology

- Encapsulated proliferation of mature adipocytes
- Lipid vacuoles single and uniform in size
- Can have necrosis, myxoid changes, calcification, fibrosis, and bone or cartilage components
- Figure 10.20b

Spindle Cell/Pleomorphic Lipoma

Key Clinical Findings

- Rare, usually older adults, predominantly male
- Common in neck and shoulder
- Superficial, similar to ordinary lipoma, can be a large mass
- Cured by local excision

Key Radiologic Findings

- Like ordinary lipomas, circumscribed and encapsulated

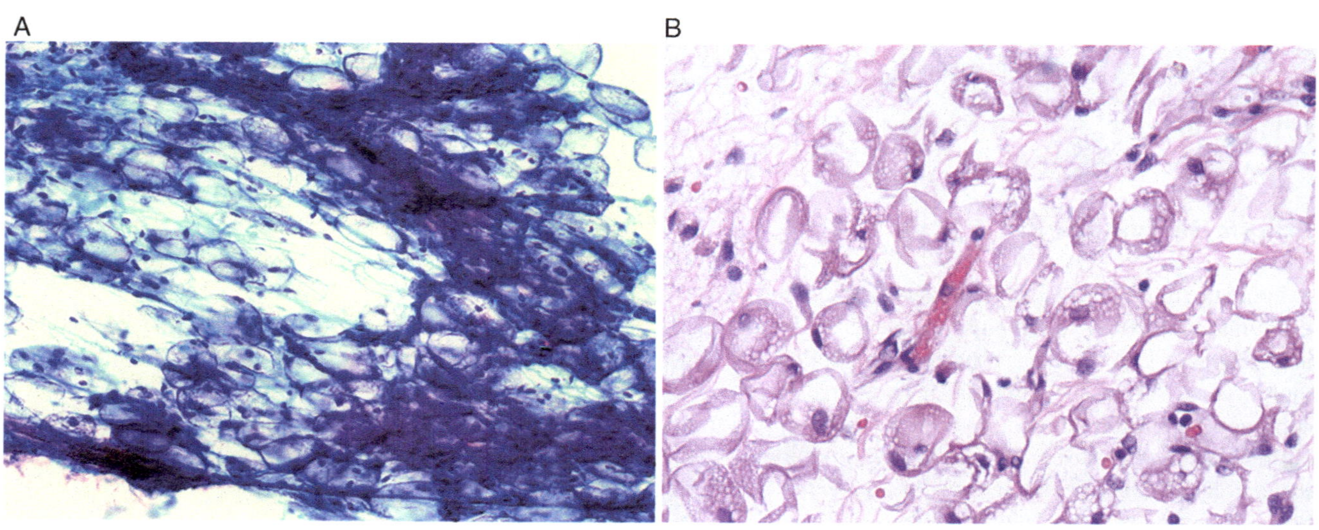

Fig. 10.19 (**a**, **b**) (**a**) Hibernoma. Cellular smear with clusters and single uniform vacuolated mature adipocytes, small bland nuclei without atypia (Papanicolaou stain). (**b**) Hibernoma. Large cells with central nuclei and cytoplasm filled with many small vacuoles containing neutral fat ranging from finely vacuolated and granular cells to more mature fat (cell block H&E)

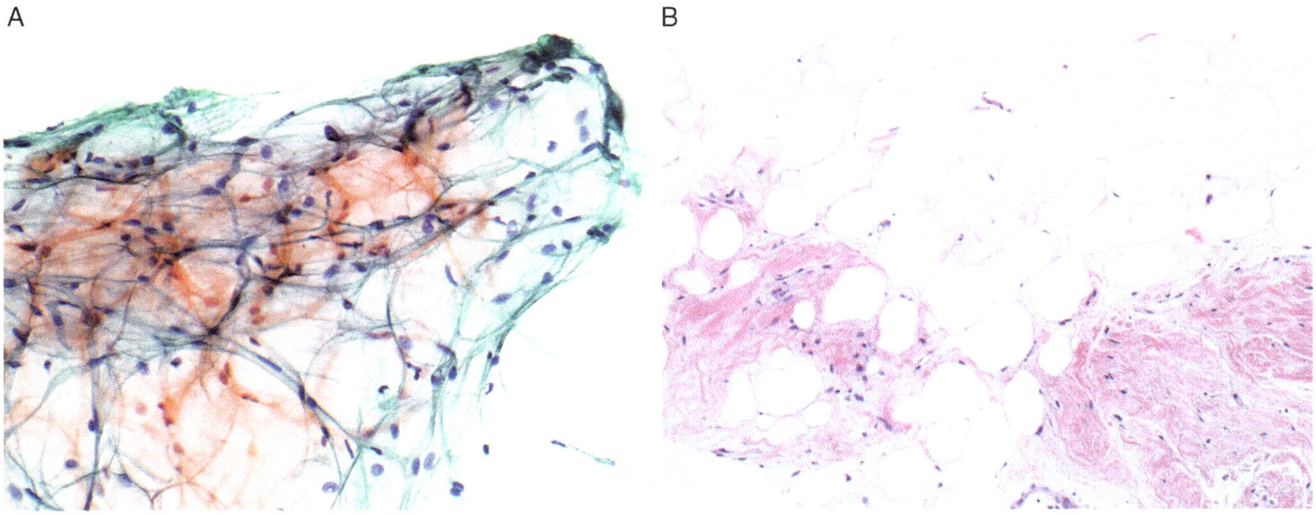

Fig. 10.20 (**a**, **b**) (**a**) Lipoma. Small clusters of uniform mature adipocytes with small, bland nuclei without atypia (Papanicolaou stain). (**b**) Lipoma. Proliferation of mature adipocytes. Lipid vacuoles single and uniform in size (H&E)

Cytopathology

- Mature adipose tissue
- Mix of spindle cell and floret-like giant cells with smudged chromatin
- Ropey collagen bundles
- Figure 10.21a

Histopathology

- Circumscribed and encapsulated mix of mature adipocytes, loose spindle cell stroma, and giant cells, including floret cells.
- The floret type cells have its nuclei in a ring at its periphery.
- Lack of prominent vascularity.
- Figure 10.21b–d.

Cytogenetics

- Like spindle cell lipoma, characterized by aberrations of the long arms of chromosomes 16 and 13
- A potential role for karyotypic analysis when distinguishing it from atypical lipoma/well-differentiated liposarcoma

Atypical Lipomatous Tumors/Well-Differentiated Liposarcoma

Key Clinical Findings

- Usually adults, typically knee, thigh, or retroperitoneum, also in the paratesticular region (most liposarcomas are of this type)
- Higher risk of recurrence and dedifferentiation in retroperitoneum versus extremities

Key Radiologic Findings

- Present mature fat density mass with mottled or streaky zones of higher density corresponding to the fibrous or sclerotic zones
- Tend to have less well-defined borders than lipomas

Cytopathology

- Variation in adipocyte size
- Atypical stromal cell nuclei
- Lipoblasts and mature fat
- Figure 10.22a, b

Histopathology

- Key cell is lipoblast and is the enlarged, hyperchromatic nucleus scalloped/indented by single or multiple vesicles of fat, may be multinucleated.
- Well-differentiated liposarcoma greatly resembles a lipoma but has lipoblasts (best found in more fibrous areas of tumor).
- Some deep-seated lesions resemble fat with scattered atypical cells yet not classic lipoblasts.
- Sclerosing variant has less fat and more dense fibrosis with scattered lipoblasts.
- Controversial as to the distinction of well-differentiated liposarcoma from atypical lipoma.
- Some authorities consider any deep-seated lesion with mature fat and lipoblasts as liposarcoma.

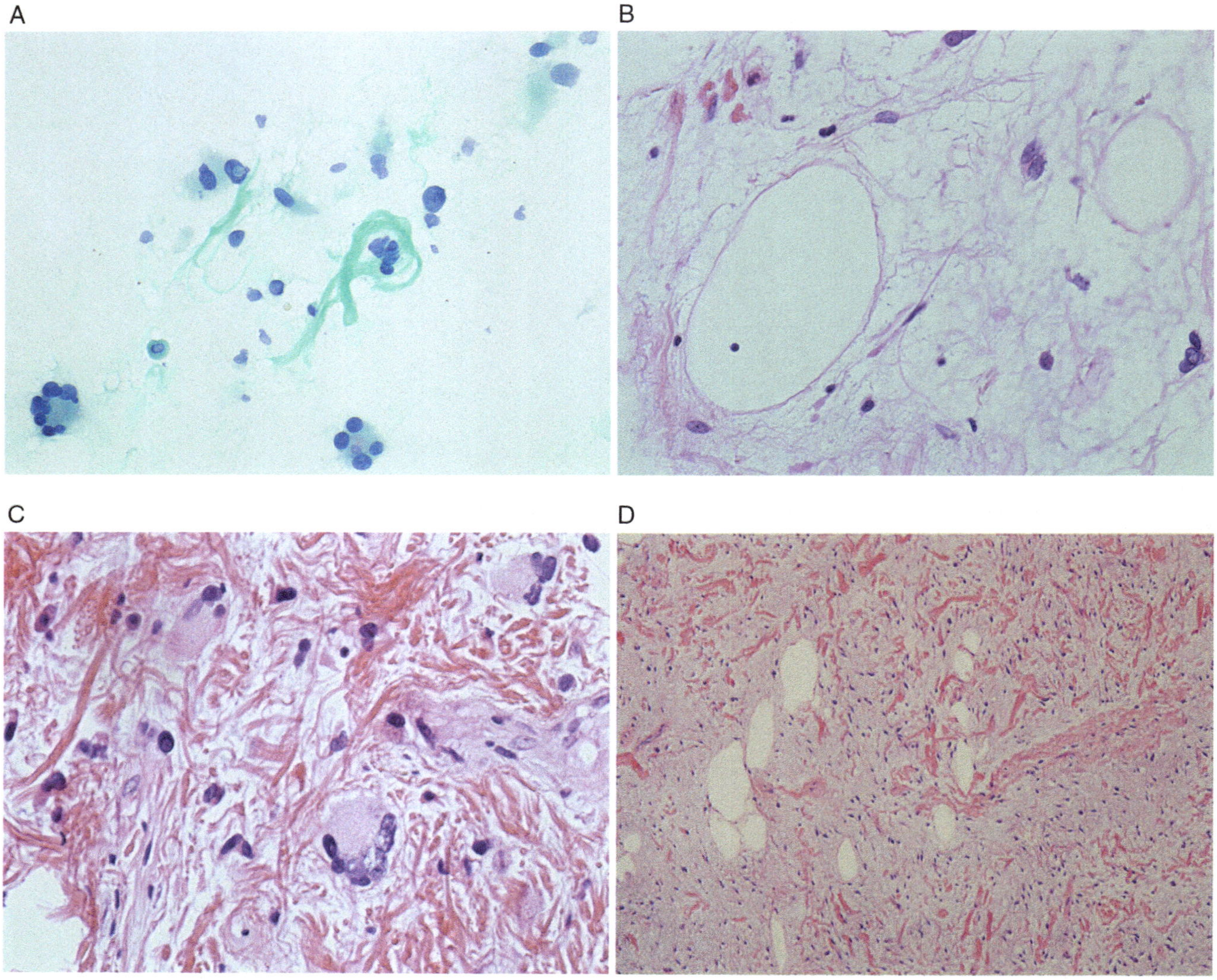

Fig. 10.21 (a–d) (a) Spindle cell/Pleomorphic lipoma. Floret-like giant cells with smudged chromatin and ropey collagen bundles (Papanicolaou stain). (b) Spindle cell/Pleomorphic lipoma. Mix of mature adipose cells and loose spindle cell stroma with degenerative nuclear atypia (H&E). (c) Spindle cell/Pleomorphic lipoma. Spindle cell stroma and giant cells with degenerative nuclear chromatin (H&E). (d) Spindle cell/Pleomorphic lipoma. Spindle cell stroma and mature adipocytes with ropey collagen bundles (H&E)

- Others consider these lesions in the extremities as atypical lipoma, yet identical lesion in retroperitoneum as liposarcoma.
- Still others consider all these lesions as atypical lipomatous tumors with a low malignant potential.
- Figure 10.22c, d.

Special Stains/Studies

- Usually S100 positive

Cytogenetics

- The defining features of ALT/WDL are the supernumerary circular (ring) and giant rod chromosomes, which contain amplification of the 12q14-15region, including the MDM2 gene, associated with co-amplification of various other chromosomal regions.
- They most often lack alpha-satellite centromeric sequences.
- Figure 10.22e

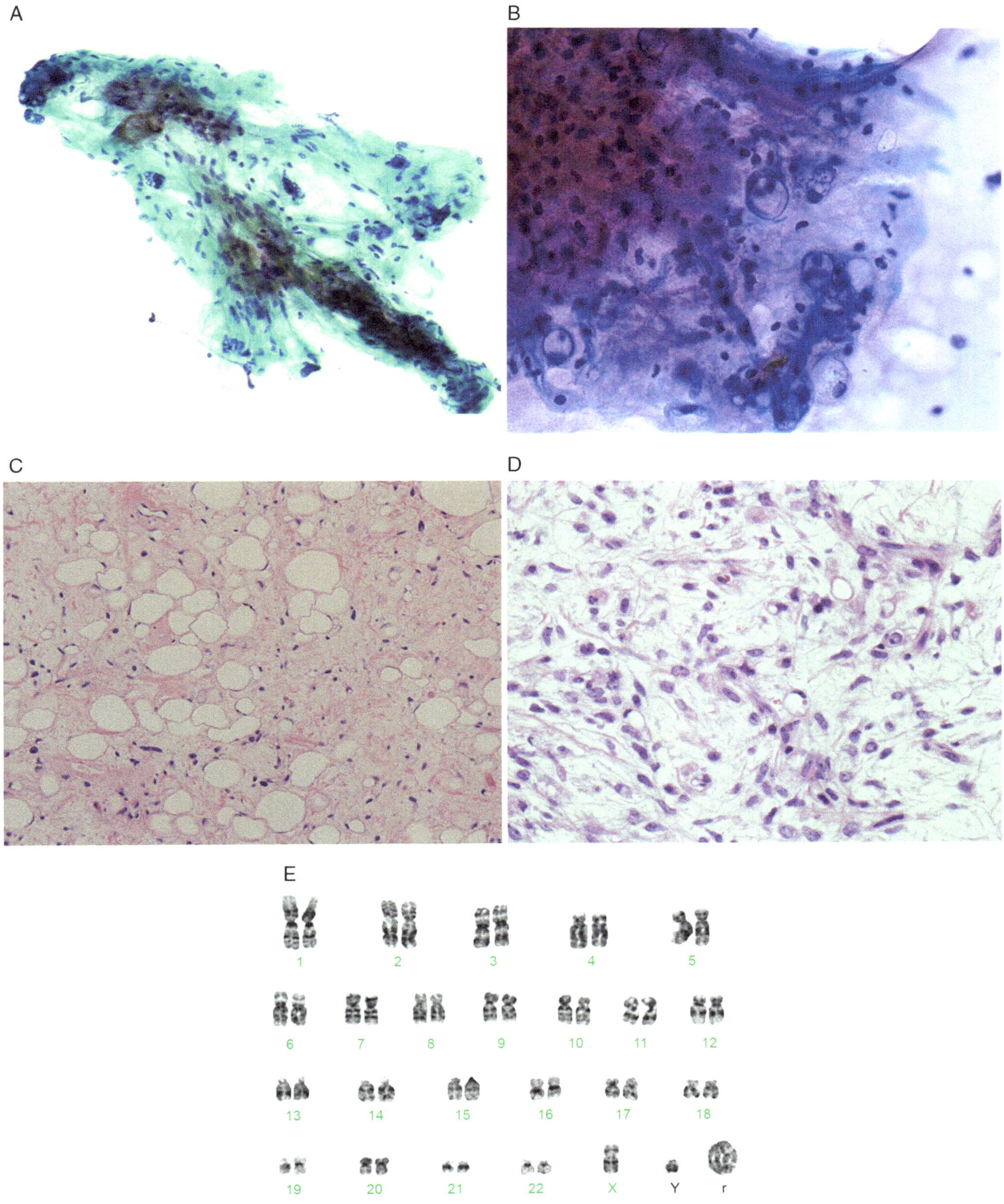

Fig. 10.22 (**a–e**) (**a**) Atypical lipomatous tumor/well-differentiated liposarcoma (ALT/WDL). Loosely cohesive cluster with variable-sized adipocytes, enlarged and hyperchromatic nuclei (scalloped/indented by single or multiple vesicles of fat-lipoblasts), and mixed with mature fat (Papanicolaou stain). (**b**) ALT/WDL. Mix of mature fat and scattered lipoblasts with single vesicle (Papanicolaou stain). (**c**) ALT/WDL. Resembles lipoma and often mixed with mature fat. Rare scattered lipoblasts with single vesicle in the more fibrous area of tumor (H&E). (**d**) ALT/WDL. Mix of mature fat and rare scattered lipoblasts with single vesicle in spindle stromal cells (H&E). (**e**) ALT/WDL. Metaphase spread showing ring chromosome

Pleomorphic Liposarcoma

Key Clinical Findings

- Least common and accounting for 5% of liposarcoma, usually adults
- Typically knee, thigh, or retroperitoneum
- Clinically dedifferentiated liposarcoma typically seen years after first diagnosis
- Poor prognosis

Key Radiologic Findings

- CT scans and MRI have areas like mature fat.
- Have areas of non-fatty tissue similar other sarcomas.

Cytopathology

- Marked nuclear pleomorphism.
- Lipoblast with cytoplasmic vacuoles vary in size.
- Rich cellular debris in the background.
- Figure 10.23a, b.

Histopathology

- Pleomorphic liposarcoma, a high-grade tumor, with giant lipoblasts with bizarre nuclei.
- The dedifferentiated subtype has poorly differentiated and well-differentiated areas in the same tumor or in the primary tumor and the recurrent tumor or metastasis.
- Figure 10.23c.

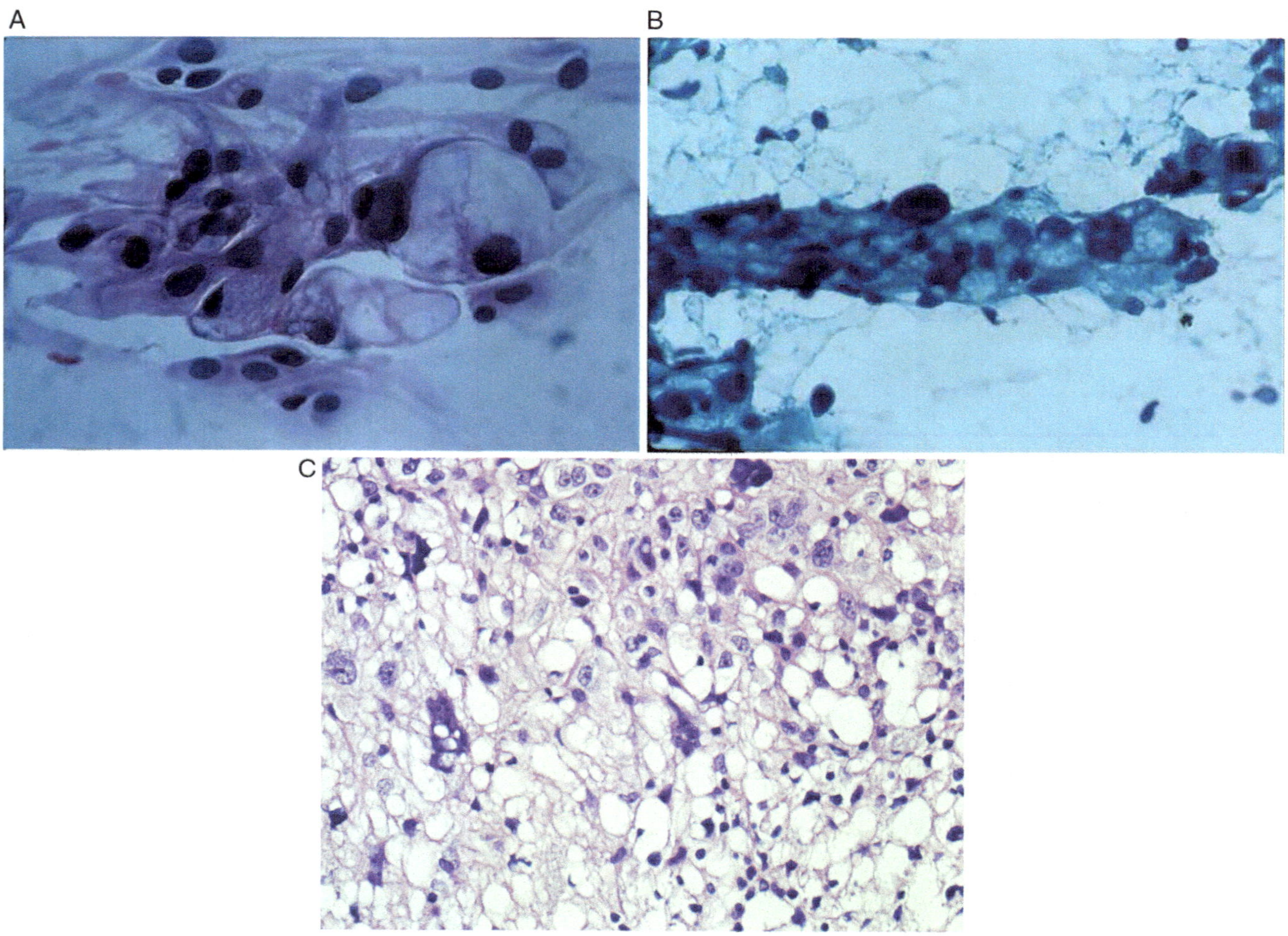

Fig. 10.23 (a–c) (a) Pleomorphic liposarcomas. Giant lipoblasts with bizarre nuclei (Romanowsky stain). (b) Pleomorphic liposarcomas. Lipoblasts with marked nuclear pleomorphism (Papanicolaou stain). (c) Pleomorphic liposarcomas. Giant lipoblasts with bizarre nuclei in the background of numerous regular lipoblasts (H&E)

Special Stains/Studies

- S100 is usually negative in poorly differentiated areas.

Myxoid Tumors

Myxoid tumors (MT) of soft tissue encompass a heterogeneous group of lesions characterized by an abundant extracellular homogeneous matrix, which is actively secreted by the tumor cells of MT, and it stains striking bluish violet with Romanowsky stains (DQ) and blue to green with Papanicolaou stain. It shows hypoechoic appearance on ultrasound, low attenuation on CT, and extremely low and high signal intensity on T1- and T2-weighted MRI, respectively. MRI is the imaging modality of choice for the evaluation of these tumors. Some key points are as follows:

- Include benign, locally aggressive, and malignant lesions and commonly affect extremities and spare the visceral organs.
- Considerable overlap in the clinical and pathologic features of these tumors.
- Most benign lesions are superficially located except intramuscular myxoma and pathologically have lower cellularity, lesser nuclear atypia.
- Most malignant lesions are deeply seated with exception of myxofibrosarcoma, and pathologically hypercellular, and more nuclear atypia.
- Lower-grade myxoid lesions can be subtyped based on cytopathologic features alone with accuracy rates up to 81%, although limited sampling may yield hypocellular smears with abundant myxoid matrix and lead to falsely low-grade assignment.
- Recent developments in genetic and molecular features led to significant advances in their classification, diagnosis, and management.
- The myxoid variant of malignant fibrous histiocytoma has been reclassified as myxofibrosarcoma, and round cell liposarcomas have been reclassified as myxoid liposarcomas because of their similar cytogenetic profile.

Intramuscular Myxoma

Key Clinical Findings

- Rare benign neoplasm, usually female adults
- Deep in muscle of extremities, especially the thigh
- Clinically multiple lesions associated with fibrous dysplasia (Albright's syndrome)
- Grossly appears circumscribed but unencapsulated yet invades muscle at periphery

Key Radiologic Findings

- Angiographic examination reveals a poorly vascularized soft tissue mass surrounded by well-vascularized muscle tissue. MRI reveals a well-defined tumor exhibiting low signal intensity relative to skeletal muscle on T1-weighted images and a hyperintense appearance relative to muscle on T2-weighted images.

Cytopathology

- Scant cellularity with stellate and spindle cells
- Uniform cells lacking pleomorphism
- Muscle fibers and no vascular component
- Background granular matrix material
- Figure 10.24a, b

A B

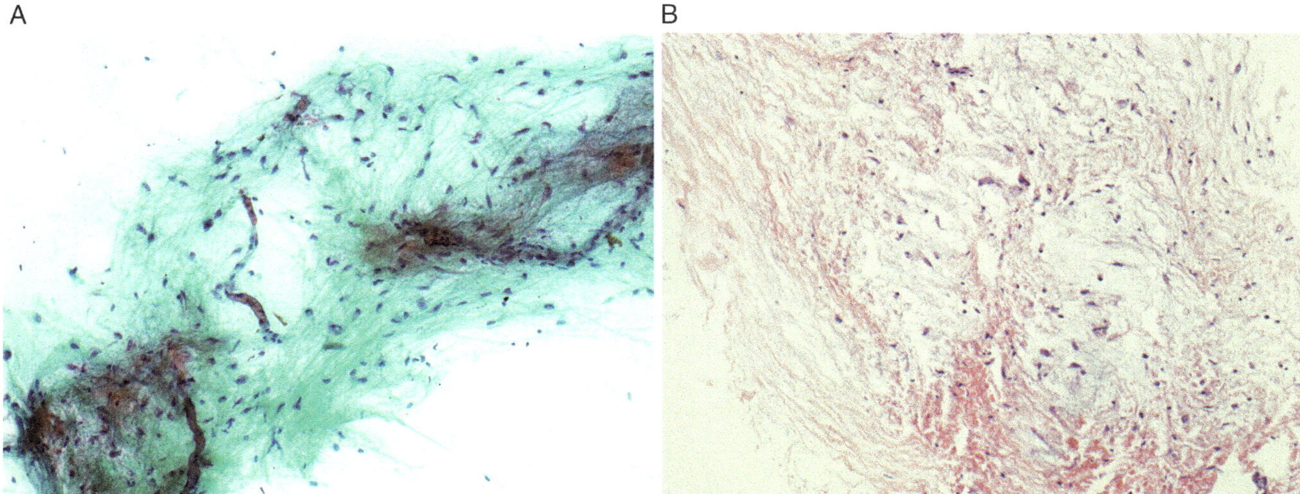

Fig. 10.24 (**a**, **b**) (**a**). Intramuscular myxoma. Scant uniform stellate and spindle cells with background granular matrix (Papanicolaou stain). (**b**) Intramuscular myxoma. Rare uniform round or stellate cells in myxoid matrix (H&E)

Special Stains/Studies

- Stellate/spindle cells S100 negative.
- A third to half of tumors have GNAS1 mutations.

Lipoblastoma/Lipoblastomatosis

Key Clinical Findings

- Rare benign tumor, almost always before age 3.
- Predominantly male, usually proximal extremities.
- Benign lipoblastoma is confined to subcutis.
- Diffuse lipoblastomatosis infiltrates subcutis and muscle.
- Grossly slowly growing circumscribed mass.

Key Radiologic Findings

- Show a well-delineated soft tissue mass with the density of adipose tissue.
- CT or MRI cannot distinguish this lesion from lipoma or liposarcoma.
- Rare postoperative recurrence and primarily restricted to the infiltrative lesions.

Cytopathology

- Cellular specimen with myxoid matrix
- Numerous bland lipoblasts and prominent vascular component
- Bare nuclei and mature adipocytes

Histopathology

- Lobules of cells divided by broad fibrous septa and prominent vasculatures. Cells show a range of differentiation from prelipoblasts, spindle or stellate, to lipoblasts.
- Figure 10.25.

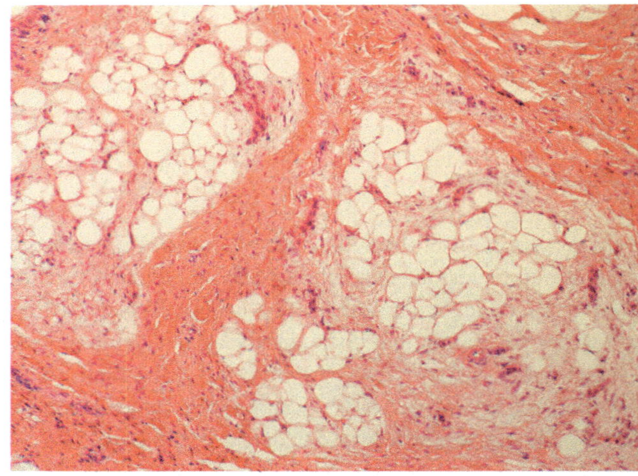

Fig. 10.25 Lipoblastoma. Lobules of cells divided by broad fibrous septa. Cells show from prelipoblasts, spindle or stellate, to lipoblasts (H&E)

Chordoma/Chondroid Chordoma

Key Clinical Findings

- Rare midline lesion at any age peaks in 50s–60s, mainly male
- The only malignant neoplasm derived from notochordal elements
- Base of skull (clivus) or sacral region. Half sacral, one third occipital/sphenoid.
- More rostral lesions occur at younger ages.
- Chondroid lesions found at the base of the skull.
- Chondroid chordomas have a longer mean survival (16 versus 4 years) than conventional chordomas.
- Both tend to be ultimately fatal, recurring locally after surgery

Key Radiologic Findings

- Radiologically osteolytic and destructive lesion

Cytopathology

- Clusters and cords of round to cuboidal cells
- Granular and fibrillary myxoid matrix
- Physaliphorous cells with abundant cytoplasmic vacuoles
- Figure 10.26a–c

Special Stains/Studies

- Positive for cytokeratin, EMA, S100

Extraskeletal Myxoid Chondrosarcoma (EMC)

Key Clinical Findings

- Usually age 30–60, at deep soft tissue of the proximal limbs, especially the thigh and popliteal fossa, and in bone, pelvis, ribs, femur, humerus, and vertebrae.
- Can be central type (medulla of diaphysis) or peripheral (or juxtacortical or periosteal) type (cortex or periosteum of metaphysis).
- Prognosis is highly dependent on initial resectability.

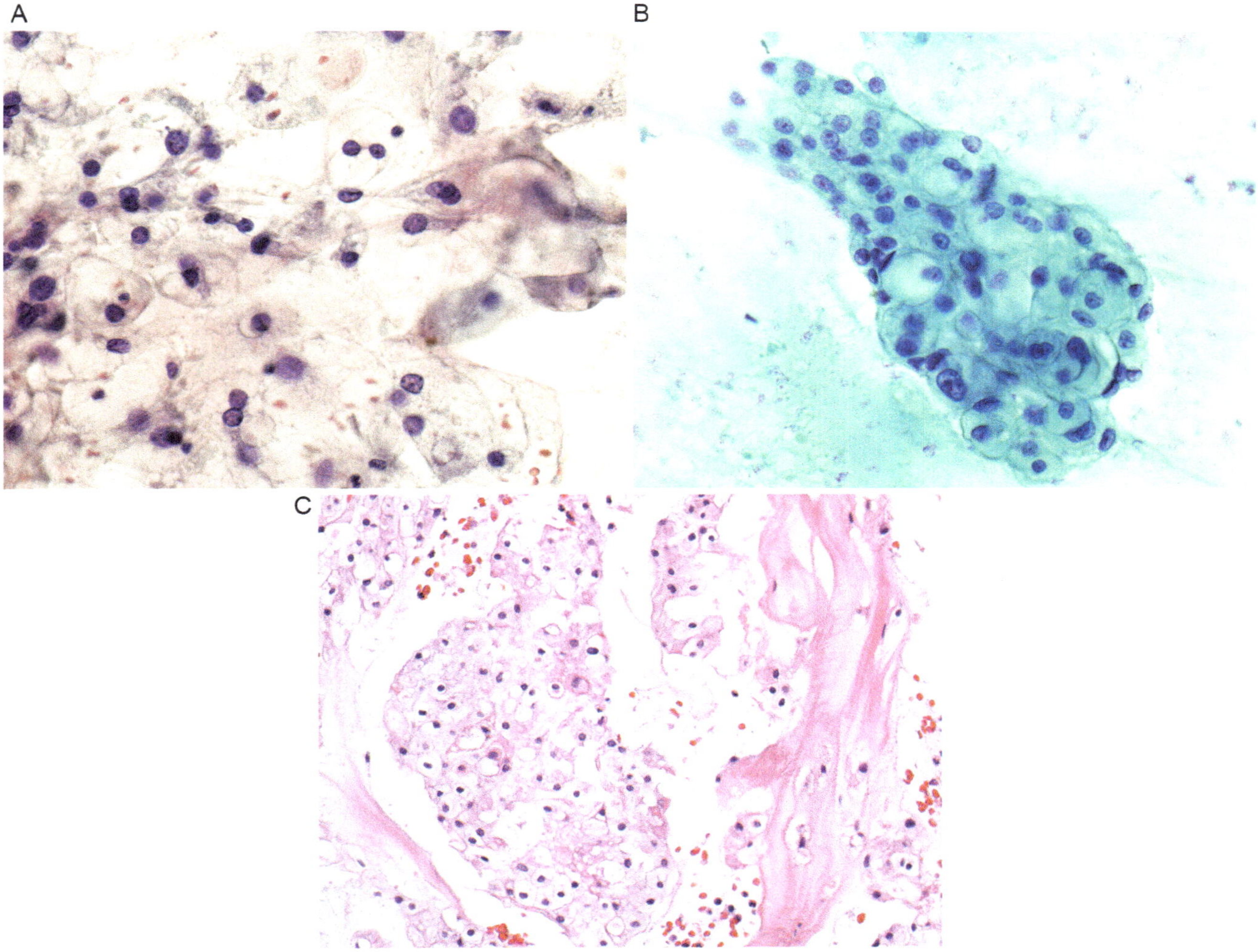

Fig. 10.26 (**a**–**c**) (**a**, **b**) Chordoma. Clusters and cords of round to cuboidal cells in fibrillary myxoid matrix (Papanicolaou stain). (**c**) Chordoma. Physaliphorous cells with abundant cytoplasmic vacuoles (H&E)

- Controversial grading tends to be based on cellularity, nuclear size and pleomorphism, mitoses, and necrosis.
- Late local recurrences and 40–50% of cases metastasize after >10 years.

Key Radiologic Findings

- Bone lesion can be large, rapidly growing, with ill-defined margins, destruction of bone.
- Partly lucent lesion with rings and/or stipples of calcification.

Cytopathology

- Fragments of fibrillar chondromyxoid matrix
- Uniform, bland, spindle tumor cells
- Long cytoplasmic tails with a lace-like appearance
- Some lacunar formation
- Figure 10.27a–d

Special Stains/Studies

- Positive for S100, leu7, lysozyme
- Negative for keratin

Myxoid Liposarcoma

Key Clinical Findings

- Myxoid and round cell liposarcoma are two ends of the spectrum of a single entity.
- Shares the same chromosomal translocation.
- Myxoid lesions form the low-grade end.
- Occurs in the third to fifth decades.
- Deep soft tissue of legs, especially the thigh.

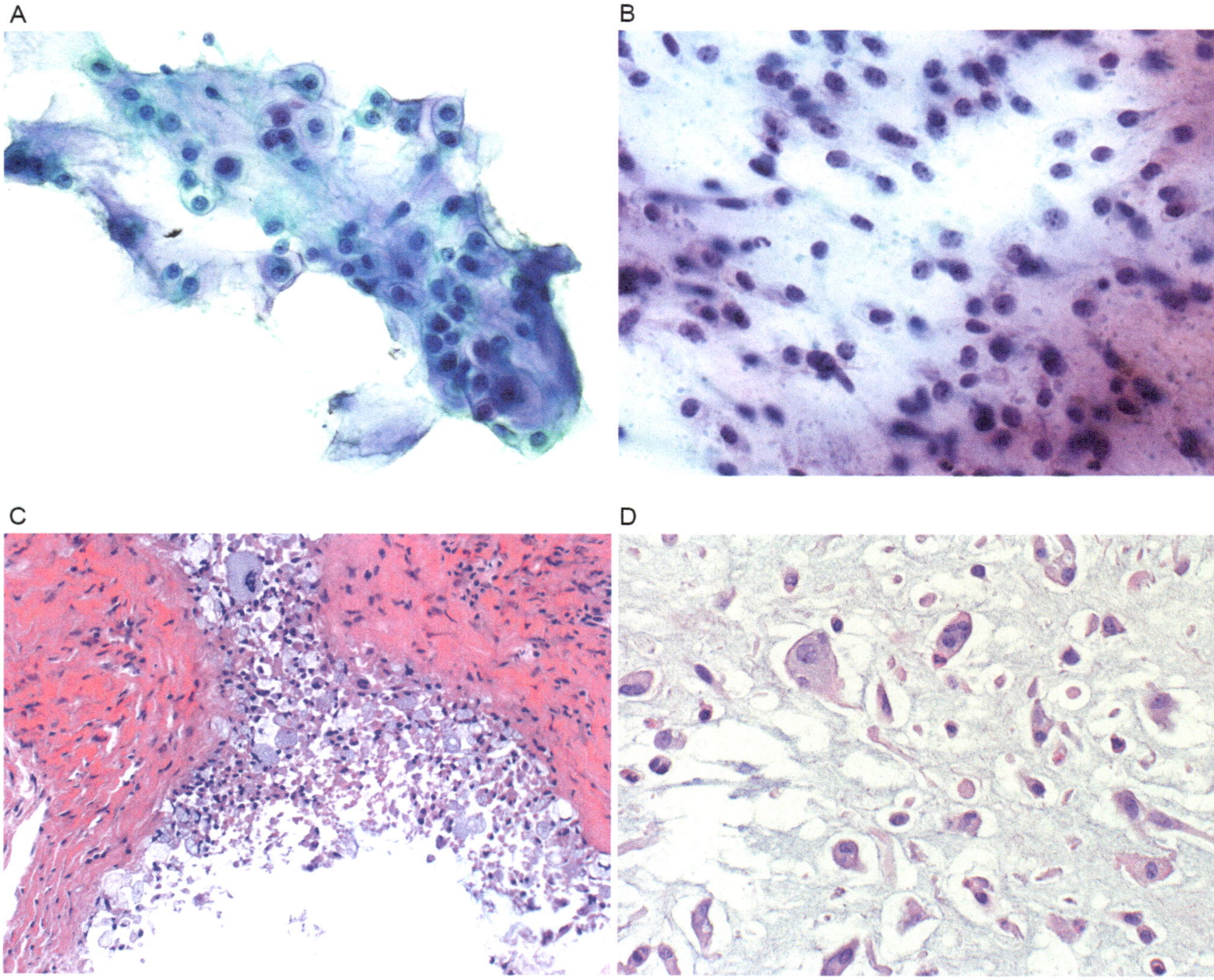

Fig. 10.27 (a–d) (a, b) Extraskeletal myxoid chondrosarcoma (EMC). Fragments of fibrillar chondromyxoid matrix with uniform, bland, spindle tumor cells, long cytoplasmic tails with a lace-like appearance and some lacunar formation (Papanicolaou stain). (c, d) Extraskeletal myxoid chondrosarcoma (EMC). Fibrillar chondromyxoid matrix with tumor cells showing long cytoplasmic tails, a lace-like appearance and some lacunar formation (H&E)

Key Radiologic Findings

- Typically appears as nonhomogeneous on CT scans.
- The attenuation values of highly myxoid lesions exceed those of normal fat but are less than that of the surrounding soft tissue.
- Round cell areas have attenuation values similar to those of other soft tissue sarcomas.

Cytopathology

- Abundant granular myxoid matrix
- Delicate, branching, thin-walled capillaries
- Uniform spindle to oval cells with monomorphic nuclei and occasional small cytoplasmic vacuoles
- Univacuolated and bivacuolated lipoblasts
- Figure 10.28a–d

Special Stains/Studies

- Positive for S100
- Chromosomal translocation; t(12:16)(q13;p11), >75%; t(12:22)(q13;q12), <5%

Myxofibrosarcoma (MFS) (Low- and High-Grade)

Key Clinical Findings

- MFS, one of the most common sarcomas of elderly patients
- During the sixth to eighth decades
- Occurs in extremities followed by retroperitoneum
- Up to 54% of cases recur locally regardless of grade and tends to become progressively higher grade with each recurrence.

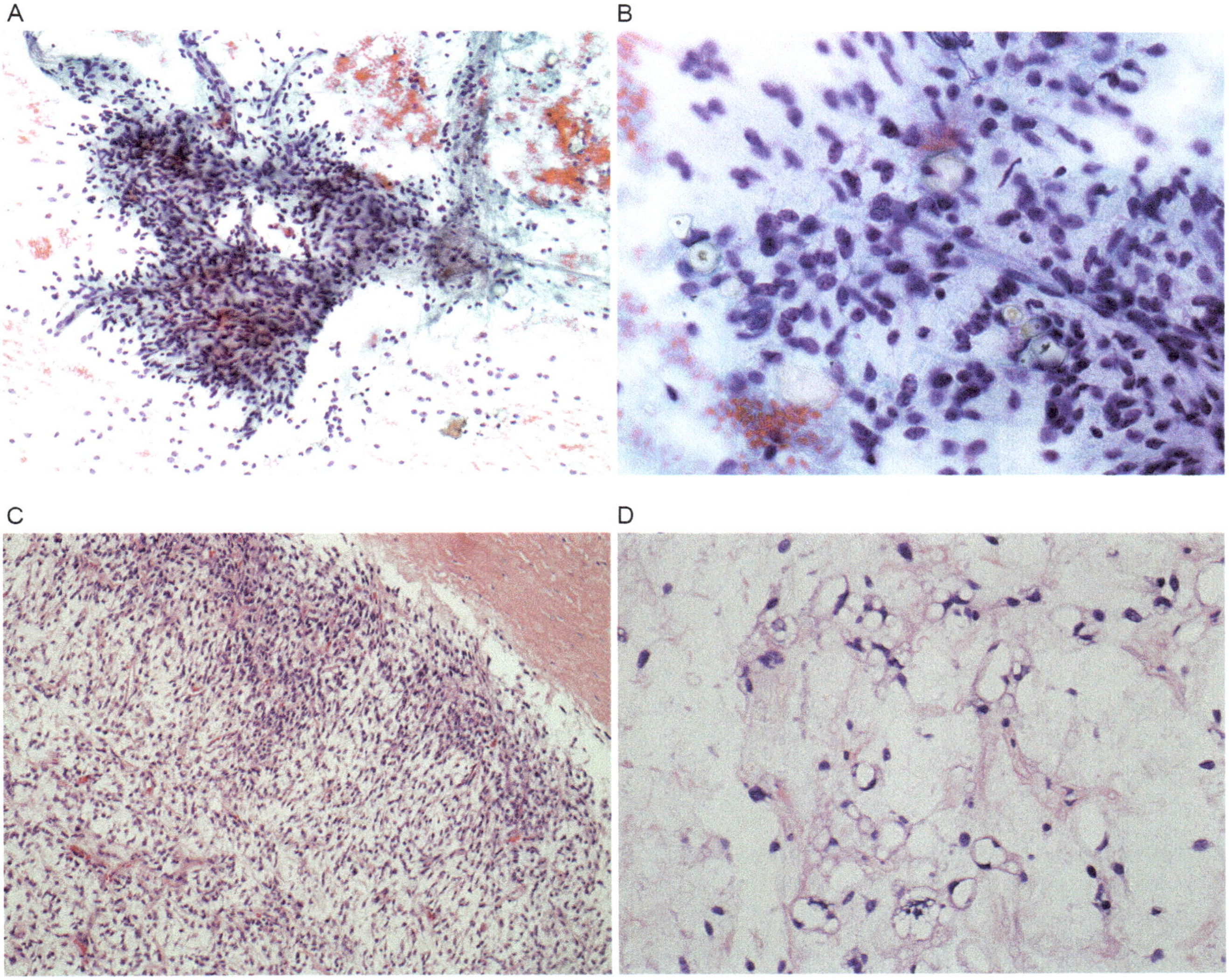

Fig. 10.28 (**a–d**) (**a**, **b**) Myxoid liposarcoma. Abundant myxoid matrix, delicate, branching, thin-walled capillaries, uniform spindle to oval cells and lipoblasts (Papanicolaou stain).(**c**, **d**) Myxoid liposarcoma. With monomorphic nuclei and occasional small cytoplasmic vacuoles. Well-demarcated lesion with myxoid matrix, delicate, branching, thin-walled capillaries, uniform spindle to oval cells, and lipoblasts (H&E)

- Only high-grade lesions have the potential to metastasize to lungs, bones, and lymph nodes. Lower metastatic rate than other variants.

Key Radiologic Findings

- CT is the method of choice in the assessment of size and extent of MFH of the soft tissues.
- When intra-arterial chemotherapy is indicated the angiograms obtained at each catheter placement may substitute CT in follow-up studies obviating additional diagnostic procedures.

Cytopathology

- Hypercellular smears
- Background myxoid matrix material
- Short segments of thick-walled vessels
- Pleomorphic spindle and stellate cells
- Binucleated and giant tumor cells
- Figure 10.29a, b

Myxofibrosarcoma-Like Dedifferentiated Liposarcoma

- Dedifferentiated liposarcoma is the most common dedifferentiated sarcoma, and up to 10% of liposarcomas, and usually retroperitoneal, limbs, testis, or spermatic cord.
- The abrupt transition between the dedifferentiated and well-differentiated components is usually present but can be gradual intermingling with pleomorphic liposarcoma.
- Most cases resemble high-grade myxofibrosarcoma or undifferentiated pleomorphic sarcoma.

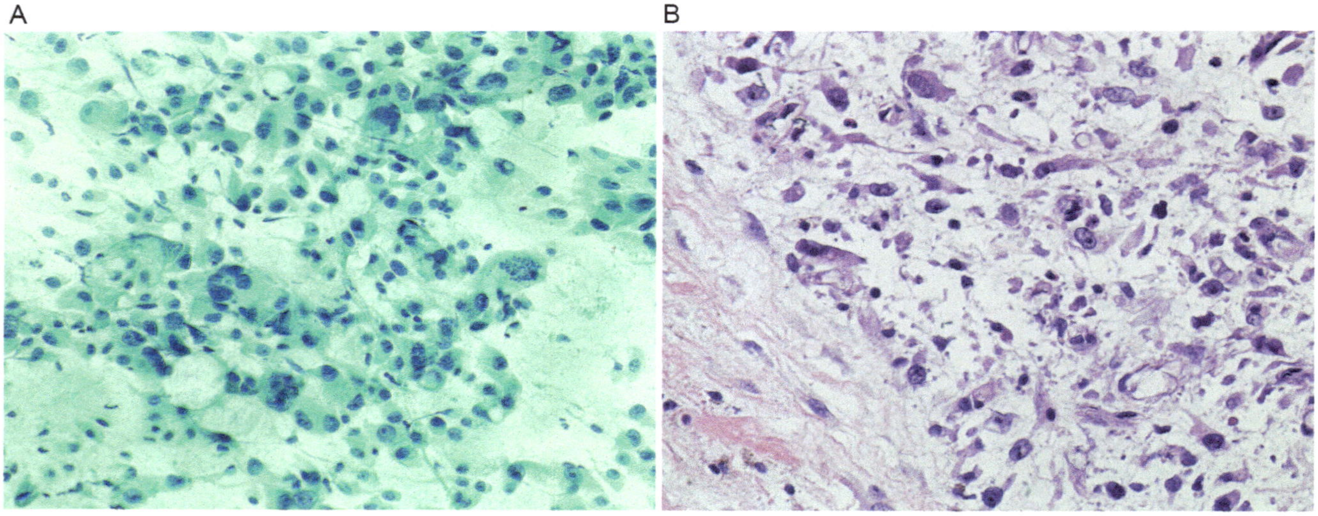

Fig. 10.29 (**a**, **b**) (**a**, **b**) Myxofibrosarcoma. Pleomorphic spindle, stellate cells, and giant tumor cells in background of myxoid matrix (Papanicolaou stain, H&E)

- Dedifferentiated liposarcoma should be in the differential diagnosis when high-grade myxofibrosarcoma is considered in the retroperitoneum.
- Cytogenetic analysis for MDM2 and positive CDK4 stain is helpful.
- Figure 10.30a–d.

Myxoinflammatory Fibroblastic Sarcoma/ Atypical Myxoinflammatory Fibroblastic Tumor

Key Clinical Findings

- Rare low-grade sarcoma, affects all age groups, both men and women equally.
- Involves the extremities, often termed "acral myxoinflammatory fibroblastic sarcoma."
- Present with a slowly growing painless mass, but some may present with pain or tenderness.
- Recurrence is common, occurring in 28–51% cases, rare metastases.

Key Radiologic Findings

- Predominantly subcutaneous but may involve dermis and synovium.
- The tumors are well defined, or ill defined and infiltrative, and are often located along the tendon sheath.
- Homogeneous or heterogeneous depending on their relative components, with the myxoid component being T2 hyperintense and T1 hypointense, and may show homogeneous or heterogeneous contrast enhancement.

Cytopathology and Histopathology

- Proliferative fibroblasts (spindle cells)
- Myxoid matrix, associated inflammatory cells
- Reed-Sternberg-like atypical giant cells

Special Stains/Studies

- Characterized by the translocation t(1;10) in the WHO 2013 classification

Low-Grade Fibromyxoid Sarcoma (Evans Tumor)

Key Clinical Findings

- Rare tumor that affects young to middle-aged adults, men and women equally
- Commonly involves the extremities, trunk, and deep soft tissue
- Recent study showing 65% recurrence and 45% metastases

Key Radiologic Findings

- On CT, tumors appear as heterogeneous with isodense and hypodense components relative to muscle, consistent with fibrous and myxoid tissue.
- Calcifications may be occasionally present.
- MRI reveals the fibrous component to be T1 and T2 hypointense and the myxoid component to be T1 hypointense and T2 hyperintense, showing mild and avid heterogeneous enhancement.

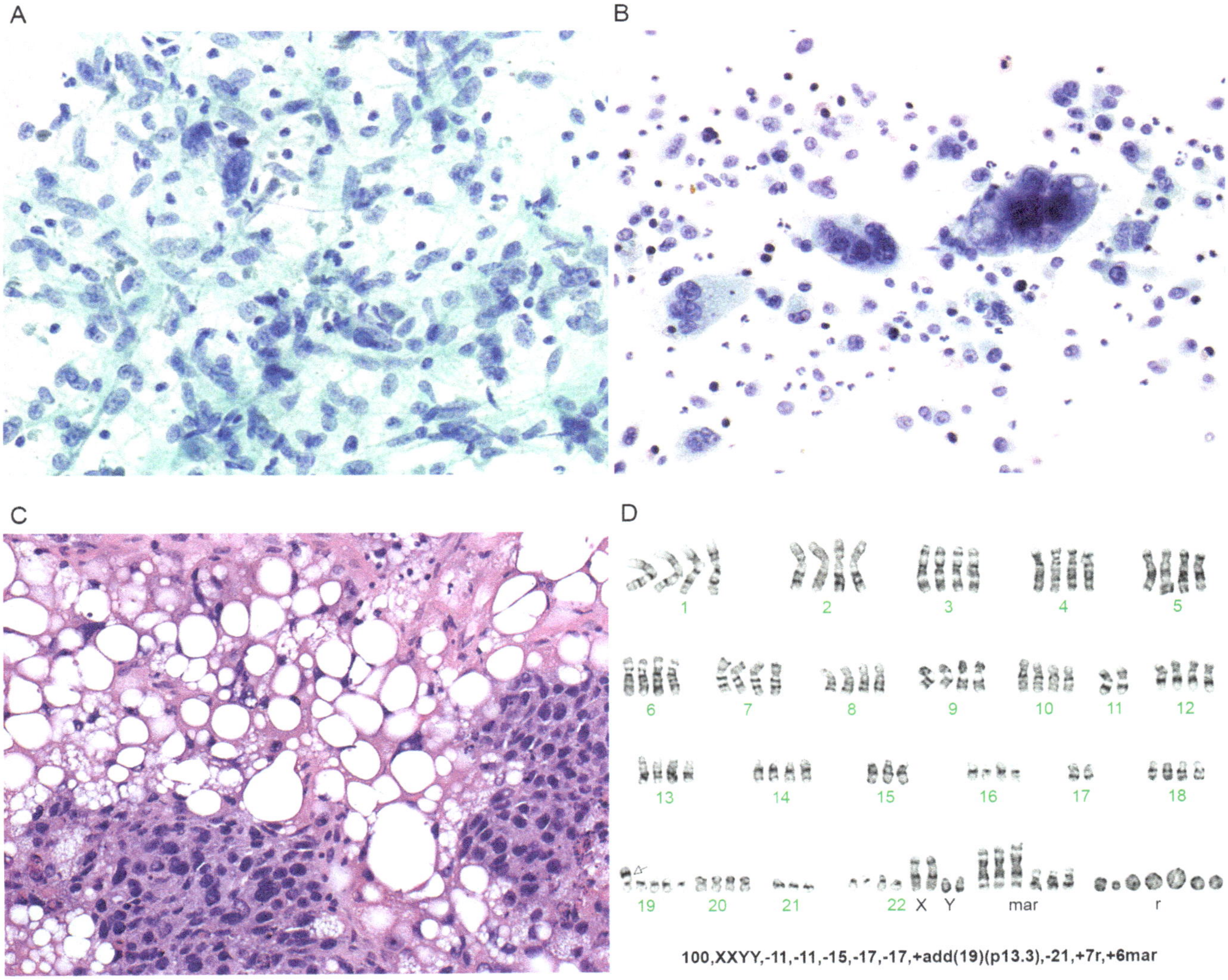

Fig. 10.30 (**a**–**d**) (**a**, **b**) Myxofibrosarcoma-like dedifferentiated liposarcoma. Pleomorphic spindle, stellate cells, and giant tumor cells in background of myxoid matrix (Papanicolaou stain). (**c**) Myxofibrosarcoma-like dedifferentiated liposarcoma. Myxoid liposarcoma with dedifferentiated liposarcoma side by side (H&E). (**d**) Myxofibrosarcoma-like dedifferentiated liposarcoma. Metaphase spread showing chromosome pattern

Cytopathology and Histopathology

- Bland spindle cells with intermixed myxoid and fibrous stroma

Special Stains/Studies

- MUC4 is a highly sensitive and specific immunohistochemical marker.
- Translocation t(7;16) leading to the formation of *FUS/CREB3L2* fusion gene.

Fibrohistiocytic Tumors

Angiomatoid Fibrous Histiocytoma

Key Clinical Findings

- Rare tumor of children and young adults with partially myoid phenotype and low metastatic potential and usually occurs in extremities.
- Clinically fever, weight loss, and anemia are common.
- Grossly circumscribed, multinodular, or multicystic hemorrhagic mass.
- Recurs locally (20%) and rarely metastases (1%).

Key Radiologic Findings

- MRI showed an intramuscular soft tissue mass.
- The tumor mass may be seen to have multiple cystic components with fluid-fluid levels.

Cytopathology and Histopathology

- Clusters of uniform cells
- Background inflammatory cells
- Endothelial and fibroblast-like or histiocyte-like cells
- Intracytoplasmic hemosiderin

Special Stains/Studies

- Positive stain for desmin, EMA, CD99, CD68; negative for SMA, myogenin
- Three characteristic translocations: t(2:22)(q33:q12) (forming the EWSR1-CREB1 fusion gene), t(12:22)(q13:q12) (forming the EWSR1-ATF1 fusion gene), and t(12:16)(q13:p11) (resulting in the FUS-ATF1 fusion gene)

Tenosynovial Giant Cell Tumor

Key Clinical Findings

- The second most common tumors of the hand; occur in patients aged 30–50 years, female-to-male ratio 3:2.
- Two types: localized (common) and diffuse (rare)
- The diffuse form is the soft tissue counterpart of diffuse pigmented villonodular synovitis (PVNS) and affects the lower extremities.
- Its anatomic distribution parallels that of PVNS, with lesions most commonly found around the knee, the ankle, and foot, and occasionally affects the hand.
- Like PVNS, occurs in young patients; 50% of cases occur in patients <40 years.
- The diffuse form is locally aggressive, and multiple recurrences are common.
- Probably represents an extra-articular extension of a primary intra-articular PVNS process.
- The mononuclear cells and giant cells present in the lesions resemble osteoclasts and suggest a bone marrow-derived monocyte/macrophage lineage.
- The polyclonal nature of the lesion suggestive of a reactive or regenerative hyperplasia associated with an inflammatory process.
- The incidence of local recurrence ranging from 9% to 44%.

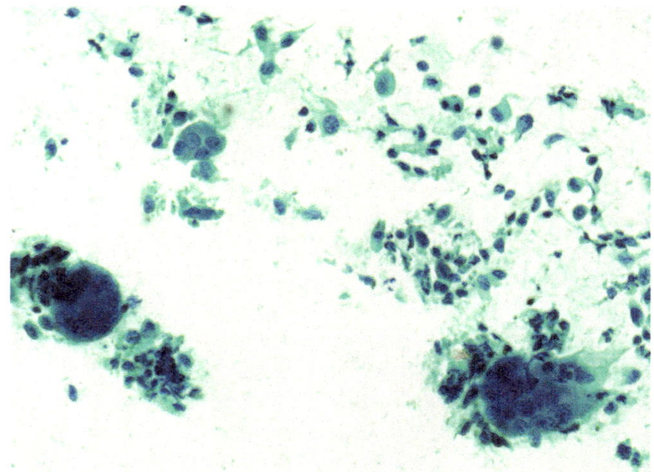

Fig. 10.31 Tenosynovial giant cell tumor. Scattered multinucleated giant cells and singly placed histiocytes and inflammatory cells (Papanicolaou stain)

Key Radiologic Findings

- No abnormal findings were found at the X-ray.
- Well-circumscribed lesion at the MR imaging.
- The lesion was hypointense on T1-weighted images and hyperintense on T2-weighted images.

Cytopathology

- Multinucleated giant cells
- Singly placed histiocytes and inflammatory cells
- Granular material in the background
- Figure 10.31

Histopathology

- Multinucleated giant cells scattered on the floor containing collagenous stroma and round mononuclear cells

Special Stains/Studies

- Positive CD68, desmin, CD45
- Chromosome translocation t(1;2)(p13;q37) carrying COL6A3-CSF1 fusion gene

Pleomorphic Tumors

Pleomorphic Rhabdomyosarcoma (PRMS)

- High-grade sarcoma composed of bizarre polygonal, round, and spindle cells that display skeletal muscle differentiation without embryonal or alveolar component

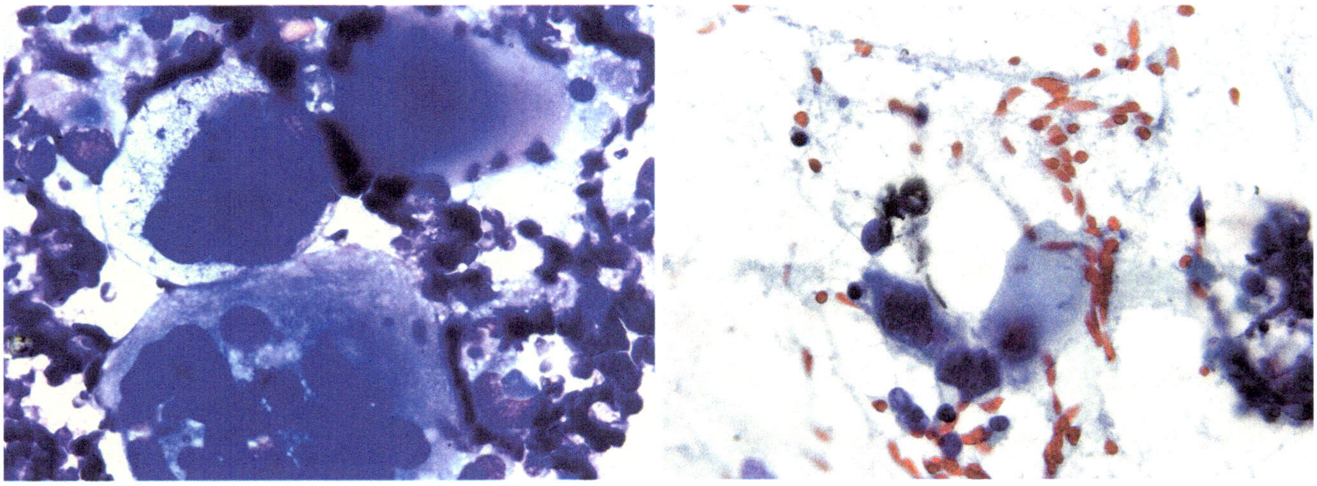

Fig. 10.32 (a, b) (a, b) Pleomorphic rhabdomyosarcoma. Multinucleated giant cells and bizarre high-grade polygonal cells with cytoplasmic inclusions (Romanowsky and Papanicolaou stain)

- Occurs in sixth to seventh decades of life, men more than women
- Deep soft tissue in limbs, chest/abdominal wall, abdomen, head, and neck
- Rapid growth painful mass

Cytopathology and Histopathology

- Sheets of large, atypical, and multinucleated polygonal eosinophilic cells or of undifferentiated round to spindle cells
- Rhabdomyoblasts with cross striations rarely seen
- Figure 10.32a, b

Special Stains/Studies

- Expressing MyoD1, myogenin, SMA, CK AE1/3, EMA
- MDM2 nuclear labeling without MDM2 amplification

Undifferentiated Pleomorphic Sarcoma (UPS)

Key Clinical Findings

- An aggressive sarcoma derived from a primitive mesenchymal cell capable of differentiating into histiocytes, fibroblasts, myofibroblasts, and osteoclasts.
- Arising from any part of the body during the sixth and seventh decades of life, clinically presenting as swelling, mass, pain, with high local recurrence and significant metastasis (the most frequent is the lung).
- Fourth most common soft tissue sarcoma with a slight male preponderance.
- The common sites: lower extremities (mainly thigh) and upper arms, retroperitoneum, viscera, head, and neck (in childhood).
- Anorexia, malaise, fever, and weight loss are present in retroperitoneal and inflammatory forms of UPS.

Key Radiologic Findings

- MRI is the imaging method of choice for limbs and shows a high signal on T2-weighted images.

Cytopathology

- Pleomorphic spindle cells with large atypical nuclei, atypical mitotic figures, necrosis, and lymphohistiocytic infiltrate. Figure 10.33a–c.

Histopathology

- Histology of biopsy specimen prior to any treatment is crucial to reach diagnosis and shows pleomorphic spindle cell population with large atypical cells frequently exhibiting numerous atypical mitotic figures, associated regions of hemorrhage, necrosis, and lymphohistiocytic infiltrate.

Special Stains/Studies

- Negative for S-100, HMB-45, CD34, and cytokeratin

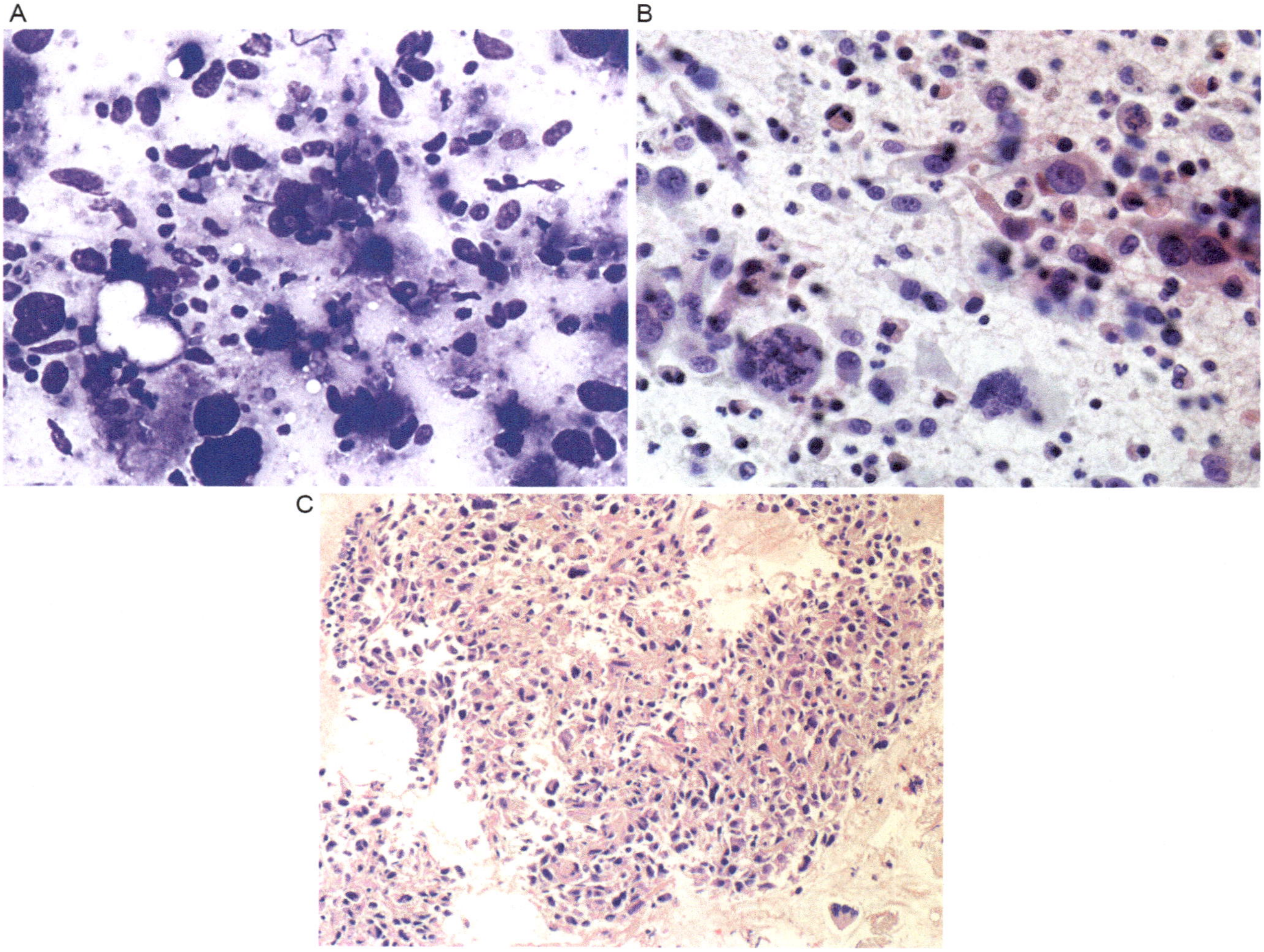

Fig. 10.33 (**a**–**c**) Undifferentiated pleomorphic sarcoma. Pleomorphic spindle cell population with large atypical cells exhibiting numerous atypical mitotic figures (Romanowsky and Papanicolaou stain and H&E)

Dedifferentiated Sarcomas (DDS)

- Dedifferentiated sarcomas include dedifferentiated liposarcoma, chondrosarcoma, and chordoma.
- Recent rapid growth in a previously stable mass is a common clinical finding, and the adjacent well-differentiated component is essential for the diagnosis.
- Dedifferentiated liposarcoma has the same giant marker and ring chromosomes as its well-differentiated counterpart. (See Myxofibrosarcoma-Like Dedifferentiated Liposarcoma.)
- Dedifferentiation of all chondrosarcomas occurs in about 10% cases and usually in patients about 10 years older than patients with conventional chondrosarcoma.
- Dedifferentiated chordoma is a very rare event resulting in a more aggressive clinical course than usual chordoma.
- The rapid FNA diagnosis: "Positive for malignancy. Cytopathologic findings consistent with high grade pleomorphic sarcoma." The final diagnosis and accurate classification defer for permanent tissue and ancillary studies.
- Cytogenetic analysis can assist with the cytopathologic diagnosis.

Fibroblastic/Myofibroblastic Lesions

Elastofibroma

Key Clinical Findings

- Rare lesion and regarded as a reactive process, occurs in mid-back and scapula of elderly
- Clinically often with history of hard manual labor and grossly with ill-defined margins
- Benign reactive condition. Does not recur

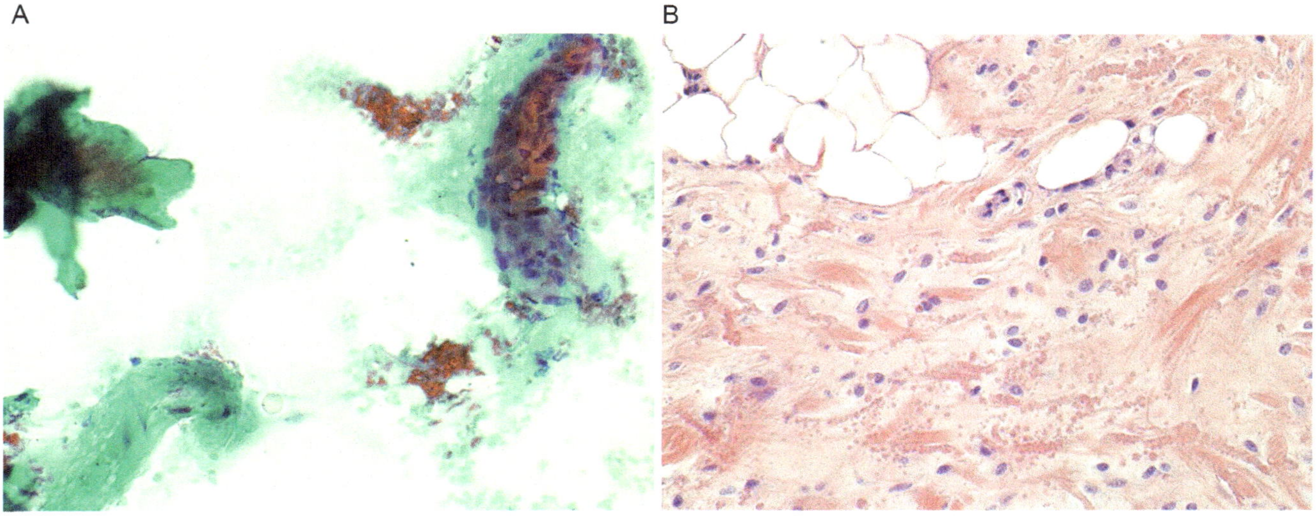

Fig. 10.34 (a, b) (a) Elastofibroma. Hypocellularity with waxy matrix, linear, serrated, rod-like structures (Papanicolaou stain). (b) Elastofibroma. Thick or coarse, deeply eosinophilic elastic fibers arranged in beaded strings or globules (H&E)

Cytopathology

- Hypocellularity with waxy matrix
- Linear, serrated, rod-like structures
- Serrated globular bodies
- Figure 10.34a, b

Special Stains/Studies

- Elastic stain markedly positive
- Positive for type 2 collagen (not normally found in this location)

Idiopathic Retroperitoneal Fibrosis/Ormond's Disease

Key Clinical Findings

- Rare enigmatic lesion affecting male adults in fourth to fifth decades of life.
- Diffuse or localized, involving retroperitoneum.
- Clinically with history of pain in lower abdomen, flank, or lower back.
- May be associated with malaise, weight loss, fever, and hypertension.
- Often encases ureters, causing hydronephrosis (fibrosing periureteritis).
- Less commonly involves aorta (periaortitis).
- May present as solid mass suggesting an enlarged lymph node or neoplasm.
- When in association with fibrosing mediastinitis, Riedel's thyroiditis, sclerosing cholangitis, and pseudotumor of the orbit, referred to as "multifocal fibrosclerosis" or "systemic idiopathic fibrosis."
- Does not metastasize but locally aggressive and often recurs after surgery.
- Spontaneous regression reported in a few cases.
- Treatment of choice is prolonged corticosteroid therapy.

Cytopathology and Histopathology

- Fragments of fibrous tissue
- Spindle fibroblastic cells
- Mixed inflammatory cells
- Prominent crush artifact

Special Stains/Studies

- Positive vimentin, SMA, negative for cytokeratin pool, caldesmon, S100, CD34, CD117, ALK-1, β-catenin, desmin, myogenin, or myoglobin. Ki67 proliferation index was always negligible.
- The bands of fibrous tissue were diffusely stained with an anti-type-I collagen antibody.

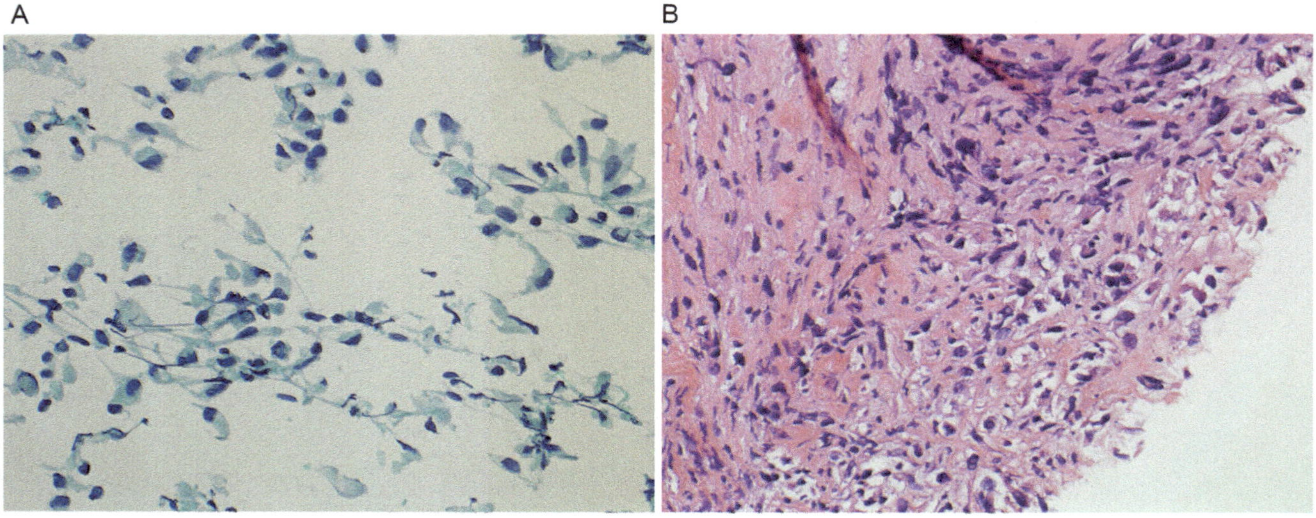

Fig. 10.35 (**a**, **b**) Metastatic sarcomatoid RCC. Singly placed and loose clusters of epithelioid, spindle, and pleomorphic sarcomatous cells on smears and in subcutaneous tissue (Papanicolaou stain and H&E)

Metastatic Sarcomatoid Carcinoma and Melanoma Involving Soft Tissue Mimicking Sarcomas

Metastatic Sarcomatoid Renal Cell Carcinoma (SRCC)

Key Clinical Findings

- Uncommon, comprise 3% of all RCCs.
- Most in association with clear cell RCC.
- Sarcomatoid transformation of chromophobe, collecting duct and papillary RCCs also occurs.
- Often has an aggressive clinical course by rapid disease progression.
- Metastasis was present in 77% of SRCC patients; median survival was 9 months.

Cytopathology and Histopathology

- Hypercellular, single, loose clusters of epithelioid, spindle and pleomorphic cells.
- Mix of typical renal cell carcinoma cells.
- Sarcomatous cells resemble melanoma, fibrosarcoma, chondrosarcoma, and osteosarcoma.
- Figure 10.35a, b.

Malignant Melanoma

Key Clinical Findings

- Any age, rare in children.
- Anywhere, though common on trunk, back, and legs.
- Pigmented nodules with irregular color and shape.
- May appear as new lesion in a preexisting nevus.
- Larger nodules may ulcerate.

Cytomorphology and Histopathology

- Single cells and loose clusters
- Epithelioid, spindle, and/or pleomorphic
- Eccentric nuclei, binucleation, single prominent nucleoli
- Intranuclear inclusions and melanin pigments
- Figure 10.36a–c

Special Stains/Studies

- HMB45, S100, melan-A, tyrosinase

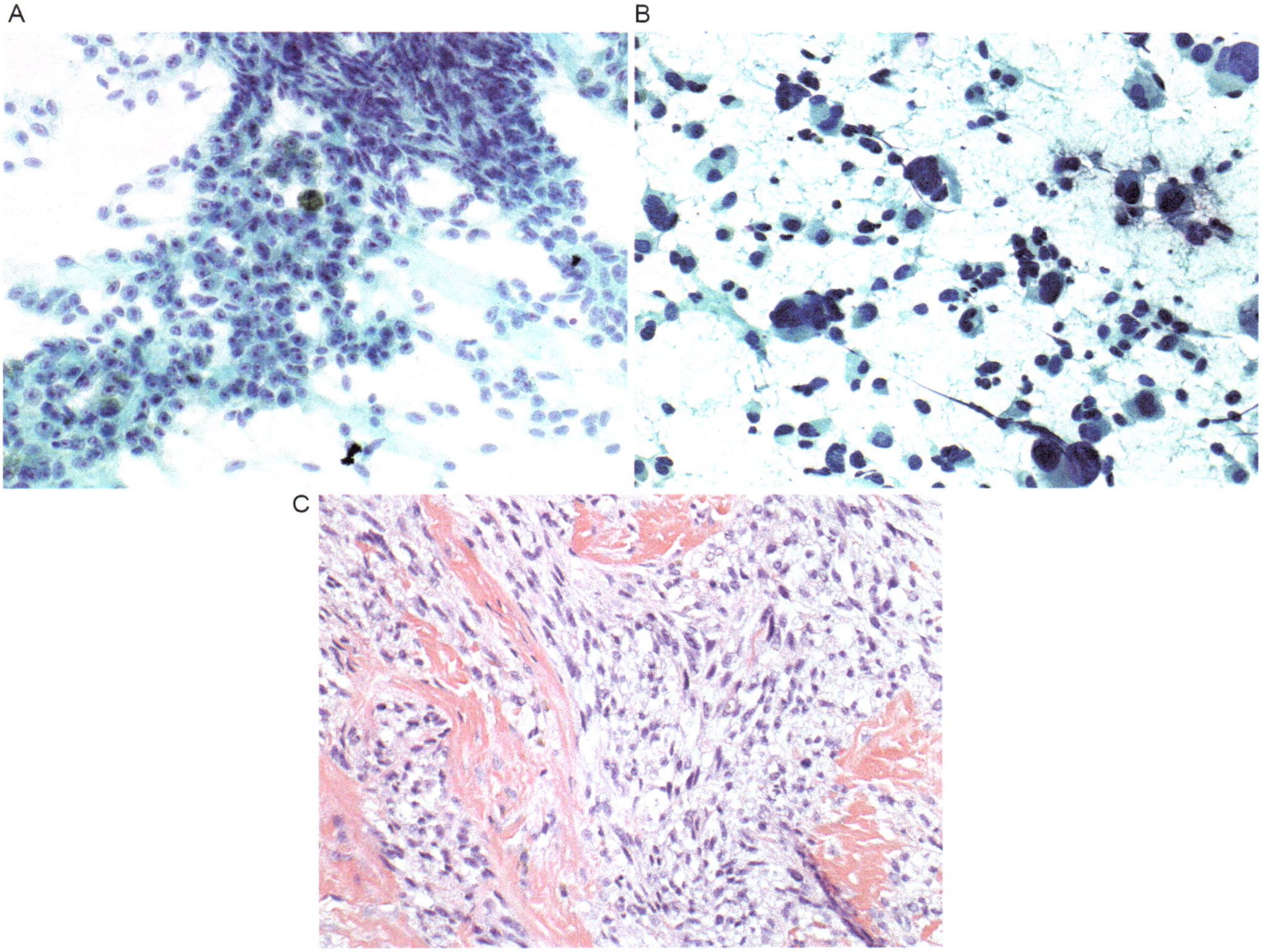

Fig. 10.36 (**a–c**) Melanoma. Singly placed and loose clusters of epithelioid, spindle, and/or pleomorphic cells with eccentric nuclei, binucleation, prominent eosinophilic nucleoli (Papanicolaou stain). (**c**) Melanoma. Infiltrative spindle cells with intranuclear inclusions and melanin pigments (H&E)

Case Presentation

Case Scenario 1

A 54-year-old male farmer, presented with a baseball-sized mass on the left elbow with recent rapid growth for 4 months. He had trauma to this area about 3 years ago. A CT scan of the chest showed several indeterminate nodules up to 2.4 cm in his bilateral lungs.

Fine needle aspiration (FNA) biopsy was done, and the smears show hypercellular specimen with discohesive, round to spindle to polygonal cells, hyperchromatic nuclei, binucleation, prominent nucleoli, and occasional intranuclear inclusions in a background of necrotic granular material in Fig. 10.1a, b.

Based on the cytopathologic features, what is the FNA preliminary diagnosis?

Step 1: Neoplastic or inflammatory reactive process?
- Hypercellularity
- Uniform spindle to oval cells

Impression: Spindle/epithelioid cell neoplasm
Step 2: Benign or malignant?

- Hypercellularity
- Discohesiveness and singly placed cells
- Nuclear hyperchromasia and atypia
- Necrotic granular background

(continued)

Impression: Malignant spindle/epithelioid cell neoplasm

Step 3: To establish the differential diagnosis including:

- Sarcomatoid carcinoma – common thing first
- Spindle cell sarcoma
- Spindle cell melanoma
- Clear cell sarcoma (malignant melanoma of soft parts)
- Epithelioid sarcoma

Step 4: To narrow down the differential diagnosis based on the cytopathologic diagnostic criteria:

- Prominent nucleoli and perinuclear clearing
- Binucleation, multinucleation, and intranuclear inclusions
- Cytoplasmic and intercellular pigments

Impression: Malignant spindle cell melanoma or clear cell sarcoma.

Tissue core biopsy shows nests of rounded or elongated cells with clear cytoplasm; some may be eosinophilic and granular, oval and vesicular nuclei, and prominent nucleoli; occasional intranuclear inclusions separated by delicate fibrovascular septa in Fig. 10.1c.

Step 5: To choose the immunohistochemical (IHC) study panel based on the differential diagnosis:

- Carcinoma-sarcomatoid differentiation?
- CK AE1/3, Oscar-CK, EMA
- Melanoma-spindle cell?
- S100, HMB45, melan-A, tyrosinase
- Sarcoma?
- SMA, desmin, myogenin, Myo D, CD34, CD31, S100

IHC panel shows positive expression for S100 (Fig. 10.1d), melan-A (Fig. 10.1e), and HMB45 (Fig. 10.1f) and no expression for the rest of the IHC panels.

Discussion: The morphologic features and IHC profile are compatible with both malignant melanoma and clear cell sarcoma.

Step 6: To choose the diagnostic molecular pathology studies (Cytogenetic Study) to nail the final diagnosis:

- >75% of the clear cell sarcomas revealed unique translocation t(12;22)(q13;q12).
- Increased copies of chromosomes 7 and 8 have been reported.
- In contrast, the gene for cutaneous malignant melanoma has been localized to 1p.

FISH performed on paraffin-embedded tissues revealed rearrangement of the EWS locus at 22q12 in 87% of cells (image demonstrated separation of EWSR1 in Fig. 10.1g).

Step 7: To establish the final diagnosis:

Discussion

- Both malignant melanoma and clear cell sarcoma have significant overlapping features, and both are strongly positive for S100, HMB45, and melan-A.
- However, the clinical and cytogenetic findings help distinguish clear cell sarcoma from cutaneous melanoma.
- Elbow mass, left, FNA/biopsy: positive for malignancy. Malignant melanoma of soft parts (clear cell sarcoma); FISH performed on paraffin-embedded tissues revealed rearrangement of the EWS locus at 22q12 in 87% of cells, supporting the above diagnosis.

Abbreviations List

Abbreviation	Full text
ALK1	Activin receptor-like kinase
BCL2	B-cell lymphoma 2
CD	Cluster of differentiation (CD15, CD31, CD34, CD45, CD56, CD68, CD99, CD117)
CEA	Carcinoembryonic antigen
CK	Cytokeratin (CK7, CK20)
COL1A1-PDGFB	Collagen type I alpha 1-platelet-derived growth factor beta
COL6A3-CSF1	Alpha(α)3(VI) chain of type VI collagen-colony stimulating factor 1
CT	Computed tomography
DQ	Diff-Quick (Romanowsky)
EMA	Epithelial membrane antigen
EWS-FLI-1	Ewing sarcoma breakpoint region-Friend leukemia integration 1
FUS-ATF1	Fused in sarcoma-cyclic AMP-dependent transcription factor
FUS-CREB3L2	Fused in sarcoma-CAMP responsive element binding protein 3 like 2
FNA	Fine needle aspiration
GNAS1	Guanine nucleotide α subunit 1
H&E	Hematoxylin and eosin
HMB45	Human melanoma black 45

Abbreviation	Full text
HMWCK	High molecular weight cytokeratin
IHC	Immunohistochemistry
INI1/ SMARCB1	SWI/SNF-related matrix-associated actin-dependent regulator of chromatin subfamily B
Leu M1	CD15
Leu 7	CD57
KIM-1	Kidney injury molecule-1
KIT	Tyrosine-protein kinase Kit
MDM2	Mouse double minute 2 homologue
MIB1	Mind bomb E3 ubiquitin protein ligase 1
MPNST	Malignant peripheral nerve sheath tumor
MRI	Magnetic resonance imaging
MSA	Muscle specific antigen
MyoD1	Myogenic differentiation 1
N/C	Nuclear-to-cytoplasmic ratio
NSE	Nonspecific esterase
Pap	Papanicolaou
PASD	periodic acid-Schiff D
PAX	Paired box gene (PAX5, PAX8)
PET	Positron emission tomography
pVHL	von Hippel–Lindau tumor suppressor
STAT6	Signal transducer and activator of transcription 6
TLE1	Transducin-like enhancer of split 1
USP6-MYH9	Ubiquitin-specific protease 6-myosin heavy chain 9
WHO	World Health Organization
WT1	Wilms tumor 1

Suggested Reading

Akhtar M, Iqbal MA, Mourad W, Ali MA. Fine-needle aspiration biopsy diagnosis of small round cell tumors of childhood: a comprehensive approach. Diagn Cytopathol. 1999;21:81–91.

Ambros IM, Ambros PF, Strehl S, Kovar H, Gadner H, Kuntschik MS. MIC2 is a specific marker for Ewing's sarcoma and peripheral primitive neuroectodermal tumors: evidence for a common histogenesis of Ewing's sarcoma and peripheral primitive neuroectodermal tumors from MIC2 expression and specific chromosome aberration. Cancer. 1991;67:1886–93.

Bale SJ, Dracopoli NC. Chromosome 9p and hereditary cutaneous malignant melanoma. J Natl Cancer Inst. 1989;81(1):70.

Burchill SA, Bradbury FM, Smith B, Lewis IJ, Selby P. Neuroblastoma cell detection by reverse transcriptase-polymerase chain reaction (RT-PCR) for tyrosine hydroxylase mRNA. Int J Cancer. 1994;57:671–5.

Cibas ES, Ducatman BS. Cytology-diagnostic principles and clinical correlates. 4th ed. Philadelphia: Elsevier, Saunders; 2013.

Costa MJ, Weiss SW. Angiomatoid malignant fibrous histiocytoma: a follow-up study of 108 cases with evaluation of possible histologic predictors of outcome. Am J Surg Pathol. 1990;14(12):1126–32.

Dave B, Shet T, Chinoy R. Desmoplastic round cell tumor of childhood: can cytology with immunocytochemistry serve as an alternative for tissue diagnosis? Diagn Cytopathol. 2005;32:330–5.

Di Grazia S, Succi G, Fragetta F, Perrotta RE. Giant cell tumor of tendon sheath: study of 64 cases and review of literature. G Chir. 2013;34(5–6):149–52.

Dias P, Parham DM, Shapiro DN, Webber BL, Houghton PJ. Myogenic regulatory protein (MyoD1) expression in childhood solid tumors: diagnostic utility in rhabdomyosarcoma. Am J Pathol. 1990;137:1283–91.

Evans HL. Low-grade fibromyxoid sarcoma: a clinicopathologic study of 33 cases with long-term follow-up. Am J Surg Pathol. 2011;35:1450–62.

Fletcher CD. The evolving classification of soft tissue tumours: an update based on the new 2013 WHO classification. Histopathology. 2014;64:2–11.

Fletcher C, Bridge J, Hogendoorn P, Mertens F. World Health Organization classification of tumours of soft tissue and bone: pathology and genetics of tumours of soft tissue and bone. 4th ed. Lyon: IARC Press; 2013.

Fletcher C, Unni K, Mertens F. World Health Organization classification of tumours: pathology and genetics of tumours of soft tissue and bone. Lyon: IARC Press; 2002.

Folpe AL, McKenney JK, Bridge JA, Weiss SW. Sclerosing rhabdomyosarcoma in adults: report of four cases of a hyalinizing, matrix-rich variant of rhabdomyosarcoma that may be confused with osteosarcoma, chondrosarcoma, or angiosarcoma. Am J Surg Pathol. 2002;26:1175–83.

Fujimura T, Okuyama R, Terui T, et al. Myxofibrosarcoma (myxoid malignant fibrous histiocytoma) showing cutaneous presentation: report of two cases. J Cutan Pathol. 2005;32:512–5.

Graadt van Roggen JF, Hogendoorn PC, Fletcher CD. Myxoid tumours of soft tissue. Histopathology. 1999;35:291–312.

Hornick JL, Dal Cin P, Fletcher CD. Loss of INI1 expression is characteristic of both conventional and proximal-type epithelioid sarcoma. Am J Surg Pathol. 2009 Apr;33(4):542–50.

Humphrey PA, Dehner LP, Pfeifer JD. The Washington manual of surgical pathology. 1st ed. Philadelphia: Lippincott Williams & Wilkins; 2008.

Kovar H, Dworzak M, Strehl S, Schnell E, Ambros IM, Ambros PF, et al. Overexpression of the pseudoautosomal gene MIC2 in Ewing's sarcoma and peripheral primitive neuroectodermal tumor. Oncogene. 1990;5:1067–70.

Layfield LJ, Glasgow B, Ostrzega N, Reynolds CP. Fine-needle aspiration cytology and the diagnosis of neoplasms in the pediatric age group. Diagn Cytopathol. 1991;7:451–61.

Mackenzie DH. The myxoid tumors of somatic soft tissues. Am J Surg Pathol. 1981;5:443–58.

Mansoor A, White CR Jr. Myxofibrosarcoma presenting in the skin: clinicopathological features and differential diagnosis with cutaneous myxoid neoplasms. Am J Dermatopathol. 2003;25:281–6.

Nascimento AF, Bertoni F, Fletcher CD. Epithelioid variant of myxofibrosarcoma: expanding the clinicomorphologic spectrum of myxofibrosarcoma in a series of 17 cases. Am J Surg Pathol. 2007;31:99–105.

Nishio J, Iwasaki H, Nabeshima K, Naito M. Cytogenetics and molecular genetics of myxoid soft-tissue sarcomas. Genet Res Int. 2011;2011:497148.

Rajwanshi A, Rao KL, Marwaha RK, Nijhawan VS, Gupta SK. Role of fine-needle aspiration cytology in childhood malignancies. Diagn Cytopathol. 1989;5:378–82.

Sahu K, Pai RR, Khadilkar UN. Fine needle aspiration cytology of the Ewing's sarcoma family of tumors. Acta Cytol. 2000;44:332–6.

Sandberg AA, Bridge JA. The cytogenetics of bone and soft tissue tumors. Austin: RG Landes Co; 1994.

Sawyer JR, Tryka AF, Lewis JM. A novel reciprocal chromosome translocation t(11;22)(p13;q12) in an intraabdominal desmoplastic small round-cell tumor. Am J Surg Pathol. 1992;16:411–6.

Silverman JF, Landreneau RJ, Sturgis CD, Raab SS, Fox KR, Jasnosz KM, et al. Small-cell variant of synovial sarcoma: Fine-needle aspiration with ancillary features and potential diagnostic pitfalls. Diagn Cytopathol. 2000;23:118–23.

Thway K, Fisher C. Angiomatoid fibrous histiocytoma. Arch Pathol Lab Med. 2015;139(5):674–82.

Walker EA, Fenton ME, Salesky JS, Murphey MD. Magnetic resonance imaging of benign soft tissue neoplasms in adults. Radiol Clin N Am. 2011;49:1197–217.

Index

© Springer International Publishing AG 2018
F. Lin et al., *Handbook of Practical Fine Needle Aspiration and Small Tissue Biopsies*, DOI 10.1007/978-3-319-57386-1

K

Printed by Printforce, the Netherlands